Nursing Practice

Nursing Practice

Knowledge and Care

Third Edition

Edited by

Ian Peate, OBE, FRCN

EN(G), RGN, DipN (Lond), RNT, BEd (Hons), MA (Lond), LLM

Senior Lecturer University of Roehampton
Visiting Professor Northumbria University
Visiting Professor of Nursing
St George's University of London and Kingston University London
Visiting Senior Clinical Fellow
University of Hertfordshire, Hatfield, UK

Aby Mitchell, RGN

BA (Hons), MA (UWL), PGCAP, FHEA

Professional Lead for Simulation and Immersive Technologies,
Senior Lecturer in Adult Nursing,
University of West London,
London, UK

WILEY Blackwell

Registered Offices
John Wiley & Sons, Inc., 111 River Street, Hoboken, NJ 07030, USA
John Wiley & Sons Ltd, The Atrium, Southern Gate, Chichester, West Sussex, PO19 8SQ, UK

Editorial Office
9600 Garsington Road, Oxford, OX4 2DQ, UK

For details of our global editorial offices, customer services, and more information about Wiley products visit us at www.wiley.com.

Wiley also publishes its books in a variety of electronic formats and by print-on-demand. Some content that appears in standard print versions of this book may not be available in other formats.

Library of Congress Cataloging-in-Publication Data applied for

Paperback ISBN: 9781119800750

Cover Design: Wiley
Cover Images: © Marko Geber/Getty Images; © Jeff J Mitchell/Getty Images; © Maskot/Getty Images; © sturti/Getty Images

Set in 9.5/11pt MinionPro by Straive, Pondicherry, India
Printed and bound by CPI Group (UK) Ltd, Croydon, CR0 4YY

C9781119800750_110223

Brief Contents

Contents

About the Editors

Ian Peate, OBE, FRCN EN(G), RGN, DipN (Lond), RNT, BEd (Hons), MA (Lond), LLM

Senior Lecturer Roehampton University, Visiting Professor of Nursing, Northumbria University, Visting Professor St George's University of London and Kingston University London, Visiting Senior Clinical Fellow University of Hertfordshire. Ian began his nursing career in 1981 at Central Middlesex Hospital, becoming an Enrolled Nurse working in an intensive care unit. He later undertook 3 years' student nurse training at Central Middlesex and Northwick Park Hospitals, becoming a Staff Nurse and then a Charge Nurse. He has worked in nurse education since 1989. His key areas of interest are nursing practice and theory, men's health, sexual health and HIV. Ian has published widely; he is Editor in Chief *British Journal of Nursing*, Founding Consultant Editor *Journal of Paramedic Practice*, Editorial Board Member *British Journal of Healthcare Assistants*. Ian was awarded an OBE in the Queen's 90th Birthday Honours List 2016 for his services to nursing and nurse education. He was made a Fellow of the Royal College of Nursing in 2017 in recognition of his contribution to the profession.

Aby Mitchell, RGN, BA (Hons), MA (UWL), PGCAP, FHEA

Aby started her nursing career in 1998 in her local general hospital, initially working within a burns and plastics and head and neck cancer unit. In 1999 she embarked on a career in district nursing with a special interest in tissue viability and palliative care. From 2014, Aby moved to work in nurse education at the University of West London where she focused on the field of adult nursing, health promotion and primary care. She also continued to work within the NHS as Senior Physical Health Lead for Community Mental Health. Aby is now professional lead for simulation and immersive technologies at the University of West London. She is a keen advocate for development of new pedagogies to enhance nurse education. Aby is a member of the *British Journal of Nursing* editorial board.

Contributors

Georgiana Assadi

MSc Health Policy, PGCert Professional Academic Practice, BSc (Hons), RMN, DipHE, FHEA

Lecturer in Mental Health Nursing, King's College London, UK.

Georgiana began her career in 2009, studying mental health nursing at Kingston University. She has had a diverse range of clinical and corporate experiences, from working in the private sector, in the NHS and within a 'Unicorn' health tech start-up. Clinically, she has worked within neurodisability and mental health, psychiatric intensive care, community secondary mental health services, crisis response, integrated care and as a clinical tutor. Georgiana started her lecturing career at the University of West London in 2018, where she went onto become college lead for inter-professional learning, before moving to King's College London in February 2022. Educationally, she teaches on several of the undergraduate nursing courses, and has developed mental health teaching on non-nursing courses such as the Paramedic Science, Social Work and Operating Department Practitioner programmes, with great success. Her areas of interest include integration within health and social care, achieving parity between mental health and physical health, wellbeing, mental health clinical skills and innovation within teaching and has published work in all of these areas.

Mary E. Braine

D Prof MSc, PGCE, BSc (Hons), DipN (Lond), RGN, FHEA

Senior Lecturer, School of Health and Society, University of Salford.

Mary completed her nurse training at University College Hospital, London, and worked initially in orthopaedic/trauma care and gastroenterology, before moving into neuroscience care. In addition to undertaking specialist education and training in neuroscience nursing, her neuroscience experience extends over 30 years, progressing through various clinical posts including ward manager, matron and practice development lead, before leaving clinical practice to start a career in nurse education and research. Mary teaches across several curricula, including BSc Pre-Registration Nursing and MSc Advanced Clinical Practice. She is author and co-author of several articles, book chapters on neuroscience nursing and nurse education, and joint author of the book *Supporting Families and Carers: a nursing perspective*. Mary is the service user and care lead in nursing at the University of Salford, working towards continuous quality improvement through providing a network of service users and carers sharing their knowledge and experiences. She is President of the British Association of Neuroscience Nurses (BANN), a member of the World Federation of Neuroscience Nurses (WFNN) and an editorial board member of the *British Journal of Neuroscience Nursing*. Her key interests include acquired brain injury and the impact of caregiving on family caregivers.

Charlotte Bramanis

MNurs, PGCert CYP, DipHE Paed Nurs, FHEA

Senior Lecturer and Course Lead in Children's Nursing, and Professional Lead for Children's Nursing and Learning Disabilities Nursing, University of West London.

Charlotte began her career in 1997 studying children's nursing at the Thames Valley University (now the University of West London), before taking up a staff nurse post at the Royal Berkshire Hospital in the general paediatric ward. In 2003, she moved to Western Australia to work in the only paediatric facility in the state, at the Princess Margaret Hospital. During that time, she worked in accident and emergency, oncology, neonatal intensive care and diagnostic imaging. After 15 years in Australia, she returned to the UK to start her career in lecturing with the University of West London. Educationally, Charlotte teaches on the Pre-Registration and Nursing Associate course at the university and has contributed to the new high-quality nursing curriculum. She has been awarded Lecturer of the Year twice in her 3-year tenure, and is currently developing a curriculum for the Masters Degree in Nursing course.

Colin Cameron

PhD, MA, BA (Hons)

Senior Lecturer, Department of Social Work, Education & Community Wellbeing.

Faculty of Health and Life Sciences, Northumbria University Colin is a senior lecturer at Northumbria University, Newcastle-upon-Tyne. He teaches sociology and philosophy on undergraduate degrees in Guidance & Counselling and Health & Social Care, and he supervises postgraduate students on various disability studies research projects. He has been active in the disabled people's movement for 30 years. He is a director of Shaping Our Lives, the national network of service user-led organisations, and an executive editor of the international journal *Disability and Society*. His Stuckist paintings have been exhibited at the Royal Academy of Arts.

Carl Clare

RN, Dip N, BSc (Hons), MSc (Lond), PGDE (Lond)
Senior Lecturer, Department of Adult Nursing and Primary Care, School of Health and Social Work, University of Hertfordshire.

Carl began his nursing career in 1990 as a nursing auxiliary. He later undertook 3 years of student nurse training at Selly Oak Hospital (Birmingham), moving to the Royal Devon and Exeter Hospitals, then Northwick Park Hospital, and finally the Royal Brompton & Harefield NHS Trust as a resuscitation officer and honorary teaching fellow of Imperial College London. Since 2006, he has worked at the University of Hertfordshire as a senior lecturer in adult nursing. His key areas of interest are long-term illness, physiology, sociology, endocrinology and cardiac care.

Nigel Davies

MSc, BSc (Hons), PGDip, Cert Ed, RN, SFHEA
Professor of Interprofessional Learning, College of Health, Medicine and Life Sciences, Brunel University, London.

Nigel graduated with a first-class Honours degree from South Bank Polytechnic in 1990. His clinical practice, across several London hospitals, was in general medicine, cardiothoracic surgery and critical care. He became a lecturer practitioner and then senior lecturer in the late 1990s and then moved into nursing management roles with responsibility for practice development and quality improvement. For over 10 years he was a director of nursing and director of infection prevention and control in two acute trusts. He has undertaken research relating to nursing policy and practice, and has published widely in peer-reviewed journals. He was head of nursing and programme lead for the BSc Nursing course at the University of East London before moving to his current role in 2021, leading interprofessional education at Brunel University London. He is also an external examiner for the Masters Degree in Nursing at the University of Sheffield.

Joanne Day

MSc Occupational Health (Policy & Practice), PGCE (Professional Education), BN (Hons), RN(A), FHEA, MInstLM
Senior Lecturer in Nursing Education, Edge Hill University.

Jo came into nursing as a mature student, having previously worked in retail and administration roles. She studied at the University of Southampton, qualifying as a registered nurse in 2007. Since qualifying, she has enjoyed the flexibility that a nursing career provided to move around while her husband served in the Armed Forces and she raised her family. She has worked in a variety of settings, including overseas. Within the NHS, she has worked in cardiothoracic (medical and surgical) and emergency care. Away from the NHS, she has also worked as a school nurse and a disability analyst. In 2017, Jo moved into an academic setting as a lecturer in practice learning followed by a role as practice lead. Educationally, Jo teaches on pre-registration courses for the university and has a strong interest in improving the clinical practice experiences for pre-registration students, particularly those with SpLD.

Hilarious De Jesus

MRes Clinical Research, PgCert (Higher Education), BSc (Nursing), RN, FHEA
Lecturer in Neonatology and Child Health, City, University of London.

Harry is an overseas-trained nurse from the Philippines. He migrated and practised in the UK as a staff nurse in 2010, working in a Level 3 neonatal intensive care unit in London. In 2012, he decided to move into clinical research, looking at nursing in paediatrics. During his time as a children's research nurse, he worked on several commercial and government clinical trials. As a research nurse, he helped facilitate the licensing of ground-breaking treatments for some chronic conditions, such as inflammatory bowel disease, Fabry disease and eczema. He eventually took up the post of senior research nurse with the North Thames Clinical Research Network. The post involves the propagation of the research portfolio within the region, improvement of access into research within diverse communities and enhancing the profile of clinical research among different stakeholders. During the pandemic, Harry served with one of the faculties that started the Nightingale Hospitals in London. He still practises as a paediatric/neonatal intensive care nurse on top of his academic role. Harry joined academia in 2020. He lectures on various nursing subjects such as healthcare law, ethics, communication and clinical skills. He has innovated practice by planning and implementing pedagogical techniques such as Socratic seminars, online debates, online peer models of learning and virtual clinical skills. His main interests are chronic conditions, participatory research methods, clinical research nursing and childhood allergy/immunology.

Julie Derbyshire

Prof Doc (Ed), MSc, PgDip Ed (Health), BA (Hons), Dip N, RGN, HEA Fellow
Director of Apprenticeships and Senior Lecturer in Nursing, Northumbria University.

Julie qualified as a registered general nurse in 1992 and specialised in neurosurgical/trauma nursing, working within the Regional Neurosciences Unit at Newcastle for 8 years. Julie moved into a specialist practice development role in 2000 and developed a keen interest in service improvement, patient safety and interprofessional learning. She commenced as a senior lecturer at Northumbria University in 2003, where she continues to work and predominantly teaches undergraduate nursing students. Julie also leads on the registered nurse degree apprenticeship programme. Julie makes a significant contribution to developing nursing curricula, advancing knowledge in her discipline, with a specialist interest in neurological conditions and works closely with NHS trust partners to develop educational practice and ultimately patient care.

Scott Elbourne

RGN
Clinical Lead in District Nursing, Berkshire Healthcare NHS Foundation Trust.

Scott completed his registered nurse education at Kingston University and St George's University of London, and his Specialist Practitioner degree at Buckingham New University. Scott's clinical experience includes working as a staff nurse in accident and emergency at Epsom and St Helier University Hospitals, and in community healthcare as a community staff nurse, district nurse and team leader for the District Nursing Service at Berkshire Healthcare NHS Foundation Trust. Scott was fortunate to undertake a 1-year secondment from practice to work at the University of West London as a lecturer in adult nursing/nursing associates. Scott currently works as a clinical lead in district nursing at Berkshire Healthcare NHS Foundation Trust. He is a specialist practitioner in district nursing and has a MSc degree in Community Healthcare. Scott's main role in practice is clinical education and performance management in all areas of community practice, although he has a specialist interest in end-of-life care and student nurse education.

Debra Fearns

MA Health & Social Policy, PGDip Teaching & Learning, BA (Hons) (Humanities), RNLD Senior Lecturer in Learning Disability Nursing, University of Hertfordshire

Debra began her career in 1983 studying learning disability nursing at West Hertfordshire College of Nursing, before taking up a staff nurse post at Scunthorpe General Hospital in the Mental Health Unit, part-time for 2 years. In 1989, she moved back to St Albans and became a staff nurse at Cell Barnes Hospital, working with people with complex needs. During that time, she became an acting ward manager and by 1990 was seconded to be the resettlement co-ordinator as part of the process of closing Cell Barnes Hospital and relocating the long-stay residents into community homes and settings. Debra held a number of secondments at Cell Barnes Hospital, including care plan co-ordinator, and was appointed as an in-service tutor in October 1981. Debra was appointed as a Senior Lecturer at the University of Hertfordshire in October 1993 when the College of Healthcare Studies merged with the University, and has worked there ever since.

Educationally, Debra teaches on both the BSc undergraduate and MSc undergraduate nursing programmes, specialising in learning disability nursing. She was also previously the programme tutor for the combined degree in Learning Disability and Social Work and for the Learning Disability nursing programme. She is currently the module lead for the cross-school interprofessional nursing education for first-year students.

Debra has published books and articles on learning disability nursing and won a University of Hertfordshire Teaching Innovation Award; the award funds were used successfully to assist combined degree students and Law School students in simulating presenting court reports. Her areas of interest include people with learning disabilities and additional mental health needs, the criminal justice system and health inequalities.

Ann Foley

MA, BSc (Hons), RGN, RSCN, RNT, FHEA
Director of Pre Qualifying Education - Nursing and Midwifery University of Manchester.

Ann undertook dual training in adult and children's nursing, working between Booth Hall Children's Hospital, Manchester and North Manchester General Hospital, qualifying in 1989. Her early career was spent working in the regional paediatric burns and plastic surgery unit in Manchester moving into a lecturer practitioner position working for Salford University and Pennine Acute NHS Trust. Ann entered full-time nurse education in 1998 and worked for the University of Salford in their Child Health team, before moving to the University of Central Lancashire (2004–2015), working initially as a principal lecturer leading the children provision and then latterly leading the undergraduate nursing programmes across all fields with a strategic lead for undergraduate recruitment and programme development . She moved to the University of Manchester in 2015 as a senior lecturer working on the Children and Young People's nursing team with a strategic lead for undergraduate admissions . In November 2019 she was appointed as director of undergraduate education with a responsibility for undergraduate Nursing and Midwifery programmes. Ann is currently completing doctoral studies which centre upon supporting student learning within the HE environment.

Annette Hand

Prof Doc (Health), MA, PGDip (CR), Dip HE, RGN
Professor of Nursing – Clinical Academic, Newcastle-upon-Tyne Hospitals NHS Foundation Trust/Northumbria University.

Annette began her nursing career in 1991, studying at the Northumbria School of Nursing. Post qualification, she worked across various settings, including orthopaedics, community nursing and palliative care. In 1998, she started her career in Parkinson's disease and progressed to nurse consultant in 2004. She continued in that role for 17 years, co-ordinating the Parkinson's service, supporting patients and their families, and managing a team of Parkinson's specialist nurses. In 2018, Annette was appointed to a national role as clinical lead for nursing with the Parkinson's Excellence Network to support services across the UK. She has continued an active research role and been involved with multiple research studies at a local, national and international level, and has published multiple articles. In 2021, she was appointed to professor of nursing – clinical academic, the first post of its type in the north east of England. Annette now divides her time between clinical practice, research and education. Educationally, Annette has been teaching within Higher Education since 2004. She currently teaches on several postgraduate courses for the university, and her interests include non-medical prescribing, Parkinson's disease, clinical research and research impact.

Barry Hill

MSc Advanced Practice, PGC Academic Practice, BSc (Hons) Intensive Care Nursing, DipHE Adult Nursing, OA Dip Counselling Skills, RN, NMC RNT/TCH, SFHEA
Programme Leader (Senior Lecturer) Adult Nursing, Northumbria University, Clinical and Commissioning Editor for the *British Journal of Nursing*.

Barry is an experienced leader, academic, educator, researcher and clinical nurse. His current role is director level and as part of the senior leadership team, as Director of Education (Employability) for the Department of Nursing, Midwifery and Health, and Programme Leader (BSc Nursing Sciences). He has a demonstrated history of working within academia, particularly in the Higher Education (HE) industry. Barry is a senior fellow (SFHEA) and an HEA mentor, a certified advanced nurse practitioner (ANP), NMC registered nurse (RN), NMC registered teacher (TCH), and an NMC registered independent and supplementary prescriber (V300). He is skilled in clinical research and clinical education, and is passionate about higher education, especially advanced clinical practice (ACP), critical care, non-medical prescribing (NMP) and pharmacology. He has been a nurse leader for more than 15 years and was trained in London's best teaching hospitals at Imperial College NHS Trust.

Barry is a strongly education-focused professional who has also published books, book chapters and peer-reviewed journal articles. He is the clinical editor and commissioning editor for the *At A Glance* and *Advanced Practice* series within the *British Journal of Nursing*. He is currently a fourth-year Doctor of Philosophy (PhD) candidate at Northumbria University, Newcastle-upon-Tyne.

Noleen P. Jones

RN, DipN, Ad Dip Management, BSc, FHEA, MEd
Acting Principal Lecturer, School of Health Studies, Gibraltar.

Noleen began her nursing career as a nursing auxiliary in 1987 before training to be an enrolled nurse, eventually qualifying as a staff nurse in 1992. She worked in critical care as a newly qualified RN until 2013, where she held the posts of senior sister and lead nurse for education and training, before she moved onto practice development for a year. It was during this time that her links to the School of Health Studies strengthened. Noleen became a lecturer with the School of Health Studies in Gibraltar in 2014. Her main role was teaching on the undergraduate nursing degree programmes. She developed a virtual case study for students as a scaffold to aid learning. The case study spans the 3 years of study and ties in with all the modules in the programme. Her key interests are cardiac care, respiratory care and teaching practice skills.

Michael Lappin

RN, EN(G), BSc (Hons), MSc, PGCE
Lecturer in Adult Nursing, University of Salford.

Mike began his career in 1976 at North Ormesby Hospital, Middlesbrough, becoming an enrolled nurse working in general medicine, respiratory medicine and coronary care. He moved to Manchester in 1988 to complete the conversion course at Trafford General Hospital. Deciding to stay in Manchester, he continued to work in coronary care as a staff nurse and then as a charge nurse at Salford Royal Hospital. He then joined the professional development team in Salford before moving to the University of Salford in April 2003 as a full-time lecturer. Mike's key areas of interest include leadership, change management, action learning and the professional development of staff. In his time at the University of Salford, he has led on many pre-registration modules and is currently module lead for the postgraduate module Leading & Managing in Complex Organisations.

Louise Lingwood

MBA, MA Ed, PGDip ANP, PGDip Ed, APMG, BSc (Hons), RNMH, FHEA
Senior Lecturer Mental Health Nursing, Northumbria University.

Louise completed her undergraduate mental health nurse education and training at Northumbria University in 2000. She has worked extensively across children and young people's mental health services (CAMHS) since qualifying and has worked as a mental health nurse, project manager and clinical manager within specialist CAMHS across the north east and nationally. She has worked clinically within forensic teams, looked after the children teams, primary mental health, CAMHS, National Deaf CAMHS, autism, eating disorder and learning disability services. Louise commenced her post at Northumbria University in 2013. She is currently the programme lead for mental health nursing and teaches pre-registration programmes across

all fields. She has a specialist interest in enhancing nurse education, anatomy, parity of esteem, autism and disability. She is involved in a number of research projects and is currently reading for her PhD.

Nadine Manfred

BSc (Hons), PGDip Physiotherapy
Unqualified Lecturer, School of Health Studies, Gibraltar.

Nadine began her career in 1995 studying physiotherapy at the University of Wales, College of Medicine (now Cardiff University), before taking up a junior rotational post at the Royal Gwent Hospital, South Wales. During her time there, she completed 2 years of general rotations before progressing onto a musculoskeletal rotational senior post. Nadine continued her progression within the musculoskeletal field, and in 2007 became a spinal clinical specialist in Cardiff & Vale NHS Trust. She left the NHS after 9 years to continue her career in the private sector and to run her own practice, specialising in musculoskeletal conditions. In 2015, Nadine moved back to her native Gibraltar and took up employment within the Gibraltar Health Authority as a rotational senior physiotherapist. In 2020, she was seconded to the post of unqualified lecturer at the School of Health Studies, Gibraltar Health Authority. During her time at the School, she has been involved in overseeing the nursing and allied health professionals through their vocational training qualifications, recruitment and interviewing for the BSc (Hons) Adult Nursing through the University of Gibraltar, as well as teaching on the undergraduate nursing degree programme.

Rosemary McCarthy

PhD, RM, RN, PGCE
Head of Global Workforce, Education and Research, Global Health Partnerships Directorate, Manchester Area, UK.

Rose is the Head of Global Workforce, Education and Research in the Directorate of Global Health Partnerships (DGHP) at Health Education England (HEE), responsible for leading the coordination of DGHPs global workforce activity to address workforce challenges in the NHS. Her background is a clinical academic, she is a registered nurse and midwife for over 30 years and maintain clinical practice at a large teaching Hospital. Rose worked in Higher Education as a lecturer, researcher, and manager for over 15 years and held the position of Deputy Director in the School of Health at the University of Salford, where she still has an Honorary Lecturer role. Her research interests focus largely on global health, global learners and learning, and the use of social and digital media to support learning.

Louise McErlean

BSc (Hons) Critical Care Nursing, MA Teaching and Learning, FHEA, RGN
Lecturer (Adult Nursing), Ulster University.

Louise commenced her career as a nurse in Glasgow and has worked across the UK, specialising in critical care nursing. Louise has worked in higher education since 2005. Her key interests are anatomy and physiology, pathophysiology, clinical simulation and nurse education.

Sara Meakin

RGN, BSc Nursing (Hons), BSc Psychology, NMP, MSc Professional Practice, FHEA

Senior Lecturer in Advanced Clinical Practice, University of West London.

Sara started her career at King's College Hospital in 1997 in neurosurgery and neuro ITU, before moving to work in accident and emergency, where her journey as an advanced nurse practitioner began. Since then, she has worked between urgent and emergency care, GP out-of-hours and primary care. Sara has been lecturing with the university since 2015; in 2019 she became a senior lecturer and is currently acting pathway lead for the MSc in Advanced Clinical Practice. She continues to work clinically one day a week as a care planning nurse practitioner, and has an interest in personalised care and support planning, as well as advanced clinical practice learning and development.

Graeme Measor

MSc Advanced Clinical Practice, PGCE LTHE, FHEA, BSc (Hons) Specialist Practitioner, BSc (Hons) Practice Effectiveness, DipN, RN

Senior Lecturer (Field Leader) in Adult Nursing, Teesside University.

Graeme began his career in 1994 studying adult nursing at the Durham and Teesside College of Health (now Teesside University), before taking up a position as staff nurse in 'scrub' in North Tees General Hospital operating theatres. He progressed to charge nurse and then became the first orthopaedic surgical practitioner in the country, recognised by the Royal College of Surgeons. During this time, he developed his knowledge of operative surgery, physical examination, diagnostics and pathophysiology. He worked autonomously, performing local anaesthetic surgeries and following patients up in outpatient clinics. He left practice after 12 years in 2009 to start his career in lecturing with Teesside University. Educationally, Graeme teaches on several pre- and postgraduate courses for the university, and has contributed to the latest NMC-approved pre-registration nursing curriculum. He leads the Physical Assessment Skills and Advanced Pathophysiology modules, developing outstanding learning materials and teaching experiences. His areas of interest include all aspects of pathophysiology and clinical examination, and he has recently commenced his doctorate, investigating anatomy and physiology learning in nursing students.

Jean Mason Mitchell

RGN, RM, MSc, PGCHER

Lecturer Midwifery, School of Health and Society, University of Salford, UK.

Jean commenced nurse education in 1980 and midwifery education in 1986. She spent 29 years in midwifery practice, team management and education. During this time she developed a passion for supporting students in practice placement and newly qualified midwives and also developed keen and diverse interests, for example developing emergency skills drills and safeguarding the unborn and vulnerable adults.

Jean joined the University of Salford in 2003 as a Lecturer / Practitioner of Midwifery and became a full time lecturer in October 2011. She is currently a level 6 lecturer and module lead for modules related to challenges in midwifery practice and complex care. She also supports students undertaking level 7 perinatal health and research modules. Her passion for supporting students and newly qualified midwives continues. She maintains strong links with clinical practice and has several publications linked to preceptorship.

Helen Paterson

EN, RN, DipN, BSc (Hons)

Matron for Elderly Care & Rheumatology, Frimley Health Foundation Trust.

Helen began her career in 1978, studying as an enrolled nurse in Dr Gray's Hospital, Elgin, Scotland. Her first role when qualified in 1980 was in a community hospital in Forres, predominantly nursing older people. Helen has taken up different posts in different venues and disciplines, such as nursing homes, maternity (military hospital in Germany), colposcopy clinics and private hospitals. She has worked as a pharmacy assistant, a discharge co-ordinator, as a falls co-ordinator for SW Surrey, and as matron for elderly care in three acute hospitals, latterly Frimley Park Hospital. This variety of positions has enabled her to acquire many transferrable skills that have enhanced her knowledge and passion in caring for the older person. In addition to her post as matron, she is also the trust lead for inpatient falls prevention. Educationally, in 2000 Helen completed the EN conversion course to RN status. Following this, she completed a DipN and BSc (Hons) in gerontological nursing. She is currently working towards her Masters. Educationally, in 2000 Helen completed the EN conversion course to RN status. Following this, she completed a DipN and BSc (Hons) in gerontological nursing. She is currently working towards her Masters.

Claire Pryor

PhD, MSc Advancing Healthcare Practice, PGC Advanced Practice (Clinical), PGC Teaching and Learning in Professional Practice, NMC Teacher (NMC/TCH), V300 Independent Prescriber, FHEA, RN

Senior Lecturer In Adult Nursing, Northumbria University.

Claire's educational interests lie predominantly in nursing care for the older person and she is module lead for non-medical prescribing. Her teaching activity spans adult pre- and postregistration professional development. Claire's specialist areas of interest include delirium and delirium superimposed on dementia, and integrating physical health and mental healthcare education and service provision. Prior to lecturing, Claire worked in a variety of primary and secondary care settings including acute medical assessment, critical care, intermediate care and as an older person's nurse practitioner in a mental health setting.

Joanna Regan

SEN, RN

Director of Nursing (Operations), Leeds Teaching Hospitals NHS Trust.

Jo began her nursing career in 1985 at Leeds Teaching Hospital, becoming an enrolled nurse, working in acute and elective orthopaedics. She later undertook a conversion course at Bradford University, continuing her career in orthopaedics as a staff nurse and ward sister. She continued her career at Leeds, working as a matron in a number of adult specialties, then as head of nursing in cardiorespiratory, neurosciences and emergency and specialty medicine, including emergency departments, acute assessment, elderly, general medicine, infectious diseases, HIV and sexual health services. Jo is particularly interested in advancing quality improvement in nursing practice, using the Leeds Improvement methodology. She also takes a keen interest in patient experience, public involvement, and staff health and well-being.

Hazel Ridgers
RN (Adult), PGCAP, MA, FHEA
Senior Lecturer, School of Sports and Health Sciences, University of Brighton.

Hazel trained as a nurse at King's College, London, and took up her first staff nurse post at Guys and St Thomas' Hospital in 2006. She developed an interest in the health and well-being of older people living with HIV and undertook sexual health and HIV specialisation courses early in her nursing career. She has worked in HIV, sexual health, research and infectious disease settings and has a keen interest in public health as well as leadership in healthcare. Hazel began her career in nursing education in 2010 and is currently a senior lecturer at the University of Brighton.

Linda Sanderson
EdD, MSc Health Professional Education, RGN Child and Adult, RNT
Head of Practice Education, Blended Learning, University of Huddersfield.

Linda trained as a nurse at Leeds Polytechnic in 1981–5. She worked as an adult nurse in medicine, renal and general surgery. Between 1988 and 1989 she trained as a children's nurse and worked between 1989 and 2004 in cancer care for children and young people at the Yorkshire specialist unit, then as a staff nurse, sister and finally as a lecturer practitioner in conjunction with Leeds University. She had a brief spell as sister of a busy children's unit at Airedale General Hospital before starting a full-time career in 2006 in education at the University of Central Lancashire (UCLan). At UCLan, Linda was a senior lecturer, course leader and eventually principal lecturer with a lead for children's nursing, international placements, admissions and business development. In 2017, Linda moved into the charity sector, working with a leading children's cancer charity, CLIC Sargent (now Young Lives vs Cancer), as their first nurse educator. She worked in the north of England, teaching health professionals about the care of children with cancer. Following redundancy due to the COVID-19 pandemic, she moved to her current post as head of practice education (blended learning) at the University of Huddersfield.

Mahesh Seewoodhary
MBE, BSc (Hons) Biological Sciences, RGN, OND (Hons), JBCNS Intensive care, FETC 730 with distinction, DN, RCNT, RNT, Cert Ed, FHEA
Senior Lecturer in Ophthalmic Nursing, University of West London.

Mahesh began his nursing career in 1971 at the West Wales General Hospital (now the Glangwili General Hospital). In 1977, he was appointed charge nurse in the accident and emergency department at Moorfields. In 1978 he was appointed clinical teacher at Moorfields and led the Ophthalmic Emergency course until 2004. He was the link teacher at Royal Berkshire Hospital, the Eye units in Windsor, and Western Eye Hospital in 2004. He is currently the link teacher for the Ophthalmic Nursing course in Jerusalem. Educationally, Mahesh has implemented a number of interactive teaching pedagogies in ophthalmic nursing. He teaches on several postgraduate courses for the university, and has contributed to the high-quality nursing curriculum in Ophthalmic Nursing and Delivering Quality Care Through Work-Based Learning. Mahesh has published widely on topics related to ophthalmic nursing and on ophthalmic medication for nurse prescribers. He was awarded an MBE in the Queen's Birthday Honours List in 2018 for services to ophthalmic nursing and for raising awareness in nursing of sickle cell disease.

Lynette Harland Shotton
EdD, MSc Health Sciences/Public Health, BSc (Hons) Community Nursing, RGN, SCPHN, Senior Fellow of Advance HE
Head of Subject, Department of Social Work, Education and Community Wellbeing, Northumbria University.

Lynette began her adult nursing career in 1995 and later qualified as a specialist community public health nurse, practising in the health visiting field. She has worked in higher education since 2008 and has contributed to a range of pre-registration and postregistration nursing provision, with particular emphasis on public health and health inequality. Her research and scholarly interests are broad, spanning public health, social care and education, connected by the common theme of inequality. Recent publications focus on research methods, educational inequality, health visiting and health literacy. As director of access and participation until September 2021, Lynette influenced educational policy at local level for under-represented university students, collaborating with key agencies across the north east and nationally. Part of this work has sought to understand and address key public health issues for students, including emotional well-being and food insecurity.

Alison Simons
Med. Learning and Teaching in Higher Education, BSc (Hons)
Cancer Care, RGN, FHEA Senior Lecturer at Birmingham City University.

Alison was a cancer nurse for 18 years within a large teaching hospital, caring for patients diagnosed with a variety of cancers. She has a passion for education and was the educational lead and a qualified NVQ assessor for nursing assistants. She went on to become a professional development sister responsible for the educational and continuing development needs of over 200 oncology and haematology nurses. Alison joined Birmingham City University in 2009 as a senior lecturer and pathway lead for cancer and haematology. She has since gone on to gain her PG Cert, PG Dip and Masters in Education. She is now course leader for the Professional Practice Programme, a postqualifying practice postgraduate course, and pathway lead for cancer and haemato-oncology. Alison's area of interest is occupational safety of handling cytotoxic chemotherapy and she has published several articles, presented at conferences, and is involved with European working groups developing legislation and policy in relation to this. She started her professional doctorate in health in September 2021.

Melanie Stephens

PhD, MA, BSc(Hons), Dip N, RGN
Senior Lecturer in Adult Nursing and Head of Interprofessional Education within the School of Health and Society, University of Salford.

Melanie is a health and social care service researcher, with specific research interests in pressure, redistributing properties of seating, tissue viability and interprofessional working and learning. She has undertaken research to provide an evidence base for products used in the 24-hour management of pressure ulcers, and affective domain development of student nurses. She co-led an amendment to the UK Tissue Viability Society Seating Guidelines with service users, and is using this work to impact policy and practice. She is currently leading a feasibility study on the impact of interprofessional student training care homes on residents, care home staff and students. Melanie is experienced in mixed methods of enquiry, working with practitioners and commerce to develop research for use in the clinical environment.

Jamie Swales

MSc Advanced Practice, NMP, BSc (Hons), RGN
Lead Advanced Clinical Practitioner and Deputy Clinical Lead, Acute Care Team, East Lancashire Hospital Trust.

Jamie started his nursing career in 2005, studying adult nursing at Manchester Metropolitan University before commencing his nursing career at Salford Royal Hospital. In 2010 Jamie moved to East Lancashire Hospital Trust, working within a variety of surgical wards before moving to the emergency department and progressing through a variety of roles including charge nurse, practice educator and senior charge nurse. Here he found a passion for managing the care of acutely deteriorating patients which resulted in him undertaking his MSc in Advanced Practice within the Acute Care Team, who manage the care of deteriorating patients across the organisation. Jamie's areas of interest include NEWS2, education of all healthcare professionals, leadership and quality improvement with the overall aim of improving patient outcomes from acute illness.

Karen Sykes

MSc Safeguarding Legislation, BSc (Hons), BA (Hons), RGN Specialist Community Public Health Nurses (HV)
Head of Nursing for Safeguarding, Mental Health Legislation, Learning Disabilities and Autism, Leeds Teaching Hospitals NHS Trust.

Karen began her career in 1986, studying adult nursing at Bury School of Nursing (now Pennine Acute NHS Trust) before taking up a staff nurse post at Fairfield General Hospital in the paediatric unit. Her career then diverted into critical care, where she worked for a number of years before commencing her specialist community nursing (health visitor) training and qualification. She worked as a health visitor for 3 years, and then began work in a multiagency adolescent substance and alcohol service in Bolton as a clinical nurse specialist. During Karen's time in these latter two posts, her interest in safeguarding grew, and in 2007 she became a safeguarding specialist nurse advisor in Bradford, progressing into a number of named nurse for safeguarding

posts in both acute and community settings. Karen completed her Masters degree in 2010 and progressed into a head of safeguarding children and adults post in a CCG in Manchester, managing a number of teams and leading on a varied portfolio. Her passion has always been working in an acute setting, and in 2015 she was appointed head of nursing for safeguarding, mental health legislation, learning disabilities and autism at Leeds Teaching Hospitals NHS Trust. Karen has contributed to both regional and local safeguarding agendas in a variety of workstreams. Educationally, she teaches on a number of courses for pre- and postgraduate students. Her areas of specific interest also include self-neglect, domestic violence and child exploitation.

Deborah Taylor

MSc Education, PGDip Leadership, PGCE, ENB998/199, PGCert Orthopaedics, Dip Applied Science (Nursing) RGN
Lead for Pre-Registration Nursing, University of West London.

Deborah initially qualified as a registered general nurse in Sydney, Australia, in 1990 and specialised in orthopaedic nursing. Relocating to London in the late 1990s, she worked briefly in the private sector before moving into the NHS. Her clinical career then focused on emergency nursing, where she became a team leader and emergency nurse practitioner. With an MSc in Education and Strategic Leadership and over 25 years of practical experience, she is highly experienced in both teaching/learning and clinical practice. She has up-to-date relevant clinical experience in emergency/critical care, managing teams, change management and mentoring/support of staff and students, and is passionate about integrating theory and practice using innovative and engaging methods both in the classroom and as part of simulated learning. Deborah's vision is to provide the NHS with inspirational and aspirational nurses who prioritise patient care within a culture of safety and support. She believes this is achievable through the application of compassionate leadership, shared vision and collaboration within the team, involving students in their learning and giving them a voice.

Luis Teixeira

MSc Bioethics, PGCert Critical Care Nursing, PGCert Professional Academic Practice, BSc (Hons) Nursing, RN, FHEA
Lecturer in Adult Nursing Complex Care, King's College London.

Luis has been a registered nurse since August 2006, with extensive clinical experience across diverse contexts in two different countries. He became a full-time lecturer in March 2018 at the University of West London, moving to King's College London in October 2021. While in clinical practice, Luis has been developing his teaching and management skills, acting as a mentor, practice educator and charge nurse. He has been leading quality improvement projects and also collaborating with nursing and healthcare schools, nationally and internationally. His clinical skills have been predominantly developed in a hospital setting, and he has become an expert in critical care nursing. Luis also has an interest in philosophy and law, and obtained a Masters degree in Bioethics linking those areas to nursing care and the decision-making process (more particularly to the contexts of acute/critical care and end-of-life care). His commitment to this subject and studies developed have contributed to important changes in Portugal, locally and nationally, by promoting bioethical discussion and legal implementation of advanced directives.

Juliana Thompson

PhD, MA, PG Cert Education for Professional Practice, SFHEA, RN, Registered Nurse Teacher

Dr Juliana Thompson is an associate professor in adult nursing at Northumbria University. Her educational and research interests lie predominantly in development of the workforce caring for older people with complex needs. She has led a number of research and evaluation studies in this area, and has published widely in international journals about workforce improvement strategies. Juliana led the development of the Enhanced Care for Older People (EnCOP) workforce strategy, which has been widely implemented in England. Prior to her career in academia, Juliana worked as a nurse in the care of older people primarily in social care settings.

Sue Tiplady

MSc Nursing Practice, BSc (Hons) Nursing Science, Independent Nurse Prescriber, PGCert Management of Long-Term Conditions, PGCert EPP, RNT, FHEA, RGN

Senior Lecturer in Adult Nursing, Northumbria University.

Sue Tiplady's teaching subject expertise centres around care of the older person and spans adult pre- and postregistration professional development. Her academic and research activities focus on the development of a workforce skilled in the health and social care of older people, integrated health and social care, development of care home placements for student nurses and the involvement of older people in nurse education. Prior to lecturing, Sue worked extensively in environments caring for older people and has held senior clinical, managerial, commissioning, and academic posts in a variety of settings across education, primary, intermediate and secondary care.

Samantha Toland

RN, BN, PGCert (Ed), FHEA

Senior Lecturer Birmingham City University and Lead Chemotherapy Nurse, Worcestershire Acute Hospitals Trust.

Sam has been a cancer/haemato-oncology nurse for 20 years, having worked initially in haemato-oncology and stem cell transplant. She then went on to become a chemotherapy nurse trainer, responsible for the chemotherapy training and education of all nursing staff in a large teaching hospital trust. During this time, she also commenced her post at Birmingham City University as a senior lecturer in haemato-oncology and chemotherapy and, more recently, non-medical prescribing. She has also had roles as a leukaemia nurse specialist and acute oncology nurse practitioner, and is currently a lead chemotherapy nurse at a large acute hospital trust and has carried out these roles in conjunction with her university post. Sam is also the Chair of the West Midlands Cancer Alliance Systemic Anti-Cancer Treatment Expert Advisory Group, and a member of the National Clinical Reference Group for Chemotherapy.

Marie Jones

RN, DipN (Adult), MSc Advanced Practice (Distinction)

Advanced Nurse Practitioner in Haematology, Manchester Royal Infirmary.

Marie has worked in haematology and stem cell transplant for over 20 years after qualifying as a nurse in Aberdeen. She worked at Aberdeen Royal Infirmary before moving to the Christie Hospital, Manchester, in 2002. After undertaking further training in oncology, haematology and transplant, she took the position of stem cell/ bone marrow transplant co-ordinator (nurse specialist) at Manchester Royal Infirmary in 2006. She then undertook an MSc in advanced practice and qualified as an ANP in 2015. Her interests include education on haematology and stem cell transplant and improving the patient experience of treatment. Additionally, Marie has teaching and honorary lecturing commitments at Manchester Metropolitan University and the University of Manchester (in conjunction with the Christie Hospital). She is currently Chair of the UK EBMT Nurses and Allied Health Professionals' Group, Nurse Representative for BSBMTCT Executive Committee and an Expert Advisor to NICE. She has presented locally, nationally and internationally at various conferences and educational meetings.

Anthony Wheeldon

MSc (Lond), PGDE, BSc (Hons), Dip HE, RN

Senior Lecturer in Adult Nursing, University of Hertfordshire.

Anthony began his nursing career at Barnet College of Nursing and Midwifery in 1992. After qualification, he worked as a staff nurse and senior staff nurse in the Respiratory Directorate at the Royal Brompton and Harefield NHS Trust in London. From 2000, he worked as a visiting lecturer for Thames Valley University (now the University of West London) and taught on postregistration cardiorespiratory courses before joining them full time in 2002. Since 2006, Anthony has worked at the University of Hertfordshire, where he has taught on BSc and MSc pre- and postregistration nursing courses. He has a broad range of interests, which include the promotion of inclusivity, success and attainment in nurse education, as well as cardiorespiratory care, anatomy and physiology, respiratory assessment, and the application of bioscience in nursing practice. He currently teaches a wide range of subjects, including communication, leadership and management, co-ordinating complex care and evidence-based healthcare.

Pamela Young

RGN, BSc(Dist) Health Studies, MSc Diabetes with Applied Education, Independent and Supplementary Prescriber, PGCE TLHE, FHEA

Lecturer in Advanced Practice and Prescribing, University of the West of Scotland.

Pam qualified in 1992 from the South-West Scotland College of Nursing and Midwifery (now University of the West of Scotland). Her first staff nurse post was in specialised orthopaedics, then intensive care. Prior to lecturing, she was a diabetes nurse specialist focusing on acute care and insulin pumps. She set up and developed the local insulin pump service and was successful in integrating technology to provide safe, equitable access to care in remote and rural areas of Dumfries and Galloway. Pam now lectures at the University of the West of Scotland in the Advanced Practice and Prescribing Team. She is also a PhD student, scoping the role of prescribing in advanced practice. She is interested in the use of technology to enhance teaching pedagogy, and now teaches via a hybrid approach following the COVID-19 pandemic.

Preface

We were delighted to have been asked to provide a third edition of the very popular text *Nursing Practice: Knowledge and Care*. Feedback from readers has enabled us to make this third edition even more user friendly. We were keen to retain the previous format used in the first and second editions.

Listening to invaluable feedback provided to us has meant that we have merged some chapters and provided a number of new chapters that reflect contemporary practice. We also welcome trainee nursing associates who as of January 2019 joined the professional register.

The text has become an invaluable resource for those who are beginning their nursing education and those who are continuing on their journey to becoming a registered nurse. The text will also be of use to individuals who educate nurses, provide supervision and preceptorship, those who are returning to practice, those already registered, for other members of the extended nursing family and individuals who have chosen nursing in the UK who are coming from other parts of the world. There are many challenges facing those who are required to keep abreast of new developments in knowledge and technologies, in the important activity of promoting health and well-being and with the provision of health and social care that has an evidence base, and all of this against a backdrop of ongoing social and economic change.

Much has changed in the field of health and social care since the second edition of this popular text was published. The ways in which health and social care are delivered will continue to change as nurses and those who provide care in order to meet the needs of others adapt their approach when striving to deliver safe and effective care. The biggest threat to humans for over a century has been the COVID-19 pandemic, closely followed by the catastrophic damage that climate change is bringing. Nursing staff locally, nationally and internationally have been at the forefront in the response to the pandemic, delivering care directly to COVID-19-positive patients and continuing to provide services across the health and care system. The world has witnessed the vital contribution of nursing to patient care day in and day out and student nurses have played their part as they stood up to the plate. The country owes you an enormous debt for the lives that you have helped to save, the care and comfort you have offered families and the significant personal sacrifices that you have made and this should never be forgotten.

The changes bring with them a number of opportunities and challenges for nurses and other health and social care professionals. The often complex needs of people with regard to their health and well-being demand that nurses are knowledgeable and up to date with current practice; the public have a right to know that the people providing their care are fit for purpose and fit for practice. This is a difficult and challenging demand given the transformations occurring within the ever-widening sphere of health and social care (wherever this may be) and the amount of knowledge that the nurse needs to amass in order to be able to say confidently and competently that they are up to date.

The content of this book has its origins in a number of sources, such as the *Standards for Pre-Registration Nursing Education* (NMC, 2018a), *Standards for Pre-Registration Nursing Associate Programmes* (NMC, 2018b), *Standards of Student Supervision and Assessment* (NMC, 2018c) and *The Code: Professional Standards of Practice and Behaviour for Nurses and Midwives* (NMC, 2018d). There are a number of themes and developments that drive strategic direction and change within and without the nursing profession and these have also had an impact on the content of the chapters within the book.

Nursing Practice: Knowledge and Care provides you with much information to enable you to develop a deeper understanding of issues that impact on the health and well-being of the people we serve. The book has been written by expert practitioners and academics who are passionate about the art and science of nursing, dedicated to the health and well-being of the public and committed to nurse education and the notion of lifelong learning.

The book is intended to be used as a reference at home or in the classroom. The art and science of nursing has been interlinked in the chapters and each unit is inter-related. The focus is on the adult field of nursing but, where appropriate, each chapter provides examples of how content can be applied to the other fields of nursing.

The early chapters in the book are 'scene-setting' chapters and we suggest that you read these first. The remaining chapters have been organised in such a way that they can be read at random; for example, if you are offering caring and support to people with cancer, it would be useful to delve into the chapter that addresses issues concerning cancer and then go on to other chapters such as the discussion of pain management and long-term conditions as related to cancer care. We all have our own learning styles and you will adopt whatever approach appeals to you.

We have continued to use a systems approach (in general); we understand that people are not systems, but we have chosen this approach in order to make your learning and the application to practice easier. There are 35 chapters. Each chapter is preceded by learning outcomes related where appropriate to the *Standards for Pre-Registration Nursing Education* (NMC, 2018a) and *Standards for Pre-Registration Nursing Associate Programmes* (NMC, 2018b).

There are a number of learning features and activities within each chapter and these are discussed in the 'How to Use Your Textbook' pages that follow the contributor's section.

Our over-riding intention is to offer you information and in doing this help you understand the important impact that you can have on the health and well-being of people. Nursing requires many skills; a large number of them are common to the care of people in hospitals and the community (primary care) setting. In the book, we indicate this aspect of commonality and in other places it should be apparent on reflection. At all times, it is understood that the provision of nursing care requires special adaptation of a general principle so the individual's, family's or community's needs are met.

We would like thank our colleagues who provided us with chapters for the second edition of the text and also Karen Wild who was a co-editor.

Once again, we have enjoyed writing this text and we hope that you find it of value as you aim to become the best possible nurse, who offers care in a confident, competent and compassionate manner.

Ian Peate, London
Aby Mitchell, London

References

Nursing and Midwifery Council (2018a) *Standards for pre-registration nursing programmes - The Nursing and Midwifery Council (nmc.org.uk)* (accessed March 2022).

Nursing and Midwifery Council (2018b) *Standards for pre-registration nursing associate programmes - The Nursing and Midwifery Council (nmc.org.uk)* (accessed March 2022).

Nursing and Midwifery Council (2018c) *Standards for student supervision and assessment - The Nursing and Midwifery Council (nmc.org.uk)* (accessed March 2022).

Nursing and Midwifery Council (2018d) *The Code: Professional standards of practice and behaviour for nurses, midwives and nursing associates - The Nursing and Midwifery Council (nmc.org.uk)* (accessed March 2022).

Acknowledgements

Ian would like to thank his partner Jussi for his ongoing encouragement and also Mrs Frances Cohen who has throughout the years been so very generous in her support.

Aby would like to thank her husband Graeme and daughters Phoebe and Lottie for all their love and continued support and dear friend Mr Barry Hill who gifted so much support and kindness over the years.

We would like to acknowledge the previous editor of the text, Karen Wild, who has now handed over the baton to Aby Mitchell.

It was and is a great pleasure to work with Karen whose contribution to the profession over the years has not gone unnoticed. Furthermore, thank you to those contributors who wrote chapters in earlier editions and to those who are contributing to this edition.

Finally, we are grateful to the team at Wiley who have supported the publication of this, the third edition.

How to Use Your Textbook

Features contained within your textbook

The **overview page** gives a summary of the topics covered in each part. Every chapter begins with a list of learning outcomes and competencies.

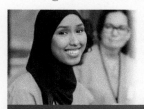

1

The Professional Nurse and Contemporary Healthcare

Deborah Taylor
University of West London, UK

Learning Outcomes
On completion of this chapter you will be able to:
- Demonstrate a knowledge of the NMC's code of professional conduct – standards for practice and behaviour for nurses, midwives and nursing associates
- Be aware of the concept of evidence-based practice
- Understand leadership styles and theories
- Have an awareness of the nurse's role in service improvement and the application of clinical governance as a quality assurance measure
- Recognise the nurse's and nursing associate's role in interprofessional working

Proficiencies
NMC Proficiencies and Standards:
- As accountable professionals, registered nurses and nursing associates act in the best interests of people, putting them first and providing nursing care that is person centred, safe and compassionate.
- They act professionally at all times and use their knowledge and experience to make evidence-based decisions about care.
- They communicate effectively, are role models for others and are accountable for their actions.
- Registered nurses continually reflect on their practice and keep abreast of new and emerging developments in nursing, health and care.

 Visit the companion website at www.wiley.com/go/peate/nursingpractice3e where you can test yourself using flashcards, multiple-choice questions and more.

 *Nursing Practice Knowledge and Care*, Third Edition. Edited by Ian Peate and Aby Mitchell.
© 2022 John Wiley & Sons Ltd. Published 2022 by John Wiley & Sons Ltd.
Companion website: www.wiley.com/go/peate/nursingpractice3e

2

What to Do If boxes give extra information on a specific topic.

What To Do If . . .

 Think about this 'Jot This Down' exercise. What would you do if a relative makes a complaint about the care home manager, saying the manager speaks to her mother in an uncivil way? What do you do next?

Jot This Down boxes are short exercises and reflective questions to get you thinking.

Jot This Down

Multimorbidity does not only include physical health conditions. Have you considered your patient's mental health, symptom complexes or any substance or alcohol history?

Make a list of some biological, social and psychological factors that may contribute to multimorbidity.

Medicines Management boxes provide information about drugs and medicines.

Medicines Management

In exceptional circumstances, where a change or addition to the administration details is required and a delay in administering a medicine (other than a Schedule 2 CD) would compromise patient care, verbal orders are used. The process is underpinned by risk assessments and organisational policy and/or procedures (RPS and RCN, 2019, p.5).

Fields boxes give further insight into the other key areas of nursing.

Nursing Fields Children's Specimens

For infants and small children, a special urine collection bag is adhered to the skin surrounding the urethral area. Once the collection is completed, the urine is poured into a collection cup or transferred directly into an evacuated tube with a transfer straw. Urine collected from a nappy is not recommended for laboratory testing since contamination from the nappy material may affect test results.

For more information see the Great Ormond Street Hospital for Children's guidelines (GOSH, 2020).

Primary Care boxes give information about how to manage issues in the primary care setting.

Primary Care

 Uniforms usually have short sleeves but often in community, social care and nursing home settings, uniform is not always worn and so thought needs to be given in these cases to ensure the 'bare below the elbows' principles can be applied if clinical care of any sort is performed. NICE has produced guidance for primary and community care which includes dress code guidance (NICE, 2017).

Red Flags highlight important points that must not be overlooked.

Red Flag

GCS may be affected if:
  · Eyes are closed due to severe swelling
  · The verbal and motor responses are absent or reduced because of intubation
· Muscle relaxants have been administered
· Sedation or other drugs such as alcohol and recreational drugs have been taken.

Practice Assessment Document boxes provide examples and innovative ways in which a student can meet the proficiencies in the PAD document.

Practice Assessment Document

Use best practice approaches to undertake nasal and oral suctioning techniques
    Certain situations such as patients who may be intubated may require suctioning to obtain sputum samples. It is important to use the correct equipment and technique in ensuring a good sample is collected. The use of normal saline prior to suctioning in some cases remains controversial. In your placement areas, ensure that you perform this procedure under expert supervision and follow the local policy regarding the use of saline.

Case Studies help to contextualise some of the theory.

Case Study Shirley

Shirley is a 42-year-old homeless woman, who currently lives in a city centre hostel. She has been suffering with a productive cough for many months. One morning she coughed up a small amount of blood, which she found frightening. She decided to go to a local accident and emergency department, where she explained to one of the nurses that in addition to the haemoptysis, she had also been experiencing night sweats. Shirley is admitted to hospital with suspected pulmonary tuberculosis. She is commenced on oral rifampicin, isoniazid, pyrazinamide and ethambutol and placed in isolation. After 10 days, Shirley begins to feel much better and is prepared for discharge back into the community.
    What advice and guidance should the nurse provide for Shirley?

The Nursing Associate boxes address issues pertaining to the trainee nursing associate.

The Nursing Associate

 The Code became effective in March 2015 for all registered nurses and midwives in the UK. In October 2018, the document was updated to reflect the regulation of nursing associates. Nursing associates are required to meet the same professional standards of practice and behaviour as nurses and midwives.

About the Companion Website

Don't forget to visit the companion website for this book:

 www.wiley.com/go/peate/nursingpractice3e

There you will find valuable material designed for both students and instructors:

- PowerPoint slides of all images from the print book for downloading
- Interactive flashcards for self-test
- Interactive multiple-choice questions
- Chapter references
- Chapter learning outcomes
- Chapter proficiencies

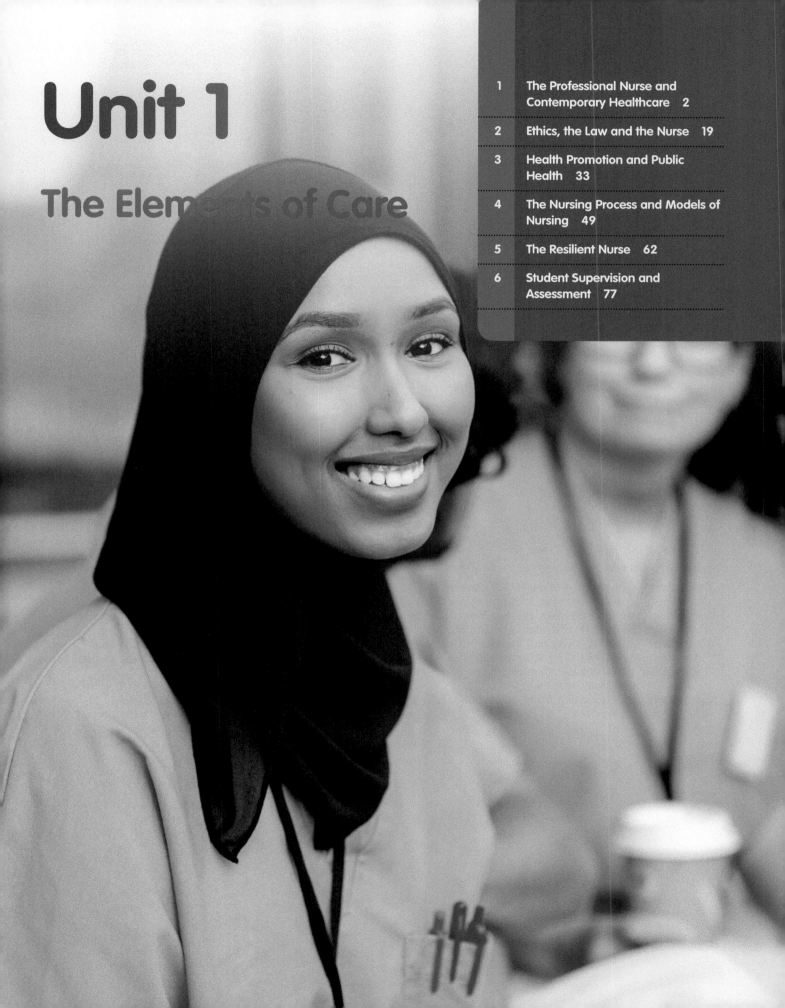

Unit 1

The Elements of Care

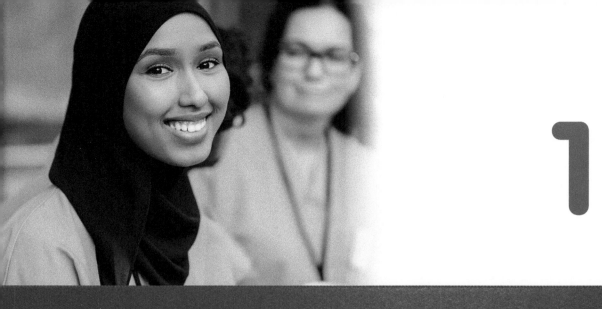

1

The Professional Nurse and Contemporary Healthcare

Deborah Taylor

University of West London, UK

Learning Outcomes

On completion of this chapter you will be able to:

- Demonstrate a knowledge of the NMC's code of professional conduct – standards for practice and behaviour for nurses, midwives and nursing associates
- Be aware of the concept of evidence-based practice
- Understand leadership styles and theories
- Have an awareness of the nurse's role in service improvement and the application of clinical governance as a quality assurance measure
- Recognise the nurse's and nursing associate's role in interprofessional working

Proficiencies

NMC Proficiencies and Standards:

- As accountable professionals, registered nurses and nursing associates act in the best interests of people, putting them first and providing nursing care that is person centred, safe and compassionate.
- They act professionally at all times and use their knowledge and experience to make evidence-based decisions about care.
- They communicate effectively, are role models for others and are accountable for their actions.
- Registered nurses continually reflect on their practice and keep abreast of new and emerging developments in nursing, health and care.

 Visit the companion website at www.wiley.com/go/peate/nursingpractice3e where you can test yourself using flashcards, multiple-choice questions and more.

Nursing Practice: Knowledge and Care, Third Edition. Edited by Ian Peate and Aby Mitchell.
© 2022 John Wiley & Sons Ltd. Published 2022 by John Wiley & Sons Ltd.
Companion website: www.wiley.com/go/peate/nursingpractice3e

Introduction

A profession can be defined by a number of key determinants; however, when asked to consider what is meant by the term 'professional', many individuals might find this a daunting task. Take, for example, the idea that a footballer may describe themselves as professional; equally, a member of the clergy will no doubt assert their professional standing within society. When considering the two examples given, it is clear how difficult defining the idea of what the term 'professional' might be. In general terms, professionals are considered to be individuals who have acquired a level of expertise or skill through formal education or training. This can be a useful starting point when describing nursing as a profession; however, it is only a small part of the criteria that can describe professional status, and the debate continues as to whether nurses fall into the true description of professional or into the category of 'semi-professional'.

Salvage (2002) describes the 'true' professions as male dominated, elitist and powerful and gives the examples of medicine and law. However, new professions and contemporary ways of working are changing how society views professional roles. An example of this is the medical profession, which is experiencing a shift in the gender balance with more equal female-to-male ratios emerging in practice. This supports the idea that ways of defining the term 'profession' are constantly shifting focus.

In general, to claim professional status or membership to a profession, certain qualities should be met and these can include:

- Being subject to a code of rigorous ethics and moral obligations
- Being governed by a regulating body with a defined membership
- The ability to perform a specialist role that requires expert skill and/or knowledge
- Being responsible for advancing knowledge and research to support the profession
- Having a minimum standard entry qualification leading to a recognised practice and academic training
- Having continuous educational development with a recognised career structure
- Having an established body of theory and evidence to underpin practice
- Commanding a salary proportionate to the level of professional responsibility.

The purpose and function of nursing have developed over time, as have the characteristics of the nurse in contemporary society. When the above criteria are mapped against the status of nursing and some of the emerging specialist roles nurses hold, then the perception of nursing as being professional in nature is clear. Examples of specialist nurses that have developed alongside technological scientific advancement include nurse endoscopists, specialist nurse practitioners, community matrons, consultant nurses, nurse prescribers and advanced nurse practitioners. This chapter explores some of the professional functions of the nurse and highlights the main issues that are important themes to the nurse as a 'professional'.

The Nurse as a Professional

Various national and international definitions of nursing exist and whilst there may be some subtle differences, the overarching themes are the same. A meta-analysis by Ghadinan *et al.* (2014) exploring what it means to be a nursing professional identified three main attributes: cognitive, attitudinal and psychomotor; in other words, knowledge, skills and attitudes. We tend to think of the latter in terms of values including integrity and honesty which are integral parts of the NMC Code of Conduct (2018d).

What can be in stark contrast is the public perception of nursing, which has been plagued with stereotypes. The historic view of nurses was as young, female, white, unmarried, virtuous and wearing white starched uniforms; selfless individuals who had dedicated their lives to working in hospitals, caring for the sick and/or dying and obeying the orders of doctors. Whilst this may have been the case at one time, modern, contemporary nursing is changing the stereotype.

What the Experts Say

> 'Nursing is more than the sum of its parts. Any health system needs nurses who are intellectually able and emotionally aware and who can combine technical clinical skills with a deep understanding and ability to care, as one human to another. This is a constant of nursing. It is the value base on which public trust rests and the profession is grounded. As a profession it is our promise to society.'
> Dame Christine Beasley (2006, p.4), Chief Nursing Officer for England 2004–2012

Most recent data from the NMC indicate that the nursing, midwifery and nursing associate workforce in the UK is becoming more diverse, with 22% of the register being from ethnic minority backgrounds, 11% of registrants identifying as male and 4% declaring a disability (NMC, 2021). Whilst this may not yet be entirely representative of the wider population, there is certainly a move in the right direction. Autonomous roles are also on the increase, with 127 366 registrants having a special or recordable qualification on the NMC register in March 2021. This includes nurse prescribers, nurse educators and other specialist practitioners and represents an increase of 1.6% over the past 4 years (NMC, 2021). What this demonstrates is that as a profession, nursing is evolving through education, research and leadership.

The Royal College of Nursing (2003) defined nursing as 'the use of clinical judgement in the provision of care to enable people to improve, maintain, or recover health, to cope with health problems, and to achieve the best possible quality of life, whatever their disease or disability, until death' (p.5). This definition draws on what are perceived as the purposes of nursing as follows:

- To promote and maintain health
- To care for people when their health is compromised
- To assist recovery
- To facilitate independence
- To meet needs
- To improve/maintain well-being/quality of life.

Whilst this and other nursing definitions are quite old, the International Council of Nursing (ICN) (2020) publication in the International Year of the Nurse explored the perceptions of nursing and attempted to define what nursing is today.

More recently, there has been an increased focus on preventing ill health and the responsibility to improve the experiences and outcomes of service users. The Five Year Forward View (NHS England, 2014) and subsequent NHS Long Term Plan (Department of Health, 2019) outlined the focus on health inequalities and prevention of ill health as priorities for healthcare professionals.

Jot This Down

Do the old definitions of nursing still stand? How would you define nursing?

Whilst thinking about this exercise, you might have considered what the role has been traditionally but also how and why it has changed. With the increased focus on nursing leadership, critical thinking, health promotion and global health, it may be time for a new definition. The NMC has gone some way to redefining what nurses do in the UK by the publication in 2018 of the Future Nurse Standards, which have expanded the expectations of the nurse's role in healthcare and society, also introducing the new role of nursing associate.

The Nursing Associate

A The Francis Report (2013) into the serious failings at the Mid Staffordshire NHS Foundation Trust was a catalyst for change throughout the NHS. System-wide failures in leadership, negative culture and poor standards of care resulted in many changes to practice spearheaded by regulatory bodies like the NMC. Numerous changes were made, including the introduction of the NHS Leadership Academy, an amended revalidation process and changes to the Code of Conduct and education standards for nurses. As part of this change, Lord Willis produced The Shape of Caring review (2015), highlighting the need for high-quality education opportunities for healthcare assistants and nurses, resulting in the development of a new role, the nursing associate. In order to build capacity within the nursing workforce and improve the quality of care being delivered, the nursing associate was introduced and is a protected title in law; the role is regulated by the NMC and is subject to the same regulatory requirements as registered nurses.

Case Study

Jackie started a nursing course in her early twenties when she had a very young family and found it overwhelming. She struggled with personal challenges and the demands of academia and reluctantly she only completed a year of the course before deciding to withdraw.

Four years later when her children were a bit older and she felt more prepared, she restarted her adult nursing degree. This time, whilst still finding it a challenge, she found the work more manageable and excelled both academically and in practice. She gained a first-class honours degree, the first person in her family to do so, and had her choice of employment, having been offered a job after almost each placement during her training.

Her first job as a newly qualified nurse was in the same ward where she did her final placement, a high-dependency surgical ward. It was fast paced and with a lot of varied cases so she was able to learn how to deliver care to patients pre- and postoperatively, work within a team, role model behaviours to others and lead her patient's care. She was already doing a lot of this as a student but needed to increase her confidence and consolidate her knowledge and skills once she became a registrant.

She was always looking for ways to improve her patients' experiences and ensure a high quality of care but after time, she decided she wanted to change to a different clinical setting to allow a better work/life balance with her children growing up and give her more opportunities to influence the care being given.

Jackie got a job as a practice nurse and began learning new skills, including childhood immunisations, travel health, cervical screening and much more, constantly expanding her patient assessment skills through further study and experiential learning. This led to Jackie running her own clinics, increasing her autonomy, making independent decisions and referrals where appropriate. After a few years she was given the role of lead practice nurse across two sites with the responsibility of supporting and educating other nurses in the practices. She was also managing chronic diseases like hypertension, diabetes and asthma, learning disability health checks and became lead for infection control. This was all done as part of her role as a nurse trained in adult nursing – influencing and leading many aspects of patient care across the lifespan for her local community.

Jackie's role required collaboration with other healthcare professionals and health and social care teams, advocating for patients and ensuring person-centred care. She challenged poor practice and began auditing performance to look for further areas requiring improvement. As a result, she led on a project which improved the cancer screening rates in her local area and was nominated for national awards as the team leader and driving force behind the initiative.

From very humble beginnings, Jackie's nursing career highlights the diverse role nurses play in society, not only in treating the ill and preventing ill health and promoting health, but responding to community needs, empowering service users and identifying innovative strategies to tackle non-engagement.

Can you see why you should never say you are 'just a nurse'?

In order to clarify the role of the nurse, midwife and nursing associate, the NMC has produced a focused Code of Conduct which drives practice and forms a professional framework against which nursing practice can be judged.

The next section focuses on the code of professional conduct for nurses and nursing associates.

The NMC Code of Professional Conduct

The Professional Standards Authority (PSA) promotes the health, safety and well-being of patients and other members of the public in the regulation of health professionals and has the job of scrutinising the work of health profession regulators such as the:

- General Medical Council
- General Optical Council
- General Osteopathic Council
- General Pharmaceutical Council
- Health and Care Professions Council
- Nursing and Midwifery Council.

Under the NHS Reforms and Health Care Professions Act 2002 and the Health and Social Care Acts of 2008 and 2012, the PSA for Health and Social Care (previously known as the Council for Healthcare and Regulatory Excellence, CHRE) has a number of powers.

- It oversees the statutory bodies that regulate healthcare professions.
- It advises on issues of professional standards in health and social care.
- It is accountable to the UK parliament.
- It shares good practice, promotes research and introduces new ideas and guidance.

Professional nursing practice is not only judged by the recipient of care – the patient – but also by the profession itself. Professionals judge other professionals with regard to the quality and appropriateness of the care they provide. One of the key ways of making such judgements is through the Nursing and Midwifery Council (NMC). People receiving nursing care must be able to trust nurses with their well-being. To justify that trust, the nursing profession has a duty to maintain a good standard of practice and care, and to support this aim the NMC has a 'code' of standards (NMC, 2018d) that registered nurses, midwives and nursing associates must uphold. There are four main categories within the code which support the values and principles of nursing and midwifery: prioritise people; practise effectively; preserve safety; and promote professionalism and trust. The following outlines the professional aspects of the Code of Conduct; please refer to Chapter 2 for sections related to law and ethics.

Professional and Legal Issues The Code: Professional Standards of Practice and Behaviour for Nurses, Midwives and Nursing Associates

Prioritise people

You put the interests of people using or needing nursing or midwifery services first. You make their care and safety your main concern and make sure that their dignity is preserved and their needs are recognised, assessed and responded to. You make sure that those receiving care are treated with respect, that their rights are upheld and that any discriminatory attitudes and behaviours towards those receiving care are challenged.

1. **Treat people as individuals and uphold their dignity**

   To achieve this, you must:
   1.1 treat people with kindness, respect and compassion
   1.2 make sure you deliver the fundamentals of care effectively
   1.3 avoid making assumptions and recognise diversity and individual choice
   1.4 make sure that any treatment, assistance or care for which you are responsible is delivered without undue delay
   1.5 respect and uphold people's human rights.

2. **Listen to people and respond to their preferences and concerns**

   To achieve this, you must:
   2.1 work in partnership with people to make sure you deliver care effectively
   2.2 recognise and respect the contribution that people can make to their own health and well-being
   2.3 encourage and empower people to share decisions about their treatment and care
   2.4 respect the level to which people receiving care want to be involved in decisions about their own health, well-being and care
   2.5 respect, support and document a person's right to accept or refuse care and treatment, and

2.6 recognise when people are anxious or in distress and respond compassionately and politely.

3. **Make sure that people's physical, social and psychological needs are assessed and responded to**

   To achieve this, you must:
   3.1 pay special attention to promoting well-being, preventing ill health and meeting the changing health and care needs of people during all life stages
   3.2 recognise and respond compassionately to the needs of those who are in the last few days and hours of life
   3.3 act in partnership with those receiving care, helping them to access relevant health and social care, information and support when they need it
   3.4 act as an advocate for the vulnerable, challenging poor practice and discriminatory attitudes and behaviour relating to their care.

4. **Act in the best interests of people at all times**

   To achieve this, you must:
   4.1 balance the need to act in the best interests of people at all times with the requirement to respect a person's right to accept or refuse treatment
   4.2 make sure that you get properly informed consent and document it before carrying out any action
   4.3 keep to all relevant laws about mental capacity that apply in the country in which you are practising, and make sure that the rights and best interests of those who lack capacity are still at the centre of the decision-making process
   4.4 tell colleagues, your manager and the person receiving care if you have a conscientious objection to a particular procedure and arrange for a suitably qualified colleague to take over responsibility for that person's care (see the note below).

5. **Respect people's right to privacy and confidentiality**

   As a nurse, midwife or nursing associate, you owe a duty of confidentiality to all those receiving care. This includes making sure that they are informed about their care and that information about them is shared appropriately. To achieve this, you must:
   5.1 respect a person's right to privacy in all aspects of their care
   5.2 make sure that people are informed about how and why information is used and shared by those who will be providing care
   5.3 respect that a person's right to privacy and confidentiality continues after they have died
   5.4 share necessary information with other healthcare professionals and agencies only when the interests of patient safety and public protection over-ride the need for confidentiality
   5.5 share with people, their families and their carers, as far as the law allows, the information they want or need to know about their health, care and ongoing treatment sensitively and in a way they can understand.

7. **Communicate clearly**

   To achieve this, you must:
   7.1 use terms that people in your care, colleagues and the public can understand
   7.2 take reasonable steps to meet people's language and communication needs, providing, wherever possible, assistance to those who need help to communicate their own or other people's needs

7.3 use a range of verbal and non-verbal communication methods, and consider cultural sensitivities, to better understand and respond to people's personal and health needs

7.4 check people's understanding from time to time to keep misunderstandings or mistakes to a minimum

7.5 be able to communicate clearly and effectively in English.

8. **Work co-operatively**

To achieve this, you must:

8.1 respect the skills, expertise and contributions of your colleagues, referring matters to them when appropriate

8.2 maintain effective communication with colleagues

8.3 keep colleagues informed when you are sharing the care of individuals with other healthcare professionals and staff

8.4 work with colleagues to evaluate the quality of your work and that of the team

8.5 work with colleagues to preserve the safety of those receiving care

8.6 share information to identify and reduce risk

8.7 be supportive of colleagues who are encountering health or performance problems. However, this support must never compromise or be at the expense of patient or public safety.

9. **Share your skills, knowledge and experience for the benefit of people receiving care and your colleagues**

To achieve this, you must:

9.1 provide honest, accurate and constructive feedback to colleagues

9.2 gather and reflect on feedback from a variety of sources, using it to improve your practice and performance

9.3 deal with differences of professional opinion with colleagues by discussion and informed debate, respecting their views and opinions and behaving in a professional way at all times

9.4 support students' and colleagues' learning to help them develop their professional competence and confidence.

10. **Keep clear and accurate records relevant to your practice**

This includes but is not limited to patient records. It includes all records that are relevant to your scope of practice. To achieve this, you must:

10.1 complete all records at the time or as soon as possible after an event, recording if the notes are written some time after the event

10.2 identify any risks or problems that have arisen and the steps taken to deal with them, so that colleagues who use the records have all the information they need

10.3 complete all records accurately and without any falsification, taking immediate and appropriate action if you become aware that someone has not kept to these requirements

10.4 attribute any entries you make in any paper or electronic records to yourself, making sure they are clearly written, dated and timed, and do not include unnecessary abbreviations, jargon or speculation

10.5 take all steps to make sure that all records are kept securely

10.6 collect, treat and store all data and research findings appropriately.

11. **Be accountable for your decisions to delegate tasks and duties to other people**

To achieve this, you must:

11.1 only delegate tasks and duties that are within the other person's scope of competence, making sure that they fully understand your instructions

11.2 make sure that everyone you delegate tasks to is adequately supervised and supported so they can provide safe and compassionate care

11.3 confirm that the outcome of any task you have delegated to someone else meets the required standard.

12. **Have in place an indemnity arrangement which provides appropriate cover for any practice you take on as a nurse, midwife or nursing associate in the United Kingdom**

To achieve this, you must:

12.1 make sure that you have an appropriate indemnity arrangement in place relevant to your scope of practice.

14. **Be open and candid with all service users about all aspects of care and treatment, including when any mistakes or harm have taken place**

To achieve this, you must:

14.1 act immediately to put right the situation if someone has suffered actual harm for any reason or an incident has happened which had the potential for harm

14.2 explain fully and promptly what has happened, including the likely effects, and apologise to the person affected and, where appropriate, their advocate, family or carers

14.3 document all these events formally and take further action (escalate) if appropriate so they can be dealt with quickly.

15. **Always offer help if an emergency arises in your practice setting or anywhere else**

To achieve this, you must:

15.1 only act in an emergency within the limits of your knowledge and competence

15.2 arrange, wherever possible, for emergency care to be accessed and provided promptly

15.3 take account of your own safety, the safety of others and the availability of other options for providing care.

16. **Act without delay if you believe that there is a risk to patient safety or public protection**

To achieve this, you must:

16.1 raise and, if necessary, escalate any concerns you may have about patient or public safety, or the level of care people are receiving in your workplace or any other healthcare setting and use the channels available to you in line with our guidance and your local working practices

16.2 raise your concerns immediately if you are being asked to practise beyond your role, experience and training

16.3 tell someone in authority at the first reasonable opportunity if you experience problems that may prevent you working within the Code or other national standards, taking prompt action to tackle the causes of concern if you can

16.4 acknowledge and act on all concerns raised to you, investigating, escalating or dealing with those concerns where it is appropriate for you to do so

16.5 not obstruct, intimidate, victimise or in any way hinder a colleague, member of staff, person you care for or member of the public who wants to raise a concern

16.6 protect anyone you have management responsibility for from any harm, detriment, victimisation or unwarranted treatment after a concern is raised.

17. Raise concerns immediately if you believe a person is vulnerable or at risk and needs extra support and protection

To achieve this, you must:

17.1 take all reasonable steps to protect people who are vulnerable or at risk from harm, neglect or abuse

17.2 share information if you believe someone may be at risk of harm, in line with the laws relating to the disclosure of information

17.3 have knowledge of and keep to the relevant laws and policies about protecting and caring for vulnerable people.

18. Advise on, prescribe, supply, dispense or administer medicines within the limits of your training and competence, the law, our guidance and other relevant policies, guidance and regulations

To achieve this, you must:

18.1 prescribe, advise on, or provide medicines or treatment, including repeat prescriptions (only if you are suitably qualified) if you have enough knowledge of that person's health and are satisfied that the medicines or treatment serve that person's health needs

18.2 keep to appropriate guidelines when giving advice on using controlled drugs and recording the prescribing, supply, dispensing or administration of controlled drugs

18.3 make sure that the care or treatment you advise on, prescribe, supply, dispense or administer for each person is compatible with any other care or treatment they are receiving, including (where possible) over-the-counter medicines

18.4 take all steps to keep medicines stored securely

18.5 wherever possible, avoid prescribing for yourself or for anyone with whom you have a close personal relationship.

Prescribing is not within the scope of practice of everyone on our register. Nursing associates don't prescribe, but they may supply, dispense and administer medicines. Nurses and midwives who have successfully completed a further qualification in prescribing and recorded it on our register are the only people on our register that can prescribe.

19. Be aware of, and reduce as far as possible, any potential for harm associated with your practice

To achieve this, you must:

19.1 take measures to reduce, as far as possible, the likelihood of mistakes, near misses, harm and the effect of harm if it takes place

19.2 take account of current evidence, knowledge and developments in reducing mistakes and the effect of them and the impact of human factors and system failures (see the note below)

19.3 keep to and promote recommended practice in relation to controlling and preventing infection

19.4 take all reasonable personal precautions necessary to avoid any potential health risks to colleagues, people receiving care and the public.

22. Fulfil all registration requirements

To achieve this, you must:

22.1 meet any reasonable requests so we can oversee the registration process

22.2 keep to our prescribed hours of practice and carry out continuing professional development activities

22.3 keep your knowledge and skills up to date, taking part in appropriate and regular learning and professional development activities that aim to maintain and develop your competence and improve your performance.

23. Co-operate with all investigations and audits

This includes investigations or audits either against you or relating to others, whether individuals or organisations. It also includes co-operating with requests to act as a witness in any hearing that forms part of an investigation, even after you have left the register.

To achieve this, you must:

23.1 co-operate with any audits of training records, registration records or other relevant audits that we may want to carry out to make sure you are still fit to practise

23.2 tell both us and any employers as soon as you can about any caution or charge against you, or if you have received a conditional discharge in relation to, or have been found guilty of, a criminal offence (other than a protected caution or conviction)

23.3 tell any employers you work for if you have had your practice restricted or had any other conditions imposed on you by us or any other relevant body

23.4 tell us and your employers at the first reasonable opportunity if you are or have been disciplined by any regulatory or licensing organisation, including those who operate outside of the professional healthcare environment

23.5 give your NMC Pin when any reasonable request for it is made.

When telling your employers, this includes telling (i) any person, body or organisation you are employed by, or intend to be employed by, as a nurse, midwife or nursing associate; and (ii) any person, body or organisation with whom you have an arrangement to provide services as a nurse, midwife or nursing associate.

24. Respond to any complaints made against you professionally

To achieve this, you must:

24.1 never allow someone's complaint to affect the care that is provided to them

24.2 use all complaints as a form of feedback and an opportunity for reflection and learning to improve practice.

25. Provide leadership to make sure people's well-being is protected and to improve their experiences of the healthcare system

To achieve this, you must:

25.1 identify priorities, manage time, staff and resources effectively and deal with risk to make sure that the quality of care or service you deliver is maintained and improved, putting the needs of those receiving care or services first

25.2 support any staff you may be responsible for to follow the Code at all times. They must have the knowledge, skills and competence for safe practice; and understand how to raise any concerns linked to any circumstances where the Code has, or could be, broken.

Source: This extract is reproduced and reprinted with permission with thanks to the Nursing and Midwifery Council: www.nmc.org.uk/ globalassets/sitedocuments/nmc-publications/nmc-code.pdf (accessed November 2021)

The Code of Conduct is not law; there is no legal imperative. It is, however, a guide which informs the general public and other professionals of the standard of conduct that they should expect from a registered nurse. Codes of conduct do not solve problems; they reflect professional morality. They operate in such a way as to remind the practitioner of the standards required by the profession. However, breaching the Code of Conduct is in effect a breach of registration and may lead to removal of the nurse's name from the register, and consequently of the right to practise.

Practice Assessment Document

Your professional values are assessed in each practice area throughout your course. These are specifically related to the Code of Conduct and assess your attitudes and behaviours. Consider how frequently turning up late or asking to leave early might be perceived in the clinical setting; does this reflect the Code?

The NMC was set up by Parliament to safeguard the public and to ensure that nurses and midwives provide high standards of care to their patients. The Nursing and Midwifery Order 2001 (SI 2002/253) established the Council, and it came into being on 1 April 2002.

Safeguarding of the public is the key concern of the NMC. It protects the public by:

- Maintaining a register listing all nurses and midwives
- Setting and monitoring standards and guidelines for nursing and midwifery education, practice and conduct
- Ensuring that registrants keep their skills and knowledge up to date
- Ensuring quality assurance related to nursing and midwifery education
- Setting standards and providing guidance for local supervising authorities for midwives
- Considering allegations of misconduct or unfitness to practise.

In March 2021, there were almost 732 000 people on the NMC register, made up of nurses, nursing associates and midwives; only those who have demonstrated that they meet the NMC standards can be registered and therefore legally allowed to practise in the UK (NMC, 2021).

Further to the Code of Conduct, the NMC has developed 'Caring with Confidence' (NMC, 2020), a resource to assist registrants with what they have identified as key aspects of the professional role.

- *Accountability*: being open to challenge and being held to account for your actions and omissions. Being able to confidently explain your decision making.

- *Professional judgement*: building confidence to make non-biased decision and use sound clinical judgement.
- *Delegation*: considering when it is appropriate to delegate and what needs to be taken into consideration.
- *Speaking up*: recognising risk and potential to cause harm and escalating concerns if something isn't right.
- *Inclusivity and challenging discrimination*: the NMC here is supporting professionals on their register to feel confident to challenge discrimination.
- *Social media*: can be used to develop professional networks, share ideas, good practice and support ongoing professional development but it is important to be aware of potential pitfalls.
- *Person-centred care*: doing what you can to show kindness and respect to all, viewing each person as unique, will lead to better care.
- *End-of-life care*: demonstrating skill and compassion in allowing people to die with dignity.
- *Professionalism*: having confidence in decisions and actions as a professional particularly in difficult circumstances.

Fitness to Practise

In addition to its regulatory powers, the NMC can also initiate investigations into a nurse's fitness to practise if they are deemed to pose a risk to public safety.

When a nurse is called before the NMC as a result of concerns about fitness to practise, there is likely to be an initial assessment of the nature of the concern to determine whether urgent action is required. An investigation can help determine if there is a case to answer and this would necessitate a hearing to adjudicate a decision. In cases where there is a serious and immediate risk to patient or public safety, an interim order to suspend or restrict the registrant from practice can be made immediately.

Fitness to practise is the nurse's suitability to be on the register without restrictions. This may mean:

- Failing always to put the patient's interests first
- Not being properly trained, qualified and up to date
- Failing to treat patients with respect and dignity
- Not speaking up for patients who cannot speak for themselves.

Jot This Down

Make a list of the reasons why you think a nurse can be investigated for fitness to practise.

While thinking about this exercise, you may have considered physical, sexual, emotional or verbal abuse; significant failure to provide adequate care; significant failure to keep proper records; failure to administer medicines safely; deliberately concealing unsafe practice; committing criminal offences; continued lack of competence despite being given opportunities to improve; theft; or a person's ill health. The NMC investigates allegations of fitness to practise that may include misconduct, lack of competence, not having necessary knowledge of English, fraudulent or criminal behaviour, and serious ill health.

A lack of competence relates to a lack of knowledge, skill or judgement of such a nature that the nurse is unfit to practise in a safe and effective manner. Some examples of lack of competence include:

- A persistent lack of ability in correctly and/or appropriately calculating and recording the administration or disposal of medicines
- A persistent lack of ability in properly identifying care needs and accordingly planning and delivering appropriate care
- Inability to work as part of a team
- Difficulty in communicating with colleagues or people in their care.

In recent years the NMC's approach to fitness to practise has been altered to have a more person-centred approach, promoting a culture of openness and learning, acknowledging that human factors can play a part in errors and as a result an attempt is made to allow the registrant to remedy concerns with perhaps a restriction to practice rather than a striking off order (NMC, 2018a).

Revalidation and Continuing Professional Development

Revalidation is the process that all registered nurses and midwives in the UK and nursing associates in England need to follow to maintain their registration with the NMC. The process takes place every 3 years and links specifically to the NMC Code (NMC, 2019).

Continuing professional development (CPD), although not a guarantee of competence, is a key component of clinical governance (discussed later in this chapter) and affects all health and social care professionals. CPD is associated with lifelong learning that will enable nurses to meet the needs of revalidation.

Professional and Legal Issues Requirements for Revalidation with the NMC

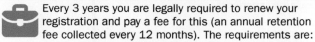 Every 3 years you are legally required to renew your registration and pay a fee for this (an annual retention fee collected every 12 months). The requirements are:
- 450 practice hours, or 900 hours if you are renewing as both a nurse and midwife
- 35 hours of CPD including 20 hours of participatory learning
- Five pieces of practice-related feedback
- Five written reflective accounts
- Reflective discussion
- Health and character declaration
- Professional indemnity arrangement
- Confirmation.

The NMC's Revalidation Requirements

1. That nurses, midwives or nursing associates have worked for a minimum of 450 hours in practice over the last 3 years (those with dual nurse and midwife registration must have worked 900 hours). The practice hours must reflect the practitioner's current scope of practice, but do not necessarily need to relate to the original field of practice on first registration. Hours worked may include direct care, managing teams, teaching others, or running and shaping care services.

2. The CPD standard requires the registrant to have recorded CPD activities during the 3-year period prior to renewal of registration. In order to meet this standard, the nurse must:
   (a) Undertake at least 35 hours of CPD activity relevant to his or her practice during the 3 years prior to renewal of registration, of which 20 hours must have included participatory learning (e.g. workshops, conferences, training courses, updates)
   (b) Maintain a record of CPD activities which must contain:
       (i) The CPD method
       (ii) A description of how the learning relates to practice
       (iii) Relevant dates
       (iv) Number of hours
       (v) Identifies which part of the Code most relates to the learning
       (vi) Evidence of participation.
   The way in which this standard is met is up to the individual nurse. The person who is required to demonstrate CPD activities is the best person to decide what learning activities are needed to comply with the standard. It is essential that learning activities are documented in a way that conveys evidence that the learning activity you have undertaken has informed and influenced your practice and directly links to the NMC Code. Having developed skills in professional portfolio management as students, many nurses continue to use this format as ongoing evidence that can be provided if requested by the NMC. Templates are available from the NMC website with examples if needed.

3. That you have obtained five pieces of practice-related feedback in the 3-year period since last registration. This may be in the form of written, verbal or formal feedback. It may be feedback that you receive in your appraisal meetings. Consideration of how you have used or responded to the feedback can be applied to the online templates provided by the NMC.

4. Five reflective accounts are required and for this you must utilise the format provided by the NMC. These can be directly related to the CPD activities, or can be feedback related, or related to practice experience. In this requirement, you must be able to provide documentation regarding the learning activities that you have completed within the 3 years prior to renewal of your registration. You will need to demonstrate what and how.
   (a) What the nature of the learning activity was concerned with and what you learned from the experience.
   (b) How the learning influenced or informed your practice, and how it related to your practice and to the NMC Code.
   An element of reflection is called for when considering what you have learned and how this has informed and developed your practice.

5. You must have discussed your reflective accounts with another NMC registrant who in turn will sign and verify your accounts. The NMC provides online resources for this.

6. A health and character declaration is a formal requirement of revalidation.

7. Formal arrangements for indemnity have to be declared.

8. The NMC also requires a 'confirmer' to look at the evidence that you have collected and to confirm that you have met the requirements for revalidation.

The next section highlights some of the processes that support the reflective practitioner.

Reflective Practice

Nursing is predominantly a practice-based discipline, where the aim of care is to be effective and competent; reflection can be a tool through which practice and knowledge about practice are communicated and validated. Reflecting on practice can provide nurses with an opportunity to learn from experience, and has the potential to help the nurse become, among other things, a lifelong learner. In addition, the learning that occurs through the process of reflection supports knowledge, skills and behavioural development and ultimately augments care provision. Don't forget this also links to the NMC requirement for revalidation so is an important practice to develop.

In support of the process of reflection, a number of models have been produced to provide a framework which, when applied, allows the nurse to reflect systematically and logically. The ultimate goal of reflection is to help the nurse bring meaning to situations both 'in' and 'on' practice. To be able to reflect on and in practice, the nurse must engage in an active and conscious process when encountering problematic aspects of care provision and attempt to make sense of them. Reflective practice is a process that can be used to engage in lifelong learning.

According to Schön (1983), there are two constituents to reflection.

- *Reflection-in-action*: this type of reflection is created from an experience and involves thinking about what is occurring while actually doing it.
- *Reflection-on-action*: this type of reflection evolves when the nurse revisits the experience after the event.

In addition to the two constituents of reflection identified by Schön (1983), there is the notion of a third component, that of 'reflecting before action' to reduce the risk of errors prior to engaging in practice, as identified by Greenwood (1993). There have been many attempts at defining the concept of reflection. Reflective learning is learning from experience formally or informally, allowing the learner to consider his or her practice honestly and critically (Moon, 2004). The outcome may be a deeper understanding of personal skills, enhanced self-awareness and individual learning needs. Nurses can develop further and enhance their understanding of practice through reflection by questioning what they do and, more importantly, why things are done, whether the outcome is as intended, and how things might be done more effectively next time.

There are a number of definitions of reflection within the nursing and wider literature and, because of this, there may be confusion about what constitutes reflection.

- Boud et al. (1985) suggest that reflection occurs when individuals engage in activities that aim to explore their experiences in order to lead to new understanding and appreciation of the situation(s). The suggestion here is that you must learn through practice.
- Johns (2000) states that reflection is a window allowing practitioners to view themselves within the context of their own lived experience. By doing this, practitioners can confront, understand and work towards resolving issues that arise in practice.

Models of Reflection

A range of models exist to support the process of reflection, and just as there are a number of definitions of reflection, so too are there a number of reflective frameworks or models. While they are similar in the overall principle that they promote, they differ in the level of complexity and detail.

Driscoll (2007) considers three stages in his approach to reflection.

- What? – describes the event by returning to the situation
- So what? – analyses the event, by understanding the context
- Now what? – proposes actions after the event to modify future outcomes.

Driscoll's model represents a very simple framework with which to order reflection.

Gibbs Reflective Cycle

Gibbs (1998) enables those who engage in reflective activity to consider events in a cyclical manner. Gibbs' model promotes a simple approach to reflection in sequential steps (Figure 1.1). Gibbs (1998) points out that deep learning takes place when reflective practice is used. The starting point is a description of an event, and through the process of reflection, the nurse produces an action plan for future practice.

Jot This Down
What would you say are the triggers that provide a stimulus for your personal reflection?

In this exercise, you may have thought about some of the events in your nursing experience that have triggered some kind of thought process. These are often called 'significant events' or 'critical incidents'. Triggers for such events might include:

- A negative/positive experience
- A crisis or emergency situation
- Feedback from a mentor or patient
- Learning experience.

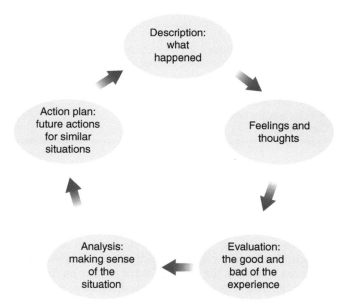

Figure 1.1 **Gibbs reflective cycle.**

The analysis of an event or incident helps the nurse to make sense of their role within the healthcare setting and the many therapeutic and working relationships that take place there.

Johns' (1994) Model of Structured Reflection

This model of reflection offers cues to nurses to support the concept of accessing, making sense of, and learning from the experiences they have. To achieve this, the nurse is encouraged to 'look in' on thoughts and emotions about events and 'look out' at the situation experienced. Over time, Johns has revised this model in an attempt to offer more in-depth reflection.

Reflexivity

Whilst sounding similar to reflection, the term 'reflexive practice' has a slightly different aim. Reflexivity is concerned more with personal reflection with the aim of developing greater self-awareness rather than dissecting specific episodes of care. This can be done through a number of techniques, including performing a SWOT (strengths, weaknesses, opportunities and threats) analysis but can also include external sources of feedback like appraisals. This activity is important and links to the Code of Conduct principle of Promoting Professionalism and Trust.

Practice Assessment Document

Part of your PAD is the opportunity to get feedback from members of the MDT, nurses, peers, patients and carers. This feedback can be used as part of your reflective practice to gain greater insight into how you are viewed and help identify your strengths and weaknesses. It is important to embrace constructive criticism and areas for development as opportunities to learn and improve your practice.

Leadership Styles and Theories

Nurses lead in a variety of ways, and in a variety of settings, and as a consequence there are a number of differing styles and theories that underpin the way that individuals as leaders direct, plan and influence the behaviour of other people. In nursing, we often use the phrase 'ward manager' when referring to the so-called leader of a team in the clinical setting. But can we use the term 'manager' to truly reflect the meaning of 'leader'? Consider the following quote from Grohar-Murray and DiCroce (2003): 'The authority of leadership is derived from the ability of the leader to influence others to accomplish goals, whereas the authority of management is derived from the manager's position in the organisation' (p.17). The quote implies that managers can hold authority from a hierarchical perspective, whereas leaders possess innate qualities to support their abilities as a leader. Leadership can be thought of in terms of an individual's ability to maintain relationships with others in a way that constructively influences the way that they work.

Leadership is a complex subject, with a wealth of definitions in the literature to illustrate what is meant by the term. Many view the leader as a charismatic, powerful individual with followers at a subordinate level. More modern concepts of leadership see it as something that is shared and distributed and can be identified at all levels within organisations. Not everyone is a leader, but everyone can contribute to the leadership process.

Leadership styles can be said to be context dependent, and in Table 1.1 you can see the characteristics of many of the common styles and their potential impact on the teams or people in the work environment.

Nurses can apply leadership styles and adapt them to the ever-changing situations with which they are faced on a regular basis. An understanding of the theories that underpin leadership can guide nurses in adopting the most effective ways of working in practice.

Transactional leadership, also known as managerial leadership, focuses on the leader as supervisor, organiser and someone interested in group performance. Classically, this type of leadership is synonymous with reward and punishment. Transactional leaders are happy to keep things on an even keel, and are thus not specifically looking for change or development. Typically, this type of leader will keep an eye on followers to praise or to find fault in ways of working. When leaders who adopt this way of leading perform poorly, then there is an associated link with poor standards of patient care (Basset & Westmore, 2012).

Transformational leadership aims to enhance the development of others in the team through a number of mechanisms.

- Establishing direction
- Aligning people
- Motivating and inspiring
- Producing change
- Where you are going (vision)
- Effective communicators

These types of leaders are inspirational, and act as role models to their followers. They are very much in tune with the skills of their followers, and they take a genuine interest in them as people and can align tasks that enhance their performance. Followers are encouraged to identify with the organisation, taking ownership for the parts that they play.

What the Experts Say Working for a **Transformational Leader**

'For a long time, I have had an interest in developing a media-based learning tool for staff and students to develop skills in communicating with people who have dementia. My manager is really supportive, as a transformational leader, he has encouraged me to go ahead with this. He recognises my skills, not just in relation to teaching and learning, but also in time management and self-direction. He shares the vision that I have, and is a real motivator. His democratic style has encouraged the involvement and enthusiasm of the ward team, who are behind me all the way.'

(Band 6 Staff Nurse, Medical Unit)

Other forms of guidance in the development of leadership skills are available through the NHS Leadership Academy. The Healthcare Leadership Model (HLM) developed by the NHS Leadership Academy (2013) is made up of nine dimensions which encompass knowledge, skills and behaviours, its aim being to help those who work in health and social care to become better leaders irrespective of their role or discipline. They provide an online facility for self-assessment and modules of study.

Table 1.1 **Leadership styles, characteristics and potential impact.**

STYLE OF LEADERSHIP	CHARACTERISTICS	POTENTIAL IMPACT
Authoritarian	Decision maker Task orientated High standards Planning and expecting others to follow In control, maintains power over others	Positive: when instructions need to be clear and directed, e.g. in an emergency situation or when working with a novice Negative: may encourage staff dependency, and can demotivate others and stifle creativity
Democratic	Team player Sharing ideas Mutual respect of others' ideas Delegates as a means of developing others Interacts and seeks opinions of others	Positive: team approach can elicit more effective solutions. Respect from team members who feel developed Negative: in emergency situations where delay in decision making might be seen as lack of competence
Bureaucratic	Adheres to the rule book Governed by policy and regulations Follows close set of values and standards Strict disciplinarian	Positive: in situations where exact and precise ways of working are needed, e.g. high-risk areas Negative: teams may feel apathetic, powerless and frustrated
Laissez-faire	Allows others to make decisions Enables others to manage and control their own work Expects others to work autonomously, and to ask for help if needed 'Hands-off' approach	Positive: in environments where the team is highly skilled, motivated and capable of working independently Negative: in environments where the team is inexperienced. The team can become demotivated, miss opportunities for development and fall behind with deadlines
Situational	Adapts style to manage particular situations Identifies the performance, competencies and commitment of others Flexible Acknowledges the relationship between the leader's supportive and directive behaviour and the follower's competence Provides emotional support and is a good communicator	Positive: allows for contingencies, and can be effective when supporting newly qualified nurses and students Negative: focuses too much on leaders and not enough on group interaction

The HLM model emphasises the need for all clinicians to be involved in the development of leadership skills and to empower leadership in others. Each of the nine domains supports the improvement of the quality and safety of healthcare services and staff and seeks to enable clinicians to be competent in each domain. From student up to experienced practitioner, it is expected that all competencies within the framework can be achieved to varying degrees, depending on the context in which they relate to practice.

The NMC Future Nurse: Standards of Proficiency for Registered Nurses (2018b) and Standards of Proficiency for Registered Nursing Associates (2018c) have embedded the need for leadership within the pre-registration curriculum, recognising that leadership is a professional competence that must be demonstrated at the point of registration. For nurses, this includes leading patient care and a team, and for nursing associates, whilst not leading a team, they are expected to support, supervise, motivate and role model behaviours to staff, students and healthcare support workers.

What the Experts Say Leadership in healthcare

 'Collective leadership is about everyone taking responsibility not just for their own job or role, but for the success of their team and their organisation as a whole. It is about ensuring that all voices are valued and contribute to the conversations where decisions are made.'
Ruth May, Chief Nursing Officer for England

Evidence-based Practice

As a practitioner working within healthcare, you will probably hear the term 'evidence-based practice' (EBP) on a regular basis; in fact, many will claim that their practice is 'evidence based' and that they adhere to the NMC's code, which asserts that nurses should provide a high standard of safe and effective practice and care at all times, making sure that any information or advice given is evidence based. The term 'evidence based' is a concept that implies the use of the best information available to inform and question contemporary nursing practice.

Evidence-based medicine was first introduced in 1972 by Archie Cochrane, who believed that the influence of tradition and custom did little to enhance healthcare, at a time when research development was providing proof that practice was in many instances outdated and harmful. In 1997, the NHS Modernisation Agenda set out a 10-year plan to improve and standardise practice, with an emphasis on EBP and clinically effective care (Department of Health, 1997). The challenge for excellence in care does not end with the government, it also comes from the public, patients and their carers and the healthcare professions. Healthcare workers use evidence from a variety of sources; many are rooted in tradition and the perception of what evidence is will differ from person to person.

Evidence-based practice has been described as 'doing the right things right' (Muir Gray, 1997). Other descriptions include EBP as a method of problem solving to elicit the best solution, and a combination of clinical expertise with application to provide the best available evidence from systematic research. EBP is key to promoting clinical effectiveness, and clinical effectiveness is synonymous with practitioners' understanding of the effectiveness of their interventions in practice.

There are clear stages to the process of EBP, which always begins with a question. This is an important step in the process, as it helps to explore the subject and focus on the right information to provide answers to the question. However, it is not straightforward. An initial activity might be questioning one's own practice, and a starting point might be to consider *why* and *how* a decision about the treatment or care provided is made. There is an art to developing questions in order to elicit a meaningful answer, and the evidence-based process flows from the question.

PICO is a framework for formulating questions and was developed by Sackett *et al.* (1997) as a way of making questions more focused.

P Population or Patient: it may be useful to specify gender, age, disease type, morbidity. It may be useful here to stipulate the setting, for example inpatient or surgical care for information that relates to the clinical environment

I Intervention: define what you are interested in; this may be a test or exposure to something (e.g. sunlight)

C Comparison: define an alternative intervention by means of comparison

O Outcomes: define the meaningful outcome, beneficial or harmful.

Jot This Down Structuring a Search Question Using PICO

Andres got a burn that blistered. They present to the Emergency Department and tell you they burst the blister because that is what their Mum used to always do but ask you if that is OK.

Using the PICO framework, think of search terms that you might use to find information for Andres that represents the best evidence.

In this exercise, you may have included search areas such as:

P Population or Patient: *burn with blisters*

I Intervention: *deroof (burst) blister*

C Comparison: *leave blister intact*

O Outcomes: *skin healing and wound complications*

Where is the Evidence Base Found?

Finding out about best practice requires discovering what has been written about it in the literature. There are many sources of literature including:

- Books
- The internet
- Journals
- Reports
- Bibliographic/electronic databases.

It would be an impossible task to perform a manual search of the thousands of journals available in health and social care alone in order to provide answers. Electronic databases store converted journal indexes to help find relevant studies and research papers. Bibliographic databases theme articles into subject categories, where an abstract of the article can be viewed.

When trying to find evidence, the best source is a systematic review, which will summarise the results from a large number of high-quality research studies. The Cochrane Library is the first place to check for reviews in healthcare. The Cochrane Library is not a standard bibliographic database but rather a collection of a number of separate databases and is accessed via the internet. Most HEIs and NHS trusts have access to the internet version.

Useful Databases for Literature Searching

Internurse
Internurse is the online archive of peer-reviewed nursing articles from 13 high-quality journals, including the *British Journal of Nursing* and the *Journal of Wound Care*.

CINAHL
Designed specifically for academic institutions, Academic Search Premier and CINAHL are multidisciplinary full-text databases containing the full text for more than 4600 journals, including nearly 3900 peer-reviewed titles.

Science Direct
Science Direct contains over 25% of the world's science, technology and medicine, full text and bibliographical information.

MEDLINE (Ovid)
MEDLINE is a bibliographical database of life sciences and biomedical information. It includes bibliographical information for articles from academic journals covering medicine, nursing, pharmacy, dentistry and health care.

PubMed
Digital archive of life sciences journal literature, maintained by the US National Library of Medicine. Essentially, PubMed is the free version of MEDLINE.

Zetoc Alert
Set up current awareness alerts, so that you are emailed the contents pages of new issues of your favourite journals. Zetoc can also send you details of new articles on topics of your choice.

Zetoc Search
Zetoc is a vast database maintained by the British Library that you can search for details of articles, conference proceedings, etc.

The Value of the Evidence Found

Nursing exists in a complex and constantly evolving healthcare system and not all published evidence is applicable to practice. Sorting through and reviewing the wealth of evidence is complex and requires the process of critical appraisal. Critical appraisal can be used to determine whether the quality of the study is robust enough to make the results useful; what the results of the study are and what they will mean to patients; and whether the results are applicable to specific clinical settings.

Evidence can be appraised in a number of ways to take into account some of the following, as suggested by Burns and Grove (2011) and Polit and Beck (2011).

- *The report structure*: is it logical in its progression?
- *The abstract*: does it give you an insight into the theme of the study, how it was carried out and the key findings?
- *The introduction*: does it explain the *how* and *why* aspects of the study?
- *The purpose of the research*: is this established from the outset, with a rationale that is specific to address the study question?
- *The literature review*: how up to date is the literature that supports the study and is it broad enough to provide a wide review?
- *Methodology*: does this provide a step-by-step approach to the processes involved in the study?
- *Analysis of the data*: is a complete discussion of the data provided?
- *The discussion*: is this critically presented?
- *The conclusions and limitations*: are the implications for practice identified?
- *References and bibliography*: do these reflect the literature review and are they relevant to the study?

Guidelines and policies

An important element of EBP is policies and guidelines that will have done the hard work for you and appraised the research, developed by experts in the relevant field. The important thing here is making sure the guidelines and policies being applied are up to date. The National Insititute for Health and Care Excellence (NICE) provides evidence-based guidance proving clinical pathways and standards to inform best practice.

Practice Assessment Document

You are required to demonstrate applying evidence to practice. This requires the translation of theoretical 'learning' into practical 'doing'. It is important to be curious about why things are done the way they are done. Having curiosity prompts you to ask questions and seek answers. Some of this can be achieved by interacting with other members of the MDT but it is also important to read widely. Even more important is to be discerning about the sources of information you use.

Clinical Governance

Clinical governance is focused on reducing the risk and improving the quality of care for patients. It is integral to healthcare, and patient safety is a top priority for all staff. Other terms that are synonymous with clinical governance are:

- Quality assurance
- Clinical audit
- Quality enhancement
- Clinical effectiveness
- Evidence-based practice.

The 21st-century NHS aspires to be a service that is responsive to individual and local needs and, as such, must decentralise its provision and be devolved. One way of making this move towards devolution is to change the way health services are managed and run. Centralised services fail to provide care that is patient centred, and do not recognise that patients are individuals with local and individual needs. Care needs to be delivered in a meaningful manner to the people who pay for it – the patients and the public. The current government is putting patients at the heart of the NHS, through an information revolution and greater choice and control; shared decision making will become the norm: 'no decision about me without me' (Department of Health, 2012).

The introduction of clinical governance in the late 1990s was seen as one way of achieving this meaningful approach to healthcare provision. In 1997, *The New NHS: Modern, Dependable* (Department of Health, 1997) was produced with a plan to modernise healthcare provision. Clinical governance was an integral part of the 10-year plan to improve the quality of care (Department of Health, 1999). One key component of this document (a White Paper) was to bring about major improvements in the quality of care delivered to patients from a clinical perspective. For the first time, statutory duties were enforced on NHS providers regarding the quality of care they offer (Department of Health, 2000). A formal responsibility for quality has now been placed on every health organisation in the UK through arrangements for clinical governance at local level.

Quality improvement within health and social care remains high on the political agenda, and there have been high-profile cases which demonstrate failings in care, such as those at the Mid Staffordshire NHS Foundation Trust (2013), where an inquiry chaired by Sir Robert Francis heard evidence that an inadequately risk-assessed reconfiguration of services resulted in a complete breakdown in fundamental nursing care and the Trust's wider governance. The National Quality Board (2013) defines quality as having a good experience of care, treatment and support alongside clinical effectiveness and safety.

Clinical governance is central to quality. There are many different interpretations of what clinical governance means, and it has been described as making each patient's experience the best it can be, enhancing and making quality in healthcare better, and doing the right thing at the right time to the right person in the right way.

The overall aim of clinical governance is to continuously improve, strengthen and build on existing systems of quality assurance across a range of services. There are a range of activities that come under the umbrella of clinical governance, including:

- Clinical audit
- Risk management
- Significant event audit
- Evidence-based practice

- Reviewing complaints
- The involvement of users and carers
- Professional development.

In order for clinical governance to be effective, a number of points must be considered: first and foremost, it must focus on improving the quality of patient care, and it applies to all areas where care is delivered. Consideration should be given to the nature of interprofessional working and the partnerships that exist not just between staff, but also between staff and patients. Public and patient involvement is an essential requirement for effective clinical governance; feedback from users of services can support a culture that acknowledges mistakes and shares positive feedback. Although it applies to all healthcare staff, nurses have a unique role to play because of their evidence-based professional practice and their prime role in influencing the patient's experience to be the best it can be. Nurses should be focused on the needs of patients and be able to use the many facets of clinical governance to constantly evaluate and improve patient care.

It is not possible to achieve clinical governance in isolation. Structures need to be in place to support it, as well as ensuring that there are common standards, and the common public ethos is ensured. National structures are in place to underpin local clinical governance initiatives; an example in England is the Care Quality Commission whose role is to inspect and regulate services applying performance ratings to enhance patient choice. The Care Quality Commission in England has put forward its strategy for 2021, its two core ambitions being to provide 'independent assurance to the public of the quality of care in their area' and 'tackling inequalities in health and care (Care Quality Commission, 2021).

Change Management

An important part of clinical governance is identifying areas in need of improvement, redesign or innovation, which requires change management processes to be utilised. Nurses and nursing associates have a key role to play in the identification of areas for improvement and management of change; they are equipped to ensure that the principles of care and compassion in addition to consideration of access, equity and efficiency remain at the heart of any changes to service provision.

One of the difficulties faced by nurses when challenged with change in the workplace is that, like all people, they may be reluctant to modify the way they work. Hewitt-Taylor (2013) cites two aspects of altering practice – change and transition (Austin & Currie, 2003; McLean, 2011) – and concludes that both need to be considered for change to be effectively managed.

- *Change*: things that can be observed to be done differently.
- *Transition*: the experience and the way people feel about the importance of change.

It is natural for people to resist change, and this is multiplied in the workplace if the reason for change is not communicated effectively. Good nurse leadership is crucial to implementing change in the clinical setting and as demonstrated earlier in this chapter, leadership is complex and multifaceted, and not limited to the nurse's grade or position within the team.

There are many approaches to managing change, with the NHS proposing its own model specifically aimed at addressing change in healthcare rather than the more traditional models designed for use in industry and business. This model acknowledges the importance of support and engagement from strategic and operational stakeholders, whose experiences or work requirements will be affected by the proposed change. This should include patients, service users and carers, as it is increasingly important to invite the involvement of such groups in the planning and design of projects within the care setting. Often the language that is adopted in the initial planning stages can influence the way that the project is interpreted, and any proposal for change should be communicated in a simple and transparent manner.

One of the challenges to change management is how to measure the effectiveness of what has been changed. It is important that any change has clear aims and objectives which may also include establishing a baseline from which you can demonstrate or quantify the effectiveness of changes made. Gage (2013) advises consideration of measurements that are well defined, allow comparison, are easy to collect and integrate into daily work patterns, and are specific and sensitive (i.e. measure what you think you are measuring). SMART is an acronym for Specific, Measurable, Achievable, Realistic and Time-oriented objectives, and this can help in clarifying the goals of any proposed change. An action plan helps to identify who, what and when objectives are to be undertaken. Revisiting and refining action plans keep the momentum going and help those involved structure their progress. Quantitative (numerical) data are easier to measure than qualitative (descriptive) data but qualitative data can be richer and give you a better understanding of the lived experience of the service. The method of measurement will therefore depend on the nature of the change and the aims set.

Dissemination of the outcomes of the project requires project leaders to sustain and share the results of their evaluation. Outcomes are the differences between 'what we did' and 'what we do now' as a result of the change that has taken place. Opportunities to share the experience and outcome of developments in practice are numerous and in organisations that embrace a culture of improvement, nurses can share developments through meetings, teaching sessions, conference presentations and publications. Initiatives that support the quality and enhancement of care are pivotal to the notion of clinical governance, as previously discussed.

Interprofessional Working

The nurse and nursing associate are professionals continuously working in partnership and collaboration with others. This approach incorporates:

- Working in collaboration with patients and their informal carers
- Collaboration within the nursing team
- Partnership and collaboration with other professionals and interprofessional teams.

Effective interprofessional working can have the potential to improve and develop care, and where teams work well, they learn and support each other in this aim. Similar to clinical governance, the philosophy underpinning interprofessional working puts emphasis on the patient at the centre of care and acknowledges that patients often move from one professional group to another, depending on need. This is not a new phenomenon; as far back as the 1970s, the British Medical

Association (1974) referred to the term 'primary health care team'. Contemporary healthcare, with the focus on Integrated Care Systems (National Quality Board, 2021), has reinforce the key principles of sharing commitment to quality care delivery, awareness of local need, variation in provision and inequalities, involving service users in their care (co-production), clear and transparent decision making, timely and transparent information sharing and focusing on the local population's identified needs.

In order to achieve this, interprofessional collaborative working must be at the forefront. The aim is to provide the patient with a service that is seamless and joined up; there is need for co-ordination of care between groups, and continuity for the individuals who receive care.

Language used to describe interprofessional working includes 'interdisciplinary teams', 'multiagency or interagency working' and 'multiprofessional teams'. Whatever terminology is used, teams who work together to provide effective individualised person-centred care are characterised by the following.

- Care is given to a common group of patients.
- Teams share common goals or outcomes of care.
- Roles are clearly defined, and each member understands the role of others in the team.
- Information is shared among the team.
- Mechanisms exist to review care and to assess and adjust outcomes.

Jot This Down

Which agencies and health professionals are you likely to work with as an interprofessional team member? Make a list of the most common professional groups in healthcare.

In this exercise, you will probably have made a list of the most common healthcare groups: physiotherapists, paramedics, GPs, police, pharmacists, to name only a few. Each of the individual groups of health professionals has its own professional culture and unique educational programme to prepare it for practice. Just as nursing has a values system, so too will the individual professions of medicine and those allied to medicine. To work effectively within teams, nurses have to be aware of the cultures and values of other professionals. This has been highlighted in child protection cases, where sharp criticism has been levelled at the poor use of interagency working and communication.

Nursing Fields Children's Nursing

Common assessments and information sharing will be a major step forward...professionals will increasingly work alongside each other in the same team...clear lines of professional accountability should ensure that multi-disciplinary teams are able to benefit from a wide range of professionals working together, without losing the advantages of those professionals' individual specialisms.

Every Child Matters (Department for Education and Skills, 2003)

Professional and Legal Issues

Subsequent to Every Child Matters Green Paper (2003) a new statutory guidance has been issued aimed at strategic and senior leaders together with frontline practitioners from any organisation or agency that works with children and families highlighting the fundamental principles of collaborative working to minimise harm and protect the vulnerable.

Working Together to Safeguard Children (HM Government, 2018)

Working in Collaboration with Patients

The development of the NHS Constitution was one of several recommendations following Lord Darzi's report (Department of Health, 2008). It is the responsibility of all healthcare providers and commissioners of NHS care to take the Constitution (Department of Health, 2013) into account in decisions affecting care. The Constitution is made up of seven key principles that spell out the core values of the NHS. Updated in January 2021, this document identifies the first NHS value as working together for patients; it goes on to say not only should patients be put first in all that we do but that they must be involved in their care and that decisions made should be shared. Whilst this is indeed the aim for healthcare professionals, some groups in society are less likely to have their voice heard.

Caring, Dignity and Compassion

It becomes the responsibility of the nurse and nursing associate to advocate on behalf of their patients and ensure they are involved in their care, afforded autonomy and treated with respect and dignity.

Case Study

Alf is 86 years old and until recently had a clean bill of health. 'I had just turned 80 and my daughter persuaded me to go and see the doctor because of pain in my knee joints.' Alf's records showed that his last medical intervention was as a young lad; he had appendicitis and was admitted for surgery at the age of 11!

Alf was prescribed non-steroidal anti-inflammatory drugs for his joint pain and referred to the practice nurse for routine health screening. 'That was the turning point for me; until then, I assumed that I was well!' reports Alf. Routine screening revealed that Alf had type 2 diabetes and an uncommon benign disorder of the liver, Gilbert syndrome. Over the past 5 years Alf has really got to know the diabetic team that monitors his health, and despite feeling at times that he is on a merry-go-round of appointments, the service provides him with support and advice from the specialist dietician, annual retinal screening from the ophthalmic services, referrals to the podiatry service and meetings with specialist nurses to review his blood glucose levels and adjust his medications accordingly.

Six months ago, Alf was admitted to hospital with acute retention of urine caused by enlargement of his prostate. While there, he developed a urinary tract infection and was

(Continued)

really disoriented for a number of days. Communication from the primary care setting meant that nursing and medical staff in hospital were able to compare his normal state and to organise intermediate care as a step down from hospital. Here, the liaison district nurse was able to review his case, discuss the prospect of a trial without catheter (TWOC) with the urologist and, as a result, speed Alf's return home. He was assessed by the occupational therapist who came home with him on discharge to gauge his need for adjustments to his home environment. He is now the proud owner of a perching stool in his kitchen, an adapted chair for his shower, a rail to help him in and out of bed and a walking stick, which he carries to the surgery. His care is now managed between the GP and specialist diabetic care team, and he has a range of drug therapies, which the local pharmacist arranges and delivers in blister packs that are easy to read and help ensure the right dosage of drug is administered at the right time. Most importantly, he feels involved in the decisions about his care and is able to express his anxieties about his prostate problem.

Communication and information about who and when to contact the service for help have supported Alf's transition from semi-dependency within the intermediate care setting, to independence within his own home.

Conclusion

The professional nature of nursing is constantly under scrutiny and, as health professionals, nurses make every effort to inspire confidence in the people for whom they care and other healthcare professionals. Patients expect nurses to provide the best care they can and this expectation is supported through the governing body for nurses and nursing associates, the NMC.

The professional nurse and nursing associate must question and challenge practice; this requires skills in the use of evidence-based activities to interpret information and to engage in the process of change. Change to promote quality is supported within the NHS in the form of clinical governance. The Care Quality Commission in England has put forward its strategy for 2021, with the core ambitions of accessing local systems and tackling inequalities in healthcare to ensure services provide people with safe, effective, compassionate, high-quality care, and to encourage services to improve.

Healthcare organisations must promote the development of professionalism, with opportunities to develop individual professional identity and to value the professional contribution made by all within health and social care settings. Interprofessional working and learning aims to support the positive experience of patients and clients in healthcare through collaboration and placing patients at the core of that activity.

Key Points

- Nurses and nursing associates are registered professionals bound by the NMC Code of Conduct.
- Failure to adhere to the Code will result in fitness to practise proceedings.

- In order to deliver safe and effective person-centered care, nurses and nursing associates must support their practice with evidence and have the ability to discern its reliability and applicability.
- Nurses need to demonstrate leadership and collaboration by working within a multidisciplinary team and be aware of clinical governance and quality assurance which may necessitate change in the form of service improvement.

References

Austin, J. & Currie, B. (2003) Changing organisations for a knowledge economy: the theory and practice of change management. *Journal of Facilities Management*, 2(3), 229–243.

Bassett, S. & Westmore, K. (2012) How nurse leaders can foster a climate of good governance. *Nursing Management*, 19(5), 22–24.

Beasley, C. (2006) *Modernising Nursing Careers – Setting the Direction.* Department of Health, London.

Boud, D., Keogh, R. & Walker, D. (1985) Promoting reflection in learning: a model. In: D. Boud, R. Keogh & D. Walker (eds) *Reflections: Turning Experience into Learning.* RoutledgeFalmer, London.

British Medical Association (1974) *Primary Health Care Teams.* BMA, London.

Burns, N. & Grove, S.K. (2011) *Understanding Nursing Research*, 4th edn. Elsevier, Philadelphia.

Care Quality Commission (2021) *A New Strategy for the Changing World of Health and Social Care. Our Strategy from 2021.* Care Quality Commission, Newcastle upon Tyne.

Department for Education and Skills (2003) *Every Child Matters.* HMSO, London.

Department of Health (1997) *The New NHS: Modern, Dependable.* Department of Health, London.

Department of Health (1999) *Clinical Governance: Quality in the New NHS.* Department of Health, London.

Department of Health (2000) *The NHS Plan: A Plan for Investment, A Plan for Reform.* Department of Health, London.

Department of Health (2008) *High Quality Care For All: NHS Next Stage Review Final Report.* Department of Health, London.

Department of Health (2012) *Equality Analysis. Government Response to: Liberating the NHS – No Decision About Me, Without Me.* Department of Health, London.

Department of Health (2013) *The NHS Constitution: The NHS Belongs To Us All.* Department of Health, London.

Department of Health (2019) *The Long Term Plan.* Department of Health, London.

Driscoll, J. (2007) Supported reflective learning: the essence of clinical supervision. In: Driscoll, J. (ed.) *Practising Clinical Supervision: A Reflective Approach for Healthcare Professionals*, 2nd edn, pp. 27–50. Elsevier, Edinburgh.

Francis, R. (2013) Report of the Mid Staffordshire NHS Foundation Trust Public Inquiry. Executive summary. https://assets.publishing.service.gov.uk/government/uploads/system/uploads/attachment_data/file/279124/0947.pdf (accessed November 2021)

Gage, W. (2013) Using service improvement methodology to change practice. *Nursing Standard*, 27(23), 51–57.

Ghadinan, F., Salsali, M. & Cheraghi. M.A. (2014) Nursing professionalism: an evolutionary concept analysis. *Iranian Journal of Nursing and Midwifery Research*, 19(1), 1–10.

Gibbs, G. (1998) *Learning by Doing: A Guide to Teaching and Learning.* Further Education Unit, Oxford Brookes University.

Greenwood, J. (1993) The apparent desensitization of student nurses during their professional socialization: a cognitive perspective. *Journal of Advanced Nursing*, 18(9), 1471–1479.

Grohar-Murray, M.E. & DiCroce, H.R. (2003) *Leadership and Management in Nursing*, 3rd edn. Prentice Hall, Upper Saddle River, NJ.

Hewitt-Taylor, J. (2013) Planning successful change incorporating process and people. *Nursing Standard*, 27(38), 35–40.

HM Government (2018) *Working Together to Safeguard Children. A Guide to Inter-Agency Working*. Crown Copyright, London

International Council of Nurses (2020) *Nurses: A Voice to Lead. Nursing the World to Health*. ICN, Geneva.

Johns, C. (ed.) (1994) A philosophical basis for nursing practice. In: *The Burford NDU Model: Caring in Practice*. Blackwell Scientific Publications, Oxford.

Johns, C. (2000) *Becoming a Reflective Practitioner: A Reflective and Holistic Approach to Clinical Nursing, Practice Development and Clinical Supervision*. Blackwell Science, Oxford.

McLean, C. (2011) Change and transition: what is the difference? *British Journal of School Nursing*, 6(2), 78–81.

Moon, J. (2004) *A Handbook of Reflective and Experiential Learning*. Routledge, London.

Muir Gray, J.A. (1997) Evidence-based practice is about 'doing the right things right'. In: *Evidence-based Healthcare: How to Make Health Policy and Management Decisions*. Churchill Livingstone, Edinburgh.

National Health Service (2013) *Healthcare Leadership Model. The Nine Dimensions of Leadership Behaviour*. NHS Leadership Academy, London.

National Health Service (2014) *Five Year Forward View*. NHS, London.

National Quality Board (2021) *A Shared Commitment to Quality for Those Working in Health and Care Systems*. Department of Health, London. www.england.nhs.uk/wp-content/uploads/2021/04/nqb-refreshed-shared-commitment-to-quality.pdf (accessed November 2021).

Nursing and Midwifery Council (2018a) *Ensuring Public Safety, Enabling Professionalism*. NMC, London.

Nursing and Midwifery Council (2018b) *Future Nurse: Standards of Proficiency for Registered Nurses*. NMC, London.

Nursing and Midwifery Council (2018c) *Standards of Proficiency for Registered Nursing Associates*. NMC, London.

Nursing and Midwifery Council (2018d) *The Code. Professional Standards of Practice and Behaviour for Nurses, Midwives and Nursing Associates*. NMC, London.

Nursing and Midwifwery Council (2019) *Revalidation. How to Revalidate with the NMC*. NMC, London.

Nursing and Midwifery Council (2020) *Caring with Confidence: The Code in Action*. www.nmc.org.uk/standards/code/code-in-action/ (accessed November 2021)

Nursing and Midwifery Council (2021) *The NMC Register 1 April 2020 – 31 March 2021*. NMC, London.

Polit, D.F. & Beck, C.T. (2011) *Nursing Research: Generating and Accessing Evidence in Nursing Practice*, 9th edn. Lippincott Williams & Wilkins, Philadelphia.

Royal College of Nursing (2003) *Defining Nursing*. RCN, London.

Sackett, D.L., Richardson, W.S., Rosenburg, W. & Haynes, R.B. (1997) *Evidence-based Medicine: How to Practise and Teach EBM*, 2nd edn. Churchill Livingstone, London.

Salvage, J. (2002) *Rethinking Professionalism: The First Step for Patient Focussed Care*. Institute for Public Policy Research, London.

Schön, D. (1983) *The Reflective Practitioner: How Professionals Think in Action*. Basic Books, New York.

Willis, Lord (2015) *Raising the Bar. Shape of Caring: A Review of the Future Education and Training of Registered Nurses and Care Assistants*. Health Education England, London.

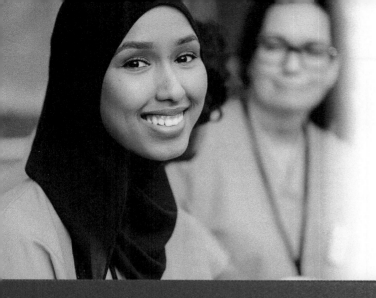

2

Ethics, the Law and the Nurse

Charlotte Bramanis[1] and Luis Teixeira[2]

[1]Senior Lecturer (Children's Nursing), Registered Nurse, UK and Australia
[2]Lecturer (Adult Nursing), Registered Nurse, UK and Portugal

Learning Outcomes

On completion of this chapter, you will be able to:

- Discuss how ethical approaches and theories contribute to the decision-making process in nursing practice
- Understand how the legal frameworks guide nursing practice
- Identify the ethical and legal principles to be applied in the different contexts of nursing practice
- Recognise the importance of accountability in nursing practice.

Proficiencies

NMC Proficiencies and Standards:

- At the point of registration, registered nurses will be able to understand and apply relevant legal, regulatory and governance requirements, policies and ethical frameworks, including any mandatory reporting duties, to all areas of practice, differentiating where appropriate between the devolved legislatures of the United Kingdom.

 Visit the companion website at www.wiley.com/go/peate/nursingpractice3e where you can test yourself using flashcards, multiple-choice questions and more.

Nursing Practice: Knowledge and Care, Third Edition. Edited by Ian Peate and Aby Mitchell.
© 2022 John Wiley & Sons Ltd. Published 2022 by John Wiley & Sons Ltd.
Companion website: www.wiley.com/go/peate/nursingpractice3e

Introduction

The ethical and legal issues in nursing practice are complex and varied. This chapter aims to provide the reader with an introduction to the ethical and legal context in which nursing takes place. As such, it will endeavour to explore the theories that can be used in decision making when nursing professionals face complex dilemmas in caring and provide opportunities to think about and develop skills in ethical practice. A number of the chapters in this book relate specifically to ethical and legal aspects of care that focus on the themes within that chapter. Moreover, the boxes 'Professional and legal issues' and 'Caring, dignity and compassion' across the main chapters will guide the reader through a reflection within the ethical and legal frameworks that are specific for that context of nursing practice.

Nursing professionals need to demonstrate that they understand and can apply codes of professional behaviour that support all patients and clients, with no exception. A 'standard' is a statement or criterion that can be used by a profession and by the general public to measure quality of practice. Established standards of nursing practice make each nursing professional accountable for practice. This means that each nursing professional providing care has the responsibility or obligation to account for their own behaviours within that role. Professional nursing organisations develop and implement standards of practice to help clarify the nursing professional's responsibilities to society. In the United Kingdom, the Nursing and Midwifery Council (2018a) has identified standards of conduct (as set out in Box 2.1); it also identifies standards of performance and ethics for nurses, midwives and nursing associates.

Box 2.1 Professional Standards for Practice and Behaviour for Nurses, Midwives and Nursing Associates (NMC, 2018a) and Future Nurse: Standards of Proficiency for Registered Nurses (NMC, 2018d)

The Code contains a series of statements that taken together signify what good nursing and midwifery practice looks like. It puts the interests of patients and service users first, is safe and effective, and promotes trust through professionalism.

Prioritise people
- *Treat people as individuals and uphold their dignity*
- *Listen to people and respond to their preferences and concerns*
- *Make sure that people's physical, social and psychological needs are assessed and responded to*
- *Act in the best interests of people at all times*
- *Respect people's right to privacy and confidentiality*

Practise effectively
- *Always practise in line with the best available evidence*
- *Communicate clearly*
- *Work co-operatively*
- *Share your skills, knowledge and experience for the benefit of people receiving care and your colleagues*
- *Keep clear and accurate records relevant to your practice*
- *Be accountable for your decisions to delegate tasks and duties to other people*

- *Have in place an indemnity arrangement which provides appropriate cover for any practice you take on as a nurse or midwife in the United Kingdom*

Preserve safety
- *Recognise and work within the limits of your competence*
- *Be open and candid with all service users about all aspects of care and treatment, including when any mistakes or harm have taken place*
- *Always offer help if an emergency arises in your practice setting or anywhere else*
- *Act without delay if you believe that there is a risk to patient safety or public protection*
- *Raise concerns immediately if you believe a person is vulnerable or at risk and needs extra support and protection*
- *Advise on, prescribe, supply, dispense or administer medicines within the limits of your training and competence, the law, our guidance and other relevant policies, guidance and regulations*
- *Be aware of, and reduce as far as possible, any potential for harm associated with your practice*

Promote professionalism and trust
- *Uphold the reputation of your profession at all times*
- *Uphold your position as a registered nurse or midwife*
- *Fulfil all registration requirements*
- *Cooperate with all investigations and audits*
- *Respond to any complaints made against you professionally*
- *Provide leadership to make sure people's wellbeing is protected and to improve their experiences of the healthcare system*

The standards of proficiency for registered nurses were reviewed in 2018 by the NMC. These standards (NMC, 2018d) help not only nurses but also the public in understanding the skills and knowledge required and expected from registered nurses. The standards have been organised in seven platforms.
1. *Being an accountable professional*
2. *Promoting health and preventing ill health*
3. *Assessing needs and planning care*
4. *Providing and evaluating care*
5. *Leading and managing nursing care and working in teams*
6. *Improving safety and quality of care*
7. *Coordinating care (NMC, 2018d)*

All seven platforms are linked to the Code (NMC, 2018a). However, platform 1 underpins platforms 2–7 from an ethical and legal perspective, by stipulating the following:
'*Registered nurses act in the best interests of people, putting them first ['Prioritising people'] and providing nursing care that is person-centred, safe and compassionate ['Preserve safety']. They act professionally at all times and use their knowledge and experience to make evidence-based decisions about care ['Practise effectively']. They communicate effectively, are role models for others, and are accountable for their actions ['Promote professionalism and trust']. Registered nurses continually reflect on their practice and keep abreast of new and emerging developments in nursing, health and care.*' (NMC, 2018a, 2018d).

Nursing associates have their own standards of proficiency (NMC, 2018e). These are organised in six platforms.

1. *Being an accountable professional*
2. *Promoting health and preventing ill health*
3. *Providing and monitoring care*
4. *Working in teams*
5. *Improving safety and quality of care*
6. *Contributing to integrated care* (NMC, 2018e)

Similarly to the analysis made regarding the standards of proficiency for registered nurses and its link to the Code (NMC, 2018a), platform 1 of the standards of proficiency for nursing associates is underpins the remaining the platforms from an ethical and legal perspective.

One of the key components for competency in pre-registration education in nursing is the importance of ethical practice. It recognises that an established code of ethics is one criterion that defines a profession and acknowledges that an ethical code is an essential feature of nursing care. The Code provides an excellent frame of reference to support nursing professionals in ethical behaviour. Ethics are principles of conduct, and ethical behaviour is concerned with values, moral duty, obligations and the distinction between right and wrong. This chapter contains different sections that will enable you to understand your accountability as a nursing professional from an ethical and legal perspective.

Morals, (bio)Ethics and (bio)Law: Clarifying Concepts

When promoting a reflection and discussion about **morals**, **ethics** and **law** *in* and *for* nursing practice, it is paramount to have these different, but also similar, concepts clarified. Etymology helps us to understand the meaning of words from their creation to their contextual changes. Thus, we propose you start this chapter by navigating through these three concepts from a brief etymological perspective.

Morals is originally derived from the Latin *moralis*, which is associated with proper 'manners' and 'behaviour'. Moral(s) can be thought of as standards of conduct that reflect ideal human behaviour, for example an expectation that in society, truth and honesty will apply to all situations, regardless of negative consequences. It is usually linked to individual values; values that have been acquired and developed by the individual under the influence of their specific sociocultural contexts and circumstances, such as family, friends and school (Kohlberg and Hersh, 1977). Just as an individual has values, it is sensible to assume that they will have some kind of moral code underpinning behaviour. The complexity of moral development, the means of learning what is right and wrong and what should or should not happen, begins in childhood and continues through life (Piaget, 1965; Kohlberg, 1971).

Jot This Down

Think about the values that you hold to be important. Where have these come from, and what influences your values?

Similarly to morals, **ethics** is also related to 'behaviour/human action'. However, when it comes to ethics, we are referring to a set of principles and values that are agreed and shared collectively (i.e. by a group of people); an example of this is the professional group comprising nurses, midwives and nursing associates and *The Code – Professional Standards of Practice and Behaviour for Nurses, Midwives and Nursing Associates* (NMC, 2018a). The known history of ethics theories begins with ancient Greek philosophers such as Socrates, Plato and Aristotle. Since then, 'virtue' and 'excellence' have been associated with the meaning and theory of ethics. Nonetheless, those theories and their application to nursing and healthcare practice have changed through time.

In the last century, nursing professionals have been confronted with drastic changes, not only in the sociocultural contexts where they are required to perform their duties but also within their scope of scientific practice and knowledge demands. Historical events such as World War II and its multiple crimes against humankind, which were then followed by the Declaration of Human Rights in 1948 and the technological revolution in the 1950s, have largely contributed to new and unprecedented challenges for ethical practice and debate within the healthcare context. Indeed, access to (presumably) inexhaustible knowledge and clinical resources to treat patients, combined with the emergence of patient rights to actively participate in decisions regarding their own health, have created an illusion of 'no limits'. This notion has led to some degree of artificialisation of human life, although not always with positive outcomes for patients, healthcare professionals/sector and society in general. 'Bioethics' emerged in the 1970s as an attempt to address such challenges with a contemporary ethical approach (Sándor, 2012).

Bioethics is about asking ourselves whether something that can be done, should be done or should not be done regarding someone's life. Some answers can be considered more socially or morally acceptable than others, depending on the context. When applied to the care setting, this decision making can be influenced by our opinions and personal values, a sense of what is right or wrong, our understanding of our obligations and duties as registered professionals and the subsequent consequences of our actions. In nursing practice, this can be challenging; however, an insight into the ethical principles and how these relate to nursing ethical frameworks can guide nursing professionals in difficult situations. The next sections of this chapter will guide you on this with more detail: section 2 provides an overview of the different approaches to ethics; section 3 is focused on one of the main bioethical models and its principles, which can be used as a framework to support the decision-making process in nursing practice.

Law comes from the Old English *lagu* which is linked to 'regulation' and 'rule prescribed by authority'. Indeed, law can be viewed as a system of rules that aims to regulate the behaviour of groups or individuals, as well as defining the rights and obligations that arise as a consequence of those rules. When it comes to a juridical reflection and legislative initiative within the healthcare sector/practice, 'biolaw' is the most appropriate term to use. **Biolaw** focuses on the capacity for human intervention in the artificialisation of life, aiming at its regulation. In section 4 of this chapter, we will discuss common aspects related to biolaw and nursing practice.

Approaches to Ethics

The actions taken by nursing professionals on a daily basis have a direct influence on the well-being of those in their care and it is often a challenge to identify all actions as being morally significant or morally neutral.

Applied ethics is the term used to describe an approach to ethical decision making which uses moral theories and principles to examine and address practical issues in everyday professional life. This approach acknowledges that ethics is not just about extreme issues, such as those linked to the limits of life and death. In nursing practice, everyday approaches to care should reflect an ethical stance. Just as nursing professionals are encouraged to reflect on the care they deliver, they are also encouraged to reflect ethically on actions that they engage in on an ongoing basis. Thus, applied ethics helps us to find the moral ground from which we can view the issues in public life. It helps us to identify morally acceptable approaches (and therefore supports nursing professionals in recognising when actions are not ethical) in the care environment.

There are three common approaches to the process of ethical thinking.

- Rules based (deontology)
- Outcomes based (utilitarianism)
- Virtue based.

Deontology

Rules-based ethics is often described as 'duty based' and is concerned with the idea that some actions are right and some are wrong. As a result of this, people have a duty to act accordingly, regardless of the consequences of the act; whether an action is ethical depends on the intentions behind the decision, rather than the outcome. Deontological ethics (deontology) considers what actions are right and has fundamental moral rules, such as: it is wrong to kill, to steal and to tell lies, and it is right to keep promises. One of its main founders was Immanuel Kant.

Generally, deontologists are bound by constraints. There are, however, complexities to the notion of deontology, because ideas of duty and what is right can vary among individuals from a variety of cultural backgrounds. Strict utilitarians, in contrast, recognise neither constraints nor options, and the aim of the utilitarian is to maximise the good by any and all means necessary.

Utilitarianism

A useful way of describing the utilitarian perspective is 'the greatest good for the greatest number' – this can be interpreted as always acting in such a way that will produce the greatest overall amount of good in the world. The value of the act is determined by its usefulness, with the main emphasis on the outcome or consequence. The focus or the moral position arising from utilitarianism is to put aside our own self-interest for the sake of all. It is often referred to as consequentialism and is based on the notion that in ethical decision making, the person should choose the action that maximises good consequences. Jeremy Bentham and John Stuart Mill were two of the main founders of this approach to ethics.

Utilitarianism can be considered as 'cost and benefit' and deciding which alternative courses of action can produce the best overall outcomes. If a nursing professional uses a utilitarian approach with regard to truth telling, for example, he or she would have to take into account, when making a decision, the consequence or outcome of truth telling, and whether the act (telling the truth) would produce more happiness than unhappiness. In this circumstance, even if a decision is made to tell the truth in order to arrive at the greatest good for the greatest number, this may not necessarily be the morally correct theory to justify the action. A deontological approach may prove to be more appropriate (Peate, 2012).

> **Jot This Down**
>
> A person in your care requires drug therapy. The prescription says to administer this parenterally, but you know that the drug can be just as effectively administered orally. What would be the difference of approach from a deontological and a utilitarian stance on this?

The attraction of a utilitarian approach within large organisations such as the NHS lies in its ability to apply the greatest benefits to the greatest numbers, i.e. to address the health needs of the majority of the population. This can be problematic as it does not necessarily allow for individual differences. An example of this may be the need for treatment of a rare condition, which may not be included in the resource allocation that is geared to the more common health problems.

Virtue Ethics

The ideology behind virtue ethics lies in the idea that it is person rather than action based; it is not so much about what we should do but more focused on how we should be. Thus, it is not the consequences of actions or the duties and rules that govern actions, but rather the moral character of the person carrying out the actions that is important. The great philosophers such as Plato and Aristotle would ponder over how a virtuous person would act in certain circumstances to draw conclusions about the nature of moral behaviour.

The traditional list of cardinal virtues includes prudence, justice, bravery and self-control (Plato, 2007). However, simply adopting these virtues to behave in an ethical way is criticised because although it sends out positive messages about how to be a good person, it does not provide clear guidance on what to do in certain situations where dilemmas occur.

A combination of intellectual and moral ethics is required for what Aristotle termed 'practical wisdom' (Thompson *et al.*, 2006). Practical wisdom comes with experience and is concerned with how to act in certain circumstances. An example is honesty; knowing how to be honest without causing pain or offence requires experience, the ability to reflect and the social skills to practise in ways that are suitable in each situation.

Ethical Principles

Ethics is relevant to all areas of nursing practice and the wider aspects of research, management and education fall under this umbrella. Active involvement in ethical decision making is an integral part of being a nursing professional, in part because the primary aims of caring are to do good (**beneficence**) and to minimise harm (**non-maleficence**). These two fundamental considerations when engaging in caring are significant overarching ethical principles. Combined with the principles of **justice** (fairness and equality) and **respect for autonomy** (individual rights and preferences), these four principles form the widely used and accepted bioethical model in healthcare practice called principlism. Principlism is a model founded by Beauchamp and Childress in 1979, being continuously reviewed and adapted; its latest version is from 2019 (Beauchamp and Childress, 2019). This model has been widely used and accepted by healthcare professionals because it:

- Provides an accessible and useable approach
- Is culturally neutral and accepted worldwide
- Ensures a degree of consistency
- Has a stronger counter to moral relativism
- Has a flexible approach (adapted from Herring, 2020).

Respect for Autonomy

The term 'autonomy' is derived from the Greek and is broadly defined as self-determination or self-rule (Dickenson *et al.*, 2010). It is the ability to make one's own decisions and have the right to choose. It recognises the uniqueness of individuals and that the person has the right to self-determination (even if the decisions taken by individuals lead to harm).

Patient autonomy and the principle of respect for a patient's autonomy are central to the nursing professional–patient relationship. As such, respecting a person's autonomy means that the nursing professional values a patient's right to make choices (including the right to refuse treatment), even if the nursing professional feels that a choice may not be in the patient's best interest. It also recognises the need to seek consent from an individual for treatment and care. Patients with **capacity to decide** (as per the Mental Capacity Act 2005) should always be allowed to choose, based not only on their own system of values, preferences and beliefs but also on the best information given: the notion of **informed consent**. We will visit the legal concepts of 'capacity to decide' and informed consent' later in this chapter.

Autonomy is a counterpoint of paternalism. Paternalism can be said to be acting for another person without their agreement or consent. The person acting paternalistically is assuming that they know best and that their actions are in the patient's best interests. Autonomy may be over-ridden or not respected when a person acts paternalistically.

Beneficence

The principle of 'doing good' in a healthcare context can be linked to a duty to avoid doing harm (non-maleficence). Nursing professionals have an obligation to do good for patients and individuals in their care and to act in a way that benefits patients. It can be argued then that beneficence is a duty of care.

The principle of beneficence means acting in the best interest of patients and clients, based on a professional skilled assessment of them. It can be said to encompass the need to:

- Make sure that any information or advice given is evidence based, including information relating to using any healthcare products or services

- Maintain the knowledge and skills you need for safe and effective practice
- Gather and reflect on feedback from a variety of sources, using it to improve your practice and performance
- Accurately assess signs of normal or worsening physical and mental health in the person receiving care.

An obligation to act in the best interest of a person may become paramount when the nursing professional is working with individuals whose capacity for autonomy is compromised, for example by immaturity, extreme distress and mental or physical incapacity.

Non-maleficence

Non-maleficence means to 'do no harm' and works with the principle of beneficence. At face value, this seems a simple mantra to follow but, in reality, it can be complicated. However, nursing professionals should never intentionally cause harm. Beauchamp and Childress (2019) point out the difficulty in defining the nature of harm.

There are many types of harm, ranging from physical and emotional injury to deprivation of property or violation of rights. Harm is a subjective entity and can mean different things to different people. In healthcare, harm can have a narrower definition, including pain, disability, emotional harm or death. Some levels of harm may have to be accepted in order to bring about good, for example when administering painful injections to deliver life-saving treatment.

Justice

Justice is often referred to as fairness and being fair and right is something that most people would wish to aim for. When justice is discussed in the healthcare arena, there are many factors that will influence whether we are being fair and right. Other definitions that are associated with justice are:

- Justice as a means of punishment or retribution. Punishment or retribution has more to do with the law than with health. Crime is punishable by society through the judicial system. This so-called legal justice is derived from morally acceptable laws
- Justice as fairness (fair distribution of resources)
- Justice as entitlement or right (rights-based justice).

Beauchamp and Childress (2019) suggest that justice is the fair, equitable and appropriate treatment of all people. Being fair and equitable will also depend on what society feels is owed to others – it is therefore subjective and can be loaded with values and judgements. Justice to individuals also implies care that does not discriminate on the basis of sexual orientation, gender, race or religion, age or illness (physical and psychological).

The underpinning principle associated with justice, therefore, is that everyone is valued equally and treated alike. It can be argued that equality is at the heart of justice; however, this is a difficult concept to tackle within the healthcare setting. Philosophical approaches to care may include Aristotle's quote that equals must be treated equally, and unequals must be treated unequally (Aristotle, 2020). This representation of formal justice allows for different approaches to care based on needs.

There are three perspectives associated with justice (Seedhouse, 2014).

- *Egalitarian*, concerned with the distribution of healthcare resources in accordance with individual need. In this perspective, individual need should be met by equal access to services.
- *Libertarian* perspective relates to liberty and choice and is associated with how hard an individual has worked in order to earn healthcare; they are judged on merit.
- *Rights* imply that the state has an obligation to provide care and that the patient should suffer no harm as a result of that provision. People's rights have to be upheld in order to meet the criteria associated with a rights perspective.

Jot This Down

Review the Code (NMC, 2018a) to identify which statements relate specifically to each ethical principle from the Beauchamp and Childress (2019) principlism model.

Legal Perspectives

There are very few areas of healthcare that are exempt from the law; however, it is only an adverse event that makes nursing professionals consider the legal implications of the care they provide. Involvement with the legal process may occur at any time during a nursing professional's career, even years after care commenced or ceased; as a nursing professional therefore, there is a legal obligation to ensure that your daily practice is in line with trust and government guidelines. We also need to consider the patient's capacity, age and cognitive ability.

Practice Assessment Document (PAD)

The PAD is a legal document and must be kept for a period of 5 years post qualifying and be used as evidence with the NMC if required. Therefore, the document, like any nursing documentation, may not be defaced or edited in any way.

Legal Frameworks

From an early age, we begin to learn the rules of what is generally described as acceptable and unacceptable behaviour. For every child, this varies, dependent on our parents' or carers' beliefs; just as our ethical stance is governed by our values, so too is our respect for authority and the law. UK law has evolved over hundreds of years based on tradition, social morals and politics. For the law to be effective, there must be a system to punish those who fail to adhere to the set rules; within the UK there is a well-established court system to ensure fairness to all. Within nursing, the Nursing and Midwifery Council has a legal framework governing how it operates, with the Department of Health at the centre of the legislation (NMC, 2019b).

In the care setting, patients are legally protected because of their rights, and as nursing professionals we have a responsibility to be aware of how the law protects patients' rights and how to safeguard them from others who may encroach on those rights. As nursing professionals, we are obliged to follow not only the UK law but also those imposed by the NMC, which ensures that registrants understand the implications of protecting patients of all ages and abilities.

Sources of Law

The UK legal system is made up of four principal sources of law: legislation, common law, European Union law and the European Convention on Human Rights. Parliament is the UK's principal source of law, and passes law through England, Wales, Scotland and Northern Ireland. Common law is developed by judges and courts and makes up part of the UK's unwritten constitution, known as the Court of Appeal and the Supreme Court. Common law is called on when the courts cannot turn to a relevant statute. This may be because a particular Act of Parliament concerning the specific area of law under deliberation has not been made. In case law, the courts look to precedent, considering previous cases to determine how a decision has been made and how statute has been interpreted.

Healthcare Law

The UK established the National Health Service on 5 July 1948, and since its inception, the British public have expected that healthcare provision should be free. In the years following, the NHS has been under immense pressure due to an increasingly ageing population and an increase in co-morbidities in healthcare. In an attempt to ensure the NHS can withstand the ever-changing requirements placed upon it, in 1977 and again in 2006, the legislation was revised to place more responsibility on the Secretary of State, who sets out the structure of the NHS in England. In 2012, the Health and Social Care Act of 2008 was revised, and is one of the most recent Acts of Parliament to influence the provision and organisation of care within the UK. The Public Interest (Social Value) Act 2012 further ensures that social, economic and environmental issues are considered in the procurement of well-being, as social determinants of health are key to ensuring the British public are given the best care based on their personal circumstances (NHS, 2020).

In the aftermath of the SARS-CoV-2 pandemic, the Department of Health and Social Care has released a White Paper to ensure that the NHS is better prepared in the future to cope with the fast-changing world, focusing on population health and appropriate resources. The paper is entitled 'Integration and innovation: working together to improve health and social care for all', and the first implementations for change are due to commence in 2022 (DHSC, 2021).

Human Rights Act 1998

The primary aim of this Act is to give the courts greater powers to protect some fundamental rights. It introduced the European Convention on Human Rights from 1950 into British domestic law. The most important principle of the legislation is that everyone's life shall be protected by law. There are six specific Articles in the Human Rights Act (1998) that impinge on nursing.

- Article 2: Right to life
- Article 3: Prohibition of torture
- Article 5: Right to liberty

- Article 6: Right to a fair trial
- Article 8: Respect for private and family life
- Article 9: Freedom of thought, conscience and religion

These Articles should influence the way that care is delivered by nursing professionals, as the principles underpinning human rights apply to all nursing professionals in that they should:

- Maintain dignity
- Promote and protect autonomy
- Practise in a non-discriminatory manner.

Nursing and Midwifery Council Standards

The Code ensures that the healthcare laws are integrated into the care we provide our patients; this comes under Domain 2: Professional and ethical practice. This domain ensures that the health and safety of the patient is foremost, including raising concerns such as safeguarding issues.

The Nursing Associate

 The Code became effective in March 2015 for all registered nurses and midwives in the UK. In October 2018, the document was updated to reflect the regulation of nursing associates. Nursing associates are required to meet the same professional standards of practice and behaviour as nurses and midwives.

The NMC regulates nursing performance, with registrants being required to revalidate their registration every 3 years; this allows the NMC to ensure that registrants are safe.

The revalidation process requires the registrant to meet with a senior member of the team and demonstrate what they do to ensure patient safety. If there are any concerns about a registrant's ability to perform their tasks effectively, the NMC can call the registrant in for a Fitness to Practise hearing. Reasons for concern include misconduct, lack of competence, not having the necessary knowledge of English, criminal behaviour and serious ill health. At a Fitness to Practise hearing, the panel hears the allegations against the registrant, and makes a decision based on the protection, promotion and maintenance of the health, safety and well-being of the public.

Practice Assessment Document (PAD)

 The PAD is used within placement settings for students to ensure they are able to achieve proficiencies in a timely manner in order to be a competent professional. Alongside these proficiencies are professional values; these professional values are linked to The Code and students are expected to act in a manner that upholds the integrity of the profession from the first time they begin placement. Failure to meet these requirements will have an impact on the student's ability to successfully register as a professional at the end of their course.

Medicines Management

 In 2019, the Nursing and Midwifery Council withdrew its Standards for Medicines Management, as more nurses were prescribing medicines and more healthcare professionals were involved in medicines management. Therefore, all professionals involved in the safe and secure handling of medicines should now follow the guidance published by the Royal Pharmaceutical Society (RPS, 2018). Furthermore, nursing professionals should also follow administration guidelines from the Royal College of Nursing, who work with the RPS to ensure safe practice (RPS and RCN, 2019).

Duty of Care and Duty of Candour

The Code emulates the Health and Social Care Act (2012) by ensuring that nursing professionals work within the Act and have a duty of care to their patients. This legal obligation to take reasonable care to avoid a breach of duty is explicitly spelled out within the first section of The Code, 'Prioritise People', which states:

'You put the interests of people using or needing nursing or midwifery services first. You make their care and safety your main concern and make sure that their dignity is preserved and their needs are recognised, assessed and responded to. You make sure that those receiving care are treated with respect, that their rights are upheld and that any discriminatory attitudes and behaviours towards those receiving care are challenged'.

(NMC, 2018a)

Negligence

Negligence relates to any act or omission on the part of the nursing professional which results in injury, harm or loss. Such acts or omissions can result in a civil claim for compensation or a criminal prosecution.

Jot This Down

When treatment is undertaken by an individual, there is a potential claim for damages if all the elements of negligence are present. Think of examples of clinical negligence that can occur in practice.

The NMC requires that all registrants caring for patients or clients have professional indemnity insurance; this is in the interest of clients, patients and registrants in the event of a claim for professional negligence. In general, within the NHS, it is the NHS trust that will be sued by the courts; however, a claim may also be brought against the nursing professional, especially in private practice.

For a successful claim of negligence, the following must be proven in a court of law.

- A duty of care is owed.
- The duty of care is breached.
- The breach of that duty has caused harm.
- Damage or other losses have resulted from that harm.

Ethical and Legal Issues in Nursing Practice

In nursing, ethical decision making, using ethical and legal guidelines, ensures that the correct moral actions are taken when providing care. Nursing professionals face moral decision making on a daily basis, most commonly around confidentiality, a person's rights and advocacy. Ethical decision making is usually making a choice between two or more unpleasant, ethically troubling alternatives. Nursing professionals face these predicaments almost daily, commonly involving confidentiality, a person's rights and issues of dying and death. The nursing professional must use ethical and legal guidelines to make decisions about moral actions when providing care in these and in many other situations. However, it should be acknowledged that no one profession is responsible for ethical decisions, and it is important in a complex care situation for all caregivers to be involved in decisions.

Consent

All adults must be presumed to have the mental capacity to agree to or refuse treatment. As such, any competent patient can decline any examination, any investigation or any proposed treatment, even if this treatment is considered life saving. It is imperative that the person consents before any treatment, care or examination. If a person refuses an intervention but it still goes ahead, then this is a civil or criminal wrong, so-called 'trespass against the person', and practitioners could be accused assault and battery and be called to account by the NMC. Harm in this situation can result in an accusation of negligence on the part of the nursing professional.

Patients and clients may give what is known as *implied consent*. For consent to be valid, there are three key principles that have to be satisfied.

- Consent is *informed*.
- The individual is *competent*.
- Consent is *voluntary*.

Informed Consent

The process of obtaining consent is important and is underpinned in The Code (NMC, 2018a) when it states: *'Make sure that you get properly informed consent and document it before carrying out any action. Individuals need to be given clear information about the nature and purpose of even basic treatments, and failure to provide sufficient information would invalidate consent. Where consent has been given, then no charge of trespass of the person can take place. Appreciations of legal cases that illustrate past examples are useful for understanding the consequences of consent'.*

Voluntary Consent

Consent must be given freely and voluntarily, without any pressure or undue influence being exerted on the patient. If the nursing professional feels the patient is being pressurised into agreeing to (or refusing) treatment, he or she should arrange to see the patient alone to ascertain if the decision is truly that of the patient.

Coercion invalidates consent. If a patient is being treated in an environment where he or she is being involuntarily detained, for example a psychiatric hospital, a psychiatric unit or a prison, care must be taken to ensure that the patient is not being coerced (Department of Health, 2009).

What the Experts Say

'Patients attending the clinic, by the very nature of them turning up for their appointment, implies that they are willing to discuss and consider the treatments that can take place. Nonetheless, it is my responsibility to respect their right to autonomy. A patient might roll up their sleeve for a blood test, but it is always important to provide information and to make sure that the patient understands the procedure and is happy to go ahead with investigations or treatment.'
(District Nursing Sister)

Confidentiality

All nursing professionals are bound by the duty of confidentiality. The Code states that:

As a nurse, midwife or nursing associate, you owe a duty of confidentiality to all those who are receiving care. This includes making sure that they are informed about their care and that information about them is shared appropriately.

To achieve this, you must:

- *respect a person's right to privacy in all aspects of their care*
- *make sure that people are informed about how and why information is used and shared by those who will be providing care*
- *respect that a person's right to privacy and confidentiality continues after they have died*
- *share necessary information with other healthcare professionals and agencies only when the interests of patient safety and public protection override the need for confidentiality, and*
- *share with people, their families and their carers, as far as the law allows, the information they want or need to know about their health, care and ongoing treatment sensitively and in a way they can understand.*

Jot This Down

Disclosure means the giving of information. Under what circumstances can nursing professionals be required to disclose patient/client information?

Nursing professionals are responsible for protecting the confidentiality and security of the individual's health information. A duty of confidence, which is derived from common law and statute law, arises when one person discloses information to another party where it is reasonable to expect that the information shared will be held in confidence. Imagine the nurse–patient relationship; information is shared and the patient expects confidentiality and treatment based on the information. Nursing professionals protect the rights of the individual. This is identified in Article 8 of the Human Rights Act (1998), which asserts that we all have a right to privacy, and that right can only be over-ruled in the interest of national security, public safety, prevention of crime, the protection of health and morals or the protection of the rights and freedom of others. The Caldicott Review developed a revised list of principles, the Caldicott Principles, that should be adhered to.

1. Justify the purpose(s): every proposed use or transfer of personal confidential data should be defined, scrutinised and documented.
2. Do not use personal confidential data unless it is absolutely necessary: the need for patients to be identified should be considered.
3. Use the minimum necessary personal confidential data: when this is deemed essential, consider and justify so the minimum amount of personal data is transferred.
4. Access to personal confidential data should be on a strict need-to-know basis.
5. Everyone with access to confidential data should be aware of their responsibilities.
6. Comply with the law: organisations must comply with legal requirements.
7. The duty to share information can be as important as the duty to protect patient confidentiality: this supports the notion of the best interests of the patient in line with professional, employer and regulatory bodies (Department of Health, 2013).

Patient/client records hold a great deal of personal information that can easily identify them. Data such as name, date of birth and so on are necessary components to apply care within a safe framework. Records also contain additional information about a person's health, lifestyle and past and current health issues.

Red Flag

It is not acceptable for nursing professionals to:
- Discuss matters related to the people in their care outside the clinical setting
- Discuss a case with colleagues in public where they may be overheard
- Leave records unattended where they may be read by unauthorised persons.

Capacity and Competency
Competent Patients

We care for patients with the assumption that all competent adults have the absolute right to refuse or to withdraw from treatment, even if this decision means that the individual will suffer or die as a result. The Code reinforces this for nurses, midwives and nursing associates when it states, 'You must respect and support people's rights to accept or decline treatment and care' (NMC, 2018a).

Alongside this, individuals need to be aware of and understand the consequences of refusing treatment. Three elements emerge associated with capacity.

- Understanding and the ability to retain information.
- Knowledge of the consequences of refusing treatment.
- Evaluation of the facts in making a decision.

Mental Health

A person's control over their life when their competency or mental capacity has been altered occurs through the use of advance directives (referred to as an advance decision to refuse treatment in the Mental Capacity Act (2005)). The Code demands that nursing professionals are aware of the legislation regarding mental capacity, ensuring that people who lack capacity remain at the centre of decision making and are fully safeguarded. The Mental Capacity Act (2005) defines mental capacity. It sets out the legal requirements for assessing whether or not a person lacks the capacity to make a decision. Where a person lacks the capacity to make a decision for themselves, any decision must be made in that person's best interests. The Mental Capacity Act (2005) is enforced in England and Wales and is applicable to all those working in health and social care, who are involved in the care, treatment and support of those aged 16 or over who may lack the capacity to make decisions for themselves.

Nursing Fields   Learning Disabilities

The patient must be able to communicate his   or her decision to the healthcare team. The nursing professional should never underestimate the patient's ability to communicate regardless of physical or psychological condition. For example, in the case of a patient with learning disabilities, the nursing professional must make use of all resources available to facilitate communication, and this may include taking time to explain to the individual the issues in simple language, employing visual aids and, if appropriate, signing. It may be advisable for the nursing professional to engage the support of those who know the patient, for example the family, carers and staff from statutory and non-statutory agencies. There are many legal routes to be explored before a decision is made exclusively by healthcare professionals.

Consent in Children

Nursing professionals working with children and young people must work within the legal framework for consent and capacity. When obtaining consent, the nursing professional should consider whether the child is legally competent, and children as a rule should be involved in decisions about their care as much as possible. Gaining consent from this age group will be the same as it is for adults. In England and Wales, children under the age of 16 are generally considered to lack the capacity to consent or to refuse treatment. Those under 16 years of age who have sufficient understanding and intelligence to enable them to fully understand what is involved in the proposed intervention may have the capacity to consent to that intervention (Department of Health, 2009). Children who possess these abilities are said to be 'Gillick competent'.

The term 'Gillick competent' comes from a court case, Gillick v. West Norfolk and Wisbech Area Health Authority in 1985. This concerned a teenage girl's right to consent to medical treatment without her parents' knowledge. The outcome of the hearing permitted children under 16 to consent to medical treatment if they understand what is being proposed. The decision is based on whether the child has the maturity and intelligence to fully understand the nature of the treatment, the options, the risks involved and the benefits. This decision is made by the doctor caring for the patient. Some of the questions that need to be considered are:

- Does the child understand the proposed treatment, his or her medical condition, the consequences that may emerge if he or she refuses or agrees to treatment?
- Does he or she understand the moral, social and family issues involved in the decision he or she is to make?
- Does the mental state of the child fluctuate?
- What treatment is to be performed? Does the child understand the complexities of the proposed treatment and potential risks associated with it?

Following the Gillick court case in 1985, the Fraser Guidelines were introduced to law in 2006; these guidelines specifically relate to contraception and sexual health only. They are named after one of the Lords responsible for the Gillick judgement but who went on to address the specific issue of giving contraceptive advice and treatment to those under 16 without parental consent. Practitioners using the Fraser guidelines should be satisfied of the following.

- The young person cannot be persuaded to inform their parents or carers that they are seeking this advice or treatment (or to allow the practitioner to inform their parents or carers).
- The young person understands the advice being given.
- The young person's physical or mental health or both are likely to suffer unless they receive the advice or treatment.
- It is in the young person's best interests to receive the advice, treatment or both without their parents' or carers' consent.
- The young person is very likely to continue having sex with or without contraceptive treatment.

Nursing Fields Children's Nursing

- Children under the age of 16 are generally considered to lack the capacity to consent or to refuse treatment; however, as nursing professionals, we have to consider Gillick competence and the Fraser Guidelines.
- For children and young people deemed competent to give consent, it is good practice to involve parents in the discussions.

Advocacy in Nursing

Individuals who are receiving care may be unable or unprepared to make independent decisions. However, patients as consumers are better educated about options for care and may have very definite opinions. The nursing professional as an advocate actively promotes the person's rights to autonomy and freedom of choice. By speaking for the person, she or he mediates between the person and others, and/or protects the person's right to self-determination or autonomy. Advocacy, empowerment,

patient-centred care and patient involvement in their care are principal themes of the Royal College of Nursing (RCN, 2021).

As a nursing professional, you must practise advocacy founded on the belief that individuals have the right to choose treatment options without coercion, based on information about the outcome of accepting or rejecting the treatment. The nursing professional must also accept and respect the decision of the individual, even though it may differ from the decision the nursing professional would make. According to Mind, the National Association for Mental Health, 'An advocate is someone who can both listen to you and speak for you in times of need' (Mind, 2021).

Being an advocate requires you to listen to your patient, discuss their wishes, and work with the medical team to ensure that the patient is listened to and is involved in their own care. Advocacy can range from discussing medication options, to ensuring a Do Not Attempt To Resuscitate order is adhered to.

Case Study

Qadira, a 13 year old, presented to the hospital with lethargy, decreased eating and easy bruising. Healthcare professionals undertook a full assessment of Qadira and it was found that she had acute lymphoblastic leukaemia. After admission to the children's oncology ward for treatment planning, Qadira suggested she did not want to undergo treatment as she would lose her hair, and would be really ill and not see her friends. Her father advised her that if she did not want treatment, he would support her decision. Both Qadira and her father were spoken to in depth by the medical team and were advised that Qadira had a greater than 90% chance of survival if she had treatment, and no survival without treatment. Qadira still insisted she would rather die than lose her hair and be ill with no friends.

Before continuing, pause and consider the following.

- Do you assess Qadira as Gillick competent?
- Why do you think parents allow their children to refuse treatment?
- How does this make you feel?
- What are the ethical and legal implications when a parent or patient does not want treatment, yet healthcare professionals can demonstrate the high chance of survival?

In this scenario, healthcare professionals had to consider Qadira's ability for making her own health choices; although she is within the right age range to be deemed Gillick competent, the team have to decide if she is aware of the risks associated with not receiving treatment. As Qadira appeared to not comprehend the enormity and finality of end of life, it was deemed that Qadira was not Gillick competent. The decision was made based on Qadiras' objections – the loss of hair and being ill can be addressed with medications and treatments, and not seeing friends can be addressed with technology. With a 90% survival rate, it is in the patient's best interest that they receive treatment (Human Rights Act 1998, Article 2).

Once the healthcare team had made this decision, they then had to discuss with Qadira's father his reasons for agreeing to her not receiving treatment. The team met with Qadira's father away from Qadira's bedside and allowed him to openly discuss his concerns. It became apparent that

Qadira's cousin had also had cancer, and was extremely unwell for almost 2 years before passing away. The cousin suffered a lot of pain and discomfort and spent a long time in hospital when he could have been home with family celebrating what was left of his life. The team identified that the cancer was different, with a lower survival rate, and this would have affected the outcome for the cousin. The team explored cultural and religious beliefs with Qadira's father, and it became apparent that he also did not want treatment, partly due to his beliefs but mostly due to his nephew not surviving cancer.

Think about the following sections from this chapter, and relate this to the case study. What do you think should have been the outcome for Qadira's treatment?

· Beneficence
· Human Rights Act
· Duty of Care
· Advocacy in Nursing
· Principles of nursing practice (Box 2.2) – principles E & G.

Accountability

Nursing professionals are involved in decision making on a constant basis, in a wide variety of settings and often under pressure to do so. Indeed, they are responsible for making the best decisions based on the evidence for best practice and can be called to account to justify the decisions that they make. As such, accountability is seen as integral to professional practice.

Historically, the definition of accountability was not always clear. In an attempt to clarify this concept within nursing practice, the NMC has defined accountability as 'the principle that individuals and organisations are responsible for their actions and may be required to explain them to others' (NMC, 2018b). If a nursing professional is asked to deliver care which they consider is unsafe or harmful to the individual, they should carefully consider options and raise concerns with the appropriate person. Nursing professionals are mainly accountable to four entities: the patient; the public; the NMC; the employer.

Accountability in Professional Practice

The need for nursing professionals to demonstrate accountability is paramount. To support accountability in practice, nursing professionals must:

• Ensure that they perform competently
• Inform a senior member of staff when they are unable to perform competently
• Have the ability (knowledge and skills) to perform the activity or intervention
• Accept the responsibility for carrying out the activity
• Have the authority to perform the activity within their role, through delegation and the policies and protocols of the organisation (RCN, 2017a).

The RCN, in partnership with the Department of Health and the NMC, developed the *Principles of Nursing Practice* (RCN, 2013). These principles guide the profession in relation to what people can expect from nursing practice, whether they are colleagues, patients or the families or carers of patients (Box 2.2).

Box 2.2 Principles of Nursing Practice (RCN, 2013) and links to Future Nurse: Standards of Proficiency for Registered Nurses (NMC, 2018d)

· **Principle A:** nurses and nursing staff treat everyone in their care with dignity and humanity – they understand their individual needs, show compassion and sensitivity, and provide care in a way that respects all people equally. (linked to Platforms 1, 3, 4 from the NMC, 2018d)
· **Principle B:** nurses and nursing staff take responsibility for the care they provide and answer for their own judgements and actions – they carry out these actions in a way that is agreed with their patients, and the families and carers of their patients, and in a way that meets the requirements of their professional bodies and the law. (linked to Platforms 1 and 7 from the NMC, 2018d)
· **Principle C:** nurses and nursing staff manage risk, are vigilant about risk, and help to keep everyone safe in the places they receive healthcare. (linked to Platforms 2 and 6 from the NMC, 2018d)
· **Principle D:** nurses and nursing staff provide and promote care that puts people at the centre, involves patients, service users, their families and their carers in decisions and helps them make informed choices about their treatment and care. (linked to Platforms 1, 3, 4, 5 and 7 from the NMC, 2018d)
· **Principle E:** nurses and nursing staff are at the heart of the communication process: they assess, record and report on treatment and care, handle information sensitively and confidentially, deal with complaints effectively, and are conscientious in reporting the things they are concerned about. (linked to Platforms 1, 3, 4, 5 and 7 from the NMC, 2018d)
· **Principle F:** nurses and nursing staff have up-to-date knowledge and skills, and use these with intelligence, insight and understanding in line with the needs of each individual in their care. (linked to Platforms 1, 5, 6 and 7 from the NMC, 2018d)
· **Principle G:** nurses and nursing staff work closely with their own team and with other professionals, making sure patients' care and treatment are co-ordinated, are of a high standard and have the best possible outcome. (linked to Platforms 5, 6 and 7 from the NMC, 2018d)
· **Principle H:** nurses and nursing staff lead by example, develop themselves and other staff, and influence the way care is given in a manner that is open and responds to individual needs. (linked to Platforms 1, 5 and 7 from the NMC, 2018d)

Within the Practice Assessment Documents (PADs) regardless of the part, all the proficiencies and professional values link to these principles and platforms.

Professional accountability involves assessment of the best interests of the patient, and the use of professional judgement and nursing skills to make the best decision and to enable the professional to account for that decision based on the best evidence available to them. Occasionally, and on behalf of the public interest, the NMC will investigate complaints made about the professional conduct or the fitness to practise of nurses, midwives and nursing associates on the professional register.

Accountability for Students and Practice Assessors/Practice Supervisors

Students are exposed to a variety of practice settings and are involved in observation and participation in care activities. The expectation is that, over time, the student will become more involved in providing care. Students have a responsibility to participate in practice activities only within their level of understanding and competence. This should always be under the supervision of 'NMC registered nurses, midwives, nursing associates and other registered health and social care professionals' (NMC, 2018c).

Although the student is supernumerary (they are additional to the workforce requirement and staffing figures), they should make an active contribution to the work of the practice area to enable them to learn how to care for patients (RCN, 2017b). This in itself implies accountability, but it is the practice assessor and/or practice supervisor who is professionally responsible for the consequences of any acts or omissions on the student's part.

Red Flag

Although students may not be called to account by the NMC for any acts or omissions in practice, this does not mean that they are immune from blame and can be called to account both in law and by universities via the 'fitness for practice' route.

Practice assessors and practice supervisors are registered professionals supporting the education and development of students in clinical practice. This mandatory requirement of the NMC ensures that all students on approved programmes of study have practice assessors and practice supervisors in place. Practice assessors, in collaboration with practice supervisors, make judgements about the performance of the student, their fitness for practice and ultimately for registration. As such, they are involved in determining a student's competence and ability to practise safely. Any delegation of duties to a student by practice assessors and practice supervisors must take place under supervision. As a practice assessor/practice supervisor, the registered professional's accountability is to ensure that the individual who undertakes the work is able to do so.

What the Experts Say

'I was asked to pass a urinary catheter on a woman who was having gynaecological surgery, but I had only seen this done in the simulation lab at university. I explained this to my practice supervisor, and she was great, talking me through the principles and allowing me to observe her when she passed the catheter. She explained that, as a second-year student she assumed I would have the skills needed to complete this task; however, I had not yet come across this in practice. My accountability was to the patient and non-maleficence.'

(Student Nurse, year 2)

Delegation

The ability to delegate, assign tasks and supervise is an essential competency for all registered nursing professionals. Decisions relating to delegation by these professionals must be based on the fundamental principles of safety and public protection. When delegating, the following should be considered.

- Delegation does not harm the interests of people in their care.
- The task is within the other person's scope of competence.
- The person they are delegating to understands the boundaries of their own competence and is clear about the circumstances.
- Those delegating are ultimately responsible to take reasonable steps to monitor the outcome of the delegated task (adapted from NMC, 2018b).

Nursing professionals are accountable for the decision to delegate care and care should be delegated only to a person who has had appropriate training and is deemed competent to perform the task. Where another, such as an employer, has the authority to delegate an aspect of care, the employer becomes accountable for that delegation. However, and in accordance with the Code (NMC, 2018a), the nurse, midwife or nursing associate must act without delay if they believe a colleague or anyone else may be putting someone at risk.

Red Flag

If an aspect of care is delegated, the nursing professional allocated to that patient remains accountable for the overall management of the person in their care (this includes going on a break).

The Nursing Associate

The Nursing and Midwifery Council has published information supplementary to The Code about delegation and accountability, aiming to 'help people think about situations when they are delegating tasks, or being given tasks to do by colleagues' (NMC, 2018b).

Case Study

Abdul qualified as a nursing associate 3 months ago and now works on a medical ward with adult patients. Today, he is responsible for looking after six patients, working closely with Sarah (a registered nurse) and Francine (a healthcare assistant) on a 12-hour shift. One of the patients in Abdul's care is Steve, who has type 2 diabetes. Steve is due his fast-acting insulin at 12.30, immediately before his lunch. Abdul checks Steve's preprandial glycaemia (7.1 mmol/L), as per the care plan for this patient, and Steve asks for his insulin injection, as prescribed. Sarah, the registered nurse with Abdul, started her hour-long lunch break at 12.15.

Before continuing, pause and reflect about the following.

- Could Abdul administer the insulin to Steve in Sarah's absence or should he wait for Sarah to arrive from her break?
- Who would be accountable for this clinical procedure?
- What has supported your decision?

Nursing associates are a recent professional group in England, and are an integral part of the care and nursing workforce. This professional group became regulated by the Nursing and Midwifery Council in 2018 and is under the scrutiny of The Code (NMC, 2018a), with specific standards of proficiency (NMC, 2018e). The standards of proficiency for registered nursing associates (NMC, 2018e) stipulate that these professionals have the knowledge and skills to administer subcutaneous injections to patients under their care. To meet these standards, training has been given by an approved Higher Education Institution, providing them with the required learning opportunities and assessment strategies to become proficient in this clinical procedure when qualified and entering the register. Therefore, Abdul won't need to wait for Sarah to arrive from her break to administer the fast-acting insulin to Steve, and Steve will not need to delay his lunch because of Sarah's absence.

Abdul is accountable for this procedure, as he has been trained appropriately. Nonetheless, as a newly qualified registered nursing associate, Abdul should feel confident in proceeding with the administration of insulin to Steve, asking for support from another registered nurse if not confident. Abdul's employer should also have clear local protocols and instructions regarding medicines administration by nursing associates so the entire multidisciplinary team has a clear understanding about the role of this recent professional group in this type of clinical procedure.

Candour

Sometimes referred to as the seventh 'C', candour is the professional responsibility of healthcare professionals to be honest with people in their care when things go wrong. In association with the General Medical Council, the NMC published guidance on the professional duty of candour, which includes:

- Telling the patient (or the patient's advocate or carer) when something has gone wrong
- Apologising, saying sorry, to the patient
- Putting matters right – providing an appropriate remedy
- Giving a full explanation of the short- and long-term effects of what has happened (adapted from General Medical Council and Nursing and Midwifery Council, 2015).

In addition, nursing professionals have a duty of candour to their co-workers and any associated agencies, providing information and raising concerns where appropriate. A culture of openness and honesty is recommended, where mutual support of raising concerns is adopted.

Candour is also part of the professional standards of practice and behaviour for nurses, midwives and nursing associates. Indeed, The Code (NMC, 2018a) states that, as a nurse, midwife and nursing associate, 'you make sure that patient and public safety is not affected. You work within the limits of your competence, exercising your professional "duty of candour" and raising concerns immediately whenever you come across situations that put patients or public safety at risk. You take necessary action to deal with any concerns where appropriate'.

Raising Concerns in Practice

Because of the duty of care that nursing professional have for their patients, they are obliged to put the interests of the people in their care first and to act to protect them if they are considered to be at risk (NMC, 2018a). No matter in what care environment nursing professionals work, they must make themselves aware of the local policy for raising concerns and for whistleblowing in practice. Local safeguarding policies should also be considered in order to protect patients and service users from abuse.

Raising and escalating concerns early can prevent minor issues becoming major ones. The key points to consider when faced with concerns include the following.

- Take immediate action.
- Protect client confidentiality.

- Refer to local policies on whistleblowing.
- Record concerns and actions taken (adapted from NMC, 2019a).

Concerns might include aspects related to the delivery of care to individuals or groups of people. There may be risks to health and safety with, for example, the incorrect use of harmful substances. Nursing professionals might find themselves in an environment of care that they feel is harmful to patients, such as one that presents a risk of infection or the use of outdated, deficient clinical equipment.

The publication of the Public Interest Disclosure Act (1998) aimed to provide protection for those who honestly raise genuine concerns about wrongdoing or malpractice in the workplace. The protection has been extended to employees who, as a result of escalating genuine concerns, are victimised or dismissed for doing so.

All senior staff and clinical leaders in nursing should make available appropriate systems for raising concerns in practice and should ensure that concerns are investigated promptly with a full objective assessment of the situation. Senior staff who investigate concerns should protect staff who raise concerns from unwarranted criticisms and keep them informed of the progress and outcomes (NMC, 2019a).

Conclusion

Nursing is structured by codes of ethics and standards, and an individual can be held accountable in a court of law for failure to comply; the standards set help define the roles of nursing professionals and are critical to moral decision making. Values underpin our decisions as nursing professionals and these values and behaviours are demonstrated in the 6Cs (caring, compassion, competence, communication, courage, commitment).

A variety of approaches in nursing underpin ethical decision making; these include the rules that we believe to be right, the consequences of our actions and the moral codes that we live by. The ethical principles of not harming, doing good, allowing choice and being fair also underpin nursing approaches.

Legal dilemmas exist in healthcare, and nursing professionals are responsible by law for their actions. In addition, people have the right to refuse treatment and to complain if treatment is poor or puts them at risk. To meet the rights of individuals in their care, nursing professionals are accountable for their actions when delivering care to patients, their families and carers, in a way that meets the requirements of their professional body and the law. To support this, UK and European law influences people's rights in healthcare situations. Furthermore, the duty of care that nursing professionals have extends to alerting others in positions of management to situations where they have concerns regarding colleagues or patient care being given.

A helpful resource for the nursing profession is The Code (NMC, 2018a), which highlights standards of conduct, performance and ethics for nurses and nursing associates.

Key Points

- Nursing practice is structured by ethical and professional standards, by which an individual can be held accountable in a court of law for failure to comply.
- The ethical and professional standards are essential to moral decision making and define the roles of nursing professionals.

- The NMC Code emphasises the standards of conduct, performance and ethics for nursing professionals.
- Values underpin our decisions and behaviours and are demonstrated in the 6Cs (caring, compassion, competence, communication, courage, commitment).
- A variety of approaches support ethical decision making; these include the rules that we believe to be right, the consequences of our actions and the moral codes that we live by.
- Ethical principles of beneficence, non-maleficence, justice and respect for autonomy are core in the nursing decision-making process.
- Legal dilemmas exist in nursing practice and nursing professionals are responsible and accountable by law for their actions.
- Patients/service users have the right to refuse treatment and to complain if treatment is poor or puts them at risk.
- Patients/service user are legally protected because of their rights and nursing professionals are obliged to follow not only UK law but also those principles imposed by the NMC.

References

Aristotle (2020) *Nicomachean Ethics* (trans. A. Beresford). Penguin Classics, London.

Beauchamp, T.L. & Childress, J.F. (2019) *Principles of Biomedical Ethics*, 9th edn. Oxford University Press, Oxford.

Department of Health (2009) *Reference Guide to Consent for Examination or Treatment*, 2nd edn. Department of Health, London.

Department of Health (2013) *Information: To Share or Not to Share? The Information Governance Review*. Department of Health, London.

Department of Health and Social Care (2021) *Policy Paper: Integration and Innovation: Working Together to Improve Health and Social Care for All*. www.gov.uk/government/publications/working-together-to-improve-health-and-social-care-for-all/integration-and-innovation-working-together-to-improve-health-and-social-care-for-all-html-version (accessed November 2021).

Dickenson, D., Huxtable, R. & Parker, M. (2010) *The Cambridge Medical Ethics Workbook*, 2nd edn. Cambridge University Press, Cambridge.

General Medical Council and Nursing and Midwifery Council (2015) *Openness and Honesty When Things Go Wrong: The Professional Duty of Candour*. www.nmc.org.uk/globalassets/sitedocuments/nmc-publications/openness-and-honesty-professional-duty-of-candour.pdf (accessed November 2021).

Health and Social Care Act 2012, c. 7. www.legislation.gov.uk/ukpga/2012/7/contents/enacted (accessed November 2021).

Herring, J. (2020) *Medical Law and Ethics*, 8th edn. Oxford University Press, Oxford.

Human Rights Act 1998, c. 42. www.legislation.gov.uk/ukpga/1998/42/contents (accessed November 2021).

Kohlberg, L. (1971) Stages of moral development as a basis for moral education. In: C.M. Beck, B.S. Crittenden & E.V. Sullivan (eds) *Moral Education: Interdisciplinary* Approaches, pp. 23–92. University of Toronto Press, Toronto.

Kohlberg, L. & R.H. Hersh (1977) Moral development: a review of the theory. *Theory into Practice*, 16(2), 53–59.

Mental Capacity Act 2005, c. 9. www.legislation.gov.uk/ukpga/2005/9/contents (accessed November 2021).

Mind (2021) *The Mind Guide to Advocacy*. Mind (National Association for Mental Health), London.

National Health Service (2020) *Key Legislation*. www.england.nhs.uk/about/equality/equality-hub/resources/legislation/ (accessed November 2021).

Nursing & Midwifery Council (2018a) *The Code: Professional Standards of Practice and Behaviour for Nurses, Midwives and Nursing Associates*. www.nmc.org.uk/standards/code/ (accessed November 2021).

Nursing & Midwifery Council (2018b) *Delegation and Accountability: Supplementary Information to the NMC Code*. www.nmc.org.uk/globalassets/sitedocuments/nmc-publications/delegation-and-accountability-supplementary-information-to-the-nmc-code.pdf (accessed November 2021).

Nursing & Midwifery Council (2018c) *Realising Professionalism: Standards for Education and Training. Part 2: Standards for Students' Supervision and Assessment*. www.nmc.org.uk/globalassets/sitedocuments/education-standards/student-supervision-assessment.pdf (accessed November 2021).

Nursing & Midwifery Council (2018d) *Future Nurse: Standards of Proficiency for Registered Nurses*. www.nmc.org.uk/globalassets/sitedocuments/standards-of-proficiency/nurses/future-nurse-proficiencies.pdf (accessed November 2021).

Nursing & Midwifery Council (2018e) *Standards of Proficiency for Nursing Associates*. www.nmc.org.uk/globalassets/sitedocuments/standards-of-proficiency/nursing-associates/nursing-associates-proficiency-standards.pdf (accessed November 2021).

Nursing & Midwifery Council (2019a) *Raising Concerns: Guidance for Nurses, Midwives and Nursing Associates*. www.nmc.org.uk/globalassets/blocks/media-block/raising-concerns-v2.pdf (accessed November 2021).

Nursing & Midwifery Council (2019b) *Our Legal Framework*. www.nmc.org.uk/about-us/governance/our-legal-framework/ (accessed November 2021).

Peate, I. (2012) *The Student's Guide to Becoming a Nurse*. Wiley Blackwell, Chichester.

Piaget, J. (1965) *The Moral Judgment of the Child*. Free Press, New York.

Plato (2007) *The Republic* (trans. D. Lee), 2nd edn. Penguin Classics, London.

Public Interest Disclosure Act 1998, c. 23. www.legislation.gov.uk/ukpga/1998/23/contents (accessed November 2021).

Public Services (Social Value) Act 2012, c. 3. www.legislation.gov.uk/ukpga/2012/3/enacted (accessed November 2021).

Royal College of Nursing (2013) *Engaging with the Principles of Nursing Practice: Guided Reflection for Nursing Students*. www.rcn.org.ukprofessional-development/publications/pub-004432 (accessed November 2021).

Royal College of Nursing (2017a) *Accountability and Delegation: A Guide for the Nursing Team*. www.rcn.org.uk/professional-development/publications/pub-006465 (accessed November 2021).

Royal College of Nursing (RCN) (2017b) *Helping Students Get the Best from Their Practice Placements: A Royal College of Nursing Toolkit*. www.richmondtraininghub.net/wp-content/uploads/2017/10/PUB-006035.pdf (accessed November 2021).

Royal College of Nursing (RCN) (2021) *Duty of Care*. www.rcn.org.uk/get-help/rcn-advice/duty-of-care (accessed November 2021).

Royal Pharmaceutical Society (RPS) (2018) *Professional Guidance on the Safe and Secure Handling of Medicines*. www.rpharms.com/recognition/setting-professional-standards/safe-and-secure-handling-of-medicines/professional-guidance-on-the-safe-and-secure-handling-of-medicines (accessed November 2021).

Royal Pharmaceutical Society and Royal College of Nursing (RPS/RCN) (2019) *Professional Guidance on the Administration of Medicines in Healthcare Settings*. www.rpharms.com/Portals/0/RPS%20document%20library/Open%20access/Professional%20standards/SSHM%20and%20Admin/Admin%20of%20Meds%20prof%20guidance.pdf?ver=2019-01-23-145026-567 (accessed November 2021).

Sándor, J. (2012) Bioethics and basic rights: persons, humans and boundaries of life. In: M. Rosenfeld & A. Sajó (eds) *The Oxford Handbook of Comparative Constitutional* Law, pp. 1142–1165. Oxford University Press, Oxford.

Seedhouse, D. (2014) An ethical perspective: how to do the right thing. In: J. Tingle & A. Cribb (eds) *Nursing Law and Ethics*, 4th edn, pp. 192–200. Wiley Blackwell, Oxford.

Thompson, I.E., Melia, K.M., Boyd, K.M. & Horsburgh, D. (2006) *Nursing Ethics*, 5th edn. Churchill Livingstone, Edinburgh.

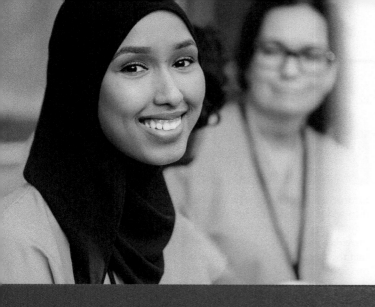

3

Health Promotion and Public Health

Lynette Harland Shotton

Northumbria University, UK

Learning Outcomes

On completion of this chapter you will be able to:

- Have insight into the historical development of public health and health promotion in the United Kingdom
- Understand and explore some of the key concepts in contemporary public health:
  - Health
  - The determinants of health
  - Inequalities in health
  - Health protection
  - Health promotion
  - Health improvement
  - Prevention
- Demonstrate knowledge of the professional and policy landscape in contemporary public health
- Consider the role of nurses and nurse associates in addressing and improving public health

Proficiencies

NMC Proficiencies and Standards:

- Registered nurses are actively involved in the prevention of and protection against disease and ill health and engage in public health, community development and global health agendas, and in the reduction of health inequalities.

 Visit the companion website at www.wiley.com/go/peate/nursingpractice3e where you can test yourself using flashcards, multiple-choice questions and more.

Nursing Practice: Knowledge and Care, Third Edition. Edited by Ian Peate and Aby Mitchell.
© 2022 John Wiley & Sons Ltd. Published 2022 by John Wiley & Sons Ltd.
Companion website: www.wiley.com/go/peate/nursingpractice3e

Introduction

The purpose of this chapter is to explore the complex nature of public health and apply this to contemporary nursing practice. Public health is defined by the World Health Organization (WHO, 2020) as: 'the art and science of preventing disease, prolonging life and promoting health through the organised efforts of society'.

The key features of contemporary public health practice will be explored in more detail throughout this chapter, focusing on how health and public health are conceptualised, as well as the nursing role in health protection, health improvement and the provision of high-quality care.

According to the RCN (2020), nurses play an essential role in identifying and minimising the impact of illness. Public health is considered everyone's responsibility and all nurses (and nursing associates in England) and midwives in the UK are responsible for promoting health and using their nursing skills to provide meaningful public health interventions across all health and social care settings, as part of the provision of person-centred, holistic nursing care.

Our professional responsibility is outlined clearly in The Code, which outlines the professional standards that nurses, midwives and nursing associates (in England) must uphold (NMC, 2018a) alongside specific guidance for nursing associates. It is vital that all nurses, nurse associates and midwives understand and embed public health principles and practice within their work in order to comply with NMC standards of proficiency.

Red Flag

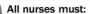

All nurses must:

2.1 work in partnership with people to make sure you deliver care effectively

3.1 pay special attention to promoting wellbeing, preventing ill-health, and meeting the changing health and care needs of people during all life stages

3.3 act in partnership with those receiving care, helping them to access relevant health and social care, information, and support when they need it

7.3 use a range of verbal and non-verbal communication methods, and consider cultural sensitivities, to better understand and respond to people's personal and health needs

5 Provide leadership to make sure people's wellbeing is protected and to improve their experiences of the health and care system

The Code (NMC, 2018a)

Red Flag

Nurse associates must:

2.1 understand and apply the aims and principles of health promotion, protection and improvement and the prevention of ill health when engaging with people

2.2 promote preventive health behaviours and provide information to support people to make informed choices to improve their mental, physical, behavioural health and wellbeing

2.4 understand the factors that may lead to inequalities in health outcomes

2.6 understand and explain the contribution of social influences, health literacy, individual circumstances, behaviours and lifestyle choices to mental, physical and behavioural health outcomes

Standards of Proficiency for Nursing Associates (NMC, 2018b)

The Code highlights specific areas relating to the nurses public health role, outlined below.

The Historical Development of Public Health in the UK

Efforts to improve public health in the UK are sometimes divided into waves of time and activity. Whilst this is an oversimplified way of considering the history of public health, it is also useful to provide a brief insight into this complex agenda. It must be noted that the waves of activity are not successive but overlap and build on each other, and are still important principles and practices in the contemporary field of public health (NHS Careers, 2021).

First wave

The first wave occurred in the nineteenth century and was driven by social changes linked to the Industrial Revolution, which started in the early 1700s. The Industrial Revolution dramatically changed the way people lived and worked and was characterised by mass migration of people from rural areas to take up work in towns and cities in factories, which produced goods that were transported and marketed across the world (Brain, 2021). As industrial Britain flourished in the 19th and 20th centuries, populations grew, and the health and welfare of the workforce deteriorated. Between 1801 and 1841, the population of London doubled. In the industrial north, with its trade in textiles, the population of the city of Leeds in Yorkshire tripled. With the increase in population numbers, combined with poor living conditions, disease and poor health became widespread. This led to greater awareness and emphasis on the need to tackle population health.

Much public health activity in the first wave was concerned with improving environmental conditions through the provisions of clean drinking water, disposal of sewage and improving working conditions (NHS Careers, 2021). There were also significant achievements in this period, including the work of John Snow.

During the nineteenth century, severe cholera epidemics posed a threat to the population of London. It was believed at the time that the spread of cholera was linked to 'bad air' and London fogs. However, Dr John Snow argued that cholera was actually a water-borne disease. In 1854 around 500 people died of cholera in the Soho area of London. To understand and explain the deaths further, Dr Snow plotted a map showing where those who were diagnosed with or died from cholera lived. In doing this, Snow identified that the water pump on Broad Street was a key link between the cases; most of the deaths occurred in those living in close proximity to the pump and frequently using it as their main source of water. Snow ordered the handle of the pump to be removed, after which there was a significant reduction in incidence, further supporting his theory. Snow is now considered to be the father of epidemiology, having shown the importance of using simple statistics and mapping to trace the distribution of cholera and causes of health-related events in the population of London (Stewart, 2017).

During this time, Florence Nightingale also championed the principles of public health to inform the practice of nursing when she published *Notes on Nursing*, which detailed her views on healthcare reform gained from her experience during the Crimean War (Nightingale, 1859).

Second wave

The second wave, dated to around 1890–1950, saw further interest and activity in public health and sanitary reform. There was an increasing body of evidence to support the idea that epidemic disease, spread through inadequate water and sanitary provision, coupled with poor housing, affected all layers of the social spectrum. As a result, state reform and intervention drove the development of public health policies. During this wave of activity, emphasis was placed on preventing and treating disease using vaccines and antibiotics (NHS Careers, 2021).

In Britain, community healthcare in the early part of the 20th century focused its attention on the welfare of mothers and children, and the health of school children. With this focus, public health nursing began to emerge. In 1909, a government examination of the Poor Law brought about the introduction of a unified state medical service. This important change in the way that medicine and healthcare were provided led to the development of the National Health Service Act of 1946.

Jot This Down

Imagine working as a nurse during the development of the NHS in 1946. What kind of public health problems do you think you might have been involved in supporting?

In this exercise, you may have thought about some of the serious communicable diseases around at the time, including common infections such as diphtheria, polio and measles. Now, owing to the development of vaccination, these infections, once life-threatening to the postwar population, are rare and treatable. However, we can still see pockets of the population not heeding campaigns to prevent outbreaks of infections and vaccine hesitancy is considered a key threat to global health. A prime example of this hesitancy is the outbreak of measles across England in 2018, where 913 laboratory-confirmed cases of measles were recorded (Public Health England (PHE), 2018). Whilst the reasons behind this are multifaceted and include the spread of transmission from Europe, there is also a legacy of poor uptake, related to unfounded claims in 1997 that there was a link between the measles, mumps and rubella vaccine (MMR) and autism and Crohn's disease (PHE, 2014). Whilst the possible links between MMR and autism and Crohn's disease were both investigated and refuted by Public Health England, the legacy of the scare and the ensuing media coverage meant that vaccination coverage fell to an all-time low in 1997. Uptake levels declined from around 92% in 1995, before the adverse publicity, to around 80% in 2003 and 2004 (PHE, 2014). Arguably, the effects of this are still being felt today, with explanations for the recent outbreaks being partially attributed to teenagers and young adults who were not vaccinated when they were young (PHE, 2018).

Red Flag

Vaccines save lives
Central to the success of both historicak and contemporary vaccination programmes is patient confidence. Healthcare professionals remain the most trusted source of vaccination information and this is a central feature of our public health role.

Vaccinations continue to feature heavily in UK public health policy and current information detailing the current routine immunisation schedule across the lifespan is provided by Public Health England (2020). Vaccinations are considered one of the most important things we can do to protect ourselves against ill health and are thought to prevent up to 3 million deaths globally every year. However, some people, for example those without a fully working immune system, those on chemotherapy, people who are either too young or very elderly, may not be able to be vaccinated. In these cases, it is vital that those who can be are vaccinated as this produces herd or population immunity, protecting the individual as well as reducing transmission of disease in the population. Herd or population immunity requires a certain percentage of the population to be vaccinated. The challenge is that those who do not get vaccinated tend to cluster together in communities. So, if a disease outbreak does occur, it is more likely to spread within these communities, Equally, herd immunity does not work for all diseases and so vaccination remains essential (Oxford Vaccine Group, 2020).

Third wave

This phase dated roughly from 1940 to 1980 and saw significant improvements in our understanding of the link between lifestyle and disease. For example, the links between smoking, hypertension and hyperlipidaemia were recognised as risk factors for coronary heart disease (NHS Careers, 2021). This generated focused activities to target those considered to be at risk with information in the form of health education to promote lifestyle changes.

Fourth wave

This period overlaps with the third wave, occurring from the 1960s. Here there was a shift from purely providing information and health education to also working on the social and economic determinants of health.

What the Experts Say

Professor Viv Bennett (2019) (Public Health England's Chief Nurse) says in her blog:
'Each year in England, millions of doses of vaccines are administered to eligible groups as part of national immunisation programmes. This would not be possible without the commitment and clinical skills of practice nurses, school immunisation nurses, midwives, health visitors and others. Using evidence of vaccine safety and efficacy, these health professionals are at the forefront of vaccine administration and advocacy, their contribution to population health should not be underestimated'.

The first comprehensive public health strategy in the UK was published in 1992 by the then Conservative government. *The Health of the Nation* (Department of Health, 1992) highlighted the major health concerns of the time, including cancers, accidents, smoking, heart disease and sexual health. Subsequent strategies of the Labour government included *Saving Lives, Our Healthier Nation* (Department of Health, 1999) and *Choosing Health: Making Healthier Choices Easier* (Department of Health, 2004). These strategies proposed targets for reducing the incidence of morbidity and mortality, and specifically used health promotion to facilitate health improvement and enable individuals to make healthy choices. These targets also addressed the wider issues of inequalities in health and environmental issues.

The following Conservative government in 2010 emphasised health improvement and prevention of ill health, with the need for individuals to make healthy choices and take more responsibility for their own health. *Healthy Lives, Healthy People: Our Strategy for Public Health in England* (Department of Health, 2010) moved away from the notion of the so-called 'nanny state' where people expect the state to take care of their health with the overall aim of:

'helping people live longer, healthier and more fulfilling lives; and improving the health of the poorest, fastest . . . tackling the wider social determinants of health. This new approach will aim to build people's self-esteem, confidence and resilience right from infancy'. (Department of Health, 2010b, p.4)

Alongside this, the Marmot review, *Fair Society, Healthy Lives*, re-emphasised the need to address enduring inequalities in health and well-being across the UK (Marmot, 2010), focusing on a range of measures, including the following six priorities:

1. giving every child the best start in life
2. enabling all children, young people and adults to maximise their capabilities and have control over their lives
3. creating fair employment and good work for all
4. ensuring a healthy standard of living for all
5. creating and developing sustainable places and communities
6. strengthening the role and impact of ill health prevention.

This phase of activity underlines the need for shared responsibility for healthier behaviours, where individuals are encouraged to value their health, but are also helped to make healthy choices more easily through public policy.

Contemporary Public Health: The Fifth Wave?

Contemporary public health continues to build on the historical approaches outlined previously. The discipline draws heavily on medical science and research evidence with a particular focus on providing the right circumstances for health. Public health is therefore concerned with a range of activities, which include provision of better housing and living conditions, alongside better access to healthcare and vaccination to protect against infectious illness, thereby promoting conditions under which people can maintain and improve their health and well-being, as well as prevent deterioration of health (WHO, 2020). Public health includes supporting individuals but extends beyond this to also support organisations, communities and wider society to identify and address preventable disease, mortality and disability. Public health has a broad remit and relies on the co-operation and collaboration of individuals, populations and organisations across society.

Contemporary public health practice in the UK is initiated at governmental level, as well as being influenced by the devolved governments in Scotland, Wales and Northern Ireland. Key agencies involved in this agenda place different emphases on the foci of activity. According to the Faculty of Public Health (2021), there are three essential domains of contemporary public health activity.

- *Health protection*: here, the focus is on surveillance and monitoring of infectious disease, emergency response and immunisation.
- *Health improvement/promotion*: here, the focus is on health education and commissioning services to meet specific health needs.
- *Health services*: here, the focus is on prioritisation and commissioning of health and social care services, as well as ensuring equity and quality of provision.

Across the four nations of the UK, the key domains of health protection and health improvement are emphasised, but also recognised is the need to improve the wider determinants of health and to implement preventive measures to reduce the incidence of ill health and support healthier lifestyles in order to reduce premature mortality (PHE, 2019; Institute of Public Health in Ireland (IPHI), 2021; Public Health Scotland (PHS), 2021; Public Health Wales (PHW), 2021). Public health intelligence, research and teaching and developing the public health workforce are central to these areas and provide the cornerstones of effective action to protect and improve health and well-being (PHS, 2021). These key areas will be considered in more detail later in this chapter.

The Role of Government

The global Covid-19 pandemic has promoted increased recognition of the need for the UK government to review and strengthen the public health system. Indeed, in March 2021 the policy paper 'Transforming the public health system: reforming the public health system for the challenges of our times' (Department of Health and Social Care (DHSC), 2021) outlined the plan to emphasise two key functions across the UK.

- Health security
- Health improvement

This policy created the UK Health Security Agency (UKHSA), whose key focus is on protecting against infectious diseases and external health threats, underpinned by use of data, digital technology and genomic surveillance. These will form part of our national defences and whilst the government recognises that this agency has emerged during a time of global crisis, the aim is for the agency to maintain vigilance and protect against future threats.

Health improvement is equally important, and this is emphasised in the newly established Office for Health Promotion within the Department of Health and Social Care. This office will focus on embedding promotion of good health across the work of the whole government and the NHS. The role of government in supporting and addressing public health will be considered in more detail throughout the chapter.

What is Health?

In any discussion around public health, there is a need to establish what we mean by the term 'health'.

Jot This Down

- Take some time to think about what health means to you.
- Now think about an older, more dependent person who you know and consider what health might mean to them.
- Are there differences in the types of perception that you have for the two exercises?

Lay Perceptions of Health

Health is a subjective concept, and you will find from completing the 'Jot This Down' exercise that health can be seen in the light of one's experiences, self-esteem, social status and level of individual control. An older, more dependent individual may view health differently from a younger independent individual, based on, for example, their level of physical need. Very often, lay concepts of health are associated with the absence of symptoms, feeling physically fit and well, having good relationships and being able to carry out one's usual tasks and activities (Naidoo and Wills, 2016). According to Evans *et al.* (2017), these are some lay perceptions of health.

- In terms of not being ill
- In the context of fitness
- In terms of control and risk
- In terms of not having a health problem which interferes with daily life
- In the context of social relationships
- As a psychosocial well-being

In this sense, there may be great diversity in the way that individuals view their health. Lay perceptions of health may be viewed differently by individuals of different social classes. Evans *et al.* (2017) indicate that working-class people may see health as being able to function physically whilst those from higher socioeconomic groups might focus more on psychosocial aspects of health. Health is also influenced by gender and age. It is important for healthcare professionals to consider personal views of health in order to understand what is important to the individual, and to identify whether there are any tensions between the lay perspective and the professional view of health.

Professional Concepts of Health

The Medical Model

It is important to note that health professionals may view health differently from their patients or service users. It is widely accepted that in modern Western societies, a narrow view of health often prevails, often referred to as the medical or scientific model of health. This view of health is characterised as:

- Biomedical – health is assumed to be a property of biological things
- Reductionist – health and disease are reduced to smaller and smaller constitutive components of the biological body
- Mechanistic – the body is a machine, in which all parts are interconnected but capable of being separated and treated separately
- Allopathic – if something is wrong with the body, treatment consists of applying opposite forces to correct this, i.e. using medicines
- Pathogenic – this focuses on why people become ill
- Dualistic – the mind and body can be treated as separate entities.

This model arose in the Enlightenment period which was characterised by a dramatic shift away from reliance on religion as the dominant means of understanding. During this time, there was an increase in scientific knowledge, equipment and treatments for diagnosed ailments, including antibiotics and immunisations. The pathogenic focus of the medical model led to an emphasis on risk factors to health, but also the notion that the more disease a person has, the further away he or she is from health (Naidoo and Wills, 2016).

As the medical model became more embedded, there was increased acceptance of professional definitions of health, whereby illness was professionally diagnosed and therefore sanctioned. This led to criticism that medicine is a form of social control, whereby medical professionals have power to categorise people as healthy or sick, mad or deviant, but equally have control in decisions about the beginning and end of life, which extends the power of medicine beyond its legitimate area of operation. Medicine also produces tensions in terms of conditions that have taken a long time to be recognised, chronic fatigue syndrome for example, but also diagnoses that may be identified through screening, when the individual feels healthy. Illich (1975) highlights the clinical, social and cultural harm (iatrogenesis) of medicine in relation to side-effects of medicines and dependency on them, as well as erosion of the ability to cope with pain and suffering or to self-care produced by reliance on and unrealistic expectations generated by medicine.

It has also been argued that modern medicine is not as effective as is often claimed and that many of the fatal diseases of the nineteenth century had actually disappeared before the arrival of antibiotics or immunisation programmes. Indeed, seminal work by McKeown (1976) claims that many advances in health are a direct result of improved sanitation, nutrition and general living conditions and not medicine. Whilst McKeown's work is contested, there is a growing recognition that the contribution of medicine is minor, when compared to the impact of improved environmental conditions. In recent years, our ability to deal with the global Covid-19 pandemic has been a key example of combining significant social changes to control the environment with medical advances in producing a vaccination capable of protecting individuals and societies against infectious disease.

The Holistic Model

One of the most prominent and widely cited definitions is that of the World Health Organization (1948) in which health is defined as 'a state of complete physical, mental and social wellbeing and not merely the absence of disease or infirmity'. Later, the WHO sponsored work published as the Ottawa Charter for Health Promotion (WHO, 1986), where this definition was revisited. Here, health was seen as a resource for everyday life, and not purely the objective of living. In this definition, health is considered to be a positive concept where social and personal resources, as well as physical capabilities, are valued and emphasised.

The holistic model expands on the medical model of health by embracing the combination of physical, emotional, mental and social aspects of health and moves away from viewing health as simply the absence or presence of disease. However, holistic definitions have been criticised for conflating happiness with health and for failing to recognise that some of the dimensions of health may be in tension with each other. Equally, the aspirational nature of the definitions fails to acknowledge that absolute health is, for many, unattainable and few of us will have complete physical, mental and social well-being all the time. Therefore, the concept has been developed further to temper the absolute and aspirational definitions of health and instead to consider health as the extent to which an individual is able to realise aspirations, as well as to cope with interpersonal, social, biological and physical environments.

Equally, many of us suffer from temporary episodes of ill health and a growing number of people live with chronic health conditions and disabilities. In this sense, health is not static and changes not only throughout the day, for example we may feel differently at different times of the day, but also over time (Evans *et al.*, 2017). Health and poor health do not occur as a dichotomy, but more as a continuum (McCartney *et al.*, 2019). Huber *et al.* (2011) suggest we should consider health as the ability to adapt and to self-manage and that this is dependent on the individual's view of health and their health needs, as well as their personal situation. Therefore, health is subjective and contextually defined by societal norms and so our definitions of health evolve over time.

The Wellness Model

Some suggest that whilst physical health is not always attainable for everyone at all times, everyone can enjoy wellness, even in the presence of physical disease, impairments or disability (Pellegrino *et al.*, 2012). The wellness model of health builds on the holistic model and is seen as a positive approach to conceptualising health that emphasises the need to improve quality of life for all people regardless of their health status. This therefore includes those who are healthy as well as those with diagnosed physical and mental health conditions and those with disabilities. This model highlights the need to foster resilience and adaptation to life changes that influence health and well-being. As healthcare professionals, our role is, therefore, to be an enabler, and to support quality of life by helping individuals self-manage their health/illnesses, develop problem-solving skills and increase their self-esteem (Evans *et al.*, 2017).

Wellness is multifaceted and involves a number of interrelated dimensions, often referred to as the dimensions of wellness. In the literature, six or seven dimensions are identified. However, the eight important dimensions of wellness below are adapted from Naidoo and Wills (2016) and Evans *et al.* (2017).

- *Physical*: how your body functions; this can often be in terms of measuring physical parameters, e.g. blood pressure monitoring, body mass index (BMI) measurement, developmental assessment of motor development in children. Optimal physical wellness requires eating well, exercising and avoiding lifestyle behaviours that are harmful to health, such as smoking.
- *Emotional*: recognition and appropriate expression of feelings, plus the ability to cope with stress. Optimum emotional well-being is enhanced by monitoring our thoughts and feelings, identifying obstacles to emotional well-being and finding solutions to them. Optimism, trust, self-esteem, satisfying relationships and ability to share our feelings are some of the qualities associated with emotional well-being.
- *Intellectual*: clear and coherent thinking; here cognitive abilities can be measured, for example in children's developmental assessment, and in the elderly who may be suffering dementia. Intellectual wellness can be supported by maintaining an active mind, engaging in creative activities and those that stimulate critical thinking.
- *Social*: the ability to make and maintain relationships with others, feeling included and valued in society. Satisfying relationships are an intrinsic feature of physical and emotional health and social wellness relies on our ability to participate in and contribute to our community and world.

- *Occupational*: occupational wellness is characterised by being able to exert some control over our working lives, being challenged and supported to learn new skills, to develop and be recognised for occupational achievements.
- *Spiritual*: being at peace with oneself through a system of beliefs. Spiritual wellness involves the capacity for love, compassion, forgiveness, joy and fulfillment. Those who enjoy spiritual wellness possess a set of guiding beliefs, principles and values that give meaning and purpose to their lives. This does include but is not exclusively associated with religion.
- *Environmental*: this dimension is increasingly important when we consider the impact of our environment on individual and population health. Here, the individual acknowledges their role in conserving natural resources, being mindful of consumption, as well as appreciating the impact of the environment on health and well-being. This aspect of health is also about the physical environment in which people live and the importance of good housing, transport and sanitation.
- *Sexual*: this dimension focuses on the ability and freedom to establish intimate, loving relationships, as well as choice and availability of procreation.

Determinants of Health

The link between social factors and health has gained increasing recognition in the last few decades and social models of health emphasise the biological as well as the social, political and environmental factors that influence health. Social models encourage us to have a deeper understanding of health that moves away from the focus on biology, physiology and anatomy. There is also emphasis on addressing structural features of society, including the distribution of wealth, income, housing and employment, with growing recognition that the more equal a society is, the better the health status of its citizens (Naidoo and Wills, 2016).

The wider determinants of health include the genes we inherit, the conditions in which we live, the choices we make and the services we are able to access to support health. Ill health is not randomly distributed, nor is it inevitable. Our ability to avoid, manage and survive disease is influenced by lifestyle behaviours, the job we do, the air we breathe and the neighbourhoods we live in. We can act, as individuals and collectively, in ways that will help us live longer lives in good physical and mental health (DHSC, 2021). At an individual level, we all want longer, healthier and more independent lives for ourselves and our families and it is increasingly recognised that positive physical and mental health allows us to participate more fully in society. Equally, at a wider social level, good health is vital to the economy, not only boosting income and productivity but also reducing pressures on the NHS, social care and other public services (DHSC, 2021). Therefore, it is increasingly emphasised that there is both a personal and a wider societal/governmental responsibility for health.

According to the King's Fund (2021), the broader determinants of health are influenced by a complex interaction between individual characteristics, lifestyle factors and social and economic environmental factors. The King's Fund (2021) outlines the following key messages.

- *Health is determined by a complex interaction between individual characteristics, lifestyle and the physical, social and economic environment. Most experts agree that these 'broader determinants* of health' are more important than healthcare in ensuring a healthy population.

- *Economic hardship is highly correlated with poor health.* The current economic downturn – the deepest since the Great Depression – threatens individual and family well-being, especially for the unemployed and those experiencing wage and benefit cuts.
- *Increased levels of education are strongly and significantly related to improved health.* Recent rises in the overall number of people in higher education and more people from poorer background in higher education should have long-term benefits for population health. However, there is uncertainty about whether improvements in access will continue.
- *Work-related illness is decreasing, particularly among people with manual occupations.* Employers are also showing a growing interest in the health of their workforce. While these trends may continue, the economic environment could exacerbate work-related stress and have a negative impact.
- *Improved housing conditions and greater access to green spaces should have a positive impact on health.* However, the future outlook is uncertain for the most disadvantaged.
- *Climate change is predicted to have both positive and negative implications for health in England.*

Importantly, the King's Fund (2021) also recognises that there are key social uncertainties that will fundamentally determine the health of individuals and our population in the future.

- *Wider economy.* It is difficult to predict how the UK and global economy will develop in the next 20 years, and the overall effect on employment and income.
- *Work environment.* Pay and working conditions could deteriorate markedly during the economic downturn. However, some large employers are recognising the benefits of investing in their staff's welfare and could act positively to improve their employees' health.
- *Education.* Recent increases in the number of people going to university may stall over time. Following the introduction of higher tuition fees, applications for English universities in 2021 are down 10%.
- *Environmental change.* Carbon reduction targets are likely to drive technological and social change, with significant health implications. There is, however, considerable uncertainty around the scale and timing of these effects.

Factors that affect health can be broadly divided into two areas.

- Intrinsic or non-modifiable factors.
- Extrinsic or modifiable factors.

Jot This Down

Think of two individuals whom you have cared for recently in the clinical setting. Jot down a list of intrinsic (non-modifiable) and extrinsic (modifiable) factors that you think have influenced their health status.

You may have considered how each person's genetic make-up influences health status throughout life. Genetic make-up affects personality, temperament, body structure, intellectual potential and susceptibility to the development of hereditary alterations in

health and, in the main, these kinds of intrinsic influences are non-modifiable. Examples of chronic illnesses associated with genetic make-up include sickle cell disease, haemophilia, diabetes mellitus and cancer. Other intrinsic factors might include age, gender and developmental factors. Cardiovascular disorders are relatively uncommon in young adults, but the incidence increases after the age of 40. Myocardial infarctions (MIs) are more common in men than women until women are past the menopause. Some diseases occur only in one gender or the other (e.g., prostate cancer in men and cervical cancer in women). The older adult often has an increased incidence of chronic illness and increased potential for serious illness or death from infectious illnesses, such as influenza and pneumonia.

Health Inequalities

The concept of health inequality is not new and has been considered in features of the public health movement, outlined at the beginning of this chapter. However, by the early 1970s in academic and health policy circles, there was renewed emphasis on addressing the differences in health status across the UK. A key publication by Hart (1971) referred to the inverse care law, whereby those who were the worst off or poorest in society faced disproportionate barriers to the NHS. This generated a range of political discussions that led to an independent inquiry into inequalities in health chaired by Sir Douglas Black and initiated by the Labour government at the time. The Black Report (1980) was eventually released under Margaret Thatcher's Conservative government.

The key findings of the report were that the poorer health experience of lower occupational groups was apparent at all stages of life and that the gap between the lower and higher occupational groups was widening. The report made a number of recommendations including improving the material circumstances of the poorest members of society, as well as addressing lifestyle behaviours that impact on health by improving access to preventive services and primary care. Whilst the report is now considered pivotal in the historic development of policy to address health inequality, it was not well publicised by the government, with only 260 copies produced and its recommendations being largely ignored.

The Acheson Report of 1998 echoed many of the issues raised in the Black Report and noted that whilst as a population, there had been significant improvements in health, these were not equally distributed. Thirty years on from the Black Report, it was evident that despite a number of policy reports, inequalities persisted. The Marmot Report (2010) noted the social gradient in health, whereby health improves as social status goes up. Whilst there was continued recognition of the link between poverty and health, Marmot (2010) suggested that a wider effort was needed to create healthy and sustainable communities and address climate change, but also that policy should be influenced by proportionate universalism where the steepness of the gradient in health requires concentrated action according to deprivation.

There are four major models used to explain social class inequalities in health (Bartley and Blane, 2008).

- *Behavioural model*: differences in the prevalence of health damaging behaviours/health enhancing behaviours among different social and cultural groups are the fundamental cause of health inequality. This model has been contested and the differences in health behaviour are thought to only explain one-third of social class differences in mortality.

- *Materialist model*: material conditions have a direct impact on health inequalities. This includes absolute and relative poverty, how wealth is distributed across societies and the gap between those with the most and those with the least, as well as factors relating to social and economic position, including good-quality, affordable housing and secure employment. While most experts in public health agree that materialist explanations play a role in explaining health inequalities, many find a simple materialist model to be insufficient. In the UK, relatively disadvantaged people receive various kinds of state help (rent, school meals, etc.) which, some argue, makes diet or poor housing unlikely to account for all inequalities in health outcomes. Furthermore, in the UK and internationally, inequalities in health tend to follow a steady gradient, rather than there being poor outcomes for the most disadvantaged and equally good outcomes for the rest of society.

- *Psychosocial model*: this suggests that exposure to poor social conditions produces a physiological stress response, which predisposes the individual to physical health conditions, such as heart disease. Psychosocial risk factors include social support, control and autonomy at work, the balance between home and work, and the balance between efforts and rewards. Evidence shows that people who have good relationships with family and friends, and who participate in their community, have longer life expectancies than those who are relatively isolated.

- *Life-course model*: the life-course approach to studying health inequality suggests that the biological and social beginnings of life produce important implications for adult health potential. This begins from preconception and it is thought that disadvantage accumulates across the life-course. The life-course approach was emphasised by the Marmot Review (2010) where action to reduce inequality before birth and throughout childhood is considered the best way to break the links between early life disadvantage and poor outcomes in adulthood. Similarly, the Welsh Adverse Childhood Experiences (ACE) Study (Bellis *et al.*, 2015) highlights the impact of adverse childhood experiences on individuals' risks of developing health-harming behaviours in adult life. ACEs are stressful experiences occurring during childhood that directly harm a child (e.g. sexual or physical abuse) or affect the environment in which they live (e.g. growing up in a house with domestic violence).

Despite policy recognition, it is concerning that the health gap is widening and according to Marmot (2020), increases in life expectancy have slowed since 2010 and there has been a significant increase in the percentage of life spent in ill health. Marmot (2020) reinforces the following key areas to address health inequality.

- *Give every child the best start in life* – early childhood is a critical time for development of later life outcomes. The recommendation is to increase spending on early years provision, reduce child poverty, improve access to early years services and improve pay and qualifications of the childcare workforce.

- *Enable all children, young people and adults to maximise their capabilities to have control over their lives* – here, the emphasis is on ensuring equitable access to education and training and increasing funding.

- *Create fair employment and good work for all* – this requires investment in labour market policies, addressing in-work poverty, increasing apprenticeships and in-work training, as well as reducing poor-quality work and precarious employment. There is also a need to support healthy living through increases to the National Living Wage and redesign of Universal Credit and the taxation system.

- *Create and develop healthy and sustainable places and communities* – through investment in economic, social and cultural resources in the most deprived communities, aim for zero carbon emissions by 2030 and invest in good-quality, affordable housing and transport.

The aim of all governmental policies should be to level up, for everyone to enjoy the good health and well-being of those at the top of the social hierarchy.

Health Protection, Health Improvement/Promotion and Prevention

The remainder of this chapter will focus on the transformation of public health in the UK and consider the three key areas of health protection, health improvement/promotion and prevention, and how health services, including nurses and nurse associates, contribute to this agenda.

Health Protection

Health protection is a central feature of public health activity. As with many public health concepts, the term is used in different ways. In health promotion literature, it often refers to wider social measures designed to protect population health. For example, Tannahill (2009) considers health protection to involve legislation, policy and fiscal measures to promote health and well-being. The first Public Health Act of 1842 brought about measures to improve living conditions of the poorest, including sanitation and housing. Since then, a raft of legislation and policies has been introduced focused on transforming healthcare provision, working and living conditions and in the late twentieth century measures focused on addressing lifestyle risks to health. The greatest achievements in the twenty-first century so far are listed below.

- The smoking ban
- The soft drinks industry levy ('sugar levy')
- Marmot review into health inequalities and understanding of the social determinants of health
- Sure Start children's centres (2000–2010)
- Minimum Unit Pricing on alcohol in Scotland
- HPV vaccination for boys and girls
- Congestion charge and ultra-low emission zone
- Decriminalisation of abortion in Northern Ireland
- Wellbeing of Future Generations Act in Wales
- Tobacco advertising bans
- Traffic light labelling on prepackaged food
- Transferral of public health into local authorities
- Scores on the Doors food hygiene ratings
- The Time to Change Campaign, run by Mind and Rethink Mental Illness
- Fixed-odds betting terminals stake limit reduced to £2

- Introduction of childhood flu vaccine
- Reduction in homelessness between 2003 and 2009
- Junk food advertising ban during kids' TV and across London transport network
- Drug safety testing at festivals and nightclubs
- Cancer screening improvements (Royal Society for Public Health, 2019)

As part of the UK government's transformation of public health, the National Institute for Health Protection was operationalised in the UK in 2021, taking over from Public Health England. The agency was introduced in response to the global Covid-19 pandemic and brings together existing public health responsibilities alongside NHS Test and Trace (to identify and trace the contacts of those diagnosed with Covid-19) and the Joint Biosecurity Centre. The primary focus is to ensure as a population that we have the best capability to control infectious disease and to deal with pandemics or health protection crises using research evidence, surveillance and epidemiology. The UK Health Security Agency will co-ordinate across the UK, building strong collaborations with public health agencies for Scotland, Wales and Northern Ireland, and will operate internationally for the UK to help understand, prevent and respond to global threats to health, as well as to provide guidance about managing communicable diseases, heatwave and cold weather plans, unusual illnesses and any other significant risks to public health.

Health protection teams across the UK are made up of nurses, practitioners, doctors, surveillance, epidemiologists and administrative staff who work closely across primary and secondary care, as well as local authorities. Every team has an on-call service which provides support to healthcare professionals and members of the public and responds to any urgent health protection needs. Some of the key areas of expertise include immunisation, gastrointestinal infections, water-borne diseases, environmental hazards, travel-associated infections, infection control/hospital-acquired infections and respiratory infections, including tuberculosis (RCN, 2021). All healthcare professionals have a duty to support health protection activities and as nurses and nurse associates, our work with patients means we may be the first to identify potential health protection threats. This is highlighted in the following case study which draws on information from the RCN (2021).

Case Study

Why notify a case of measles?

Measles is a highly infectious vaccine preventable infection. One in 10 children who catch measles need hospital care and the disease can result in serious complications including pneumonia and encephalitis. Measles is a notifiable disease and medical professionals have a statutory duty to report cases/suspected cases to the designated officer at their local council or local health protection team.

It is vital that cases are reported to the health protection team (HPT) as soon as they are suspected. The HPT can:

1. Attempt to prevent future cases by advising unvaccinated/partially vaccinated contacts to receive the vaccine
2. Advise other vulnerable contacts of the case and assess whether there is a need for intervention (this may include antibody testing or administration of human immunoglobulin to provide protective antibodies)
3. Advise contacts more widely to try to prevent tertiary cases. This may include sending letters to potential contacts alerting them to confirm their MMR status with a healthcare provider and if necessary be advised to seek an MMR vaccination as soon as possible
4. Early vaccination can assist the HPT to take public health action to prevent further cases.

Epidemiology and Health Protection

Epidemiology is the study of how diseases are dispersed between groups of populations and the factors that influence this distribution. As such, the rate of disease, its timing and place, and the people who are affected can suggest a pattern to epidemiologists, who will be involved in predicting the development of disease amongst the wider population.

Jot This Down

Think about the factors that an epidemiologist might consider when an outbreak of influenza spreads within a community.

In this exercise, you will have probably thought about the key risk factors (or conditions) that might lead to an outbreak of influenza, and in particular those for whom the infection will be most risky. Epidemiologists will want to establish such things as:

- Does the outbreak coincide with climate conditions/seasonal changes?
- Are there certain geographical patterns?
- Which age groups are most commonly affected?
- Do lifestyle and habit affect the vulnerability to contracting the illness?
- What preventive strategies might there be available?

These considerations were pivotal in dealing with the recent Covid-19 pandemic, where epidemiologists and scientists across the world worked to identify the source of the outbreak, monitor and track the disease using a range of surveillance systems to understand new cases, hospitalisations, deaths, demographic information such as age, race/ethnicity or sex and also symptoms and treatments. The disease was also studied to find out more about how long someone with Covid-19 is contagious, risk factors for severe illness and which medical treatments are most effective. This information was used to develop advice to slow the spread of the disease and lessen its impact.

Epidemiologists are interested in the health experiences of groups, as opposed to the health of individuals. The nature and cause of disease (the aetiology) is the focus of attention, alongside the study and distribution of disease. Data derived from population studies, the incidence of birth and death, lifestyles, and the health behaviours of populations, alongside the sociological determinants of health, all contribute to the study of epidemiology.

Epidemiologists categorise information in relation to patterns of health and disease in two ways.

- **Descriptive** epidemiology, which describes the patterns of distribution of health and disease, as well as the determinants of disease.

- **Analytical** epidemiology, which explores the 'cause-and-effect' relationship between determinants and health/disease (often multiple causes and multiple effects).

The public health system in the UK is geared towards this type of disease surveillance. Doctors in both the community and hospital setting are responsible for notifying the occurrence of the most communicable diseases. Directors of public health collate the evidence to support the planning of health services in response to trends.

Health Improvement/Promotion and Prevention

Health promotion is about improving the health status of individuals and the population generally and is an integral feature of public health practice. The discussion presented in the early part of this chapter is essential in informing our health promotion role, where practice is underpinned by knowledge of concepts of health and understanding the complex nature of the determinants of health.

The health promotion agenda gained momentum in the latter part of the twentieth century as a process to shift healthcare provision away from hospital settings. Early efforts were orientated towards disease and infection prevention, focusing on providing expert-led advice and government direction to educate individuals and direct their behaviour. The Ottawa Charter (WHO, 1986) was pivotal in driving forward the health promotion agenda and producing some of the principles of health promotion that are relevant today, which include building healthy public policy, creating supportive environments, strengthening community action, developing personal skills and reorienting health services to focus more on prevention of illness and promotion of wellness (covered in the first part of the chapter). The current emphasis is influenced by 'bottom-up' approaches where individuals and communities are involved in decision making and planning processes around health. This is underpinned by recognition that health behaviours are influenced by a complex range of factors (the determinants of health) and rejection of the victim-blaming approach of early health promotion efforts, that blamed individuals for failing to conform to health education messages. This approach accepts that individuals have varying levels of control over their health and that whilst individual approaches to health improvement are important, there also needs to be wider societal change across all determinants of health to make healthy behaviours more accessible for all.

The Covid-19 pandemic has underlined significant inequalities in health across the UK and as part of the UK government's commitment to address these, a new Office for Health Promotion has been established within the Department of Health and Social Care, operationalised in the autumn of 2021. The office will be a dynamic, multidisciplinary unit that oversees policy development, expert advice and implementation on prevention of ill health across national and local government, the NHS and wider health system (DHSC, 2021). The office will track the wider determinants of health and implement policies and strategies to address these, tackling important public health issues including obesity and nutrition, mental health across all ages, physical activity, sexual health, alcohol and tobacco, as well as a range of other important current and emerging public health issues. The aim is to improve the health of the population.

The terms 'health promotion' and 'health improvement' are sometimes used interchangeably. The King's Fund (2019) suggests that health improvement focuses on a population approach to promoting public health and involves addressing four key pillars: the wider determinants of health, the places and communities we live in and with, developing an integrated health and care system, and focusing on our health behaviours and lifestyles. Central to this, the government has outlined national strategies including 'Prevention is better than cure' (DHSC, 2018) and the 'Long-term plan for the NHS' (NHS, 2019) where the focus is on expanding community services and integrated working across health and social care. This will be managed by Integrated Care Systems, which will bring together a range of health, social care and community agencies to address health need at local level. There is also emphasis on prevention of illness and working with individuals and communities to address the most significant causes of ill health.

Prevention

Prevention is about helping people stay healthy, happy and independent for as long as possible. It focuses on stopping problems from arising in the first place. At an individual level, the everyday decisions we make can help us to improve our physical health as outlined in the key prevention messages published by the DHSC (2018).

- Don't smoke.
- Limit sugar and salt intake.
- Eat five portions of fruit and vegetables each day.
- Eat plenty of high-fibre foods.
- Get regular exercise.
- Limit alcohol intake.

Prevention can be primary, secondary or tertiary.

- *Primary prevention* – universal measures are taken that reduce lifestyle risks and their causes or by targeting high-risk groups. An example of this is the influenza vaccine for older people or those who are vulnerable. Primary prevention involves educating people about health risks as well as producing legislation to protect health.

Nursing Fields Child: Nursing Practice and Decision Making, Communication and Interpersonal Skills

Primary prevention: immunisation session in a secondary school for girls and boys aged 12–13 against the human papilloma virus (HPV)

The school health advisor (school nurse) sees each pupil individually and there is an opportunity to give opportunistic health information; she connects with the pupils at their level, explaining the terminology and using a range of written and visual materials to explain why the vaccine is given and how it protects against HPV-related cancers.

The health promotion role of the nurse here includes:

- Primary prevention in the form of the provision of immunisation
- The opportunity to discuss health issues, such as healthy eating
- Acting as a source of information
- Listening and talking (generally finding out how well the pupils are)
- Picking up on cues related to ill health or risky health behaviour.

- *Secondary prevention* – where emphasis is on detecting health or care needs early and managing them effectively. This can be through screening programmes, such as cancer screening. Cancer is the leading cause of avoidable death, but if detected in the early stages when a tumour is small, survival rates are significantly higher (DHSC, 2018). Screening is the process of identifying individuals who may have an increased chance of a disease or condition in those who are apparently healthy and often symptom free. Screening does not guarantee protection and in any screening programme there are false positives, where individuals are wrongly reported as having the condition, and false negatives, where individuals are wrongly reported as not having the condition (PHE, 2021). As nurses and nurse associates, it is important to understand when individuals may be offered screening as identified in the NHS population screening timeline (PHE, 2021). This can help you to provide information and encourage uptake of screening at appropriate stages of the life-course.

Secondary prevention also includes reducing the impact of illness through health promotion to encourage behaviour change or intervention such as treatment for the condition.

Alongside the screening activities outlined in the NHS population screening timeline (PHE, 2021), the NHS also offers a health check every 5 years to adults in England who are aged 40–74 and who do not have any of the following pre-existing conditions: heart disease, chronic kidney disease, diabetes, hypertension, atrial fibrillation, transient ischaemic attacks, familial hypercholesterolaemia, heart failure, peripheral arterial disease, stroke. This is in recognition that as we age, our risk of some health conditions increases, and early detection is likely to produce better health outcomes (NHS, 2021). Therefore, a key feature of our nursing role is raising awareness about and encouraging uptake of screening opportunities.

Nursing Fields Adult Health: Nursing Practice and Decision Making, Communication and Interpersonal Skills

Secondary prevention: patient on a surgical ward

The nurse is engaged in assessing a presurgical patient for risk of venous thromboembolism (VTE) postoperatively. Risk factors for developing VTE depend on the condition and/or surgical procedure as well as age, obesity and any concomitant conditions

The health promotion role of the nurse or nurse associate for non-pharmacological prevention here includes:

- Teaching the person to perform leg exercises to shorten or reduce the impact of disease
- Adhering to local policy in applying antiembolism stockings
- Building up coping skills in the patient, for example how to recognise early signs of VTE
- Acting as a source of information.

- *Tertiary prevention* – here, the aim is to reduce the impact of ongoing illness or injury by helping people to manage long-term, often complex health problems and injuries. The aim is to improve their ability to function, quality of life and life expectancy.

Nursing Fields Mental Health: Nursing Practice and Decision Making, Communication and Interpersonal Skills

Tertiary prevention

People with established mental health problems may not notice symptoms of physical disease and may be reluctant to seek help. The unwanted side-effects of medication can also affect the person's health, for example weight gain.

Nurses can support tertiary prevention by understanding the links between psychological health and physical health. The health promotion role of the nurse here includes:

- Monitoring the person's health, e.g. nutritional assessment, BMI measurement and exploring the use of coping strategies to maintain health. This may include accessing support available within the community, for example community support groups
- Carefully monitoring the side-effects of medications and promoting concordance
- Encouraging the person not to ignore physical symptoms, and to seek support and diagnosis.

Case Study

Mrs Smith attends her GP surgery and sees the practice nurse for her cervical screening test. The practice nurse notices that Mrs Smith is now 42 years of age.

Here, it is important that the nurse checks whether Mrs Smith has had an NHS health check. As Mrs Smith has not had the check, this is an important opportunity to:

- Provide information about the value of the check
- Give information about what it involves
- Encourage Mrs Smith and her spouse, if eligible, to make an appointment for the check
- Provide information about healthy living and resources such as NHS health apps and trackers.

Nurses as Educators

As nurses, a central feature of our role is patient education in order to help individuals to stay healthy, to use health services appropriately, but also to help them manage their own health and well-being (Blevins, 2018). Platform 2 outlines the nurse's role in the promotion of health and proficiency 2.6 for nursing associates and 2.7 for adult nurses specifically relate to health literacy (NMC, 2018a).

Education is a key social determinant of health and those with lower levels of literacy, numeracy and language skills are much more likely to experience the worst health outcomes and also show higher rates of use of healthcare services. Whilst this is partially attributed to these individuals being more likely to be living in disadvantaged socioeconomic circumstances, some of the adverse effects on health are also related to being less able to manage long-term health conditions and also being less receptive to and responsive to health education and intervention (Rowlands & Nutbeam, 2013).

Health literacy influences the extent to which individuals interact with providers of health services, manage their own health and that of others and, importantly, their ability to engage in discussions with health professionals about their health (NHS Scotland, 2017). It also determines ability to make judgements

44

and decisions in everyday life concerning healthcare, disease prevention, management and health improvement throughout the life-course (Rowlands *et al.*, 2020). There is a direct link between low levels of literacy and risk of engaging in behaviours that harm health and increase risk of morbidity and mortality, such as smoking and alcohol misuse, alongside increased use of health services, emergency care and hospitalisation, compounded by reduced ability to self-care, as outlined above (Protheroe *et al.*, 2017).

Berry (2016) suggests that the financial cost of low levels of health literacy are between 3% and 5% of the annual UK health budget, therefore it is not surprising that improving health literacy is a key priority. Trueland (2012) quotes two examples of the consequences of poor health literacy when she states, 'You can give the best medicine in the world, but if the patient does not understand how it should be taken then it can be useless, or even dangerous. Similarly, if a new mother cannot read the instructions on mixing formula, then her baby will not thrive'.

Nursing Fields Learning Disabilities

Gwen is admitted to the women's health unit for investigations for suspected breast cancer. Gwen has a learning disability and has brought her hospital 'traffic light assessment' (hospital passport) with her to the ward.

In Gwen's scenario, she is faced with complex investigations and a treatment regimen for her breast cancer. As part of the learning disability toolkit, Gwen has her 'hospital passport' with her.

Caring, Dignity and Compassion

What elements of Gwen's life do you think will be highlighted in the traffic light assessment booklet?
- Red signals issues that staff must know about.
- Amber signals things that are important to Gwen.
- Green signals Gwen's likes and dislikes.

Why might this be important in your role as a nurse or nurse associate?

In this exercise, you may have highlighted aspects in the amber signal that can help you to support Gwen's understanding of her treatment and care while she is being investigated and treated. There will be information about how to communicate with her and, importantly, how to help her understand things. This is an

---

What the Experts Say

'Even the smallest thing can have an impact on the experience my son has whilst in hospital, for example he won't eat and will be distressed if he doesn't have his 'special' adapted knife and fork. The traffic light assessment document is really helpful to give the nurses and staff a real insight into his daily activities, and to prevent any upset or further complications in his health and well-being'.

(Ruth, a carer for her grown-up son with learning difficulties)

---

essential feature of our role and offering choice 'demonstrates respect, enhances autonomy and provides evidence of individualized care' (NMC, 2018a,b).

Nurses need to think carefully about how to educate patients and this includes ensuring enough time to get to know the patient, considering the environment and ensuring privacy, as well as planning enough time to communicate and facilitate discussion. It is also important to consider any barriers such as learning disability, as well as embarrassment, limits on ability to process and remember information, particularly in the presence of health conditions and during times of stress. Equally, simple measures must be considered, such as ensuring the individual is able to see and hear well and any devices, such as glasses and hearing aids, are worn and functioning properly. It is also important to determine the individual's primary language and whether a translator service is required. Where possible, any written information should be provided in the person's primary language (Blevins, 2018). The NHS website can provide access to online translation, as well as health information in other languages. Often health professionals use complex terminology and jargon, and this can confuse some patients or alienate them; this can be avoided by using simple language and carefully explaining terms (Evans *et al.*, 2017).

What To Do If . . . you are educating a patient about their diagnosis

NHS Scotland (2021) provides a range of resources for healthcare professionals and suggests the following methods are useful when communicating with service users.

- *Teach back* – this approach confirms that the information provided has been understood by asking the individual to 'teach back' what has been discussed or demonstrated.
- *Chunk and check* – this can also be used alongside teach back, where information is broken down into small chunks during consultations and the nurse checks for understanding along the way.
- *Use simple language* – explain terminology.
- *Use pictures* – some concepts are difficult to explain, and graphics or pictures may work well to support other forms of communication.
- *Help with paperwork* – it is not always obvious that individuals have problems with paperwork or understanding written health information. Therefore, we should routinely offer help.

Often, as nurses and nurse associates, we use a range of resources to support health education. Written information is usually in the form of patient information leaflets, but care must be taken to ensure that this meets individual needs, the content is accurate, balanced and evidence based. As with verbal communication, the language should be clear, easy to understand and jargon free. It is also vital that the information is current, and appropriate for the target audience. For example, it is important to consider language, culture and special group needs, for example, those with a learning disability (NHS Wales, 2021). This is also true when referring patients to electronic media.

It is widely accepted that many people now rely on the internet for sources of health information. However, one of the challenges is that many websites do not offer accurate, evidence-based information. In order to address this, the NHS website and NHS app, which is owned and run by the NHS, provide reliable information about health, living well and NHS services and offer a range of formats, languages and services for those with specific needs, i.e. learning disability (NHS, 2021).

Health Promotion/Improvement and Behaviour Change

All health improvement/health promotion activity has the aim of promoting health behaviour change. As outlined earlier, health behaviours are influenced by a range of factors including our social and cultural experience, our beliefs, our education, as well as the environment we live in, our social contacts, religion and income (Evans *et al.*, 2017). The government's transformation of public health services outlines the need to strengthen design and delivery of behaviour change interventions and programmes using innovative and evidence-based behaviour change and public engagement activity (DHSC, 2021). It is too early to envisage how this will move the health promotion agenda forward but it is likely that the role of nurses and nursing associates will be pivotal.

In recent years, the value of opportunistic delivery of consistent and concise healthy lifestyle information and conversations about health has been underlined and embedded in the Making Every Contact Count (MECC) approach (Health Education England, 2021) and the framework of evidence for healthcare professionals 'All our Health: personalised care and population health' which introduced a range of resources and e-learning focused on 25 key public health issues for all health and care professionals. These provide bite-sized information and signposting to trusted sources of helpful evidence, guidance and support to inform health promotion activity (e-learning for Healthcare, 2021). Embedding the principles of MECC within our work is essential and this approach underlines that all staff have a responsibility to improve health and deliver health promotion messages. Key to this is brief intervention for behaviour change. According to the National Institute for Health and Care Excellence (NICE, 2014), this can take the following forms.

- *Very brief intervention* – which can take from 30 seconds to a couple of minutes. This form of intervention follows an 'ask, advise, assist' structure. If we focus on smoking, using this approach, we would ask about smoking status, record smoking status and then advise about smoking cessation services and assist the individual to access these if they show interest in changing their behaviour. This is about giving people information or directing them where to go for further help.
- *Brief intervention* – usually takes no more than a few minutes for basic advice to be given. This usually involves discussion, encouragement, possibly supported by written materials or directions to other sources of information and support and/or follow-up.
- *Extended brief intervention* – this usually lasts more than 30 minutes and consists of an individually focused discussion over a single or multiple brief sessions. The emphasis is on providing advice, information, encouragement and support, as well as feedback about progress.

The aim here is to be solution focused and keep the brief session focused on behaviour change. Brief intervention approaches are important, but it is necessary to acknowledge that behaviour change is complex. It is here where the COM-B model, outlined by Michie *et al.* (2011), is of use and notes that the following must be addressed for behaviour change to occur.

- *Capability* – the person must be both physically and psychologically capable of performing the necessary actions to change their behaviour.
- *Opportunity* – they must have the physical and social opportunity. This reflects the fact that there are many barriers to behaviour change, which include access to healthy food, green spaces to exercise, public transport, etc.
- *Motivation* – the person must be motivated to adopt the new behaviour.

Therefore, behaviour change may also require motivational interviewing techniques. These are informed by four key principles outlined by Evans *et al.* (2017, p.36).

1. Express empathy with the problem and the need to change.
2. Develop discrepancy (make people understand the differences and the pros and cons) between current behaviour and desired change.
3. Accept resistance to change as normal.
4. Support self-efficacy and autonomy in changing behaviour.

Motivational interviewing is widely used by healthcare professionals and works by showing understanding that change is needed, accepting that many are reluctant to change, but also building confidence in the person that they can make healthy changes to their lifestyle.

Practice Assessment Document

Nurses and nurse associates have a key responsibility to promote health.

Think about a recent contact with a service user. Did you use this as an opportunity to Make Every Contact Count? If yes, think about how you went about this. If you missed this opportunity, take time to think about how you might MECC in future contacts with service users using brief intervention and motivational interviewing. Now refer to your PAD document and identify those that relate to MECC. These might include competencies that focus on promoting health and well-being, appropriate communication skills, being aware of your own values and how they might influence your practice. Below is an example of applying the Ask, Advise Assist approach in practice.

- *Ask*: asking patients about their health behaviour relies on your ability to develop and use appropriate communication strategies. Sometimes patients feel embarrassed and so you will need to think about their privacy, as well as avoiding judging them. You will need to record health status in the patient record – so think about proficiencies that relate to accurate record keeping.
- *Advise*: when advising patients you will need to make sure you use up-to-date and accurate information – this links to competencies focused on using research findings and evidence to inform your practice. Think about different communication strategies, but also your patient. You will need to ensure your approach to educating and providing information considers age, mental, physical and cognitive ability. This links to competencies focused on promoting health and particularly health literacy.
- *Assist*: this involves referring to agencies, for example smoking cessation. This will link to competencies focused on partnership working and knowledge of when to refer.

Understanding the reasons behind individual health behaviour is the focus of health psychology and the models below can help inform our health promotion practice.

The health belief model (Becker, 1974) suggests that behaviour change is dependent on the person's beliefs about how susceptible they are to a disease, how severe that illness might be and the pros and cons of any changes to health behaviour. Understanding these beliefs can help us to determine the likelihood of behaviour change.

Bandura's (1977) social cognitive theory also provides insight into understanding and predicting behaviour change. Bandura suggests that behaviour change is governed by:

- *Self-efficacy* – an individual's confidence that they can carry out behaviour change
- *Expectancy* – the belief that certain actions will result in the desired outcome
- *Incentives* – that behaviour is linked to the value the individual places on the perceived outcome.

Prochaska and DiClemente's (1982) model incorporates many aspects of health psychology and as such is referred to as a transtheoretical model. It outlines a number of stages involved in behaviour change.

- *Precontemplation* – where the individual is not thinking of behaviour change. The individual may not see the advantages of change or deny they have a problem. Here, our role as nurses or nurse associates is important, as we can use opportunities to identify health risks and provide information, but also explain that resistance to change is natural. This may help the person progress to the next stage of the model (RCN, 2019).
- *Contemplation* – at this stage the person is considering change. Many people remain in this stage for a long time and so we can help them to formulate clear plans for change and confirm the benefits of change. We can also provide a range of options for behaviour change.
- *Preparation* – at this stage the person has realised change is beneficial and possible and has plans to make a change in the near future. Here, we can provide positive feedback, approval and sources of information. Negotiating a start date can also be helpful, as can focusing on the strengths the individual possesses that are likely to help with behaviour change.
- *Action* – at this stage there is clear evidence of behaviour modification. In this phase it is important to reinforce the positive change in order to encourage the person to continue.
- *Maintenance* – this is a challenging phase where individuals must deal with barriers to continuing their change in behaviour. Here, we can offer support by discussing ways to maintain change and cope with temptation.
- *Relapse* – this phase is common and many who are changing behaviour experience relapse. It is important to acknowledge that this can lead to feelings of failure or disappointment. Here, we can reassure individuals that this is common, but that they can recommence their journey and perhaps consider other approaches.

Models such as this can be helpful in supporting service users to understand the stages of behaviour change and to help them set realistic goals, as well as dealing with relapse. It is helpful for us to consider which stage of behaviour change the individual is at in order to tailor our support effectively.

Caring, Dignity and Compassion and Your PAD Competencies

Take time to think about the last time you used health information to educate a service user.

1. What strategies did you use? (This may have included discussions about health, provision of written/pictorial information, reference to digital information via websites.)
2. Did you consider the person's background, cultural characteristics?
3. Did you consider the person's stage of life, the presence of any mental, physical, cognitive and behavioural health challenges?
4. Did you focus on providing person-centred and sensitive care?
5. Did you identify personal strengths and support the individual to make informed choices about their health and well-being?
6. Did you document your interaction in the patient's records?
7. Did you make any referrals?

Now refer to your PAD document and identify the specific competencies that relate to platforms 1 and 2.

Platforms 1 and 2 outline the need to provide person-centred care, to focus on strengths-based approaches to support and enable people to make informed choices about their care and their health and well-being. Providing information in accessible ways is essential. When engaging in these activities, it is essential you document your interaction accurately and record any referrals.

Nurses as Healthy Role Models?

Platform 1 – Proficiency 1.6 for Nurses and Nurse Associates (NMC 2018a, b)

At the point of registration, the registered nurse and nurse associate will be able to understand the professional responsibility to adopt a healthy lifestyle to maintain the level of personal fitness and well-being required to meet people's needs for mental and physical care (NMC, 2018a,b).

Whilst there is a professional duty for nurses and nurse associates to adopt a healthy lifestyle, Darch *et al.* (2017) suggest that this regulatory requirement is not always consistent with the reality of the health status of many nursing professionals. Indeed, a study by Keele (2019) suggests that whilst nursing staff are knowledgeable about the benefits of a healthy lifestyle, many nurses experience the same struggles, if not more so, than the general public, and that across the nursing profession a significant number are overweight/obese, smoke, do not take adequate nutrition or exercise regularly. This is partly attributed to the stress associated with providing nursing care, as well as working shifts and long hours (Darch *et al.*, 2017). Nurse education providers should support nurses of the future to prioritise their own health and help them to develop health-enhancing coping mechanisms to deal with the pressures of their working lives.

Whilst many in the nursing profession aspire to be healthy, opinion is divided over whether being the perfect role model might inspire patients or make them feel inferior or that behaviour change is unattainable for them. Perhaps the 'imperfect' role model is more helpful, and patients can relate to professionals who are encountering the same challenges (Darch *et al.*, 2017). It is clear that being a healthy role model extends beyond being physically health, to demonstrating positive role-modelling behaviours, which include being caring, non-judgemental and supportive. Equally, whilst as nurses we may not be perfect, what we can model is having accurate facts and ability to help service users understand the risks to health and to signpost them to sources of help (Evans *et al.*, 2017).

Conclusion

This chapter has provided an overview of some of the key features of contemporary public health policy and practice. All nurses and nurse associates are responsible for engaging in public health activity and working with others to promote well-being, prevent ill health and work in partnership with individuals to ensure they are able to access relevant information and services to support their health and well-being. To do this effectively, it is essential that nurses and nurse associates understand the complex nature of health and the wider determinants of health, as well as ensuring they make every contact count as an opportunity to identify actual or potential risks to health and well-being, offer advice and support for behaviour change and signpost to relevant health and social care services.

Key Points

- Health is subjective and personal views must be considered in order to provide person-centred care. It is important to understand relevant theories of health, including those which focus on medical, holistic and wellness approaches, to inform our practice.
- Health is influenced by wider determinants, which include the genes we inherit, the conditions in which we live, the choices we make and the services we are able to access to support health. Ill health is not randomly distributed, nor is it inevitable. The aim of all governmental policies should be to level up, for everyone to enjoy the good health and well-being of those at the top of the social hierarchy.
- All nurses and nurse associates have a key role in identifying and minimising the impact of illness.
- Nurses and nursing associates in the UK are responsible for promoting health and providing meaningful public health interventions.
- A central feature of the nursing role is health education to support individuals to stay healthy, to use health services appropriately and to manage their health and well-being. We can make every contact count to identify and provide support and signposting to relevant health services, as well as acting as healthy role models.

References

Acheson, D. (1998) *Independent Inquiry into Inequalities in Health.* https://assets.publishing.service.gov.uk/government/uploads/system/uploads/attachment_data/file/265503/ih.pdf (accessed December 2021).

Bandura, A. (1977) Self-efficacy: toward a unifying theory of behaviour change. *Psychological Review*, 84, 191–215.

Bartley, M. & Blane, D. (2008) Inequality and social class. In: G. Scambler (ed.) *Sociology as Applied to Medicine.* Elsevier, Edinburgh.

Becker, M.H. (ed.) (1974) *The Health Belief Model and Personal Health Behavior.* Slack, New Jersey.

Bellis, M.A., Ashton, K., Hughes, K., Ford, K., Bishop, J. & Paranjothy, S. (2015) *Welsh Adverse Childhood Experiences (ACE) Study. Adverse Childhood Experiences and Their Impact on Health-Harming Behaviours in the Welsh Adult Population.* www2.nphs.wales.nhs.uk:8080/PRIDDocs.nsf/7c21215d6d0c613e80256f490030c05a/d488a3852491bc1d80257f370038919e/$FILE/ACE%20Report%20FINAL%20%28E%29.pdf (accessed December 2021)

Bennett, V. (2019) *The Role of Nurses in Delivering Successful Immunisation Programmes.* https://ukhsa.blog.gov.uk/author/viv-bennett/ (accessed December 2021).

Berry, J. (2016) *Does Health Literacy Matter?* www.england.nhs.uk/blog/jonathan-berry/#:~:text=Jonathan%20Berry%2C%20Personalisation%20and%20Control,it%20can%20have%20for%20patients (accessed December 2021).

Black, D. (1980) *The Black Report.* www.sochealth.co.uk/national-health-service/public-health-and-wellbeing/poverty-and-inequality/the-black-report-1980/ (accessed December 2021).

Blevins, S. (2018) The art of patient education. *MedSurg Nursing*, 27, 401.

Brain, J. (2021) *Timeline of the Industrial Revolution.* www.historic-uk.com/HistoryUK/HistoryofBritain/Timeline-Industrial-Revolution/ (accessed December 2021).

Darch, J., Baillie, L. & Gillison, F. (2017) Nurses as role models in health promotion: a concept analysis. *British Journal of Nursing*, 26(17), https://doi.org/10.12968/bjon.2017.26.17.982

Department of Health (1992) *The Health of the Nation.* Department of Health, London.

Department of Health (1999) *Saving Lives: Our Healthier Nation.* Department of Health, London.

Department of Health (2004) *Choosing Health: Making Healthier Choices Easier.* Department of Health, London.

Department of Health (2010) *Healthy Lives, Healthy People: Our Strategy for Public Health in England.* Department of Health, London.

Department of Health and Social Care (2018) *Prevention is Better Than Cure. Our Vision to Help You Live Well for Longer.* https://assets.publishing.service.gov.uk/government/uploads/system/uploads/attachment_data/file/753688/Prevention_is_better_than_cure_5-11.pdf (accessed December 2021).

Department of Health and Social Care (2021) *Transforming the Public Health System: Reforming the Public Health System for the Challenges of Our Times.* www.gov.uk/government/publications/transforming-the-public-health-system/transforming-the-public-health-system-reforming-the-public-health-system-for-the-challenges-of-our-times (accessed December 2021).

e-learning for Healthcare (2021) *About the All our Health Programme.* www.e-lfh.org.uk/programmes/all-our-health/ (accessed December 2021).

Evans, D., Coutsaftiki, D. & Fathers, C.P. (2017) *Health Promotion and Public Health Nursing for Students*, 3rd edn. Sage, London.

Faculty of Public Health (2021) *Functions and Standards of a Public Health System.* www.fph.org.uk/media/3031/fph_systems_and_function-final-v2.pdf (accessed December 2021).

Hart, J.T (1971) The inverse care law. *Lancet*, 297(766), 405–412.

Health Education England (2021) *Making Every Contact Count.* www.makingeverycontactcount.co.uk (accessed December 2021).

Huber, M., Knottnerus, J.A., Green, L., *et al.* (2011) How should we define health? *British Medical Journal*, 343, d4163.

Illich, I. (1975) *Medical Nemesis, Part One.* Calder and Boyers, London.

Institute of Public Health Ireland (2021) *Who We Are.* https://publichealth.ie/who-we-are/ (accessed December 2021).

Keele, R. (2019) To role model or not? Nurses' challenges in promoting a healthy lifestyle. *Workplace Health and Safety*, 67(2), 584–591.

King's Fund (2019) *What Does Improving Population Health Really Mean?* https://kingsfund.org.uk/publications/what-does-improving-population-health-mean (accessed December 2021).

King's Fund (2021) *Broader Determinants of Health: Future Trends.* www.kingsfund.org.uk/projects/time-think-differently/trends-broader-determinants-health (accessed December 2021).

Marmot, M. (2010) *Fair Society, Healthy Lives.* www.parliament.uk/globalassets/documents/fair-society-healthy-lives-full-report.pdf (accessed December 2021).

Marmot, M., Allen, J., Boyce, T., Goldblatt, P. & Morrison, J. (2020) *Health Equity in England: The Marmot Review 10 Years On.* www.health.org.uk/publications/reports/the-marmot-review-10-years-on (accessed December 2020).

McCartney, G., Popham, F., McMaster, R. & Cumbers, A. (2019) Defining health and health inequalities. *Public Health*, 172, 22–30.

McKeown, T. (1976) *The Role of Medicine: Dream, Mirage or Nemesis?* www.nuffieldtrust.org.uk/research/the-role-of-medicine-dream-mirage-or-nemesis (accessed December 2021).

Michie, S., van Stralen, M.M. & West, R. (2011) The behaviour change wheel: a new method for characterising and designing behaviour change interventions. *Implementation Science*, 6, 42.

Naidoo, J. & Wills, J. (2016) *Foundations for Health Promotion*, 4th edn. Elsevier, London.

National Health Service (2019) *The NHS Long Term Plan.* www.longtermplan.nhs.uk/wp-content/uploads/2019/01/the-nhs-long-term-plan-summary.pdf (accessed December 2021).

National Health Service (2021) *NHS Health Check.* www.nhs.uk/conditions/nhs-health-check/ (Accessed 24.5.2021)

National Health Service Careers (2021) *A Brief History of Public Health.* www.healthcareers.nhs.uk/career-planning/resources/brief-history-public-health (accessed December 2021).

National Health Service Scotland (2017) *Making It Easier. A Health Literacy Action Plan for Scotland.* www.gov.scot/binaries/content/documents/govscot/publications/strategy-plan/2017/11/making-easier-health-literacy-action-plan-scotland-2017-2025/documents/00528139-pdf/00528139-pdf/govscot%3Adocument/00528139.pdf (accessed December 2021).

National Health Service Scotland (2021) *The Health Literacy Place.* www.healthliteracyplace.org.uk/tools-and-techniques/techniques/ (accessed December 2021).

National Health Service Wales (2021) *Framework for Best Practice. The Production and Use of Health Information for the Public.* www.wales.nhs.uk/sites3/Documents/420/framework_bestpractice_e1.pdf (accessed December 2021).

National Institute for Health and Care Excellence (2014) *Behaviour Change: Individual Approaches.* www.nice.org.uk/guidance/ph49/chapter/1-Recommendations (accessed December 2021).

Nightingale, F. (1859) *Notes on Nursing: What It Is and What It Is Not.* Wilder Publications, Virginia.

Nursing & Midwifery Council (2018a) *The Code.* www.nmc.org.uk/globalassets/sitedocuments/nmc-publications/nmc-code.pdf (accessed December 2021).

Nursing & Midwifery Council (2018b) *Standards of Proficiency for Nursing Associates.* www.nmc.org.uk/globalassets/sitedocuments/standards-of-proficiency/nursing-associates-proficiency-standards.pdf (accessed December 2021).

Oxford Vaccine Group (2020) *Herd Immunity (Herd Protection).* http://vk.ovg.ox.ac.uk/herd-immunity (accessed December 2021).

Pellegrino, R.J., Saffici, C. & Pellegrino, K. (2012) *What is Wellness? A New Measure of General Wellness for the Social Sciences.* http://asbbs.org/files/ASBBS2012V1/PDF/P/PellegrinoR.pdf (accessed December 2021).

Prochaska, J.O. & DiClemente C.C. (1982) Transtheoretical therapy: toward a more integrative models of change, *Psychotherapy: Theory Research and Practice*, 20, 161–173.

Protheroe, J., Whittle, R., Bartlam, B., Estacio, E.V., Clark, L. & Kurth, J. (2017) Health literacy, associated lifestyle and demographic factors in adult population of an English city: a cross-sectional survey. *Health Expectations*, 20, 112–119.

Public Health Act (1842) www.parliament.uk/about/living-heritage/transformingsociety/towncountry/towns/tyne-and-wear-case-study/about-the-group/public-administration/the-1848-public-health-act/ (accessed December 2021).

Public Health England (2014) *Measles, Mumps, Rubella (MMR): Use of Combined Vaccine Instead of Single Vaccines.* www.gov.uk/government/publications/mmr-vaccine-dispelling-myths/measles-mumps-rubella-mmr-maintaining-uptake-of-vaccine (accessed December 2021).

Public Health England (2018) *Measles Outbreaks Across England.* www.gov.uk/government/news/measles-outbreaks-across-england (accessed December 2021).

Public Health England (2019) *Public Health Outcomes Framework 2019-2022. At a Glance.* https://assets.publishing.service.gov.uk/government/uploads/system/uploads/attachment_data/file/862264/At_a_glance_document2.pdf (accessed December 2021).

Public Health England (2020) *The Routine Immunisation Schedule.* https://assets.publishing.service.gov.uk/government/uploads/system/uploads/attachment_data/file/899423/PHE_Complete_Immunisation_Schedule_Jun2020_05.pdf (accessed December 2021).

Public Health England (2021) *NHS Population Screening Explained.* www.gov.uk/guidance/nhs-population-screening-explained#printable-screening-information-resource (accessed December 2021).

Public Health Scotland (2021) *Our Areas of Work.* www.publichealthscotland.scot/our-areas-of-work/ (accessed December 2021).

Public Health Wales (2021) *Welcome to Public Health Wales.* https://phw.nhs.wales (accessed December 2021).

Rowlands, G. & Nutbeam, D. (2013) Health literacy and the 'inverse information law'. *British Journal of General Practice*, 63(608), 120–121.

Rowlands, G., Tabassum, B., Campbell, P., *et al.* (2020) The evidence-based development of an intervention to improve clinical health literacy practice. *International Journal of Environmental Research and Public Health*, 17(5), 1513.

Royal College of Nursing (2019) *Understanding Behaviour Change.* www.rcn.org.uk/clinical-topics/supporting-behaviour-change/understanding-behaviour-change (accessed December 2021).

Royal College of Nursing (2020) *The Role of Nursing Staff in Public Health.* www.rcn.org.uk/clinical-topics/public-health/the-role-of-nursing-staff-in-public-health (accessed December 2021).

Royal College of Nursing (2021) *Health Protection.* www.rcn.org.uk/clinical-topics/public-health/health-protection (accessed December 2021).

Royal Society for Public Health (2019) *Top 20 Public Health Achievements of the 21st Century.* www.rsph.org.uk/about-us/news/top-20-public-health-achievements-of-the-21st-century.html (accessed December 2021).

Stewart, J. (ed.) (2017) *Pioneers in Public Health. Lessons from History.* Routledge, London.

Tannahill, A. (2009) The Tannahill Model revisited. *Public Health*, 123(5), 396–399.

Trueland, J. (2012) Read this carefully. *Nursing Standard*, 27(8), 20–21.

World Health Organization (1948) *Constitution of the World Health Organization.* WHO, Geneva.

World Health Organization (1986) *Ottawa Charter for Health Promotion.* WHO, Geneva.

World Health Organization (2020) *WHO Definition of Public Health.* www.publichealth.com.ng/who-definition-of-public-health/ (accessed December 2021).

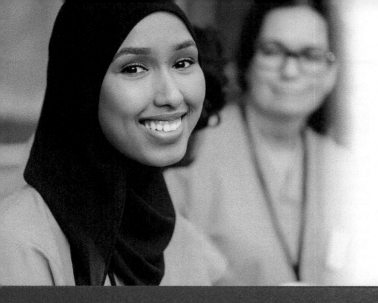

4

The Nursing Process and Models of Nursing

Michael Lappin

University of Salford, UK

Learning Outcomes

On completion of this chapter you will be able to:

- Gain an awareness of the concept (philosophy/principles) of the Nursing Process
- Have an understanding of the stages of the Nursing Process: Assessment, Diagnosis, Planning, Implementation and Evaluation (ADPIE)
- Gain an insight into the importance of the nursing diagnosis
- Have an overview of nursing models with particular emphasis on the most widespread model in the UK: the Roper, Logan and Tierney activities of living (ALs) model
- Recognise how a nursing model links to patient-centred care, safety and enhanced quality for your patient.

Proficiencies

NMC Proficiencies and Standards:

- Must appreciate the value of evidence and promote health and best practice
- Build partnerships and therapeutic relationships
- Use the full range of communication methods
- Maintain accurate, clear and complete records, including the use of electronic formats, using appropriate and plain language
- Use up-to-date knowledge and evidence to assess, diagnose, plan, deliver and evaluate (ADPIE) care
- Carry out comprehensive, systematic nursing assessments
- Work in partnership with service users, carers, families, groups, communities and organisations
- Build partnerships and therapeutic relationships through safe, effective and non-discriminatory communication
- Use a range of communication skills and technologies to support person-centred care and enhance quality and safety.

 Visit the companion website at **www.wiley.com/go/peate/nursingpractice3e** where you can test yourself using flashcards, multiple-choice questions and more.

Nursing Practice: Knowledge and Care, Third Edition. Edited by Ian Peate and Aby Mitchell.
© 2022 John Wiley & Sons Ltd. Published 2022 by John Wiley & Sons Ltd.
Companion website: www.wiley.com/go/peate/nursingpractice3e

Introduction

On nursing. . . 'A distinct profession, providing direct assistance to individuals in whatever setting they are found for the purpose of avoiding, relieving, diminishing, or curing the individual's sense of helplessness.'

(Ida Jean Orlando, who first described the four stages of the Nursing Process in 1958)

If you were to be admitted to hospital or in need of nursing care in any setting, you would expect the nurses caring for you to be gentle, considerate, compassionate and concerned for your well-being. The care you receive should be personal and centred around you as an individual. The Nursing Process and nursing models have been advocated by many nurses as a means of moving nursing from depersonalised, task-focused and a traditional style of nursing towards an individualised, patient-centred philosophy of care (Walsh & Ford, 1994, p.181). In any caring environment this should be a given; however, it is worth remembering that for nurses to practise their art, they require a number of tools to allow this. The Nursing Process is one such tool that assists nurses to plan care; it is a framework that helps the nurse to focus on the 'person' and will help set a pathway leading to a world of patient comfort, rehabilitation and recovery, depending on the observable conditions. Similarly, the humanistic model of care first proposed in 1956 (Paterson & Zderad, 2007) placed an emphasis on the nurse–patient relationship, where both influence the outcome of nursing practice. At this time, the authors stressed that the purpose of holism should demonstrate the vital role of the patient's healing as much as the medical interventions. It's about the developing connection between the two and the impact this has on both the physical and mental health of the patient.

Patricia Benner (2001) believed that the finest nurses develop their skills over a period of time. Her 'Novice to Expert' continuum went on to highlight how experience helps to contribute to a nurse's development, allowing an understanding of what it means to provide high-quality patient care. The degree of quality also links to patient empowerment, patient self-care and the promotion of patient participation where the nurse guides the patient to better health, rehabilitation and progress. An article by Ozdemir (2019) discusses the work of others, highlighting that personalised care is considered a gauge for the quality of care due to positive patient outcomes. The appropriate use of nursing theories and nursing models guides nursing staff during the assessment process; key questioning will lead to the proper nursing interventions and collaborative decision making, ensuring that the nurse–patient relationship is unique.

Another nurse theorist, Jean Watson (1991), postulated her 'Philosophy and Theory of Transpersonal Caring'. This mainly concerns how nurses care for their patients, and how the caring progresses into better plans to promote health and wellness, prevent illness and restore health. In the theory of Jean Watson, the essence of nursing involves caring. A large component of a nurse's role is to not only help restore the patient to optimal health but to help them find meaning in their illness or suffering to help promote a harmonious balance (Lukose, 2011, p.27).

The whole concept of 'holism' and the holistic approach to care when nursing your patient clearly demonstrates the benefits of the therapeutic relationship and shows how vital this is when combined with the medical treatment required. Vinje *et al.* (2016) refer to Aaron Antonovsky's development of salutogenesis, a medical approach that concentrates on aspects that support healthiness rather than pathogenesis – the causes of disease. This model concerns itself with the relationship between human health, stress and the individual's self-management of health. Like the Nursing Process, it looks towards problem solving and using the resources available. Over the years, this framework has become a recognised concept in public health and health promotion. Pelikan (2017, p.261) highlights that salutogenesis guides health promotion interventions in the practice setting whilst Rizk & Almond (2013) suggest that Sense of Coherence (SOC) links to a person's general attitude of the world and can assist the individual to enhance their health and help them manage the traumatic issues associated with ill health. In the conclusion to their literature review (p.9), they state that it is unclear to what extent a high SOC improves self-management in the diabetes patient but it may improve their psychological well-being. However, there seems to be no doubt that it is an alternative tool for nurses to understand the non-compliance, depression and apprehension that people with a long-term condition experience. The introduction of this instrument may enhance our nursing practice further and help nurses in their assessment of patients in pursuit of a higher quality service.

De Bronkart & Sands (2018) quote Warner Slack, the visionary physician who wrote that the patient is the 'largest and least utilised resource in healthcare'. He insisted on patients being informed and empowered. It would seem, then, that as nurses, we are in an exclusive position in promoting excellence in healthcare. As we apply the tools of our trade, including the Nursing Process and the full employment of specific models of nursing, and practise a salutogenic approach, we can feel more fulfilled and with heightened self-confidence we can build a therapeutic relationship, using this all-inclusive approach and allowing the patient to be a partner in their care.

Practice Assessment Document (PAD)

The PAD highlights that the student is required to deliver safe, patient-centred care utilising the appropriate skills. The student must understand that it is their professional responsibility in the promotion of a healthy lifestyle when caring for patients. When undertaking precise nursing assessments, the student must accurately process the assembled information to identify the patient's needs. A well-developed patient-centred care plan will guide the student as they prepare to deliver the essential care necessary for that individual.

Requesting 'spoke' placements whilst in practice will give you an opportunity to observe a variety of assessments in action and a range of care plans specific to each clinical area. This will help to develop your knowledge and skills further. If you get an opportunity to work in the community. it will allow you to observe care plans that foster partnerships with the family and carers of your patient, encouraging shared decision making to help them manage their own care when appropriate.

Ask your practice assessor (PA) or practice supervisor (PS) about each area within the specific field to discover how assessments and care plans are utilised in that division.

Defining Nursing

Before introducing the concept of the Nursing Process and how we utilise the framework, it is important to define what nursing is. There are many definitions of nursing; the Royal College of Nursing (RCN, 2003, pp.5–7) highlights many of these, including the classic description by Florence Nightingale and that of the World Health Organization (WHO). However, the most often quoted and widely used classification comes from Virginia Henderson and was taken up by the International Council of Nurses (ICN) in 1960. In it she describes the 'unique function of the nurse' as:

'... to assist the individual, sick or well, in the performance of those activities contributing to the health or its recovery (or to peaceful death) that he would perform unaided if he had the necessary strength, will or knowledge ...'

(Henderson 1966, quoted in Aggleton & Chalmers, 1986, p.18)

The RCN (2003, p.6) quite rightly points out that this is only the first part of Henderson's definition and only one part of nursing, and it is unfortunate that it is often used as if it were the full definition. The RCN stresses the continuation:

'In addition, she helps the patient to carry out the therapeutic plan as initiated by the physician, and she also, as a member of a team, helps others as they in turn help her, to plan and carry out the total programme whether it be for the improvement of health, or recovery from illness, or support in death.'

Hall & Ritchie (2009, pp.6–7) put forward a number of reasons for creating a clear definition of what nursing is. It enables nurses to describe nursing to people who do not understand it, it helps to clarify the role within the multidisciplinary (MDT) team, it will influence the policy agenda at both local and national level and it will develop educational curricula and identify areas where research is needed to strengthen the knowledge base of the profession. It will also inform decisions about whether and how nursing work should be delegated to others and support negotiations at local and national level on issues such as nurse staffing, skill mix and nurses' pay.

The Evidence

Experience shows that patients are basically unaccustomed to the way we organise our work. In 2006, Christine Beasley, the then Chief Nursing Officer (CNO) for England, rightly pointed out:

'Nursing may not be easy to describe but patients know when they get good nursing and when they do not. Nursing requires a high-level set of skills and understanding which taken separately may seem commonplace and undemanding but combined as a whole is far more complex and powerful.'

(Department of Health, 2006, p.4)

Since taking up the post as CNO for England in January 2019, Ruth May has emphasised the need to firmly establish the value and importance of our profession. Raising the profile of the work that nurses do and presenting the breadth of the role will increase understanding of the job. Highly skilled, educated professionals need to tackle the entrenched stereotypes of nursing.

Grimette (2021) conducted an interview with Dr Rebecca Garcia of the Open University who pointed out that despite the extent of a nurse's knowledge and skills, the public perception has been tainted by media coverage, portraying the nurse as a subordinate 'handmaiden' to the doctor. Prior to March 2020, the majority of the public had little awareness of the true roles of the nurse (Girvin et al., 2016). However, in late 2019 the world was hit by the coronavirus pandemic and from this calamitous situation, the media began reporting the reality of what nurses actually do. The variety of settings were on view to the public, from working in acute settings and highly technical areas such as intensive care to the care of residents in nursing homes. In a time of anguish and great distress, nursing was now positioned as a fundamental role in patient care. Posters and signs were now prominent commending nursing staff and those from other professions. The weekly hand-clapping became a representation of the public's appreciation of the status now held by nurses.

Together with this new-found standing, it remains crucial that nurses continue to utilise the structure the Nursing Process offers to continue to deliver appropriate nursing interventions based on a sound assessment and plan of care. Your patient may not be aware of the systems we use but they will certainly garner the benefits of the arrangements we put in place.

Jot This Down

- Take some time to think about your personal definition of nursing.
- Discuss this with your colleagues and maybe ask your patient what nursing means to them.

How does the perception of one differ from the other? What have you learned from the patient's description of nursing?

Ask your patient if their perception of the nurse's role has changed in any way since the pandemic.

You may be interested to find out what a student nurse's perception of nursing was before they entered the profession and whether it has changed since the COVID-19 contagion.

No doubt, you will find from completing this exercise that each individual will come up with a different definition of nursing. This obviously depends on where the person is placed at that time.

Long before the inception of the Nursing and Midwifery Council (NMC) in April 2002, guidance was provided to registrants by the United Kingdom Central Council for Nursing, Midwifery and Health Visiting (UKCC). This was set up in 1983 and like the NMC, its primary function was to underscore the principles required for nurse registration and thus present a method through which the organisation would pursue its main purpose of protecting the public. It is hard to believe that in 1999, the UKCC remained uncertain about the value of trying to come up with a definition of nursing and concluded that: 'A definition of nursing would be too restrictive for the profession'.

In nursing practice, however, some measurement is necessary for the intention of formulating guidelines, designing nursing services and the advancement of programmes of nurse education. As Clark & Lang (1992) pointed out: 'If we cannot name it, we cannot control it, finance it, research it, teach it, or put it into public policy'.

Nursing is:

'the use of clinical judgement in the provision of care to enable people to improve, maintain, or recover health, to cope with health problems, and to achieve the best possible quality of life, whatever their disease or disability, until death'.

(RCN, 2003, p.3)

The RCN (2003, p.3) list six defining characteristics of nursing: the promotion of health, healing and growth, modes of intervention, people's physiological/psychological/social/cultural or spiritual response to health and illness and the commitment to the nurse–patient partnership. Point 4 describes the focus of nursing on the whole person and the human response rather than one particular aspect of the person or a particular pathological condition. Whilst all the characteristics are connected in some way to the overall concept of the Nursing Process, it is point 4 that stands above the rest in terms of the holistic approach to care and the nursing judgement and interventions that follow a medical diagnosis.

The RCN (2003, p.4) continued to highlight the difficulties associated with grading the work of nurses and nursing. we will all experience nursing in some shape or form and yet, it is still very complicated to explain; even nurses find it difficult to articulate an adequate definition when asked to do so.

In 1859 Florence Nightingale wrote: 'The elements of nursing are all but unknown' (Skretkowicz, 1992). Even today, this declaration rings true. Nursing can be allied to the physical tasks we deliver at the bedside, ensuring that the patient is treated as an individual in an environment that is clean, safe and comfortable.

Jot This Down

- Think about the public's awareness of nursing and the role nurses play.
- What do *you* think is the public perception of our work as nurses?

You may find that from completing this exercise that each individual will have common perceptions of the profession but there will be many variations amongst the group. This may depend on the person's experiences of healthcare and nursing.

As previously stated, nursing is seen by some as supporting medicine and the physicians by carrying out work coupled to the medical management of patients. Of course, these are fundamental aspects of our practice, but the idea that nursing consists of these elements alone ignores the wider contribution of professional nursing to healthcare, and will result in a service which does not offer its full potential (RCN, 2003, p.4). Ford *et al.* (2004, pp.3–6) have examined much of the existing research evidence that demonstrates that skilled nursing makes a difference.

Once again, Ruth May (2018), the Chief Nursing Officer for England, recognised the proficiencies of the nursing workforce, highlighting innovative practice that offers cutting-edge techniques with scientific and academic rigour, all delivered with care and compassion.

The NMC Code (NMC, 2015, updated October 2018 to reflect the regulation of nursing associates) emphasises putting the patient at the heart of care. Whilst this could be regarded as nothing new as it is considered a sense of duty, the Code follows four themes: Prioritise people, Practise Effectively, Preserve Safety and Promote Professionalism and Trust. The themes are not only there to guide nurses but to help patients and others to understand what nurses do and explain to them that the profession is aiming to meet their expectations in a safe environment. It highlights to the patient how important they are in this partnership and allows both partners to recognise each other's part in the process. We know that not all nursing is done by qualified nurses, any more than all law enforcement work is done by trained police officers. A patient's relatives, unofficial carers and a variety of support workers and healthcare assistants will also carry out this work. Their involvement is precious for the patient, but it does differ from that of the registered nurse.

It is almost 20 years since the RCN (2003) highlighted the distinction between professional nursing and the nursing undertaken by other people, stating that it does not lie in the type of task performed, nor in the level of skill required to perform a particular task. As for all professional practice, the difference lies in:

- the clinical judgement inherent in the processes of assessment, diagnosis, prescription and evaluation
- the knowledge that is the basis of the assessment of need and the determination of action to meet the need
- the personal accountability for all decisions and actions, including the decision to delegate to others
- the structured relationship between the nurse and the patient which incorporates professional regulation and a code of ethics within a statutory framework (RCN, 2003, p.4).

The RCN (2010) published a further guide specific to nursing students, highlighting the need for understanding of the eight principles of nursing practice. The aim of the guide is to help nurses relate the principles to their practice.

You will no doubt observe in practice that qualified nurses do work in a different way when caring for their patients. For example, whilst assisting a patient to the toilet, the support worker will deal with the task in the appropriate manner, with care and consideration for the patient. However, the qualified practitioner will carry out the same task but will be mindful of many other aspects associated with that individual, as constant assessment and reassessment often takes place sometimes without the nurse really thinking about it. For instance, the nurse may be assessing their patient's mobility, asking about their diet, whether they have pain or breathlessness, as well as assessing their psychological status and asking about their home circumstances and how their family will manage when it's time for discharge. This is all done with the steps of the Nursing Process and a nursing model in mind; what is a fundamental aspect of care now becomes a holistic approach to the actual and potential needs of the patient. Clearly, the qualified nurse has been prepared for this through their education and development, and is also conscious of the underlying principles and evidence base for the care they deliver. With the task completed and with the new information gathered, the nurse will now revisit the care plan and update it accordingly.

In January 2019, the NMC set up the regulation of nursing associates (NA). A member of the nursing team, the NA helps to bridge the gap between health and care assistants and registered nurses. Their work is diverse; caring for people across all ages in various settings, their role contributes to the fundamental aspects of nursing, freeing up registered nurses (RN) as they concentrate on more complex clinical care. Regarded as a stand-alone role, for some it provides a platform into graduate-level nursing. The Standards of Proficiency (NMC, 2018) highlights six platforms that include aspects linked to promoting health and preventing ill health whilst providing and monitoring care. Similar to their RN colleagues, the NA is expected to contribute to the ongoing assessment of patients, identify their needs, implement nursing care and evaluate the care in a patient-centred approach. This is an ideal opportunity for individual progression; employing their care planning skills and using the Nursing Process will add to the quality of the care delivered.

The Standards of Proficiency

- Platform 1 Being an accountable professional
- Platform 2 Promoting health and preventing ill health
- Platform 3 Providing and monitoring care
- Platform 4 Working in teams
- Platform 5 Improving safety and quality of care
- Platform 6 Contributing to integrated care (NMC, 2018)

What the Experts Say

Ann-Marie is a student nurse in her second year; she is currently working on an acute medical ward. Her mentor tells her that the Nursing Process and nursing models is 'a complete waste of time and it's just a lot of unnecessary paperwork'.

Ann-Marie is currently working on a patient-centred essay that requests that she use a Nursing Process approach. Her mentor's statement is the last thing she wants to hear if she is to remain motivated to complete the essay.

In the scenario above, Ann-Marie is faced with a dilemma; she has completed a lot of reading, including numerous analyses of the Nursing Process, so she is shocked by her mentor's sweeping statement and is disheartened by the opinion put forward.

Jot This Down

- What do you think Ann-Marie should do?
- How should she approach the issue with her mentor?

In this exercise you may have highlighted Ann-Marie's need to speak to her mentor (in a professional manner) to establish exactly what she meant by the comments. This may be an opportunity for both practitioners to discuss their own views and explain their judgements to each other. This makes for a healthy debate and gives them both an opening for reflection. This can be done in an informal manner, over a coffee break perhaps.

Florence Nightingale's focus on the promotion of health and healing as distinct from the cure of illness, and the harmony of the person, health and the environment, remain central to modern definitions of nursing (Skretkowicz, 1992). This too can be linked to the process of nursing, as person-centred nursing allows for recovery, rehabilitation or comfort of people who present with any illness or condition. Planning care for these people helps them to deal with the situations, needs or requirements associated with their circumstances. The RCN (2003, p.7) echoes the sentiment, stressing that the task of nursing in society is to help individuals, their families and groups to find their physical, mental and social potential. Care plans and the application of models permit the nurse to engage in the art and science of nursing and allow them to deliver a quality service for the patient population.

Looking back at Ann-Marie's experience and her mentor's rather negative view, it would appear that there are criticisms of the Nursing Process. Walsh & Ford (1994, p.186) highlight the many criticisms and the notion that it is a waste of nursing time, with endless paperwork and a ritualistic, task-centred process. However, it can be argued that a model underpins the delivery of care via the Nursing Process and can be fully implemented within a primary nursing system. It gives structure to the assessment and guides the nurse away from irrelevant areas (Walsh & Ford, 1994, p.206). This is clearly one of the key advantages of the Nursing Process; using the documentation appropriately will help the nurse to see that from a robust assessment comes the identification of key patient-centred goals. This in turn will lead to important nursing interventions, ensuring that valuable nursing time is administered without the distractions of more extraneous issues. What we see here is true patient-centred care and when the Nursing Process is used in combination with an appropriate nursing model, it results in an empowered workforce who can prioritise care, manage time, solve problems and make decisions about their patient and ultimately influence the quality of care in practice.

The Nursing Process

The Influence of Nursing from the USA

During the early part of the 1960s, the nursing profession began to press forward in the education of its workforce, stressing the need to further develop the knowledge base and competencies of nursing students and those already in practice. This was the case especially in the USA, leading to new explanations and theories as nurse lecturers and researchers were finding ways of explaining the nature of nursing to new entrants on the programmes offered. The aim of such theories was to make the work of nurses understandable and guide nursing education and training. Theorists such as Peplau, Orem, Henderson, Neuman and, in the UK, Roper, Logan and Tierney (as cited in Aggleton & Chalmers, 1986) highlighted different features of the patient which included their biological, social and psychological needs. From the 1950s onward, the development of the 'nursing process', and the concept of nursing diagnosis, focused attention on the identification of patient problems that nurses know about and treat. As nursing began to develop in universities in countries such as the USA, Canada, Australia and the Netherlands, the development of nursing science (the discipline-specific knowledge base of nursing) in these countries rapidly accelerated and was incorporated into definitions of nursing (RCN, 200,3 p.8).

The UK Picture

In the UK, things were more measured and the uptake of these theoretical concepts was a lot slower. The development of a body of 'nursing science' was disappointingly unhurried and the notion of the 'nursing diagnosis' was rarely (if ever) used in practice. In fact, the medical model of care was still very much in use at this time. Aggleton & Chalmers (1986, p.11) point out that for many years, the medical model formed the basis not only of medical training but of most nurse training as well. The model focuses on anatomical, physiological and biochemical causes of ill health.

On commencing nurse training in 1976, the author found that this was very much at the heart of his learning. It's difficult to imagine now, 45 years later, that a nurse would be using this model. As a student back then, patients were nursed according to their medical diagnosis; what you had was a set of guidelines and strategies associated with each diagnosis and it was not unusual for patients to be referred to the 'appendix in bed 6' or 'the coronary in bed 2'. The way we delivered nursing care for surgical patients, for instance, would be linked to where the patient was situated in the days postoperatively. The initial guidelines were carried out preoperatively with some common features applied but there would be a degree of uniqueness associated with the individual operation planned. The first day post surgery (day 1) would direct the nurse to a set of responsibilities; each one was different depending on whether the patient had returned from theatre having had a cholecystectomy, a gastrectomy or toenail removal. To some extent, this is where the distinctiveness of the care delivered was evident but overall, it was this set of rigid guidelines that stifled the nurse–patient relationship.

Definition

A shift away from the medical model was not too far away, and it was the introduction of the Nursing Process that helped to achieve this movement. However, the Nursing Process alone does not provide nurses with complete understanding about people and their health-related needs around which to plan and deliver care. This stems from the fact that while the Nursing Process suggests that nurses should assess, plan, intervene and evaluate, it does not indicate what should be the focus of such activities (Aggleton & Chalmers, 1986, p.15). When used alongside nursing models, the Nursing Process helps us to focus on the individual, their specific characteristics and their health-related requirements.

Jot This Down

Take a look at the definition of the medical model (above) and how nursing differs from it. Imagine using the 'medical model' in practice, where the patient is referred to by his medical diagnosis and his bed number; individualised nursing care was virtually non-existent and the nursing contribution to patient care was directed by this method. Nurses at the time were often regarded as 'physicians' assistants' and there needed to be a clear move towards enhancing the nursing profession's contribution to healthcare.

Take some time to discuss this situation with your mentor and peers; you may like to think about how valuable the Nursing Process and care planning are and how they contribute to the quality of your nursing practice. Miller (1985, p.63) found a reduction in length of hospital stay and patient dependency and a better chance of surviving the hospital stay after implementation of the Nursing Process. It is a truly worldwide concept; a South American study (Pokorski *et al.*, 2009) highlighted that active application of the Nursing Process leads to improved quality of care for patients whilst inspiring nurses to construct their academic and scientific knowledge in an effort to inform their clinical practice. This individualising of patient care leads to less dependent patients who could be discharged earlier. Walsh & Ford (1990, p.147) point out that any statement refuting the merits of the Nursing Process is therefore a myth.

Practice Assessment Document (PAD)

In the Assessment of Performance section of the PAD, it's quite clear that the student must maintain consistent, safe and person-centred practice based on the best available evidence. Precise, clear and understandable documentation of all facets of the care delivered is vital. Where appropriate, digital technologies should be employed – digitised care plans are now more commonly used in practice. The student is able to access the patient's care plan on the move, cutting time spent on examining paperwork and sitting at a desk away from the patient. Care planning encourages partnership working and shared decision making with your patient, their family and carers. The process directs nursing interventions and supports the person's potential for self-management.

Because feedback is a crucial part of the learning process, it is important that you seek regular evaluations of your care planning skills. The goals you write and the decisions you make regarding the required nursing interventions following your assessment should be discussed with your PA and PS during your time in each placement. You should also take the opportunity to discuss the Nursing Process, care planning and nursing models with your peers, sharing ideas and thoughts about the systems used. You may want to use this feedback and the skills and knowledge accrued to teach others who have less experience. Finally, the student should reflect on their progress, identifying strengths and areas for development.

A Systematic Approach

Hall & Richie (2009, p.67) comment that the Nursing Process offers a systematic approach to planning and delivering nursing care using a problem-solving cycle in which the needs of the individual patient are taken into account. Howatson-Jones *et al.* (2012, p.55) highlight that this systematic method integrates assessment information with decisions made about care. It includes critically thinking about potential nursing interventions to develop a care strategy and then evaluating the outcomes of the care provided.

Jot This Down

Think about the care plans you've observed and used in practice.

· What sort of information do you look for when assessing your patient?
· What information is important?
· As you collect the data, are you already beginning to think about a plan for this individual?
· Are you thinking about nursing interventions and the evaluation of your actions?

You may have thought about objective data such as the symptoms associated with the patient's condition. If a patient is admitted to your ward with pyrexia or a swollen calf muscle or nausea and diarrhoea, this can be seen immediately and is quite clearly a symptom of an underlying condition. On the other hand, there is subjective data to be collected, which is personal to the patient, and it is necessary to question the patient (at the appropriate point) about their experiences to assemble a more complete picture of them. Both sets of data complement each other, and the assessment is also a time for establishing a meaningful nurse–patient relationship although this may not be the most immediate action possible if the patient's health problem is critical (Holland *et al.*, 2008, p.14).

Case Study

A 45-year-old male patient presents with a history of palpitations, light-headedness and a feeling of weakness and low energy for the past 4 weeks. His pulse is irregular and you can feel 'missed beats' when recording his pulse. When determining his apex beat, it always sounds louder when an ectopic impulse is evident. The patient seems to get more breathless at night when he lies down to sleep. He admits to a 'fluttering' in his chest, which radiates to his throat and he's feeling more breathless when mobilising. This has increased his anxiety levels and he's afraid that he may collapse and die at any minute. He is normally an outgoing person but the situation is now beginning to affect his mood and he feels depressed. He stopped socialising with his friends because of the way this makes him feel and he is concerned that it may be serious; he is now very frightened of what may happen and he has not wanted to talk about it to anyone. Although it has been difficult, he has continued to go to work. He is troubled that it may have had an effect on his productivity. If his boss notices this and given the current climate, he fears the company may sack him or look at making him redundant.

You can see from the above case study that it first draws attention to the patient's symptoms, the objective data, whereas the subjective data that follow expand on the information and add greatly to the information already assembled. The symptoms described provide us with the physiological response to what sounds like a cardiac arrhythmia (perhaps frequent atrial ectopics or atrial fibrillation). The individual's experience also describes symptoms but tells us much more. You not only have physiological data; you now have a measurement of the patient's psychological

well-being and the effect this condition is having on his work and social life. You can see how the two sets of data broaden the overall assessment and can help the nurse to lay down a suitable plan of action for the patient.

The four key steps of the Nursing Process have been illustrated in many texts over the years (Yura & Walsh, 1978; Roper *et al.*, 1985, p.14; Holland *et al.*, 2008, p.12; Howatson-Jones *et al.*, 2012, p.56). The main stages of this process are:

· **Assessment**
· **Planning**
· **Implementation**
· **Evaluation.**

Habermann & Uys (2005, p.3) went on to expand on the four phases:

· Collecting the information and assessing the patient
· Planning the care and defining the relevant objectives for nursing care
· Implementing actual interventions
· Evaluating the results.

They also considered that in some areas, further stages need to be added to these, one of which is 'making a diagnosis', and that all the stages 'guide the production of nursing care plans and documentation of care in all fields of nursing'. Matthews (2010, p.5) also points to the steps of the Nursing Process but includes the 'nursing diagnosis', placing it between assessment and planning. Assessment, Planning, Implementation and Evaluation (APIE, see Figure 4.1) now becomes Assessment, **D**iagnosis Planning, Implementation and Evaluation (ADPIE, see Figure 4.2).

Figure 4.2 represents a continuous loop and is a progression of actions that continually recycle as patient problems and priorities change or resolve (Matthews, 2010, p.7).

Myra Estrin Levine was said to be the first person to question the idea of the 'nursing diagnosis'. Marriner-Tomey & Alligood (1998) pay tribute to her work as a nursing theorist, whilst Bullough & Sentz (2000, p.179) go further, pointing to where she began her scholarly activities and her contribution to the concept of the

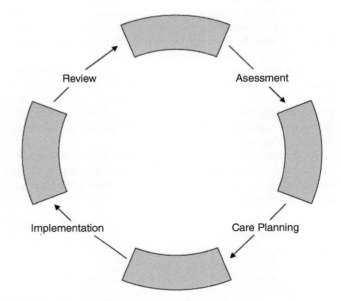

Figure 4.1 **The four phases of the Nursing Process.**

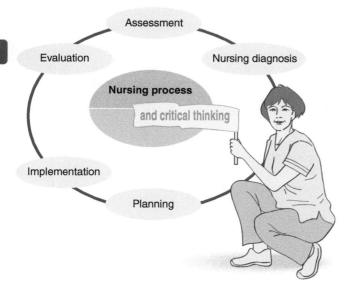

Figure 4.2 The four phases plus the nursing diagnosis. *Source:* Reproduced with permission from Matthews (2010)/Wolters Kluwer.

nursing process. As an author and principal investigator of a surgical dressing project at the University of Chicago (1952–3), Levine went on to contribute in 1966 to the concept of 'trophicognosis', a term she coined to replace 'diagnosis' which she felt to be incorrect and legally unsound when applied to nursing. She defined 'trophicognosis' as a nursing care judgement arrived at by the scientific method. 'Trophico' is derived from the Greek words *trophikos techne* and translates as the art of nursing, while 'gnosis' literally means knowledge. Trophicognosis is seen, then, as the applicatio of science n to resolve an individual's nursing care needs, suggested as an alternative to the term 'diagnosis'. Whether you want to call it a nursing diagnosis (ADPIE) or trophicognosis (ATPIE) is not a major issue; what Levine has highlighted here is the importance and significance of the art and science of nursing.

It is the nurse's task to bring a body of scientific principles on which decisions depend into the precise situation which is shared with the patient. Sensitive observation and the selection of relevant data form the basis for an assessment of nursing requirements. The essence of Levine's theory is that:

'When nursing intervention influences adaptation favourably, or toward renewed social well-being, then the nurse is acting in a therapeutic sense; when the response is unfavourable, the nurse provides supportive care. The goal of nursing is to promote adaptation and maintain wholeness'. (Levine quoted in Marriner-Tomey & Alligood, 1998, p.199)

At the beginning of the 1990s, Walsh & Ford (1990, p.144) commented that experience shows that many nurses still do not understand how to devise a care plan. The theory of care planning is simply not practised, they said.

Jot This Down

- Do you think this is still the case today?
- If so, why do you think this is?
- When using a care plan, do you tend to include and document information that is not relevant?
- Do you think it's all become a ritual?

You may have thought about the documentation you have used and that you have felt obliged to robotically complete all sections on the care plan. You may have become frustrated at the fact that you did not have the time or opportunity to sit down with the patient to identify their problems, whether they were actual or potential. For a lot of nurses, this becomes a source of irritation and switches the attention from the patient. The nurse wants to sit with the patient and discuss 'patient' problems so that they can collaborate and work in partnership and the patient can see from this that you place a value on their well-being and recovery.

Case Study

A 75-year-old man with a known history of ischaemic heart disease but no history of a previous myocardial infarction (MI) was admitted to the ward suffering from a sudden onset of severe angina; this was the worst pain he had ever suffered. On admission, he was very anxious with slight breathlessness. He was pain free having had a dose of nitrate (GTN) therapy whilst in the A&E department. The patient lives alone, his wife having died some years ago, and his only child, a daughter, now lives in Canada. Once I had settled him into bed and given him a cup of tea, I asked him if he had any worries. Thinking that he would share his fear that this time it may be a heart attack and the impact this may have on him being able to get back home and live a 'normal' life, I was surprised at his response to my question.

'My only worry at the moment', he said, was 'who is going to look after my dog? He is on his own in the house and will need feeding and taking out for his walk this evening.'

I immediately called his next-door neighbour (who he was very friendly with and holds a spare key to his house). She had already taken his dog to her house and wanted me to pass on the message that everything was fine and that the dog would be staying with her until he was discharged and well enough once more.

I passed on the message and the patient was extremely grateful and then said, 'I have no more worries, just do what you need to do and I can get home as soon as possible.'

Registered nurse, care of the elderly ward

Think about this case study, the registered nurse had presumed that the patient would share thoughts and feelings related to his medical condition and the symptoms he had been admitted with. However, his anxieties were completely different in terms of priority; this is unmistakably a patient-centred problem and is of no less concern.

Nursing Models

In their seminal work, Walsh & Ford (1990) demonstrated the rituals of clinical practice, examining the patient's day and comparing it to the nurse's day. They made recommendations for good practice, including an evaluation of the routine tasks we carry out and the need to ask patients what they want in order to improve their hospital stay and develop patient-centred care further. It was argued that many of the rituals that take place are staff centred, as getting the job done within a specific window of time was more important than dealing with the patients' needs on an individual basis. It seemed more more important to complete all the work before the staff on the late shift arrive rather than considering any wishes that the patient may have had. Not everyone wants to be woken at 6.30am to be given their medication; the patient may not want to be bathed first thing in the morning, opting instead for a bath during the afternoon or early evening.

Jot This Down

- What rituals have you noticed in practice?
- How should we deal with these issues for the benefit of the patient?
- Is the care on your ward/area patient centred or staff centred?

In this box you have been asked a number of key questions with relation to the way nursing work is organised. You may have thought about the habitual experience at office handover – a group of nurses huddled together for 20–40 minutes. In this time, we are expected to write down the important facts associated with the mass of information given to us. If you have four nurses in the office during handover, 20 minutes equates to almost 1.5 hours and 40 minutes becomes 160 minutes (in excess of 2.5 hours) of nursing time. Think about it!

Is it any wonder that when nurses on the late shift finally emerge from the handover, they spend the next few hours playing 'catch up', possibly missing a much-needed break later due to the obligation to recover that lost time? Walsh & Ford (1990, p.119) declare that a much more efficient use of time would be to have a bedside report for a group of patients for which one nurse is responsible. That way you have three or four reports going on at the same time but in the process, you cut the time down to 10–15 minutes, thus saving several nursing hours. This is also an opportunity to involve the patient in the process; patients will become part of the handover, contributing to the dialogue that takes place at the bedside. This is true patient-centred care, and much more resourceful, thus giving nurses the time to get on with other work.

Case Study

I was admitted to a rheumatology ward for treatment of my osteoporosis. I have managed to monitor and take my medication with no problems for the past 4 years. However, on arrival to the ward, the staff insisted on taking all my medication from me, telling me that from now on the staff will administer my tablets at the stipulated times on my medication sheet. I was not happy about this and I asked to speak to the nurse in charge. From their reaction to me, I think the staff are beginning to think I'm going to be a 'difficult' patient.

Female patient, aged 59 years

In the above scenario, what is your verdict? It is based on fact and you may want to reflect on it before you come to a conclusion. You could possibly think that this is perfectly reasonable and you may have witnessed this in practice. However, I think we need to ask ourselves a couple of questions here. Why do we need to take a patient's medication from them as soon as they are admitted to the ward? Do we need to be in control and thus deprive the person of patient-centred care? If the patient has been in control of her medication regime for that length of time without any problems, why remove their individual responsibility? What right have we to strip people of their uniqueness, dignity and independence? We must ensure that their self-determination is left intact and that they have the freedom to govern their lives. In fact, one of the chief recommendations of the Francis Report (2013, p.4) is the need to foster a common culture, shared by all in the service, of putting the patient first. Through collaboration, an improved recognition of the patient's contribution to self-care and open communication between nursing staff and patients, we can go some way to achieving this recommendation and help the patient seize control, safe in the knowledge that they have expert support available if necessary.

History and Principles

Walsh & Ford (1994, p.205) stated that much has been written about conceptual models of nursing, ranging from outright rejection of them as just another North American import we can do without, through to total slavish acceptance of a one-model-only approach. However, nursing models have also been seen as a set of frameworks based on the environment of care, the people involved in nursing activity, the health status of the patient or service user and the nursing capabilities and knowledge of the practitioner (Hinchcliff *et al.*, 2008). Howatson-Jones *et al.* (2012, p.80) argue that the nursing approach to care must vary according to the specialty of practice – nursing a patient with intensive care unit (ICU) needs is different from nursing a patient in an ambulatory care environment or in the community.

You can see that this chapter asserts that the patient is a unique individual with a series of differing healthcare needs. The use of a 'one-size-fits-all' model is therefore neither desirable nor practical. Fawcett (1992) observed that many nursing models lack a clear linkage to the clinical practice they seek to guide. As a model is tried in practice, staff should be reflecting on its strengths and weaknesses, changing and adapting the model, perhaps grafting and attaching sections of another model if it is philosophically consistent. Models would then be seen as more vibrant and forever evolving in reaction to the real world of nursing.

Jot This Down

Think about the model(s) of nursing you have used and been exposed to in practice.

- Did the model fit well within that specialty?
- Did you find it easy to use or understand?
- If you had no framework to help you focus, how would this affect your practice?

> **Box 4.1** The 12 activities of living (Roper, Logan and Tierney, 1985)
>
> 1. Maintaining a safe environment
> 2. Communication
> 3. Breathing
> 4. Eating and drinking
> 5. Controlling body temperature
> 6. Working and playing
> 7. Expressing sexuality
> 8. Elimination
> 9. Personal cleansing and dressing
> 10. Mobilising
> 11. Sleeping
> 12. Dying/Fears for the future*
>
> * The final activity of living is dying; this is not always relevant when dealing with the individual. However, when assessing patients against the 12 activities it will always be relevant to gauge and consider any fears that the patient may have. It's true, he may fear death or he may be apprehensive about his impending operation or medical condition. In any event, the nurse must ascertain any angst the patient presents with. As has been highlighted in this chapter, it may be the smallest of issues that has the most profound effect on the patient. More often than not, the nurse can easily deal with such issues and alleviate the worries and so minimise the patient's fears.

You may have used the most familiar framework here in the UK – the Roper, Logan and Tierney (1980, 1981, 1983) model of nursing. You may possibly have applied Orem's self-care model (1980, 1985) or perhaps Roy's adaptation model (1980, 1984) or a combination of models (all cited in Aggleton & Chalmers, 1986). Thinking back, if you used Roper, Logan and Tierney's model, for example, it may have helped you to understand each of the 12 activities of living (Box 4.1) – assisting patients to return to an independent state using the dependence to independence continuum (Roper *et al.*, 1985; Holland *et al.*, 2008).

The Roper, Logan and Tierney Model

The use of the Roper, Logan and Tierney activities of living model helped me to both appreciate and focus on the individual patient. When using the model in my everyday practice, it became clear that no matter what the patient's medical condition, it was the nursing model that helped to shape my nursing practice. It allowed for true patient-centred care and when applied, the 12 activities of living meant that the patient's requirements and needs were dealt with in an efficient manner.

Jot This Down

Imagine you are getting up for work. From the moment your alarm clock rings, the 12 activities of living will become noticeable, but it will not enter your consciousness as these things have become a part of your everyday life.

If you were to think consciously about the 12 activities as you wake up and get ready for work, what would you discover about them and how much they influence everything we do?

To illustrate this, I'd like you to think about the 12 activities (see Figure 4.3) as they relate to you as an individual.

This may seem like a pointless exercise but it should become clearer once you've done it. To put the activities into this context may help you appreciate your patients' needs in both health and illness.

So, you awake (**sleeping**), you'll take your first breath of the day (**breathing**, of course this is an unconscious response), you may say good morning to a loved one (**communication**), you'll get out of bed (**mobilising**) and go to the bathroom (**elimination and personal cleansing and dressing**). After this you may go back to the bedroom to put on your uniform (**personal cleansing and dressing**), you will probably put some make up on and brush your hair or if you're a male, you may have shaved in advance (**expressing sexuality**). Once ready, you'll go to the kitchen to prepare some breakfast and make a hot drink (**eating and drinking**). You may be thinking about the day ahead and the visit to the gym after work (**working and playing**). Breakfast over, it's time to get your coat on; the weather outside will dictate your choice of clothing as you will want to be comfortable for the journey to work (**controlling body temperature**). Depending on your mode of transport, you will be mindful of a safe trip and what is required when driving, cycling or simply crossing the road (**maintaining a safe environment**). Finally, you may be thinking about certain anxieties related to specific issues in your social life, family relationships or work (**fears for the future**).

It could be argued that nursing models, when used correctly, can assist nurses, providing a sound structure and, as Walsh & Ford (1994, p.206) point out, guiding the nurse away from irrelevant areas, whilst directing their attention to the way problems are understood and goals are set. They should also influence how interventions are carried out and evaluated.

> **Case Study**
>
> A 38-year-old man in the community has recently been diagnosed with diabetes; he is a heavy smoker, overweight and eats a lot of convenient/fast foods. He lives alone, is unemployed and has a family history of heart disease. His blood pressure is within a normal range at 130/78 mmHg but his cholesterol is above the normal level. He does very little exercise due to a previous back injury sustained in his last job when working on a building site as a hod carrier. Given this short history, using Roper, Logan and Tierney's model, what are the key factors to consider from a nursing perspective?
>
> Discuss this with your colleagues and your mentor.

From a 'universal self-care' perspective, it is clear that the patient's standard of living puts him at risk for impaired cardiovascular functioning and perhaps this is related to lack of knowledge about the connection between his current lifestyle and the potential threat of a myocardial infarction or stroke. He may also have little understanding of his increased vulnerability caused by the onset of diabetes. The 'self-care deficit' is the difference between his knowledge base and his life choices, all of which increase the undoubted risk to his cardiovascular health. A salutogenic plan of care must include interventions that will help him to reduce the risks to his well-being.

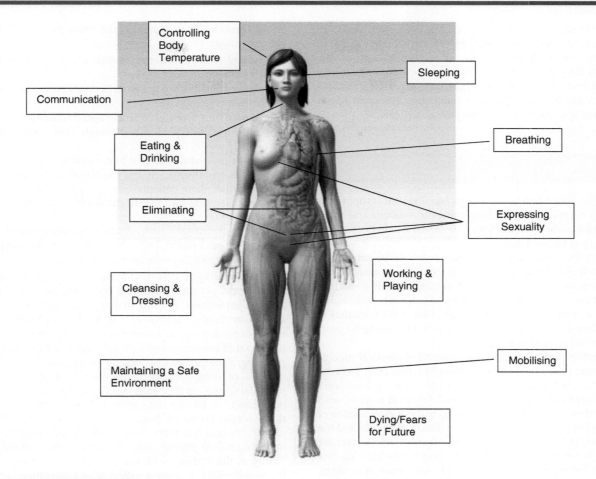

Figure 4.3 The 12 activities of living.

The nurse will aim to develop an agreement with him to help reduce his cholesterol level.

Asking the patient to keep a food diary, teaching him about foods high in fats and the effect that this has on the cardiovascular system will allow him to think about foods that have a lower cholesterol content. The importance of gentle exercise and reducing his smoking habit will be discussed and he will be encourage to think about what he can do to achieve his goals. Strategies will be considered and examined together, the nurse assisting the patient in his decision making and allowing him to manage the situation. You can see from this that the nurse directs and guides the patient, teaching him along the way, providing psychological support and ensuring that it is done in a sympathetic environment.

Jot This Down

Think about how the model helps you deliver consistent care. What evidence do you think about and use to inform your practice when writing down the nursing interventions section of your care plan?

You may have thought about the importance of communicating with your patient, educating and informing him and understanding the importance of building a nurse–patient relationship.

The NHS Plan (Department of Health, 2000) emphasises the importance of patient-centred care and service user involvement. Crawford *et al.* (2002) highlight that in England and Wales the involvement of patients is central to current efforts to improve the quality of healthcare. The belief generally is that putting patients at the centre of care will lead to more services that are available and will help to develop the health and quality of life of patients. Ward (2011) comments that:

'We as nurses have a responsibility to tend to our patients' needs, but we have an equal responsibility to teach. Providing "care" means ensuring that patients are fully educated about their condition and their proposed treatments. Through education, patients can be made aware of their disease process and potential treatment options'.

Furthermore, she highlights that through teaching and empowering our patients, we are giving them the tools they need to manage their disease process and that managing the disease process will result in fewer hospitalisations and an improved quality of life. The positive results of effective communication are well documented and are essential in achieving, amongst other things, increased recovery rates, a sense of safety and protection, improved levels of patient satisfaction and greater adherence to treatment options. Aside from these, successful communication through a patient-centred approach also serves to reassure relatives that their loved ones are receiving the necessary treatment. Within the nursing field, such skills are considered indicative of best practice (McCabe & Timmins, 2006). You can see that such models allow nurses to focus on exactly what skills the patient possesses and what he actually knows to care for himself. Once the nurse uses their expertise in assessment, they can then put into place the appropriate approach to support and lead patients down the path to self-care.

Conclusion

This chapter shows that when using a Nursing Process approach to care, all nurses can benefit from using the structure and when combining a nursing model with this method, it helps support the delivery of high-quality care.

Many critics have judged nursing models to be excessively abstract, with little place in modern nursing. Wimpenny (2002) examines many of the criticisms of nursing models and highlights features such as their complexity of language, inflexibility and lack of rigorous testing. Others add that nursing models as promoted by theorists and educators have made little or no positive impact on clinical practice.

Wimpenny points to the suggestion that theoretical models may be more valuable as tools for thought rather than tools for use. Kaplan (1964) comments on the fact that nursing models are often presented as some final truth and defended as such, with the result that they attract pros and cons without examination of their worth or limitations. Numerous critics in the media and the general public have declared on many occasions that nurses are spending too much valuable time away from the bedside, placing too much emphasis on the input of data onto ward computers. Add to this the feeling that nursing students spend a lot of their time studying and that this could be better utilised with their patients.

It's easy to criticise the design of the way we organise care; perhaps the answer to this lies in the way we apply nursing models and the Nursing Process in practice. The framework helps to support our nursing practice but we need to make sure we use it to our advantage. Nurses need to be more confident when using care plans and models. The framework is like a skeleton, it provides an outline, and the essential action for nurses is to build the muscle, sinew and exterior around the frame in an attempt to enhance our assessment of patients and deliver excellence in healthcare. For student nurses, a model provides a comprehensive guide to each stage of care planning. The more experienced you become, the more you will be able to develop your own ideas based on the theoretical concepts, which will help free you from the limitations that some authors so often highlight.

When beginning my nurse education and training in the 1970s, I experienced a system that was largely based on directives from such things as the procedure manual, the bath book and the dressings book. During my time as both a student nurse and a newly qualified practitioner, it was quite clear that nursing was considered as supplementary to the medical team, and was not thought of as an independent profession. The introduction of the Nursing Process and nursing models seemed to emancipate a lot of nurses at the time (including me) and although many colleagues regarded them as vague and unclear, the benefits seemed to be clear to many.

As nurses began to appreciate the whole process, the benefits shone through.

- It helped to support communication between the nurse and their patients
- It allowed patients to participate in decisions made about them and their ongoing care
- It allowed the nurse and patient to spend valuable time together
- It improved safety of care through open communication channels
- It was a very useful education tool, especially for student nurses
- It enhanced information and the nurses had better access to information about patients
- Patients felt that staff valued them and dealt with their individual needs
- The time spent with patients was used appropriately helping them to understand their condition and the preparation required to give them the best care available.

If we are using models and the Nursing Process appropriately, assessing the person against their individual needs and requirements, then why are we using so many risk assessment questions and an increasing number of risk assessment tools when the model of nursing should include all of these factors? The key is to develop staff awareness and for them to extend their skills in care planning; a comprehensive ongoing assessment linked to patient activities of living, for instance, should help the nurse to identify potential dangers to their safety and in doing this we can take the opportunity to involve the patient fully in the process to avoid the potential for harm. Regular, active patient involvement in identifying care that meets their needs should cover all aspects, including risk to patient safety, comfort, health and well-being. Sitting at the bedside with the care plan and engaging more frequently with your patient will result in a more meaningful dialogue, not just chitchat but something much more –a therapeutic partnership, one that is supportive and compassionate, putting the patient at the centre of everything we do, which is the measure of quality.

Key Points

- This chapter has provided the reader with an understanding of the Nursing Process and nursing frameworks, with a particular emphasis on the Roper, Logan and Tierney 12 Activities of Living model.
- It has highlighted the importance of the key stages of the Nursing Process, a systematised assessment and the influence of a robust nursing diagnosis.
- The use of the 12 Activities of Living model contributes to a solid nursing assessment, allowing the patient to be seen as an individual, thus adding to the safe delivery of care and contributing to the quality agenda.
- The nurse will also begin to understand how this method enhances the nurse–patient partnership through good communication skills, helping to build a therapeutic relationship.
- The promotion of patient healthiness and well-being is also emphasised through salutogenesis, which focuses on the relationship of health, stress and the person's self-management of health. Used in tandem with the Nursing Process, salutogenesis looks towards problem solving using the resources presented.

References

Aggleton, P. & Chalmers, H. (1986) *Nursing Models and the Nursing Process*. Macmillan, London.

Benner, P. (2001) *From Novice to Expert: Excellence snd Power in Clinical Nursing Practice*. Prentice Hall, Upper Saddle River, NJ.

Bullough, V.L. & Sentz, L. (eds) (2000) *American Nursing: A Biographical Dictionary*, vol. 3. Springer, New York.

Clark, J. & Lang, N.M. (1992) Nursing's next advance: an international classification for nursing practice. *International Nursing Review*, 38(4), 109–112.

Crawford, M.J., Rutter, D., Manley, C., *et al.* (2002) Systematic review of involving patients in the planning and development of health care. *British Medical Journal*, 325, 1263.

de Bronkart, D. & Sands, D.Z. (2018) Warner Slack: 'Patients are the most underused resource'. *British Medical Journal*, 362, k3194.

Department of Health (2000) *The NHS Plan: A Plan for Investment, A Plan for Reform*. Stationery Office, London.

Department of Health (2006) *Modernising Nursing Careers: Setting the Direction*. HMSO, London. www.nursingleadership.org.uk/publications/settingthedirection.pdf (accessed December 2021).

Fawcett, J. (1992) Conceptual models and nursing practice: the reciprocal relationship. *Journal of Advanced Nursing*, 17(2), 224–228.

Ford, P., Heath, H., McCormack, B. & Phair, L. (2004) *What a Difference a Nurse Makes: An RCN Report on the Benefits of Expert Nursing to the Clinical Outcomes in the Continuing Care of Older People*. RCN, London.

Francis, R (2013) *Report of the Mid Staffordshire Foundation Trust Public Enquiry*. Stationery Office, London.

Girvin, J., Jackson, D. & Hutchinson, M. (2016) Contemporary public perceptions of nursing: a systematic review and narrative synthesis of the international research evidence. *Journal of Nursing Management*, 24, 994–1006.

Grimette, H. (2021) Has COVID-19 changed the public perception of nursing? https://ounews.co/education-languages-health/health/has-covid-19-changed-the-public-perception-of-nursing/ (accessed December 2021).

Habermann, M. & Uys, L. (eds) (2005) *The Nursing Process: A Global Concept*. Elsevier Churchill Livingstone, Edinburgh.

Hall, C. & Ritchie, D. (2009) *What is Nursing? Exploring Theory & Practice*. Learning Matters, London.

Hinchcliff, S., Norman, S. & Schober, J. (eds) (2008) *Nursing Practice and Health Care*, 5th edn. Hodder Arnold, London.

Holland, K., Jenkins, J., Solomon, J. & Whittam, S. (2008) *Applying the Roper, Logan and Tierney Model in Practice*, 2nd edn. Churchill Livingstone, Edinburgh.

Howatson-Jones, L., Standing, M. & Roberts, S. (2012) *Patient Assessment and Care Planning in Nursing*. Learning Matters, London.

Kaplan, A. (1964) *The Conduct of Inquiry, Methodology for Behavioral Science*. Chandler, San Francisco, CA.

Lukose, A. (2011) Developing a practice model for Watson's theory of caring. *Nursing Science Quarterly*, 24(1) 27–30.

Marriner-Tomey, A. & Alligood, M.R. (1998) *Nursing Theorists and their Work*, 4th edn. Mosby, St Louis, MO.

Matthews, E. (2010) *Nursing Care Planning Made Incredibly Easy!* Wolters Kluwer/Lippincott, Williams and Wilkins, London.

May, R. (2018) *The Future is Here and Nursing is Ready*. www.england.nhs.uk/2018/05/the-future-is-here-and-nursing-is-ready/ (accessed December 2021).

McCabe, C. & Timmins, F. (2006) *Communication Skills for Nursing Practice*. Palgrave Macmillan, Basingstoke.

Miller, A. (1985) Nurse patient dependency: is it iatrogenic? *Journal of Advanced Nursing*, 10(1), 63–69.

Nursing & Midwifery Council (2015) *The Code: Professional Standards of Practice and Behaviour for Nurses and Midwives*. NMC, London.

Nursing & Midwifery Council (2018) *Standards of Proficiency for Registered Nursing Associates*. www.nmc.org.uk/standards/standards-for-nursing-associates/standards-of-proficiency-for-nursing-associates/ (accessed December 2021).

Ozdemir, N.G. (2019) The development of nurses' individualized care perceptions and practices: Benner's Novice to Expert Model Perspective. *International Journal of Caring Sciences*, 12(2), 1279–1285.

Patterson, J. & Zderad, L. (2007) *Humanistic Nursing*. www.gutenberg.org/ebooks/25020 (acccessed December 2021).

Pelikan, J.M. (2017) The application of salutogenesis in healthcare settings. In: M. Mittelmark, S. Sagy & M. Eriksson (eds) *The Handbook of Salutogenesis*, pp.261–266. Springer, Cham.

Pokorski, S., Moraes, M.A., Chiarelli, R., Costanzi, A.P. & Rabelo, E.R. (2009) Nursing process: from literature to practice. What are we actually doing? *Rev Latino-am Enfermagem*, 17(3), 302–307.

Rizk K. & Almond, P. (2013) Salutogenesis and Antonovsky's Sense of Coherence Scale: a literature review in relation to self-management of diabetes. *Working Papers in Health Sciences*, 1(5), 1–11.

Roper, N., Logan, W.W. & Tierney, A.J. (1985) *The Elements of Nursing*, 2nd edn. Churchill Livingstone, Edinburgh.

Royal College of Nursing (2003) *Defining Nursing*. RCN, London.

Royal College of Nursing (2010) *Engaging with the Principles of Nursing Practice: Guided Reflection for Nursing Students*. RCN, London.

Skretkowicz, V. (ed.) (1992) *Florence Nightingale's Notes on Nursing* (Revised with additions). Scutari Press, Middlesex.

Vinje, H.F., Langeland, E. & Bull, T. (2016) Aaron Antonovsky's development of salutogenesis, 1979 to 1994. In: M. Mittelmark, S. Sagy & M. Eriksson (eds) *The Handbook of Salutogenesis*, pp.25–40. Springer, Cham.

Walsh, M. & Ford, P. (1990) *Nursing Rituals: Research and Rational Action*. Heinemann Nursing, Oxford.

Walsh, M. & Ford, P (1994) *New Rituals for Old: Nursing through the Looking Glass*. Butterworth Heinemann, Oxford.

Ward, J. (2011) How to educate patients. www.nursingtimes.net/roles/nurse-educators/how-to-educate-patients-25-05-2011/ (accessed December 2021).

Watson, J. (1991) *Watson's Philosophy and Theory of Transpersonal Caring*. | Nurse Key https://nursekey.com/7-watsons-philosophy-and-theory-of-transpersonal-caring/ (accessed December 2021).

Wimpenny, P. (2002) The meaning of models of nursing to practising nurses. *Journal of Advanced Nursing*, 40(3), 346–354.

Yura, D. & Walsh, M.B. (1978) *The Nursing Process: Assessing, Planning, Implementing and Evaluating*. Appleton Century Crofts, New York.

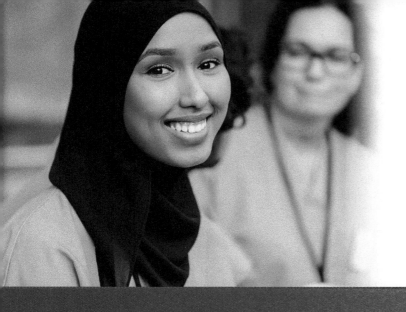

5

The Resilient Nurse

Georgiana Assadi

King's College London, UK

Learning Outcomes

On completion of this chapter, you will be able to:

- Develop an understanding of the concept of resilience
- Be able to differentiate between recovery and resilience within the context of health and social care
- Improve your awareness of the importance of resilience within your own nursing professional practice
- Understand the link between resilience, personal health and the ability to provide person-centred care as highlighted by the NMC
- Apply strategies and approaches in order to develop your own levels of resilience.

Proficiencies

NMC Proficiencies and Standards:

- Demonstrate resilience and emotional intelligence and be capable of explaining the rationale that influences their judgments and decisions in routine, complex and challenging situations
- Acknowledge the need to accept and manage uncertainty, and demonstrate an understanding of strategies that develop resilience in self and others.

 Visit the companion website at www.wiley.com/go/peate/nursingpractice3e where you can test yourself using flashcards, multiple-choice questions and more.

Nursing Practice: Knowledge and Care, Third Edition. Edited by Ian Peate and Aby Mitchell.
© 2022 John Wiley & Sons Ltd. Published 2022 by John Wiley & Sons Ltd.
Companion website: www.wiley.com/go/peate/nursingpractice3e

Introduction

Healthcare is an ever-evolving field that faces as many challenges as it does successes. Advances in healthcare and support have meant changes in population demographics, showing an ageing population within the UK (Office for National Statistics, 2019), treatment advances meaning that long-term conditions are also on the rise (Department of Health, 2012), and the use of technology being part of innovation within healthcare (Department of Health and Social Care, 2018). Yet, despite the growth occurring within the last decade, healthcare remains a complex area, with many current challenges such as staffing issues (NHS England, 2020), the Covid-19 pandemic, and a demand for services superseding what can be delivered by the NHS at present. Therefore, to survive and thrive within a nursing role, there is a developing demand that individuals need to be resilient in order to be caring, competent and provide excellent levels of care and support for the populations accessing services.

What is Resilience?

Definitions of resilience within the literature often use the word as an overarching term, without acknowledging its intersected nature. Therefore, definitions and understandings of resilience need to be contextualised and discussions should be focused on defining resilience as being a trait, a process or an outcome (Southwick et al., 2014). Table 5.1 shows how resilience as a trait process or outcome may be defined. Regardless of the context, a key underlying factor is that resilience is a continuum; it may be more or less evident, in varying levels across numerous aspects of an individual's life (Pietrzak & Southwick, 2011). When relating resilience to the health and social care environment, it can be described as the ability of an individual, group, community or population to endure and adapt in the face of adverse circumstances (World Health Organization, 2017); however, this ability (whether it be individual skill, process or outcome) is dynamic and fluid in nature.

Jot This Down

Reflecting on your own resilience, do you think it is a trait, a process or an outcome for you and why?

Table 5.1 **Defining areas of resilience.**

RESILIENCE AS A:	DEFINITION
Trait	A quality a person has which helps them execute an action successfully. This can be innate or a quality that is developed through learning
Process	When a series of actions or steps are taken to adapt and promote optimal levels (for the individual) of mental and/or physical health despite adversity
Outcome	When mental or physical health and well-being are maintained despite adversity

Resilience is not something 'extraordinary' that is born of rare occurrences in life; in fact, it can develop from everyday living and can be shaped and influenced by the individual and their exposure to risk during their lives and ability to function in a positive manner despite this. It is also influenced by the environment and the societal ecosystem (including culture) (Shean, 2015) that a person is surrounded by. Therefore, everyone has some level of resilience; however, the degree of resilience varies from person to person based on the situational challenges presented (both negative and positive) in their lives. Some individuals may be more resilient than they are aware of, and others may be resilient to particular types of stresses and not so much or at all with others (Bonanno, 2004). Furthermore, access to resilience may be greater at certain points in their lives compared to others due to varying factors such as the economic, social or cultural technological resources able to the individual and how these are utilised (Southwick et al., 2014).

Resilience and Health

Resilience is also closely linked to concepts relating to health, whether this be on an individual (micro) or a population (macro) level. When looking at this relationship, health can be defined as 'the ability to adapt and self-manage in the face of social, physical, and emotional challenges' (Huber et al., 2011), with a focus being on the individual and their health. Health and the notion of resilience are interlinked, and it is key to take a holistic approach by understanding that there is a plethora of bio-psycho-social factors that may be impacting an individual's life in a positive or negative way and therefore shaping levels of resilience. In order for an individual to develop their own resilience levels, their behaviours, thoughts and feelings need to be reflected on, developed and nurtured, as they form part of the personal aspects which can achieve positive health and well-being outcomes.

Resilience and Recovery: Is It the Same?

Within healthcare, there is often mention of the importance of 'recovery', which refers to an individual having a life that has meaning to them (Rethink Mental Illness, 2021). Recovery is underpinned by the control, hope and opportunities an individual has after a period of poor/undesired health or poor/undesired well-being. This therefore suggests that in order for someone to 'recover', their health and well-being must have deviated from their norm at some point, causing some change in the individual's ability to function in their 'normal' manner. This is different from the notion of resilience, which is when an individual is able to endure and adapt in the face of adverse circumstances, so despite the challenges the individual faces, they are able to maintain a stable equilibrium (Bonanno, 2004) through the harnessing of internal or external means. The focus of recovery therefore differs greatly from that of resilience, and so when evolving understandings of resilience it is helpful to think of it as 'a stable trajectory of healthy functioning' (Southwick et al., 2014) after an adverse event, with the 'healthy functioning' being individual to each person and how they moved forward despite what they have experienced.

Understanding Resilience: Models and Approaches

Historically, three main models were developed which aimed to explain resilience, from an ecological perspective (Garmenzy *et al.*, 1984). The protective, compensatory and challenge models all explore the dynamic influences that make up an individual's resilience levels. The protective model explores the relationship between a protective factor counteracting a risk factor that is present, reducing the likelihood that the outcome is negative. In the compensatory model, a resilience factor works in the opposite direction of a risk factor, which in turn has an effect on the outcome. Lastly, the challenge model shows a curvilinear connection between a risk factor that is present and an outcome. It details that exposure to high and low levels of risk is linked with poorer outcomes for an individual, whereas moderate-risk levels are linked to less negative or less positive outcomes for the individual. Table 5.2 provides some real-life examples of each model contextualised within the healthcare environment.

The work by Garmenzy *et al.* (1984) underpins each model with the understanding that there are individual traits that form part of resilience, as well as familial support and support

Table 5.2 Contextual examples of each model in the healthcare environment.

MODEL TYPE	REAL-LIFE EXAMPLE
Compensatory model	A child being exposed to a high-conflict home environment but who has a loving and close relationship with a grandparent. Resilience may be influenced by the relationship with the grandparent compensating for the difficult home environment
Protective model	A family may be living below the poverty threshold but have a loving, supportive home environment, where family members support each other to achieve. The family dynamic interacts with the poverty to reduce risk
Challenge model	Student nurses being exposed to moderate levels of risk, e.g. a medication error being fixed by their practice assessor in the first year of practice before the patient is given medication, are confronted with enough of the risk factor to learn how to overcome it, but are not exposed to so much of it that overcoming it is impossible, e.g. the patient being given the medication error and perhaps dying, which then can negatively affect the student and perhaps cause them to stop their course

available to individuals and families within the community or wider society. Protective or positive factors are also key aspects that inter-relate dynamically to help an individual navigate adversity in some way, regardless of how big or small, and therefore underpin the notion that resilience is something that can be developed and that everyone can access in their lives.

Resilience: Protective Factors

Protective factors are one of the most importance aspects of resilience building. A protective factor can be individual in nature, can stem from family and loved ones (and the relationships built) or can be as a result of the community and environments people find themselves in (Fleming & Ledogar, 2008). Protective factors are therefore particular conditions, attributes or resources that an individual, family, community or society can access to help to manage adversity and contribute to developing resilience in a positive manner.

The use of protective factors can aid the growth of resilience to strengthen the individual's ability to overcome adversity. Protective factors may also contribute to the notion of resilience itself and be integrated in nature to help people grow through adversity, or be something innate which helps people to continue to develop their resilience in a dynamic manner (Fleming & Ledogar, 2008). This highlights that resilience can be promoted on an individual, community or population level and also the benefits of preventive approaches in developing resilience even before adversities may be experienced.

As the research around the notion of resilience continues to be developed, there is no unanimous list of protective factors that promote resilience, but there are key themes that are often cited in the literature and which can be grouped into individual-level protective factors, family-level factors and community or societal-level factors. Fleming & Ledogar (2008) offer an adapted list of key components and resources available at the varying levels to promote resilience (Figure 5.1, Tables 5.3 and 5.4).

Jot This Down

Considering the individual, family and community/societal resources that can promote resilience, what protective factors help you manage when you feel you are having a 'bad' day?

Resilience from an Individual Perspective

On an individual level, the development of resilience is positive for the individual but it is also a process that is inter-related with external factors such as family dynamics, societal influences and the type of adversity faced. With this inter-related approach to developing resilience, a link between Maslow's Hierarchy of Needs (Maslow, 1943) (Figure 5.2) and resilience can be established. Through the fulfilment of the varying stages of need, a positive effect can be felt by the person, even when the achievements have

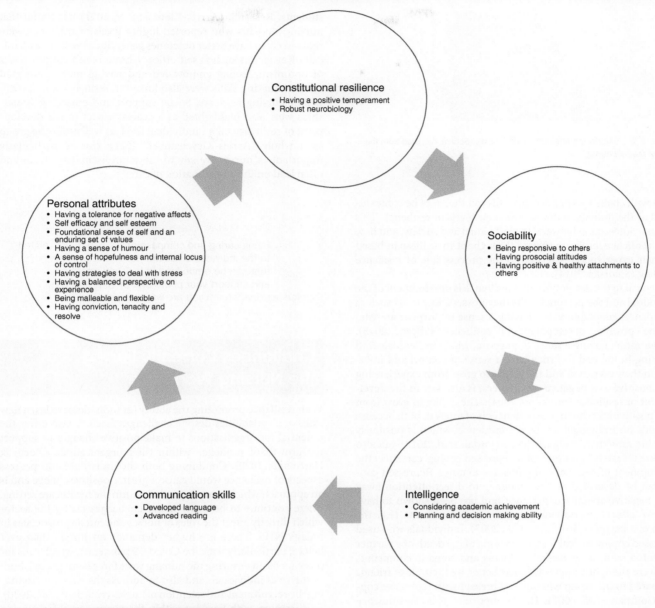

Figure 5.1 **Individual resources to promote resilience building.**

Table 5.3 **Family-level resources to promote resilience building.**

Supportive families	Parental warmth, encouragement and assistance
	Cohesion and care inthe family
	Having a close relationship with a caring adult
	A non-blaming environment
	Support between partners
	Having talents or hobbies valued by others
Socio-economic status	Having access to material resources needed

Table 5.4 **Community or societal-level resources to promote resilience building.**

School experience
· Having supportive peers
· Having positive teacher influences
· Experiencing success (academic or other)
Supportive communities
· Belief in the individual
· Non-punitive in nature
· Provisions and resources available to assist belief in the values of society
Cultural resources
· Traditional activities

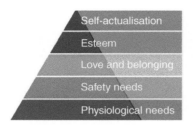

Figure 5.2 Maslow's Hierarchy of Needs. *Source:* Adapted from the work of Maslow (1943).

come with challenges or adversity; this can therefore be contextualised as the individual developing their levels of resilience. This dynamic interaction between the individual and society, and how their resilience levels are shaped throughout their lifespan based on their experiences, is related to the process side of resilience building (Sikorska, 2014).

Central to the development of resilience is development of the individual and the personal traits they possess. Key traits such as confidence, adaptability and having a sense of purpose are vital in the positive development of resilience (Shean, 2015). Furthermore, having a sense of purpose, where individuals find meaning in life and feel they have a sense of control and influence in their own lives and the ability to grow from experiencing both positive and negative experiences, is also key in the development of resilience (Bonanno, 2004). The ability to grow from both positive and negative experiences is of interest, both because it builds on individual levels of confidence, which is positively linked to growth in resilience levels (Jordan *et al.*, 2018), but also because research has shown that 'repressed coping' can affect the development of resilience in a positive manner. Repressed coping can be described as 'the tendency to direct attention away from negative affective experience' and has been shown to have positive effects in individuals after traumatic events (e.g. the death of a partner) (Coifman *et al.*, 2007). Individuals who used repressed coping to deal with the trauma of the death of a partner presented with fewer health problems and somatic complaints and were thought to have adjusted better by their close friends compared to the group who did not present with repressive coping (Coifman *et al.*, 2007). This is important as it can influence the interventions and approaches in building resilience that individuals may attempt.

Psychosocial resilience is made up of individual protective factors paired with the social resources the individual can access at any given time to allow them to mentally or emotionally cope with an adversity or challenge. Those noted to have higher levels of resilience, even when exposed to negative experiences, are able to disengage from the emotions created by those experiences more quickly than those with lower levels of resilience (Yi *et al.*, 2020). This is beneficial as the individual is able to protect themselves from feeling worse in light of the emotions they experience in the negative situation, and it prevents the escalation of those emotions reaching a point where they might feel overwhelmed, which is what occurs for individuals with lower levels of resilience.

Intertwined with the individual, process and outcome aspects of resilience is the importance of education, which has been shown to improve the development of resilience in nursing students. Research (Arries-Kleyenstüber, 2021) has found that nursing students who reported higher levels of resilience were more likely to have better outcomes generally, as well as academically. Key factors such as self-efficacy, levels of self-esteem, levels of optimism, feeling empowered and having more developed critical thinking skills were also linked to resilience and growth within nursing students. Social support and emerging friendships were also highlighted as a crucial aspect in the development of resilience on an individual level, as well as for the group as a whole (Arries-Kleyenstüber, 2021); this is particularly important as nurses are key to the multidisciplinary team and often lead on the co-ordination of care.

Caring, Dignity and Compassion

Being caring and compassionate is not just related to the individuals you are nursing; it is something that can be embedded in how you approach and support your peers and members of the multidisciplinary team you are working with.

Challenges Currently Facing the Nursing Workforce

With resilience promoting the ability for individuals to learn new skills and capabilities despite challenges faced, it also offers the potential for organisations to make positive changes to support the growth of resilience within their organisations (Hoegl & Hartmann, 2020). Combining both the individual and process aspects of resilience would cause a greater positive change and is an approach which is much needed within the healthcare setting. There continue to be many major challenges facing the sector which directly affect the roles of nurses and nursing associates in today's NHS. There are higher demands on nurses than ever before, particularly with the Covid-19 pandemic, which calls for more focus on ensuring the nursing workforce is supported, both to thrive as individuals and also to address the issues surrounding the recruitment and retention of nurses (Henshall *et al.*, 2020). Furthermore, with burnout within the nursing workforce being an issue (Marangozov *et al.*, 2017) and the link to how an individual is able to manage their stress levels (Evans *et al.*, 2020), the time is ripe to ensure the nursing workforce is resilient and given every opportunity to thrive and provide excellent levels of care. One way of doing this is through education and preparing the workforce of tomorrow (nursing students and nursing associate students) whilst also offering training and support for qualified nurses in relation to resilience (Reyes *et al.*, 2015).

Why Resilience is Important within the Nursing Profession

As one of the largest workforces within the NHS and growing since the introduction of nursing associates, those within the nursing profession (students included) are the professional group who spend the most time overall with individuals who access support from health and social care services. This is both a privilege and a challenge in the current health and social care climate because of the issues presented by working in today's NHS.

The nursing workforce (and the NHS) are experiencing many changes which directly relate to the nursing workforce such as the following.

- Integrated care being at the forefront of how the NHS works and will continue to be shaped, meaning new ways of working (NHS, 2019).
- An increase in demand for health services occurring at a time when nursing workforce numbers are not at optimum levels (NHS England, 2020).
- Advances in technology and access to information being readily available to the populations nurses look after, which is beneficial as well as challenging (Hutchings, 2020).
- Recent changes have occurred to the proficiencies expected of nursing students, as well as qualified nurses, meaning not just new expectations of the workforce but also new ways of supporting student nurses and nursing associates within the theoretical and practical aspects of their training (NMC, 2018a).

Jot This Down

Considering some of the challenges that the nursing workforce might face, what examples have you come across within clinical areas and how have they been managed? Can you think of any other challenges which you have seen or experienced on your placement that have affected the nursing workforce? Write down your thoughts and reflections.

Resilience and The Nursing and Midwifery Council Code of Conduct

The Nursing and Midwifery Council Code of Conduct (NMC, 2018c) details the professional standards that UK nurses, midwives and nursing associates must uphold. The NMC is also the regulatory body for nurses, midwives and nursing associates practising within the UK. There are four main areas into which standards are grouped.

1. Prioritise people
2. Practise effectively
3. Preserve safety
4. Promote professionalism and trust

Nurses must practise in line with the Code of Conduct and should not deviate away from the professional standards detailed above, as this could result in anything from a caution to a sanction, to conditions of practice being put into place or complete removal from the NMC register, meaning an individual is no longer allowed to work as a qualified, registered nursing professional in any setting.

The NMC Code aligns well with the 6 Cs (Figure 5.3), which when initially revealed were for the nursing workforce only

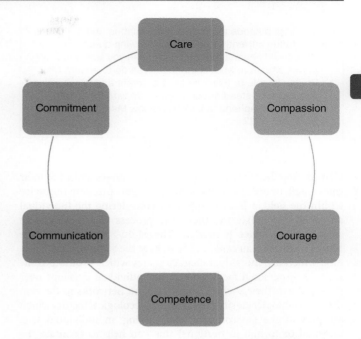

Figure 5.3 **The 6 Cs.** *Source*: Adapted from NHS England (2012).

(NHS England, 2012) but have since been rolled out for the whole NHS workforce.

The 6 Cs are:

1. Care
2. Compassion
3. Competence
4. Commitment
5. Courage
6. Communication.

There are key themes across both the NMC Code and the 6 Cs that can be directly linked to the ability of an individual to be resilient in their nature and approach. However, contextualising resilience and what that may look like for nurses and nursing associates is complex because of the uniqueness that comes with training and practising as a nurse. In order to be an 'excellent nurse', one must be analytical, communicative, co-operative, co-ordinating, be able to disseminate information effectively, be knowledgeable, empathic, evidence driven, innovative and introspective (Paans *et al.*, 2017).

Case Study

Saphena is a newly qualified nurse working on an inpatient unit for older adults and one of the people admitted to the unit, Ms Brogan, has a diagnosis of vascular dementia and a suspected UTI (urinary tract infection). Saphena walks over to ask how Ms Brogan how she is feeling and administer her morning medication. When Saphena arrives to the bedside, she is confronted with Ms Brogan telling her to 'Get lost! I don't even like you, you've got no idea what the hell you are talking about, how can you, you're a child half my age!'

Ms Brogan needs to have here medication and the unit is short-staffed currently. Answer the following questions.
- How would hearing that outburst make you feel and why?
- In this situation, what could the nurse do to ensure Ms Brogan is able to focus on her treatment and her morning medication instead of her displeasure with the nurse?
- Who could Saphena talk to about how Ms Brogan has made her feel?

Considering the variety of expectations of nurses and what their roles entail, in order to understand what may promote resilience within the field, a holistic approach considering the individual and how they relate to others, the process and the outcome aspects of resilience is needed. The Multi-Systems Resilience Model (MSRM) (Liu *et al.*, 2017) looks at the intraindividual factors, which are individual characteristics which promote resilience; interpersonal factors which an individual develops over time through their social interactions and networks to develop their psychological resilience; and socio-ecological factors which are part of the environment surrounding an individual (e.g. informal or formal institutions) that can help to facilitate the development of resilience and is representative of wider community influences. Considering this model, it can be deduced that the intraindividual and intrapersonal factors are areas that a nurse can focus the development of their resilience on, as the socio-ecological factors, whilst they may have significant influences, cannot always be changed as readily. Some examples of socio-ecological factors which might affect the individual are challenges the NHS faces at scale, the policies and approach of varying institutions like the NMC or the NHS or the trust they work for, perceived social status, or the influence of the media on the nursing workforce and public perceptions.

Therefore, the following are proposed as the six key areas (detailed in Table 5.5) which the nurse or nursing associate can work on to develop their own levels of resilience.

1. Confidence
2. Adaptability
3. Having a sense of purpose
4. Cultivating meaningful social connections
5. Managing one's emotions, both independently of others and in relation to interacting with others
6. Having a sense of hope and capability

What the Experts Say

'I was supposed to finish work at 20:00 hrs, but I ended up finishing at 21:30 hrs. I felt mentally and physically exhausted and had to move the dinner plans I had with my partner which made me feel awful. When I got home, I just wanted to sleep. The next day me and my partner spoke about my long day at work the day before. I remember him saying 'How can you look after patients if no one is looking after you?'. He was right, and that was the push I needed to go into work and ask my manager to give me/the team an update on the concerns we had raised over the short-staffing issue.'

Registered mental health nurse, working in a psychiatric intensive care unit.

Table 5.5 **Six areas for promoting resilience within the nursing workforce.**

AREA	DESCRIPTION
Confidence	Having confidence in yourself and your ability in general, but also in being able to overcome adversity
Adaptability	Being able to easily change to suit different conditions or situations that may arise. If the situation is new and one does not know how to adapt, the willingness to learn is key
Having a sense of purpose	Being consciously aware of what gives purpose and meaning to your life
Cultivating meaningful social connections	Forming and maintaining good-quality relationships from which you can draw learning and support and in return provide support to others
Managing one's emotions, both independently of others and in relation to interacting with others	For both positive and negative experiences, be able to adapt your emotional response to match whatever the situation demands, e.g. if an individual you are caring for has said something hurtful to you, manage your emotions, remain professional and maintain your composure in the moment and find an appropriate outlet for your emotions outside this interaction
Having a sense of hope and capability	Adopt an encouraging outlook in which you feel you can achieve a constructive outcome for yourself in any given situation, despite the challenges presented. Where you lack the capability to do this, you reflect and enhance your knowledge to help you thrive in the future

Within the NMC Code of Conduct there are key aspects which are expected of nurses and nursing associates that are directly linked to the underpinnings of resilience.

8.7 Be supportive of colleagues who are encountering health or performance problems. However, this support must never compromise or be at the expense of patient or public safety. *This is linked to cultivating meaningful social connections in light of difficulty.*

13.4 Take account of your own personal safety as well as the safety of people in your care. *This is linked to cultivating meaningful social connections and managing emotions, as emotions can affect how a nurse behaves, which in turn can affect the emotions and behaviours of those interacting with the nurse (such as individuals being supported) (Bergquist, 2009).*

20.3 Be aware at all times of how your behaviour can affect and influence the behaviour of other people. *This is linked managing one's emotions, both independently of others and in relation to interacting with others, as emotions can affect how a nurse behaves, which in turn can affect the emotions and behaviours of those interacting with the nurse (such as individuals being supported by nurses, or those working alongside them) (Bergquist, 2009).*

20.9 Maintain the level of health you need to carry out your professional role. *This is linked to having a sense of hope and capability, as if your health is affected, you can reflect and/or enhance your knowledge to help you continue to thrive.*

25 Provide leadership to make sure people's well-being is protected and to improve their experiences of the health and care system.

25.1 Identify priorities, manage time, staff and resources effectively and deal with risk to make sure that the quality of care or service you deliver is maintained and improved, putting the needs of those receiving care first.

25.2 Support any staff you may be responsible for to follow the Code at all times. They must have the knowledge, skills and competence for safe practice, and understand how to raise any concerns linked to any circumstances where the Code has been, or could be, broken.

The above three areas (25, 25.1 and 25.2) are linked to cultivating meaningful social connections and managing emotions in yourself and supporting others to develop their own levels of resilience.

Red Flag

If a colleague appears to be struggling, burnt out and/or non-responsive to the expectations of their role, this can affect patient care and should be escalated and managed immediately.

Today's Nurse and Nursing Associate

2018 was a transformational year for the nursing workforce as this was when the NMC reviewed and updated the standards of proficiency for registered nurses and nursing associates (NMC, 2018a,b). Within these two documents, the NMC highlighted the domains, skills and behaviours expected of nurses and nursing associates in today's healthcare environment. A common theme that runs between both documents is the parity between physical health and mental health and taking a person-centred approach to care regardless of the field of practice a nurse or a nursing associate is working in. This is a positive as it means all nurses and nursing associates will have the same foundations, which they can then build on within their own fields of practice as students and once they become registered. This will result in a workforce which is more adaptable to the needs of service users.

A further positive of this is that in the current climate where there are fewer nurses than desired, particularly within the mental health and learning disabilities field (Nuffield Trust, 2018), nurses within the child and adult nursing fields can still offer some basic level of care in relation to the mental health needs of individuals across the lifespan and have some insight into the challenges for those living with diverse neurological conditions. Moreover, mental health and learning disabilities nurses, whose skills and training are focused on building meaningful therapeutic relationships with people experiencing mental health difficulties or those with diverse learning needs, can now ensure that they promote the physical health of the individuals they build relationships with to a basic standard.

This approach builds on the ethos of integration and hopes to reduce the lack of personalisation in care that individuals with multifaceted and complex needs are often faced with when they navigate the NHS for help and support. It also means that individuals with diverse neurological conditions and those experiencing challenges with their mental health will have better outcomes in relation to their lifespan and quality of life, which has been an ongoing issue when compared to the general population (Kinnear *et al.*, 2018; Cullen *et al.*, 2020).

Within both documents there are key platforms, skills and procedures that are closely linked to the notion of resilience within nurses and nursing associates. Both documents also align to how student nurses and nursing associates are assessed when they are in the clinical aspects of their courses through their practice assessment documents (PADs) and ongoing achievement records (OARs). There is a clear emphasis on the accountability of the individual in that 'they must be emotionally intelligent and resilient individuals, who are able to manage their own personal health and well-being, and know when and how to access support' (NMC, 2018a). Considering the six areas where a nurse or nursing associate can develop resilience detailed above in Table 5.5, Table 5.6 depicts the platforms, skills and procedures that can be aligned to the importance of resilience within the workforce.

In addition to the platforms linked to resilience detailed in Table 5.6, other platforms can be linked to resilience in a more complex manner. If the nurse or nursing associate is resilient, they are inherently more likely to be reflective in their mindset, which is linked to greater levels of knowledge and the potential to educate the individuals they are looking after to improve their own knowledge and levels of resilience in the face of adversity (health, well-being, environmental or societal).

This is also true of all the Annex A communication and relationship management skills and Annex B procedural skills of the Future Nurse proficiencies. For Annex A, the ability to competently execute the communication and management skills listed is linked with one's resilience and ability to cultivate meaningful social connections (with individuals being cared for as well as peers from the multidisciplinary team). For Annex B, the ability to competently execute the procedures required is linked with one's ability to form a robust therapeutic relationship, whereby an individual trusts a clinician (student or qualified), or a clinician is able to pick up on cues to support the assessment, planning and management of appropriate care. This links back to resilience and the ability to cultivate meaningful social connections (with individuals being cared for).

Table 5.6 Platforms that nurses and nursing associates are expected to have proficiency in which align to being resilient. *Source:* Adapted from NMC, 2018a,b).

PLATFORMS LINKED TO RESILIENCE	NURSING OR NURSING ASSOCIATE
Platform 1.6 Understand the professional responsibility to adopt a healthy lifestyle to maintain the level of fitness and well-being required to meet people's needs for mental and physical care	Nursing
Platform 1.10 Demonstrate resilience and emotional intelligence and be capable of explaining the rationale that influences their judgements and decisions in routine, complex and challenging situations	Nursing
Platform 6.11 Acknowledge the need to accept and manage uncertainty, and demonstrate an understanding of strategies that develop resilience in self and others	Nursing
Platform 1.6 Understand the professional responsibility to adopt a healthy lifestyle to maintain the level of personal fitness and well-being required to meet people's needs for mental and physical care	Nursing associate
Platform 1.8 Understand and explain the meaning of resilience and emotional intelligence, and their influence on an individual's ability to provide care	Nursing associate
Platform 5.9 Recognise uncertainty and demonstrate an awareness of strategies to develop resilience in themselves. Know how to seek support to help deal with uncertain situations	Nursing associate

Practice Assessment Document

PAD example of a proficiency that student nurses are assessed on in the second part of their nursing course: *Demonstrates awareness of strategies that develop resilience in themselves and others and applies these in practice, e.g. solution-focused therapies or talking therapies.*

What you can do: take the learning you do in relation to solution-focused therapies, cognitive behavioural approaches or mindfulness (just some examples) and do not just advise the people you are supporting to do it to promote their health and well-being, try it yourself as a way of helping you develop your own well-being and resilience levels!

Jot This Down

Choose a skill from Annex A or a procedure from Annex B and link it back to any of the six domains of resilience (see Table 5.5). Can you see the link between what you do professionally and your own personal health and well-being?

Resilience and Emotional Intelligence

Resilience and emotional intelligence (EI) are themes which are detailed in the NMC's views of what the nursing workforce should be (NMC, 2018a,b), as well as being something that is needed in ensuring the NHS is able to fulfil its promise of improving the experiences of those working within the NHS and those accessing support from the NHS (NHS, 2019).

Emotional intelligence can be defined as 'The ability to monitor one's own and others' feelings, to discriminate among them, and to use this information to guide one's thinking and action' (Salovey & Mayer, 1990, p.189). It focuses on how an individual is able to perceive, understand, use and manage emotions; for the most part their own, but in some areas those of others, e.g. perception of another's emotions as a cue to understand what the individual may be going through (Salovey & Grewal, 2005). Initially theorised in the 1990s by Salovey & Mayer (1990), it was further developed and conceptualised by Goleman (1995) who highlighted five key areas which an individual who is emotionally intelligent possesses: self-awareness, self-regulation, motivation, empathy and social skills.

Emotional intelligence can be used in a prosocial manner or an antisocial manner, which means emotionally intelligent people have the opportunity to use their abilities in a positive or negative way (Salovey & Grewal, 2005). Being emotionally aware allows individuals to regulate their own emotions, which within a challenging area such as healthcare is vital for developing the personal health and well-being of nurses and nursing associates despite the challenges faced. It also allows the building of constructive relationships founded on clinicians being responsive to the emotions of the individuals they are supporting, whilst being able to regulate emotions to ensure that they do not affect professionalism or the care being provided regardless of the challenge (Box 5.1).

Box 5.1 Five key areas of emotional intelligence (EI) adapted from the work of Daniel Goleman (1995)

1. *Self-awareness*: being aware of your emotions and how they may impact others.
2. *Self-regulation*: having control over your emotions and being able to redirect unhelpful impulses and gain a level of control, which allows you to think before taking action.
3. *Motivation*: having the ability to face obstacles and achieve your goals.
4. *Empathy*: being able to sense and understand the emotions of others, which can then help you understand their needs.
5. *Social skills*: being able to constructively manage relationships with others by listening and responding fittingly.

The Benefits of Emotional Intelligence Within Healthcare

Emotional intelligence has many benefits, some of which can be directly linked to providing better levels of care. It can promote positive experiences for student nurses, as well as encourage professional development and better communication skills (Judge *et al.*, 2018). It has also been aligned to nurturing collaboration (Judge *et al.*, 2018), which when working within new integrated systems is a significant benefit (and need) as the nursing workforce works closely alongside other members of the multidisciplinary team, the individuals being cared for and their families in a collaborative manner as a key aspect of person-centred care.

Caring, Dignity and Compassion

Remember that you may be a member of the nursing workforce at one point in your career and then at another point you may need to access support from health and social care services. It is important you are caring, competent and professional always, as that is what you will be expecting of those looking after you!

How is Emotional Intelligence Linked to Resilience?

To be resilient, an individual must be able to manage their own emotions, be reflective, form meaningful relationships with others and have a sense of purpose (Ledesma, 2014). Emotional intelligence contributes to the protective factors that help build resilience by aiding an individual to manage their own emotions effectively, reflect on themselves and others, develop their planning and management skills when faced with issues, contribute to how they solve problems in a situation that may arise and promote self-esteem (Ledesma, 2014).

Case Study

Reuben is on placement with a palliative care team in the community. He is on a home visit with an occupational therapist (OT) to reassess Mr Abdullah's mobility and install aids to promote mobilisation. Mr Abdullah has a diagnosis of stage 4 metastasised lung cancer and has been told that his prognosis is between 3 and 6 months to live at the most. The OT and Reuben arrive at the house to find paramedics giving CPR (cardiopulmonary resuscitation), as there was no DNA CPR in place. Reuben starts to feel overwhelmed by this and is on the verge of tears, as Mr Abdullah is only 37 years old and had his whole life ahead of him. He is married and has a young child.

Explore the following issues.

· Death is something that healthcare professionals are exposed to as part of their role. What have been your experiences of death and bereavement so far?
· Is it OK for Reuben to cry whilst out on that home visit? Yes or no, and why do you think that?
· Are there certain types of death that you are more comfortable with processing than others and why is that?
· What could Reuben do to help manage his emotions during and after the home visit?
· What do you do to help you process difficult issues?

Good social relationships are proven to improve well-being in individuals, and to help develop resilience as a nurse or nursing associate, so having meaning relationships that are supportive, whilst also being able support others (e.g. people accessing services), is key (Kansky & Diener, 2017). To cultivate these constructive relationships both within the professional remit and in personal life, an individual must have social skills and the ability to communicate effectively with others, which is linked back to being emotionally resilient and emotionally intelligent.

Caring, Dignity and Compassion

If you develop your emotional intelligence, this will help you provide better care to the individuals you support as you will become more self-aware, in control of your own emotions and less likely to act in an emotional manner without thinking, which could affect a therapeutic relationship with someone in need of support. Remember, being ethical and professional but also emotionally intelligent is a difficult balance within nursing, but it is an essential part of the role!

Approaches to Developing Resilience

Knowing that there is a clear link between resilience and an individual's health and well-being, it is therefore imperative that nurses, nursing associates and students look after themselves in order to be able to provide excellent levels of care. Whilst approaches to developing resilience are personal and individual in nature, this section will offer a variety of strategies that any nurse, nursing associate or student can try (and suitably adapt) to enhance their own levels of resilience. A proactive, two-pronged approach will be taken that considers the personal and professional ways in which resilience may be developed.

The Development of Resilience on a Personal Level

The six areas for promoting resilience within the nursing workforce that were proposed earlier (see Table 5.5) will be used as a means of exploring potential approaches and strategies to developing resilience on a personal level.

Building Confidence

Working within healthcare can add more challenges to an already busy life. Practising mindfulness, individually and in a group setting, has been shown to increase baseline levels of self-esteem (Pepping *et al.*, 2013). There are many self-directed or teacher-directed mindfulness sessions you can go to on your own or as part of a group. If you want to practise a bit of mindfulness, try this 3-minute breathing space meditation or hourglass meditation (adapted from the work of Williams & Penman, 2011) to help you be a little more mindful of what you are feeling, thinking and experiencing at any moment.

Step 1: Becoming Aware Get yourself comfortable in your seat. You can move around or adjust your position at any point during the meditation to help you feel comfortable.

You are welcome to close your eyes or lower your gaze – do whichever feels comfortable for you.

72

Take a moment to focus on your breath and consciously be aware of where you feel your breath the most. Is it in your chest, perhaps with an inhalation or exhalation, or do you feel your breath in your mouth, or is it felt most in your nostrils? Make a note of wherever it is felt for you. Remember not to try and change your breath in any way; the idea is to be mindful in this moment.

Now, imagine you have a wide field of awareness, both inside and outside your body. Take a moment to notice what you are feeling in this moment. What are your thoughts? What body sensations are you experiencing? Be curious. Observe things in a non-judgemental way. Take a mental note of any of these.

Step 2: Focusing Your Attention Take a moment to refocus on your breath and consciously be aware of where you feel your breath the most. Remember not to try and change your breath in any way; the idea is to be mindful in this moment and give you the opportunity to anchor yourself to the here and now with each breath.

If your mind wanders, that is OK. Non-judgementally escort your attention back to your breath each time this happens.

Step 3: Expanding Your Attention Now, expand your conscious awareness, from focusing on your breath alone to focusing your breath into your whole body. What do you notice by doing this? Whilst you are exploring the sensations you are experiencing, remember to befriend them and try not to change them in any way.

See if you can be aware of a sense of wholeness or completeness in yourself, fully accepting and non-judgemental, remembering that it is OK to be just who you are in this moment. Take a few seconds to slowly prepare yourself to open your eyes and continue with your day. Stretch if you find that comfortable and take the time you need before opening your eyes or re-engaging your gaze and ending the meditation.

What the Experts Say

" 'It was difficult for me to adapt during the peak of my mental illness. The negative thoughts far superseded the positive ones, and I was left fearing even my own thoughts. That being said, my inner optimism to return to "normal" kept pushing me towards recognising my strengths and doing things to take care of myself and my mental health. Music and meditation and being mindful were the defining factors as they allowed me to either change my thoughts or release them entirely. Without that hint of optimism, I wouldn't have acknowledged my self-worth and wouldn't have made such a speedy recovery.'

Expert by experience: person with a lived experience of first-episode psychosis

---

Being Adaptable and Having a Sense of Hope and Capability

Adaptability is a multifaceted state but the link between being adaptable and better health and well-being outcomes can be underpinned by one's outlook on life; the use of positive psychology is noted to reduce health risks in healthy individuals in the short term (Park *et al.*, 2016). One way to develop adaptability on a personal level is to have a constructive outlook on life, which entails acknowledging that there are challenges in life (both on a personal and a professional level) which you can address to some extent in a positive manner. This may be by choosing to accept

there is nothing further you can do in a situation or seeking out support to work out a new path or doing some research or reading to broaden your knowledge base as a means of cultivating new ways of addressing challenges you are faced with.

Jot This Down

Think about something that you feel that you cannot do and write it down. Next write down the reason why you 'cannot' do that thing. Afterwards write down anything you have tried to do to overcome the challenge; if you have tried nothing, just write 'nothing'. Finally, present the problem to other people as a hypothetical case and see what they would do and make a note. Or do some research on the challenge area and see what studies, field experts or evidence you can find on the challenge you are facing and decide on one new way of attempting to overcome your challenge that you have not tried before.

Having a Sense of Purpose

The ability to be consciously aware of what gives purpose and meaning to your life is something that can promote resilience in the face of adversity, whilst also improving aspects of mental health like the ability to better manage anxieties and worries (Schippers & Ziegler, 2019). 'Life crafting' (Schippers & Ziegler, 2019) is a tangible way in which an individual can consciously explore aspects of their lives as a way of promoting the development of a sense of meaning, purpose and direction.

Using the structure detailed in Figure 5.4, adapted from the work of Schippers and Ziegler, you can consciously nurture what meaning and purpose you want in your life. You have the choice to use any medium to help you 'life craft': writing lists, writing in a journal, creating a visual artefact like a vision board, creating a mind map of your vision, or perhaps collating pictures, words and to-do lists all in one place like a collage.

Cultivating Meaningful Social Connections

Forming and maintaining good-quality relationships, from which you can draw learning and support and in return provide support to others, is key for building resilience. Even in the face of trauma (such as going to war), the research shows that individuals with meaningful social connections are more resilient (Pietrzak & Southwick, 2011). Whilst working in nursing differs from fighting in a war, there are some similarities in the challenges faced, including experiencing high levels of stress within the work environment, being at the forefront of the loss of human life and having to navigate an ever-changing environment where there are multiple competing demands.

An approach which can help develop constructive relationships in your personal life is to be sure to actively listen when you are communicating with people. The skill of active listening is both an art and science. Active listening is a two-way, active form of communication founded on being empathetic, paying attention, respecting the other person and making a conscious effort to listen to what is being said (taking into account non-verbal cues) with the sole intention of understanding them and their viewpoint. It is key to avoid the temptation to think of your response whilst the other person is actively speaking to you, thus promoting being fully present in that moment (Weger *et al.*, 2014).

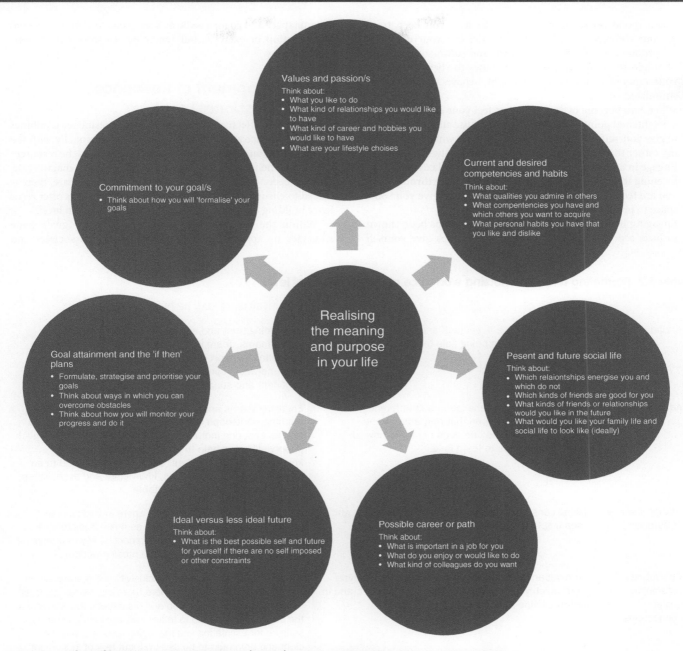

Figure 5.4 Life crafting your way to purpose and meaning. *Source:* Modified from Schippers & Ziegler (2019).

Managing Your Emotions

Being able to adapt your emotional response to match whatever the situation demands, regardless of whether the feeling/emotion is positive or negative, will develop your ability to process things rationally and therefore respond or behave in a constructive way. There are a variety of ways in which to become more emotionally intelligent with regard to managing emotions.

- Reflect on the impact of your emotions by picking a situation and reflecting on what happened. Think about how you felt and how you behaved. Reflect on why you felt the way you did and if your behaviour was constructive or destructive in that situation. Lastly, think of one or two ways in which you might react differently or what might help you cope better with what you are feeling if the same situation, e.g. someone shouting at you unfairly, happens again. It helps to think of these options when you are not emotionally stimulated.

- Remember that managing your emotions is not about ignoring them or pretending they do not exist. Sometimes our bodies can give us cues about how we are feeling, so if you cannot 'name' the emotion, think about what you are feeling in your body or mind. Are you feeling tense? Or are you feeling 'blank' mentally'? Reflecting on this will help you navigate why you might be feeling that way.

- Accept your emotions because it is OK to have feelings, no matter how horrible or difficult they might be.

- Use a mood board or mood diary to help you keep track of your feelings and what may be affecting your emotions to promote your own reflection and ultimately growth in understanding yourself and how to better regulate your emotions and how you might behave when you are stimulated.
- When you become overwhelmed or feel your emotions are at a heightened point, do not be afraid to pause and take a breath to give yourself a moment or two to 'sit' with what you are feeling rather than acting/behaving instantaneously.
- Engage in activities or hobbies that generally relax you such as listening to music, reading, gardening or talking through how you are feeling with someone else as these can give you some space to process your emotions.
- Engaging in some degree of physical activity has been shown to have a positive effect on mood, so perhaps give yourself

some space and go for a walk, do some yoga or some movement meditation or exercise, but remember to work within your own ability.

The Development of Resilience on a Professional Level

In order to be effective, the development of resilience combines the self-resilience an individual can develop personally with the environments and societies in which people live and the resources available to help the development of resilience on a macro scale. Therefore, considering the challenges within healthcare, there is a need to ensure workplaces and professional settings offer resilience building on a team, community and population level.

Within the healthcare environment, Table 5.7 gives some strategies or approaches that nurses, nursing associates and

Table 5.7 Promoting a resilient nursing workforce at the professional level.

AREA	DESCRIPTION	HOW RESILIENCE CAN BE PROMOTED AT WORK
Confidence	Having confidence in yourself and your ability in general, but also in being able to overcome adversity	By building trust and a sense of shared responsibility within teams. Team building days, staff meetings and a mentoring/support ethos within the workplace can help build individual confidence within the team, as well as a confident and supportive team overall
Adaptability	Being able to easily change to suit different conditions or situations that may arise. If the situation is new and one does not know how to adapt, willingness to learn is key	Engaging teams and individuals in postincident debriefs, learning workshops and reflective practice sessions, as well as ensuring individual case management supervision, can help to promote the sharing of knowledge and techniques, which in turn can add to an individual's 'tool kit' of skills, knowledge and approaches, thus making them more adaptable
Having a sense of purpose	Being consciously aware of what gives purpose and meaning to your life	Prioritising supervision sessions where individuals can discuss their current role, as well as other aspects such career goals and plans for development, is key to promoting resilience and retention within the nursing workforce
Cultivating meaningful social connections	Forming and maintaining good-quality relationships from which you can draw learning and support, and in return provide support to others	Actively nurturing a culture of inclusivity and respect within the workplace is a priority. Where there are issues, such as bullying, poor team cohesion and disrespect, this can affect the care being provided to individuals accessing services, so lines for escalating and managing issues should be clear and promoted to be used without fear of judgement
Managing one's emotions, both independently of others and when interacting with others	For both positive and negative experiences, have the ability to adapt your emotional response to match whatever the situation demands, e.g. if an individual you are caring for has said something hurtful to you, manage your emotions, remain professional and maintain your composure in the moment and find an appropriate outlet for your emotions outside this interaction	Facilitation of clinical team supervision where individuals can be honest about how they feel and why and others actively listen can help promote relationships within the workplace which are constructive despite differences Individuals being able to take breaks within the workplace regardless of the demands
Having a sense of hope and capability	Adopt an encouraging outlook in which you feel you can achieve a constructive outcome for yourself in any given situation, despite the challenges presented. Where you lack the capability to do this, you reflect and enhance your knowledge to help you thrive in the future	Utilising official and unofficial means of support is key to enhancing knowledge and awareness. This can be via engaging with a practice assessor, practice supervisor or academic assessor (for students), seeking support from lecturers (for students), having an allocated coach or mentor in the workplace, or approaching a peer for mutually agreed mentorship or coaching informally

students can access as a means of developing resilience within themselves, as well as encouraging the organisations and cultures in which they work to effectively address issues. Once again, the examples listed will be aligned to the six areas for promoting resilience within the nursing workforce presented earlier in the chapter (see Table 5.5).

Why Resilience Within the Nursing Workforce is Needed Now More Than Ever

With the ethos of integrated care being at the forefront of the NHS and the delivery of healthcare, healthcare is a changing landscape which brings new challenges with how the nursing workforce work within their own field, and also how nurses lead on and support the co-ordination of care in partnership with the multidisciplinary team and beyond. Paired with integration is the drive for technology to form an active part of care and so the nursing workforce has to be receptive and resilient to deal with technological challenges such as misinformation, use of applications, data sharing and public views on the use of technology within healthcare. Another topically relevant area is the effects of the Covid-19 pandemic and its suspected after-effects, such as a potential growth in mental health needs of the population, physical and mental health complications of 'long Covid' and the burnout potential for staff increasing due to the longevity of the pandemic. These continued challenges create a need for resilience across the workforce in order to survive and thrive during these challenging times.

Staff shortages within nursing have been an endemic issue spanning the last 20-plus years and are unlikely to be rectified within the next 5 years. Therefore, nurses and nursing associates will have to work smarter and be able to make difficult decisions based on the challenges that face them. It is therefore important that individuals build their own resilience levels as they will have to (when needed) be advocates for those accessing services by holding organisations and the government accountable for fulfilling promises on care expectations, staffing issues and system changes, as these directly affect patient care and safety.

Changes in the nursing profession since 2018 mean the qualified workforce and students have to adapt to new approaches and requirements in regard to teaching and learning. This means, for those already qualified, self-development and continuing professional development, which can add further to the time pressure challenges already faced by nurses and nursing associates when working clinically.

Lastly, as resilience is something that can be continually developed, nurses, nursing associates and students being resilient themselves means that they are 'experts' in their own well-being. This means they are even better placed to share their knowledge, the approaches and processes related to developing resilience as part of the education and health promotion work they do when supporting individuals accessing services within their fields of practice.

Key Points

- Resilience is key on an individual level, as well as on a societal level, but has been defined in many ways to date.
- This chapter highlighted that a resilient nurse is only as effective as the working environment they are part of, therefore it is important that the organisation has an ethos of resilience and acts upon making this ethos a reality.
- Nurses need to be resilient to effectively support others with their well-being. However, it is also the role of the nurse or nursing associate to educate others on promoting their own resilience.
- The chapter has offered some approaches to developing resilience on an individual level, but it is key to note that resilience and its development are individual in nature and the same approach does not work for everyone – so find what works for you!

References

Arries-Kleyenstüber, E.J. (2021) Moral resilience in nursing education: exploring undergraduate nursing students perceptions of resilience in relation to ethical ideology. *SAGE Open Nursing*, 7. doi: 10.1177/23779608211017798.

Bergquist, W. (2009) The Johari Window: exploring the unconscious processes of interpersonal relationships and the coaching engagement. *International Journal of Coaching in Organizations*, 7(3), 73.

Bonanno, G.A. (2004) Loss, trauma, and human resilience: have we underestimated the human capacity to thrive after extremely aversive events?' *American Psychologist*, 59(1), 20–28.

Coifman, K.G., Bonanno, G., Ray, R. & Gross, J. (2007) Does repressive coping promote resilience? Affective-autonomic response discrepancy during bereavement. *Journal of Personality and Social Psychology*, 92(4), 745–758.

Cullen, W., Gulati, G. and Kelly, B.D. (2020) Mental health in the COVID-19 pandemic. *Quarterly Journal of Medicine*, 113(5), 311–312.

Department of Health (2012) *Long Term Conditions Compendium of Information*, 3rd edn. Department of Health, London.

Department of Health and Social Care (2018) *The Future of Healthcare: Our Vision for Digital, Data and Technology in Health and Care*. Department of Health and Social Care, London.

Evans, K., Nizette, D. & O'Brien, A. (2020) *Psychiatric and Mental Health Nursing in the UK*. Elsevier, Oxford.

Fleming, J. & Ledogar, R.J. (2008) Resilience, an evolving concept: a review of literature relevant to Aboriginal research. *Pimatisiwin*, 6(2), 7–23.

Garmenzy, N., Masten, A.S. & Tellegen, A. (1984) The study of stress and competence in children: a building block for developmental psychopathology. *Child Development*, 55, 97–111.

Goleman, D. (1995) *Emotional Intelligence: Why It Can Matter More Than IQ*. Bloomsbury, London.

Henshall, C., Davey, Z. & Jackson, D. (2020) Nursing resilience interventions – a way forward in challenging healthcare territories. *Journal of Clinical Nursing*, 29(19–20), 3597–3599.

Hoegl, M. & Hartmann, S. (2020) Bouncing back, if not beyond: challenges for research on resilience. *Asian Business and Management*, 20, 456–464.

Huber, M., Knottnerus, J., Green, L., *et al.* (2011) How should we define health? *BMJ (Online)*, 343(7817), 1–3.

Hutchings, R. (2020) *The Impact of Covid-19 on the Use of Digital Technology in the NHS*. www.nuffieldtrust.org.uk/files/2020-08/the-impact-of-covid-19-on-the-use-of-digital-technology-in-the-nhs-web-2.pdf (accessed December 2021).

Jordan, G., MacDonald, K., Pope, M., *et al.* (2018) Positive changes experienced after a first episode of psychosis: a systematic review. *Psychiatric Services*, 69(1), 84–99.

Judge, D.S., Opsahl, A. & Robinson, D. (2018) Collaboration between two schools of nursing: emotional intelligence education for prelicensure students. *Teaching and Learning in Nursing*, 13(4), 244–246.

Kansky, J. & Diener, E. (2017) Benefits of well-being: health, social relationships, work, and resilience. *Journal of Positive Psychology and Wellbeing*, 1(2), 129–169.

Kinnear, D., Morrison, J., Allan, L., *et al.* (2018) Prevalence of physical conditions and multimorbidity in a cohort of adults with intellectual disabilities with and without Down syndrome: cross-sectional study. *BMJ Open*, 8(2), 1–9.

Ledesma, J. (2014) Conceptual frameworks and research models on resilience in leadership. *SAGE Open*, 4(3). doi: 10.1177/2158244014545464.

Liu, J.J.W., Reed, M. & Girard, T.A. (2017) Advancing resilience: an integrative, multi-system model of resilience. *Personality and Individual Differences*, 111, 111–118.

Marangozov, R., Huxley, C., Manzoni, C. & Pike, G. (2017) Royal College of Nursing Employment Survey 2017. www.rcn.org.uk/professional-development/publications/pdf-007076 (accessed Decembe 2021).

Maslow, A.H. (1943) A theory of human motivation. *Psychological Review*, 50(4), 370–396.

National Health Service (2019) *The NHS Long-Term Plan*. NHS, London.

National Health Service England (2012) *Compassion in Practice: Nursing, Midwifery and Care Staff. Our Vision and Strategy*. NHS, London.

National Health ServiceEngland (2020) *We are the NHS: People Plan 2020/21 – Action for Us All*. www.england.nhs.uk/wp-content/uploads/2020/07/We-Are-The-NHS-Action-For-All-Of-Us-FINAL-March-21.pdf (accessed December 2021).

Nuffied Trust (2018) *The NHS Workforce in Numbers. Facts on Staffing and Staff Shortages in England*. www.nuffieldtrust.org.uk/resource/the-nhs-workforce-in-numbers#3-what-do-the-shortages-mean-for-hospital-staffing (accessed December 2021).).

Nursing & Midwifery Council (NMC) (2018a) *Standards of Proficiency for Nursing Associates*. NMC, London.

Nursing & Midwifery Council (NMC) (2018b) *Future Nurse: Standards of Proficiency for Registered Nurses*. NMC, London

Nursing & Midwifery Council (NMC) (2018c) *The Code*. NMC, London.

Office for National Statistics (2019) *Living longer: Caring in Later Working Life*. www.ons.gov.uk/peoplepopulationandcommunity/birthsdeathsandmarriages/ageing/articles/livinglongerhowourpopulationischangingandwhyitmatters/2019-03-15 (accessed December 2021).

Paans, W., Robbe, P., Wijkamp, I. & Wolfensberger, M. *et al.* (2017) What establishes an excellent nurse? A focus group and delphi panel approach. *BMC Nursing*, 16(1), 1–10.

Park, N., Peterson, C., Szvarca, D., *et al.* (2016) Positive psychology and physical health: research and applications. *American Journal of Lifestyle Medicine*, 10(3), 200–206.

Pepping, C.A., O'Donovan, A. & Davis, P.J. (2013) The positive effects of mindfulness on self-esteem. *Journal of Positive Psychology*, 8(5), 376–386.

Pietrzak, R.H. & Southwick, S.M. (2011) Psychological resilience in OEF-OIF veterans: application of a novel classification approach and examination of demographic and psychosocial correlates. *Journal of Affective Disorders*, 133(3), 560–568.

Rethink Mental Illness (2021) *Recovery, Fact Sheets*. www.rethink.org/advice-and-information/living-with-mental-illness/treatment-and-support/recovery/ (accessed December 2021).

Reyes, A.T., Andrusyszyn, M., Iwasiw, C., *et al.* (2015) Resilience in nursing education: an integrative review. *Journal of Nursing Education*, 54(8), 438–444.

Salovey, P. & Grewal, D. (2005) The science of emotional intelligence. *Current Directions in Psychological Science*, 14(6), 281–285.

Salovey, P. & Mayer, J.D. (1990) *Emotional Intelligence. Imagination, Cognition, and Personality*. http://citeseerx.ist.psu.edu/viewdoc/download?doi=10.1.1.385.4383&rep=rep1&type=pdf (accessed December 2021).

Schippers, M.C. & Ziegler, N. (2019) Life crafting as a way to find purpose and meaning in life. *Frontiers in Psychology*, 10, 2778.

Shean, M. (2015) *Current Theories Relating to Resilience and Young People: A Literature Review*. Victorian Health Promotion Foundation, Melbourne.

Sikorska, I. (2014) Theoretical models of resilience and resilience measurement tools in children and young people. In: Ostrowski, T. & Sikorska, I. (eds) *Health and Resilience*,. Jagiellonian University Press, Cracow.

Southwick, S.M., Bonanno, G., Masten, A., *et al.* (2014) Resilience definitions, theory, and challenges: interdisciplinary perspectives. *European Journal of Psychotraumatology*, 5, 1–14.

Weger, H., Bell, G., Minei, E. & Robinson, M. (2014) The relative effectiveness of active listening in initial interactions. *International Journal of Listening*, 28(1), 13–31.

World Health Organization (2017) *Strengthening Resilience: A Priority Shared by Health 2020 and the Sustainable Development Goals*. WHO, Geneva.

Yi, F., Li, X., Song, X. & Zhu, L. (2020) The underlying mechanisms of psychological resilience on emotional experience: attention-bias or emotion disengagement. *Frontiers in Psychology*, 11(September), 1–12.

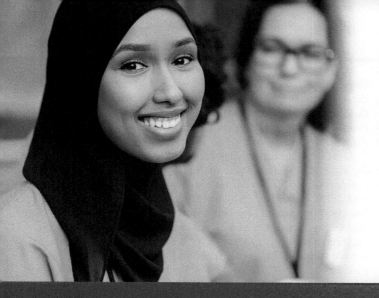

6

Student Supervision and Assessment

Joanne Day

Edge Hill University, UK

Learning Outcomes

On completion of this chapter, you will be able to:

- Understand the evolution and regulation of nursing education in the United Kingdom
- Understand the role of the student nurse in clinical practice
- Be aware of the roles to support your supervision and assessment in practice (NMC, 2019a)
- Be able to identify the different assessment requirements of your Practice Assessment Document (Pan London Practice Learning Group, 2019)
- Be able to identify processes to resolve concerns in practice (NMC, 2018a)
- Start to engage with coaching approaches and collaborative learning models

Proficiencies

NMC Proficiencies and Standards:

- Demonstrate evidence-based, best practice communication skills and approaches for working with people in professional teams
- Demonstrate effective supervision, teaching and performance appraisal through clear instructions and explanations when supervising, teaching or appraising others

 Visit the companion website at www.wiley.com/go/peate/nursingpractice3e where you can test yourself using flashcards, multiple-choice questions and more.

Nursing Practice: Knowledge and Care, Third Edition. Edited by Ian Peate and Aby Mitchell.
© 2022 John Wiley & Sons Ltd. Published 2022 by John Wiley & Sons Ltd.
Companion website: www.wiley.com/go/peate/nursingpractice3e

Introduction to Nursing Education in the Clinical Setting

The first documented reference to the profession of nursing was dated to approximately 300 AD when the Romans were attempting to provide hospitals in every city they controlled (Smith, 2019). Since that time nursing care has been provided throughout history, predominantly through religious orders, and was regarded as a vocation. Yet, we tend to consider the beginning of the modern nursing profession as stemming from the work of Florence Nightingale in the Crimean War and the opening of the first school of nursing at St Thomas' in 1860. Following these developments, nursing became a more socially acceptable occupation and was regarded as a profession; training was provided through hospital-based schools of nursing with the majority of the teaching and learning having a practical focus and being ward based. The British Nurses Association was created in 1887 and nurses began looking for professional registration. This was achieved in 1919 when the Nurses Act established the first professional register held by the General Nurses Council (GNC). The first professional qualification in nursing was formalised with the recognition of the state enrolled nurse following a 2-year training period in 1940.

The next substantial changes for the nursing profession came with the Briggs Committee in 1972 which introduced the concept of practice based on research and a recognised preparation for nurses. The Briggs Report recommended an 18-month shared foundation course leading to a certificate in nursing practice, with the ability to then complete a further 18 months of more advanced or specialised study resulting in a higher certificate of nursing practice. Briggs also advocated that student nurses should not be included in the workforce since they required supervision and leaving students unsupervised could have a detrimental effect on patient care. This was consolidated with the new professional register set out in 1983 by the UK Central Council for Nursing, Midwifery and Health Visiting (UKCC) which identified four branches of nursing recognised as Adult, Child, Mental Health and Learning Disability; these would later be called fields of nursing rather than branches following later reviews.

The Judge Report in 1985 considered the high attrition rate for student nurses and identified that nurse education should have a broader curriculum and move into the higher education sector (Ousey, 2011). The introduction of the diploma level Project 2000 programme in 1986 moved nurse education into universities while continuing to have a close relationship with nursing practice. Following a government review into the regulation of nurses in 1998, the UKCC was disbanded and the current regulator, the Nursing and Midwifery Council (NMC), was established in 2002 with a new professional register. In 2009, all nursing courses became degree level and the NMC Standards for Pre-Registration Nursing Education were published in 2010, with specific standards for competence for each of the four fields, divided into four domains:

- Professional values
- Communication and interpersonal skills
- Nursing practice and decision making
- Leadership, management and team working.

Under these standards, students were supervised in practice in clinical settings by mentors and worked a minimum of 40% of their clinical hours with their designated mentor (NMC, 2010), making the support, development and assessment of the student dependent upon the one individual mentor.

Over time, concerns were raised about how the mentor model could be maintained; criticisms were levelled that there was a problem with 'failing to fail' poorly performing students (Cassidy *et al.*, 2020; Honkavuo, 2020; Lee & Chiang, 2020), that there was too much opportunity for bias in assessments and that this created undue pressure for clinical staff acting in the role of mentor. Huybrecht *et al.* (2011) argue that the roles of mentor and assessor are incompatible given the environment of friendship and guidance which is inherent in the mentor–student relationship. In addition, the one-to-one model of working between mentor and student restricts the opportunity to increase placement capacity to meet the increasing workforce needs of the wider healthcare sector.

The most recent review of educational standards for NMC-approved programmes occurred in 2018 with the release of new standards of competence and new standards for education. In recognition of the increasing breadth and advanced clinical skills of registered nurses, *Future Nurse: Standards of Proficiency for Registered Nurses* (NMC, 2018c) sets out the level of competence expected for registered nurses across seven platforms.

1. Being an accountable professional
2. Promoting health and preventing ill health
3. Assessing needs and planning care
4. Providing and evaluating care
5. Leading and managing nursing care and working in teams
6. Improving safety and quality of care
7. Co-ordinating care

In addition, there were two annexes:

- Annexe A: Communication and relationship skills
- Annexe B: Nursing procedures.

The new standards were supported by three other significant documents: *Standards Framework for Nursing & Midwifery Education* (NMC, 2019c), *Standards for Pre-Registration Nursing Programmes* (NMC, 2019) and *Standards for Student Supervision and Assessment* (SSSA) (NMC, 2019b). These three documents in combination with the new standards for registration resulted in modernisation of pre-registration curriculums, Practice Assessment Documents (PAD) and the methods by which students are supervised and assessed in practice. Although the four fields of nursing are still recognised as separate specialties, they no longer have differing requirements in the standards for registration. There is a recognition that mental health nurses still need to be able to meet the physical care needs of their service users, and adult nurses still need to be able to recognise emotional distress and poor mental health. These transferable skill requirements apply across all four fields, hence the need for a shared curriculum where all four fields explore the same topics across the 3 years. This is enhanced by considering any field-specific implications of a given topic.

In addition to the changed curriculum and requirements for registration, the standards also provide a seismic cultural change in how students are supported in practice, with a move to a more team-based approach and separation of the supervision and assessment roles. The new standards allow for more innovation in local practice areas to improve the quality of student placements and help to support increases to capacity and more interdisciplinary working. The new standards formalise the requirement from the Code of Conduct (NMC, 2018a) that registered nurses:

> '9.4 support students' and colleagues' learning to help them to develop their professional competence and confidence'.

The emphasis is on the whole team in a clinical placement area being responsible for supporting the student's learning and development. There is also a formalisation of the need for the Approved Education Institute (AEI) to work in partnership with practice areas when assessing students' performance and ensuring that assessment processes are followed correctly, and judgements are evidence based.

The Nursing Associate

The NMC became the legal regulator for the role of nursing associate in 2018 and opened the Nursing Associate part of the register in January 2019. This was accompanied by the publication of the *Standards of Proficiency for Nursing Associates* (NMC, 2018b). The educational and supervision standards apply to all NMC-approved programmes and therefore are applicable to the Nursing Associate Programme. The standards of proficiency are also divided into six platforms with two annexes.

1. Being an accountable professional
2. Promoting health and preventing ill health
3. Providing and monitoring care
4. Working in teams
5. Improving safety and quality of care
6. Contributing to integrated care
   - Annexe A: Communication and relationship management skills
   - Annexe B: Procedures

These complement the requirements for Registered Nurses.

Importance of Clinical Practice Experience

The *Standards for Pre-Registration Nursing Programmes* (NMC, 2019a) sets out the requirement that the training curriculum will include an equal balance of theory and practice learning, with pre-registration students expected to experience a variety of practice settings and the full range of working hours of a registered nurse. The clinical placements are designed to provide students with a range of clinical experiences which will allow them to meet all the required assessment outcomes, but also to gain insight into the role of the registered nurse as part of the wider healthcare team to deliver patient-centred care (Baker-Armstrong, 2020; Lee & Chiang, 2020; Williamson *et al.*, 2020). Some of the major events in recent healthcare history such as the Francis Report (Mid Staffordshire NHS Foundation Trust Public Inquiry, 2013) and the Gosport War Memorial (Gosport Independent Panel, 2018) have also highlighted the need for high-quality nursing education to improve patient safety and prevent such failings in the future.

The clinical placements student nurses undertake are just the start of a professional journey of development and it is through these experiences that students will understand and embrace their own professional identity as well as the role of the registered nurse within the wider multidisciplinary team. However, students still report feeling unprepared for their new role after completion of their training programmes and placement dissatisfaction is acknowledged as a significant factor in attrition when students withdraw from their studies before completion (Coutts, 2016). Given the significance of clinical placements within the wider aspect of nursing education, it is therefore essential that students are well supported but also have clear expectations of what is expected in practice, in terms of their own learning and behaviours but also how they will be supported and what the assessment processes are. In summary, the clinical placements that students undertake as part of their programme are just as important to understand and prepare for as the academic modules.

Preparation for Clinical Placement Experiences

It is important for students to consider how to prepare for clinical placements. Most people will usually consider aspects such as refreshing their knowledge of anatomy and physiology or researching the conditions they are likely to encounter within that clinical setting. However, there are some more general factors that should be considered for all placements.

For each clinical placement, students should:

- take the time to get to know the assessment documentation (Drew, 2020)
- understand what they need to achieve within that placement and what skills and proficiencies they need to demonstrate. Are they generic skills or quite specific, requiring exposure to a particular client group? Will they be able to achieve them in the placement setting they are allocated to?
- make contact with the practice setting and introduce themselves well in advance of the placement commencing. This is their opportunity to identify what the specialty is, which assessments can be accommodated within the setting and to explore how students are supported
- ask questions such as do they have a dedicated education team, do they utilise collaborative learning opportunities, are there opportunities to spoke out to other services to gain a wider understanding of the specialty? Ask what is expected of students before starting the placement. For example, they may be asked to review the anatomy and physiology of the cardiovascular system or ensure that they are familiar with safeguarding and legislation relating to mental health and deprivation of liberties. It will depend upon the clinical setting, but this is the student's first opportunity to demonstrate their willingness to develop and to start to identify areas of weakness that will require more support.

Jot This Down

Take some time to perform a SWOT analysis (Strengths, Weaknesses, Opportunities, Threats) regarding how you learn best and how this will apply in a clinical setting.

By doing the research and identifying the specialty of the practice area, students can start to be proactive in their learning journey, for example looking into the types of caseloads cared for by that practice environment, identifying the terms and language used, what processes are utilised and what they want to learn more about. This will help to shape the initial interview when starting a placement.

What To Do If . . .

What if I call my placement and they're not expecting me? First, contact the placements office at your AEI to check that there hasn't been a late change to your placement (the placements team try to avoid this but sometimes it can't be helped because of staff shortages or changes in service provision). Once you have confirmed that you have the correct current details for your placement, contact them again and tell them politely that your university has confirmed that you are allocated to them for placement. Ask them when a good time would be to make contact again to discuss learning opportunities and rotas, etc. Be aware that while we all advocate contacting your placements as early as possible, in many cases they will be very busy and supporting a continuous stream of students, so they may ask you to wait until closer to the start of your placement.

The initial interview will usually cover all the health and safety requirements of a placement setting such as where the fire exits are, how to access relevant policies and procedures, etc. But it is also, more importantly, the opportunity for a student to explore what can be achieved within the placement and to identify any concerns and who they need to speak to if they have any difficulties. It is particularly important to set out in this meeting if there are specific proficiencies that they need to achieve, particularly if it is something that the student may not have much exposure to within that setting. Discussing this at the start of a placement allows time for a plan to be developed, whether that is arranging a short visit to another area in the organisation or highlighting to other members of the team that the student needs to be assessed while inserting a catheter, for example, so that they can be allocated to those service users. If a student has specific assessments to complete within a placement and does not communicate this until late in the placement, they may not be able to achieve that assessment and progress through the nursing programme.

Another important aspect in planning for placements, in addition to identifying what needs to be achieved, is to identify what barriers may exist to reaching these goals. Consider time management: students need to have time to undertake independent study to improve their clinical practice whilst working full-time clinical hours, will they also have academic assignments to complete while in placement and are there any other demands on their time? Consider if there is any additional support that may be required.

Students should think about the practicalities of getting to the placement, check out the routes to drive or the public transport provision to ensure prompt arrival for shifts, and make sure they have childcare in place if the student is a parent. Things can always go wrong so make sure there are back-up plans. The less obvious preparation includes thinking about how the student will cope with new experiences; are they prepared to be with someone when they are given bad news or to work with a trauma patient coming into the emergency department? In many cases, we will not know how we are going to react to a situation, so it is important to identify what support is available before someone is in that situation. Check what support is available from the AEI such as personal tutor support, student services and counselling, etc. as well as what can be provided by the placement area; will there be an opportunity to talk things through at the end of the shift and have a debrief to process events?

Additionally, students should think about tools that could improve resilience and help to cope with stresses in normal day-to-day life. For example, do they go running or bake cakes or just spend time with family and friends? It is important that students factor in how they are going to maintain these hobbies whilst on clinical placement. It is easy to fall into the trap of just working the placement hours and not taking the opportunity to follow usual pastimes, but it is important to maintain some of these activities to maintain health and well-being. This is reflected in the assessment of professional values where students will be expected to recognise the impact of their own health and well-being on the care they provide for patients and colleagues.

When thinking about support structures, remember to consider how students can utilise their peers. It is useful to be able to share experiences to help put things in perspective and to learn from each other and many student forums on social media will be useful in providing this support. However, students need to make sure that they are familiar with the NMC guidance on the use of social media and the AEI's own policies. Remember, students will only be assessed against the assessment requirements of the Practice Assessment Document, not by a comparison against other students. A student's clinical practice experience is exactly that! It is personal to them and to that clinical area.

What the Experts Say

I have lost count of the occasions where I have supported a student who is struggling, and they have highlighted another student as being a role model who is performing excellently in practice, without being aware that I was also supporting that role model student and they weren't coping as well as everyone perceived them to be. Share your highs and your lows and seek support from each other by all means but do keep things in perspective and don't fall into the trap of thinking of everything as a competition.

Liz, university practice learning lecturer

Supporting Additional Needs in Practice

The Code (NMC, 2018a) states:

'19. Be aware of, and reduce as far as possible, any potential for harm associated with your practice.'

Students are also required to annually self-declare that they are of good health and good character. In some cases, this can cause students to feel reluctance to disclose underlying health conditions or disabilities because they are frightened it will preclude them from undertaking their chosen professional role in nursing. However, the definition of good health in this context does not require an absence of disability or underlying condition. Students are declaring that they have sufficient physical and mental ability to be able to deliver excellent quality nursing care practising safely and effectively. As with any other employment, the profession of nursing is still legally obligated to provide reasonable adjustments under the Equality Act (2010) and this still applies to students (Ramluggun *et al.*, 2021).

Twenty percent of the UK working population report that they have a disability as defined by the Equality Act (Powell, 2021). With such a high percentage of people with disability in the population, it is reasonable to imagine that there will be a similar proportion amongst the population of nursing students. Disabilities will range from physical disabilities and long-term conditions, through specific learning difficulties and mental health conditions. Students need to have the self-awareness to recognise when disabilities or conditions prevent them from being able to carry out safe and effective practice and this should be discussed with personal tutors. However, they should expect to be supported to continue their studies when they recover or to have reasonable adjustments made to help them to achieve despite their conditions. It is important to note that 'reasonable adjustments' do not include altering the level of performance needed to achieve. Students still need to meet the level of competency required by the NMC for registration, but there may be coping strategies or specialised equipment that can be used to support them in their clinical practice (Ramluggun *et al.*, 2021; Salkeld, 2016; Coutts, 2016).

Because of the rules around maintaining confidentiality, the education provider will not usually disclose this information to the practice area, so the student will need to inform them directly or they can ask academic staff for support with this. That is not to say that they must disclose this information to everyone in the clinical area, or that they need to disclose every detail of their condition. But students certainly need to consider how this would impact on their practice and what support they would need from the practice assessor, team manager and clinical staff that they are working closely with.

Although students may have clear strategies to assist with learning in the academic environment, such as using a computer or having extra time in assessments, this may not always transfer easily to the clinical environment where they may not have access to adaptive equipment such as voice recorders and will be required to provide accurate information quickly. Salkeld (2016) suggests an open approach to supporting students in practice. The four domains of the OPEL model are:

- Openness and transparency
- Planning and organisation
- Evaluation and reflection
- Learning and feedforward.

While the focus of Salkeld's (2016) work was to support student nurses with a diagnosis of dyslexia, this model can be utilised to support all students with additional needs. The principles of utilising a tripartite approach between the student, academic staff and clinical staff to discuss and explore difficulties in an open and supportive manner to help plan and organise support for the student's placement would still apply regardless of the nature of the additional need.

It is important to recognise that unless it is a significant risk to patient safety, the decision to disclose additional needs remains at the discretion of the student, so they can choose not to disclose. However, if they choose not to inform the clinical area of any additional needs, area staff will not be able to provide additional support and any difficulties experienced may be perceived as poor performance, resulting in unsatisfactory assessment results. If a student chooses not to disclose additional needs to the practice area, they are potentially disadvantaging themselves when it comes to successfully completing the clinical requirements of the course.

Changes to Student Supervision and Assessment in Practice with the New NMC Standards

In 2018, the NMC produced updated standards for student supervision and assessment with a key factor in the standards being the formalisation of a team-based approach to supporting students. The new standards state that all registered nurses are responsible for supporting the learning and development of students and colleagues. This has already been written into the Code (NMC, 2018a), but now forms an essential tenet of student supervision and assessment in the clinical area.

The new standards allow for more flexibility working with students and encourage the use of new models of collaborative working which utilise coaching approaches and peer learning alongside more traditional mentorship styles. The new standards recognise the importance of the wider multidisciplinary team and the registered nurse's role within the organisation through the recognition that all registered healthcare professionals can act as supervisors for students following an NMC-approved programme of preparation. This in turn opens the possibility to explore new areas of practice which have not traditionally supported nursing students, such as therapy-led teams.

It is hoped that the new standards will help to increase capacity for placements for student nurses. However, the requirements for high-quality placements are not just a question of capacity. The AEIs and their practice partners also need to consider the quality of the learning experiences for the student and the support provided for practice supervisors and assessors as well as for the student. The NMC standards specify that the learning environment must be safe for the student to learn in, both from a health and safety point of view but also within the culture of the practice setting. In a good-quality practice area, the student should feel safe to ask questions, seek support and raise concerns. This includes operating within a culture of openness, transparency and candour with a recognition that while learning, the student also must work within their professional code and has a duty of care for the safety of patients and colleagues. Students should feel supported to question practice and should not be made to feel that there will be a detrimental effect to their assessment and development if they raise concerns. With the culture of peer learning highlighted by the Francis Report (2013), it is important that registered staff recognise that they have as much to learn from the process of supporting students as the students themselves will.

Case Study

Sarah was on her second placement as a first-year student nurse on a surgical ward. While documenting notes at the nursing station, she observed a healthcare support worker interacting with the patients in one of the bays. She heard the support worker speaking very abruptly to the patients and noted that she appeared quite rough in her handling of the patients when assisting them to move in the bed. She didn't think the behaviour was appropriate but did not feel she could speak up as a student. She later went into the bay to take observations and provide assistance to some of the patients. The patients spoke to Sarah about how they had been treated by the support worker and how much this had upset them. Sarah went to speak to the ward manager about this. The ward manager was very supportive. She spoke with the patients and listened to their concerns before addressing the issues with the support worker.

On reflection, Sarah felt guilty that she had not spoken up immediately when she witnessed the behaviour; she knew it was unacceptable, but did not feel it was her place to say anything until the patients had reported their distress directly to her.

How do you think you would react in this situation?

To support a student to develop into a confident and competent practitioner, it is essential that an overarching systematic approach is taken when considering their learning experiences in the clinical setting (van de Mortel *et al.*, 2021). One aspect of this is to ensure that there is a co-ordinated approach to the student's learning and development from all the staff in the clinical area and a sufficient level of supervision to ensure students can practise their clinical skills and communication without being put in situations which are beyond their capability. There is an expectation that the clinical environment will value learning and ensure that all members of the team will understand their role in supporting students to develop their nursing practice. There also needs to be an understanding of the differing roles within the interdisciplinary team and a recognition of how they interact and support each other, not just the registered healthcare staff but also the administrators, housekeepers and porters, etc., promoting teamworking and professional respect across all areas of specialty.

Academic Assessor, Practice Assessor and Practice Supervisor Roles (Table 6.1)

It is quite common for students to want the safety blanket of working with the same person all the time so that they know who to go to with questions and feel supported. Indeed, it is good practice to have one individual identified to work with regularly to ensure the continuity of support for a student. However, there are also some inherent weaknesses in this way of working. Different individuals will use different approaches to communication and teamworking and it is useful for students to experience this variety in approaches to help them develop their own style of communication and teamworking. In addition, one individual may not possess all the skills and competencies that the student is required to demonstrate in that placement, so the student will need to work with others who do hold those skill sets, whether that is working with a physiotherapist to learn chest auscultation or working with social workers to follow the processes involved with safeguarding referrals. Universities will therefore encourage and support placement partners to provide a balanced approach between exposing students to diverse ways of working, but also ensuring continuity of support and development for the student.

An advantage of this approach is that it develops a whole-team approach to supporting students and encourages all members of the practice team to provide support and feedback for a student's development.

In placement students will be expected to work across the whole team to experience a variety of ways of working. Any registered healthcare professional who works with students to support their practice and development is a practice supervisor. However, there should always be one person who is designated to oversee their assessments and co-ordinate their placement to ensure they have the best opportunity to achieve the required learning outcomes; this will be the practice assessor. There are differences between these two roles of practice assessor and practice supervisor.

The X Factor

One explanation is to compare this to the team on the talent show X Factor. The student takes the same role as the competitor, trying to make the most of their opportunity to shine and show how competent they can be in the workplace. The team of choreographers, vocal coaches and wardrobe assistants who contribute to the impact of the contestant's performance each week can be equated to our team of practice supervisors (PS) who will come from a variety of backgrounds and professions, and will help the student to experience new clinical skills and develop better understanding of delegation and interprofessional working.

Students are encouraged to seek out a variety of PSs to work with to experience differing communication techniques and leadership styles as well as benefiting from a more diverse range of clinical skills. Students need to seek regular feedback from their PS to help them to develop their practice. While the workload is not likely to allow PSs the time to write a 12-page testimonial for students, they should be able to comment on the student's attitude and approach to learning as well as their competency with clinical skills and teamworking. While it is very pleasant to receive feedback such as 'She's very pleasant and hardworking, asks appropriate questions and will be a lovely nurse when she qualifies', think about whether this guides and supports the student's development. All students will have areas they can improve upon and if they receive the very pleasant but generic feedback quote above, the risk is that they will not be able to identify their weaker areas of professional practice to improve and develop. Ideally, students should ask supervisors to give them more personalised specific feedback. It is entirely appropriate to give positive feedback: 'You communicated well with Mrs Jones today and were able to assist her to mobilise using a Zimmer frame', for example. The next step might be 'It would be useful for you to

Table 6.1 Practice assessment.

ASSESSMENT	DESCRIPTION	STUDENT ROLE	PRACTICE SUPERVISOR ROLE	PRACTICE ASSESSOR ROLE
Professional values	These are aligned to the Code Prioritise people Practise effectively Preserve safety Promote professionalism and trust These must be achieved in every placement	Understanding the professional values and ensuring that they practise with these in mind	Role model good practice Provide feedback on student's performance in relation to professional values	Role model good practice Review feedback on student's performance in relation to professional values Make evidence-based judgement about whether the student has demonstrated the required professional values
Proficiencies	Clinical skills which form the building blocks of the seven platforms described in the NMC Standards These will increase in complexity as students progress through the course Required proficiencies must be achieved in each part of a programme A small number of proficiencies have flexibility to be completed in either Part 2 or Part 3 depending on clinical opportunities	To identify which proficiencies need to be completed in each placement To seek out opportunities to practise To raise concerns early if worried they will not have opportunity to complete required proficiencies	To role model good practice To support student to practise proficiencies To assess whether student has demonstrated safe and effective delivery of the required proficiency	To role model good practice To support student to practise proficiencies To assess whether student has demonstrated safe and effective delivery of the required proficiency
Medicines management	An assessment to demonstrate the student can safely and effectively administer and monitor the effectiveness of medications. This includes drug calculations, safety-critical procedures and an understanding of the pharmacology of the prescribed medications	Ensure that they have sufficient opportunity to practise drug calculations Learn as much as possible about commonly prescribed medications Ensure a patient-centred holistic approach to the administration and management of medications	Practice supervisors cannot sign off this assessment, it must be completed by the practice assessor Role model good practice Support student in the development of their medicines management knowledge and practice. Provide feedback to practice assessor on student's performance	Role model good practice Support student in the development of their medicines management knowledge and practice Assess the student dispensing and administering medications to an appropriate caseload of patients or service users Make evidence-based decision about whether student has demonstrated the required assessment outcomes
Episodes of care	This is a reflective assessment. The student will reflect upon the care they have given and how they have learned from it to improve their practice. This will begin with meeting an individual's needs at the start of the programme and progress through to demonstrating leadership and management towards the end of their course of study	Engage with the reflection process Work with supervisors and assessors to identify appropriate episodes of care Identify the required learning outcomes that must be demonstrated	Practice supervisors cannot sign off this assessment, it must be completed by the practice assessor Support student to identify appropriate episode of care Provide feedback to practice assessor on student's performance	Review the student's reflection Review feedback from practice supervisors Understand the required learning outcomes to be demonstrated Make an evidence-based assessment on whether the student has demonstrated the required learning outcomes

spend some time working with the physiotherapy team to gain a better understanding of how mobility is assessed, and the rationale used to support a patient to be more independent with their mobility needs'.

You can see from this example how constructive feedback can be used to identify new areas of study and ideas to develop practice further, while still acknowledging where students are doing well.

The student will need to be assessed based on whether they are meeting their required outcomes. This is where the practice assessors (PA) come in, performing the same role as the panel of judges on the X Factor to look at your performance and decide whether you have achieved sufficiently to progress. The PA is expected to have an overall understanding of the learning and development needs within a student's clinical placement and to help them to achieve the required assessments. The PA will be a registered nurse with extensive current experience within the clinical setting. The PA will co-ordinate with the PS to ensure that students have consistent support and exposure to the required clinical skills, communication and teamworking. They will ensure that they spend enough time working with a student or observing them to be able to assess their practice and will review the feedback from the PS as supporting evidence to assess progress. The PA will also work in partnership with the academic assessor (AA) (Donaldson, 2019; Drayton & Edmonds, 2020; Walsh, 2014).

Academic Assessor

The AA is a member of staff from the AEI who is responsible for liaising with the PA and reporting the student's progress within the educational setting. They should have a good understanding of where the student is in their learning and the assessment requirements for each placement. They will liaise with the PA at regular points during a placement to review the available evidence and discuss whether the student is performing at the required levels. They will help the PA to ensure that the correct assessment processes are followed and will share the decision making on evidence-based assessments with the PA.

Although the AA is from the AEI, students will work with a variety of AAs throughout their studies since they are not allowed to work with the same student across consecutive parts of the programme. While the way the AA is allocated and works with practice may vary from one AEI to another, the principal focus of the role remains the same – to support the development and assessment of the student in their clinical practice and ensure they are making sufficient progress in both the academic and clinical settings to meet the NMC requirements for registration.

The Nursing Associate

The standards for student supervision and assessment (NMC, 2019b) also apply to the nursing associate programme, but the PA for a nursing associate student can be either a registered nurse or a registered nursing associate.

The Role of the Pre-Registration Nursing Student in Clinical Practice

Pre-registration nursing students are expected to hold supernumerary status while they are in clinical placement, so it is important to understand how supernumerary status works. This status means that the student is not counted in the staffing numbers for the clinical area and that service users would still receive a high standard of care regardless of whether the student was there or just the regular clinical staff. However, this is not to say that the role of the student is purely observational. With the newer collaborative learning models which are being utilised in practice, students are much more likely to take the responsibility for planning and delivering hands-on patient care for a designated group of patients, increasing in complexity as they progress through their studies.

- Students are expected to demonstrate competence in clinical skills as well as teamwork and leadership, so are expected to take a hands-on role in delivering and evaluating the care given to service users.
- Students are expected to work alongside all members of the multidisciplinary team, and it is important to remember that the clinical staff supervising and assessing will have a good oversight of what a student needs to achieve throughout their course of study and what is required in the role of a registered nurse.
- It is quite common for students to become very focused on achieving their clinical skills at the expense of developing their fundamental nursing care. Whilst the clinical proficiencies are an important requirement of the clinical assessment, it is equally important to develop professionalism and teamworking with softer skills such as communication and emotional intelligence. Honkavuo (2020) reports that the relationship between clinical supervisors and their students is a caring relationship based on the ethics and ethos of caring as well as communication and co-operation to support the student's professional growth.
- In addition, those involved with supervising and assessing students will be viewed as 'gatekeepers' to the profession, ensuring that students are able to deliver safe and effective patient-centred care upon registration. Students are therefore expected to approach each clinical placement with an open mind and a willingness to learn.

Practice Assessment Document

The introduction of new competencies for registration in 2018 and new standards for nursing education also precipitated a review of the Practice Assessment Document (PAD) used to record a student's progress in the clinical area. Although each AEI will use its own PAD, they will broadly cover the same assessments and proficiencies although the format may differ. Most AEIs now use the Pan London Practice Assessment Document 2.0 which was originally developed by the Pan London Practice Learning Group (PLPLG) (2019) and has been widely adopted and adapted across the other regions of the UK. The PAD and Ongoing Achievement Record (OAR) are the student's supporting evidence to prove that they have met the clinical requirements for registration. The development of clinical progress is mapped through parts of a programme, each part being identified as a progression point in accordance with the NMC standards (2019a–c). Within a standard pre-registration course, there are three parts to the programme. It is important to clarify when each part of the programme needs to be completed, because this will impact on when a student needs to achieve their clinical assessments.

Professional Values

Clinical placements are as much about learning the professionalism in the role of the registered nurse and how it interacts with others, as it is about clinical skills. Because the professional values are so closely tied to the Code (NMC, 2018a) students will be expected to demonstrate the professional values to an acceptable level in all placements. A large body of evidence for how students are performing in professional values will be drawn from their attitude and communication with others as well as their ability to receive and develop upon constructive feedback. These values will also cover aspects such as punctuality, time management, professional image and being able to act as a role model to others.

Jot This Down

Think about how this relates to you as a student and your supernumerary status. You may think that you can simply swap the shift you are working because there is a learning opportunity elsewhere that you want to attend but consider how this impacts on the clinical area.

If there is a pattern of chopping and changing shifts, this may give the impression that a student is unreliable, and this would not comply with the professional values relating to promoting professionalism and trust. This is not to say that students cannot take advantage of opportunities to visit other areas and make the most of clinical learning opportunities, but as with all things, this must be negotiated with the practice area.

In addition to general behaviours and professionalism in their practice setting, students will also need to write a reflection on an experience during the placement, relating this to how they comply with the Code (NMC, 2018a). Please remember that a reflection is a tool to show how the student has developed and grown in their practice because of their experience, and even the very best students will still have areas where they can improve their practice. This is where reflection time is so important.

Assessment of Proficiencies

The clinical proficiencies or essential skills develop in number and complexity as students progress through the course. The proficiencies can be assessed by any PS, which includes other professions within the MDT if they have a registration with a healthcare regulatory body (NMC, 2019b). It is important to remember that the PS assessing a student must already hold enough competency within this skill to be able to assess their ability to demonstrate safe practice and underpinning

knowledge related to the proficiency. Students should ensure that they have read and understood all the proficiencies before starting a clinical placement. If the placement is their final clinical experience in a part of the programme, they will need to ensure that all the required assessments have been completed by the end of the placement. Students need to be aware of what they need to complete before starting the initial interview in a placement to allow for a discussion about how this can be achieved.

If the student does not discuss their requirements with the PA at the start of their placement, they risk missing learning opportunities to successfully achieve the proficiencies. Another aspect to consider is making sure that both student and assessor/supervisor understand what the proficiency is asking the student to be able to demonstrate. The proficiencies are written in such a way that they can be applied across all clinical settings and all four fields of nursing, which can sometimes make them appear vague in their descriptions. Please take time to read and interpret the proficiencies that need to be achieved before starting clinical placements. AAs can provide guidance about what is required in any of the proficiencies.

What the Experts Say

If you are on a placement in a GP practice, you may only have limited opportunities to insert and manage an NG tube, for example. If you discuss this with your PA at the start of your placement, they may be able to pair you up with a team responsible for managing NG tubes in the community or in a nursing home that they support, for example. If you understand the proficiencies that you need to achieve, and you have done your research about the specialism of your placement, you should be able to identify with your practice assessor which proficiencies are more easily achieved in each placement.

Fiona, practice assessor and GP practice nurse

Medicines Management Assessment

The next area of assessment is the medicines management assessment which must be successfully achieved in each part of the programme. The medicines management assessment will cover the practical skills needed to deliver medication and the safety checks required as well as the ability to perform drug calculations. Whilst it is essential to understand all the steps in administration of medication, such as the 'seven rights' and checking expiry dates, etc., it is also important that students demonstrate knowledge of the pharmacology of commonly used medications. It is not enough to know how we give a medication to the patient; we need to understand why that medication is prescribed and how it works to ensure that the efficacy of the treatment can be evaluated and to consider any possible side-effects or supplemental treatments or dietary warnings that may be required. The PA will observe the student giving medications to an appropriate caseload of patients or service users and will ask questions to assess underlying knowledge in all aspects of medicines management. The student is then also asked to reflect upon their performance in the assessment, which is an opportunity to identify how they can develop and improve.

Episodes of Care Assessment

The final area of assessment to consider is the episodes of care. Students will be asked to complete episodes of care in each part of the programme. These will increase in complexity as they progress through their studies. In the first part, students would be asked to reflect upon an episode of care where they met the needs of one individual patient; by the second part, this progresses to meeting the needs of a group of individuals, through to reflecting upon leadership and management and teaching and coaching in the final part. As already mentioned, a reflective assessment is an opportunity to demonstrate learning and development. Students need to review reflective models to help guide their development as a reflective practitioner (Johns, 2017).

Students work with their PA to identify an appropriate episode of care, carefully consider the learning outcomes that they are being asked to demonstrate within the reflection and whether the episode of care will give sufficient opportunity to meet those outcomes. Make sure that all aspects of the episode are considered, not just a factual description. The student should explore how they felt. Did they feel prepared? Did they feel anxious? As students progress through the questions in the episode of care, they will be asked to consider what worked well, what they could have done differently and what learning they will take forward from this experience. The PA will use the evidence from the reflection and their observations of the student's practice to make an evidence-based decision about whether they have demonstrated the required learning outcomes.

This section has covered the formal assessment aspects of the PAD, but students also need to consider how the wider aspects of the PAD can be used to support their development in clinical placements.

Placement Interviews

The aim of the initial interview is to identify learning goals for the placement and for the PA and PS to identify what support may be needed to achieve the required outcomes. It is good practice to have an idea in mind of what learning opportunities may be available in that clinical area but these must be guided by the PA/PS since they will be very experienced in the clinical area and will have a clearer view of what can or cannot be achieved by a student in that setting.

At the midpoint interview, students will work with their PA to reflect on and review their progress so far and identify any areas that need further support and development. To get the most out of this interview, students need to prepare for it in advance. Review the original learning plan from the initial interview and, utilising a reflective approach, consider what progression has been made towards the learning goals. Students should by now be able to identify whether there are any learning goals that were not considered in the initial interview. The midpoint interview is designed to be a collaborative approach to ensure that both the student and the clinical practice team agree about the student's progress and plans to move forwards in the placement. Do not forget that the AA is also likely to be involved with this process since they need to liaise with the PA at regular intervals.

At the end of the clinical placement, students will meet with their PA to complete the final interview. This is very much a reflective interview where all evidence will be reviewed to decide whether the student has achieved the practice learning requirements of the placement. As with the midpoint interview, students should prepare for this meeting by reflecting upon their practice throughout the placement, identifying what they have experienced and learned and how they will use this to improve their practice. Likewise, the PA and AA will review the available evidence, including feedback from the PS, notes taken during assessments and their observations of the student working in practice to make an objective evidence-based decision about their progression within the clinical area and provide feedback about how they can continue to develop. As part of this final interview, the PA and AA will also complete the OAR, providing a summary of the student's performance in the clinical area. If the student is at the end of a part, the PA and AA will also complete the relevant section for the end of that part in the OAR, confirming whether the student has successfully completed the required assessments and providing their recommendation about whether the student should be allowed to progress to the next part of the programme, or to the NMC register if at the end of the programme.

Red Flag

If your practice supervisors and practice assessors are not completing your documentation in a timely fashion, this needs escalating. The whole purpose of your clinical placement is to promote your learning and development so the feedback and assessment processes are an essential aspect of this. If you do not receive feedback, you do not know where you need to improve and you can't reflect upon your practice and identify support to develop further. In the first instance, ask your practice assessor to set a time to complete the documentation and keep a record of this. If it is cancelled once, ask for a new appointment; if you are delayed again, please raise concerns with your AA and/or the clinical education team and ask them for support to speak to your PA/PS to ensure time is put aside to complete your documentation. Do not carry on without making sure your documentation is completed since you may not have time to address any concerns if they are not reported early enough.

The Role of an Action Plan

Many students will mistakenly view an action plan in a negative light and regard it as a sign of failure if they are asked to engage with an action plan while in clinical placement. By contrast, action plans can be regarded as a sign that things are going well, and a student is receiving a high level of support in practice. It is important to recognise that an action plan is a tool designed to provide personalised specific support to help a student to achieve successfully in practice and to become a competent and confident practitioner (Figure 6.1). At any point in a placement, if the PS or PA has concerns about a student's practice or their ability to successfully achieve the assessments, they should start the process of developing an action plan in partnership with the student and their AA. The aim of the action plan is to help guide the student and practice area staff to develop very targeted and individualised support to help a student to achieve.

An action plan is required when a student's performance causes concern
The Practice Assessor must liaise with the Academic Assessor and senior practice representative
The **SMART** principles should be used to construct the Action Plan.

Placement Name	Date action plan initiated:				
Nature of concern **Refer to Professional Value(s), Proficiency and/or Episode of Care** (Specific)	**What does the student need to demonstrate;** *objectives and meaure of success* **(Measurable, Achievable and Realistic)**	**Support available and who is responsible**	**Date for review** (Timed)	**Review/feedbak**	
				Date: **Comments:**	
Student's Name:	Signature:		Date:	**Practice Assessor Name:**	
Practice Assessor's Name:	Signature:		Date:		
Academic Assessor's Name:	Signature:		Date:	**Signature:**	

PLPAD 2.0 Master Part 1 (Version 40) Final Print Version SAMPLE 13.05.19 JF KW IGR   63

Figure 6.1 Pan London Practice Learning Group Action Plan Template 2021. https://plplg.uk/wp-content/uploads/2019/06/PLPAD-2.0-Master-Part-1-Version-40-Final-Print-Version-13.05.19-JF-KW-IGR.pdf

Action Plan Stages

- *Stage 1*: The first stage of the process is to identify the nature of the concerns, with specific examples; these must be linked to the required assessments in the PAD. So, for example, a concern might be raised about confidentiality which relates to the section of the professional values on promoting professionalism and trust. The concern would be identified as problems maintaining confidentiality, with specific examples given of when the student breached confidentiality.
- *Stage 2*: Identify what behaviour change needs to be observed, i.e. what does success look like? These need to follow the principle of SMART targets; they should be clearly identifiable and measurable and should be realistic to achieve in the time remaining in your placement.
- *Stage 3*: The support is available and who is responsible need to be considered, which will invariably require input from both student and practice staff. Using our example of confidentiality, the clinical staff should discuss the obstacles to a student observing confidentiality; for example, do they have quiet spaces for students to ask questions and are they available to have discussions in a quiet area? However, from a student

perspective, it would be reasonable to ask the student to consider what confidentiality means and where is the most appropriate place to have discussions to aid learning and reflect on their personal actions.
- *Stage 4*: The final stage is to identify a period over which the action plan will run before it is reviewed; this needs to be sufficiently long enough for the required support to be put in place and for the student to demonstrate the required improvement.

The development of an action plan is therefore very much a partnership process which needs to fully engage PAs and PSs as well as the student. The student needs to be able to understand the feedback they are being given and to accept the support to improve their performance. If at any point the student is unsure what is being asked of them, they should ask their assessors to explain it again. A useful tool is to try repeating their concerns in your own words or paraphrasing the action plan to check understanding. At the end of the day, if the student is at all unclear about what is expected of them, they are unlikely to be able to demonstrate the required change in their behaviours and practice, so they need to make sure that they have clearly understood everything discussed.

Case Study

Sarah was in her second placement of Part 1. The practice assessor Sue contacted her academic assessor Jack to raise concerns that Sarah was not meeting Professional Value 1 which relates to maintaining patient confidentiality in accordance with the NMC Code (NMC, 2018a).

A tripartite meeting was arranged so that Jack could facilitate a discussion and support Sarah when the concerns were addressed. In the meeting, Sue reported that although Sarah would always move away from the bay of patients to the nursing desk to discuss patient care and ask questions to support her development, she spoke quite loudly, and her conversations could be heard clearly at the other end of the ward. Sarah was very distressed and had no idea that her voice could carry so much in the ward area. On discussion, it transpired that she came from a large family and there was always lots of conversation in her home, so she was used to having to make herself heard and did not recognise how loud she was or how much her voice carried. Sarah was keen to work with the feedback to ensure she was maintaining confidentiality but needed to develop more self-awareness of when her voice was becoming raised or could be heard further than she intended. An action plan was agreed where the clinical staff of the ward would highlight to Sarah when they could hear her conversations in the patient care area and Sarah would embrace this feedback to try to adjust her speech. Over time, Sarah became more aware of when the volume of her conversation was rising, usually when she was enthusiastic about a learning opportunity, and was able to work with the clinical staff to develop a more professional tone and volume, ensuring that she achieved all her required outcomes by the end of the placement.

Jot This Down

Reflect on the case study above and consider how you would have reacted if you were this student. How can you improve your resilience to positively accept constructive feedback?

What to Do When a Placement Does Not Go to Plan

Sometimes, regardless of the preparation a student has put in or their expectations of the placement area, things can just start going wrong. Students do have a duty to raise concerns if they witness or are exposed to unprofessional behaviour, poor practice, any risk to public protection or patient safety and any behaviour which is contrary to the Code (NMC, 2018a). The AEI and practice areas will have clear processes around how to raise concerns and will ensure that these are investigated, and students are supported through this process, so students need make sure they are aware of these policies and who to speak to. Students will often be very reluctant to raise concerns because they are worried they will not be believed, or it will somehow have a negative impact on their assessments or just that it is not their place as a student. However, if the concerns have been raised in an appropriate

manner, they will always be taken seriously and investigated. Sometimes this will provide a learning opportunity for the student to understand why a particular action is taken or how things are prioritised.

In most instances, students will be encouraged to raise concerns with their practice supervisors and assessors or a nominated person in the clinical environment in the first instance. This direct approach allows for misunderstandings to be cleared up quickly and for supervisors and assessors to have a clear idea of how to support the student.

In some circumstances, the student may not feel that they can discuss their concerns in the clinical environment, for example of they have witnessed inappropriate behaviour or poor practice. In these instances, students may be supported by the education team within the placement organisation or their AEI, or a combination of both. It is important that the student familiarises themselves with their AEI's policies for raising concerns in practice.

The first and most important stage in this situation is to take a breath and try to get some perspective on the situation. Students can ask themselves the following questions:

Jot This Down

Reflect upon the advice given regarding personal resilience in Chapter 5. What steps can you take to understand the situation and what can you learn from this?

Is my perception of the situation correct? Do I have any other stressors away from the placement that are affecting my perspective and my levels of resilience?

What the Experts Say

Practice assessors and supervisors are very experienced staff who want to share their knowledge and expertise with students to help them to develop.

Students need to identify exactly what the clinical staff mean in their feedback. Often a student may become defensive because they feel that they are completing a task successfully, but this can be because the student is focused on the physical task and the assessors and supervisors are identifying gaps in their knowledge or how they apply theory in practice. One useful piece of advice for students is to listen to the feedback and pause before responding to consider the information given. The initial reaction will tend to be an emotional response, so by pausing to get past the emotional response, a student can start to process the information they are being given in the feedback.

Helen, practice educator

One of the biggest causes of poor performance in practice is unclear expectations and miscommunication on the part of both student and practice staff. Usually the practice assessor/supervisor is unaware that the student is feeling unhappy and unsupported and is quite distressed when they find out. Most clinical staff are keen to support students and want to help them develop so they are very disappointed if they feel that they have somehow let the student down. Students can take steps to resolve a negative placement experience by reflecting on the situation, advocating for themselves and trying to provide constructive solutions (Rawson, 2021). Here are some simple tips to guide students when they are proactive in addressing placement concerns.

- Meet with the practice assessor.supervisor.
- Explain how you are feeling.
- Use non-judgemental statements – 'I feel. . .' rather than 'You did. . .'.
- Actively listen to the practice assessor/supervisor.
- Try not to respond from an emotional reaction; take a breath and reflect on the information.
- Ask for clarification if unsure.
- Ask for support in the meeting if needed.

It can be a difficult balance for students to strike when asking for support to be proactive in trying to meet their learning needs versus being aggressive and demanding, which can be perceived as unprofessional. If students do not feel comfortable or confident to have that conversation, they should seek support from their AA or the clinical education team to help to facilitate that conversation. In any interaction, there are always at least two perceptions of how the interaction commenced and progressed

---

Case Study

June started her first clinical placement during the second wave of the Covid-19 pandemic in January 2020. She correctly raised concerns that the ward she was placed on appeared untidy. Several patients on the ward reported that they had not been washed since their admission and there didn't seem to be enough staff on shift at any one time.

June raised concerns by contacting her AA Sam and the organisation's clinical education team. Once these concerns were raised, a meeting was arranged with the ward manager; June was supported by Sam, and the clinical education team from the trust also sent a representative. The meeting was very positive, with good learning opportunities for both sides. The ward manager explained that 24 hours before June started her placement, the ward had changed from a rehabilitation unit with a small number of stable patients to a Red Covid Cohort ward with an increased number of patients, and these were not medically stable. Due to these circumstances, care had to be prioritised to deliver safe and effective care rather than the high-quality person-centred care they would usually aim to deliver. The ward looked untidy because of the infection control measures which had been implemented. There was a very productive discussion which was similar to those held in many other clinical areas about the difference between good care and safe care and the effects the Covid pandemic had on healthcare. Once the patients had been stabilised and the ward staff had adjusted to the new status as a Covid Cohort ward, the delivery of care could be reviewed, and patients were assisted with personal hygiene and a more patient-centred model of care was able to be followed.

Following this meeting, June understood the rationale for the care being delivered on the ward and felt more able to integrate as part of the team, looking for ways in which she could help to support the delivery of care. At the end of the placement, she reported that this had been a very positive learning experience despite the concerns raised initially.

---

and the truth is usually somewhere in the middle. In order to move forwards with a positive and constructive relationship, there is usually an element of adjustment or compromise required from both sides.

Another cause of confusion in communication between students and clinical staff is the expectation of how learning is supported. Students often expect to be told the information and instructed to complete tasks, but there is now more of a movement to encourage students to find the answers for themselves through a coaching and questioning technique to support learning, which can lead to some friction when students do not understand the benefits of the coaching approach.

The Role of Coaching

Throughout the history of nursing education, there has been a tendency to teach students their practice through directions and instruction. This encourages students to learn through muscle memory and learning by rote, but it does not promote a deeper understanding or encourage them to question the practice and how it links to theory. In modern nursing, clinical staff are required to understand the evidence base behind the care they deliver and to be able to question poor practice. The older system of mentorship started to develop this approach in the one-to-one relationship between students and mentors who shared their clinical experience and aided students to make the links between their theory and clinical practice.

Mentoring is described as the process by which an individual is supported and encouraged to manage their own learning to improve their performance and maximise their potential (Passmore, 2016). In this example, the mentor will guide the student to identify possible learning opportunities and will develop a supportive relationship with them, with some aspects of coaching to help them to progress. However, once qualified as registered nurses, those students will be expected to be able to work as independent practitioners and will need to understand the decision-making processes required in planning and evaluating patient care.

The new standards for student supervision and assessment (NMC, 2019b), in addition to formalising a whole-team approach to supporting students, are accompanied by a cultural move towards more of a coaching approach to support student learning. Parsloe & Leedham (2009) and Passmore (2016) describe coaching as a process to release the self-knowledge and potential that is inherent in everyone. There is a difference between mentoring and coaching. In a mentoring relationship, the mentor has specialised expert knowledge which they will impart to the student, acting as a guide and teacher. In a coaching approach, the coach will assist the students to unlock their own knowledge and skills so they can become their own guides and teachers.

This involves the student on the receiving end of coaching taking responsibility for their learning and developing their own self-awareness of their performance, strengths and weaknesses. The coaching approach encourages the student, through a process of active listening, clarification and questioning, to develop their own self-directed learning to improve performance. In this approach, the practice supervisor or assessor will support the student by questioning them in a supportive and guiding manner rather than instructing them. This encourages the student to consolidate their knowledge further by applying theory to practice and helps them to identify for themselves the gaps in their own knowledge and skills. The student needs to be able to trust in the relationships with their supervisors that they are being supported to develop rather than feeling that they are somehow being tested or put on the spot. The questioning is designed to improve their learning, not to catch them out in their weaker areas. There are several models of coaching which can be used, but it is important for students to recognise that if a supervisor asks them questions rather than giving them the information directly, this is not a resignation of their responsibilities to support the student.

One of the most widely established coaching models is GROW (Goal, Reality, Options, Will) which was developed in the 1980s (Passmore, 2016). In this model, coaching is a cyclical process which incorporates a reflective approach to identify what the student wants to achieve, where they are now and what their choices are to progress before identifying which option to use. Following this process, the coaching cycle starts again by continuing back through the stages of goal, reality, options and will.

Another process that could be followed for coaching in the clinical setting is a solution-focused approach. In this approach, the coach supports the student to identify constructive solutions rather than barriers and the expectation is that the student will follow their own self-directed learning to achieve a positive action and outcome.

What the differing coaching models do have in common is the identification of a goal through supportive questioning and the use of active listening and clarification to help the student to identify how those goals will be achieved, especially through exploring SMART targets.

It is important to understand the principles of coaching because this will affect how practice supervisors and assessors interact with students within the clinical setting. If a student asks their practice assessor or supervisor a question, they are highly likely to respond by asking another question. This is not intended to be difficult or awkward but is designed to get the student thinking about the theory they have been taught and how to apply it to the current situation. Rather than giving an instruction to go and call the doctor to escalate a NEWS2 score of 5 or more, the supervisor is more likely to ask what is the significance of such a high score, what needs to happen next and why, what information the doctor will need to know, is there anything else that needs to be done? The reason for adopting this approach is because it has been shown to improve students' confidence and helps to consolidate knowledge as well as developing a critical questioning approach to clinical practice to ensure the care given is evidence based (Crozier *et al.*, 2021).

New Approaches to Collaborative Learning in a Clinical Setting

The move towards a new coaching approach and the new NMC standards (2018a–c) have been accompanied by innovations in the way students are allocated and supported in clinical placements. Collaborative learning models put students and self-directed peer learning at the heart of clinical practice experiences

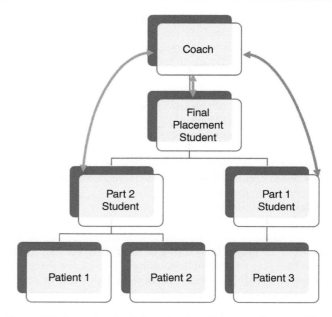

Figure 6.2 Example of collaborative learning scenario in practice.

(Figure 6.2). Although there are many models being developed, such as GM Synergy, Collaborative Learning in Practice (CLiP) and the Collaborative Assessment and Learning Model (CALM) (Crozier *et al.*, 2021; Elliott, 2021; Wareing *et al.*, 2018; Williamson *et al.*, 2020), they all share the same basic principles. You will most frequently hear them being referred to as CLiP models, but this is identifying a specific model of practice and the more correct generic term is collaborative learning models.

The use of collaborative learning models continues the theme of utilising all members of the multidisciplinary team to facilitate the clinical education of nursing students. This in turn matches the ethos of the new NMC standards which state that the support and development of learning is the responsibility of every registrant. The collaborative learning model allows for an increase in placement capacity while also delivering a high-quality learning experience for students and improving patient outcomes and satisfaction. The model relies on a skills mix of students with a coach overseeing the group. Due to the increased number of students working in a clinical area and supporting each other under the supervision of a registered nurse, patients have constant contact and support providing a high level of individualised care.

The group of students will be responsible for a cohort of patients each day. At the start of their shift, they will meet with their coach and discuss the handover notes for their cohort of patients, working as a team to rank the priorities of care for the day and identify any available learning opportunities. Within the group, they will identify which students are responsible for which tasks and how they can help each other to develop. Ideally, there would be a mixture of students from different parts of the programme. For example, in a bay of six patients, there might be two part 1 students concentrating on the care of a single individual patient being supported by two part 2 students who are taking the care of the remaining four patients between them. In addition, you would have a part 3 student overseeing the care of all the patients for the day and ensuring appropriate delegation of tasks.

Table 6.2 Coaching conversations.

TYPE OF QUESTION	EXAMPLE
Questions for clarification	What is the rationale for using aseptic non-touch techniques? How does this relate to our previous conversation about medicines management?
Questions that probe assumptions	How else could we interpret that behaviour? How can you verify or disprove that assumption? Why aren't we questioning that care plan?
Questions that probe reason and evidence	Why do you think Mrs Smith fainted? Do you think that providing risk assessment training has reduced the number of falls in our area? Is it worth investing in more training?

This is in effect a 'mini-ward' structure; the part 1 students take the role of a Band 5 staff nurse, the part 2 students are equivalent to Band 6, overseeing the work of the part 1 students and helping them to develop, while the Part 3 student sits in the same role as the ward manager, all under the supervision and support of the registered nurse who is acting as their coach for that shift.

Collaborative learning utilises coaching conversations to support students to explore and express their own understanding while developing clinical decision-making processes rather than being directed and instructed in tasks (Table 6.2).

The idea is that by asking questions and getting the student to consider the possible solutions, the student is more able to link theory to practice and will develop greater confidence and competence than if they were 'just' following instructions. There is a limited base of research to evaluate the implementation of collaborative learning across the UK so far, but the initial responses have reported that the collaborative learning approach helps to reduce student anxiety when entering their first clinical placement, enhances clinical competence and competence in students across all parts and improves preparation for supervision and leadership in part 3 students (Van de Mortel et al., 2021). Peer teaching and learning is a valuable tool to improve self-efficacy with a reported improvement in clinical skills and preparation for real-life scenarios.

Conclusion

Clinical practice is a significant factor in a student's journey to becoming a competent registered nurse. The aim is to develop a good understanding of teamworking, leadership and the professional role of the nurse as well as clinical skills and communication approaches. To ensure the best outcomes from clinical practice, students need to prepare effectively for their placements by developing a sound understanding of their PAD requirements and considering how these will be met in differing practice environments.

An equally important factor in the success or failure of clinical placements is the support and supervision provided for students in clinical practice. It is the responsibility of the whole team in a clinical area to support student learning. Most team members will work as practice supervisors demonstrating diverse ways of working and providing support and assessment for specific clinical skills as required. The practice assessor will work with both practice supervisors and academic assessors to review the student's progress and make evidence-based judgements about their progression. The practice assessor will also have an overarching view to ensure that there is consistent co-ordinated support provided for the student to achieve their goals.

The practice assessors and academic assessors will also work together to support a student with action plans and development needs if concerns are raised during a clinical placement.

To support students' professional development and confidence, there is also a move towards using coaching methods (both peer and expert coaching) when supervising students in practice. The coaching approaches have been shown to enhance students' confidence and competence as they approach registration and use of these approaches is now starting to expand across practice settings.

Key Points

- Students need to research their placement areas and make contact early to understand the learning opportunities.
- There is a whole-team approach to supporting students in placement.
- Students are entitlted to reasonable adjustments in their placements if they disclose additional needs.
- Students need to be proactive in managing their documentation and identifying learning opportunities.
- Concerns need to be escalated as early as possible to ensure that appropriate support can be put in place.
- Student supervision and assessment is a shared responsibility between academic and clinical staff.

References

Baker-Armstrong, J. (2020) Building nurses' resilience. *Nursing New Zealand*, 26(3), 31.

Cassidy, S., Coffey, M. & Murphy, F. (2020) Transparency of assessment decision-making when students are not meeting required levels of proficiency in clinical practice. *Nurse Education in Practice*, 43, 102711.

Coutts, A. (2016) Supporting student nurses. *Gastrointestinal Nursing*, 14(10), 12–15.

Crozier, K., Lobo, C. & Paul, R. (2021) *Collaborative Learning in Practice: Coaching to Support Student Learners in Healthcare*. Wiley, Chichester.

Donaldson, I. (2019) From mentor to supervisor and assessor: changes in pre-registration programmes. *British Journal of Nursing*, 28(1), 64.

Drayton, L. & Edmonds, M. (2020) Understanding the role of the academic assessor. *Nursing Standard*, 35(9), 41–45.

Drew, L. (2020) Getting the most out of your practice placement. https://rcni.com/nursing-standard/students/getting-most-out-of-your-practice-placement-171361 (accessed December 2021).

Elliott, T. & East Suffolk and North Essex NHS Foundation Trust (2021). Implementation of Collaborative Assessment & Learning Model (CALM). www.rcn.org.uk/professional-development/practice-based-learning/innovations-from-around-the-uk/implementation-of-collaborative-assessment-and-learning-model

Gosport Independent Panel (2018) *The Panel Report*. www.gosportpanel.independent.gov.uk/panel-report/ (accessed December 2021).

Honkavuo, L. (2020) Nursing students' perspective on a caring relationship in clinical supervision. *Nursing Ethics*, 27(5), 1225–1237.

Huybrecht, S., Loeckx, W., Quaeyhaegens, Y., de Tobel, D. and Mistiaen, W. (2011) Mentoring in nursing education: perceived characteristics of mentors and the consequences of mentorship. *Nurse Education Today*, 31(3), 274–278.

Johns, C. (2017) *Becoming a Reflective Practitioner*, 5th edn. Wiley Blackwell, Chichester.

Lee, N.P.M. & Chiang, V.C.L. (2020) The mentorship experience of students and nurses in pre-registration nursing education: a thematic synthesis of qualitative studies. *Nursing & Health Sciences*, 23(1), 69–86.

Mid Staffordshire NHS Foundation Trust Public Inquiry (2013) *Report of the Mid Staffordshire NHS Foundation Trust Public Inquiry: Executive Summary*. https://assets.publishing.service.gov.uk/government/uploads/system/uploads/attachment_data/file/279124/0947.pdf (accessed December 2021).

Nursing & Midwifery Council (2010) *Standards for Pre-Registration Nursing Education*. NMC, London.

Nursing & Midwifery Council (2018a) *The Code:Professional Standards of Practice and Behaviour for Nurses, Midwives and Nursing Associates*. NMC, London.

Nursing & Midwifery Council (2018b) *Standards of Proficiency for Nursing Associates*. NMC, London.

Nursing & Midwifery Council (2018c) *Standards of Proficiency for Registered Nurses*. NMC, London.

Nursing & Midwifery Council (2019a) *Standards for Pre-Registration Nursing Programmes*. NMC, London.

Nursing & Midwifery Council (2019b) *Standards for Student Supervision and Assessment*. NMC, London.

Nursing & Midwifery Council (2019c) *Standards Framework for Nursing and Midwifery Education*. NMC, London.

Ousey, K. (2011) The changing face of student nurse education and training programmes. *Wounds UK*, 7(1), 70–75.

Pan London Practice Learning Group (2019) *Pan London Practice Assessment Document (PLPAD 2:0)*. Pan London Practice Learning Group, London.

Parsloe, E. & Leedham, M. (2009) *Coaching and Mentoring: Practical Conversations to Improve Learning*, 2nd edn. Kogan Page, London.

Passmore, J. (2016) *Excellence in Coaching: The Industry Guide*, 3rd edn. Kogan Page, London.

Powell, A. (2021) *Disabled People in Employment*. House of Commons Library, London.

Ramluggun, P., Jackson, D. & Usher, K. (2021) Supporting students with disabilities in preregistration nursing programmes. *International Journal of Mental Health Nursing*, 30(2), 353–356.

Rawson, R. (2021) *How to Integrate into a Clinical Placement Team*. https://rcni.com/nursing-standard/students/clinical-placements/how-to-integrate-a-clinical-placement-team-175976 (accessed December 2021).

Salkeld, J. (2016) A model to support nursing students with dyslexia. *Nursing Standard*, 30(47), 46–51.

Smith, Y. (2019) *History of Nursing*. www.news-medical.net/health/History-of-Nursing.aspx (accessed December 2021).

Van de Mortel, T. F., Needham, J. & Henderson, S. (2021) Facilitating learning on clinical placement using near-peer supervision: a mixed methods study. *Nurse Education Today*, 102, 104921.

Walsh, D. (2014) *The Nurse Mentor's Handbook: Supporting Students in Clinical Practice*, 2nd edn. Open University Press, Maidenhead.

Wareing, M., Green, H., Burden, B., *et al.* (2018) Coaching and Peer-Assisted Learning (C-PAL) – the mental health nursing student experience: a qualitative evaluation. *Journal of Psychiatric and Mental Health Nursing*, 25(8), 486–495.

Williamson, G.R., Kane, A., Plowright, H., Bunce, J., Clarke, D. and Jamison, C. (2020) 'Thinking like a nurse'. Changing the culture of nursing students' clinical learning: implementing collaborative learning in practice. *Nurse Education in Practice*, 43, 102742.

92

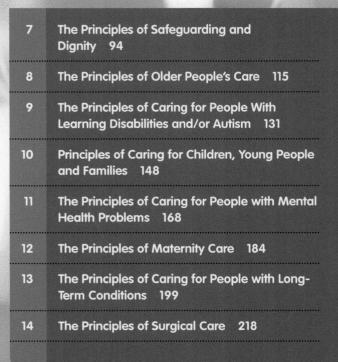

Unit 2

The Principles of Care

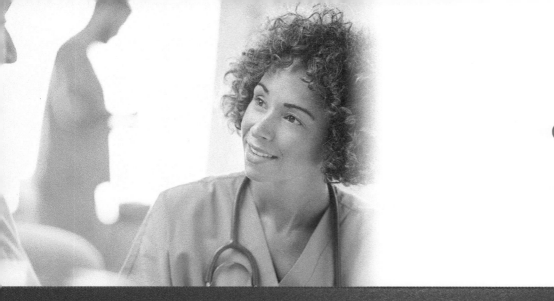

7

The Principles of Safeguarding and Dignity

Joanna Regan and Karen Sykes

Leeds Teaching Hospitals NHS Trust, UK

Learning Outcomes

On completion of this chapter you will be able to:

- Define what is meant by the terms 'safeguarding' and 'dignity'
- Consider how safeguarding and dignity are key concepts that can affect people you care for and offer support to
- Demonstrate an understanding of the legislative frameworks that help monitor and support safeguarding and dignity
- Gain insight into the application of the principles concerning safeguarding and dignity
- Demonstrate an awareness of the dignity challenges and framework
- Have an insight into dignity action planning and influencing

Proficiencies

NMC Proficiencies and Standards:

- Understand and apply the principles of courage, transparency and the professional duty of candour, recognising and reporting any situations, behaviours or errors that could result in poor care outcomes. (1.3)
- Demonstrate the skills and abilities required to support people at all stages of life who are emotionally or physically vulnerable. (1.12)
- Recognise and assess people at risk of harm and the situations that may put them at risk, ensuring prompt action is taken to safeguard those who are vulnerable. (3.9)

(Continued)

Nursing Practice: Knowledge and Care, Third Edition. Edited by Ian Peate and Aby Mitchell.
© 2022 John Wiley & Sons Ltd. Published 2022 by John Wiley & Sons Ltd.
Companion website: www.wiley.com/go/peate/nursingpractice3e

Proficiencies (Continued)

- **Demonstrate an understanding of how to identify, report and critically reflect on near misses, critical incidents, major incidents and serious adverse events in order to learn from them and influence their future practice. (6.8)**

- **Apply an understanding of the differences between risk aversion and risk management and how to avoid compromising quality of care and health outcomes. (6.10)**

Visit the companion website at www.wiley.com/go/peate/nursingpractice3e where you can test yourself using flashcards, multiple-choice questions and more.

Introduction

This chapter will support your learning about the key principles of 'safeguarding adults at risk' and of 'dignity in care', and help you examine how these can and do causally relate to your practice and practice setting. Important issues such as consent and human rights will be explored.

The Nursing Associate

The nursing associate delivers hands-on, person-centred care as part of a multidisciplinary team in a range of different settings. As registered healthcare professionals, they have a key role to play in ensuring adults at risk are safeguarded and also to guarantee dignity in care regardless of care setting.

Because of the media coverage associated with poor care and practices in several settings, for example the Mid Staffordshire Inquiry (Francis, 2013), safeguarding and dignity of individuals is more widely recognised than ever before. As such, it is essential for all those working within health and social care to have a sound knowledge and understanding of safeguarding and dignity and to practise conscientiously and professionally in relation to professional and legislative frameworks.

What is Safeguarding?

'Safeguarding' is an umbrella term that includes the concepts of promoting the welfare and well-being of an individual, as well as protecting from harm (Social Care Institute for Excellence, 2012).

Safeguarding and providing dignity and respect are the highest priority for people in your care. This means making sure that individuals are actively involved in any planning, decisions and implementation of care and support they are receiving.

Safeguarding should not be seen as a negative or restrictive option, but rather a positive way of promoting individualised care and support. Organisations have policies and procedures in place, highlighting the roles and responsibilities of individual practitioners for safeguarding an individual.

Safeguarding of adults aims to ensure that each individual maintains (to the best of their abilities):

- Dignity and respect
- Quality of life
- Health
- Choice
- Control
- Safety.

To Whom Does Safeguarding Apply?

Safeguarding could and may apply to any 'adult at risk'. This term itself could apply to a wide range of people, some for a short period of time and some for a substantial period or indefinitely.

Anyone with a condition or illness that affects their ability to maintain their own safety, well-being or interests and express their views could be included in safeguarding principles and procedures. For example, a young person who has been involved in a motorcycle accident and is temporarily incapacitated both physically and mentally due to injuries and condition, or a person who has a dementia, learning disability or mental health condition that can fluctuate in mental capacity, could require the principles of safeguarding applied to their care.

Principles of Safeguarding

The Department of Health (2011) issued a Statement of Government Policy on Adult Safeguarding that outlined six principles of safeguarding adults; these are now embedded in the Care Act 2014 and are detailed in Box 7.1.

Box 7.1 Principles of safeguarding adults.	
Empowerment	This includes a belief that the individual has been involved in person-led decisions and informed consent
Protection	This includes the support and interpretation of those in utmost need
Prevention	This includes the anticipation and avoidance of situations before harm could occur
Proportionality	This includes a balanced and least restrictive option and response, which is fitting to the risk identified

| Partnership | This includes working within local communities, to prevent, identify and report any signs of neglect or harm to an individual |
| Accountability | This includes the need to be accountable for all actions, transparent with care and support for individuals and while taking part in safeguarding |

Source: Modifiled from Department of Health (2011).

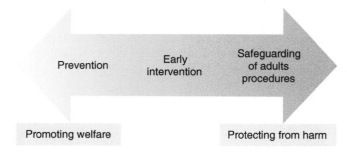

Figure 7.1 Safeguarding continuum. *Source*: Social Care Institute for Excellence (2013a). Reproduced with permission of SCIE.

Safeguarding Continuum

Safeguarding of adults should never be viewed in isolation or as a single act once safeguarding procedures have commenced. It should be viewed as a two-way continuum that travels from promoting welfare and well-being to protecting from harm. Figure 7.1 highlights how the continuum of safeguarding is envisaged by multiple local authorities and safeguarding boards (Social Care Institute for Excellence, 2013a).

Safeguarding in Action

The six principles of safeguarding (see Box 7.1) can be applied in practice and will include similar guidelines to those listed here.

- Service provision should be suitable for the individual, and non-discriminatory.
- Allow individuals to make their own decisions as far as possible and support or offer advocacy support to make choices.
- Presume that adults do have the mental capacity to make informed decisions about their lives, unless they have been assessed as not having capacity at that point in time.
- Provide information, advice and support to any identified adult at risk, in a format that they can understand, and ensure that their wishes and chosen outcomes are central to any safeguarding decision made about them and their lives.
- Ensure that any decision by health or social care professionals about an individual's life is taken in a timely fashion, is reasonable, justified and proportionate to the risks identified.

As well as the six principles of safeguarding included in the organisational policy, there are some other inclusions which you will be able to locate within the opening statement or throughout the document.

- A statement that the individuals you care for are kept safe and lead lives that are rewarding.
- Information on the staff's responsibilities.

- Evidence that your organisation is taking its responsibilities about safeguarding seriously.
- Legal disclaimers to protect staff members and the organisation.
- Early intervention.
- Identify routes of referral that a professional body or safeguarding authority may take, and the circumstances associated with these.
- Compliance with legislation and regulations, including good practice guidance and evidence-based support.

Who is an Adult at Risk?

The 'No Secrets' guidance from the Department of Health and Home Office (2000) offers definitions on who might be an adult at risk and exists to protect and support some of the most vulnerable adults in society. Adults at risk are defined as:

'Any adult over the age of 18, who is or may be in need of community care services by reason of mental or other disability, age or illness; and who is or maybe unable to take care of him or herself, or unable to protect him or herself against significant harm or exploitation'.

(Department of Health and Home Office, 2000)

Jot This Down

- Think of some of the *characteristics* that might make someone more at risk of harm.
- Think of some of the *factors* that might make someone more at risk of harm.

Case Study

Rishi is employed as a nursing associate (TNA) at a stepdown care facility for people with learning disabilities. This social care facility provides care for people with learning disabilities across all age ranges.

'My role requires me to work with a variety of health and care professionals as well as working and liaising across agencies, such as housing, education and the police. The main aspect of my role is to help individuals to rehabilitate in an assisted living environment. As a nursing associate, I am called upon to discuss health and care issues about those who I offer care and support to. As I have become much more experienced, I am now able to recognise more potential causes for risk or harm and I now know the right channels and processes that have to be adhered to so I am acting in the best interest of the residents I work with. I am able to act as an advocate on their behalf in a competent and confident way.'

What Does 'Mental Capacity' Mean?

In a safeguarding situation, mental capacity is the ability of an individual to:

- Understand the potential implications of their situation and the risks to themselves
- Take appropriate measures to protect themselves against abuse
- Take part in any decision-making process involving them as individuals, to the fullest extent, regardless of it relating to everyday matters or significant life events.

Table 7.1 Principles of the Mental Capacity Act and Adults with Incapacity (Scotland) Act.

MENTAL CAPACITY ACT 2005	ADULTS WITH INCAPACITY (SCOTLAND) ACT 2000
Principle 1: Assumption of capacity	**Principle 1:** Benefit
Principle 2: Support to make decisions	**Principle 2:** Least restrictive option
Principle 3: Right to make unwise decisions	**Principle 3:** Take account of the wishes of the person
Principle 4: Best interests	**Principle 4:** Consultation with relevant others
Principle 5: Least restrictive option	**Principle 5:** Encourage the person to use existing skills and develop new skills

The Mental Capacity Act 2005 (MCA) and the Adults with Incapacity (Scotland) Act 2000 are both based on five principles, which are detailed in Table 7.1. You will see from Table 7.1 that there are some differences between both elements of law relating to mental capacity. Ultimately they are both in place to ensure the safety and well-being of individuals and prevent the likelihood of harm or exploitation.

Principle 1: Assumption of Capacity

Everyone, even those with a diagnosis of an illness or condition, has the right to make their own decisions and must be assumed to have capacity, unless it is proved otherwise. This requires a 'balance of probability' test initially, where we need to ensure that 'a reasonable person' would think that there is evidence of an individual understanding the required decision and its consequences.

Following this, a two-stage functional test of capacity is required to decide if an individual has capacity to make a decision (Social Care Institute for Excellence, 2010).

- *Stage 1.* Is there an impairment or disturbance in the functioning of a person's mind or brain? If so,
- *Stage 2.* Is the impairment or disturbance sufficient that the person lacks the capacity to make a particular decision?

Following this functional test of capacity, the MCA states that an individual is not able to make their own decision if they cannot achieve one or more of the following.

- Understand and retain the information given to them to be able to make a decision.
- Process the information that has been made available to them to make the decision.
- Communicate their decision.

Health and social care professionals cannot solely consider verbal communication as a valid communication method and every effort should be made to establish ways of communicating with someone before making a decision that they lack capacity. It is essential to document all findings and how you have concluded that their capacity is lacking for the particular decision.

Who should Assess Mental Capacity?

The answer to the question in the 'Jot This Down' exercise is dependent on who is directly involved in care delivery and who is immediately involved in the outcome from that decision. This means that everyone on the list you have made above, including yourself, will be involved in assessing an individual's capacity at different times and for different decisions.

The Nursing Associate

 Nursing associates play an important role in the multidisciplinary and multiagency workforce. They work alongside care assistants, registered nurses, social workers and other staff to provide safe and effective care and support to those who may be vulnerable or at risk of abuse.

Principle 2: Support to Make Decisions

Some individuals can make decisions when supported in doing so. Any adult at risk must receive all the help and support possible to make decisions before anyone presumes that they cannot do so.

The Department for Constitutional Affairs (2007), in the *Mental Capacity Act 2005 Code of Practice*, identifies several items to be taken into consideration to ensure that a person has been supported to make a decision and these should be followed as part of the overall assessment of the individual's abilities.

- Has the individual received all significant information to make a decision?
- If there are alternatives available, has the individual been given the information on all alternatives?
- Would the individual be able to understand or process the information better if it were presented differently?
- Does the individual demonstrate a better understanding at different times of the day?
- Does the individual feel more comfortable in different places, and therefore able to make decisions better?
- Does the decision have to be made now or can it be delayed until the conditions are different, allowing the individual to make the decision?
- Does the individual need anyone else to help them to make their choices or views known?

Principle 3: Right to Make Unwise Decisions

Any adult has the right to make decisions that others might consider unwise or eccentric. This also applies to adults at risk, and the person cannot be treated as lacking capacity because of these reasons. However, if someone repeatedly makes unwise decisions that place them at significant risk, this might be grounds to question and assess their capacity.

Red Flag

Throughout the considerations within Principle 3, it is important to remember that everyone has their own values, beliefs and preferences, which may not be the same as yours. People cannot be treated as lacking in capacity because they hold different values, beliefs or preferences from those that healthcare professionals hold.

As members of the health and social care team, it is essential to try to understand, to the best of our abilities, the beliefs and values of the person whose capacity to make decisions is under question. Evidence can be found in things such as:

- Cultural background
- Religious beliefs
- Political convictions
- Past behaviour or habits.

Some people set out their beliefs and values in a written statement while they still have capacity.

Principle 4: Best Interests

If it is essential to decide on behalf of someone who has been assessed as lacking capacity, then whatever the decision, it must be in the person's best interests. The term 'best interest' is not defined within the Mental Capacity Act 2005 as the Act deals with so many different types of decisions and actions.

Principles Governing 'Best Interest' Decisions

When working out what is in the best interests of the person who lacks capacity to decide or act for themselves, decision makers must consider all relevant factors that would be reasonable, not just those that they think are important.

The following principles should be applied while making a 'best interest' decision on behalf of a person who is lacking capacity.

- Do not discriminate. Do not make assumptions about someone's best interests merely on the basis of their age or appearance, condition or any aspect of their behaviour.
- Take into account all relevant circumstances.
- If faced with a particularly difficult or contentious decision, it is recommended that practitioners adopt a 'balance sheet' approach (weighing up the advantages and disadvantages of each option in turn).
- Will the person regain capacity? If so, can the decision wait?
- Involve the individual as fully as possible.
- Take into account the individual's past and present wishes and feelings, and any beliefs and values likely to have a bearing on the decision.
- Consult as far and as widely as possible.

Principle 5: Least Restrictive Option

If a best interest decision is made on behalf of someone who is judged to be lacking capacity, it is important that you make the choice that least restricts the person's liberty.

It is also essential that you record your decision given the evidence-based approach required by the Mental Capacity Act, so that you have an objective record should your decision or decision-making process later be challenged. This should be in line with local policy and procedure.

What is Meant by Deprivation of Liberty Safeguards?

The Deprivation of Liberty Safeguards (DoLS) is an amendment to the Mental Capacity Act 2005. It applies to England and Wales only. The MCA allows restraint and restrictions to be used, but only if they are in the person's best interests. Extra safeguards are needed if the restraint and restrictions will deprive a person of their liberty and they do not have the capacity to consent; these are called the Deprivation of Liberty Safeguards (Royal College of Psychiatrists, 2015).

Red Flag

Liberty Protection Safegaurds (LPS)
From April 2022, it is proposed that Liberty Protection Safeguards will replace Deprivation of Liberty Safeguards. This was announced in a Mental Capacity (Amendment) Bill passed into law in May 2019.

LPS will provide protection for people aged 16 and above who have been or need to be deprived their liberty, but who lack capacity to consent to this aspect of their care. Examples may include individuals with autism, dementia and learning disabilities.

Source: DHSC (2021a)

The DoLS may only be used if the person will be deprived of their liberty within a care home or hospital setting. Ways in which a person's freedoms may be curtailed can include:

- Using locks or keypads, which stop a person going out or into different areas of a building
- The use of certain medications, for example to calm a person
- Close supervision in the clinical setting
- Requiring a person to be supervised when out
- Restricting contact with family, friends and acquaintances, including if they could cause the person harm
- Physically preventing a person from doing something that might cause them harm
- Removing items from a person that could cause them harm
- Holding a person so that they can be given care or treatment
- The use of bedrails, wheelchair straps or splints
- The person having to stay somewhere against their wishes
- The person having to stay somewhere against the wishes of a family member.

Members of the health and social care teams need to ensure that they are using the least restrictive alternative and have sought the permission of the correct supervisory body. The *Mental Capacity Act 2005 Code of Practice* (Department for Constitutional Affairs, 2007) provides a checklist of common factors that must always be considered by anyone who needs to decide what is in the best interests of a person who lacks capacity in any particular situation. This is only the starting point; in many cases, extra factors will need to be considered.

Case Study

Applying the DoLS in practice

Edith, a 68-year-old woman with early-onset Parkinson disease and dementia, is admitted to a care home for respite. During her admission, Edith has repeatedly wandered out of

(Continued)

the home and has sustained several falls, due to her poor mobility. During the last episode, she was found on the main road near the home by a member of the public.

These episodes occur despite Edith being regularly monitored by staff, but she becomes aggressive when they try to persuade her to stay. She cannot leave the home unattended and now requires constant supervision. The home manager feels that it will be necessary to start using the lock on the main door to ensure Edith's safety.

Do you think that Edith is being deprived of her liberty? List your examples and the rationale to support your responses. What are the factors that must be considered in this case?

What is Abuse or Harm?

The terms 'abuse' and 'harm' are often interchangeable and, depending on the location of your studies, may be included in the country's laws and legislation. The Adult Support and Protection (Scotland) Act 2007, for example, uses the term 'harm' to adults at risk, rather than 'abuse'. For the purposes of this chapter, the term 'abuse' will be used.

'Abuse' in its broadest sense relates to the misuse or application of power and control over one individual by another and can take place in virtually any environment within society, regardless of circumstance. The Royal College of Nursing (2015) suggests abuse is a violation of a person's human and civil rights by any other person or persons.

Abuse does not always require motive or to be intended, and can be considered in terms of the impact of the harm caused on the individual.

The Social Care Institute for Excellence (2011) states that early legal or police involvement in any suspected or alleged abuse is essential and should be a key consideration in any circumstances, although not all cases of reported abuse escalate to legal or criminal proceedings.

The Nature of Abuse

Unfortunately, abuse is not as straightforward in practice, as the misuse of power or control over an individual and several complexities come into play within this arena. There are four main themes to consider. Table 7.2 highlights the nature of the abuse which can take place.

Consent

When considering abusive acts and reporting and dealing with such, consent from the individual must be a consideration within the process. The application of the Principles of the Mental Capacity Act and the Adults with Incapacity (Scotland) Act, which have already been described, would need to be a consideration at these times.

While considering if consent was given, attention should be paid to whether it was given under duress, for example through intimidation, fear and for potential outcomes or gain for other family members. If consent was given in any of these circumstances, it is likely to be regarded as non-consensual and action can be taken against the perpetrator.

Table 7.2 The nature of abuse. *Source*: Modified from Social Care Institute for Excellence (2011).

NATURE OF ABUSE	DESCRIPTION
A single act or repeated acts	Abuse may take place in a single act or a series of acts, both large and small
Unintentional	Causing harm may have been unintentional and not wilful, but harm has been caused and abuse has taken place
An act of neglect or a failure to act	Neglect or failing to act may still cause harm to an individual and would require a response under the safeguarding procedures
Multiple acts	The individual receiving care and support may be experiencing several forms of abuse at the same time, some more discreet than others

99

Types of Adult Abuse

Safeguarding requires the nurse and nursing associate to understand various types of abuse and neglect. There are numerous types and indicators of abuse.

- *Physical abuse* may involve violence, misuse of medicines, inappropriate sanctions or restraints.
- *Domestic violence or abuse* includes physical, financial, sexual, emotional and honour-based violence.
- *Sexual abuse* includes rape, sexual assault and any sexual activity that the person lacks the capacity to consent to.
- *Psychological or emotional abuse*, threats, deprivation, humiliation, controlling, blaming, intimidation, harassment, online abuse.
- *Financial or material abuse* including theft, exploitation, fraud, misuse or misappropriation of property, possessions and benefits. The misuse of an enduring power of attorney or a lasting power of attorney, or appointeeship (NHS England, 2015).
- *Modern slavery* includes human trafficking, domestic servitude and forced labour.
- *Discriminatory abuse* including racist or sexist abuse or abuse based on age or disability.
- *Organisational or institutional abuse* include poor care and neglect within a health or social care setting.
- *Neglect or acts of omission* include failing to meet physical or medical care needs, failing to provide access to health and social care and education, withholding basic needs such as food and warmth, withholding medication.
- *Self-neglect or harm* The Mental Health Foundation (2019) estimated that 400 in every 100 000 of the population self-harm. It is often seen as a cry for help or as a means of coping with stress or emotion that is overwhelming and out of control for individuals. Other examples include neglecting to care for personal hygiene or behaviours such as hoarding.

Jot This Down

What impact do you think the COVID-19 pandemic has had on safeguarding adults in society?

In the Jot This Down exercise, you might have reviewed the types and indicators of abuse to help you to address this question. The Social Care Institute for Excellence published the following statement.

'We can assume that the greatest opportunity for abuse during the COVID-19 crisis is financial. With additional pressures on services, normal service reductions, fear and isolation, the window is open to those who may seek to exploit those who may be vulnerable. There were early reports of a 400 per cent increase in fraud reporting in March relating to the COVID-19 crisis. The Chartered Trading Standards Institute has warned the public not to open their doors to bogus healthcare workers claiming to be offering "home-testing" for COVID-19. The BBC reported on:

- online sales of sanitation equipment that is never delivered
- links to a fake daily newsletter for COVID-19 updates
- fake insurance schemes and trading advice
- fake government emails offering tax refunds.

Other types of abuse have escalated during this time – domestic abuse being a prominent example. Some living with an abusive partner or family member have seen an escalation in abuse due to the added tensions and frustration caused by the whole family having to stay indoors. The tensions can be further increased where families are living in cramped, temporary accommodation. The abuser may experience additional anxiety about, for example, supplies of food, alcohol, medication and illicit drugs. The consequences of this could be escalated abuse of those around them. People who are experiencing abuse may be less likely to ask for help as they know that emergency services are stretched. Fewer visitors to the household may mean that evidence of physical abuse goes unnoticed.' (Social Care Institute for Excellence, 2021)

Identifying Abuse

Your level of contact with and support of an individual can affect how abuse can be identified. If you are supporting the individual with personal care, you might notice signs more readily than someone who is providing support in a social capacity. Potential or actual abuse is not always obvious and it can often go unnoticed for long periods.

The identification of abuse can be split into three potential indicator groups.

- *Physical signs*: does the individual show any physical changes or signs that may indicate abuse taking place?
- *Behavioural signs*: are there any changes in the individual's behaviours that may lessen or increase your concerns? Are the behaviours significantly different from usual?
- *Other factors*: are there any historical influences that need to be considered, and do they increase your concern or reduce it?

Jot This Down

Can you list three potential signs of abuse for each of the following types?
- Physical abuse
- Emotional/psychological abuse
- Sexual abuse
- Institutional abuse
- Discriminatory abuse
- Financial abuse
- Neglect and acts of omission
- Domestic abuse
- Modern slavery

Safeguarding is Everybody's Business

Safeguarding is everybody's business. However, your responsibilities may vary depending on your role, which may include being a family member, friend, volunteer, health and social care worker, professional, safeguarding professional or manager.

There are six key principles of safeguarding that are applicable to all roles, which everyone should be aware of.

1. *Empowerment*: presumption of person-led activities and informed consent.
2. *Protection*: support and representation for those in greatest need.
3. *Prevention*: it is better to take action before harm occurs.
4. *Proportionality*: proportionate and least intrusive response appropriate to the risk presented.
5. *Partnership*: local solutions through services working with their communities (communities have a part to play in prevention, detection and reporting of neglect and abuse).
6. *Accountability*: accountability and transparency in delivering safeguarding.

Policy Framework for Safeguarding Adults

Adult safeguarding is framed in terms of the responsibilities of local authorities and partners in the NHS, police forces and other emergency services, with the Safeguarding Adults Boards managing the delivery of services across all agencies.

The Centre for Public Scrutiny and the Improvement and Development Agency (2010) published *Adult Safeguarding Scrutiny Guide*, which recognised the need for safeguarding to be everybody's business, and identified four main work streams involved in adult safeguarding. In 2013, the above guide was reviewed and evidence was presented that older people are the main group receiving adult safeguarding, followed by people with learning disabilities, physical disabilities and sensory impairment, and people with mental health conditions. In addition, physical abuse, and multiple abuse involving physical abuse, are the most frequent forms of reported abuse. The review also stated that physical abuse is the most frequent type of reported abuse in residential settings, whilst financial abuse is the most frequent type of reported abuse in domiciliary settings (Institute for Public Care, 2013). Since then, the picture remains constant. More recent evidence identifies an increase in neglect and acts of omission, and the most common location of risk was the person's own home. Safeguarding concerns during the 2019–20 period showed an increase of 14.6% on the previous year (NHS Digital, 2020).

Prevention and Awareness Raising

It is always better to act before harm occurs. Local policies and procedures will be in place detailing agreed ways of working when it comes to prevention and raising awareness of issues associated with safeguarding. These incorporate ways to improve the general well-being of everyone, to support communities to look out for each other, and to assist the public in knowing what to do if they think someone may be being harmed or abused.

Inclusion

Activities are explicitly designed to ensure that providers of community safety activities and other services are attentive to and include 'vulnerable' adults and that they also identify and support people who, for one reason or another, are vulnerable to poor life circumstances and outcomes from services.

Personalised Management of Benefits and Risks

This involves specific actions taken by those responsible for the commissioning, design and delivery of services to people at risk. Personalised management ensures the identification and support of people to help them to protect themselves and make informed decisions about action.

> ### Jot This Down
> Make a list of ways in which the possibility of abuse can be reduced by managing risk and concentrating on prevention.

Specialist Safeguarding Services

Where issues concerning safeguarding arise, it is important the individual concerned is at the centre of any investigation. This will involve specific action to ensure that people who lack capacity are supported through advocates and processes to ensure that their best interests are pursued. It also includes ensuring that justice is facilitated where people at risk are the victims of crime.

> **Caring, Dignity and Compassion**
>
> Be sensitive to the emotions that you think a person might be feeling when considering whether to talk about abuse.
>
> What might they be looking for or wanting from the person they are disclosing to? How can you demonstrate compassion and dignity when supporting an abused individual?

If someone chooses to disclose abuse to you, it is because they trust you. If someone confides in you, no matter what position you hold or your relationship to the person making the disclosure, you must act. Your responsibility is not to decide whether they are being abused; that is the responsibility of the relevant social work and safeguarding teams.

From the two activities completed concerning abuse and disclosure, you may have identified that a person who is disclosing abuse to you could potentially be feeling:

- Sad
- Lonely
- Angry
- Frightened
- Guilty
- Confused
- Worried

- Anxious
- Worthless.

They may be looking for any of the following from the person they are disclosing to.

- To be listened to
- To be believed
- Reassurance
- Help
- Support
- Empathy
- Privacy
- Understanding
- Kindness
- To make it stop

Responding to Disclosures

If an individual chooses to disclose harm or abuse to you, you will need to be aware of the feelings they could be experiencing and what they may be looking for by disclosing to you – which can be identified from the preceding lists.

Other guidelines should be followed when responding to an at-risk adult who is disclosing to you.

- Assure the individual that you are taking them seriously.
- Listen carefully to what they are telling you, stay calm, get as clear a picture as you can, but avoid asking too many questions at this stage.
- Do not give promises of being completely confidential.
- Explain that you have a duty to tell your manager or other designated person, and that their concerns may be shared with others who could have a part to play in protecting them.
- Reassure the individual that they will be involved in decisions about what will happen.
- Explain that you will try to take steps to protect them from further abuse or neglect.
- If they have specific communication needs, provide support and information in a way that is most appropriate to them.
- Do not be judgemental or jump to conclusions.

Northway (2013), in her work with people with learning disabilities who disclose or seek support, identified three key issues.

- Listen to us and do not ignore us.
- Believe us, believe what it is that we are saying.
- Do something to help to change things.

Immediate Action

Everyone who witnesses abuse or has abuse disclosed to them needs to know what immediate action to take. It is vital to become familiar with the local organisation's policies and procedures, so responses are made in line with these documents.

If no policy or procedure is in place or available, the following steps should be utilised as a framework for response in an emergency.

- Make an immediate evaluation of the risk and take steps to ensure that the adult is not in immediate danger
- If there is need for emergency medical treatment, contact the emergency services where you are located. If you suspect that the injury is non-accidental, alert the ambulance staff so that

appropriate measures are taken to preserve possible forensic evidence. Wherever possible, establish with the adult at risk the action they wish you to take.

- Consider contacting the police if a crime has been or may have been committed. Professional staff should alert their safeguarding lead or deputy, as they will be the people who will involve the police.
- Do not disturb or move articles that could be used in evidence, and secure the scene, for example by locking the door to a room.
- Contact the children and families' department if there is also or you suspect that there is also a child at risk.
- As far as possible, make sure that others are not at risk.

Case Study

Mary is a 29-year-old mum of two, who is attending the emergency department with her two young children and her partner Roberta after she slipped on a toy and fell down a flight of stairs and sustained a soft tissue injury to her right leg. When you are alone with Mary, she becomes very distressed and discloses to you that she is a victim of domestic abuse and her partner Roberta is the perpetrator. She tells you that Roberta pushed her down the stairs and that she did not slip accidentally. She is very frightened and wants help, but she asks you not to tell anyone.

- What should you do?
- Jot down the next steps and actions you would take.
- What are the main issues in this case scenario?

What to Do If a Criminal Offence is Suspected

The first concern of everyone must be to ensure the safety and well-being of the alleged victim.

It is the responsibility of the police to gather and preserve evidence in order to pursue criminal allegations against people causing harm and they should be contacted immediately. However, the victims themselves and other people and organisations play a vital role in the preservation of evidence to ensure that vital information or forensics is not lost. In some situations, it is important that you do not touch anything, so resist the natural inclination to tidy up or wash away blood or other forensic materials. It may also contaminate evidence if the victim eats, drinks or smokes a cigarette, so think carefully about what the individual is doing.

Professional and Legal Issues

Evidence in criminal investigations is based on the Criminal Justice Act 2003 and the Police and Criminal Evidence Act 1984. The classes of evidence you are likely to come across are:

- direct evidence
- circumstantial evidence
- primary and secondary evidence
- forensic evidence
- expert evidence.

Source: Home Office (2020)

Resist the temptation to take pictures of the scene with your phone. Your pictures are unlikely to be of sufficient quality to be submitted to court as part of a prosecution case; the police will also confiscate your phone. The preferred option is to leave the scene undisturbed and allow a police photographer to capture the evidence.

Police are required to obtain oral (spoken) evidence in specific ways. Questioning the alleged victim at this stage runs the risk of contaminating their oral evidence and a defence lawyer may be able to allege that the victim was coached by you.

Red Flag

Preventing abuse means doing three things.
- Listening to people and their caregivers.
- Intervening when you suspect abuse.
- Educating others about how to recognise and report abuse.

Making a Record

Anybody who is witness to or is alerted to a situation of abuse should make a written record of any incident or allegation of crime as soon as possible, and keep a signed, dated and timed copy.

The record must reflect, as accurately as possible, what was said and done by the people initially involved in the incident (the victim, suspect and potential witnesses). Use the words spoken and not a sanitised version of them – this is important. This record is an account of what was observed, disclosed or witnessed at the time and not an investigation. Investigation is the responsibility of the safeguarding professionals.

The notes must be kept safe, as it may be necessary to make records available as evidence and to disclose them in court.

Key Stages of the Adult Safeguarding Process

There are seven key stages in the adult safeguarding process. Brief information will be given on all the stages but this chapter focuses on the first two stages, as the later ones require further specialist training.

- Stage 1: Raising an alert
- Stage 2: Making a referral
- Stage 3: Strategy discussion or meeting
- Stage 4: Investigation
- Stage 5: Case conference and protection plan
- Stage 6: Review of the protection plan
- Stage 7: Closing the safeguarding adult's process

Stage 1: Raising an Alert

Everyone has a responsibility for safeguarding adults. If you are raising a concern within an organisation, then the concern should be passed immediately to the person responsible for dealing with safeguarding adults. If there is no organisation involved, the person raising the alert should contact the local Social Services Department directly.

Stage 2: Making a Referral

The decision to make a referral will normally be made by the person responsible for dealing with safeguarding. Alternatively, the person who is concerned can make a referral directly to the local Social Services Department.

Stage 3: Strategy Discussion or Meeting

This is a multiagency meeting convened and coordinated by the safeguarding adults manager (SAM) in the local authority, who will discuss the allegations with a range of professionals (usually including the police, where appropriate) to:

- Consider the wishes of the adult at risk
- Agree whether an investigation will take place and, if so, how it should be conducted and by whom
- Undertake risk assessment
- Agree an interim protection plan
- Make a clear record of the decisions
- Record what information is shared
- Agree an investigation plan with timescales
- Agree a communication strategy
- Consider whether a child (under 18 years) may also be at risk
- Circulate decisions to all invitees within 5 days, using the appropriate pro forma.

Stage 4: Investigation

The nature of the investigation is decided by those at the strategy meeting, who will also appoint an investigating officer. The purpose of the investigation is to:

- Establish the facts and contributing factors leading up to the referral
- Identify and manage risk and ensure the safety of the individual and others.

Stage 5: Case Conference and Protection Plan

The aim of a case conference is to:

- Consider the information contained in the investigating officer's report(s)
- Consider the evidence and, if substantiated, plan what action is indicated, or alternatively:
  - Plan further action if the allegation is not substantiated
  - Plan further action if the investigation is inconclusive
- Consider what legal or statutory action or redress is indicated

- Make a decision about the levels of current risks and a judgement about any likely future plans
- Agree a protection plan
  - Agree how the protection plan will be reviewed and monitored.

Stage 6: Review of the Protection Plan

The purpose of the review is to ensure that the actions agreed in the protection plan have been implemented and to decide whether further action is needed, including any service improvements.

Stage 7: Closing the Safeguarding Adults Process

The adult safeguarding process may be closed at any stage, if it is agreed that an ongoing investigation is not needed or if the investigation has been completed and a protection plan has been agreed and put in place. In most cases, a decision to close the process is taken at the case conference or protection plan review.

Timescales of the Key Stages of the Adult Safeguarding Process

It is vital that each of the stages of the adult safeguarding process takes place within the stipulated timescale and with certain tasks and responsibilities being completed at each of the stages. This allows the correct systems to be in place and utilised and ensures the safety and welfare of the individual who might be subject to the safeguarding process.

Stage 1: Raising an Alert

Raising an alert means passing on a concern. Everyone has a responsibility for safeguarding adults. If you are raising a concern within an organisation, then the concern should be passed immediately to the person responsible for dealing with safeguarding alerts (the 'alerting manager').

If an Adult is on the Receiving End of Abuse

An adult at risk may find it difficult to identify their vulnerabilities and to respond to neglect or ill treatment by others.

You must contact your local Social Services Department. If it is difficult for you to do this directly, speak to someone you trust – a family member, friend or professional not involved in the abuse – and ask them to do this for you.

You should expect a response from Social Services within 24 hours. If the situation is an emergency, call the emergency services and the police will ensure that your concerns are passed onto Social Services and that you get an immediate response.

If You are a Friend or Family Member

Discuss with the adult concerned the need to involve Social Services. As adults, we have the right to make our own decisions, even unwise ones, so always try to obtain the consent of the person involved before contacting the local Social Services Department.

However, you may contact the department without gaining the individual's consent if:

- You doubt their capacity to understand the consequences of their decision to take no action
- You fear for the safety of others
- You feel there is an immediate danger.

When contacting Social Services, explain your fears and the fact that the adult concerned did not want you to involve them. They will decide how best to take matters forward.

If you are a Professional (Including All Healthcare Students), Care Worker or Volunteer

If you are concerned that a member of staff has abused an adult at risk, you have a duty to report these concerns. You must inform your line manager immediately; as a student, it can be difficult to identify who your line manager is; while on practice placements, this would be your link lecturer or university tutor.

If you are concerned that your line manager has abused an adult at risk, you must inform a senior manager in your organisation, or another designated manager for safeguarding adults, without delay.

If you are concerned that an adult at risk may have abused another adult at risk, inform your line manager immediately.

Practice Assessment Document (NMC Competency 3.9)

There is an opportunity here for the healthcare student to demonstrate awareness, understanding and application of where to find policies and key protocols causally related to safe practice.

For example: safeguarding in practice and escalating concerns when abuse is suspected.

List the policies and protocols and make notes on each; share these with your practice supervisor so they can see how informed you have become.

Responsibilities of the 'Alerting Manager'

An 'alerting manager' is the person within an organisation designated to make safeguarding adult referrals. The alert may be made to them by the adult at risk, their family or friends, care workers, volunteers or other professionals. They must decide without delay on the most appropriate course of action.

If you are a staff member or a volunteer it is your responsibility to find out who is the designated person within your organisation to make a safeguarding referral.

Jot This Down

What areas do you think, as a student nurse or trainee nursing associate, you may need to consider when making someone aware of a safeguarding matter? List your thoughts.

Depending on the circumstances, the alerting manager needs to consider the adult's immediate:

- *Health needs*: have they sustained an injury or does the neglect they have experienced warrant medical attention?

- *Forensic needs*: if they need to see a doctor, should it be someone competent to collect forensic evidence? If the matter is to be referred to the police, the alerting manager should discuss any potential forensic considerations, particularly if the abuse is thought to be of a sexual nature
- *Legal needs*: has a crime been committed? If so, immediate consultation with the police is necessary
- *Safety needs*: are they at continued risk in their current home? What additional support is necessary? Do they need to be provided with alternative services or accommodation?

If the person causing the harm is also an adult at risk, an arrangement should be made for a member of staff to make a parallel referral to Social Services to address their needs.

If a staff member is suspected of causing the abuse, their manager should consider suspending the staff member (or otherwise removing them from the person at risk) in line with their organisation's safeguarding policy.

Responsibilities to the Alleged Abuser

The alerting manager should also consider the action they need to take in relation to the person alleged to have caused harm. It is always worth considering liaising with the police regarding the management of any risks.

Where the allegation is against a staff member, the first consideration should be whether to separate the member of staff from the person at risk. This may involve suspending them, without prejudice, pending further investigation; however, the staff member has a right to know that allegations have been made against them (the details of the allegation should not be shared at this stage). The strategy meeting (identified in Stage 3 of the seven-stage adult safeguarding process) will decide on what will be shared and when. Consideration must also be given to the risks, if any, to other service users and staff members, particularly if the conduct of the staff member came to light as the result of whistle-blowing. NHS England (2015) has produced guidance regarding managing and safeguarding allegations against staff.

Speaking to the Adult at Risk

The alerting manager may feel that it is appropriate to speak to the adult at risk before contacting Social Services. Consideration must be given to the at-risk adult's communication needs as well as their capacity to understand the information they are being provided with and their ability to make decisions. Specifically, the alerting manager should:

- Speak in a private and safe place to inform the adult at risk of the concerns
- Obtain their views on what has occurred and what they want done about it
- Provide information regarding the adult safeguarding process and how it can help to make them safer
- Ensure that they understand the limits of confidentiality
- Explain how they will be kept informed, particularly if they have communication needs
- Consider how the abusive experience could impact on the ongoing delivery of services, particularly personal care arrangements and access arrangements
- Explore their immediate protection needs.

Stage 2: Making a Referral

The consent of the adult at risk is a significant factor in deciding what action to take in response to an allegation but this in turn will depend on the capacity of the adult to make a decision.

When considering whether to refer or not and assessing the person's capacity, the following questions need to be included as part of the overall assessment.

- What do they understand about the abuse they have experienced?
- What do they think will be the consequence of making or not making a referral, both in terms of their immediate safety and in the longer term?
- What outcome do they want?
- What action do they think will be taken and by whom?
- What is their ability to protect themselves from future harm?

What If the Adult at Risk Decides Not to Refer?

The safeguarding processes assume capacity and the right of the individual to make their own choices, even unwise ones. In situations where the adult alleging abuse decides they do not want action taken:

- Give information about where to get help if they change their mind or if the abuse or neglect continues
- The referrer/alerting manager must assure themselves that the decision to withhold consent is not made under undue influence, coercion or intimidation
- A record must be made of the concern, the at-risk adult's decision and the decision not to refer, along with both your and their reasons
- A record should also be made of what information/advice they were given in a separate part of the individual's file or record that is clearly labelled 'safeguarding'.

Over-riding the At-Risk Adult's Decision

Where the referrer/alerting manager believes that there is an over-riding public interest or if gaining consent would put the individual at further risk, a referral must be made and the views of the individual over-ridden.

The key issue in deciding whether to make a referral is the harm or risk of harm to the adult at risk and any other individual who may have contact with the person who could have caused harm. Be especially vigilant where the person who could have caused harm remains in contact with the same organisation, service or care setting. This would include situations where:

- Other people or children could be at risk from the person causing harm
- It is necessary to prevent crime
- There is a high risk to the health and safety of the adult at risk
- The person lacks capacity to consent.

Preventing the Abuse of Adults at Risk

In recent years, the debate about prevention in safeguarding has been assisted and developed further with the introduction of the personalisation agenda and the self-directed care initiatives and schemes. It is important to achieve a balance between the

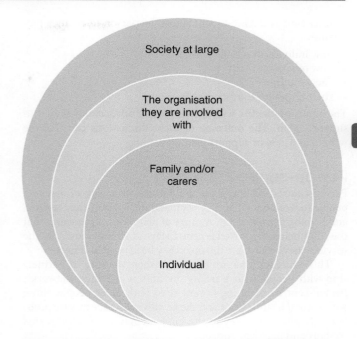

Figure 7.2 Multidimensional approach to preventing abuse or neglect. *Sources:* Social Care Institute for Excellence (2011) and New Jersey Task Force on Child Abuse and Neglect.

individual's rights to make choices for themselves and the duty of those caring and supporting the individual to keep them free from harm. In practice, this means not being overprotective or risk averse, but rather promoting empowerment and positive risk taking within any care setting.

The prevention of the abuse or neglect of the vulnerable in our society requires a multidimensional approach. Figure 7.2 represents the people and services that any individual may reasonably expect to 'look out' for them.

The Right to be Free from Abuse

Everyone needs to know that they have the right to be free from abuse. Some adults need support in exercising this right. This might mean ensuring they have access to advocacy services.

Empowerment and Choice

Many people at risk have reported wanting help to deal with situations in their own way; specifically, they want to do their own safeguarding. People want help with information, options, alternatives, suggestions, mediation, talking to others in a way that helps them get what they want, and so forth. What they do not want is decisions being made for them.

The 'personalisation' agenda provides one such environment within which to exercise choice and, despite the potential for the financial exploitation of vulnerable adults, there is a range of strategies identified that can help empower adults to make their own decisions (Carr, 2011).

Person-centred Practice

There is much written about person-centred practice throughout the nursing and care literature but the main features can be summarised as talking to and about the person to create a picture of:

- How individuals see themselves
- How others see them
- Their routines
- Their hopes for the future.

The aim is to identify with them (or their advocate) how best to support them. The outcome of these discussions can then be written as a care or support plan.

Person-centred Planning

Person-centred planning can be defined as a way of assisting people to work out what they want and the support they require, and helping them to get it. A range of planning tools ensures that the adult being supported is centre stage at all times and that the services they receive are the ones they both want and need.

This approach was initially used when working in partnership with people with learning disabilities and their networks. Person-centred planning is now used with older people, those with mental health issues and those with substance misuse problems. It has become key to the implementation of self-directed support and personal budgets.

Approaches differ in the way in which information is gathered and whether emphasis is on the detail of day-to-day life or longer-term plans for the future. However, all start with who the person is and end with specific actions to be taken.

A range of techniques is employed in person-centred practice, many of which use graphic or pictorial approaches. Some practitioners favour 'maps' as assessment and engagement tools and are outlined in Box 7.2.

Box 7.2 Maps Assessment Tools	
Relationship map	Identifies who is important to the person and could contribute to the planning process or identify the balance of family, friends and paid workers in the person's life to help maintain the person at the centre
Places map	Shows where the person goes and how they spend their time, so as to identify time spent in segregated and community places and illustrate opportunities for increasing the time spent in the community
Background map	Can be useful in understanding the experiences in a person's life that should be celebrated and those which need to be avoided, enabling the identification of positive experiences to build on
Preferences map	Describes what the person likes and dislikes. This map can show what the person enjoys and is good at, and can contribute to identifying things that the person may want to do more often or to show what situations and experiences should be avoided
Dreams, hopes and fears map	Helps to identify future goals and the barriers to achieving them. This map is useful to get a sense of how someone would like their life to be and to identify what the person is most afraid of happening, and can help to set the agenda for the planning meeting
Choices map	Shows what decisions the person makes and which are made by others. This map can help to establish what autonomy the person has, so as to indicate the areas in which the person could have more control
Health map	Describes what helps and what damages the person's health. This map can help to specify aspects of the person's health that need attention or to show what makes the person healthier and needs to be continued or developed

Source: McCormack & McCance (2017)

Prevention and Families

Where the adult at risk has a family or social network, efforts should be made to involve them in the planning and support, assuming that this is what the person concerned wants. There may be some difficulties faced when thinking about involving the family of an adult at risk. Each of these is listed here with a discussion on how it can be potentially problematic for those involved.

- *There is no involved family*: the person may be isolated and benefit from increased involvement with their local community.
- *The family may be intentionally or unintentionally harming the individual*: getting to know the family helps to understand the problem, the risks and how best to intervene.
- *The person may not want their family involved*: the person has the right not to involve others but an exploration of the reasons will give a better understanding of their perspective and occasionally may assist reconciliation.
- *The family may not understand that the person has a right to make choices so long as they have capacity and should be supported to do so*: getting involved with the family is the best way to help them understand that the person has the right to make choices.
- *Involving the family takes time*: involving the family potentially has the effect of empowering them and their relatives, making them more independent of services. It is likely to improve the quality of the provision being made.

Often, the family are concerned about the welfare of the adult at risk and have a meaningful contribution to make. However, in some situations, their actions contribute to risk or harm to the individual. Even then, it is important to have a dialogue with them to understand how best to intervene, particularly because carers who feel isolated may be more likely to be abusive. Wherever possible, involving the family should be done with the consent of the person at risk.

Promoting Resilience

The consequences of experiencing abuse or neglect can vary from person to person, depending on their resilience. Resilience is that quality in us all which helps us withstand adversity better. It has been described as 'the ability to cope with life's knocks' or 'the ability to pick yourself up and dust yourself off and start all over again' (Social Care Institute for Excellence, 2013b).

How resilient we are depends on a number of factors: the personal attributes we were born with, the sort of parenting we received and the amount and nature of the supports available to us. However, there are core components which are listed in Box 7.3.

> **Box 7.3 Core Components of Promoting Resilience**
> · Multiple social roles
> · Good relationships with family, friends and others
> · Positive leisure pursuits
> · Taking care of others
> · Making the most of educational opportunities
> · Stability
> · Spirituality
> · Involvement in the creative or expressive arts
>
> *Source*: Social Care Institute for Excellence (2013b) and Department of Health and Public Health England (2015)

What is Dignity?

In recent years, a considerable amount of literature has been produced on the subject of dignity in care, both in professional reading and in the media and on the internet. Despite the coverage, there has been no formal decision on the definition of what 'dignity' is.

It can often be easier to describe what dignified care is not, as there are examples highlighted within the media on a regular basis; for example, the Francis Report (2013) and the Winterbourne View inquiry (Department of Health, 2012) discovered that the quality of dignified care being delivered in many of the health and social care settings across the UK was unacceptable.

The Royal College of Nursing (2008) offers a definition of dignity related to how individuals might think, feel or behave as to their own worth and value, as well as that of others. It also offers insight into treating someone in a respectful manner.

A number of perspectives are evident, despite the term being used in overlapping ways, depending on the groups of individuals being discussed. Key perspectives associated with dignity include the following (Health and Social Care Advisory Service, 2010; RCN, 2014).

- *Dignity is a quality of the way we treat others*: dignity is one *quality* of our behaviour and actions towards others (e.g. 'the person was treated with dignity').
- *Dignity is a quality of a person's 'inner self'*: everyone has psychological needs and these are related to feelings of self-respect, self-esteem and self-worth.
- Dignity respects a person's autonomy.

The term 'dignity' can be used in more complex ways, as follows.

- *Expectations of being treated with dignity*: people want to be treated with dignity and most people have a very individual, finely tuned sense of whether they are being treated with the dignity they believe they deserve. Some vulnerable adults have considerable expectations, with feelings of self-worth associated with previous achievements or status.

- *Appearing and acting dignified*: the outward appearance or behaviour of a person may be a direct indication of how they feel about themselves (self-esteem). Maintaining a dignified appearance may be a major contribution to whether a person is treated with dignity by others.
- *Dignity of the human being*: this type of dignity is based on the principles of humanity and the universal worth of human beings and their inalienable rights, which can never be taken away. This is a moral approach, which considers that we all have a moral obligation to treat other human beings with dignity because of the belief that all human beings have 'nobility' and 'worth' and people need to be treated with dignity as part of fulfilling their human lives. Various international conventions and legal instruments define this in terms of human rights and how all human beings ought to be treated. This brings with it other ideas such as equality where, for example, it is expected that all people merit treatment as human beings on an equal basis, whoever they are, whatever their age, whatever their background, how they are behaving or whatever they may be suffering from.
- *Dignity of personal identity*: this form of dignity is related to personal feelings of self-respect and personal identity, which also provides the basis for relationships with other people. Most people have a self-image and wish to be treated by others in the manner they believe they deserve. Most people, even those who have learning disabilities or mental health issues, have a sense of self and whether they are being treated in a dignified and respectful matter. On the other hand, it is relatively easy to damage a person's perception of their self-esteem and self-worth with a few harsh words or physical mistreatment.
- *Dignity of merit*: this form of dignity is related to a vulnerable adult's status. Many vulnerable adults may have held positions in society, been awarded honours and had significant achievements in their lifetime. Uniforms, awards, badges and titles all bring to the owner a level of respect and dignity in society. People have a reasonable expectation of continued recognition for their achievements.
- *Dignity of moral stature*: this is a variation of dignity of merit, where people had status as they stand out because of the way they lead their lives according to their principles. This form of dignity is exceedingly difficult to appreciate because the meaning and value of 'stature' will vary and unlike awards or honours, 'moral stature' is not something everyone recognises. For example, an unelected 'community leader' may well carry considerable moral stature and be treated with the dignity the role demands by members of their community. Yet to others, this unelected individual may seem to have no legitimate right to represent anyone and just be ignored. This has many implications for the care of at-risk adults with dignity and the maintenance of their perceptions of themselves.

What is Respect?

'Respect' is a term which is very closely related to dignity. 'Respect' as a verb is probably the most important action word used to describe how dignity works in practice.

107

Respect is a difficult concept but can be defined as:

- Paying attention to
- Honouring
- Avoiding damaging, insulting or injuring
- Not interfering with or interrupting
- Treating with consideration
- Not offending.

The NMC supports this through the Code of Conduct (NMC, 2018) as well as its publication *Care and Respect: What You Can Expect From Nurses* (NMC, 2012).

Dignity is brought to life by the level of *respect* given to people's:

- Rights and freedoms
- Capabilities and limits
- Privacy, personal space and modesty
- Culture
- Habits and values
- Freedoms
- Individual beliefs of self-worth
- Personal merits
- Reputation
- Personal beliefs.

What The Experts Say

Respect and dignity

We value every person – whether patient, their families or carers, or staff – as an individual, respect their aspirations and commitments in life, and seek to understand their priorities, needs, abilities and limits. We take what others have to say seriously. We are honest and open about our point of view and what we can and cannot do.

DHSC (2021b)

Thinking About and Understanding Dignity

When thinking about dignity in practice and trying to understand how dignity in care can be applied to practice, it can create emotions and reflections on situations we have already been in, personally and professionally.

This is where a clear framework is useful when thinking about and understanding the subject of dignity in care, and it is recommended that the idea of dignity is considered from two linked points of view:

- Human rights
- Human needs.

Human Rights

The framework for human rights has been present within society for many years, although it is only more recently that it has had a larger presence within everyday practice and life in general. Figure 7.3 demonstrates how human rights, along with the relevant laws and legislation within the UK, have been developed from wider declarations.

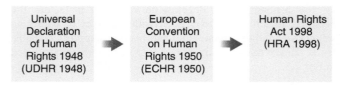

Figure 7.3 **Universal Declaration of Human Rights 1948.**
Source: Based on Health and Social Care Advisory Service (2010).

In 1948 the Universal Declaration of Human Rights was adopted by the United Nations General Assembly because of the experience of the Second World War. With the end of that war, and the creation of the United Nations, the international community vowed never again to allow atrocities such as those that occurred in that conflict.

European Convention on Human Rights 1950

Following on from the United Nations' work on human rights, the European Court of Human Rights (ECHR) was established and the publication of the European Convention on Human Rights 1950 followed, being fully implemented by 1953.

Human Rights Act 1998

The Human Rights Act 1998 was formulated as a 1997 White Paper 'Rights Brought Home' by the UK Government. This underpinned the need for UK domestic law on maintaining and overseeing the application of the European Convention of Human Rights closer to home.

There is a direct correlation between the Universal Declaration of Human Rights, the European Convention on Human Rights and the Human Rights Act, with the 16 human rights in UK law being taken from the ECHR (Box 7.4). Some of the articles in Box 7.4 are more applicable than others within a health and social care setting. Examples of some of the potential breaches to the articles are displayed in Box 7.5.

Box 7.4 Summary of the Human Rights Act 1998

Article 1	Introduction
Article 2	Right to life
Article 3	Prohibition of torture, and inhuman, degrading or humiliating treatment (abuse)
Article 4	Prohibition of slavery and forced labour
Article 5	Right to liberty and security
Article 6	Right to a fair trial
Article 7	No punishment without law
Article 8	Right to respect for private and family life
Article 9	Freedom of thought, conscience and religion
Article 10	Freedom of expression
Article 11	Freedom of assembly and association
Article 12	Right to marry
Article 14	Prohibition of discrimination
Article 16	Restrictions on political activity of aliens
Article 17	Prohibition of abuse of rights (unless objective reasons)
Article 18	Limitation on use of restrictions on rights
Protocol	Protection of property
Additional protocols	Right to education
	Right to free elections
	Abolition of the death penalty

Box 7.5 Examples of Potential Article Breaches

Article 2	Right to Life	No proper assessment of needs
Article 3	Prohibition of torture or degrading treatment (abuse)	Not being given enough diet or fluids
Article 5	Right to liberty and security	Individuals being given sedatives, tranquillisers and being physically restrained
Article 8	Right to respect for private and family life	Going through someone's belongings without permission
Article 9	Freedom of thought, conscience and religion	Restricting access to places of worship
Article 10	Freedom of expression	An individual being too frightened to complain
Article 14	Prohibition of discrimination	Restricted access to health or social care services because of discrimination
Protocol	Protection of property	Disposal of personal property without proper consent or permission

Source: Health and Social Care Advisory Service (2010) and Age UK (2020)

Other UK Legislation Relating to Human Rights

There are a number of other key pieces of UK legislation that directly relate to the protection of human rights; some have already been discussed in this chapter, others will require you to undertake some additional reading to develop your knowledge and understanding of them, including:

- Mental Capacity Act 2005
- Adults with Incapacity (Scotland) Act 2000
- Equality Act 2 010
- Safeguarding Vulnerable Groups Act 2006
- Mental Health Act 2007
- Mental Health (Care and Treatment) (Scotland) Act 2003
- Health and Social Care Act 2012.

Human Needs

We all have complex overlapping personal needs, each of them relating to dignity and respect as part of normal life. Maslow's hierarchy of needs, published in 1954, explores the needs of a human being in five sections, each having relevance and direct connections to providing dignified care to individuals. His theory stems from his initial work in 1943, where his developmental psychology theory focused on the successful growth of humans (Maslow, 1943).

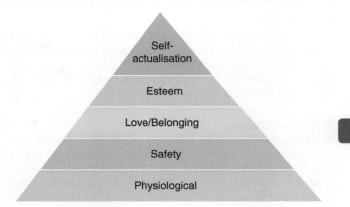

Figure 7.4 **Maslow's hierarchy of needs (Maslow, 1954).**

Figure 7.4 illustrates Maslow's hierarchy of needs. It is often represented as a pyramid, with the most fundamental needs at the bottom and the greater needs at the top (Giddens, 2017). The hierarchy of needs is based on the successful fulfilment of the lower levels initially, then rising up the framework to reach self-actualisation.

Jot This Down

List three aspects of each need, and how these can be supported within health and social care practice: physiological needs; safety needs; love/belonging; esteem; self-actualisation.

Physiological Needs

These are the most basic of human needs and requirements. Physiological needs include the need for air, water and food along with clothing, shelter and protection from the elements. They are essential for human survival, and if not met the human body will not function properly, ultimately leading to illness, disease or death. These needs should be met first, as they are considered the most important.

Safety Needs

With an individual's physical needs being met or relatively satisfied, safety needs take priority. Safety and security needs could potentially include personal safety, financial safety, health and well-being, and safety net against accidents/illness.

Love and Belonging Needs

Once the physiological and safety needs have been met, there is a requirement for a sense of belonging and acceptance within an individual's social groups. The term 'social groups' can be used to cover a wide range of circumstances, including family members, loved ones and friends, as well as wider communities like social groups or clubs.

Every human has the need to be loved and to love, in both a sexual and non-sexual way, and many people may become prone to loneliness, social isolation and potentially depression if there is an absence of this love or belonging need.

Esteem

We all have a need to feel respected, and this includes the need for self-esteem. The overall need is to be accepted and valued by others. Maslow did identify that the relationship between this and the lower levels of the hierarchy is not completely separated, but more gently blended from one to the other.

Self-actualisation

This is the final level of the hierarchy, where the individual realises what their full potential is and achieves it. Maslow believes that for this to be achieved, the previous levels have to be mastered rather than just met. This level can often be described as: the desire to accomplish everything that one can, to become the most that one can be (Maslow, 1954).

When relating the hierarchy of needs to dignity and respect within a health and social care setting, there are five main needs that can be drawn from all the levels to complement existing thoughts and practices.

- The need to have personal identity, self-respect, self-esteem, self-worth and resilience.
- The need to feel respected by others.
- The need to be treated as an individual.
- The need to have independence, choice and control in personal lives.
- The need to develop and maintain interpersonal relationships.

If personal needs remain unfulfilled, this can often lead to unhappiness and frustration and a poor quality of life. Adults at risk can potentially have more complicated personal needs than others.

Dignity from a human needs perspective is difficult to define, but the term which is often used in this way is to describe the *quality* of the way people:

- Treat other people with 'dignity', which affects a person's feelings of self-esteem and self-worth
- Behave and look, and so deserve to be treated with dignity.

The 'human rights' and 'human needs' points of view can provide a clear framework for:

- Understanding the current problems, and wider challenges associated with dignity
- Considering the dignity challenges that face you in day-to-day practice
- Delivering care practices with a deeper awareness of dignity
- Identifying local dignity in care problems and make action plans to resolve them.

Types of Dignity

A study completed by the European Commission and University of Cardiff (European Commission, 2004) merges the human rights and needs of individuals along with the types of dignity into one framework, allowing easier application of theory into practice, regardless of the setting or client group that is being provided with care and support. Figure 7.5 demonstrates the merged concepts of human rights and needs.

Following on from the combined human rights and human needs approach, further exploration can be made into each of the types of dignity, with some concepts of application and consideration being introduced. Table 7.3 demonstrates this.

Dignity in Care Campaign

The Dignity in Care campaign was launched following a number of consultations and frameworks. A number of factors were identified, establishing the absence of the focus of dignity in care before this time, such as poor management, absence of training and education and rapid turnover of staff within some health and social care settings (Social Care Institute for Excellence, 2013c). The campaign was updated in 2015 (National Dignity in Care Council, 2021).

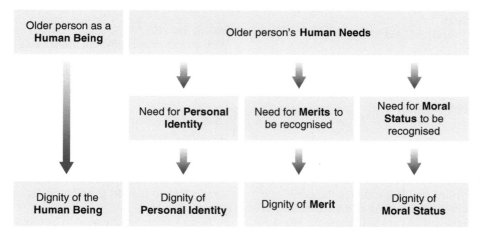

Figure 7.5 Combined framework of human rights and needs. *Source:* Based on Health and Social Care Advisory Service (2010).

Table 7.3 Concepts and considerations towards application to practice. *Source:* Health and Social Care Advisory Service (2010). Reproduced with permission of HASCAS.

DIGNITY OF HUMAN BEING	DIGNITY OF PERSONAL IDENTITY	DIGNITY OF MERIT	DIGNITY OF MORAL STATUS
Conventions and laws	Personal identity	Achievements	People's moral principles
Right to life	Self-respect	Rank and seniority	Religious faith
No abuse	Self-esteem	Place in society	Community membership
Justice	Resilience	Honours and awards	Leadership
Privacy	Personal relationships	Employment	Recognised roles
No discrimination		Knowledge and skills	
Freedoms/respect		Experience	
		Qualifications	
		Financial worth	
		Success in life	
		Independence	

The National Dignity in Care Council leads the campaign, maintaining the focus of having 'dignity in our hearts, minds and actions' (Social Care Institute for Excellence, 2013d). Part of the Dignity in Care campaign was the creation, launch and embedding of 10 dignity challenges, discussed later in the chapter.

The campaign now has thousands of registered dignity champions who work both locally and nationally on raising the profile of the campaign and improving outcomes for individuals receiving care and support (National Dignity in Care Council, 2021). Education and sharing of best practice was another theme of the campaign, with the creation of key learning materials and messages for all to utilise.

The 10-point Dignity Challenges

The Dignity in Care campaign launched the 10-point dignity challenges for all health and social care organisations and practitioners to meet and exceed, each having their own rationale, definitions and requirements.

1. **Abuse:** *have zero tolerance of all forms of abuse.* Respect for dignity is highlighted as a priority for most health and social care organisations.
2. **Respect:** *support people with the same respect you would want for yourself or a member of your family.* Individuals should receive care in a courteous and considerate manner, allowing time to get to know the individual. Individuals should be encouraged and supported within this challenge to manage their care as independently as possible.
3. **Person-centred care:** *treat each person as an individual by offering a personalised service.* This is seen as an essential behaviour and attitude at all levels of service provision. Although each service will have standards to meet in relation to their regulatory requirements, care delivery for each individual should not be standardised and is customised to their care needs.
4. **Autonomy:** *enable people to maintain the maximum possible level of independence, choice and control.* Any indi-

vidual receiving care and support from a health or social care service should be encouraged to participate in daily life and be involved in decisions about their care and support.

5. **Communication:** *listen to and support people to express their needs and wants.* This challenge includes all aspects of providing information relating to care delivery, including seeking agreement in care planning, and seeking valid consent for any care and support taking place.
6. **Privacy:** *respect people's right to privacy.* People's personal space is essential for the provision of dignified care and support. Ensuring that it is accessible and available demonstrates a commitment to dignity.
7. **Complaints:** *ensure people feel able to complain without fear of retribution.* Any individual receiving care and support from a health and social care organisation should be provided with information and advice that they need to pass comment on the service provision as well as the quality markers and standards that each service is regulated on. The provision of or access to advocacy services would be included within this challenge.
8. **Care partners:** *engage with family members and carers as care partners.* Family members, informal carers and significant others should be kept fully informed on care needs of their loved one in a timely fashion. Everyone involved in the care and support of an individual should feel engaged and listened to when accessing health and social care services.
9. **Self-esteem:** *assist people to maintain confidence and positive self-esteem.* Individuals should be supported in a manner that promotes confidence and self-esteem, which in turn would support and promote health and well-being.
10. **Loneliness and isolation:** *act to alleviate loneliness and isolation.* Any individual receiving care and support should be offered the opportunity to engage in age-appropriate, enjoyable and stimulating activities that hold personal meaning for them.

What the Experts Say

Despite a renewed focus on conquering loneliness amongst the older generation, there is still a stigma attached to admitting being lonely.

Loneliness and social isolation can affect everyone but older people are particularly vulnerable after the loss of friends and family, reduced mobility or limited income.

Services that aim to reduce loneliness and social isolation can be divided into one-to-one interventions, group services and wider community engagement. The number of services and the different ways of measuring their success make it difficult to be certain what works for whom. Those services that look most promising include befriending schemes, social group schemes and community navigators.

Dame Esther Rantzen

Dignity Challenges Framework

The majority of these 10 challenges can be 'fitted' into one of two headings: treating individuals as human beings or meeting individuals' human needs. Figure 7.6 demonstrates how the 10 challenges can be fitted into the framework model.

Meeting older people's human needs

Respect
Support people with respect as you would want yourself

Abuse	Self-esteem
Zero tolerance of abuse	Assist people to maintain confidence and self-esteem

Privacy	Loneliness and isolation
Respect people's right to privacy	Act to alleviate people's loneliness and isolation

Autonomy	Communication
Enable maximum levels of independence, choice and control	Listen and support people to express their views

Person-centred care	Ability to complain
Offer personalised services to preserve individuality	People feel able to complain without fear of retribution

Care partners
Engage with family members as care partners

Figure 7.6 **Dignity Challenges Framework.** *Source:* Health and Social Care Advisory Service (2010). Reproduced with permission of HASCAS.

Jot This Down

Identify, from your practice experiences so far, examples of where you have been able to demonstrate aspects of meeting each of these 10 dignity challenges.
- Respect
- Zero tolerance of abuse
- Privacy
- Autonomy
- Person-centred care
- Confidence and positive self-esteem
- Communication
- Complaints
- Engage with family and carers.

What To Do If . . .

Think about this 'Jot This Down' exercise. What would you do if a relative makes a complaint about the care home manager, saying the manager speaks to her mother in an uncivil way? What do you do next?

Influencing Dignity in Care Practice

Every member of the health and social care workforce should hold dignity at the heart of everything that they do, regardless of practice setting, job role or discipline, and so be in the optimal position to influence dignity in care. You do not have to be 'a person of influence' to be influential.

Dignity can be influenced by a number of factors (RCN, 2013), but ultimately can be placed into three themes: place, people and process (RCN, 2009). In its guidance, the RCN elaborates on each point.

- **Place** relates to the physical environment where the services are delivered.
- **People** relates to the behaviours and attitudes of others and the organisational culture in which you are practising.
- **Process** relates to the way the care and support are actually delivered.

Influencing dignity in care does not need considerable changes in practice or organisational policy but can be done on a singular basis, relating to a specific area of practice. In a more recent document focused on fair care for trans and non-binary people, the RCN has reaffirmed the need to 'always treat trans and non-binary patients in a respectful way, as you would any other patient or client' (RCN, 2020).

Any goal or influence that you establish should be able to demonstrate the main characteristics for action plans or objectives. The characteristics that are required allow for SMART action plans or objectives.

Practice Assessment Document (NMC Competency 4.1)

Demonstrate safe, basic, person-centred care, under supervision, for people who are unable to meet their own physical and emotional needs.

(Continued)

When considering what (if any) change is needed in relation to dignified care practice, the following points might be useful to consider.
· Who is affected?
· Why are they affected?
· How do you know they are affected?
· What effects are being experienced by the individual?
Once you have established the answers to these, you will be in a position to discuss the matter with your practice assessor. It will also allow you to demonstrate how you establish some dignity action plans and goals relating to the influences or changes that you have identified.

- **S**pecific: including clear statements of what is to be achieved, using terms and phrasing relating to the individual or organisation to which it relates.
- **M**easurable: this is probably the most important consideration, as being able to measure the response or influence will allow you to evidence the effects that it is having, both positive and negative.
- **A**chievable: the influence that you are planning must be achievable – there is little point in starting a change if it is not likely to be completed.
- **R**ealistic: the influence or change that you have identified must be realistic, both within your scope of practice and organisation.
- **T**imed: any influence or change that has been identified should be timed, providing a focus for the tasks in hand, along with allowing for a balance of optimism and pessimism.

Along with these required characteristics, others can be considered when looking at influencing practice or completing dignity action plans, resulting in the objectives being SMART*IES*.

- **I**nspiring: will the action plan or objective encourage and inspire other people to change their practice, attitudes or behaviours relating to dignity in care?
- **E**nthusiastic: will the action plan or objective excite and enthuse other people?
- **S**ustainable: will the objective be maintained in the long term?

Conclusion

This chapter has provided an understanding of the principles of safeguarding 'adults at risk' and the different types of abuse that may present within a health or social care setting. The application of this knowledge to nursing practice will be essential when recognising the potential physical and behavioural signs of abuse, and what to do if abuse is suspected.

As a healthcare student, you are an essential and vital part of the health and social care team, providing direct care and support to a number of adults who may be vulnerable in all your practice placement settings. Practice placements give you the practical skills required to register as a nurse, and to develop further your knowledge and understanding of working in partnership with families, friends and other professionals, all central to the protection and safeguarding of vulnerable adults.

Abuse can take place in a number of environments and these include health and social care settings. You may at times recognise these situations and you will be required to report these to the appropriate people, including your mentor, university tutor, manager and the organisation. This chapter has focused on the patient, who is central to all that is done, as well as identifying how to respond to a disclosure of abuse, and some of the general processes that are there to assist you to do this, regardless of setting or role.

Key Points

· In all parts of society there are vulnerable individuals who should be afforded dignity, protection and safeguarding against abuse or inequality.
· This chapter has focused on the older person, but the principles discussed may be applied to all fields of nursing.
· Key terms have been defined and discussed, considering how safeguarding and dignity can directly impact on care and support.
· There are a number of legislative frameworks concerning safeguarding and dignity and these have been outlined.
· The chapter has offered insight into the application of the principles relating to safeguarding and dignity.
· Supporting and promoting the principles of safeguarding and dignity in care, among other things, requires the nurse to apply the principles of the Mental Capacity Act in a capacity assessment, and encourage and advocate the application of the dignity challenges and practice framework.
· When nurses participate in the delivery of safe and dignified care, offering support to individuals in any care setting, they must practise within the Nursing and Midwifery Council (2015) Code of Conduct.

References

Age UK (2020) *Factsheet 78. Safeguarding Older People from Abuse and Neglect.* www.ageuk.org.uk/globalassets/age-uk/documents/factsheets/fs78_safeguarding_older_people_from_abuse_fcs.pdf?epslanguage=en-GB?dtrk=true (accessed December 2021).

Care Act (2014) Chapter 23. www.legislation.gov.uk/ukpga/2014/23/pdfs/ukpga_20140023_en.pdf (accessed December 2021).

Carr, S. (2011) Enabling risk and ensuring safety: self-directed support and personal budgets. *Journal of Adult Protection*, 13(3), 122–136.

Centre for Public Scrutiny and the Improvement and Development Agency (2010) *Adult Safeguarding Scrutiny Guide.* Centre for Public Scrutiny and Improvement and Development Agency, London.

Department for Constitutional Affairs (2007) *Mental Capacity Act 2005 Code of Practice.* Stationery Office, London.

Department of Health (2011) *Statement of Government Policy on Adult Safeguarding.* Department of Health, London.

Department of Health (2012) *Transforming Care: A National Response to Winterbourne View Hospital.* Department of Health, London.

Department of Health and Home Office (2000) *No Secrets: Guidance on Developing and Implementing Multi-agency Policies and Procedures to Protect Vulnerable Adults from Abuse.* Department of Health, London.

Department of Health and Public Health England (2015) *Promoting Emotional Wellbeing and Positive Mental Health of Children and Young People.* https://assets.publishing.service.gov.uk/government/uploads/system/uploads/attachment_data/file/1020249/Promoting_ children_and_young_people_s_mental_health_and_wellbeing.pdf (accessed December 2021).

Department of Health and Social Care (2021a) *Liberty Protection Safegaurds: What They Are*. www.gov.uk/government/publications/liberty-protection-safeguards-factsheets/liberty-protection-safeguards-what-they-are (accessed December 2021).

Department of Health and Social Care (2021b) *The NHS Constitution for England*. www.gov.uk/government/publications/the-nhs-constitution-for-england/the-nhs-constitution-for-england (accessed December 2021).

European Commission (2004) *Educating for Dignity: The Dignity and Older Europeans Project*. European Commission and University of Cardiff, Cardiff.

Francis, R. (2013) *Report of the Mid Staffordshire NHS Foundation Trust Public Inquiry*. www.midstaffspublicinquiry.com/report (accessed December 2021).

Giddens, J.F. (2017) *Concepts for Nursing Practice*, 2nd edn. Elsevier, St Louis, MO.

Health and Social Care Advisory Service (2010) *Dignity through Action (Vulnerable Adults) Resource 2: Dignity Workshop Pack*. Health and Social Care Advisory Service, London.

Home Office (2020) *Evidence in Criminal Investigations*. https://assets.publishing.service.gov.uk/government/uploads/system/uploads/attachment_data/file/919630/evidence-in-criminal-investigations-v5.0.pdf (accessed December 2021).

Institute for Public Care (2013) *Evidence Review - Adult Safeguarding*. https://ipc.brookes.ac.uk/docs/Evidence_Review_-_Adult_Safeguarding.pdf (accessed December 2021).

Maslow, A. (1943) A theory of human motivation. *Psychological Review*, 50(4), 370–396.

Maslow, A. (1954) *Motivation and Personality*. Harper, New York.

McCormack, B. & McCance, T. (2017) *Person-Centred Nursing and Health Care: Theory and Practice*. Wiley Blackwell, Oxford.

Mental Health Foundation (2019) www.mentalhealth.org.uk/a-to-z/s/self-harm (accessed December 2021).

National Dignity in Care Council (2021) *The Dignity in Care Campaign*. www.dignityincare.org.uk/About/Dignity_in_Care_campaign/ (accessed December 2021).

NHS Digital (2020) *Safeguarding Adults, England, 2019–20*. https://digital.nhs.uk/data-and-information/publications/statistical/safeguarding-adults/2019-20 (accessed December 2021).

NHS England (2015) *Safeguarding Policy*. www.england.nhs.uk/publication/safeguarding-policy/ (accessed December 2021).

Northway, R. (2013) Responding to abuse. *Learning Disability Practice*, 16(3), 11.

Nursing & Midwifery Council (2012) *Care and Respect: What You Can Expect From Nurses*. NMC, London.

Nursing & Midwifery Council (2018) *The Code. Professional Standards of Practice and Behaviour for Nurses, Midwives and Nursing Associates*. www.nmc.org.uk/globalassets/sitedocuments/nmc-publications/nmc-code.pdf (accessed December 2021).

Royal College of Nursing (2008) *The RCN's Definition of Dignity*. www.dignityincare.org.uk/_assets/RCN_Digntiy_at_the_heart_of_everything_we_do.pdf (accessed December 2021).

Royal College of Nursing (2009) *Small Changes Make a Big Difference: How You Can Influence to Deliver Dignified Care*. RCN, London.

Royal College of Nursing (2013) *Dignity in Healthcare for People with Learning Disabilities*. RCN, London.

Royal College of Nursing (2014) *Defining Nursing*. RCN, London.

Royal College of Nursing (2015) *Safeguarding Adults: Everyone's Responsibility*. RCN, London.

Royal College of Nursing (2020) *Fair Care for Trans and Non-Binary People. An RCN Guide for Nursing and Health Care Professionals*. www.rcn.org.uk/news-and-events/news/uk-updated-rcn-guidance-aims-to-ensure-fair-care-for-trans-patients-191120 (accessed December 2021).

Royal College of Psychiatrists (2015) *Deprivation of Liberty Safeguards*. www.rcpsych.ac.uk/mental-health/treatments-and-wellbeing/deprivation-of-liberty-safeguards (accessed December 2021).

Social Care Institute for Excellence (2010) *Mental Capacity Act 2005 at a Glance*. SCIE, London. www.scie.org.uk/mca/introduction/mental-capacity-act-2005-at-a-glance#:~:text=The%20Mental%20Capacity%20Act%20(MCA)%202005%20applies%20to%20everyone%20involved,vulnerable%20people%20who%20lack%20capacity (accessed December 2021).

Social Care Institute for Excellence (2011) *SCIE Report 39. Protecting Adults at Risk: London Multi-Agency Policy and Procedure to Safeguard Adults from Abuse*. SCIE, London.

Social Care Institute for Excellence (2012) *Guide 45: Safeguarding and Quality in Commissioning Care Homes*. SCIE, London.

Social Care Institute for Excellence (2013a) *1.3 Safeguarding Continuum*. SCIE, London.

Social Care Institute for Excellence (2013b) *5.1.1 Promoting Resilience*. SCIE, London.

Social Care Institute for Excellence (2013c) *Adult Services Guide 15: Dignity in Care*. SCIE, London.

Social Care Institute for Excellence (2013d) *The Dignity in Care Campaign*. SCIE, London.

Social Care Institute for Excellence (2021) *Safeguarding Adults During the COVID-19 Crisis*. www.scie.org.uk/care-providers/coronavirus-covid-19/safeguarding-adults (accessed December 2021).

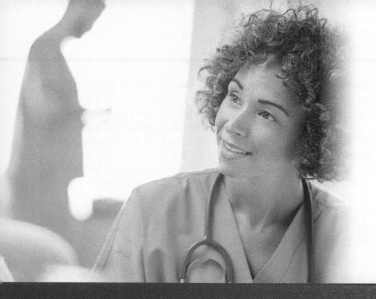

8

The Principles of Older People's Care

Helen Paterson

Frimley Park Hospital, UK

Learning Outcomes

On completion of this chapter, you will be able to:

- Define communication and appreciate why effective communication is essential when offering care to older people
- Understand the importance of maintaining and respecting dignity when providing care to older people
- Understand the importance of effective and timely assessment of an older person's nutritional needs
- Demonstrate insight concerning the critical role of the nurse in the assessment of risk and the reduction of falls in the older person
- Gain an understanding of the discharge and transfer process

Proficiencies

NMC Proficiencies and Standards:

- Communicate effectively so that appropriate information is shared in a timely manner
- Provide individual, evidence-based care to older people
- Carry out competent assessment of an older person's nutritional needs
- Identify factors associated with the potential development of pressure ulcers
- Perform a timely falls risk assessment in order to identify those at risk of falls
- Identify different types of communication
- Ensure that the older person has a structured discharge plan tailored to their individual needs

 Visit the companion website at **www.wiley.com/go/peate/nursingpractice3e** where you can test yourself using flashcards, multiple-choice questions and more.

Nursing Practice: Knowledge and Care, Third Edition. Edited by Ian Peate and Aby Mitchell.
© 2022 John Wiley & Sons Ltd. Published 2022 by John Wiley & Sons Ltd.
Companion website: www.wiley.com/go/peate/nursingpractice3e

Introduction

One of the main challenges of the healthcare system is the increasing number of elderly patients with unique and complex needs. Caring for older people is a specialty that requires highly skilled nurses who can deal with complex health and social care needs an older person can present with (NMC, 2009a).

Essential skills required by professionals working with older people are extremely diverse, necessitating the ability to be astute in their observations of older people, through continuously assessing function and health status.

As the older population increases, so does the need for greater understanding of the specific needs of older people (NMC, 2009a). The Compassion in Care strategy was built on the values of the 6Cs: Care, Compassion, Competence, Communication, Courage and Commitment. The purpose of the 6Cs was to ensure patients are looked after with care and compassion, by professionals who are competent and communicate well, have the courage to make changes that improve care and can deliver the best and commit to delivering this all day, every day (Department of Health, 2010b). This supports the NMC (2018) standard specifying the knowledge and skills that registered nurses must demonstrate when caring for people of all ages and across all settings.

It is important to remember that in order to offer care that is safe, effective and person centred, nurses are required to work in partnership with the person, their relatives and other care providers in the statutory, independent and voluntary sectors. Understanding the roles and responsibilities of practitioners in each domain, older people, and their relatives and how they work in partnership will enable individuals to manage their own health and well-being with the support they need and choose.

When a multidisciplinary/interdisciplinary team approach is advocated, it facilitates an environment of ever evolving practice services based on the changing needs of the older person. This integrated care requires professionals and practitioners from different sectors to work together around the needs of older people, their families and communities. Communicating effectively is an absolute prerequisite to achieving the best outcome for the older person which requires appropriately utilising knowledge, skills and best practice from multiple disciplines and across service provider boundaries, e.g., health, social care or voluntary and private sector providers, to redefine, rescope and reframe health and social care delivery issues and reach solutions based on an improved collective understanding of complex patient need(s) (NHS England, 2014). Some members in a multidisciplinary team (MDT) are outlined in Figure 8.1.

This chapter provides you with an insight into the ways in which the nurse can excel at care provision for older people.

Attitudes and Stereotyping

The number of people aged 65 and over will increase by more than 40% within 20 years, and the number of households where the oldest person is 85 and over is increasing faster than any other age group (Office for National Statistics, 2017). With the global trend towards an increasingly frail ageing population, we need to rethink old age, and move from a reactive approach to managing frailty to a more proactive approach (Welford *et al.*, 2010). Additionally, people living with frailty are at greater risk of hospitalisation, long hospital stays, unplanned readmission to hospital, care home admission or mortality. Indeed, for those living with severe frailty, the annual risk of hospitalisation, care home admission or death is over four times greater (NHS England, 2018a). Consequently, care of older people will become an increasingly important part of nurses' remit.

Chrisler *et al.* (2016) suggest that there is a widespread negative attitude toward older people and old age among physicians, medical students and nurses. Therefore, all healthcare professionals should be made aware of their influence on the attitudes of student nurses towards older people; good practice includes the ability to demonstrate that older people in hospital settings are valued.

Sadly, ageism, defined as stereotyping, prejudice or discrimination toward people based on age, is a mounting international concern with important health implications (Officer *et al.*, 2016). Yet little is known about the effectiveness of strategies to reduce ageism (Burnes *et al.*, 2019). Worryingly, ageism has broad and far-reaching negative consequences. It can have a negative impact on physical and mental health, and influence whether older patients receive treatment at all, and the duration, frequency and appropriateness of that treatment (Chang *et al.*, 2020). Therefore, it is important that registered nurses have the skills and knowledge to meet the person-centred, holistic needs of the people they encounter in their practice (NMC, 2018b). This underlines the importance of the skills and knowledge of the nursing workforce, starting from nurse training, to reflect the ageing population and facilitation of a positive nursing attitude (Rush *et al.*, 2017).

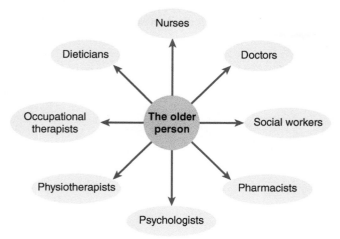

Figure 8.1 **Some members of the multidisciplinary team.**

The Nursing Associate Student Nurses

To ensure student nurses are prepared successfully to meet the *Future Nurse: Standards of Proficiency for Registered Nurses* (NMC, 2018b), they are required to complete a Practice Assessment Document (PAD) on each placement. This has been developed to ensure students can demonstrate that they are able to

(Continued)

provide care to those with complex mental, physical, cognitive and behavioural care in any healthcare setting, in addition to providing and promoting non-discriminatory, person-centred and sensitive care.

At every placement, the student will have an assessor/mentor who will enable the student to identify their learning opportunities, facilitate completion of the learning objectives and provide regular feedback.

The student is obligated to take responsibility for their own learning and know how to access support whilst engaging positively with all learning opportunities. The student also needs to understand the assessment requirements, work with and receive written feedback from a range of staff. This will give the student the opportunity to demonstrate their learning objectives for each placement that meet the required standards and proficiencies (NMC, 2018a).

The practice assessor will provide feedback based on the student's reflection, their observation of the student in practice and discussions of the episode of care. These standards of proficiency will be graded on the PAD as fail/satisfactory/good/very good or excellent. An integral component of this assessment is the student reflection on the delivery of patient-centred care.

The Nursing Associate

 Nursing associates (NA) need to complete both academic and work-based learning that will prepare them to work with people of all ages and in a variety of settings in health and social care.

The standards of proficiency represent the knowledge and skills that a NA will need to meet in order to be considered by the NMC as capable of safe and effective nursing associate practice. These standards have been designed to apply across all health and care settings. These proficiencies set out what pre-registration training will equip NAs to know how to provide care for people of all ages and from different backgrounds, cultures and beliefs, in addition to providing care for people who have mental, physical, cognitive and behavioural care needs, those living with dementia, the elderly and for people at the end of their life.

Nursing associates are expected to apply evidence-based best practice across all procedures, and have the ability to carry out these procedures safely, effectively, with sensitivity and compassion, while demonstrating that communication and relationship is crucial to the provision of person-centred care. These proficiencies must be demonstrated with an awareness of variations required for different practice settings and for people across their lifespan.

This will be evidenced in their work-based proficiency files which are completed with their assessor as well as reflective discussions. This must be carried out in a way that reflects cultural awareness and ensures that the needs, priorities, expertise and preferences of people are always valued and taken into account.

Similar to student nurses, the assessor will provide feedback and complete their work books, taking into account the NA's reflections, observation of the NA in practice and professional discussions.

This will enable the associate to gain further insight into how they can ensure they are providing patient-centred care through various placements and experiences that will enable them to assist nurses with a greater range of care-giving responsibilities, that will be patient centred and be an advocacy for patients.

Effective Communication

The Department of Health (2010b) defines communication as a process that involves a meaningful exchange between at least two people, to convey facts, needs, opinions, thoughts, feelings or other information, through both verbal and non-verbal means, including face-to-face exchanges and the written word.

Effective communication is an essential aspect of nursing practice and requires professional competence and engagement. Ineffective communication can lead to older people feeling inadequate, disempowered and helpless (Jack *et al.*, 2019). Nurses have a duty to ensure that older people feel they are being listened to and that their concerns are being validated in a non-judgemental way (NMC, 2018a).

Communication is an important characteristic of nursing care and much of nurses' duties, such as providing physical care, emotional support, and exchanging of information with patients, cannot be performed without communication (Fahkr-Movahedi *et al.*, 2011). Moreover, the quality of communication in interactions between the nurse and patient has a major influence on patients' outcome (Sibiya, 2018). Ironically, when people think of communication, listening is not the first thing that comes to mind, yet it is an incredibly important skill for a clinician to develop.

Conversely, despite the emphasis on teaching communication skills over the past two decades, there is recognition that such skills are not always evident, and nurses do not always communicate well with patients, family members and colleagues (Sibiya, 2018). Ineffective communication among healthcare professionals is one of the leading causes of error and patient harm (Quinn & Thomas, 2017), highlighting that it is essential for nurses to promote effective communication with older people to ensure they have a positive experience during their journey from admission to discharge.

Jot This Down

- How do you ensure service users' communication needs are met?
- How do you check service users' understanding through communication?
- Identify specific communication strategies and the obstacles that can prevent effective communication, particularly when working with older people.

What the Experts Say

 Admission to and treatment in hospital is almost invariably a time of great anxiety, not only for the patient but also for those closest to him or her. Patients and those closest to them naturally require to be kept informed of developments and will be worried if they are denied this or if they have to make great efforts to find out what they want to know. It is of the very essence of modern medical care that it is provided in partnership with the patient and always subject to the consent of the patient or authorised representative, following the provision of the information needed to make decisions. This requires a continual professional conversation with the patient and those authorised by him or her to receive treatment information, so

(Continued)

that those involved are thoroughly informed of the current position and enabled to play their full part in the process. Communication in a hospital setting is not a one-way process. It is as vital that patients and their relatives are listened to – for in many ways they are the experts on the patient and his or her needs – as it is for hospital staff to provide information (Francis, 2013).

It is important to remember that nonverbal messages may perhaps be more powerful than words; nurses observing a patient's body language can be just as important as looking for clinical outcomes (Ali, 2017).

The Nursing Associate Student Nurses

Effective communication is central to the provision of safe and compassionate person-centred care. Proficiency 2.5 in the NMC (2018b) Future Nurse standards requires students to be able to identify the need for and manage a range of alternative communication techniques. Nurses in all fields of practice must be able to demonstrate the ability to communicate and manage relationships with people of all ages with a range of mental, physical, cognitive and behavioural health challenges.

Student nurses will be assessed during their PAD discussion, observation in practice and the student's own reflections to demonstrate that the student is able to utilise a range of communication skills to effectively engage with the person receiving care, their family/carers and members of the multidisciplinary team in the provision and evaluation of care. An example could be reflection on what communication skills they utilised to communicate with a patient with dementia who was getting very distressed and agitated.

The Nursing Associate

Nursing associates need a diverse range of communication skills and strategies to ensure that individuals, their families and carers are supported to be actively involved in their own care wherever appropriate, and that they are kept informed and well prepared.

During the assessor's feedback sessions, it is important for nursing associates to demonstrate when communicating with patients/relatives/carers that they consider cultural awareness to ensure that the needs, priorities, expertise and preferences of people are always valued and taken into account.

They also need to demonstrate awareness of those who have special communication needs or a disability, which would require reasonable adjustments. This could entail the provision of pictures boards for those who are unable to communicate their needs verbally that enable the person to point to a picture that depicts their specific need such as a toilet or cup for a drink.

This will provide the assessor with assurances that the NA is able to provide and share information in a way that promotes good health and health outcomes and does not prevent people from having equal access to the highest quality of care.

Types of Communication

There are four main types of effective communication.

- *Verbal communication*: exchanging information using speech. Your choice of words and tone is important.
- *Non-verbal communication*: facial expressions, posture, gestures and movements (can sometimes be misinterpreted).
- *Written communication*.
- *Visual communication*.

It is vital that all nurses are aware of potential barriers to communication, and reflect on their own skills and how their workplace environment affects their ability to communicate effectively with patients (Ali, 2017).

Barriers to Effective Communication

Ineffective communication comes down to two areas: problems relating to message being given and/or problems relating to message being received.

- *Poor listening skills*: communication can become difficult if a listener does not appear to be interested in what the older person is saying or does not give them adequate time to say what they want to say. Some older people may have memory problems, so it may take them a little longer to process what it is they are trying to communicate.
- *Environmental*: remember that a hearing aid amplifies the background noise, as well as speech. Some fluorescent strip lighting emits a humming noise, which can be distracting to hearing aid wearers. Poor lighting and telephones can make communicating with the older person difficult. Noise and other distractions can impede communication with patients with dementia and other cognitive impairments, who find concentration challenging (Ali, 2017), as it can be easy for the older person to become distracted.
- *Staffing time constraints*: a busy ward/clinical environment, together with poor staffing or skill mix, can restrict the time nurses spend with patients (Department of Health, 2010b).
- *Patients' ability to communicate effectively*: may also be affected by their condition, medication, pain and/or anxiety (Ali, 2017).
- *Medical jargon*: using technical jargon and clinical acronyms; even though the patient may not understand, they may not ask you for a plain English translation (Ali, 2017).
- *Compulsory face covering*: due to COVID-19, all staff must wear a facemask the whole time they are at work. This can affect communication with an older person, especially if they have some cognitive impairment or are hard of hearing. Covering the mouth also eliminates the possibility of using lip-reading cues to support understanding, which are particularly valuable in substantiating the acoustic signals required for auditory comprehension in patients with communication difficulties (Dupuis, 2011).

What the Experts Say

I am 78 years of age, I still have all of my faculties, my left leg is a bit dodgy but I'm all there. To be addressed by the nurses as love, dear, sweetie really irks me. For me, this is a lack of respect. I think they should ask me what I would like to be called, this way I am still being seen as an individual.

Miss Mary O'Leary

Handover

Handovers are an essential part of everyday nursing practice and play a key part in ensuring patient safety (Pearce, 2018). According to the WHO (2007), the primary purpose of handover is to convey information. Handover is considered key to taking over the responsibility for a patient's care and enables continuity of care (Lin *et al.*, 2011). Problems typically arise at shift or patient handovers and may involve ambiguous or poorly recorded information in patient files (JCR, 2007). Debatably, this is because many handovers happen at the end of a shift when staff are tired and waiting to go home (Pearce, 2018). Manias *et al.* (2016) found that poor handovers were often associated with adverse events or a near miss. Handovers can often occur in distracting contexts, such as interruptions from staff, patients/relative or environmental factors such as equipment alarms (Spooner *et al.*, 2015).

One way in which we could improve communication during handovers is to use briefing tools such as SBAR (**S**ituation, **B**ackground, **A**ssessment and **R**ecommendation). The SBAR communication tool supports common language among team members. It promotes shared decision making and conflict resolution which will probably improve patient satisfaction and outcomes (Lees & Delpino, 2007). However, this will require a culture change to adopt and sustain structured communication formats by all healthcare providers (Shahid & Thomas, 2018) to ensure person-centred care.

Jot This Down

- Perform a literature review of clinical handover.
- Compare the methods described with what you have experienced on your placements or your place of work if already qualified.
- Would a change in practice enhance the quality of information provided during handover?
- If yes, consider discussing this with the ward manager with a rationale of the need for change.

Person-centred Care

Person-centred care is usually described as 'individualised care'; some say 'it's all about the person' while many struggle to be more specific (Butterworth, 2012). The phrase 'person-centred care' is often encountered when reading about how older people should be supported and involved in any decision making relating to their care (Pope, 2011).

National Voices (2017) describes person-centredness and person-centred thinking as 'a philosophy, a way of thinking or mindset which involves viewing, listening to and supporting a person based on their strengths, abilities, aspirations and preferences and supporting their decisions to maintain a life which is meaningful to them'.

Person-centred care supports people to develop the knowledge, skills and confidence they need to more effectively manage and make informed decisions about their own health and healthcare. If an individual has capacity, it is their choice to make. Person-centred care is co-ordinated and tailored to the needs of the individual and, crucially, ensures that people are always treated with dignity, compassion and respect. Conceptually, person-centred care is a model in which healthcare providers are encouraged to partner with patients to co-design and deliver personalised care that provides people with the high-quality care they need and improves healthcare system efficiency and effectiveness (Santana *et al.*, 2018).

The Health Foundation (2016) has identified a framework that comprises four principles of person-centred care.

1. Affording people dignity, compassion and respect.
2. Offering co-ordinated care, support or treatment.
3. Offering personalised care, support or treatment.
4. Supporting people to recognise and develop their own strengths and abilities to enable them to live an independent and fulfilling life.

Responding to individual needs and respecting individual choices can help to demonstrate that nurses respect the needs of the older person and their families.

Jot This Down

Describe what person-centred care means to you. Can you write an example of when you have seen good patient-centred care? How did it compare to other care you have seen?

What the Experts Say

High-quality care is care where patients are in control, have effective access to treatment, are safe and where illnesses are not just treated but prevented (Department of Health, 2008).

Personalised Care

The Health and Social Care Act 2012 imposes a legal duty for NHS England and clinical commissioning groups (CCGs) to involve older people in their care. Personalisation of service provision is central to achieving improved services for people that meet their needs as individuals, regardless of health and social services boundaries (Department of Health, 2008). Articulated in the *NHS Long Term Plan* (2019) are six principles of providing personalised care so that it becomes 'business as usual' across the health and care system by 2023–24. The six principles are:

1. Personalised support and care planning (PSCP)
2. Shared decision making
3. Enabling choice, including legal rights to choose
4. Social prescribing and community-based support
5. Supported self-management
6. Personal health budgets and integrated personal budgets.

Fundamentally, personalisation places an emphasis on providing social care services tailored to the needs of the user, rather than fitting people into existing services that may not deliver the right kind of support for their particular circumstances (Harlock, 2010, p.371).

What the Experts Say

Personalisation reinforces the idea that the individual is best placed to know what they need and how those needs can be best met. It means that people can be responsible for themselves and can make their own decisions about what they require, but that they should also have information and support to enable them to do so. In this way services should respond to the individual instead of the person having to fit with the service (Department of Health, 2008).

Dementia

Worldwide, around 50 million people have dementia, and there are nearly 10 million new cases every year, projecting to reach 82 million in 2030 and 152 in 2050 (WHO, 2017). In the UK the rate of emergency admissions to hospital for people with dementia in 2017–18 was 3609 per 100^000 population aged 65 years and over, an increase on 2016–17 (3482). Furthermore, the proportion of these admissions being for one night or less (short stay) increased to 28.9% from 28.2% in 2016–17 (PHE, 2019).

Bale & Jenkins (2018) found that nursing students and registered nurses often feel underprepared for their roles in dementia care. Hartung *et al.* (2020) suggest that this could be due to new graduate nurses experiencing a phenomenon called reality shock when they do not feel prepared for the reality of nursing. Reality shock can lead to nurse turnover and poor retention rates. In order to address this issue, their findings suggest that providing effective training to students on dementia communication during clinical placements may help prepare nurses to care for this patient population.

This training would give students the knowledge and skills that they need to demonstrate their understanding of the importance of therapeutic relationships in providing an appropriate level of care for people with mental health, behavioural, cognitive and learning challenges, i.e. an older person with dementia.

Dignity

Dignity in provision of care includes maintaining privacy of the body, providing spatial privacy, giving sufficient time, treating patients as a whole person and allowing patients to have autonomy (Lin & Tsai, 2011). Patients are vulnerable to loss of dignity in hospital, as staff behaviour and the hospital environment can influence whether dignity is lost or upheld. To address these barriers to providing dignified care, the Department of Health (2006a) launched the Dignity in Care Campaign in 2006. It aims to address the lack of dignity in health and social care services by stimulating national debate around dignity in care and inspiring people to act. Yet, despite this campaign, other reports highlight that there are still cases of undignified care of older people in our hospitals and care homes; in too many instances, people have been let down when they were most vulnerable (Berry, 2012).

The RCN publication *Defending Dignity* (2008a) suggests nurses reflect on their practice to ensure they embed the practices highlighted in the Francis Report (2013) when caring for the older person. Box 8.1 outlines a number of principles that may be applied to improve the care of older people with an emphasis on dignity and respect following the Francis Report.

Box 8.1 Principles of Care

- All patients are individuals with their own backgrounds, needs, interests and wishes for which they are entitled to recognition and respect.
- No patient should ever be referred to by a name other than that which he or she wishes to be called.
- Staff should be readily identifiable by name and grade.
- If, for whatever reason, a patient has received less than acceptable care, every effort must be made to recognise the effects on the patient, remedy them and explain to the patient the reason for what has happened.

- Sensitive information, particularly concerning diagnosis and prognosis, must be given to patients in privacy, and within earshot only of those people the patient agrees to being present.
- The patient's right to physical privacy should be respected wherever possible, and in no circumstances should a patient be left in an undressed state visible to those passing by the bed.Source: Francis (2013)/Crown Copyright/Public Domain.

The Older Person's Nutritional Needs (Malnutrition and Dehydration)

Providing food and nutritional care in hospitals is integral to patient-centred care (Yinusa *et al.*, 2021). Having enough to eat and drink is one of the most basic human needs (Department of Health, 2006a) yet for some vulnerable people this need is not always met (Department of Health, 2009). The nurse is well placed to identify those patients with poor appetite, identify and treat any underlying cause of malnutrition and dehydration, and use various strategies to help older people improve their appetite and the adequacy of their diet (Pilgrim *et al.*, 2015). Undernutrition remains poorly detected by nursing and medical staff and although nutritional care in hospitals is highly prioritised, it can be inconsistent in terms of routines, lack of time and extensive use of temporary staff (Cooke *et al.*, 2012; Hestevik *et al.*, 2019). Nutritional problems among older patients are often complex and are determined by physiological, psychological and social changes which lead to poor appetite, insufficient food intake and poor health (Hestevik *et al.*, 2019).

To deliver safe nursing care to this group of patients demands skill and time. For example, to provide double-handed care for people who are acutely ill and immobile; to spend 30 minutes or more helping a person who has swallowing difficulties to take food and drink safely; to establish communication with someone who has both sensory and cognitive impairments (RCN, 2012). In addition, there is a high incidence of delirium (which can develop very quickly) resulting in high risks for patients, challenging behaviour and unpredictable needs for additional nursing support.

Malnutrition

There is no universally accepted definition of malnutrition, but Elia (2015) defines it as:

'. . . a state of nutrition in which a deficiency or excess (or imbalance) of energy, protein, and other nutrients causes measurable adverse effects on tissue/body form (body shape, size and composition) and function, and clinical outcome'.

Malnutrition affects every system in the body and results in increased vulnerability to illness and complications, which can lead to prolonged hospital stays, more visits to the doctor and, in some cases, death (British Dietetic Association, 2020). The main consequences of malnutrition are:

- Fatigue and lethargy
- Falls
- Difficulty coughing, which increases the risk of chest infection

- Heart failure
- Anxiety and depression
- Reduced ability to fight infection (British Dietetic Association, 2020).

Older people are at higher risk of malnutrition if they are ill, live alone or have difficulty eating. COVID-19 infection negatively impacts nutritional status on many levels, increasing nutritional requirements induced by pyrexia, sepsis and dyspnoea, and reducing nutritional intake due to excessive coughing, dysphagia and chronic fatigue. The detection and management of malnutrition in patients with COVID-19 are therefore of fundamental importance (Cawood *et al.*, 2020).

Healthcare professionals have a key role to play in the recognition and prevention of malnutrition by ensuring patients have their nutritional status assessed and nutritional intake monitored regularly, to ensure they are receiving adequate nutrition (Avelino-Silva *et al.*, 2017). Failure to do this is tantamount to professional misconduct.

NICE (2012) recommended that:

- All hospital inpatients on admission should be screened (weighed, measured and have their body mass index [BMI] calculated)
- Screening should be repeated weekly
- A clear process should be established for documenting the outcomes of screening and the subsequent actions taken if the patient is recognised as malnourished or at risk of malnutrition.

Screening for malnutrition is an important step in recognising and identifying risk of or diagnosis of malnourishment (Volkert *et al.*, 2019) The Malnutrition Universal Screening Tool (MUST) (BAPEN, 2020) is the most commonly used in hospital. The MUST is simple to complete with a few details, is useful for identifying if someone is malnourished or at risk of becoming so and can guide toward the appropriate referral to a dietitian. However, assessments should be reviewed regularly, either weekly or if the patient's condition changes, and any risks addressed, including making timely referrals for nutritional advice or treatment (Care Quality Commission, 2012). It must be emphasised that this tool must support, not replace, clinical judgement.

Chapter 17 discusses nutrition in more detail. In this section of the chapter, nutritional needs are related to the older person, with a focus upon their specific needs.

Jot This Down

Why is it so important to ensure older people have their nutritional status assessed within 4 hours of being admitted to hospital and what are the aims of nutritional interventions in older patients?

Despite malnutrition being high on the professional, political and media agenda, the Care Quality Commission (2013) review of various hospitals supported the findings from the Francis Report (2013). For example, when older people are malnourished, their basic health and social care outcomes are significantly affected, making malnutrition an important patient safety issue.

Specific common themes that emerged from the Francis Report (2013) and the Care Quality Commission (2013) inspections were:

- Lack of choice in the menus
- Inappropriate food given to patients in light of their condition
- Patients not provided with a meal
- Patients' meals placed out of reach and taken away even though they had not been touched
- No assistance provided to patients to unwrap a meal or cutlery
- No encouragement to patients to eat
- Relatives and other visitors denied access to wards during mealtimes
- Visitors prevented from helping patients with feeding.

Malnutrition continues to be both underdetected and undertreated. demonstrating that multidisciplinary care approaches benefit from the engagement of the different disciplines, including volunteers, patients and relatives (Yunisa *et al.*, 2021).

There are many initiatives around the country aiming to improve the way that older people are provided food in hospitals (Department of Health, 2010b).

- Protected mealtimes for all non-urgent activity. This allows patients to eat their meals without being interrupted by other activity and gives ward staff the time needed to assist those who need help with eating (Age UK, 2010).
- Use of a red tray to easily identify patients who require assistance to eat/drink (Age UK, 2010).
- Many organisations encourage family and carers to come in at mealtimes to assist their relative with eating and drinking. This is good practice, particularly for patients with dementia or learning disabilities, as they may be more willing to accept help from a person they know (Anderson, 2017).
- Verbal prompting by nursing staff to encourage patients to eat and drink can have a significant impact on increasing oral intake (Anderson, 2017).
- Use of the MUST and personalised dietary care plans (Department of Health, 2010d).

When older people decline food, this must be recorded by nurses as the patient's choice. However, some older people, including those with mental health needs such as dementia, need encouragement to eat, especially in the strange environment of a hospital ward (Age Concern, 2010). This highlights a need to ensure that the older patient's food intake is recorded and acted upon if concerns are raised, indicating a referral to a dietitian, nurse swallow assessment or just simply asking relatives to assist the patient to fill in their menu card. Furthermore, it is important to remember when completing the food charts that you do not just document 'patient declined'; you need to record what strategies were tried to encourage the patient to eat, i.e. offer milky drink or finger food.

What the Experts Say

It is a national scandal that six out of 10 older people are at risk of becoming malnourished, or their situation getting worse, in hospital.

Malnourished patients stay in hospital for longer, are three times more likely to develop complications during surgery and have a higher mortality rate than well-fed patients. Ending the scandal of malnourished older people in hospitals will save lives (Age Concern, 2010).

122

Jot This Down

Undertake an audit of nutrition and fluid charts of patients who are at risk of malnutrition or dehydration. Discuss with the team, including a dietitian, whether you are adequately recording intake and output. Reflect on the implications of this; what could you do to improve this practice?

Dehydration

Dehydration can be defined as a 'state in which a relative deficiency of fluid causes adverse effects on function and clinical outcome' (NICE, 2012). Water is an essential nutrient in the maintenance of human health. When net loss of body water exceeds input, dehydration occurs. While hospital food and malnutrition are often in the news, dehydration is also a growing hospital concern. This has a substantial impact on clinical outcomes for older people, leading to prolonged bed days, failed discharges and ultimately an increase in mortality (NHS, 2015). Preventable dehydration in care settings, whether residential or hospitals, is an indicator of poor-quality care. The risk of dehydration is exacerbated by co-morbidities, polypharmacy and physical and mental disability (El-Sharkawy *et al.*, 2014). McMillen & Pitcher (2010) found that the main causes of dehydration are inadequate fluid intake, excessive fluid loss or both. The likelihood of dehydration may also be exacerbated by medications including diuretics and laxatives. Importantly, incontinence predisposes to dehydration as people may limit their fluid intake to manage symptoms (BNF, 2021).

The following are potential signs that could indicate that a person is becoming dehydrated.

- Thirst
- Dry mouth, lips, and eyes
- Tiredness
- Dry skin
- Low blood pressure
- Confusion
- Headaches
- Dark urine or producing small amounts of urine

What the Experts Say

My examination of the medical records of many patients suggested that proper records of fluid balance and nutritional intake were not maintained. In many cases, charts would be started but not continued, or filled in for some days but not others, allowing no picture to be built up of patients' progress. I very much doubt that such incomplete records would be of any significant assistance in assessing patients' continuing nutrition and hydration needs (Francis, 2013).

Box 8.2 outlines some examples of records and nutrition which are accurate and fit for purpose. Box 8.3 provides examples of records that are not accurate or fit for purpose.

Being aware of the nutritional and hydration needs of older people and their individual preferences is an essential nursing duty that requires skill and a multidisciplinary approach including engagement from different disciplines, including volunteers, patients and relatives (Yunisa *et al.*, 2021).

Box 8.2 Examples Where Records Concerning Nutrition Are Both Accurate and Fit for Purpose

- Multidisciplinary records demonstrate that patients have had their nutritional risk assessed on admission and this was reviewed on a regular basis. Appropriate referrals were made to other healthcare professionals (e.g. dietitians).
- Patients' weights are recorded and monitored if required.
- Records of patients' food intake and fluid balance are accurately completed.
- Working records, for example fluid balance charts, are kept near to the patient, and other nursing and medical notes holding confidential information are held securely but within easy reach of staff.

Source: Adapted from Care Quality Commission (2015)

Box 8.3 Examples Where Records Concerning Nutrition Are Not Fit for Purpose

- Staff concentrate on delivering the food in a timely manner, but patients are not always positioned in a way that helped them to eat without assistance.
- Food is left for patients who are lying in bed, by the bedside table.
- Person is slumped in bed and the table is not near enough to the patient.
- Care assistants remove trays without asking if the patient has finished.
- The food charts are not always completed for evening meals.
- Food charts are not reviewed to ensure that people's nutritional needs are regularly updated.
- Insufficient evidence to inform clinical decisions about treatments and interventions in order to ensure people are protected from inadequate nutrition and hydration.

Source: Adapted from Care Quality Commission (2015)

Shahin *et al.* (2010) found a significant relationship between malnutrition parameters such as weight loss, BMI <18.5, poor nutritional intake and patients developing pressure ulcers. It is important for nurses to recognise the link between hydration and nutrition for tissue repair and pressure ulcer management (Saghaleini et al., 2018).

Case Study

Mrs Mir was admitted from home due to a deterioration in mobility, loss of appetite/fluid intake and suspected urinary tract infection. Primary diagnosis of an acute kidney infection (AKI 2) and symptomatic with dizziness when standing. Medication included ramipril and furosemide. Past medical history included Alzheimer's, macular degeneration, heart failure and hip replacement. She lives alone with a twice-a-day package of care and daily support from the daughter. Mrs Mir's daughter raised concerns that her mother's appetite had reduced considerably over the past 6 months, and over the past few weeks she also noted her mother was not drinking very much or able to mobilise as well as she used to. Your initial impression was that the patient appeared undernourished and dehydrated.

On admission to the ward, the nurse/NA caring for this patient should ensure that she is weighed, and her BMI calculated. If the assessment concludes that a referral to the dietitian is indicated, this must be completed accordingly.

They should then commence a food and hydration chart so that this can be monitored and would also assist the dietitian with a management plan when they review the patient. The patient would benefit from utilisation of a 'red tray' system which highlights to staff that she requires assistance/encouragement to eat and drink. It would also be beneficial to encourage a family member or someone very familiar with the patient to come in and provide support during mealtimes.

What could be causing the dizziness? Performing a lying and standing blood pressure check could confirm there is a notable deficit suggesting hypotension. If this is the case, it is important to ensure the doctor is made aware of the findings. There could be a simple solution, such as the nurse/NA encouraging the patient frequently throughout the day to drink more. Finding out from the daughter what drinks her mother enjoys would ensure you were not trying to get her to drink anything she would not normally drink.

It is important to ensure the patient is kept as mobile as possible, so they do not decompensate muscle tone. It is too easy for a normally mobile frail older person to be admitted with reduced mobility and then become bed bound. Early mobilisation is important with early referral to a physiotherapist.

Jot This Down

What is meant by 'decompensating'?

Look up Brian Dolan's 'End PJ Paralysis' (**https://endpjparalysis.org/**). Could this be something you could initiate in your placement to reduce the risk of older people decompensating? What do you think would be the barriers and what could you do to overcome this?

Pressure Ulcers

Chapter 18 considers skin integrity, and the reader is advised to read that chapter to learn more. In this section, a brief consideration of pressure ulcer prevention in the older person is discussed.

Pressure area care is an essential component of nursing practice, with all patients potentially at risk of developing a pressure ulcer (NICE, 2014). Pressure ulcers remain a concerning and mainly avoidable harm associated with healthcare delivery (NHSI, 2018). Despite extensive prevention programmes, in the UK, over 700^000 patients are affected by pressure ulcers each year, and 180^000 of those are newly acquired each year (Wood et al., 2019). The prevalence of pressure ulcers, particularly in the frail older adult population, continues to be high and very costly, especially in those suffering from chronic diseases (Jaul et al., 2018), suggesting that the occurrence of pressure ulcers in healthcare remains a challenge for care providers (Fletcher & Hall, 2018). It is crucial that pressure injury prevention remains a nursing priority to improve patient health outcomes and reduce preventable harm (Oozageer et al., 2020).

Jot This Down

What do you think are the main causes of pressure ulcers in older patients?

What are the pressure ulcer points on the body?

Those Most at Risk

People most at risk of pressure ulcers have medical conditions that limit their ability to change positions or cause them to spend most of their time in a bed or chair. Ulcers can develop over hours or days. Haleem et al. (2008) suggested that the risk was higher in patients with an extracapsular neck of femur fracture and those with an increased time interval between admission to hospital and surgery. Their study indicated that while co-morbidities constitute a substantial risk in an elderly population, the increase in incidence of pressure sores can be reduced by minimising delays to surgery. Age alone is not a risk factor; rather, it is the problems common in older people that are associated with pressure ulceration (hip fractures, faecal and urinary incontinence, smoking, dry skin, chronic systemic conditions, and terminal illness) (PHE, 2015).

Areas at Risk of Developing a Pressure Ulcer

The most common places for pressure ulcers to occur are over bony prominences (bones close to the skin), such as the sacrum, heel and elbow, ankle, shoulder, back (bony prominences) and the back of the head (occipital) (NICE, 2014) (Figure 8.2).

Many pressure ulcers can be prevented when the right interventions are utilised and could be avoided through simple actions by staff, individuals and their carers (Department of Health and Social Care, 2018).

Pressure Ulcer Assessment Tools

A risk assessment tool is a formal tool that uses a point scale or traffic light system to rate a selection of known risk factors (Young & Fletcher, 2019). Identifying an older person's risk of developing pressure ulcers is considered the first step in prevention and forms the basis for planning, implementing and evaluating pressure ulcer prevention care (Balzer et al., 2014 cited in Young & Fletcher, 2019). Although a validated risk assessment tool gives a logical and structured assessment, which is easily documented and reviewed, these must be used alongside clinical judgement (Moore & Patton, 2019 cited in Young & Fletcher, 2019).

The skin assessment and care element of the new education framework, SSKIN, is based on this principle (NHS Improvement, 2018) that provides practitioners with the knowledge they need to be able to do this (Fletcher, 2019). SSKIN enables healthcare professionals to effectively assess key factors associated with the prevention and management of pressure ulcers, including:

- *Surface*: assessment of the appropriateness of mattresses and/or cushions and review of the functionality and integrity of equipment intended to reduce risk of pressure ulcers
- *Skin inspection*: assessing pressure areas and monitoring skin reddening
- *Keep moving*: assessment of regularity of movement intended to prevent pressure ulcers or deterioration of existing pressure ulcers
- *Incontinence/increased moisture*: assessing bowel and bladder function and control, and other body fluids on the skin
- *Nutrition*: ensuring the right diet, fluids and supplements (NHS Improvement, 2018).

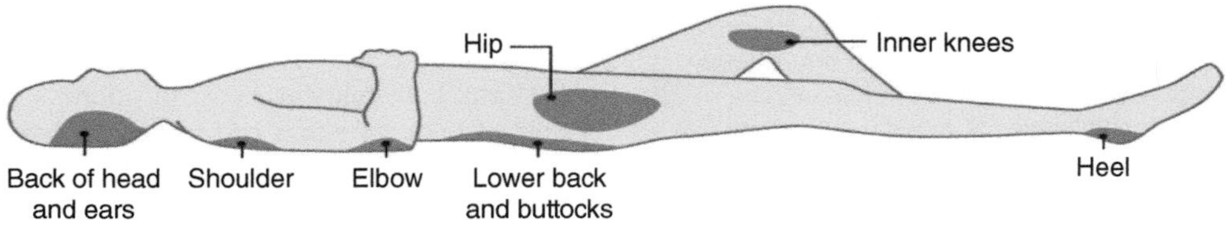

Figure 8.2 **Pressure ulcers: early inspection means early detection.**

124

Jot This Down

Review the assessment scores on a patient who has developed a pressure ulcer in the care environment you are currently caring for. Is there evidence to support that continued assessment is being carried out?

The three tools most commonly used to predict pressure ulcer risk are the Braden Scale, Waterlow and Purpose T assessment scores. Review the assessment tools used in your area of work and perform a literature review. What are the advantages and/or disadvantages of each tool?

Do you think the right one is being utilised in your workplace?

Preventive Measures

Pressure-relieving Mattresses

NICE (2014) recommends using a high-specification foam mattress for all adults who are admitted to secondary care or at high risk of developing a pressure ulcer in primary and community care settings. High-specification foam mattresses should be used for adults who have a pressure ulcer (NICE, 2014). One way of preventing pressure sores is by using pressure-redistributing devices, which allow capillaries to refill. These include specially designed mattresses or cushions (Nixon *et al.*, 2019). However, some older people ask for the alternating pressure mattress to be changed to a foam mattress due to discomfort. In some cases, this type of mattress also makes rehabilitation difficult as it can restrict therapist movements compared with foam (Nixon *et al.*, 2019).

Positional Changes

Pressure ulcers are caused by sustained pressure on tissue so keeping patients moving and the use of repositioning are important elements in pressure ulcer prevention (Fletcher, 2020). Current guidelines state that all patients at risk of pressure ulcers should be repositioned, unless otherwise contraindicated, following an individualised schedule (European Pressure Ulcer Advisory Panel, 2019; NICE, 2014). Patients should be repositioned at least every 6 hours and every 4 hours for those at high risk (NICE, 2014). If possible, patients should not be turned onto reddened areas; redness is an indication that the body has not recovered from previous pressure-loading conditions (Mitchell, 2018). Given the limited data from economic evaluations, it remains unclear whether repositioning every 3 hours using the 30° tilt versus 'usual care' (90° tilt) or repositioning 3–4-hourly versus 2-hourly is less costly relative to nursing time (Gillespie *et al.*, 2020).

Falls and Their Impact on Older People

Falls are the most common single reason for older people to present to urgent care. Furthermore, falls among hospital inpatients are the most frequently reported safety incident with more than 250^000 recorded annually in England and Wales (Morris & O'Riordan, 2017). Inpatient falls in older people are a frequent complication of hospital care that results in significant morbidity and mortality, including serious injuries, prolonged hospitalisation, increased hospital financial liability, decreased quality of life and increased risk for placement in nursing homes (Twibell *et al.*, 2015).

The NICE (2015) definition of a fall is as follows: 'A fall is defined as an unintentional or unexpected loss of balance resulting in coming to rest on the floor, the ground, or an object below knee level'.

Currently, nurses are caring for more adults over 65 than any other patient population and hospital admission. Acute illness, particularly in frail older people or those recovering from serious injury or surgery, increases the risk of a fall in hospital. Patients are vulnerable to delirium, dehydration and deconditioning, all of which affect balance and mobility, especially in unfamiliar surroundings (RCP, 2020). Also, older people are more prone to fractures due to frailty, osteoporosis and associated co-morbidities (Arafa *et al.*, 2020).

The Royal College of Physicians (RCP) National Audit of Inpatient Falls (RCP, 2020) report confirms that patients who fall and fracture their hip in hospital are the 'oldest old' and the 'frailest frail' and perhaps challenges ideas about where injurious falls occur, with only 21% occurring in elderly care wards. It is therefore essential that all specialties caring for older people need to be fully signed up to falls prevention.

A further influence on the importance of falls prevention has been highlighted during the recent COVID-19 pandemic. Arafa *et al.* (2020) identified that older people with hip fractures were a particularly vulnerable group with regard to mortality when they were positive for the COVID-19 virus. Prior to this pandemic, the mortality rate of older people with a hip fracture was 6.1% but this increased to 30% within 12 months (Arafa *et al.*, 2020). The pandemic has also had a significant impact on falls prevention services which have ceased delivery for large parts of the pandemic. This includes exercise programmes to encourage older people to exercise as well as provision of education on what they can do to prevent falls such as exercise, diet intake and pacing what they do (PHE, 2021). Ultimately, the key goals of healthy ageing, where older people are supported to remain mobile, have their needs met, continue to learn, develop and maintain relationships and contribute to society, are deliverable at least in part through proactive falls and fracture prevention (PHE, 2017).

The Impact of a Fall for an Older Person

Falls among inpatients are the most frequently reported safety incident in NHS hospitals; 30–50% of falls result in some physical injury and fractures occur in 1–3%. No fall is harmless, with psychological sequelae leading to lost confidence, delays in functional recovery and prolonged hospitalisation (Morris & O'Riordan, 2017l Age UK, 2012). The psychological impact of falling can be devastating, with lower levels of confidence and independence, fear of falling, reduced quality of life and well-being, increased isolation and depression inhibiting prompt recovery, even if a fall does not result in serious consequences (Age UK, 2012). The unfamiliar hospital setting coupled with concomitant acute physical and/or mental illness serve to amplify the risk of falls for hospitalised older people (Morris & O'Riordan, 2017).

> ### Jot This Down
>
> Falls in hospital are the most commonly reported patient accident in the country (Patient Safety Observatory, 2007).
>
> People may fall in hospital for a variety of reasons. What do you think they are?
>
> Review the notes of some older patients who have fallen. What are the main contributing factors causing them to fall?

Causes of Falls

The causes of having a fall are multifactorial – a fall is the result of the interplay of multiple risk factors. These include:

- Muscle weakness
- Poor balance
- Visual impairment
- Polypharmacy and the use of certain medicines
- Environmental hazards
- Some specific medical conditions (PHE, 2020).

A patient who is *not allowed* to walk alone will quickly become a patient who is *unable* to walk alone (Healey, 2010). Training needs to provide an overview of legislation, including the Mental Capacity Act 2005 and professional guidance, including the Royal College of Nursing's *Positive and Proactive Care: Reducing the Need for Restrictive Interventions* (RCN, 2016).

Older adults are susceptible to polypharmacy and higher risk of falls (WHO, 2019). Even though the patient's fall risk may be scored on admission, the medication-induced fall risk may be ignored (Michalcova et al., 2020). A leading mechanism for increased risk can be sedation which slows reaction time and causes orthostatic hypotension, syncope, dizziness, drowsiness and blood pressure change or impaired balance (Walgers et al., 2017). Furthermore, drugs reducing blood pressure are associated with fall risk because of their hypotension effect. Thus, adjusting antihypertensive medication may reduce syncope and falls (Luiting et al., 2019).

Red Flag Drugs which affect the central nervous system

Falls are associated with cardiovascular medications, psychotropic medications, sedative hypnotics, antipsychotics, antidepressants, benzodiazepines, antiepileptic medication, anticholinergics and anti-Parkinson medications (Bradley et al., 2014). Psychotropics including anxiolytics/sedative-hypnotics, antipsychotics, antidepressants, anticonvulsants, and narcotic pain medications typically increase risk due to their effects on cognitive function, resulting in sedation, slower reaction times and impaired balance (Coggins, 2020). Furthermore, antipsychotic medications, including haloperidol, olanzapine, quetiapine, aripiprazole and risperidone, can increase fall risk due to syncope, sedation, slowed reflexes, loss of balance and impaired psychomotor function (Coggins, 2020).

Preventive Measures in Falls Prevention

When older people are identified as having a risk of falls, it is essential that a 'falls prevention care plan' is initiated, and preventive measures put in place, such as the following.

- Ensure the patient is being nursed in an observable area.
- They should be nursed on a bed that goes right to the floor (high-low bed).
- Consider using a falls prevention sensor alarm, which is placed under the patient so that if they move off the sensor pad, an alarm sounds to alert staff that the patient is at risk of falling, so they attend straight away. However, these alarms do not stop falls from occurring, but they do alert the staff member that the patient is trying to get out of bed/chair unassisted. The aim is for the staff member to attend to the patient as soon as the alarm goes off, to increase the likelihood of preventing a fall.
- If the patient is very confused, it may necessitate the use of one-to-one enhanced supervision to ensure the patient's safety is maximised.
- Ensure the doctors/pharmacist have performed a medication review.
- Ensure there has been a multifactorial review of the patient.

Given the many different causes of falls in hospital patients, engagement of all the multidisciplinary team is needed and will be most effective if nurses, doctors, therapists, pharmacists, housekeeping staff and relevant others work together to develop key aspects to reduce older people falling in hospital (Boushon et al., 2012).

Assessment of Those at Risk of Falling

The NICE updated pathway review (CG161; NICE, 2013) recommends not to use fall risk prediction tools to predict inpatients' risk of falling in hospital. Instead, practitioners should regard the following groups of inpatients as being at risk of falling in hospital:

- All patients aged 65 years and/or
- Patients aged 50–64 years who are judged by a clinician to be at higher risk of falling because of an underlying condition.

However, most trusts continue to use a form of falls assessment to identify those at risk of falls, to ensure that a trigger mechanism is in place, as it is imperative to ensure interventions have been implemented to prevent a fall/further falls. Nevertheless, it is important to note that there are some older people who will fall, regardless of whatever interventions are put in place.

126

Initiatives to Prevent an Older Person Falling

- Ensure environment is free from clutter.
- Ensure they have adequate footwear that fits properly.
- Ensure walking aids are near them.
- Ensure the call bell is within reach.
- Ensure a medication review has occurred to reduce any unnecessary hypnotics or sedatives.
- Ensure they have been assessed by the physiotherapist for an appropriate walking aid and assessment of their balance and gait.
- Consider the use of equipment, such as a falls prevention sensor alarm.
- Consider the use of a high-low bed.
- Ensure those high at risk of falls are in observable bays.
- Ensure one-to-one monitoring/observation is in place if an older person is unsafe to be left unsupervised.

Introducing 'safety huddles', which are short multidisciplinary team briefings that describe the current status of each patient and attempt to identify clinical and non-clinical opportunities to improve patient care and safety (Morris & O'Riordan, 2017), has been associated with a reduction in falls in some hospital (Cracknell *et al.*, 2016).

After a Fall

Immediate Checks

A medical examination should take place immediately if the patient displays an altered Glasgow Coma Scale score, possible signs of fracture/spinal/head injury or new pain, confusion or distress (NICE, 2019). It is essential that practitioners ensure they are familiar with their employer's falls prevention and management policy and follow the guidance accordingly.

Unwitnessed Fall/Suspected Head Injury

Staggs *et al.* (2014) found that unwitnessed falls were associated with higher odds of injury than witnessed falls, including higher odds of minor, moderate and major injury. If the patient is unable to verbalise why they fell, it is important to rule out that a head injury may have occurred, even if there are no visible signs of injury. Furthermore, the practitioner needs to note frequency and duration of neurological observations for all patients where head injury has/may have occurred or cannot be excluded (NICE, 2019).

Discharge Planning

The goal of efficient discharge planning is to improve an older person's quality of life by ensuring continuity of care and to reduce the rate of unplanned readmissions and/or complications, which may decrease the financial burden on the healthcare system (Gonçalves-Bradley *et al.*, 2016). Older people may require complex support networks, both formal and informal, to support them in their own homes, so comprehensive discharge planning is crucial to ensure that the individual's problems have been addressed, so they can return safely to their own home (Shepperd *et al.*, 2013; Heath *et al.*, 2010). Furthermore, older people with more complex needs, such as multimorbidity or frailty, may need additional input from other professionals such as social workers, pharmacists, transport, care packages and therapists provided by external agencies (NICE, 2018).

The involvement of additional services, staff and specialties makes prior co-ordination and planning even more critical (Department of Health, 2010c). This is of particular importance in the frail elderly and those patients with mental health issues (NICE, 2018), requiring adequate and timely information to be shared between services whenever there is a transfer of care between individuals or services (Cooke *et al.*, 2012). These patient groups are vulnerable to poor communication and co-ordination which can have a disproportionate impact on the discharge processes (NICE, 2018). Effective collaboration is the key to successful discharge planning (Patel & Bechmann, 2020).

A crucial part of effective discharge planning is to ensure the older person, and where appropriate their carers and families, are involved in the decision-making process around assessment and management of ongoing and future care, and self-care (Cooke *et al.*, 2012). The NMC (2008) stipulates that: 'You must be aware of the legislation regarding mental capacity, ensuring that people who lack capacity remain at the centre of decision-making and are fully safeguarded'. This is a key element in working with the older person and their family when considering discharge planning.

Francis (2013) found that patients and their families had raised some concerns with regard to discharge.

- Premature discharge from wards resulting in readmission to hospital.
- Protracted process of discharge.
- Failure to communicate discharge arrangements to patients and their families.
- Discharge at an inappropriate time or in an inappropriate condition.
- Failure to ensure appropriate support.
- Lack of communication about changes in discharge plans.

Jot This Down

What is your experience of the discharge process?
As a nurse, how can you influence the discharge process and what are your responsibilities to ensure a safe and effective discharge is achieved?

What the Experts Say Nurses' Responsibilities

- Listen to people in their care and respond to their needs and preferences.
- Share with people the information they want and need to know about their health and care in a way they understand.
- Share information with colleagues and keep them informed.
- Work effectively as part of a team.
- Ensure that patient consent is gained before intervention.
- Act as advocate for patients (NMC, 2008).

The MDT needs to develop an understanding of how the patient managed prior to admission, for example with activities of living, mobility, issues concerning continence, nutrition and any concerns the older person or significant others may have with regard to discharge planning.

Involvement of Carers/Significant Others

Families and carers can play a significant role in helping adults with social care needs return home after a hospital admission (NICE, 2016). They can provide information about the person's needs and circumstances beyond medical conditions or physical needs (NICE, 2016). However, nurses should not assume that a person's carer will necessarily be able to, or want to, continue in a caring role (Tuffrey-Wijne *et al.*, 2013). Nevertheless, is important that they are involved in decisions about the person's discharge plan (NICE, 2016).

Primary Care

It is important to ensure the GP receives a full summary of the admission to hospital to ensure continuity of care.

If the older person has complex needs or a long-term condition, consider a referral to the community matron to assess the patient post discharge.

District nurses will require a referral if the patient needs medication to be administered by them, catheter care or dressings to wounds (ensure they have at least 3 days' supply of dressings on discharge, as it takes time for the district nurse to get a prescription from the GP for the appropriate dressing, especially if it is a newly acquired wound).

Case Study

An older person is due to be discharged – he is excited and very keen to be going back home with his wife. His wife has called you aside to say that she no longer feels able or willing to care for her husband at home. She feels the burden is too great, as she herself has a number of health issues that restrict her physically. What will your next steps be?

It is important for the nurse/NA to find out what the wife's main concerns are around not being able to continue to provide care for her husband on discharge. The wife could then be advised of what support would be available from occupational therapists (OT) and Social Services to reduce the burden of caring for her husband. The OT would assess his care needs and make recommendations and order any necessary equipment to help maintain his independence as much as possible when home, whilst reducing the burden on the wife. If the patient has the means to pay privately for the care, he would still have the support of the OT and Social Services. It is also worth noting that if the patient has capacity, still wants to go home and the house is in joint names, he is entitled to return with the identified support, despite his wife stating she does not want to have him home.

This emphasises the importance of the nurse/NA gaining collateral history on admission of how the wife was coping, whilst providing an opportunity for her to raise any concerns early so that the MDT can put actions in place to address those concerns. This would hopefully ensure the wife felt supported and involved with any discharge planning for a timely and effective discharge and reduced length of stay.

There are occasions when an older person will decide against the need for a care package identified by the MDT and want to be discharged accordingly. As long as they have the mental capacity to make that decision, the nurse and other MDT members must respect their decision, despite how unwise it may appear to them.

Older people who do not have the capacity to make decisions are given their rights and obligations under the Mental Capacity Act (Department of health, 2005). Where the patient cannot represent themselves, the next of kin, carer, relative or an independent mental capacity advocate (IMCA) must be involved. Their role is to represent the patient's interests, and to challenge any decision that does not appear to be in the best interest of the patient.

Understanding how the discharge process works and any potential issues would ensure the nurse/NA involves the older person and their next of king, whilst focusing on providing a seamless and effective journey through the hospital to discharge destination.

Key Points

- The chapter has emphasised the importance of communication in the older person setting and also when communicating with older people and their families. Key issues associated with all aspects of care have been discussed, including dignity and respect. The need to ensure that people are treated as individuals has been highlighted.
- It is imperative that care planning is (when possible) done with patients, reflecting and respecting their individual needs.
- When undertaking an assessment of individual needs, a holistic approach must be adopted. The person undertaking the assessment of needs must be deemed competent and confident in this important aspect of care. Assessment tools must be used judiciously, be fit for purpose and be relevant.
- There are a number of tools available to assess the older person's nutritional needs. Assessment of need concerning nutrition has been discussed.
- Falls are a major cause of morbidity and mortality in the ageing population. Undertaking a detailed and patient-centred assessment can identify those at risk and help to prevent a fall occurring.
- Caring for people in their own homes in a safe and effective manner will require the nurse to plan the discharge in such a way that the patient is at the centre of any decisions being made. A multidisciplinary team approach has been advocated.

References

Age UK (2010) *Still Hungry to Be Heard – in London.* www.ageuk.org.uk/bp-assets/globalassets/london/documents/campaigns/still-hungry-to-be-heard.pdf (accessed December 2021).

Age UK (2012) *Stop Falling: Start Saving Lives and Money.* www.ageingwellinwales.com/Libraries/Documents/Stop-Falling---Start-Saving-Lives-and-Money.pdf (accessed December 2021).

Ali, M (2017) Communication skills 2: overcoming barriers to effective communication *Nursing Times,* 114(1), 40–42.

Anderson, L. (2017) Assisting patients with eating and drinking to prevent malnutrition. *Nursing Times,* 113, 23–25.

Arafa, A., Mohamed, A., Saleh, L., *et al.* (2020) Psychological impacts of the COVID-19 pandemic on the public in Egypt. *Community Mental Health Journal,* 57, 64–69.

Avelino-Silva, T.J. & Jaluul, O. (2017) Malnutrition in hospitalized older patients: management strategies to improve patient care and clinical outcomes. *International Journal of Gerontology,*11, 56–61.

Bale, L. & Jenkins, C. (2018) Nursing students' experiences of delivering dementia friends sessions to peers. *Nursing Older People,* 30, 32–37.

Berry, L. (2012) University courses should stress the value of dignity. *Nursing Older People,* 24(6), 5.

Boushon, B., Nielsen, G., Quigley, P., *et al.* (2012) *How-to Guide: Reducing Patient Injuries from Falls.* Institute for Healthcare Improvement, Cambridge, MA.

Bradley, M.C., Motterlini, N., Padmanabhan, S., *et al.* (2014) Potentially inappropriate prescribing among older people in the United Kingdom. *BMC Geriatrics,* 14(1), 72.

British Association for Parenteral and Enteral Nutrition (BAPEN) (2020) Malnutrition Universal Screening Tool. www.bapen.org.uk/pdfs/must/must_full.pdf (accessed June 2021).

British Dietetic Association (2020) *Malnutrition in Older People.* www.bda.uk.com/resource/malnutrition-in-older-people.html (accessed December 2021).

British Nutrition Foundation (BNF) (2021) *Dehydration in older people.* www.nutrition.org.uk/life-stages/older-people/malnutrition-and-dehydration/dehydration-in-older-people/ (accessed December 2021).

Burnes, D., Sheppard, C., Henderson, C.R. Jr, *et al.* (2019) Interventions to reduce ageism against older adults: a systematic review and meta-analysis. *American Journal of Public Health,* 109(8), e1–e9.

Butterworth, C. (2012) How to achieve a person-centred writing style in care plans. *Nursing Older People,* 24(8), 21–26.

Care Quality Commission (2012) *The State of Health Care and Adult Social Care in England in 2011–2012.* Care Quality Commission, London.

Care Quality Commission (2013) *Time to Listen in NHS Hospitals. Dignity and Nutrition Inspection Programme 2012 Summary.* Care Quality Commission, London.

Care Quality Commission (2015) *Consultation: CQC's Code of Practice on Confidential Personal Information.* Care Quality Commision. London

Cawood, A.L., Walters, E.R., Smith, T.R., *et al.* (2020) A review of nutrition support guidelines for individuals with or recovering from COVID-19 in the community. *Nutrients,* 12, 3230.

Chang, E.S., Kannoth, S., Levy, S., Wang, S.Y., Lee, J.E. & Levy, B.R. (2020) Global reach of ageism on older persons' health: a systematic review. *PLoS One,* 15(1), e0220857.

Chrisler, J.C., Barney, A. & Palatino, B. (2016) Ageism can be hazardous to women's health: ageism, sexism, and stereotypes of older women in the healthcare system. *Journal of Social Issues,* 72(1), 86–104.

Coggins, M.D. (2020) Medication monitor: medications that increase fall risk. *Today's Geriatric Medicine,* 11, 30.

Cooke, M., Oliver, D. & Burns, A. (2012) *Quality Care for Older People with Urgent and Emergency Care Needs.* http://aace.org.uk/wp-content/uploads/2012/06/SILVER_BOOK_FINAL.pdf (accessed December 2021).

Cracknell, A. Lovatt, A. Winfield, A., *et al.* (2016) Huddle up for safer healthcare: how frontline teams can work together to improve patient safety. *Future Hospital Journal,* 3(Suppl 2), s31.

Department of Health (2005) *Mental Capacity Act.* HMSO, London.

Department of Health (2006a) *Dignity in Care Campaign.* Department of Health, London.

Department of Health (2006b) *National Service Framework: Next Steps.* Department of Health, London.

Department of Health (2008) *High Quality Care For All. NHS Next Stage Review Final Report.* Department of Health, London.

Department of Health (2009) *Final Report on the Review of the DOH 2006 Dignity in Care Campaign.* Department of Health, London.

Department of Health (2010a) *Nutrition, Patients, Person-Centred Care, Quality Assurance, Standards, Assessment, Care Planning, Choice; Practice Guidance.* Department of Health, London.

Department of Health (2010b) *Essence of Care 2010: Benchmarks For Communication.* Department of Health, London.

Department of Health (2010c) *Essence of Care. Communication, Promoting Health and Care Environment.* Department of Health, London.

Department of Health (2010d) *Ready to Go? Planning the Discharge and The Transfer of Patients from Hospital and Intermediate Care.* Department of Health, London.

Department of Health and Social Care (2018) *Safeguarding Adults Protocol. Pressure Ulcers and the Interface with a Safeguarding Enquiry.* https://assets.publishing.service.gov.uk/government/uploads/system/uploads/attachment_data/file/756243/safeguarding-adults-protocol-pressure-ulcers.pdf (accessed December 2021).

Dupuis, K. (2011) *Bimodal Cueing in Aphasia: The Influence of Lipreading on Speech Discrimination and Language Comprehension.* University of British Columbia. https://open.library.ubc.ca/collections/ubctheses/24/items/1.0071733 (accessed December 2021).

Elia, M. (on behalf of the Malnutrition Action Group of BAPEN and the NIHR Biomedical Research Centre (Nutrition) Southampton) (2015) *The Cost of Malnutrition in England and the Potential Cost Savings from Nutritional Interventions (Full Report).* https://www.bapen.org.uk/resources-and-education/publications-and-reports/malnutrition/cost-of-malnutrition-in-england (accessed December 2021).

El-Sharkawy, A.M., Sahota, O., Maughan, R.J. & Lobo, D.N. (2014) The pathophysiology of fluid and electrolyte balance in the older adult surgical patient. *Clinical Nutrition*, 33, 6–13.

European Pressure Ulcer Advisory Panel (2019) *Prevention and Treatment of Pressure Ulcers/Injuries: Quick Reference Guide.* www.nursingtimes.net/clinical-archive/tissue-viability/pressure-ulcer-education-5-keeping-patients-moving-13-01-2020/ (accessed December 2021).

Fakhr-Movahedi, A., Salsali, M., Negarandeh, R. & Rahnavard, Z. (2011) Exploring contextual factors of the nurse–patient relationship: a qualitative study. *Koomesh*, 13(1), 23–34.

Fletcher, J. (2019) Pressure ulcer education 3: skin assessment and care. *Nursing Times*, 115, 26–29.

Fletcher, J. (2020) Pressure ulcer education 5: keeping patients moving. *Nursing Times*,116, 2.

Fletcher, J. & Hall, J. (2018) New guidance on how to define and pressure ulcers. *Nursing Times*, 114, 41–44.

Francis, R. (2013) *Independent Inquiry into Care Provided by Mid Staffordshire NHS Foundation Trust.* www.gov.uk/government/publications/report-of-the-mid-staffordshire-nhs-foundation-trust-public-inquiry (accessed December 2021).

Gillespie, B.M., Walker, R.M., Latimer, S.L., *et al.* (2020) Repositioning for pressure injury prevention in adults. *Cochrane Database of Systematic Reviews*, 6, CD009958.

Gonçalves-Bradley, D.C., Lannin, N.A., Clemson, L.M., Cameron, I.D. & Shepperd, S. (2016) Discharge planning from hospital. *Cochrane Database of Systematic Reviews*, 1, CD000313.

Haleem, S., Heinert, G. & Parker, M.J. (2008) Pressure sores and hip fractures. *Injury*, 39, 219–223.

Harlock, J. (2010) Personalisation: emerging implications for the voluntary and community sector. *Voluntary Sector Review*, 13, 371–378.

Hartung, B., Freeman, C., Grosbein, H., *et al.* (2020) Responding to responsive behaviours: a clinical placement workshop for nursing students. *Nurse Education in Practice*, 45, 102759.

Healey, F. (2010) A guide on how to prevent falls and injury in hospital. *Nursing Older People*, 22(9), 16–22.

Health Foundation (2016) *Person-centred Care Made Simple. What Everyone Should Know About Person-Centred Care.* Health Foundation, London.

Heath, H., Sturdy, D. & Cheesly, A. (2010) *Discharge Planning: A summary of the Department of Health's guidance, Ready to go? Planning the discharge and the transfer of patients from hospital and intermediate care.* RCN Publishing, Harrow.

Hestevik, C.H., Molin, M., Debesay, J. *et al.* (2019) Healthcare professionals' experiences of providing individualized nutritional care for older people in hospital and home care: a qualitative study. *BMC Geriatrics*, 19, 317.

Jack, K., Ridley, C. & Turner, S. (2019) Effective communication with older people. *Nursing Older People*, 31. doi: 10.7748/nop.2019.e1126.

Jaul, E., Barron, J., Rosenzweig, J.P., *et al.* (2018) An overview of co-morbidities and the development of pressure ulcers among older adults. *BMC Geriatrics*, 18, 305.

JCR (2007) *Improving Hands-Off Communication.* Joint Commission Resources, Illinois.

Lees, L. & Delpino, R. (2007) Facilitating an effective discharge from hospital. *Nursing Times*, 103(29), 30–31.

Lin, Y.P. & Tsai, Y.F. (2011) Maintaining patients' dignity during clinical care: a qualitative interview study. *Journal of Advanced Nursing*, 67(2), 340–348.

Luiting, S., Jansen, S., Seppälä, L.J., Daams, J.G. & van der Velde, N. (2019) Effectiveness of cardiovascular evaluations and interventions on fall risk: a scoping review. *Journal of Nutrition, Health and Aging*, 23(4), 330–337.

Manias, E., Geddes, F., Watson, B., Jones, D. & Della, P. (2016) Perspectives of clinical handover processes: a multi-site survey across different health professionals. *Journal of Clinical Nursing*, 25, 80–91.

McMillen, R. & Pitcher, B. (2010) The balancing act: body fluids and protecting patient health. *British Journal of Healthcare Assistants*, 5, 117–121.

Michalcova, J., Vasut, K., Airaksinen, M., *et al.* (2020) Inclusion of medication-related fall risk in fall risk assessment tool in geriatric care units. *BMC Geriatrics*, 20, 454.

Mitchell, A. (2018) Adult pressure area care: preventing pressure ulcers. *British Journal of Nursing*, 27, 1050–1052.

Moore, Z.E.H. & Patton, D. (2019) Risk assessment tools used for the prevention of pressure ulcers. *Cochrane Database of Systematic Reviews*, 1, CD006471.

Morris, R. & O'Riordan, S. (2017) Prevention of falls in hospital. *Clinical Medicine*, 17(4), 360–362.

National Institute for Health and Care Excellence (2012) *Nutrition Support in Adults. QS24.* www.nice.org.uk/guidance/qs24 (accessed December 2021).

National Institute for Health and Care Excellence (2013) *Falls in Older People: Assessing Risk and Prevention Clinical Guideline. CG161.* NICE, London.

National Institute for Health and Care Excellence (2014) *Pressure Ulcers: Prevention and Management. CG179.* www.nice.org.uk/guidance/cg179 (accessed December 2021).

National Institute for Health and Care Excellence (2015) *Falls in Older People. QS86.* www.nice.org.uk/guidance/qs86 (accessed December 2021).

National institute for Health and Care Excellence (2016) *Transition Between Inpatient Hospital Settings and Community or Care Home Settings for Adults with Social Care Needs. QS136.* www.nice.org.uk/guidance/qs136/chapter/quality-statement-5-involving-carers-in-discharge-planning. (accessed December 2021).

National Institute for Health and Care Excellence (2018) *Discharge planning: Emergency and Acute Medical Care in Over 16s: Service Delivery and Organisation.* www.nice.org.uk/guidance/ng94/evidence/35.discharge-planning-pdf-172397464674 (accessed December 2021).

National Institute for Health and Care Excellence (2019) *Head Injury: Assessment and Early Management. CG 176.* www.nice.org.uk/guidance/cg176/chapter/Introduction (accessed December 2021).

National Voices (2017) *Person-centred care in 2017: evidence from service users.* www.nationalvoices.org.uk/sites/default/files/public/publications/person-centred_care_in_2017_-_national_voices.pdf (accessed February 2021).

NHS Choices (2012) *Pressure Ulcers.* www.nhs.uk/conditions/pressure-sores/ (accessed December 2021).

NHS England (2014) *Safe, Compassionate Care for Frail Older People Using an Integrated Care Pathway.* www.england.nhs.uk/wp-content/uploads/2014/02/safe-comp-care.pdf (accessed December 2021).

NHS England (2015) *Guidance – Commissioning Excellent Nutrition and Hydration 2015–2018.* www.england.nhs.uk/wp-content/uploads/2015/10/nut-hyd-guid.pdf (accessed December 2021).

NHS England (2018) *Ageing Well and Supporting People Living with Frailty.* www.england.nhs.uk/ourwork/clinical-policy/older-people/frailty/ (accessed December 2021).

NHSI (2018) *Pressure Ulcers: Revised Definition and Measurement Framework.* www.england.nhs.uk/pressure-ulcers-revised-definition-and-measurement-framework/ (accessed December 2021).

Nixon, J., Smith, I.L., Brown, S., *et al.* (2019) Pressure relieving support surfaces for pressure ulcer prevention (PRESSURE 2): clinical and health economic results of a randomised controlled trial. *EClinicalMedicine*, 14, 42–52.

Nursing & Midwifery Council (2008) *Performance and Ethics for Nurses and Midwives*. NMC, London.

Nursing & Midwifery Council (2009) *Guidance for the Care of Older People*. NMC, London.

Nursing & Midwifery Council (2018a) *The Code: Professional Standards of Practice and Behaviour for Nurses, Midwives and Nursing Associates*. NMC, London.

Nursing & Midwifery Council (2018b) *Future Nurse: Standards of Proficiency for Registered Nurses*. NMC, London.

Nursing & Midwifery Council (2018c) *Standards of Proficiency for Nursing Associates*. NMC, London.

Nursing & Midwifery Council (2020) *The Code: Professional Standards of Practice and Behaviour for Nurses, Midwives and Nursing Associates*. NMC, London.

Office for National Statistics (2017) *UK Population 2017*. www.ons.gov.uk/aboutus/transparencyandgovernance/freedomofinformationfoi/ukpopulation2017 (accessed December 2021).

Officer, A., Schneiders, M.L., Wu, D., Nash, P., Thiyagarajan, J.A. & Beard, J.R. (2016) Valuing older people: time for a global campaign to combat ageism. *Bulletin of the World Health Organization*, 94(10), 710–710A.

Oozageer, N., Brooke, J., Hutchinson, M. & Jackson, D. (2020) Embedding skin tone diversity into undergraduate nurse education: through the lens of pressure injury. Journal of Clinical Nursing, 29, 4358–4367.

Patel, P.R. & Bechmann, S. (2020) *Discharge Planning*. www.ncbi.nlm.nih.gov/books/NBK557819/ (accessed December 2021).

Patient Safety Observatory (2007) *Slips, Trips and Falls in Hospital*. www.mtpinnacle.com/pdfs/slips-trips-fall-2007.pdf (accessed December 2021).

Pearce, L. (2018) *How to Make Handovers More Effective*. https://rcni.com/nursing-standard/features/how-to-make-handovers-more-effective-141126 (accessed December 2021).

Pilgrim, A.L., Robinson, S.M., Sayer, A.A. & Roberts, H.C. (2015) An overview of appetite decline in older people. *Nursing Older People*, 27(5), 29–35.

Pope, T. (2011) How person-centred care can improve nurses' attitudes to hospitalised older patients. *Nursing Older People*, 24(1), 32–36.

Public Health England (2015) *Pressure Ulcers: Applying All Our Health*. www.gov.uk/government/publications/pressure-ulcers-applying-all-our-health/pressure-ulcers-applying-all-our-health (accessed December 2021).

Public Health England (2017) *Falls and Fracture Consensus Statement*. https://assets.publishing.service.gov.uk/government/uploads/system/uploads/attachment_data/file/586382/falls_and_fractures_consensus_statement.pdf (accessed December 2021).

Public Health England (2019) *Statistical Commentary: Dementia Profile*. www.gov.uk/government/statistics/dementia-profile-updates/statistical-commentary-dementia-profile-april-2019-data-update (accessed December 2021).

Public Health England (2020) *Falls: Applying All Our Health*. www.gov.uk/government/publications/falls-applying-all-our-health/falls-applying-all-our-health (accessed December 2021).

Public Health England (2021) *National Falls Prevention Coordination Group Progress Report*. www.gov.uk/government/publications/national-falls-prevention-coordination-group-progress-report/national-falls-prevention-coordination-group-progress-report (accessed December 2021).

Quinn, B. & Thomas, K. (2017) Using the Gold Standards Framework to deliver good end of life care. *Nursing Management*, 23, 20–25.

Royal College of Nursing (2008) *Defending Dignity: Challenges and Opportunities for Nurses*. Royal College of Nursing, London.

Royal College of Nursing (2012) *Safe Staffing for Older People's Wards*. Royal College of Nursing, London.

Royal College of Nursing (2016) *Positive and Proactive Care. Reducing the Need for Restrictive Interventions*. Royal College of Nursing, London.

Royal College of Physicians. (2020) *National Audit of Inpatient Falls Report 2020*. RCP, London.

Rush, K.L., Hickey, S., Epp, S. & Janke, R., (2017) Nurses' attitudes towards older people care: an integrative review. *Journal of Clinical Nursing*, 26, 4105–4116.

Saghaleini, S.H., Dehghan, K., Shadvar, K., Sanaie, S., Mahmoodpoor, A. & Ostadi, Z. (2018) Pressure ulcer and nutrition. *Indian Journal of Critical Care Medicine*, 22(4), 283–289.

Santana, M.J., Manalili, K., Jolley, R.J., Zelinsky, S., Quan, H. & Lu, M. (2018) How to practice person-centred care: a conceptual framework. *Health Expectations*, 21(2), 429–440.

Shahid, S. & Thomas, S. (2018) Situation, Background, Assessment, Recommendation (SBAR) communication tool for handoff in health care – a narrative review. *Safety in Health*, 4, 7.

Shahin, E.S., Meijers, J.M., Schols, J.M., Tannen, A., Halfens, R.J. & Dassen, T. (2010) The relationship between malnutrition parameters and pressure ulcers in hospitals and nursing homes. *Nutrition*, 26(9), 886–889.

Shepperd, S., Lannin, N.A., Clemson, L.M., McCluskey, A., Cameron, I.D. & Barras, S.L. (2013) Discharge planning from hospital to home. *Cochrane Database of Systematic Reviews*, 1, CD000313.

Sibiya, M.N. (2018) *Effective Communication in Nursing*. www.intechopen.com/chapters/59779 (accessed December 2021).

Spooner, J., Corley, A., Chaboyer, W., Hammond, N.E. & Fraser, J.F. (2015) Measurement of the frequency and source of interruptions occurring during bedside nursing handover in the intensive care unit: an observational study. *Australian Critical Care*, 28, 19–23.

Staggs, V.S., Mion, L.C. & Shorr, R.I. (2014) Assisted and unassisted falls: different events, different outcomes, different implications for quality of hospital care. *Joint Commission Journal on Quality and Patient Safety*, 40(8), 358–364.

Tuffrey-Wijne, I., Giatras, N., Goulding, L., et al. (2013) *Identifying the factors affecting the implementation of strategies to promote a safer environment for patients with learning disabilities in NHS hospitals: a mixed-methods study*. www.ncbi.nlm.nih.gov/books/NBK259498 (accessed December 2021).

Twibell, R.S., Siela, D., Sproat, T. & Coers, G. (2015) Perceptions related to falls and fall prevention among hospitalized adults. *American Journal of Critical Care*, 24(5), e78–85.

Volkert, D., Beck, A.M., Cederholm, T., *et al.* (2019) ESPEN guideline on clinical nutrition and hydration in geriatrics. *Clinical Nutrition*, 38(1), 10–47.

Walgers, J.J., Ruiter, S.C., Germans, T., Kat, M.G., Ruiter, J.H. & Jansen, R.W.M.M. (2017) Psychiatric symptoms and use of psychotropic medication in elderly fall and syncope patients. *European Geriatric Medicine*, 8(5–6), 419–423.

Welford, C., Murphy, K., Wallace, M. & Casey, D. (2010) A concept analysis of autonomy for older people in residential care. *Journal of Clinical Nursing*, 19, 1226–1235.

Wood, J., Brown, B. & Bartley, A., *et al.* (2019) Reducing pressure ulcers across multiple care settings using a collaborative approach. *BMJ Open Quality*, 8, e000409.

World Health Organization (2007) *Communication during Patient Hand-overs*. www.who.int/patientsafety/solutions/patientsafety/PS-Solution3.pdf (accessed December 2021).

World Health Organization (2017) *Global Action Plan on the Public Health Response to Dementia 2017–2025*. https://apps.who.int/iris/bitstream/handle/10665/259615/9789241513487-eng.pdf (accessed December 2021).

Yinusa, G., Scammell, J., Murphy, J., Ford, G. & Baron, S. (2021) Multidisciplinary provision of food and nutritional care to hospitalized adult in-patients: a scoping review. *Journal of Multidisciplinary Healthcare*, 14, 459–491.

Young, C. & Fletcher, J. (2019) Pressure ulcer education 2: assessing patients' risk of pressure ulcers. *Nursing Times*, 115, 20–22.

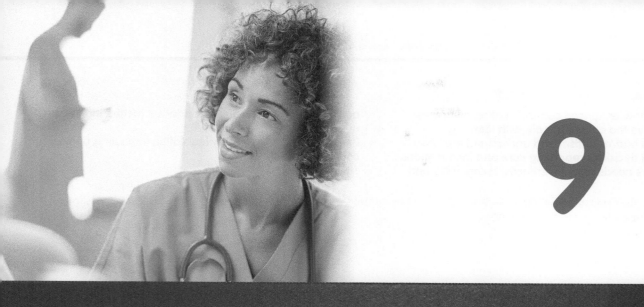

9

The Principles of Caring for People With Learning Disabilities and/or Autism

Debra Fearns

University of Hertfordshire, UK

Learning Outcomes

On completion of this chapter you will be able to:

- Understand the nature, causes and prevalence of learning disabilities
- Have a greater understanding of why people with learning disabilities and/or autism are more susceptible to inequalities in healthcare and demonstrate an understanding of, and the ability to challenge, discriminatory behaviour
- Provide information in accessible ways to help people understand and make decisions about their health, life choices, illness and care
- Provide and promote non-discriminatory, person-centred and sensitive care, reflecting on people's values and beliefs, diverse backgrounds, cultural characteristics, language requirements, needs and preferences, taking account of any need for adjustment
- Gain an insight into the role of the learning disability nurse

Proficiencies

NMC Proficiencies and Standards:

- The outcome statements for each platform of the NMC Standards of proficiency have been designed to apply across all four fields of nursing practice (adult, children, learning disabilities, mental health) and all care settings.

Nursing Practice: Knowledge and Care, Third Edition. Edited by Ian Peate and Aby Mitchell.
© 2022 John Wiley & Sons Ltd. Published 2022 by John Wiley & Sons Ltd.
Companion website: www.wiley.com/go/peate/nursingpractice3e

Introduction

This chapter is designed to meet the learning needs of nurses and nursing associates coming in direct contact with patients with learning disabilities and/or autism. Kinnear *et al.* (2018) identified that 98.7% of people with learning disabilities have two or more health conditions in addition to their learning disability; therefore, they are more likely to attend, and be admitted to, acute general hospitals. Reports consistently highlight the poorer experience and poorer health outcomes, including premature and avoidable deaths, of people with a learning disability in general hospital services (Mencap 2007, 2012; Michael & Richardson, 2008; Heslop *et al.*, 2017). These are seminal reports that highlighted the unequal treatment and needless deaths of people with a learning disability and brought them to the attention of the national press and government, ensuring that these poor standards of care and treatment could not go on unnoticed and unchallenged. *Death by Indifference* (Mencap, 2007) exposed and highlighted instances of very poor practice surrounding the deaths of six people with learning disabilities while they were in the care of the NHS.

While many positive changes have occurred in the care of people with learning disabilities, there is still a long way to go and far more progress to be made when providing NHS services and the COVID pandemic has once again highlighted these deficiencies (Courtenay & Perera, 2020). Mencap (2007) suggested that people with learning disabilities, their families and carers were facing institutional discrimination in healthcare services; the subsequent report of an independent inquiry, *Healthcare for All*, led by Sir Jonathan Michael (Department of Health, 2008) exposed the unequal healthcare that people with learning disabilities often receive within the NHS.

In 2012, Mencap published a further report, *Death by Indifference: 74 Deaths and Counting*, which commented on the progress made following the recommendations in *Death by Indifference* (Mencap, 2007) and made further suggestions to the government, including that healthcare professionals understand and apply key legislation such as the Mental Capacity Act 2005 and the Equality Act 2010. These reports continue to raise awareness of the discrepancies in healthcare experienced by people with learning disabilities and/or autism. Recent data estimate that there are 1200 avoidable deaths in the NHS each year (Mencap, 2018) so much still needs to be done.

COVID-19 has exacerbated the inequalities people with a learning disability and/or autism face and in June 2020 Mencap published a report which stated that:

> *'The devastating impact of COVID-19 on our community is shocking, but sadly not surprising, when we have long been warning that the healthcare rights of people with a learning disability are under threat like never before. Throughout this crisis, we have repeatedly challenged discriminatory healthcare guidance and practice, and we continue to support people with a learning disability and their families to access the treatment and support they have a right to'* (Mencap, 2020).

This was in part due to the government's position on testing, which excluded people with a learning disability and/or autism as they were not eligible for testing in the same way that home care residents aged over 65 were. The Office for National Statistics revealed in June 2020 that nearly 60% of deaths from coronavirus in the UK were of people with disabilities (Jackson, 2020).

Albert (2020) revealed that in one month in 2020, government statistics showed that there was a 175% increase in unexpected deaths of people with learning disabilities and/or autism compared to the same period a year earlier.

On 24 February 2021, it was announced that 150 000 adults with learning disabilities would be prioritised to receive the COVID vaccine, following advice from the Joint Committee on Vaccination and Immunisation, later than healthy individuals aged 65 and over, despite their increased risk. This is a significant step forward but there are approximately 1.5 million people with a learning disability and/or autism, many of whom will need advice and support to access the vaccines.

Access to mainstream services is the way forward in ensuring that people who have a learning disability and/or autism are treated properly within the NHS. There are 1.13 million adults with a learning disability in the UK. The total number of adults aged 18–64 with learning disabilities in England receiving long-term social care in 2017–18 was 131 415 (PHE, 2016, 2020).

Many people with a learning disability and/or autism have greater healthcare needs than the general population. The LeDeR programme was established in 2015 and reports annually on deaths (mortality) of people with learning disabilities and/or autism that have been notified as needing to be reviewed so that lessons can be learned in how to improve services and reduce health inequalities. The LeDeR Programme Report of 2018 found that, on average, men and women with a learning disability die 20 years and 27 years younger, respectively, than men and women in the general population.

This chapter recognises that having a greater knowledge and understanding of people with learning disabilities and/or autism will enable nurses and nursing associates to provide a level of care that is at least of the same standard for all patients. It provides an overview of the classification and causes of learning disabilities and identifies some of the key health needs of this population group.

This chapter also explores patients with learning disabilities whose needs are more complex due to an associated mental health problem, autistic spectrum disorder or the inability to verbally communicate pain and other needs. Communication is at the heart of effective nursing care and there is no better example of this than when a nurse or nursing associate is faced with a patient whose communication skills are significantly impaired. Some quick and easy skills will be identified that can have an impact on the success of care and interventions. The legalities of working with people who find it difficult to communicate their needs and desires can be complicated and this chapter will assist in making lawful and beneficial decisions regarding their care.

Definitions of Learning Disabilities

Defining learning disabilities can be tricky, as the tendency is to explain it in a very clinical way that would suggest that it is an illness, which it is not. It is a lifelong condition, beginning before, during or after birth, or as a result of a brain injury in very early childhood, which can affect a person's ability to learn and communicate effectively. While the condition cannot be 'cured', it is possible for someone with a learning disability to lead an independent life or, with support, develop new skills and progress.

The terminology used may be confusing. For example, the media use the term 'learning difficulty' when reporting on a person with a learning disability. A person with learning difficulties is normally considered to have educational needs, such as dyslexia, dyspraxia or hyperactive disorders. Learning disabilities is not the same as mental illness, although 40% (28% if problem behaviours are excluded) of adults with learning disabilities experience mental health problems and it is estimated that 36% (24% if problem behaviours are excluded) of children and young people with learning disabilities experience mental health problems. These rates are much higher than the general population (NICE, 2016).

The International Classification of Disease (ICD)-11 (WHO, 2018) lists Intellectual Disability (ID) (the term preferred to 'learning disabilities', currently used in England; Department of Health, 2001) as neurodevelopmental disorder, highlighting the importance of adaptive functioning. The reduction in intellectual functioning on standardised IQ assessment is two or more standard deviations below the mean.

The *Diagnostic Statistical Manual -V* (DSM-V; APA, 2013) defines it as a significantly subaverage intellectual functioning: an intelligence quotient (IQ) of approximately 70 or below, with concurrent deficits or impairments in adaptive functioning in at least three areas: social skills (e.g. communicating with others), conceptual skills (e.g. reading and writing ability) and practical ability (e.g. clothing/bathing one's self).

It is also important to think about groups of people within the wider learning disability context; for example 75–80% of people with autistic spectrum disorders will have a measured IQ of below 70 and therefore are diagnosed as also having a learning disability. Approximately 20–30% of this population are more likely to experience mental health problems (NHS England and NHS Improvement, 2019).

Jot This Down

Think about the terms you may have heard being used to describe people with learning disabilities. Note them down and consider how they would sound to a person with learning disabilities.

Think about the terms you may have heard used to describe people with learning disabilities. Note them down and consider how they would sound to a person with learning disabilities?

In the 'Jot This Down' exercise above, you might have identified several negative labels that have been associated with people with learning disabilities. In 'What the Experts Say' below, you can see how this kind of behaviour affects the emotional and social health of a person with learning disabilities and/or autism.

What the Experts Say

Mohammad is a man in his 30s who has learning disabilities and autism; he has struggled to cope with day-to-day living all his life, but now attends college regularly. Mohammad explains below the impact of some of the name calling he experiences from the teenagers in the college.

'When I am at college, some of the people would call me names, and laugh at me because I am different. They have called me freak, geek, monster and a few more that I wouldn't want to repeat. I feel very vulnerable and I am not able to stop it; instead I try and act as "normal" as possible so I can fit in and not stand out from the crowd. But I am rubbish at this and it causes me a lot of stress when I can't do it. I don't want to involve the staff at college, because then I would be a grass as well as odd!'

Autistic Spectrum Disorders Defined

The variation in presentation of autistic spectrum disorders (ASD) is wide; therefore, the intervention and support required are clearly varied and can be different from person to person. Despite this, there are three consistent traits that all people with an ASD diagnosis share.

- Social interaction.
- Communication.
- Lack of flexibility in thinking and behaviour.

Outline of the Autistic Spectrum Criteria defined by DSM-V

A. **Persistent deficits in social communication and social interaction across multiple contexts, as manifested by the following, currently or by history.**
   1. Deficits in social-emotional reciprocity
   2. Deficits in non-verbal communicative behaviours used for social interaction

3. Deficits in developing, maintaining and understanding relationships

B. **Restricted, repetitive patterns of behaviour, interests or activities, as manifested by at least two of the following, currently or by history.**
   1. Stereotyped or repetitive motor movements, use of objects or speech
   2. Insistence on sameness, inflexible adherence to routines, or ritualised patterns or verbal or non-verbal behaviour
   3. Highly restricted, fixated interests that are abnormal in intensity or focus
   4. Hyper- or hyporeactivity to sensory input or unusual interests in sensory aspects of the environment

C. **Symptoms must be present in the early developmental period (but may not become fully manifest until social demands exceed limited capacities or may be masked by learned strategies in later life).**

D. **Symptoms cause clinically significant impairment in social, occupational or other important areas of current functioning.**

E. **These disturbances are not better explained by intellectual disability (intellectual developmental disorder) or global developmental delay. Intellectual disability and autism spectrum disorder frequently co-occur; to make co-morbid diagnoses of autism spectrum disorder and intellectual disability, social communication should be below that expected for general developmental level.**

There is a growing body of research analysing the hypersensitivities that people with ASD experience to some sounds, smells and visual simulation, which can affect their behaviour as outlined in DSM-V. Knowing this is crucial to the care of someone with ASD in a hospital setting, as ward environments can be overstimulating. Later in this chapter, 'reasonable adjustments' are discussed and services are challenged to consider alterations that can be made to existing services to help people with different needs. Awareness of hypersensitivities for people with ASD can make a huge impact on their general anxiety levels while they are in hospital and out of their usual, more controlled environment. Strobe lighting, the smell of cleaning products and constant noises from machines are very common stressors for people with ASD.

> Nurses are required to assess comfort levels, rest and sleep patterns, demonstrating understanding of the specific needs of the person being cared for. Being aware of these factors may help you understand how the environment can be stressful for people with ASD and/or learning disabilities and to think of things you can do to make small, but significant, 'reasonable adjustments', for example, turning off overhead lights in the evening where possible.
>
> Working with your practice assessor, you could prepare a list of specific needs that you have identified, discuss these and in so doing you may be able to provide evidence to the assessor that you are aware of key issues.

The DSM-V criteria mean that when people go for a diagnosis in the future, they will be given a diagnosis of 'autism spectrum disorder'. Some people with Asperger syndrome are not happy with this change of terminology.

What the Experts Say

Malcolm was diagnosed with Asperger syndrome 20 years ago. Now in his 40s, he feels that his diagnosis is an essential part of his identity.

'The term Aspie or Asperger's is who I am, I do not want to be called anything else and they are suggesting changing it to autistic something or other. Firstly, I am autistic, but I don't like to use the terminology, because people are ignorant and automatically think I have a learning disability and treat me very differently. I don't have a learning disability, not that there is anything wrong with that, it's just not me, I have an above average IQ and many people know this about Aspies and respect us for it. Besides, people on the spectrum hate change, so please don't change our identities!'

Prevalence and Causes of Learning Disabilities

The causes of learning disability are multifaceted and can be complex. The causative factors can be divided into two parts: first, *heredity*, i.e. the transmission of genetic characteristics from parents to offspring, and second, *environmental*, for example childhood infections that could cause brain injury and consequently lead to a child being diagnosed with a learning disability. Additionally, we can consider these two causative factors within periods of time: preconceptual, prenatal, perinatal and postnatal.

The main causes of learning disability can be considered as follows.

- Preconceptual
  - Heredity – parental genotype
  - Environmental – maternal health
- Prenatal
  - Heredity – genetic conditions such as Down syndrome
  - Environmental – infection, maternal health, nutrition and toxic agents
- Perinatal
  - Environmental – prematurity and injury during birth
- Postnatal
  - Environmental – infection, trauma, toxic agents, sensory and social deprivation, brain injury and nutrition.

Genetic abnormalities are estimated to be the cause of 50% of learning disabilities.

People with severe or profound learning disabilities are more easily recognised, diagnosed and recorded as requiring service interventions. Accurate reporting of mild to moderate learning disabilities is more difficult, with people not being diagnosed until much later in their lives or not at all.

Classification of Learning Disability

It is important to note that great care must be taken not to make assumptions on what a person can or cannot achieve based upon their classification and 'label' of learning disabilities; for example, the majority of people with mild learning disabilities have the potential to communicate well, be able to address their own personal care needs and, to a degree, be independent. As the person's IQ diminishes, usually the ability to communicate and be independent does too. This chapter explains how information regarding the person's needs can be obtained efficiently and how this can help you care for the individual.

An 'IQ' score is derived from one of several standardised tests designed to assess intelligence. The average test score for much of the population (95%) will be between 70 and 130. Below 70 will indicate significant intellectual/learning disability. The 5% who can reach scores of above 130 are considered to have an above average IQ. A number of these extremely intelligent people may also have an ASD, normally people with Asperger syndrome, which is positioned on the higher end of the autistic spectrum disorders.

Disease Classifications

The ICD-11 and DSM-V divide learning disability into four categories.
1. Mild: IQ 50–70
2. Moderate: IQ 35–49
3. Severe: IQ 20–34
4. Profound: IQ below 20

These IQ measures are often used primarily to decide on access criteria for services and taken on their own do not present a rounded picture of the person's capabilities, strengths and needs. A holistic approach to measuring how the person adapts and manages daily living skills is a more realistic assessment of the impact their learning disability has on them and what support they may need.

Inequalities in Healthcare

The learning disability population have poorer health than the general population and are more likely to experience mental illness, epilepsy, physical disability and sensory impairments, as well as chronic health problems (Cooper et al., 2015). Respiratory disease and circulatory disease are the leading causes of death in people with learning disabilities (O'Leary *et al.*, 2018). Yet, they are less likely to access healthcare in a way that the rest of us take for granted. The co-existence of learning disability and autism also has a significantly adverse effect on their health (Dunn et al., 2019). Of the deaths reviewed by the LeDeR Programme in its 2018 annual report, 93% of those who died had at least one long-term health condition (LeDeR Programme, 2019).

Philips (2019) states that:

'Nurses have a responsibility to ensure reasonable adjustments are made to the care of people with learning disabilities. Equality of care for people with learning disabilities does not necessarily mean they need to receive exactly the same service as anyone else (which is why some prefer the term "equity of care"). To achieve a positive outcome, the person may need additional and/or alternative methods of support. These additional and alternative methods of support are "reasonable adjustments"'.

Mencap states in *Death by Indifference* that '. . .it is Mencap's belief that there is institutional discrimination within the NHS against people with a learning disability – leading to neglect and, as we have shown, to premature death' (2007, p.18).

A range of barriers to accessing healthcare and other services have been identified. These include:

- Scarcity of appropriate services
- Physical and informational barriers to access
- Unhelpful, inexperienced or discriminatory healthcare staff
- Increasingly stringent eligibility criteria for accessing social care services
- Failure of healthcare providers to make 'reasonable adjustments' in light of the literacy and communication difficulties experienced by many people with learning disabilities
- 'Diagnostic overshadowing' (e.g. symptoms of physical ill health either being mistakenly attributed to a mental health/behavioural problem or as being inherent in the person's learning disabilities).

The mortality rates among people with moderate to severe learning disabilities are three times higher than in the general population (O'Leary *et al.*, 2017); despite this, people with learning disabilities are less likely to receive regular health checks and access to screening opportunities, which are routine. In 2015–16 less than half of the patients on GP registers known to have a learning disability received an annual health check (NHS Digital, 2017).

Some people with a learning disability and additional complex or profound physical disabilities will require health professionals from mainstream and specialist learning disability services to work in partnership with them, in order to use medical technology and access essential therapeutic assessments and interventions, thus helping to assess needs and plan care. Similar partnership arrangements are also needed to ensure that people with more complex needs gain access to the best care and treatment and the full range of health services, from maternity services through to end-of-life care (Department of Health, 2009).

Their health needs can be perceived as complex, which can add to accessibility issues. These complexities are too intricate to address within a regular appointment with the GP, with the average appointment time only lasting 10 minutes. Additionally, hospital outpatient appointments are usually scheduled for the same amount of time. It is difficult in this limited time to fully understand some of the interactions that people with learning disabilities may present with; therefore behavioural, physical and mental health issues can appear to be difficult to interpret and may cause illness to be overlooked, so that serious conditions can present too late for prevention or cure. This is called 'diagnostic overshadowing' and may lead to some healthcare professionals not investigating symptoms early enough and can contribute to ongoing health inequalities (Javaid *et al.*, 2019).

Practice Assessment Document

Proficiency 7 – Takes appropriate action in responding promptly to signs of deterioration or distress considering mental, physical, cognitive and behavioural health.

Spend some time with your practice assessor and reflect on how you may respond promptly to signs suggesting that a person's health and well-being are deteriorating. Then describe the actions you could take to mitigate or relieve the deterioration or distress.

A person with significant communication problems will express pain in different ways; this can often be through changes in their behaviour and commonly, aggression may increase, or the person may become significantly quieter than usual. To reduce the risk of 'diagnostic overshadowing', checking for physical causes for changes in behaviour is an essential first step. To exemplify these complexities, read 'What the Experts Say'.

What the Experts Say

A community learning disability nurse's attempts to gain equitable mental healthcare for a service user in her care

Prisha is a 53-year-old woman with Down syndrome and moderate learning disability, who for the past 5 years has lived in supported-living accommodation. Prisha's support mechanisms consist of a 24-hour call-out support network, provided by an outreach team, and 2 hours a week support with her weekly budgeting and shopping provided by a social support worker.

Prisha works in a charity shop 2 days a week, though her time in the shop is mostly spent sorting and tidying in the back, as her speech is too quiet and unclear to communicate effectively with customers.

Until recently, Prisha has always appeared a quiet and contented lady, preferring to keep herself to herself, but in the last few weeks, she has been seen exhibiting some strange behaviours. One neighbour, Tom, said he saw a very 'red-faced' Prisha talking loudly and aggressively to herself while fiddling with her door key and when he approached her, she spat at him. Her colleagues in the shop have also reported Prisha to be vague and uninterested in her work and far from being her normal punctual self, she has been arriving late for work and inappropriately dressed for the cold weather.

Her social support worker, Queenie, has also noticed that Prisha's flat is uncharacteristically untidy and Prisha still in her nightwear, complaining of being too hot, in the afternoon. Queenie is concerned and contacts Prisha's GP practice. Prisha is seen by a doctor whom she has never met before and despite Queenie explaining that Prisha is normally able to communicate her feelings in a more coherent manner, the doctor has read her notes and appears to have made up his mind that all these behaviours are due to Prisha's learning disability. The GP tells Queenie to contact Social Services if she feels that Prisha needs more support.

Unsatisfied with the GP's assessment, Queenie contacts the local Community Learning Disability Team. A nurse in the team carries out their own assessment and finds clear evidence that Prisha is beginning to show signs of dementia. Knowing that there is a direct link between Alzheimer and Down syndromes, the psychiatrist in the team agrees that a formal diagnostic assessment should follow. Within weeks, a formal diagnosis is in place and Prisha's care package is reviewed in the likelihood that her condition could deteriorate further.

Jot This Down

The GP clearly found this case to be complex, why?
What would you have done differently if you were the nurse or nursing associate?

In the 'Jot This Down' exercise above, you may have considered the complexity of the case by thinking about the similarities that can exist between dementia and moderate learning disability. Both can manifest in a variety of ways and a baseline of Prisha's intellectual abilities needs to be determined so that differences can be more easily noted and documented, so the nurse can evidence the changes when engaging with a GP or a psychiatrist.

The Royal College of General Practitioners website has guidance and a toolkit on annual health checks for people with learning disabilities in its Clinical Toolkits section (RCGP, 2021). The introduction of annual health checks is important for improvements to health outcomes: to help identify and treat medical conditions early; to screen for health issues particular to people with learning disabilities and specific conditions; to improve access to generic health promotion in people with learning disabilities; and to develop relationships with GPs, practice nurses and primary care staff, particularly after comprehensive paediatric care finishes at the age of 18.

Understanding of the increased prevalence of physical health issues for those with learning disabilities and those with genetic or chromosomal abnormalities has improved greatly. Annual health checks by GPs will assess for health needs which are very common to those with specific chromosomal syndromes. For example, there is an increase in the prevalence of ophthalmic problems (cataract, glaucoma, keratoconus and refractive errors) in people with Down syndrome, therefore annual health checks should include an eye test. However, in 2016–17, only 53% of people with a learning disability and on the GP register had an annual health check, so just under 47% did not (NHS, 2018).

Nursing Fields

As adult, children's or mental health nurses or nursing associates, you need to be aware of the health issues pertinent to those with specific chromosomal abnormalities, to assist with the assessment and diagnosis of the patient and understand their experience. Gaining knowledge of a person's condition is essential to improving health outcomes for the individual.

Attitudes Towards People with Learning Disabilities

Cummings (2012) stated there is a lack of 'basic values' in the way that the nursing profession cares for its patients. The 3-year strategy 'Compassion in Practice' involved senior nurses undertaking training courses to learn how to promote care and compassion among their teams of nurses and support workers (Department of Health, 2012). This strategy, involving the Royal College of Nursing and the Department of Health, emerged from repeated complaints from patients and those close to them regarding issues of neglect and people being stripped of their dignity. The strategy cited the abuse of the residents with learning disability at Winterbourne View, which became infamous after the BBC 'Panorama' programme in 2012 (BBC, 2012). The strategy was evaluated and published by O'Driscoll *et al.* (2018) which highlighted that this 'top-down' strategy did not fully understand the service limitations on nursing staff which hindered compassionate care and that compassion also needed to be demonstrated towards nurses.

The BBC's 'Panorama' showed patients at a residential care home near Bristol being slapped and restrained under chairs, having their hair pulled and being held down as medication was forced into their mouths. The victims, who had severe learning disabilities, were visibly upset and were shown screaming and shaking. One victim was showered while fully clothed and had mouthwash poured into her eyes.

Scandals have continued to emerge in the media, such as Whorlton Hall in County Durham, England (BBC Panorama, 2019) and Muckamore Abbey in County Antrim, Northern Ireland (BBC News, 2020).

Health Care for All (Department of Health, 2008) states that: *'The health and strength of a society can be measured by how well it cares for its most vulnerable members. For a variety of reasons, including the way society behaves towards them, adults and children with learning disabilities, especially those with severe disability and the most complex needs are some of the most vulnerable members of our society today'.*

Supporting Access to Services

The Equality Act (2010) recognises the importance of 'reasonable adjustments' to support people accessing services. Key ways in which services can implement 'reasonable adjustments' include the following.

- Using people who have specific roles in supporting people with learning disabilities to access and support the service; this may include roles such as health liaison nurse, hospital liaison nurse and health facilitator.
- Engaging with any health-related documents the person may have such as health action plans, hospital passports or person-centred plans.

Health Liaison Nurse, Hospital Liaison Nurse and Health Facilitator

The learning disability nurse has a pivotal role in supporting other nurses and nursing associates to develop their specialist skills and champion the needs of people with learning disabilities (Mason-Angelow, 2020). These roles exist to ensure the needs of the person with a learning disability are met either on admission to an acute hospital or attending outpatient appointments by facilitating:

- Open and easy access to the various wards and departments by considering and adapting the care environment
- Access to care through arrangement and adjustment of appointments
- Work with the person and their family or carers to help prepare for hospital admission
- Accessible, easy-to-read information.

The health facilitator/health liaison role will provide similar support but within community settings, for example GP or dental practices. In each of these roles, the nurse will liaise with an array of clinicians and services in both hospital and community settings, identifying and offering training (formal and informal) and, where appropriate, providing training support alongside specialist nursing advice. It requires extensive close communication and involvement with individuals, family, carers and others during preadmission, admission and discharge, actively engaging with hospital staff to assist and empower them to provide care that meets the needs of people with learning disabilities and those who support them. This is the opportunity to 'mind the gap' which is present for those with a learning disability, with the nurse having a pivotal role in achieving 'reasonable adjustments' (Brown, 2020). These roles help people with complex health conditions to access assessment, treatment and investigations in acute hospitals (Glover et al., 2019).

These learning disability nursing roles will be useful resources to support the discharge process, ensuring that people have the necessary support when they leave hospital. It should not be assumed that people with learning disabilities live in homes which are staffed 24 hours per day; the majority have minimal additional support coming into their homes. Understanding the specific support a person had prior to admission and ensuring what is needed at discharge is in place will significantly reduce the risk of a person going home to inadequate care provision.

137

Care, Dignity and Compassion

The role of the liaison nurse can be summarised as follows.

Advocate
- An ambassador for people with a learning disability, fostering equal care through recommending reasonable and achievable adjustments at a local and strategic level
- Representing the views of patients and carers to hospital staff
- Ensuring recognition of and adherence to specific legislation and sensitive policies such as 'do not resuscitate' orders

Collaborator
- Often providing the connection between individuals, their families and services

Communicator
- Enabling information flow across healthcare sectors, professionals and between health staff and carers
- Advising hospital staff on specific communication issues and methods

Educator
- Through induction, updates, continuing professional development programmes and skill development (formal)
- Opportunistic learning opportunities and role modelling; sharing information (informal)
- Educating across professional groups, including input for medical staff
- Offering advice and support on the Mental Capacity Act 2005 and safeguarding
- Contribution and development of accessible healthcare resources

Mediator
- Networking with key individuals, departments, services and agencies
- Translating information between the person with a learning disability and hospital staff
- Removing barriers to appropriate healthcare. Forming effective working relationships with clinicians and ward teams

(Continued)

Facilitator
- Creating and using accessible information
- Supporting reasonable and achievable adjustments; reasonable adjustments may mean a greater use of accessible information
- Demonstrating new ideas and explicitly explaining what is required
- Actively engaging with hospital staff to assist and empower them to provide care which meets the needs of people with learning disabilities and their carers

Key to all of this is working together to achieve positive health outcomes for people with a learning disability as this enables everyone to meet the 10 key recommendations in *Health Care for All* (Department of Health, 2008).

The responsibility of the liaison nurse is to raise the profile of the healthcare needs of people with a learning disability across secondary care provision, bridging the gap between acute clinical care areas to enable better communication and access to healthcare. The liaison nurse should be visible to healthcare staff in order to support them in the role they have in providing care. They need to be creative, minimising constraints and challenges to ensure a successful outcome for all involved, specifically the person with a learning disability. The LD nurse aims to ensure people with a learning disability receive the healthcare required to live a healthy life and have equity with others in society (Mason-Angelow, 2020). The health liaison nurse, hospital liaison nurse and health facilitator have a crucial role in supporting a person with a learning disability and the staff providing healthcare (Brown, 2020). It is suggested that local contact details are given to each ward and documented in a prominent place so that if needed staff can easily approach the service to request support.

Documents Held by People Who Have Learning Disabilities

These documents include health action plans, hospital passports and person-centred plans.

Health Action Plans

Action for Health (Department of Health, 2002) required health providers to ensure each person with a learning disability was offered a health action plan that outlined their needs, to use as a baseline of information for any health professional when the person presents for an appointment, consultation or assessment. The health action plan contains an information passport, which gives the health staff a snapshot picture to help formulate outcomes

Jot This Down

Imagine you are being asked for information about your childhood health by a healthcare practitioner. What is your history of immunisation, did you have chickenpox as a child? You will probably have something to inform you of when these were, or you can refer to your family, medical history or others for such information. Often, this can be challenging for someone who has led a life where the information is not so joined up, is missing or non-existent. The health action plan enables all this information to be brought together in one place.

with the individual, providing an increasingly cohesive picture. Everyone with a learning disability can access a health action plan, which draws together aspects of their 'health picture' into a useable framework and informs the healthcare staff they meet.

Hospital Passport

The hospital passport presents the healthcare professional with a picture of the 'whole person'. It contains information not only relevant to health but also about the individual. By owning the passport, this individual is empowered to participate further in the care they may require and will bring this with them to appointments and consultations. They vary from area to area and people often add their own personalised touches. This provides healthcare practitioners with additional information about how they can focus care and provide choices in healthcare. They can base decisions on this information and be more confident of the outcome. The increased information can enable the individual to be more involved in their decisions and this provides a safer environment for everyone. It can enable services to be flexible and responsive to individual needs.

The hospital passport will have information relating to the person's mode of communication, their likes and dislikes. It is important that staff take the time to read this information as this will enable them to develop a therapeutic relationship with the person and so may help reduce anxieties. These also enable the staff to make reasonable adjustments with the person to enable better adherence to treatment planning, admission and discharge. Northway *et al.* (2017) revealed inconsistencies and variations which could impact the effectiveness of hospital passports and recommended that a more standardised approach would benefit people with learning disabilities and/or autism and that they should be involved in making hospital passports standardised.

Person-centred Plan (PCP)

Person-centred planning discovers and acts on what is important to a person. It is a process of continual listening and learning, focusing on what's important to someone now and in the future, and acting on this in alliance with their family and friends (Ross *et al.*, 2015).

Person-centred planning is a means of ascertaining what people want, the support they need and how they can achieve it. This is empowering as it shifts the balance of power from people who work in services to those who use or participate within them to lead an independent and inclusive life. PCP aims to consider aspirations and capacities, rather than needs and deficiencies.

'People with a learning disability and/or autism, and families/carers of children in this group, should have the same rights to choice and control over different aspects of their lives as everyone else (though in some cases, for instance due to legal restrictions, there may need to be limits on the choice a person can exercise for their own safety or the protection of others). This is not simply about respecting their rights: giving people more choice and control also means they are more likely to benefit from the support they receive' (NHS England, 2015, p.8).

It should also take account of wishes and aspirations in relation to other aspects of the person's life such as housing, education, employment and leisure (Department of Health, 2001). When a person with a learning disability is accessing services, it is important for clinicians to check if the person's PCP contains any information which may be relevant to preferences around their healthcare.

Care, Dignity and Compassion

Reasonable Adjustments

The *Healthcare for All* (Department of Health, 2008) report highlights the need for nurses and nursing associates to show vulnerable people compassion, but also identified insufficient attention to making 'reasonable adjustments' to support the delivery of equal treatment, as required by the Disability Discrimination Act 2005. Adjustments are not always made to allow for communication problems, difficulty in understanding (cognitive impairment) or the anxieties and preferences of individuals concerning their treatment.

Under the Disability Equality Duty, cited in the Equality Act 2010, all public sector organisations are required to make 'reasonable adjustments' to services to ensure they are accessible for disabled people. This includes planning for people with learning disabilities. This might include:

- Making sure that information is written in a way that is accessible to people with learning disabilities – for example, by using plain English and avoiding jargon, using short sentences and pictures or symbols to illustrate meaning
- Nurses with special skills to look out for people with learning disabilities
- Giving people more time with doctors and nurses, so they have a chance to explain what is wrong or so they can be assessed comprehensively.
- www.england.nhs.uk/learning-disabilities/improving-health/reasonable-adjustments/

The Accessible Information Standard was introduced in 2016 for all health services. The intent is to help people with disabilities communicate their needs.

The Improving Health and Lives: Learning Disabilities Observatory (IHaL) was set up in April 2010 as a 3-year programme following one of the recommendations of the Report of the Independent Inquiry into Access to Healthcare for People with Learning Disabilities (Department of Health, 2008). The IHaL aimed to make information more accessible, gain more information and support commissioners and providers to use the information to improve services. The IHaL has now been archived and Public Health England (PHE) is the host website for all current and future information on reducing health inequalities for people with learning disabilities and/or autism.

Reasonable Adjustments

1. Ensure that people with learning disabilities are easily identified in records systems.
2. Foster a culture in which everyone understands reasonable adjustments and how they can help everyone when applied in a timely and appropriate manner.
3. Have a policy on accessible information and review coverage and use on a regular basis.
4. Promote the involvement of family carers in the healthcare of people with learning disabilities.
5. Continuously monitor how well the Mental Capacity Act 2005 is being implemented.
6. Develop clear and widely used protocols for service delivery and, where applicable, discharge arrangements that take account of the additional support needs of people with learning disabilities.
7. Ensure that people with learning disabilities and their family carers can influence what happens within the organisation at all levels (IHaL, 2012).

Jot This Down

Think about people with learning disabilities in general hospitals that you have worked with. Use the reasonable adjustments from the Mid Yorkshire NHS Trust in Box 9.1 and jot down any adjustments you have witnessed and consider if those would have improved the patient experience?

Being person centred should be at the heart of how we support people in hospital. This is something that takes time but will help to understand the individual and their needs. It is imperative to involve people who are important to the individual and know them well and include healthcare workers. The health liaison nurse role is part of the commitment to develop effective healthcare practices and therefore improve the quality of care for people with a learning disability.

Nurses are essential in helping to reduce inequalities of care for people with learning disabilities and/or autism. This requires nurses to understand the needs of people with a learning disability and/or autism and to have the knowledge and confidence to refer to specialist support, for example, health liaison nurses (Northway & Dix, 2019).

In November 2019, the government published Right to Be Heard in response to the consultation on proposals for introducing mandatory learning disability and autism training for health and social care staff (DHSC, 2019). It was a key recommendation from LeDeR (2019) that mandatory learning disability awareness training should be provided to all staff, delivered in conjunction with people with learning disabilities and their families. The response included a commitment to develop a standardised training package. The training will draw on existing best practice and the expertise of people with autism, people with a learning disability, family carers and subject matter experts. Health Education England and Skills for Care are co-ordinating the development of training in both health and social care.

This training should help all staff improve their communication and interactions with people with learning disabilities and/or autism.

This mandatory training is named after Oliver McGowan, whose needless death highlighted the need for health and social care staff to have better training when caring for people with learning disabilities and autism. Oliver McGowan died on 11 November 2016 at the age of 18. He was admitted to hospital following an epileptic seizure. He was given olanzapine, despite Oliver and his parents telling medical staff not to give him the drug and that he was likely to have an extreme reaction to it. They were not listened to and Oliver died in intensive care 17 days later, after a rare side-effect caused his brain to swell (neuroleptic malignant syndrome).

Box 9.1 Reasonable adjustments made by the Mid Yorkshire NHS Trust in 2012, when caring for a person with learning disabilities on a ward in their hospital (Gibb, 2012)

Orientation to the ward

Patients with learning disabilities can often feel isolated on busy wards. Please consider the following actions where appropriate to the patient.

- Orientate the patient to the ward
- Introduce them to other patients in their ward area
- Ensure that toilets and bathrooms have appropriate signage and the patient understands where they can find them if able to carry out their own personal care
- Remember that you might need to repeat information on where they can find the toilet/bathroom/rest room during their stay
- Make sure the patient and their carer, if appropriate, knows who their named nurse on duty is

Environment

- Assess the patient's clinical and individual need for a single cubicle or a ward bay
- Some patients with a learning disability will be more comfortable cared for alongside other people and may feel isolated and frightened in a single cubicle. Others with complex needs, autism or challenging behaviour will benefit from the quieter environment of a cubicle, where there are fewer distractions from the general activity of a busy ward
- Involve the patient with a learning disability and their carer/support worker in decisions regarding individual requirements
- Ensure lighting is not too bright or intrusive, as this can be stressful for a person with a learning disability and for people with ASD
- Reduce distracting noise if possible, as this can be stressful for a person with a learning disability and for people with ASD
- Reduce general clutter and objects which are not required in the provision of care, as these can distract a patient with a learning disability and make it difficult for them to visually focus on you and may become a general hazard

- Make sure that the environment is physically accessible and safe
- Use the health action plan to determine individual needs

General nursing care

- Patients with severe learning disabilities may be very dependent on ward staff. They might have difficulty expressing their needs, such as hunger, thirst, pain, distress, toilet and washing requirements, so staff should anticipate these needs and involve the carer/support workers if there are any indications or non-verbal signals the patient with learning disabilities uses to communicate their needs
- Please refer to the patient's health action plan

Ward routine

- Predictability and routine are often important to patients with a learning disability; develop a routine as soon as possible to reduce anxiety. Ask the patient's carer/support worker to help write an accessible timetable that includes mealtimes, ward rounds and other activities

Discharge planning

- Consider the need to hold a discharge planning meeting; this is particularly relevant to patients with severe learning disabilities, complex healthcare needs and patients who are vulnerable. Discharge planning meetings offer the opportunity to share important information, amend care plans and adjust support required in the community
- Inform the discharge co-ordinator, as soon as possible, whenever a patient with a learning disability is admitted to your ward. Patients with learning disabilities often experience severe delays in the discharge process if potential problems are not considered on admission
- Provide a discharge sheet with accessible 'easy read' information, covering diagnosis, treatment, when to return for follow-up appointments, any possible side-effects of medication and details of someone on the ward to contact if necessary

---

Communication

Communication is one of the most significant issues for people with learning disability when admitted to hospital. As a two-way process, communication can be affected by a person's ability to express themselves, i.e. explain their symptoms, and to receive messages and understand what is being said. It is important to note that communication may also be non-verbal and alternative methods of communication such as sign language, symbols, photographs and objects of reference are all commonplace when working with people with learning disability.

Many people with learning disabilities, and especially those with autism, have difficulty with abstract language; they have a more literal understanding of what is being said to them.

Over 21% of people with a learning disability think that healthcare staff are bad at explaining things to them when they are at the hospital; 75% of people with a learning disability said their experience of going to hospital would be improved if staff explained things in a way that was easy to understand (Mencap, 2018).

Nurses and nursing associates will need to use a range of strategies to support communication with people who have learning disabilities and should include simple techniques in face-to-face communication.

- Say your name first.
- Say what you mean and mean what you say.
- Keep language short and simple.
- Avoid or explain irony, sarcasm, jokes and metaphor.
- Be positive – avoid saying 'no' and 'don't'. Say what you want, rather than what you do not want.
- Give time for processing information.
- Be explicit – avoid inferred and implied concepts.
- Use concrete not abstract concepts.
- Look for and interpret non-verbal communication and be aware of your own.
- Listen to and involve families and/or carers.
- Take more time whenever necessary. This will save time in the long run as important information will be acquired.
- Be aware that the ability to talk does not mean that someone understands (Ainsworth et al., 2021).

Additional ways to support communication include the following.

- Try and reduce ambient noise and distractions when discussing important information.
- Use environmental clues to support what you are saying or asking. For example, show the person a medicine pot when discussing medication or make a drinking gesture when asking if they would like a drink.
- Make sure that your face and mouth are visible.

An individual's level of comprehension should always be clarified; often, people who accompany the patient with learning disabilities may make statements such as 'He understands what you say to him'. People with learning disabilities are very familiar with their own routines and notice the visual cues and clues given, which can lead to carers believing the person's understanding is greater than it may be. A person's level of comprehension can also be altered if they are anxious and being in hospital is likely to cause some level of nervousness, and if a medical procedure is being discussed, this is likely to increase anxiety further. It is always important to check that someone has understood what you have said before carrying out a healthcare intervention.

People with learning disabilities may be accompanied in hospital by a carer, a family member or perhaps a health liaison nurse from the local learning disability team. It is easy to make the mistake of talking to them instead of the patient. Whilst focusing your conversation with the patient, it is also important to include others in the discussion and if they are trusted by the patient, then they can help to keep anxiety at a level which assists in clear and concise communication. Consider the 'What the Experts Say' scenario.

Jot This Down

Consider if you would have done anything differently to manage this intervention and support his mum with explaining the procedure. Sayed was only mildly sedated; could more have been done, and should more have been done? Would you expect Sayed to be able to consent to his treatment?

In the 'Jot This Down' exercise, you may have considered the experiences of those with learning disabilities and an invasive intervention, such as the endoscopy described. There are often no right or wrong answers in these scenarios, but it is important to exhaust all avenues; using a community learning disability nurse or a health liaison nurse may have helped Sayed he to be better prepared for the very frightening insertion of the camera down into his stomach.

Effective communication is essential to reduce anxieties in order to support a person's comprehension and expressive language. Makaton is the most widely used sign and symbol system for people with learning disabilities and is used by over 100 000 people in the UK today. For those who have experienced the frustration of being unable to communicate meaningfully or

141

What the Experts Say

Sayed's Mum

Sayed is autistic and has a moderate learning disability; although he has some verbal communication skills, he uses Makaton for most of his communication. Consistent with many people with ASD, he uses communication in a very minimalistic manner, i.e. he does not tend to engage in 'small talk' and only initiates a conversation if he needs someone to help him. To support his spoken language, Sayed has a few Makaton signs which he uses regularly; some of these are shown in Figure 9.1.

Sayed was visiting outpatients to have an endoscopy as part of a gastrointestinal investigation. He had been suffering from severe chest pains, which are thought to be associated with a suspected hiatus hernia. As part of a desensitisation process, on a previous visit, Sayed and his mum were given pictures of the procedure, showing how and where the camera will be inserted and what it will show. Sayed and his mum had spent time talking about the procedure and attempting to alleviate Sayed's understandable anxiety.

The difficult part was trying to explain the discomfort as the camera was passed down into his stomach. During the procedure when this happened, Sayed reacted by standing up, pulling the camera from his throat and attacking the very shocked medical team.

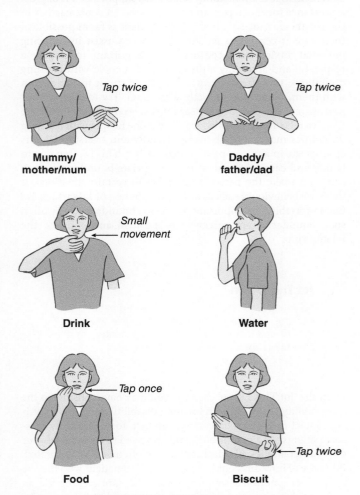

Figure 9.1 Examples of Makaton signs (https://makaton.org/TMC/Free_resources_).

142

effectively, Makaton alleviates some of that frustration and enables individuals to connect with other people and the world around them. Makaton is often taught in special schools so many people with learning disabilities would have some experience of this language system. It is important that people working with adults and children with learning disabilities undertake some specific and relevant Makaton training. The training incorporates signs and symbols acknowledging that for every Makaton sign, there is a corresponding symbol. In some hospitals, the use of Makaton is prevalent; as part of the reasonable adjustments made to enhance equality, nurses and nursing associates take advice from speech and language therapists on which signs and symbols to learn. Ideally, some training on augmentive and alternative communication systems, such as Makaton, would be included in healthcare workers' induction and ongoing training. Communication could be further enhanced by ensuring all staff are familiar with the key sign and symbols identified in their local work area.

Communication with people with learning disabilities is always easier when a relationship with the patient is made; it is only then that it is possible to understand what a person's learning disability means to them. A rapport with the patient may help them to feel understood, valued and supported; it is of great importance for the person to be considered an equal partner in the healthcare process. Involving the patient as far as possible in their care is central to its success and can assist in reducing potential anxiety and conflict. It is important to display a respectful and accepting attitude towards people with learning disabilities; too often nurses and doctors speak to the person with them, rather than directly with them. Try to change your posture and voice tone to appear more relaxed and this will help them to relax more. It is also true that some people with learning disabilities may try to be overly friendly and overstep what is appropriate in a nurse–patient relationship. This is often due to family and carers not enforcing appropriate boundaries which can then make the person vulnerable in certain situations. If there are behaviours such as attempting to hug or kiss which are uncomfortable, it is important to provide boundaries; very often such boundaries are perceived as positive and enhance the relationship.

Jot This Down

Do you feel you can be assertive with a patient with learning disabilities who attempts to give you a hug? How do you feel about giving physical contact to a patient? Is there a time when this is OK?

In the 'Jot This Down' exercise, you may have considered the vulnerability of people with learning disabilities and how physical contact in the correct context can help to significantly reassure patients. As a practitioner, you also need to be aware of your own vulnerabilities; physical contact can often be misinterpreted. Be aware of how this could be perceived by a patient who may be in need of emotional support, which they are seeking via an embrace. You can overanalyse such scenarios but be sure to be aware of any potential risks.

Legal Aspects

When a person with a learning disability needs healthcare, an area which frequently causes anxiety to the healthcare professional is capacity to consent. The following section gives an overview of legal aspects and specific issues for your consideration.

Mental Capacity Act 2005 (MCA)

Death by Indifference (Mencap, 2007) demonstrated clearly that there was a void in the understanding of people's rights in hospital and significant confusion around the MCA and its implications for decision making for those who do not have capacity. Mencap (2007) also highlighted how some people with learning disabilities had not received essential and possibly life-saving treatment as it was perceived that they would be unable to give informed consent.

The MCA is intended to provide protection to people who cannot make a decision at a particular time because their mind or brain is affected. That could be because of mental illness, injury or learning disability. The MCA affects everyone working with or caring for adults who may lack capacity and applies to everyday matters or life altering events. The MCA looks at how decisions are made concerning adults. It applies to all people who are 16 years and over in England and Wales (different rules apply to children). The Mental Capacity (Amendment) Act 2019 introduces a new system for approving deprivations of liberty in care, known as Liberty Protection Safeguards, which are due to replace DoLS in England and Wales from April 2022 (UK Parliament, 2020).

We all have a responsibility to enable people to make their own decisions wherever possible (House of Lords *et al.*, 2008) and should look to the MCA to support the decision-making process as it provides a clear framework for people to follow. In the situation where an individual is unable, at that time, to decide, others will need to step in on their behalf, but the resulting decision must then be made in what is the person's 'best interests'. Frequently, family, carers and people well known to the individual get involved but sometimes other people must make the decision. If it is a medical decision, this will be made by the doctor – but not independently from others involved. Sometimes the local authority will be involved in making decisions. Anybody making 'best interests' decisions on behalf of a person with profound and multiple learning disabilities must consult with the person's family and others who know the person well.

By following the framework laid out in the MCA, safe and legal decisions can be made either by the individual themselves or by others in their best interests.

The Five Principles of the MCA

1. Assume a person has capacity unless proved otherwise.
2. Do not treat someone as incapable of making decisions before everything practicable has been done to help them decide for themselves.
3. A person should not be treated as unable to decide merely because their decision may seem unwise.
4. Always do things, or take decisions, for a person without capacity in their best interests.
5. Before doing something to someone, or deciding on their behalf, consider how the outcome could be achieved in a way which is least restrictive of their basic rights and freedoms.

The responsibility lies with the person requiring the decision, to determine if the individual has capacity, i.e. if a patient needs surgery, then the surgeon must be satisfied that they have capacity to consent. Principle 2 expects every effort to be made to facilitate the person's understanding so that they can make informed consent. Ideally this would mean adapting how information is presented to the person to increase their comprehension and allowing time for them to process the information. For some people with learning disabilities, this could take some time, so the person proposing the treatment would have to decide on the seriousness of the person's condition and therefore what is an acceptable and safe timescale for this to be undertaken.

Professional and Legal Issues

Lacking capacity – someone lacks capacity to decide if they cannot do one or more of the following.

- Understand information given to them.
- Retain that information long enough to be able to make the decision.
- Weigh up the information available to make the decision.
- Communicate their decision.

Note: someone can lack capacity in one area of life and not in another.

If a person cannot make one decision, this does not mean that they are not able to make any decisions at all. Also, if they are not able to decide at one point in time, this does not mean they are unable to make a similar decision at another time. It is time and topic dependent (Mental Capacity Act, 2005).

Best Interests

When a person lacks capacity, then actions subsequently taken or decisions made on behalf of the individual must be done in their best interests. The person who makes the decision about what is in someone's best interest must:

- Involve, as much as possible, the individual who is lacking capacity in deciding what actions will be taken
- Explore the views and feelings of the individual, including anything they may have said or written at a time when they did have capacity, e.g. lasting power of attorney, advanced decisions, discussions and conversations with relatives or friends
- Consult other people involved in the care of the person, such as relatives and friends, and take their views into account.

If decisions are being made about serious medical treatment or significant changes of residence, and the patient is 'without friends', i.e. they have no one at all involved in their life apart from paid carers, a referral must be made to the local Independent Mental Capacity Advocate (IMCA) service, which can be accessed via the local authority.

The MCA now points out that it is a criminal offence to ill-treat or wilfully neglect a person who lacks capacity. 'Before the act is done, or the decision is made, regard must be had to whether the purpose for which it is needed can be as effectively achieved in a way that is less restrictive of the person's rights and freedom of action' (Mental Capacity Act, 2005). The decision maker must prove that they have made every effort to enable the person to be able to decide. All this evidence must be documented and, dependent on the nature of the decision, the assessment

may need to be repeated at different times of the day, so you can see when they are functioning at their optimum level.

Lasting Power of Attorney

A Lasting Power of Attorney (LPA) is a legal document and must be registered with the Office of the Public Guardian. The appointed person can be 'authorised to make decisions on behalf of the individual in relation to personal welfare which includes health' (Department of Health, 2007). Thus, an individual could have a relative or friend who is willing to make decisions about their healthcare once that individual no longer has capacity. Day-to-day care, as well as consenting to or refusal of medical treatment/examination, could be included. The appointed person is not able to consent to or refuse life-sustaining treatment unless the LPA expressly states and authorises this.

Advanced Decisions

Someone over 18 can specify, while they still have capacity, to refuse specific medical treatment for a time in the future when they may lack capacity to consent or refuse that treatment. This includes people with a learning disability, although often they are not given the opportunity. This must be valid and applicable to the current circumstances to be effective and is treated as a decision made by that individual when they had capacity. An advanced decision can be written or verbal. The exception is where there is life-sustaining treatment, when the advanced decision must be in writing and witnessed.

Court of Protection (CP)

The CP is intended to deal with decision making for individuals who may lack capacity to make specific decisions for themselves. This relates to property and affairs and can also now be applied to serious decisions affecting healthcare and personal welfare matters.

Deprivation of Liberties Safeguards (DoLS)

This became part of the MCA in April 2009, as a result of the Bournewood Inquiry, and applies to people over 18 who lack capacity. The premise here is that all care must be carried out in the 'best interest' and in the 'least restrictive' approach.

DoLS sets out the strict criteria for when a person may be deprived of their liberty.

- If you are acting in their best interest to protect them from harm.
- Proportionate action/response is taken in the event of likelihood of serious harm. Only the least restrictive alternative may be used.

This is so the person is free from harm and must not be used:

- As a form of punishment
- At the staff, carer's or organisation's convenience
- Without the appropriate DoLS assessment carried out by a best interest assessor
- Indefinitely.

Liberty Protection Safeguards will now apply to a broader range of settings than DoLS, including care homes, nursing homes, hospitals, supported living, people's own homes, day services and sheltered housing. Deprivations of liberty will need to be authorised in advance by the 'responsible body'; this may be the local authority, hospital manager, clinical commissioning group or local health board (SCIE, 2020).

Rather than six assessment criteria, there will now be three: a capacity assessment, a medical assessment and a necessary and proportionate assessment.

Consent

Consent is an individual's agreement for a health professional to provide care and may be indicated in a variety of ways. A person may show consent non-verbally, for example by presenting their arm for their pulse to be taken; consent can be given orally or in writing. For someone who has a learning disability, this is the same but the person may indicate consent in a different way, so it is important that you also refer to someone who knows the person well to understand their style of communication.

Regardless of how the person indicates consent, for the consent to be valid, the patient must:

- Be competent to take the decision
- Have received enough information to take it in
- Be able to weigh up and communicate a decision
- Not be acting under duress.

Where an adult patient lacks the mental capacity (either temporarily or permanently) to give or withhold consent for themselves, a decision may be made on their behalf. If they have a Lasting Power of Attorney (LPA), as discussed above, this would be followed. If there is no LPA, treatment can be given if it is in the patient's best interests, if it has not been refused in advance in a valid and applicable manner.

Whenever possible, people should be supported to make their own decisions by being given all the practicable help (for example, the use of simple language, photographs, drawings, sign language, interpreters) before anyone treats them as not being able to make their own decision. It must also be remembered that, like the rest of us, people with learning disabilities can make what might seem like an unwise decision. Making an unwise decision does not mean a person lacks capacity but that they have made their own choice and that this may be different to what others might have done.

Safeguarding

Each person in the health services has a responsibility for the safety and well-being of patients and colleagues. Safeguarding adults is a fundamental part of all aspects of safety and well-being. Safeguarding adults is also explicit within legislation, regulations and for delivering effective care (Care Act, 2014). These notes should be used by you as a guide to the overarching principles. If you have a safeguarding concern, they should always be used alongside your organisation's safeguarding policy and procedures.

- Living a life that is free from harm and abuse is a fundamental human right of every person and an essential requirement for health and well-being.
- Safeguarding adults is about the safety and well-being of all patients but providing additional measures for those least able to protect themselves from harm or abuse (*No Secrets*, Department of Health, 2000).

Definition of a Vulnerable Adult

Someone aged 18 years or over – who may be in need of community care services by reason of mental or other disability, age or illness; and who is or may be unable to take care of him or herself, or unable to protect him or herself against significant harm or exploitation (*No Secrets*, Department of Health, 2000).

You have a responsibility to follow the six safeguarding principles.

- *Promotion of empowerment and well-being* – presumption of person-led decisions and consent.
- *Protection* – supporting the rights of the individual to lead an independent life based on self-determination and personal choice.
- *Prevention* – from harm or abuse and reducing unacceptable risks.
- *Proportionality* –means the least intrusive response to harm or abuse and considers the person's age, culture, wishes, lifestyle and beliefs. Managing concerns in the most effective and efficient manner.
- *Partnerships* – working to implement local solutions, with communities working together collaboratively to prevent, identify and respond accordingly.
- *Accountability* – be accountable and transparent in the delivery of services, ensuring all those involved are aware of safeguarding and accountable to those the service is for – patients, public – and to their governing bodies. Working in partnerships also entails being open and transparent with the partner.

Significant Harm

'Harm should be taken to include not only ill treatment but also the impairment of, or avoidable deterioration in, physical or mental health; and the impairment of physical, intellectual, emotional, social, or behavioural development' (Law Commission, 1995).

Whistleblowing

You must always act whenever abuse is suspected, including when your legitimate concern is not acted upon. Whistleblowers are given protection under the Public Interest Disclosure Act 1998. If in doubt, contact your nominated lead for adult safeguarding.

Categories of Abuse

The Social Care Institute for Excellence (SCIE, 2015) outlines the following categories of abuse.

- *Physical abuse*, including hitting, slapping, pushing, kicking, misuse of medication, restraint or inappropriate sanctions.
- *Domestic violence*, including physical, psychological, sexual, financial and also coercive, controlling and threatening behaviour.
- *Sexual abuse*, including rape and sexual assault or sexual acts to which the vulnerable adult has not consented, or could not consent or was pressured into consenting.
- *Emotional and psychological abuse*, including emotional abuse, threats of harm or abandonment, deprivation of contact, humiliation, blaming, controlling, intimidation, coercion, harassment, verbal abuse, isolation or withdrawal from services or supportive networks.

- *Financial or material abuse*, including theft, fraud, exploitation, pressure in connection with wills, property or inheritance or financial transactions, or the misuse or misappropriation of property, possessions or benefits.
- *Neglect and acts of omission*, including ignoring medical or physical care needs, failure to provide access to appropriate health, social care or educational services, the withholding of the necessities of life, such as medication, adequate nutrition and heating.
- *Discriminatory abuse*, including racist, sexist, that based on a person's disability, and other forms of harassment, slurs or similar treatment.
- *Institutional abuse* can happen in residential homes, nursing homes or hospitals, when people are mistreated with poor or inadequate care, neglect and poor practice.
- *Modern slavery*, including human trafficking, forced labour and sexual exploitation.
- *Self-neglect*, including neglecting personal hygiene and health, inability to manage personal affairs and inability to maintain own safety.

Death by Indifference (Mencap, 2007) and *Healthcare for All* (Department of Health, 2008) both highlighted the need for good commissioning to address the quality of healthcare for people with learning disabilities. Acute services need to ensure they have effective care pathways and communication strategies for this vulnerable group of people. Key actions should include:

- Increase knowledge and confidence of staff within these services through training and education
- Provide the opportunity to work with the liaison nurses who can give guidance and role model effective approaches
- Identify and implement reasonable adjustments
- Ensure systems of support are instigated for all staff (Department of Health, 2009).

Getting it Right (Mencap, 2008) identifies the need for health professionals, healthcare authorities and others involved in the lives of people with a learning disability to work together to ensure the health needs of individuals with a learning disability are being met in a timely and equitable manner. Learning from other services, opportunities for best practice and reasonable adjustments can assist in the provision of a unified service, where we are able to share ideas, thoughts and protocols to the benefit of everyone and thus see a positive change in the future in the health status of people with learning disabilities.

Conclusion

This chapter has provided you with some insight and understanding concerning the care of adults with learning disabilities and/or autism. Working with any patient is very individual and this chapter aims to provide a guide to thinking holistically about the person and to improve their experience in healthcare. It is acknowledged that most healthcare practitioners are providing the best care possible in sometimes very difficult situations. It is also recognised that the more time you have to get to know and understand the patient, the better the experience will be for the patient. The implementation of some of the simple points in this chapter should help clarify some of those difficulties and increase confidence where needed. Effective access to mainstream services is unquestionably the way forward and people who have a learning disability will be increasing their access to these services now and in the future, therefore awareness of how to work with this group of people is crucial to the continued growth in the quality of their care.

Key Points

- This chapter has provided the reader with an understanding of the nature of learning disabilities, causes and prevalence. Gaining insight into these issues can help the nurse provide person-centred care.
- People with learning disabilities are more likely to have poorer health than the general population.
- People with learning disabilities are more susceptible to inequalities in health and social care compared with other people in society.
- Enhanced communication awareness and the use of effective communication skills have the potential to improve the health and well-being of people with learning disabilities.
- When service provision has been reasonably adjusted, the needs of the person with learning disabilities can be met more effectively.
- Legislation can impact positively on care delivery for people with learning disabilities (and their families).
- The key role of the nurse is to support and promote the health, well-being and rights of people with learning disabilities.
- Partnership with specialist learning disability services is essential when offering health and social care services to those with learning disabilities.
- The nurse is required to assess the person's physical and psychological needs using communication strategies that are appropriate and effective.
- When encouraging person-centred planning, the nurse empowers the person with regard to choices in health and social care.

References

Ainsworth, V., Ainsworth, T. & Blair, J. (2021) How to get care right for people with learning disabilities in the emergency department: ask and engage. *Emergency Nurse*. doi: 10.7748/en.2021.e2070

Albert, A. (2020) Coronavirus tests denied to people with learning disabilities despite 175% rise in their deaths. *Care Home News*. www.carehome.co.uk/news/article.cfm/id/1625875/Coronavirus-testing-denied-to-people-with-learning-disabilities-despite-huge-rise-in-their-deaths (accessed December 2021).

APA (2013) *The Diagnostic and Statistical Manual of Mental Disorders*, 5th edn. American Psychiatric Association, Washington, DC.

BBC (2012) *Winterbourne View: Abuse footage shocked nation*. Panorama. www.bbc.co.uk/news/uk-england-bristol-20084254 (accessed December 2021).

BBC (2019) *Undercover Hospital Abuse Scandal*. www.bbc.co.uk/programmes/m00059qb (accessed December 2021).

BBC News (2020) *Muckamore Abbey Hospital: Timeline of Abuse Allegations*. www.bbc.co.uk/news/uk-northern-ireland-49498971 (accessed December 2021).

Brown, M. (2020) Learning disability liaison nurses: the provision of compassionate, person-centred care for people with learning disabilities accessing acute hospital care. *Nursing Standard*, 35(10), 90–94.

Care Act (2014) Stationery Office, London.

Cooper, S.A., McLean, G., Guthrie, B., *et al* (2015) Multiple physical and mental health comorbidity in adults with intellectual disabilities: population-based cross-sectional analysis. *BMC Family Practice*, 16, 110.

Courtenay, K. & Perera, B. (2020) Covid 19 and people with intellectual disability: impacts of a pandemic. *Irish Journal of Psychological Medicine*, 37, 231–236.

Cummings, J., Chief Nursing Officer for England (2012) Compassion in practice: nursing has to change if patients are going to be treated well. *The Times*, 4 December.

Department of Health (2000) *No Secrets: guidance on developing and implementing multiagency policies and procedures to protect vulnerable adults from abuse*. Department of Health, London.

Department of Health (2001) *Valuing People: a new strategy for learning disability for the 21st century*. Department of Health, London.

Department of Health (2002) *Action for Health: health action plans and health facilitation; detailed good practice guidance for learning disability partnership boards*. Department of Health, London.

Department of Health (2007) *Putting People First: a shared vision and commitment to the transformation of adult social care*. Department of Health, London.

Department of Health (2008) *Healthcare for All. Report of the Independent Inquiry into Access to Healthcare for People with Learning Disabilities, Sir Jonathan Michael*. Department of Health, London.

Department of Health (2009) *Valuing People Now*. Department of Health, London.

Department of Health (2012) *Compassion in Practice: nursing, midwifery and care staff our vision and strategy. Department of Health*, London.

Department of Health and Social Care (2019) *Right to Be Heard*. https://assets.publishing.service.gov.uk/government/uploads/system/uploads/attachment_data/file/844356/autism-and-learning-disability-training-for-staff-consultation-response.pdf (accessed December 2021).

Dunn, K., Rydzewska, E., MacIntyre, C., *et al.* (2019) The prevalence and general health status of people with intellectual disabilities and autism co-occurring together: a total population study. *Journal of Intellectual Disability Research*, 63, 277–285.

Equality Act (2010) HMSO, London.

Gibb, M. (2012) *Guide to Caring for an Adult Patient with a Learning Disability*. Mid Yorkshire Hospitals NHS Trust, Wakefield.

Glover, G., Williams, R., Tompkins, G., *et al.* (2019) An observational study of the use of acute hospital care by people with intellectual disabilities in England. *Journal of Intellectual Disability Research*, 63, 85–99.

Heslop *et al* (2017) *The Learning Disabilities Mortality Review (LeDeR) Programme Annual Report*. www.basw.co.uk/resources/learning-disabilities-mortality-review-leder-programme-annual-report-2016-2017 (accessed December 2021).

House of Lords, House of Commons, Joint Committee on Human Rights (2008) *A Life Like Any Other? Human Rights of Adults with Learning Disabilities*. https://publications.parliament.uk/pa/jt200708/jtselect/jtrights/40/40i.pdf (accessed December 2021).

IHaL (2012) *Improving Health and Lives*. https://improvinghealthandlives.org.uk/ (accessed December 2021).

Jackson, R. (2020) Coronavirus and people with an intellectual disability: time to change our approach to the provision of social care in the UK. *International Journal of Developmental Disabilities*. www.tandfonline.com/doi/full/10.1080/20473869.2020.1845931 (accessed December 2021).

Javaid, Amir, Nakata, V, Michael, Dasari (2019) Diagnostic overshadowing in learning disability: think beyond the disability. *Progress in Neurology and Psychiatry*, 23, 8–10.

Kinnear, D., Morrison, J., Allan, L., *et al.* (2018) Prevalence of physical conditions and multimorbidity in a cohort of adults with intellectual disabilities with and without Down syndrome: cross-sectional study. *BMJOpen*, 8, e018292.

Law Commission for England and Wales (1995) *Mental Incapacity*, Report No. 231. HMSO, London.

Learning Disability Mortality Review (LeDeR) Programme (2019) *Annual Report*. www.hqip.org.uk/resource/the-learning-disabilities-mortality-review-programme-annual-report-2019/#.YbCh79DP3IU (accessed December 2021).

Mason-Angelow, V. (2020) *This is Us – This is What We Do. A report to Inform the Future of Learning Disability Nursing*. www.ndti.org.uk/assets/files/Learning-Disability-Nursing-Report-FINAL.pdf (accessed December 2021).

Mencap (2007) *Death by Indifference*. Mencap, London.

Mencap (2008) *Getting It Right*. Mencap, London.

Mencap (2012) *Death by Indifference; 74 Deaths and Counting*. Mencap, London.

Mencap (2012) *What is a Learning Disability?* www.mencap.org.uk/learning-disability-explained/what-learning-disability (accessed December 2021).

Mencap (2018) *Annual Report*. www.mencap.org.uk/sites/default/files/2018-08/2018.032%20Annual%20Report_final_online%20version.pdf (accessed December 2021).

Mencap (2020) *Mencap responds to CQC death data on people with a learning disability and calls for Government to extend priority testing to people with a learning disability*. www.mencap.org.uk/press-release/mencap-responds-cqc-death-data-people-learning-disability-and-calls-government-extend (accessed December 2021).

Mental Capacity Act (2005) HMSO, London.

Mental Capacity Amendment Act (2019) HMSO, London.

Michael, J. & Richardson, A. (2008) Healthcare for all: the independent inquiry into access to healthcare for people with learning disabilities. *Tizard Learning Disability Review*, 13(4), 28–34.

NHS (2018) *Annual Health Checks: Learning Disabilities*. www.nhs.uk/conditions/learning-disabilities/annual-health-checks/ (accessed December 2021).

NHS Digital (2017) *Health and care of people with learning disabilities: 2015–16*. www.content.digital.nhs.uk/catalogue/PUB23781/Health-care-learning-disabilities-2015-16-summary.pdf (accessed December 2021).

NHS England (2015) *Supporting people with a learning disability and/or autism who display behaviour that challenges including those with a mental health condition*. www.england.nhs.uk/wp-content/uploads/2015/10/ld-serv-model-oct15.pdf (accessed December 2021).

NHS England and NHS Improvement (2019) *Learning Disability and Autism*. www.england.nhs.uk/learning-disabilities/ (accessed December 2021).

NICE (2016) *Guideline 54. Mental health problems in people with learning disabilities: prevention, assessment and management*. www.nice.org.uk/guidance/ng54/evidence/full-guideline-pdf-2612227933 (accessed December 2021).

Northway, R. & Dix, A. (2019) Improving equality of healthcare for people with learning disabilities. *Nursing Times*, 115, 27–31.

Northway, R., Rees, S., Davies, M. & Williams, S. (2017) Hospital passports, patient safety and person centred care: a review of documents currently used for people with intellectual disabilities in the United Kingdom. *Journal of Clinical Nursing*, 26(23), 5160–5168.

O'Driscoll, M., Allan, H., Liu, L., Corbett, K. & Serrant, L. (2018) Compassion in practice. Evaluating the awareness, involvement and perceived impact of a national nursing and midwifery strategy amongst healthcare professionals in NHS Trusts in England. *Journal of Clinical Nursing*, 27(5-6), e1097–e1109.

O'Leary, L., Cooper, S.A. & Hughes-McCormack, L. (2018) Early death and causes of death of people with intellectual disabilities: a systematic review. *Journal of Applied Research in Intellectual Disabilities*, 31(3), 325–342.

Philips, L. (2019) *Learning disabilities: making reasonable adjustments in hospital. Nursing Times, 115*, 38–42.

Public Health England (2016) *Learning Disabilities Observatory. People with Learning Disabilities in England 2015, Main report.* https://assets. publishing.service.gov.uk/government/uploads/system/uploads/ attachment_data/file/613182/PWLDIE_2015_main_report_NB090517. pdf (accessed December 2021).

Public Health England (2020) *Research and Analysis. Chapter 5: adult social care.* www.gov.uk/government/publications/people-with-learning-disabilities-in-england/chapter-5-adult-social-care (accessed December 2021).

Public Interest Disclosure Act (1998) HMSO, London.

Royal College of General Practitioners (2021) *Learning Disabilities Toolkit.* www.rcgp.org.uk/clinical-and-research/resources/toolkits/ health-check-toolkit.aspx (accessed December 2021).

Ross, H., Tod, A.M. & Clarke, A. (2015) Understanding and achieving person-centred care: the nurse perspective. *Journal of Clinical Nursing*, 24 (9-10), 1223–1233.

Social Care Institute for Excellence (SCIE) (2015) *At a Glance 69: Adults Safeguarding: types of abuse and indicators of abuse.* www.scie.org.uk/ publications/ataglance/69-adults-safeguarding-types-and-indicators-of-abuse.asp (accessed December 2021).

Social Care Institute for Excellence (SCIE) (2020) *Deprivation of Liberty Safeguards (DoLS).* www.scie.org.uk/mca/dols/practice/lps (accessed December 2021).

UK Parliament (2020) *Implementation of Liberty Protection Safeguards: Statement Made on 16 July 2020.* http://questions-statements.parliament. uk/written-statements/detail/2020-07-16/HCWS377 (accessed December 2021).

WHO (2018) *ICD-11.* https://icd.who.int/en (accessed December 2021).

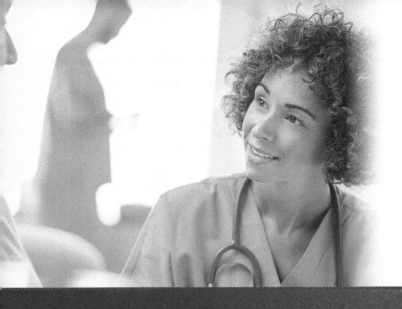

10

Principles of Caring for Children, Young People and Families

Ann Foley[1] and Linda Sanderson[2]

[1]University of Manchester, UK
[2]University of Huddersfield, UK

Learning Outcomes

On completion of this chapter, you will be able to:

- **Recognise key stages in the development of children and young people**
- **Use a range of communication skills to establish a caring relationship with children, young people and their families**
- **Recognise common physical and mental health issues associated with children and young people to promote health and prevent ill health**
- **Assess requirements of children and young people to provide person-centred nursing care**
- **Recognise and assess the risk of harm to children and young people. ensuring prompt action is taken to safeguard those who are vulnerable**
- **Assess the general health of children and young people to identify signs of deterioration and consider person-centred end-of-life care**

Proficiencies

NMC Proficiencies and Standards:

- **The outcome statements for each platform of the NMC Standards of proficiency have been designed to apply across all four fields of nursing practice (adult, children, learning disabilities, mental health) and all care settings.**

 Visit the companion website at www.wiley.com/go/peate/nursingpractice3e where you can test yourself using flashcards, multiple-choice questions and more.

Nursing Practice: Knowledge and Care, Third Edition. Edited by Ian Peate and Aby Mitchell.
© 2022 John Wiley & Sons Ltd. Published 2022 by John Wiley & Sons Ltd.
Companion website: www.wiley.com/go/peate/nursingpractice3e

Introduction

Children and young people (CYP) attend healthcare services in various settings. All registered nurses must be able to meet the person-centred care needs of people at any stage of life and who may have a range of mental, physical, cognitive or behavioural health challenges (NMC, 2018a, p.6). It is essential that CYP and their families are cared for compassionately, appropriately and confidently. Caring for CYP of different age groups is fascinating, challenging and rewarding. It is hoped that this chapter will stimulate interest and encourage exploration of the care of CYP.

Key Stages in the Development of Infants, Children and Young People

Early childhood is fascinating; it is a period of major growth and development. The child explores a world where opportunities abound. Parents and carers of children have much to offer in this process. Growth and development are affected by myriad factors, such as nutrition, sleep and maintaining safety. In addition, there are inherited attributes and the social, economic, geographic and political factors cannot be forgotten. All these factors interact and affect the overall child's development into adulthood. Within this chapter, development will be considered in the following age ranges: the baby 0–18 months, the preschool child, the school child and the adolescent.

The information contained here will not lead to expertise in child development – there are books entirely given over to this subject matter (Lightfoot *et al.*, 2018) – but it is important for nurses to know about child development so that they are able to:

- Teach and advise parents (NMC, 2018a, b, Annex A)
- Have reasonable expectations of what the child can and cannot do (NMC, 2018a, b, Platform 2,)
- Undertake suitable play activities with the child (NMC, 2018a, b, Annex A)
- Recognise where there are changes from the normal and be able to recognise disabilities and irregularities (NMC, 2018a, b, Platforms 2 & 3).

Development involves learning, physical growth and maturation, enabling the achievement of recognised, anticipated milestones (Bee & Boyd, 2014). There are differing schools of thought about what development actually is and what it is influenced by. An important debate relevant to child development is the extent to which 'nature' and 'nurture' influence the child (Lightfoot *et al.*, 2018). Proponents of the influence of 'nature' argue that behaviour and development are affected and guided by inborn and hereditary factors. Supporters of the influence of 'nurture' suggest that individual human differences reflect life experiences. These stances are polarised and child development is mainly considered to be a combination of both nature and nurture (Lightfoot *et al.*, 2018).

Child development is an amazing, complex process and nurses need to look at each child and family unit on an individual basis to consider their stage of development.

Baby 0–18 Months

Development is generally assessed by the utilisation of developmental scales in the following distinct areas.

1. *Physical*: includes growth, vision, hearing, gross motor development and co-ordination
2. *Cognitive*: language and understanding
3. *Psychosocial*: involves adapting to the society and culture to which the child belongs
4. *Emotional*: the control of feelings and emotions

It is the responsibility of the health visitor and general practitioner (GP) to undertake developmental assessments; occasionally paediatricians may also be involved. Assessments are focused on five areas.

- Gross motor development, referring to large-muscle skills
- Fine motor skills, referring to small-muscle skills
- Hearing and speech
- Vision
- Social development: feeding, dressing and social behaviour traits

Box 10.1 gives an overview of major milestones and the approximate age at which they occur. There may be individual differences in the rate and timing of specific developmental progress; for example, three healthy infants may sit unaided at 5, 6 or 9 months. However, the sequence of achievement of milestones will always be the same.

Box 10.1 Major Milestones for a Baby

- Smiles: 1–2 months
- Laughs: 6 months
- Sits (with support): 6 months
- Sits (without support): 8–9 months
- Crawls: 8–9 months
- Stands/walks: 12 months
- Pincer grip: 12 months
- Delicate pincer: 18 months
- Walks backwards: 18 months

Developmental skills of babies are achieved chronologically, e.g. head control is always developed before the baby can sit independently; crawling follows on from this and then control of the lower limbs facilitates standing and walking.

Preschool Child

When observing the preschool child, it can be noted that their growth rates relating to body and brain are considerably slower than when they were a baby. However, children's ability to control what their body can do grows enormously.

Table 10.1 identifies a vast array of skills that the preschool child masters developmentally; they also love to practise them. Watch a child in the supermarket or waiting for a bus hopping around just for the joy of it because it is a new skill. This increase in developmental skills increases the child's ability to explore and develop new ways to think and act.

School-age Child

Within this age range (5–11 years), physical changes are less obvious than in the baby and preschool child. Children are growing taller, they are changing in body shape and still adding to their

Table 10.1 Milestones in the preschool child.
Source: Sharma and Cockerill (2014).

AGE (IN YEARS)	GROSS MOTOR SKILLS	FINE MOTOR SKILLS
2	Walks well	Uses a spoon and fork
	Runs	Turns pages in a book
	Up and down stairs alone	Imitates a circle stroke
	Kicks a ball	Builds a tower of six cubes
3	Runs well	Feeds themselves well
	Marches	Puts on shoes and socks
	Rides a tricycle	Buttons and unbuttons
	Stands on one foot	Builds a tower of 10 cubes
4	Skips	Draws a person
	Can do a broad jump	Cuts with scissors (not expertly)
	Throws a ball overhand	Dresses self well
	High motor drive	Washes and dries face
5	Hops and skips	Dresses without help
	Good balance	Prints simple letters
	Rides scooter	

toolbox of skills. The height and weight of school-aged children are increasing gradually at the rate of 5 cm and 2–3 kg per year up until adolescence. Boys are on average 2.5 cm taller and 1 kg heavier than girls in the early school years but by around 12 years girls are both taller and heavier than boys in their peer group.

When assessing children look for the following.

Five year olds can:

- Write their own name, draw a person and/or a house
- Hop, skip, swing, jump, balance, climb, dance and throw a ball
- Choose their friends and be very clear who they will play with
- Undress and dress, although not able to tie laces
- Undertake play activities alone or in groups – likes imaginative play.

Six year olds can:

- Swing by the arms on monkey poles in playgrounds
- Skip with a rope.

Seven year olds can:

- Be proficient with bat and ball.

8–10 year olds can:

- Play hopscotch
- Play team games.

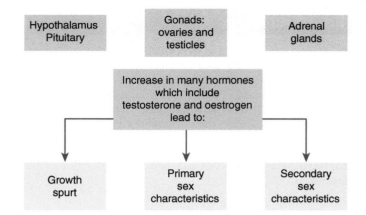

Figure 10.1 **Hormones produced in adolescence.**

Adolescence

Adolescence is triggered by a range of hormonal changes that bring about a set of physical changes (Figure 10.1). These hormonal changes are controlled by the anterior pituitary in response to a stimulus from the hypothalamus.

Puberty can begin in boys as early as 10.5 years and as late as 16 years, with the average onset at 12 years. In girls, puberty can begin as early as 7.5 years and as late as 11.5 years, with the average onset at 10 years.

During adolescence there is a rapid growth spurt. The internal organs grow and this includes the lungs and heart, which in turn increases physical endurance. The lymphoid system, which includes the tonsils and adenoids, decreases in size, which for some teenagers leads to improvements in asthma. Longer skeletal growth in boys is reflected in their greater height, with longer legs and arms. Muscle mass increases in boys and girls: for girls it peaks at menarche and then slows down; for boys it continues with the resultant leaner body mass (Coleman, 2011).

The brain continues to grow during adolescence. There is no increase in the number of neurones but the myelin sheath grows until puberty which ensures faster neural processing and resultant development of cognitive abilities.

Platform 3 of the NMC proficiencies (2018a) relates to assessing needs and planning care which should be relevant to the CYP stage of development. By watching and recording data, talking to the child and parents, nurses can begin to understand child development and contribute to the assessment of the CYP.

Case Study

Student nurse Megan was attending a baby clinic with her practice supervisor, a health visitor. A mum told Megan that she was very worried about her 9-month-old baby as he was not taking notice of his surroundings and not smiling much.

It is important to report the mother's concerns to the health visitor. A developmental assessment can be undertaken to see if the baby is reaching expected milestones. If the baby is reaching the milestones, the mother can be reassured and given suggestions about interacting with her baby to promote his interest in the environment, for example reading to the baby, describing

(Continued)

everything happening around him, helping to establish a regular sleep and rest pattern.

If the baby is not reaching expected milestones, the health visitor would refer mother and baby to the community paediatrician for a more thorough assessment of vision, hearing and neurological system.

Approaches to Communicating with CYP and Their Families

Children, young people and their families often encounter health services: health centres, neonatal units, emergency departments, outpatient clinics, acute ward areas, community nurses, school nurses. Whatever the situation, the CYP will be uncertain/anxious to openly distressed and fearful. The CYP will be asked to co-operate with care in their best interests, but which may appear to be unacceptable to the child, for example taking a medicine, passing urine into a bedpan. It is essential that the nurse uses appropriate and genuine communication to support the CYP to complete procedures that they would rather not undergo.

Alongside the CYP is often a parent or carer. The communication between parent/carer and nurse is understandably focused on the CYP. The parent/carer may feel anxious and protective of their child in a situation where the nurse is perceived to be the expert and powerful. The nurse must enable the parent/carer to support the CYP in a way which ensures they feel involved and contributing positively to their child's care.

Communication with the CYP and family is not just about passing on information. It is about building caring relationships which promote rapport, trust and openness. In such circumstances the child, young person and family are afforded their best opportunity to experience healthcare in a positive way, even in the face of difficult, even tragic, circumstances. This approach to communication is not an optional extra; it is embedded in the value set of nursing (NMC, 2018a, Annex A).

In this section, aspects of communication will be considered, particularly in relation to CYP of different ages and abilities, and their families. The reader is encouraged to reflect on their own practice and tips will be offered for communicating with CYP and their families.

Using Communication to Build Relationships

At a basic level, communication is the passage of a message from a 'sender' to a 'receiver' and possibly a reply. The ideal scenario is for the sender and receiver of the message to have the same mental image of the message and the same understanding of what is required. The potential barriers to conveying information between nurses, children, young people and their families are many and varied (Box 10.2). In Annex A (NMC, 2018a), the nurse is required to use clear language and written materials to convey information clearly, to check understanding and make reasonable adjustments where necessary.

Box 10.2 Barriers to Effective Communication

Physical: visual or hearing impairment, speech impediment, neurological impairment or other factors causing poor health status, e.g. diarrhoea and vomiting

Cognitive: age of the child, learning difficulties, stress, anxiety, mental health problems (e.g. depression, anorexia nervosa)

Environmental: noise level, temperature, seating arrangements, privacy, interruptions, time available

Personal: confidence, experience and skills in communication, perception of the power relationship between health professionals, children, young people and their families, perception of hierarchy in a relationship, culture, language

151

Effective verbal communication is one aspect of establishing a caring, trusting relationship with CYP and their families. Verbal communication, non-verbal communication, listening skills and valuing the CYP and family as fellow human beings are all vital components of effective relationship building. With this genuine approach to communication, rapport can be established and trust built between the CYP, family and nurse; this is likely to facilitate co-operation during procedures, reduce anxiety and distress and promote the CYP's developing sense of achievement and self-worth.

What the Experts Say

 'Young people with cancer want more honesty from health professionals'
Sue Morgan (2017) (Nurse Consultant, Teenage Cancer Care)

Communication and relationship formation with CYP of different ages and abilities, and their families, will now be considered.

Babies and Infants

Babies and infants are reliant on those around them to provide food, security, warmth and social interaction for them to achieve their full potential (Bee & Boyd, 2014). Social interaction with consistent caring adults is essential for the baby to learn about all aspects of communication: verbal communication and the development of language; body language, particularly facial expressions; experiencing love, security and the emotions associated with communication. The quality of early social experiences is linked to the child's mental health and well-being, particularly their resilience and ability to cope with stressors as they grow and develop.

What to Do If . . .

 Baby Sarah is 4 months old. She has been admitted to a children's ward with diarrhoea. She is likely to be on the ward for 1 or 2 days. Sarah's mum and dad visit between 1000h and 1400h each day but then leave Sarah to care for their other three children who attend nursery and school.

How would you promote communication and social interaction with baby Sarah?

In relation to baby Sarah, you might have thought about sitting down with Sarah's parents, showing that you want to listen to them by smiling, making eye contact and sitting in a relaxed way so as not to appear rushed. If you only have limited time, say this in a positive way: 'It is important for me to find out about the usual care you give Sarah, I have 10 minutes now if that is convenient for you?'

The nurse should plan and evaluate care for Sarah with her parents. For example: What is her usual routine? When Sarah's parents are there, what care would they like to give Sarah? What care would they like the nurses to give Sarah?

Make sure Sarah's parents know who will be looking after Sarah in their absence. One nurse per shift should be allocated to care for Sarah to provide as much consistency as possible. When caring for Sarah, make her feel special. Smile, coo and talk to her. Hold her closely and securely so she feels safe. This all communicates the care that she will thrive on.

Listen to Sarah: what are her cries like? Is she trying to tell you she is hungry, hot/cold, has a soiled nappy or wants comfort and security?

Even at this young age Sarah requires excellent communication.

Children

'Children' covers a large age range, from toddlers to 12 year olds; it is beyond the scope of this chapter to address communication issues related to each year group. Some aspects of child development are covered elsewhere in this chapter and a child's language develops tremendously over the period of childhood, as does their ability to communicate through body language; listening becomes more purposeful and intuitive; social interaction opportunities increase; their knowledge improves as does their ability to understand new information. In healthcare settings, all these factors, which influence the way in which messages are sent and received, must be taken into consideration to ensure the child feels involved and considered in communication about the care they are being offered. The United Nations Convention on the Rights of the Child (1989, ratified by the UK in 1992) emphasises this important point in article 12: 'When adults are making decisions that affect children, children have the right to say what they think should happen and have their opinions taken into account'.

Most children enjoy adult company and will be happy to communicate with them if the adult is genuine in the relationships they are seeking to build. Here are some tips for building relationships with children.

- Minimise the size difference between yourself and the child. Sit on a chair or on the floor so that you can make eye contact with the child and hear what they are saying.
- Play is an essential part of the child's world and can be a useful way of 'breaking the ice' with a child.
- Show an interest in what the child is doing. Invite the child to tell you what is happening rather than assuming from your perspective. 'This looks like an interesting game, can you tell me about it please?' rather than 'I used to love playing farms with my tractors, can I be the farmer?' If you make the wrong assumption, this can create an unnecessary barrier to conversation (Howard & McInnes, 2013).

Some children will not have the words to explain to you how they are feeling, or what hurts, or give you the details of an illness. Parents and carers will often fill in the details of their child's

situation but this does not mean you cannot show a genuine interest in the child and pick up on any cues that the child may present, for example 'I don't like going to the toilet at school'; respond to this and try to get more information – 'What are the toilets like at school?' This may help to explain why a child has severe constipation and abdominal pain.

Some children may find it easier to communicate whilst playing. Provide toys and dolls that represent what the child is undergoing, for example a teddy bear with a cannula, and listen to what the child is explaining to the teddy bear. Is the child explaining the benefits of the cannula to the bear or are they telling the bear that it is horrible and painful? This may indicate that you need to try a different explanation so the child can be reassured that you are trying to make them better.

Even very young children may be able to paint or draw their feelings or the situation they perceive themselves to be in. For example, some children have complex family arrangements, and it may be very important to find out who the child sees as the important people around them. Ask them to draw their family and then sit down with them and ask questions about the child's picture.

Adults who work with children on a regular basis often appear to be 'natural' in their relationships with children of different ages but for others it is a skill that needs to be developed. Watch the experienced people (e.g. children's nurses, play specialists, nursery nurses), listen to the interactions between child and adult and note some of the helpful phrases used. Prepare yourself with topics of conversation by watching popular TV programmes, reading children's literature and playing children's computer games. Another tip is to have something about you that might help to begin a conversation with a child, such as a pen with a character on, paper and pen to play a game or draw, a pack of cards to show your magician's skills. Take the opportunity to develop your skills with children by getting feedback from your practice supervisor and reflect on your relationships with children.

What the Experts Say

" Student children's nurses are given an opportunity to develop their communication skills in local primary schools when they run a 'Teddy bear clinic'. The children, aged 6 and 7 years, bring their teddy bear to school. The student nurses go to the school in uniform and take real equipment that the children are likely to encounter if they need acute healthcare, such as a stethoscope, thermometer, pen torch. This activity has been evaluated very positively by the students, and many have commented on their increased confidence in talking to children.

The teacher reported that the children had learnt about the equipment and talked about it for a long time afterwards. Some children thought they might want to be a nurse. Some Year 6 children (aged 10–11 years) reported that one of their highlights of school was the Teddy bear clinic. Ofsted (a government institution responsible for the inspection of educational institutions) visited one Teddy bear clinic and mentioned it in the school report as good practice.

The student nurses also enjoyed the Teddy bear clinic. Their evaluations include the following statements:

'I learnt that it is an important part of our role as student nurses to prepare children for hospital – in a way that is fun and age appropriate.'

(Continued)

'We still had to think about how to answer some of the questions we were asked, therefore it was reinforcing our knowledge base and developing our learning.'

'I enjoyed listening to the children's stories of their time in hospital.'

(*Source*: Sanderson, 2015)

Young people

Many of the tips for forming a relationship with children apply equally to young people, i.e. those 13–18 years, but an important point to take into consideration is the natural, increasing, independence of the young person. A barrier to communication can be created if the young person feels that their opinions are not being heard or if they perceive that information they require is not being made available to them.

What to Do If . . .

 Samantha (14 years) is awaiting a surgical review, following appendectomy, to discuss discharge plans. Samantha has been up and dressed since 0800h and it is now lunchtime. When you come onto the late shift, it is reported that Samantha has been 'slamming about' all morning, abrupt and increasingly uncommunicative.

How would you go about establishing a caring, professional relationship with Samantha?

In this scenario, it may be that Samantha is not receiving the information that she requires to stay calm; she may perceive she is being treated 'like a child'. An important step to establishing a relationship is to acknowledge her frustration but also to find an explanation. With this explanation Samantha is more likely to appreciate the situation.

It is important to find some common ground when talking to younger people. Familiarise yourself with popular music, sport, magazines, internet sites, books, films so that you can offer conversation rather than a string of questions – young people do not like to feel interrogated.

An increasingly popular way for young people to communicate is via social media. This can be used to convey important messages about health and well-being if face-to-face communication cannot be established.

Children/Young People with Problems Affecting Communication

Some CYP may not communicate as would be anticipated for their age; for example, children with hearing or visual impairments, children with developmental disorders affecting communication such as autism, and children with global developmental delay. These children require creativity when communicating with them. If a verbal approach is not possible, then other strategies must be used to convey your enthusiasm in establishing a relationship with the child.

What to Do If . . .

 Usman (aged 7 years) has profound developmental delay. He is dependent on his carers to meet all his needs. Usman cannot talk but he smiles and hears well. When you meet Usman for the first time, what can you do to communicate with him?

Take the time to get some information about Usman by talking to his parents, or other carers. What makes him happy? What makes him sad? How does he communicate that information to you? What does Usman like to do?

Approach Usman confidently, as you would with any child, sit down, smile and talk to him. Use play as a way of communicating, using sensory toys, music, books. Listen to Usman and respond to his communication with you. Is he making sounds which are conveying happiness or unhappiness?

Some children may have aids to assist with their communication, such as picture boards (Vaz, 2013). Other children may use a form of sign language such as Makaton or British Sign Language. It is useful to learn some of the signs, such as 'Hello', 'Goodbye', 'Where does it hurt?'. However, if working with children who use sign language, a more detailed course would be valuable.

> ### Jot This Down
> When meeting a parent/carer for the first time, what steps can you take to promote a rapport and minimise the formation of barriers? Make a note of your responses.

Some Tips for Developing a Rapport with Parents

Introduce yourself and your role in the team looking after the child. Sit down, make eye contact and smile. Unless it is an acute situation, make time to talk to the parents before commencing any intervention. This shows a genuine interest in the family and their child.

Find out, from the parents' perspective, why the child has come into contact with the health services and what they hope to get out of the experience. Find out about the child. Explain how you may be able to support them to care for their child, or what you can offer to participate in the care of their child.

The relationship between the parent/carer and nurse can be very effective in offering the 'best' care for a CYP but it does not 'just happen'. The professional, i.e. the nurse, may be perceived by the parent/carer as the expert and this can create a barrier for the parent; they may feel unsure about their role in caring for their child, unconfident about talking to a professional, particularly at initial meetings. Alternatively, the parent may be dismissive of the nurse, considering that the nurse does not know their child as they do, again creating a barrier to establishing a relationship.

To understand what it is like to care for a child who requires nursing support, there is an increasing body of research you may wish to access, for example Williams *et al.* (2012) and Flynn *et al.* (2020) and the seminal work of Phillip Darbyshire (1994) *Living with a Sick Child in Hospital. The Experiences of Parents and Nurses.*

When communicating with a parent/carer, there may be many influences which affect their communication. Great sensitivity and a professional approach are required to avoid unnecessary misunderstandings, even confrontation, in communication. Always sit down when talking to a parent/carer, show a willingness to listen and acknowledge the emotions the parent may be demonstrating, for example 'You seem a bit fed up today'. This approach will encourage the parent/carer to share their concerns with you and facilitate the open, honest communication necessary to offer the best care to the child.

Some Common Physical and Mental Health Problems

This section considers common physical and mental health problems for CYP and signposts have been given for further information, e.g. to the immunisation programme. Topics discussed include:

- The febrile child
- The child with a respiratory problem
- The child with a skin problem
- The child with gastroenteritis
- Mental health and well-being of young people.

Significant and beneficial effects on children's health have been seen since the introduction of immunisation programmes. See the companion website for resources giving an overview of the current immunisation programme in the UK.

The Febrile Child: Febrile Seizures

In relation to the febrile child (a child with a temperature), there are a few points to consider.

- A fever is defined as an abnormal rise in temperature, usually above 38°C, although children's temperatures are generally higher than adult temperatures.
- Children aged between 6 months and 6 years are most likely to experience a febrile seizure, usually caused by a bacterial or viral infection.
- Febrile seizures usually occur up to the age of 7 years.
- Usually last between 1 and 2 minutes and are generalised in nature.
- If they last longer (i.e. greater than 30 minutes), the child would need further investigation.

Red Flag

 'If a diagnosis of febrile seizure is suspected, assessment should include: Identifying red flag symptoms and signs suggesting a serious or life-threatening cause such as meningitis/meningococcal disease or encephalitis, and managing this appropriately.'

Source: NICE (2018)

The Child with a Respiratory Problem

Physiologically, children aged 1–4 years are more susceptible to respiratory illness due to immaturity of the respiratory system and anatomically they have narrower airways and often enlarged adenoids and tonsils.

Upper Respiratory Tract Infections

Around 80% of respiratory problems involve only the nose, ears and sinuses and thus cover several conditions such as the common cold (coryza), sore throat, acute otitis media and sinusitis (Lissauer & Carroll, 2018).

The child may present with a sore throat, fever, nasal blockage and earache; these symptoms would usually be accompanied by a troublesome cough. Management of these children is usually in the home environment with possibly a visit to the GP for advice.

This would usually centre upon antipyretics, such as paracetamol, to bring the temperature down, rest and encouraging the intake of plenty of fluids. These symptoms can precipitate a hospital admission if the child develops a febrile seizure (due to increasing temperature), becomes wheezy and has difficulties with breathing activities or develops a severe upper respiratory tract infection which may need medical and nursing interventions.

Red Flag

 Paracetamol is a commonly used medication. It is presented in many different forms, e.g. liquid, tablet, caplet, soluble tablets, and has many different proprietary names. The parents may not realise that a supermarket own-brand medicine contains paracetamol. It is essential that the healthcare professional clarifies with the parents what medication they have already given to their child before giving the child further paracetamol, to avoid overdosage.

Asthma

Asthma is a chronic inflammatory condition of the airways; the cause is still not completely understood. Airway obstruction is caused by airway inflammation and an increased airway responsiveness to a variety of stimuli. Asthma is usually reversible.

The inflammation results in a narrowing of the airway with an associated cough and wheeze. Although the cause is not completely understood, there are a variety of causative factors.

- Genetic predisposition
- Environmental factors
- Parental smoking
- Exposure to allergens in infancy
- Viral infection in infancy

Diagnosis and Management of Asthma Diagnosis in the child under 5 years is inherently difficult, mainly because wheezing and cough are prevalent in this age group. A diagnosis of asthma is considered if the child is being troubled by the following.

- Frequent episodes of wheezing, more than once a month.
- A nocturnal cough.
- Wheezing that happens in all seasons.
- Symptoms persisting after the child turns 3 years old.
- Cough which is induced by activity.

Management focuses on controlling the underlying inflammatory response, achieved by using prophylactic therapy, and breakthrough symptoms, which are generally treated by bronchodilators. It is important to highlight to the child and family that asthma cannot be cured but symptoms can be managed with the aim of the child leading a full and active life.

Medicines Management

 Find out about the drug therapy that is utilised to treat asthma:
- Bronchodilators
- Steroid therapy

The Child with a Skin Problem: Eczema

Infantile eczema is also known as atopic dermatitis or atopic eczema. The word 'eczema' has its origins in Greek and means 'to boil over'. Eczema describes itchy skin which develops into a rash of pustules which break down and leak serous fluid. It usually appears in the first year of life but can happen to children and adults at any time in their lives. The areas most affected are:

- The neck
- Flexures of the wrist and ankles
- Antecubital areas
- Popliteal areas.

Atopic eczema is an inflammation of genetically sensitive skin. Eczema is a symptom rather than a disorder. The condition in infants and children is multifactorial and indicates an oversensitivity to substances which are referred to as allergens. The allergens enter the body via the following routes.

- Digestive tract in food.
- Inhalation of dust and pollen.
- Direct contact with wool, soap and, in some cases, strong sunlight.
- Injections, some insect bites, some vaccinations.

> ### Jot This Down
> Define the following terms in relation to the child with eczema:
>   blister, erythema, excoriation, petechiae, pruritus, purpura, pustule, urticarial, vesicle.

Atopic eczema begins around 2–6 months and generally undergoes spontaneous remission by 3 years. This infant has a greater chance of developing dry skin and eczema in later life. Eczema can also occur in later childhood at 2–3 years and, in this instance, the skin is usually healed by 5 years. Adolescent eczema can begin at about 12 years of age and continue into adulthood. Some children will develop the trio of atopic eczema, asthma and hay fever (Lee *et al.*, 2016).

Signs of Atopic Eczema

- Erythema
- Vesicles that leak serous fluid
- Developing a dry crust over the vesicles as fluid leakage stops
- Scaling of the skin where the erythema and vesicles have been

Symptoms of Atopic Eczema

- Intense itching (pruritus)
- Scratching
- Irritable
- Broken sleep patterns

These signs and symptoms may worsen following immunisations and in the winter months. Extremes of temperature, humidity and sunlight can irritate the skin. The lesions caused by the eczema are easily infected by bacteria.

Principles of Care in Children with Eczema

The main principles of care are to hydrate the child's skin, reduce the pruritus and inflammation, and prevent secondary infection.

Hydrate the Skin

- Give lukewarm rather than hot baths (32–36 °C)
- Use emollient bath treatments
- Apply the emollient immediately after the bath
- Avoid bubble baths
- Pat the skin. DO NOT RUB

Red Flag

Emollients can make the bath slippery. Stay with the child to prevent accidents.

155

Relieve Pruritus

- Prevent scratching wherever possible
- Distract the child from scratching
- Keep the child's fingernails short
- May need to put cotton gloves on the young child to stop scratching
- Avoid wool
- May use prescribed sedating antihistamines at night

Reduce Inflammation

- Protect skin from excessive moisture
- Avoid overheating
- Limit exposure to dust, cigarettes smoke and pollens
- Recognise and limit emotional stressors
- Flare-ups may need pharmacological intervention: topical steroids/wet wraps

Prevent Secondary Infection

- Recognition of skin infections: seek prompt treatment
- Secondary infections can be treated by systemic antibiotics

The Child with Gastroenteritis

Acute gastroenteritis in children and young people is characterised by the sudden onset of diarrhoea and/or vomiting and a variety of other symptoms including poor appetite, fever and abdominal cramps. Many cases are caused by rotavirus, although there can be bacterial and parasitic causes too.

Gastroenteritis can be very serious, particularly in infancy and early childhood, because loss of fluid will affect the child's fluid balance. This is primarily due to an increased metabolic rate and the distribution of extracellular and intracellular fluid. Gastroenteritis should be treated with oral rehydration for around 3–4 hours, with resumption of normal feeding following this. The management of severe dehydration caused by gastroenteritis would need more intensive treatment by intravenous fluids (Freedman *et al.*, 2015).

Organisms will be transmitted quickly, particularly in areas such as nurseries and schools, but competent hand washing is a very effective method of reducing the incidence of gastroenteritis.

Table 10.2 highlights specific causative organisms and gives an overview of the presenting signs in the child.

Table 10.2 Causative organisms of gastroenteritis.

CAUSATIVE ORGANISM	SIGNS
Rotavirus	Severe diarrhoea, frequent watery stools, nausea and vomiting
Adenovirus	Diarrhoea, also linked to upper respiratory tract infection
Hepatitis A	Fever, malaise, nausea and jaundice
Campylobacter	Pyrexia, abdominal pain, watery foul-smelling diarrhoea which may contain blood
Salmonella	Rapid onset, nausea, vomiting, pain, diarrhoea contains blood and pus
Shigella	High fever, cramping pain, watery diarrhoea with mucus and blood
Escherichia coli	Gradual or sudden onset, explosive watery-green diarrhoea, pyrexia and abdominal distension
Escherichia coli 0157	Colitis, bloody diarrhoea and severe abdominal cramps

Mental Health and Well-being in Young People

Nurses from all fields will meet CYP who have challenges to their mental health, so it is important that opportunities are taken to promote mental health and well-being. Depending on the situation, mental ill health may be the prime concern to the managing healthcare team, at other times a physical issue may be the primary concern, but assessments should be holistic, and care offered in a person-centred way to support physical and mental health.

The physical development of young people (YP) was considered earlier, highlighting the rapid changes taking place during adolescence. There are other inherent pressures during adolescence: peer pressure, pressure via social media, experimentation (drugs, alcohol, smoking, sex and sexuality), examination stress, and some YP may be acting in a caring role within their family unit. There is not sufficient scope within this chapter to examine, in significant depth, the health challenges which face YP but it is useful to consider specific policy documents that influence the health and social care of YP and provide an insight into some of their health challenges.

Jot This Down

Explore some of the challenges YP face, for example alcohol misuse, eating disorders and depressive illnesses.

The main policy documents which frame the health and social care of young people are:

- *The NHS Long Term Plan* (NHS, 2019) which includes the mental health implementation plan
- *Future in Mind: Promoting, protecting and improving our children and young people's mental health and wellbeing* (Department of Health, 2015)
- *Support for Children and Young People's Mental Health* (Parkin & Long, 2021).

Health risk behaviours in YP are closely related to factors which can contribute to emotional distress and mental health problems, e.g. misuse of substances, smoking, risk-taking behaviours. In 2020, the Royal College of Paediatrics and Child Health reported 'There is a high risk of death among adolescence, with accidents and suicide being two of the highest causes of death for young people aged between 10 and 19'.

The list that follows is not exhaustive but offers examples of stressors which may affect the mental well-being of YP.

- Poverty and deprivation
- Maltreatment and neglect
- Parental mental health problems or addiction
- Long-term health conditions of parents or self
- Family disruption, or pressures of caring for others
- Bullying and social media issues
- Peer problems, relationship stresses, or pressures from substance use
- Pressures on body confidence (Association for Young People's Health, 2016)

Opportunities to provide person-centred care to YP may be brief and so it is important to establish rapport and elicit the YP's concerns; the most effective way to achieve this is to show respect and genuine interest when undertaking assessments or offering care. Effective communication skills are essential, e.g. actively listen, recognise and respond to verbal and non-verbal cues (NMC, 2018a, b). More specialised approaches to assessment and therapeutic conversations may include brief motivational interviewing and solution-focused conversations.

Poor mental health in YP can have an effect on exercise patterns, eating behaviours and sexual activities. This in turn can impact on the physical health of YP, e.g. obesity/eating disorders, substance misuse.

Red Flag Considerations when working with young people

- Depressive illnesses are very common in adolescence.
  - In early adolescence (11–14 years), there are high rates of conduct and emotional disorders.
  - Mid to late adolescence is the peak time for the onset of depressive disorders.
- Self-injury and self-harm: deliberate self-harm is common in adolescent girls. The peak age for presentation to services is 15–24 years for females.
- Eating disorders (e.g. anorexia nervosa and bulimia) affect more females than males.
- Attempted suicide: the rate is low under 14 years. It begins to occur around age 12 years and then increases in the early and mid teens. Young men are more at risk and are less likely than young women to show any distress before the suicide attempt.

Case Study

Jake is 15 years and is admitted to your unit following ingestion of alcohol and drugs. Jake's mum is not around and Jake acts as carer for his dad who suffers from a neurological disorder.

1. Consider what Jake most needs from the nurse and health agencies at this time.
2. Consider his situation and list the risk factors which may be impacting on Jake's life at present.
3. Outline short- and longer-term goals to reduce Jake's health risk behaviours.
4. Describe the role of the multiagency team who will be working with Jake.

Fundamental Care Needs

In this section, meeting the fundamental care needs of CYP is discussed. For the purposes of this chapter, the term 'fundamental care needs' refers to those needs that have to be met in order for the child to thrive. The aspects to be considered are physiological needs (i.e. air, food, water, warmth) and safety needs (i.e. security, freedom from fear) (Figure 10.2). These are loosely based on Maslow's hierarchy of needs (Maslow, 1943).

The fundamental care needs of a child are usually attended to by their parents or carers. As the child grows and develops, they take on more responsibility for meeting their own needs and the guidance from parents decreases. If there is concern that a parent/carer is not attending to the fundamental needs of the child, then the child may be considered to be neglected (HM Government, 2018). This is a serious issue, which will be discussed in more detail later in the chapter, hence the importance of nurses attending to the fundamental needs of the CYP. For the purposes of this section, it will be assumed that the CYP is an inpatient within a ward environment, possibly without a parent/carer present.

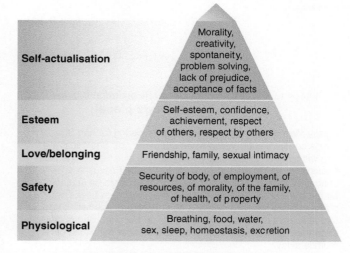

Figure 10.2 **Maslow's hierarchy of needs.** *Source:* Factoryjoe, Maslow's Hierarchy of Needs/Wikimedia Commons/CC BY-SA 3.0.

Meeting the Fundamental Care Needs of Infants

From 0 to 1 year the infant is totally dependent on their parent or carer to meet all their fundamental care needs except, usually, the need for air. The process of birth ensures that the baby very quickly becomes self-sufficient in inhaling air and exhaling the by-products of respiration. However, the airways of an infant are very small and if they have increased mucosal secretions for any reason, they may need assistance to meet the fundamental need for air, most specifically oxygen.

Very young babies breathe almost exclusively through the nose; hard, dry secretions will obstruct their tiny airway. When caring for the infant, every effort should be made to remove nasal secretions which are clearly obstructing the baby's nasal air passage. (Note: only secretions which can be removed by wiping the base of the nose with a tissue.) If it appears that the nasal passages and upper airways are becoming obstructed with secretions, suctioning may be required.

Red Flag

 Nasal and upper airway suction should only be performed by individuals who have been assessed as competent to do so. Poor technique may lead to mucosal irritation, damage and the production of further secretions (Foster et al., 2017).

Infants may also require oxygen therapy if they have an illness which means they are unable to take sufficient oxygen into their body to meet their physiological needs, i.e. hypoxia. Oxygen therapy can be delivered most effectively to young infants via an incubator. Within an incubator, the ambient oxygen concentration and humidity can be controlled. It is beyond the scope of this chapter to discuss the care of the infant in an incubator in detail, but readers are directed to Kenner et al. (2019).

As the infant gets older, beyond 5 months, an incubator may not be appropriate. In this situation, oxygen may be delivered via nasal cannula, via a headbox (Figure 10.3) and for short periods by holding an oxygen facemask close to the infant's face, for example whilst the infant is feeding or eating (Gormley-Fleming & Martin, 2018).

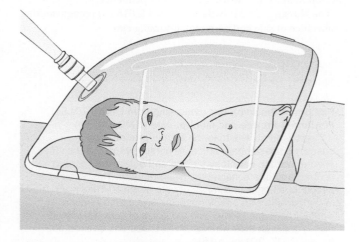

Figure 10.3 **An infant receiving headbox oxygen.**

157

Red Flag

 Oxygen is classed as a medicine and must be prescribed. The administration of oxygen must adhere to local policies and procedures.

Caring for an infant who requires oxygen demands accurate observational skills to spot signs of deterioration or distress, and these are discussed elsewhere in the chapter. Nursing assessments must be made to consider the infant's other fundamental needs whilst receiving the oxygen. For example, feeding the infant must be considered, monitoring the infant safely, attending to hygiene needs and, very importantly, ensuring the parents/carers can continue to care for and comfort the infant. If possible, care should be organised around the parent/carer availability to ensure they can participate in feeds, nappy changes and cuddles.

The focus of this section will now move to meeting the other fundamental needs that an infant may have. To facilitate this, consider the case of Maryam (Figure 10.4).

What to Do If . . .

 Maryam is 8 months old. She has been in hospital for 1 day and her condition is improving, so she is likely to go home later today. You have taken over her care at 0730h and Maryam's mother is due to arrive at 1200h. What are Maryam's fundamental care needs and how will you attend to them?

Meeting the Fundamental Care Needs of Children

During childhood (1–12 years), children begin to take a much more active role in meeting their fundamental care needs but close supervision and adult input remain an important aspect of caring for children in this age group. Whatever the age of the child, the nurse should encourage them to actively participate in meeting their fundamental needs; this is important for the child's development as they work towards independence.

The Nursing and Midwifery Council (2018a,b) recognises the importance of safe and competent nursing care.

Nursing Fields Nursing Practice and Decision making

Platform 4 Providing and evaluating care (NMC, 2018a), Platform 4 Provide and monitor care (NMC, 2018b)

Registered nurses take the lead in providing evidence-based, compassionate and safe nursing interventions. They ensure that the care they provide and delegate is person centred and of a consistently high standard. They support people of all ages in a range of care settings. They work in partnership with people, families and carers to evaluate whether care is effective and the goals of care have been met in line with their wishes, preferences and desired outcomes (NMC, 2018a, p.16).

Nursing associates provide compassionate, safe and effective care and support to people in a range of care settings. They monitor the condition and health needs of people within their care on a continual basis in partnership with people, families and carers. They contribute to ongoing assessment and can recognise when it is necessary to refer to others for reassessment (NMC, 2018b, p.9).

As with infants, the child is largely independent when meeting their requirement for air. However, one in 11 children has asthma (Asthma UK, 2021) so prompt, effective management of a wheeze in childhood is essential. This will include the administration of bronchodilating inhalers or nebulisers and the appropriate administration of prescribed oxygen.

Red Flag

 All medications must be prescribed and checked, according to the local policy and guidelines, before administering to the child.

I need food!

At 8 months Maryam will be 'weaned', she will probably have cereal or toast for breakfast, mashed food for lunch and tea. Fruit snacks in between, e.g. mashed banana. Maryam will want to feed herself with assistance. She must be supervised at all times as she will not be able to recognise food that may cause her to choke. 'I love water with my meals'. Maryam will still have baby milk (breast or formula, before bed).

I need to be warm too!

Maryam will need to be dressed in clothes that will keep her warm but also enable her to move freely. No loose buttons, no tapes or cords.

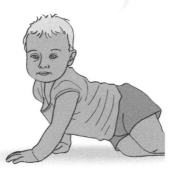

I need to feel safe and secure while my mum is away
This is a very strange place!

Ideally Maryam will have the same nurse caring for her. She needs constant supervision when out of her cot. She can crawl and will be keen to explore. When Maryam is in her cot the sides should be fully raised and securely fastened. If she is in a pushchair or highchair all of the fastenings should be in place. Maryam will enjoy sitting with her nurse, looking at books or playing, this will make her feel safe and secure. It is essential that strangers do not approach or pick up Maryam. She is totally dependent on the healthcare team to look after her whilst her mum is away.

Figure 10.4 **Maryam's fundamental care needs.**

As children get older, they are more likely to tolerate face-mask oxygen but younger children (i.e. 1–4 years) may find this very difficult, particularly when awake. The nurse needs to use their creative skills to encourage the young child to sit quietly and at least allow the oxygen to waft via oxygen tubing. Parents and carers can be very supportive; they could sit and cuddle the young child whilst the oxygen is administered. Plenty of distractions are required to occupy the young child, for example laptop computers/tablets, books, TV, bubble machines, light projection machines.

As well as the fundamental need for air the nurse also needs to consider the child's fundamental need for food, water, warmth, safety, security, freedom from fear – but the approach taken to meet them will differ with the age of the child.

What to Do If . . .

You have been allocated two children to look after. Dev is 3 years old and Aysha is 10 years old. They are both well enough to be up and about out of bed. Both children have parents who are usually on the ward.

What are Dev and Aysha's fundamental care needs and how will you attend to them (Figures 10.5 and 10.6)?

Mum or dad stay with me at night usually and then I feel safe. If they can't stay it is best if I go to sleep and have my teddies around me. If I wake up at night it is best if there is a nurse I know. They ask me to wear a bracelet so they know my name and birthday.

I am Dev and I need a little bit to eat and drink every two or three hours. I don't eat or drink much because I get fed up with it!

Mum sometimes gets a bit frustrated with me because I don't always want to eat what she gives me.

Getting dressed can be a bit of a nuisance but I always like to try and put my socks on, trouble is I get fed up and wander off to watch TV before I get my tee-shirt on!

At 3 years Dev will need guidance about what to wear but it is essential that he is offered some choice and time to try things himself.

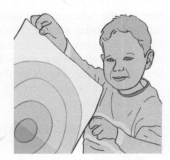

Hospital is a very strange place! I get a bit worried about some of the things I have to do such as a 'temperature' but most nurses make me giggle while they are doing it!

My favourite place is the play room because it is a bit like nursery. I get really worried if mum goes to get her tea but if she leaves her handbag and a nurse sits with me and reads me a story I can cope.

Figure 10.5 Dev's fundamental care needs.

Of course I need food and drink but I will be able to tell you what I like or if I am hungry or thirsty. I am really interested in how my body works and trying to keep healthy so if you have any information about this I would be happy to listen.

One of my friends has diabetes and she gets a bit fed up with it, she eats sweets even though she shouldn't. If she was in hospital you would really need to help her to stick to her healthy eating!

I get a bit bored in hospital if I don't have anything to do. I like it if other children are in around my own age because we can talk about school and guides and stuff. My mum lets me have my mobile so I can keep in touch with my friends.

I sometimes get nervous if there are noisy families around, that's when I really need to know where the nurses are.

My favourite nurse is Lisa. She gives me jobs to do and just seems to know when I am not feeling well, or I am in pain. If mum's not here Lisa makes sure I get ready for bed properly and turns the lights off at a good time.

At 10 years of age Aysha still likes routine to make her feel secure.

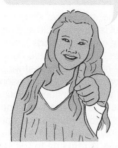

I am quite happy for mum and dad to go off the ward as long as I know where they are going, what time they will be back and who is looking after me. I don't like doing anything different when they are not here. Aysha can be trusted to sit quietly on her bed, or in the play room, or with the hospital school teacher but she should be accompanied if she wants to leave the ward area.

Figure 10.6 Aysha's fundamental care needs.

Meeting the Fundamental Care Needs of Young People

Young people from 13 to 18 years are usually independent at meeting their own care needs. They can find it extremely difficult to relinquish this independence, even when very unwell. The strong desire for independence should be encouraged and nurtured unless this is contraindicated by the young person's health needs or illness. During this age spectrum the young person is naturally decreasing their reliance on parents/carers and building strong relationships with their peers. Every effort should be made to help the young person maintain contact with their friends by allowing the use of mobile phones and internet access but the safety of all people using the healthcare services needs to be considered and sometimes an open discussion with young people is required to ensure they understand any rules that may be in place in the healthcare setting.

Young people have been acknowledged as a group with particular needs. As they move through a potentially turbulent period of their life, contact with healthcare services can be an added challenge for them. Healthcare professionals can do a lot to minimise this challenge by ensuring young people have privacy, are included in all decisions about themselves and are encouraged to express their opinions. Some services have developed teenage units in recognition of the unique needs of this age group (Teenage Cancer Trust, 2016) but Dodds (2010) argues that a lot can be done without major financial investment to offer good care to young people using healthcare services.

An important aspect of the fundamental care of young people is to ensure that they are competent to make decisions about their healthcare, i.e. to consent to or refuse treatment.

Case Study

Consider these two situations.

Paul is 16 years old and has fractured his elbow whilst playing rugby. He needs prompt surgery to stabilise the fracture. His parents are away on holiday and cannot get back for 12 hours. Paul was staying with a friend and his parents are not contactable. Could consent for the surgery be taken from Paul? What will influence your thoughts about this situation?

Naeve is 14 years old and has also sustained a fracture of her elbow, which needs prompt surgery to stabilise the fracture. Naeve has had an excessive amount of alcohol and she is refusing to tell you her parents' telephone number and insisting that she gives permission for the operation to go ahead.

Could consent for the surgery be taken from Naeve? What will influence your thoughts about this situation?

There is a legal framework which guides whether consent can be taken from a young person or not. The main considerations are as follows.

- What is in the best interest of the child? This may require consideration of what benefits will come from the procedure and what harm may be caused by the procedure.
- Is the young person cognitively competent to consent to treatment? Does the child fully understand the potential benefits of the procedure and the potential risks?

Assessments in relation to these questions largely rely on a discussion between the medical and nursing staff, the young person and the parents. This can be a complex subject and dilemmas in practice can arise. The General Medical Council (2021) has produced guidance that is a useful resource.

The fundamental care needs of CYP have been considered. The discussion has focused on children who are progressing as expected developmentally and who have a short-term illness. It is important to consider those children for whom chronological age does not correspond with their developmental age and those children with chronic illness.

Each CYP is of course unique and children with complex care needs are no exception. It is important to listen to the family about the fundamental care needs that the child may require so that appropriate nursing care can be offered.

Case Study

Imran is 12 years old. He has global developmental delay due to a rare genetic disorder. Imran has a poor swallow reflex so he has gastrostomy feeds. He has occasional seizures, moves very little and is fully dependent on his carers to meet all his needs.

How would you ensure that Imran received excellent fundamental care?

Issues you should have considered in discussion with Imran's carers include the following.

- Because of a poor swallowing reflex, Imran is vulnerable to obstructing his airway with secretions. He needs to always have suction and oxygen available.
- Imran may not be able to have any foods or drinks orally, or only drinks and foods of a particular consistency. This measure is to prevent Imran aspirating the food or drink, i.e. because of a poor swallowing reflex food and drink may enter the trachea rather than the oesophagus and lead to airway obstruction or a chest infection.
- Gastrostomy feeds must be given as per the dietitian's protocol. Staff must be deemed suitably competent in caring for a child with a gastrostomy *in situ*.
- Imran is dependent on carers to meet his hygiene needs. He will need washing, mouth care and frequent nappy area care to prevent excoriation of the skin. Always ensure that Imran has privacy and is treated with dignity when attending to hygiene needs.
- Imran is unable to move himself so he will require frequent position changes to prevent the development of pressure ulcers, to promote circulation, prevent stiffness and to ensure comfort.
- Safety must always be a priority. Imran must have sides on his bed to prevent him falling from the bed. When moving Imran from bed to chair, an appropriate hoist must be used safely. When he is sitting in his chair, all the fastenings must be made to prevent falling. Care must be taken not to have the fastenings too tight and not to trap Imran's skin or clothes when securing the fasteners.
- Anticonvulsant medication must be given as prescribed to minimise the risk of seizures. Rescue medication must be easily available in case Imran has prolonged seizures.
- Liaise with Imran's family/carers to ensure that his psychological needs are also met, e.g. what makes him happy/not happy, how does he communicate his feelings, discomfort or pleasure. Imran may have a 'health passport' which details many aspects of his specific care requirements (Together for Short Lives, 2021).

Meeting the fundamental needs of any CYP is an essential and fulfilling nursing activity. The extent to which a parent/carer, child, young person or nurse meets the child's needs must be discussed with all parties and negotiated when the child is in a healthcare setting. Nurses need to willingly learn about the fundamental care needs of each CYP so that they can participate in person-centred care.

The Importance of Acting to Protect Children and Young People

The way in which a society treats its children is perhaps the best measure of its humanity.

(Lord Laming, 2003)

Protecting CYP is everybody's responsibility. Children are the future of any society and hold the aspirations for its future. This section will provide a brief overview of the legal framework safeguarding children. Definitions of harm will be provided and the importance of parenting will be explored to enable you to recognise the importance of protecting children across the age spectrum.

Legal and Policy Framework

The NSPCC has summarised the child protection framework in the UK (NSPCC, 2021).

- 'The UK's four nations – England, Northern Ireland, Scotland and Wales – each have their own child protection system and laws to help protect children from abuse and neglect.
- Each nation has a framework of legislation, guidance and practice to identify children who are at risk of harm, take action to protect those children and prevent further abuse occurring.
- Each UK nation is responsible for its own policies and laws around education, health and social welfare. This covers most aspects of safeguarding and child protection.
- Laws are passed to prevent behaviour that can harm children or require action to protect children. Guidance sets out what organisations should do to play their part to keep children safe.
- Although the child protection systems are different in each nation, they are all based on similar principles.'

The NMC expects registrants to understand and apply the aims and principles of protection when engaging with people (NMC, 2018a, b, Platform 2). Protecting CYP is everyone's responsibility and legal frameworks guide policy within a healthcare setting. It is useful to consider that everyone approaches the protection of CYP based on a value set developed over their lifetime, their own experiences of being parented and their interactions and experiences. Some consequences from protecting children are very clear-cut, others less so.

Look at the scenarios that follow and consider whether the behaviour described gives you concerns in relation to protecting activity. Would you report this further?

- Lily is a 5 year old in reception at school and often comes to school not washed and not having had breakfast.
- Ellis is 8 years old and is often left alone to care for her mother who has a chronic illness.
- Miss Smith, a teacher in a primary school, often shouts at a child in the class, telling him he is useless.
- Fran, a 13-year-old girl, is having sex with Jane, her 17-year-old girlfriend.
- Sally is a pregnant mother and using heroin and cocaine during her pregnancy.
- Mark is a stressed dad caring for his children on his own; he hits one of his children, which causes marks and bruising.
- Sammy is 10 years old. He has hearing aids and has missed two of his appointments with the audiology team.

A student nurse/nursing associate's assessment of a situation may not correspond with that of the practice supervisor but every opportunity should be taken to discuss concerns and learn from the multidisciplinary team. Parents or guardians are entrusted to provide safety for CYP and keep them from harm. A key part of protecting CYP is judging whether the parents are 'good enough' parents.

Deciding whether parents are 'good enough' can be challenging for all staff involved with the care of CYP. Student nurses/nurse associates need to consider the concept of 'good enough parenting' but remember that the 'good enough' standard is affected by social and cultural norms. Munro (2011) points out that professionals may become accustomed to poor standards of parenting and then sometimes accept them as normal or 'good enough', with devastating consequences for children.

Case Study

You are undertaking a placement with the school nurse and attend school with the nurse to observe her role with the reception class. Kate, age 5 years, attends and you notice that she is very quiet. You also notice that she has bruising to her cheek, a couple of small bruises on her ear lobes and some bruising around her wrist. The school nurse discusses your concerns with the class teacher, who advises that Kate's mum has just started a new relationship and the man has moved into their flat.

What are your concerns?

A referral would be made by the school nurse in relation to the scenario with Kate. There are developmental pointers relating to a withdrawn quiet child and physical pointers relating to the bruises on her cheek, ear lobes and wrist.

Categories of Abuse

There are four categories of abuse: physical abuse, emotional abuse, sexual abuse and neglect. The signs and symptoms and how to recognise child abuse are fully documented by the NSPCC, please visit their website for further details (**www.nspcc.org.uk/what-is-child-abuse/spotting-signs-child-abuse/**).

Professional Advice

The following are the main organisations and individuals concerned with safeguarding and protecting children.

- Social Services
- Police
- Health visitors, school nurses, midwives, GPs and practice nurses
- Paediatricians, psychologists, nurses and allied health professionals
- Addiction services
- Named nurses for child protection
- Education: early years workers, teachers at primary and secondary school
- Voluntary organisations
- Probation Service
- Youth offending teams
- Lawyers
- Foster carers

Student nurses/nurse associates should expect to be supported with any concerns they raise whilst in the clinical learning environment. Safeguarding and protecting CYP cause anxiety to new and experienced healthcare practitioners. There have been several serious case reviews which set out messages for all healthcare professionals (Clark, 2020). These key messages highlight that all healthcare professionals should be aware of the myriad factors that could indicate a child is in need and these should always be discussed, not dismissed. The other vital key message is that all healthcare professionals should follow policies at national level and protocols at local level to make sure a full accurate picture is painted, and that support is given for a positive outcome for the child and family unit.

Practice Assessment Document

People should be able to have trust in healthcare providers in that they understand how vulnerable people (this may include CYP) can be protected from vulnerable situations and can support and protect them from harm.

It may be a challenge during a health and social care placement to take part in safeguarding meetings as the details being discussed may be limited to certain individuals and agencies. If this is the case and you are unable to take part in safeguarding meetings, gather information to share with your supervisor around the following issues.

· How you would share information with colleagues and how you might seek advice from various reputable sources that could help you if you have a concern or if there is any uncertainty regarding issues around safeguarding.
· Thinking of you, what support systems are in place that can help you manage and deal with your own emotions? How can you access support systems?

Take time to receive feedback from your supervisor regarding this activity. Doing this can demonstrate to your supervisor that you have sufficient understanding and knowledge regarding this complex topic.

Identifying Signs of Deterioration in General Health

Assessing the General Health of Children

The discussion in this section is about identifying signs of deterioration in the general health of CYP.

A previous section of this chapter discussed the fundamental health needs of CYP. In this section it is acknowledged that healthcare practitioners will often encounter CYP when they are unwell. The spectrum of 'unwell' is vast: children with asthma, diarrhoea and vomiting, appendicitis, rashes, head injury, burns – the potential list of illness is phenomenal. Most children will be supported appropriately, during their illness, by their parents/carers, GPs, paramedics or acute hospital services, and recover to full health. However, the Office for National Statistics (2021) *Child and Infant Mortality Statistics 2019* shows that infants, children and young people do still die in the UK from a variety of acute, chronic and genetic illnesses and also accidents. The prevention of childhood death is not always a realistic option; however, in the majority of cases, it is but CYP are reliant upon the people around them to recognise deterioration in their condition and respond accordingly and promptly to support them.

It is not possible to cover this entire topic in one section of a chapter so the focus will be on the nurse's role in the recognition of the deterioration of physical health in CYP with an acute-onset illness. The Nursing and Midwifery Council (2018a, b) recognises the importance of safe and competent nursing care from all nurses to all age groups. This section is concerned with the generic NMC proficiencies (2018a, b), rather than the specialist skills of the children's nurse.

The Nursing Associate Assessing Needs and Planning Care

The nursing associate will be able to 'demonstrate an understanding of human development from conception to death, to enable delivery of person-centred safe and effective care' (NMC, 2018b, 3.1)

Annex B: Part 1 (all registered nurses): Procedures for assessing people's needs for person-centred care

1. Use evidence-based, best practice approaches to take a history, observe, recognise and accurately assess people of all ages.
   1.2. physical health and well-being
      1.2.1. symptoms and signs of physical ill health
      1.2.2. symptoms and signs of physical distress
      1.2.3. symptoms and signs of deterioration and sepsis (NMC, 2018a)

Annex B, Part 1(nursing associates) are expected to recognise deterioration and act upon their observations

1.11. recognise emergency situations and administer basic physical first aid, including basic life support

In order to recognise physical deterioration in CYP, it is important to assess them at the time of admission so a 'baseline' can be recorded. From this baseline, it can be seen if the child improves, stays the same or deteriorates. Also from this baseline assessment the nurse can begin to plan and administer appropriate care, reassessing regularly to evaluate the child's response. This cycle of assessment, diagnosis, planning, intervention and evaluation is commonly known as the Nursing Process and it is a useful approach to nursing, particularly if a child's condition is changing rapidly. The whole process may be done in conjunction with other healthcare professionals but it is often the nurse and nursing associate who spend prolonged periods with the CYP and family and so it is essential that the nursing assessment (registered nurse) and monitoring (registered nurse and nursing associate) of the CYP are thorough, systematic and reliable.

Assessment is both subjective and objective; it needs to take account of the CYP's physical health, mental health, developmental achievements, usual activities of living, family situation, presenting problems and any relevant past health history. To do a thorough assessment of all these aspects of the child's health requires time and the development of a trusting relationship between the nurse, CYP and family. In the acute care situation, the nurse must prioritise their assessment approach. If a child is acutely unwell, then the nurse needs an assessment approach to quickly identify the child's physical status, i.e. their baseline – this is the priority. Having assessed the child's physical status, the nurse can alert other healthcare professionals to the findings and appropriate interventions can be put in place to support the child's physical status, with the goal of preventing deterioration. Once the child is physically stable, a more detailed general assessment can be undertaken.

A systematic approach to the assessment of an acutely ill child is suggested in Figure 10.7. This assessment is based on the ABCDE approach recommended by the Advanced Life Support Group (2016) in the care of the seriously ill child. It is not anticipated that readers of this chapter will have the knowledge and skills to perform the comprehensive assessments recommended by the Advanced Life Support Group, but they can use this approach to make a baseline assessment and summon help

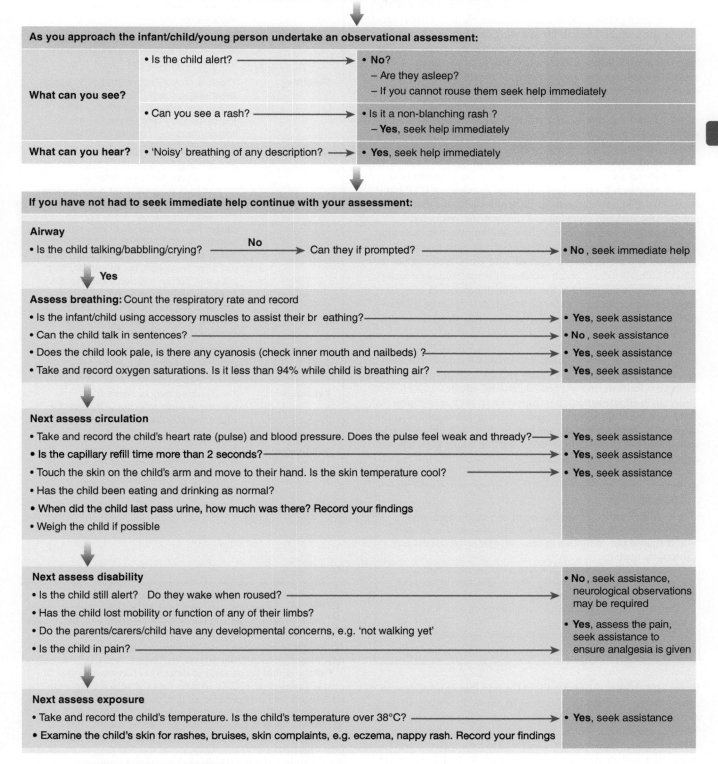

- Gain a quick insight into the infant/child/young person's current problem
- Read any available notes/letters/ask the child or parent
- Are there any significant past health problems, e.g. is the child asthmatic?

As you approach the infant/child/young person undertake an observational assessment:

What can you see?	• Is the child alert?	• **No**? – Are they asleep? – If you cannot rouse them seek help immediately
	• Can you see a rash?	• Is it a non-blanching rash ? – **Yes**, seek help immediately
What can you hear?	• 'Noisy' breathing of any description?	• **Yes**, seek help immediately

If you have not had to seek immediate help continue with your assessment:

Airway
- Is the child talking/babbling/crying? — **No** → Can they if prompted? — → • **No**, seek immediate help

Yes

Assess breathing: Count the respiratory rate and record
- Is the infant/child using accessory muscles to assist their breathing? —————→ • **Yes**, seek assistance
- Can the child talk in sentences? —————→ • **No**, seek assistance
- Does the child look pale, is there any cyanosis (check inner mouth and nailbeds) ? —————→ • **Yes**, seek assistance
- Take and record oxygen saturations. Is it less than 94% while child is breathing air? —————→ • **Yes**, seek assistance

Next assess circulation
- Take and record the child's heart rate (pulse) and blood pressure. Does the pulse feel weak and thready? —→ • **Yes**, seek assistance
- Is the capillary refill time more than 2 seconds? —————→ • **Yes**, seek assistance
- Touch the skin on the child's arm and move to their hand. Is the skin temperature cool? —————→ • **Yes**, seek assistance
- Has the child been eating and drinking as normal?
- When did the child last pass urine, how much was there? Record your findings
- Weigh the child if possible

Next assess disability
- Is the child still alert? Do they wake when roused? —————→
- Has the child lost mobility or function of any of their limbs?
- Do the parents/carers/child have any developmental concerns, e.g. 'not walking yet'
- Is the child in pain? —————→

• **No**, seek assistance, neurological observations may be required

• **Yes**, assess the pain, seek assistance to ensure analgesia is given

Next assess exposure
- Take and record the child's temperature. Is the child's temperature over 38°C? —————→ • **Yes**, seek assistance
- Examine the child's skin for rashes, bruises, skin complaints, e.g. eczema, nappy rash. Record your findings

Figure 10.7 **Assessment of an acutely ill child.**

163

quickly and appropriately if they are at all concerned by the child's physical health status.

In order to undertake a reliable assessment, it is important to use appropriate techniques when, for example, taking the heart rate of an infant (which requires a stethoscope) and assessing the pain of a young child. The Royal College of Nursing (2020) provides some useful standards for assessing children and Gormley-Fleming (2010) provides a comprehensive review of the assessment of children and the expected 'normal' values of vital signs (i.e. temperature, pulse, respiratory rate and blood pressure) for children of different ages.

An important aspect of the assessment is checking the child's effort of breathing, assessing whether the child is using their accessory muscles in order to breathe, i.e. intercostal and subcostal muscles. If they are, you will be able to see the child's head 'bobbing' and the areas between their ribs appearing to be 'sucked in'. These features are often most pronounced in the younger child.

The approach detailed here will assist in assessing CYP but it is essential that any concerns or difficulties with the assessment are documented and reported to a senior nurse or doctor.

To ensure a systematic and consistent approach to assessing CYP, and to encourage the early raising of concerns, many clinical areas now use a tool known as Paediatric Early Warning Scores (PEWS). This is a chart which facilitates the recording of a variety of observations suggested in the assessment process, in one place. From these observations, a score is achieved. If the score increases as the observations are repeated over time, this alerts the healthcare professional to a potentially deteriorating child.

If the child is acutely unwell, they can deteriorate quickly from the baseline observations, particularly if supportive measures are not put in place in a timely and appropriate manner, for example administering oxygen, fluids and medication. Having undertaken an assessment, it is important to keep reassessing the child to monitor for signs of improvement or deterioration. If the cause of the illness is known, the path of the child's illness may be anticipated but every child is individual and so the early signs of deterioration need to be identified.

Case Studies

John is 6 months old. He has been admitted with a 2-day history of diarrhoea and vomiting. On admission he is alert and smiling but continues to have several small vomits and two dirty nappies.

Sabrina is 5 years old. She has a temperature and a cough. Her voice is very husky. She is reluctant to eat and drink and she looks miserable.

Moya is 13 years old. She has abdominal pain and is reluctant to walk about.

What would alert you to the physical deterioration of these children?

Boxes 10.3, 10.4 and 10.5 highlight the possible signs of deterioration in the 'case study' children. In these three case studies, robust systematic assessment, which is ongoing from the initial baseline assessment, will assist with the successful management of the children. The assessment will lead to appropriate interventions from nurses and other members of the healthcare team. This in turn should lead to the children returning to their previous level of good health.

Box 10.3 Possible Signs of Deterioration in John, Aged 6 Months

Alert?	Will become increasingly fractious or, more worryingly, quiet and less responsive
Airway	As John is alert and smiling, his airway is open and stable. It is unlikely that this would deteriorate
Breathing	There is no suggestion that John has a breathing problem. However, deterioration in any system may initially raise the respiratory rate as part of John's compensatory or 'coping' mechanism
Circulation	John is losing fluid and electrolytes through diarrhoea and vomiting, his circulatory system may deteriorate as he has to compensate for a decreasing fluid volume in that system. His heart rate will increase out of his normal range; his blood pressure may rise slightly initially and then begin to fall out of his normal range. His fontanelle will appear sunken, his mouth dry and his urine output will decrease. He will look increasingly pale and his peripheral skin will be cooler to the touch than central skin. His capillary refill time will be more than 2 seconds
Disability	Will become increasingly fractious or, more worryingly, quiet, and less responsive. May have abdominal pain
Exposure	Temperature may increase if a gastrointestinal infection. Observe for rashes with every nappy change
Priority of management	John needs fluid and electrolyte replacement to prevent further dehydration and potential hypovolaemic shock (British Medical Association, 2018)

Red Flag

Skin assessment can be very useful to detect vasoconstriction, as with John (Box 10.3). Children with light skin tones will become increasingly pale and cooler to touch as vasoconstriction progresses (this is a physiological response to shock with the aim of directing blood flow to essential internal organs, e.g. heart, brain, liver, kidneys).

Pallor may not be as easy to detect in children with skin of colour. Lewis et al. (2020) explain that pallor in people with dark-toned skin may present as grey or ashen while people with brown-toned skin present 'more yellowish' in colour. A good place to assess the skin colour is the palm of the hands.

Ensure you touch the skin to detect changes in temperature (the extremities will become cool and this will progress towards the central body if the cause of shock is not treated).

Children with skin of colour may become grey/ashen

Box 10.4 Possible Signs of Deterioration in Sabrina, Age 5 Years

Alert?	Sabrina is alert but miserable
Airway	Sabrina has a husky voice and a temperature which could suggest an infection in her 'airway'. At 5 years it is unlikely to obstruct her airway, but it is essential that this is assessed regularly
Breathing	Sabrina is coughing, and has a temperature which may be because of a chest infection. Her respiratory rate and effort of breathing may increase as she compensates to ensure adequate oxygenation of her blood. These signs and a decreasing oxygen saturation level are signs of deterioration
Circulation	A high temperature and the increased work of breathing will raise Sabrina's heart rate out of her normal range. Blood pressure should remain stable. Reluctance to drink and increased work of breathing could cause slight dehydration, so urine output and fluid intake should be monitored
Disability	May become increasingly miserable and fractious. Increasing tiredness and becoming less responsive may be due to hypoxia. A pain assessment should be undertaken as Sabrina may be most miserable due to a sore throat
Exposure	Any developing rashes should be reported
Priority of management	The source of infection should be treated to prevent the infection developing into septic shock (Sanchez-Pinto et al., 2020). Supportive care for respiration (e.g. oxygen therapy) may be required to prevent deterioration. Adequate analgesia should be given to enable Sabrina to feel improved and to eat and drink.

Box 10.5 Possible Signs of Deterioration in Moya, Age 13 Years

Alert?	Moya is alert
Airway	No suggestion of a problem with Moya's airway. Regular conversations with her will enable ongoing assessment
Breathing	No suggestion of a problem with Moya's breathing. Increasing pain may raise the respiratory rate above the normal range
Circulation	Increasing pain may raise the heart rate and blood pressure, particularly if there is an infectious or inflammatory underlying cause (e.g. appendicitis)
Disability	Pain is the main problem and increasing pain will increase Moya's reluctance to move. Moya needs regular pain assessment and observation of her body posture to spot deterioration due to pain
Exposure	Temperature may increase
Priority of management	Pain assessment and management, referral to surgical team for assessment

Best Practice Relating to End-of-Life Care

It is not always possible for children to recover from an acute illness. For those children who cannot recover, the goal of care becomes a dignified and pain-free death. The family are central to the nursing care offered at these distressing times and another important goal of care is to assist the family to have positive memories of their child's final days until the time of death.

The death of a child is a significant event for the parents/carers and all their family. The minute details of the events leading up to the death of a child can be engrained on the minds of the families forever, so it is essential that the potential for unnecessarily distressing memories is minimised. It may be that a child is brought into the resuscitation room of an emergency department. Shaw et al. (2011) provide a useful literature review which highlights the debate and discussion about whether parents/carers should be witnesses to the resuscitation of their child. Some parents need to witness that everything possible has been done for their child. Other parents may find the whole situation too distressing to be involved in. The main issue here is to communicate openly with the family, explain the options and offer them a choice, respecting the decision made and offering the support of a caring nurse.

Another important aspect when caring for a dying child is to remember to include the parents and wider family in the care that is offered the child, for example washing the child, changing clothes. Again, choices should be given and the parent's decision respected. In the final days and hours, the family may want privacy but also the reassurance that a nurse is close by. The parents may want time alone, away from the child, but the confidence that a nurse will stay with their child so he or she is not alone. Care of the dying child requires compassion and a willingness to communicate openly and honestly with the parents. The nurse also needs to work closely with other health professionals to avoid offering conflicting information to the parents.

A big decision for parents concerns the environment where the child might receive their end-of-life care: in hospital, at home or in a hospice. There may not always be the opportunity to offer all these choices if the child is so acutely ill that they die in the resuscitation room or on intensive care, but if possible the options should be discussed with the parents so they can make an informed choice. The RCN (2021) provides a valuable resource concerning palliative and end-of-life care for CYP.

A selection of topics have been discussed related to a child's end-of-life care. There are many other important aspects to

165

consider, such as the child's age and understanding of their imminent death, the care and support that can be offered to siblings at the end of life, and the care that can be offered to the whole family following the death of their child. These are all fascinating topics but beyond the scope of this chapter. There are several excellent resources which will support further understanding of these issues.

Key Points

- The care and communication shared with children and young people (CYP) should be appropriate to their developmental stage.
- Parents and carers are, in the majority of situations, fundamental to the well-being of CYP. Healthcare professionals must establish an open, professional relationship with the CYP's carers if they are to offer holistic, person-centred care.
- An infant, child or young person's health can deteriorate rapidly. Healthcare professionals must be alert to subtle changes in the CYP and any concerns raised by the child's parent/carer.
- Care offered to CYP should be relevant to all aspects of their well-being: physical, emotional, social and spiritual.
- Protecting CYP is everyone's responsibility.

References

Advanced Life Support Group (2016) *Advanced Paediatric Life Support. The Practical Approach*, 6th edn. Wiley Blackwell, Oxford.

Association for Young People's Health (2016) *A Public Health Approach to Promoting Young People's Resilience*. AYPH, London.

Asthma UK (2021) *What is Asthma?* www.asthma.org.uk/advice/understanding-asthma/what-is-asthma/ (accessed December 2021).

Bee, H.L. & Boyd, D.R. (2014) *The Developing Child*, 13th edn. Pearson, Harlow.

British Medical Association (2018) *Volume depletion in children*. https://bestpractice.bmj.com/topics/en-gb/706 (accessed December 2021)

Clark, M. (2020) *2019 Triennial Analysis of Serious Case Reviews: Health Professionals*. Research in Practice, Devon.

Coleman, J. (2011) *The Nature of Adolescence*, 4th edn. Routledge, Hove.

Darbyshire, P. (1994) *Living with a Sick Child in Hospital. The Experiences of Parents and Nurses*. Chapman & Hall, London.

Department of Health (2015) *Future in Mind: Promoting, protecting and improving our children and young people's mental health and wellbeing*. www.england.nhs.uk/blog/martin-mcshane-14/ (accessed December 2021)

Dodds, H. (2010) Meeting the needs of young people in hospital. *Paediatric Nursing*, 22(9), 16–20.

Flynn, A., Whittaker, K., Donne, A.J., Bray, L. & Carter, B. (2020) Holding their own and being resilient: narratives of parents over the first 12 months of their child having tracheostomy. *Comprehensive Child and Adolescent Nursing*. doi: 10.1080/24694193.2020.1785046 (accessed December 2021).

Foster, J.P., Dawson, J.A., Davis, P.G. & Dahlen, H.G. (2017) Routine oro/nasopharyngeal suction versus no suction at birth. *Cochrane Database of Systematic Reviews*, 4(4), CD010332.

Freedman, S.B., Pasichnyk, D., Black, K.J., *et al.* (2015) Gastroenteritis therapies in developed countries: systematic review and meta-analysis. *PLoS One*, 10(6), e0128754.

General Medical Council (2021) *0–18 years: Guidance for all Doctors*. www.gmc-uk.org/ethical-guidance/ethical-guidance-for-doctors/0-18-years/introduction (accessed December 2021).

Gormley-Fleming, E. (2010) Assessment and vital signs: a comprehensive review. In: A. Glasper, M. Aylott & C. Battrick (eds) *Developing Practical Skills for Nursing Children and Young People*. Hodder Arnold, London.

Gormley-Fleming, E. & Martin, D. (eds) (2018) *Children and Young People's Nursing Skills at a Glance*. Wiley, Oxford.

HM Government (2018) *Working Together to Safeguard Children. A Guide to Inter-agency Working to Safeguard and Promote the Welfare of Children*. https://assets.publishing.service.gov.uk/government/uploads/system/uploads/attachment_data/file/942454/Working_together_to_safeguard_children_inter_agency_guidance.pdf (accessed December 2021).

Howard, J. & McInnes, K. (2013) *The Essence of Play*. Routledge, Oxford.

Kenner, C.P., Altimier, L.D. & Boykova, M.V. (eds) (2019) *Comprehensive Neonatal Nursing Care*, 6th edn. Springer, New York.

Laming, Lord (2003) *The Victoria Climbie Inquiry*. http://webarchive.nationalarchives.gov.uk/20130401151715/https:/www.education.gov.uk/publications/eOrderingDownload/CM-5730PDF.pdf (accessed December 2021).

Lee, J.H., Son, S.W. & Cho, S.H. (2016) A comprehensive review of the treatment of atopic eczema. *Allergy, Asthma & Immunology Research*, 8(3), 181–190.

Lewis, G., Addison, A., Machingaifa, F. & McGuire, R. (2020) *Identifying AEFI in Diverse Skin Colour*. https://mvec.mcri.edu.au/references/identifying-aefi-in-diverse-skin-colour/ (accessed December 2021).

Lightfoot, C., Cole, M. & Cole, S. (2018) *The Development of Children*, 8th edn. Worth, New York.

Lissauer, T. & Carroll, W. (2018) *Illustrated Textbook of Paediatrics*, 5th edn. Elsevier, Philadelphia, PA.

Maslow, A.H. (1943) A theory of human motivation. *Psychological Review*, 50(4), 370–396.

Morgan, S. (2017) *Young people with cancer want more honesty from health professionals*. https://rcni.com/nursing-standard/opinion/comment/sue-morgan-young-people-cancer-want-more-honesty-health-professionals-91916 (accessed December 2021).

Munro, E. (2011) *The Munro Review of Child Protection: Final Report. A Child-centred System*. www.gov.uk/government/publications/munro-review-of-child-protection-final-report-a-child-centred-system (accessed December 2021).

National Institute for Health and Care Excellence (2018) *Febrile Seizure*. https://cks.nice.org.uk/topics/febrile-seizure/ (accessed December 2021).

NHS (2019) *NHS Long Term Plan*. www.longtermplan.nhs.uk/ (accessed December 2021).

NSPCC (2021) *Child Protection System in the UK*. https://learning.nspcc.org.uk/child-protection-system (accessed December 2021).

Nursing & Midwifery Council (2018a) *Future Nurse: Standards of proficiency for registered nurses*. www.nmc-uk.org/ (accessed December 2021).

Nursing & Midwifery Council (2018b) *Standards of proficiency for nursing associates*. www.nmc-uk.org/ (accessed December 2021).

Office for National Statistics (2021) *Child and Infant Mortality in England and Wales, 2019*. www.ons.gov.uk/peoplepopulationandcommunity/birthsdeathsandmarriages/deaths/bulletins/childhoodinfantandperinatalmortalityinenglandandwales/2019#child-and-infant-mortality-(accessed December 2021).

Parkin, E. & Long, R. (2021) *Support for Children and Young People's Mental Health*. https://commonslibrary.parliament.uk/research-briefings/cbp-7196/ (accessed December 2021).

Royal College of Nursing (2020) *Standards for Assessing, Measuring and Monitoring Vital Signs in Infants, Children and Young People*. RCN Publishing, London.

Royal College of Nursing (2021) *Palliative and End of Life Care*. www.rcn.org.uk/clinical-topics/children-and-young-people/palliative-and-end-of-life-care-nursing (accessed December 2021).

Royal College of Paediatrics and Child Health (2020) *Adolescent Mortality*. https://stateofchildhealth.rcpch.ac.uk/evidence/mortality/adolescent-mortality/ (accessed December 2021).

Sanchez-Pinto, L.N., González-Dambrauskas, S., Jabornisky, R., *et al.* (2020) Sepsis hysteria? Not for children. *Lancet*, 396(10259), 1332–1333.

Sanderson, L. (2015) Developing a Teddy bear clinic: a framework for involving child service users in a nursing curriculum. In: G. Brewer & R. Hogarth (eds) *Creative Education, Teaching and Learning*. Palgrave Macmillan, London.

Sharma, A. & Cockerill, H. (2014) *Mary Sheridan's from Birth to Five Years: Children's Developmental Progress*, 4th edn. Routledge, London.

Shaw, K., Ritchie, D. & Adams, G. (2011) Does witnessing resuscitation help parents come to terms with the death of their child? A review of the literature. *Intensive and Critical Care Nursing*, 27(5), 253–262.

Teenage Cancer Trust (2016) *A Blueprint of Care for Teenagers and Young Adults with Cancer*, 2nd edn. Teenage Cancer Trust, London. www.teenagecancertrust.org/sites/default/files/BlueprintOfCare_2nd Edition.pdf (accessed December 2021).

Together for Short Lives (2021) *Editable Hospital Passport Template*. www.togetherforshortlives.org.uk/resource/editable-hospital-passport-template/ (accessed December 2021).

United Nations Convention on the Rights of the Child (1989) www.gov.uk/government/publications/united-nations-convention-on-the-rights-of-the-child-uncrc-how-legislation-underpins-implementation-in-england (accessed December 2021).

Vaz, I. (2013) Visual symbols in healthcare settings for children with learning disabilities and autism spectrum disorder. *British Journal of Nursing*, 22(3), 156–159.

Williams, L., Eilers, J., Heermann, J. & Smith, K. (2012) The lived experience of parents and guardians providing care for child transplant recipients. *Progress in Transplantation*, 22(4), 393–402.

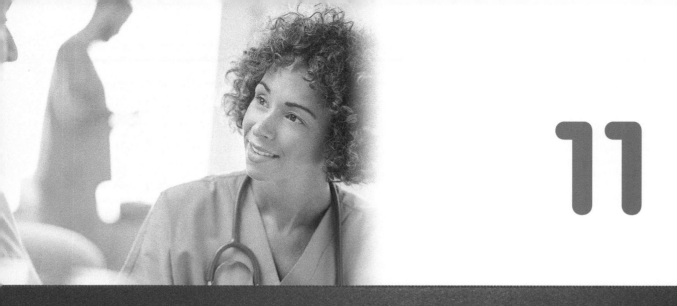

11

The Principles of Caring for People with Mental Health Problems

Louise Lingwood and Colin Cameron

Northumbria University Newcastle, UK

Learning Outcomes

On completion of this chapter you will be able to:

- The policy context for contemporary mental health nursing care and of the contexts for mental health care, including settings for care and legal contexts
- The various approaches to understanding mental health issues
- The principles of the 'recovery' approach
- The principles of holism in the delivery of nursing care for people with mental health issues
- The impact of mental health on physical health and well-being
- The principles of nursing care for people experiencing emotional disturbance and their carers, including assessment, management and therapeutic nursing care

Proficiencies

NMC Proficiencies and Standards:

- Demonstrate and articulate through reflection an understanding of and the ability to challenge discriminatory behaviour
- Provide and promote non-discriminatory person-centred and sensitive care at all times, reflecting on people's values and beliefs, diverse backgrounds, cultural characteristics, language requirements, needs and preferences, taking account of any need for adjustments
- Discuss how health inequalities may impact on the health and well-being of the individual and their choices
- Recognise and assist in the assessment of people who may be at risk of harm and the situations that may put them at risk, escalating concerns as appropriate to safeguard those who are vulnerable

 Visit the companion website at www.wiley.com/go/peate/nursingpractice3e where you can test yourself using flashcards, multiple-choice questions and more.

Nursing Practice: Knowledge and Care, Third Edition. Edited by Ian Peate and Aby Mitchell.
© 2022 John Wiley & Sons Ltd. Published 2022 by John Wiley & Sons Ltd.
Companion website: www.wiley.com/go/peate/nursingpractice3e

Introduction

Nurses will encounter service users who experience emotional disturbance or mental health issues across all fields of nursing and in all settings. Mental health issues may not always be recognised or acknowledged and may go unaddressed and escalate in seriousness. This can lead to a deterioration of a person's emotional and physical health, have a negative impact upon their quality of life and cause a person's overall health and safety to potentially become severely compromised. Mental health issues affect one in four people and half are established by the age of 14. One in 10 children and young people has a diagnosable mental health issue and three-quarters of the population receive no help at all in relation to their mental health (Mental Health Task Force, 2016).

Globally there is a well-established link between the mental health of children of adults with mental health issues, as they are often diagnosed with disorders such as bipolar, depression, post-traumatic stress and anxiety (Landstedt & Almquist, 2019). Mental health issues not only affect the mother's health and well-being but may have long-term implications for their children's emotional, social and cognitive development and health (Mental Health Taskforce, 2016).

Data from the Office for National Statistics (ONS) warns of a looming crisis in terms of mental health demand and access to services (Health Foundation, 2021). People in marginalised groups, including black, Asian and minority ethnic (BAME) people, lesbian, gay, bisexual and transgender people, disabled people, children and young people and those who face unemployment and poverty are at the greatest risk of developing mental health issues (Mental Health Task Force, 2016). There is a financial cost of mental health issues to the UK economy and the indirect and direct costs of mental health issues are growing. In 2014, the Organisation for Economic Co-operation and Development estimated this at £70 billion and that 40% of all new claimants for disability benefit each year are accounted for by mental health issues. In 2020, the cost in England alone is estimated to be almost £119 billion a year, a sharp increase when compared to calculated costs from 2010 of £105 billion (Centre for Mental Health, 2020).

Nurses work in partnership with people who experience chronic, complex and perhaps long-term needs associated with mental health issues, in conjunction with co-morbid physical illnesses, learning disabilities and difficulties. Some mental health issues can be persistent and episodic in nature. Presentations can vary in acuteness, where at one end of a continuum (acute crisis) high-intensity person-centred care and support from interprofessional teams is needed and, at the other end of the continuum, low-intensity ongoing support (i.e. when symptoms have abated or resolved).

Policy Context

Service user involvement in all aspects of their care is a mandatory requirement of current mental health policy. Similarly, service users have been increasingly involved in sustainable quality improvement, the co-production of research and the commissioning of clinical services. The mental health strategy for England, *No Health Without Mental Health* (Department of Health, 2011), sought to improve the mental health of people with existing mental health issues. The policy identified six priority areas to address, outlined in Box 11.1. *Every Mind Matters* (NHS, 2019) was the first NHS mental health online platform and built on the action campaigns of *Time to Change*, *Rethink* and *Mental Health First Aid* in urging people to move from talking about the issues of mental health to taking action to address the stigma present. In addition, the impact of the COVID-19 pandemic and the restrictions on people's everyday lives has been well publicised, raising the profile of mental health globally. In the UK, the *NHS Long Term Plan* (Department of Health, 2019) recognised the pressures on mental health services across the NHS. This policy places an emphasis on moving from 'one size fits all' to a tailored individualised approach to care.

> **Jot This Down**
> - Think about the implications of these mental health objectives in your field of practice.
> - Considering these objectives, what contribution can you make to the health and well-being of people with mental health issues?

The strategy is both a public mental health strategy and a strategy for social justice (Department of Health, 2011, p.3), and recognises the link between mental health and social inequalities (such as lack of employment prospects, poor housing, social exclusion, discrimination and so forth) and that they contribute to the way people experience mental health.

> **Box 11.1 Six High-level Mental Health Objectives**
> 1. More people will have good mental health
> 2. More people with mental health problems will recover
> 3. More people with mental health problems will have good physical health
> 4. More people will have a positive experience of care and support
> 5. Fewer people will suffer avoidable harm
> 6. Fewer people will experience stigma and discrimination
>
> *Source:* Department of Health (2011)

The 2011 Mental Health Strategy went some way to encouraging people to access services. However, many services faced low staffing numbers and inadequate funding to meet the new demand. Concerns emerged related to the quality and safety of mental healthcare, increased pressures on services and the increase in suicide rates. A report from the independent Mental Health Taskforce (2016) concluded that those inequalities are still present, reiterating that people are marginalised and stigmatised because of attitudes towards their mental health. In a pledge of commitment to change, the Independent Task Force set a 10-year vision to address what service users identified as their priorities. Service users stated they wanted to have equal opportunities, prevention, access, integration, quality and a positive experience of care.

In the policy *Choosing Health: Supporting the Physical Health Needs of People with Severe Mental Illness* (Department of Health, 2006), attention was focused on the tendency for people who experience mental health issues to be at increased risk of developing serious physical health issues. The *NHS Long Term Plan* (Department of Health, 2019) indicated that those with serious mental health issues are at higher risk than the general population of developing diabetes, cardiovascular and respiratory disease and obesity. The parity of esteem principle, which mandates equal importance of mental and physical health, was protected in law by the Health and Social Care Act 2012.

The use of medication traditionally employed to manage mental health issues (Faulkner & Layzell, 2000) has been de-emphasised in recent times and a focus placed on the provision of social and psychological care that is hopeful, optimistic and positive. The *NHS Long Term Plan* sought to turn the vision of transforming services into 'a reality'. The achievement of this continues to be reliant on tackling stigma and inequality (Box 11.2).

The term 'recovery' has traditionally had its roots in the biomedical model and often has been understood as the return to some former health status or the absence of symptoms caused by ill health. This understanding has historically been accepted by both the public and those working within health and social care settings. In recent years, biomedical definitions have been challenged on an international scale and there has been a shift of understanding about what recovery means within the field of mental health.

The lens has moved from a view of clinical recovery to one of personal recovery that is subjective in nature and whilst some overlap may be evident in the experiences of individuals, people's understanding of their own recovery journey may change over time (Slade *et al.*, 2014). The focus is on living life to the full regardless of the clinical recovery that has occurred. The emphasis is on acceptance of self and mastery of the decisions people make in their own lives (Anthony, 2000).

This recovery approach has found expression in mental health policies, for example *The NHS Plan* (Department of Health, 2000) and *The NHS Long Term Plan* (Department of Health, 2019). Both emphasise the importance of supportive, collaborative therapeutic alliances and shared decision making between service users and healthcare professionals in the shaping of policy and practice. There is a recognition that people have strengths, talents and abilities as well as needs and issues. However, abuses of the recovery frameworks occur to justify cuts in mental health provision (Slade *et al.*, 2014). The themes most

important to personal recovery are connected to what is important to us as humans. These include connectedness, hope, identity, meaning and empowerment (CHIME factors). These CHIME factors are intrinsically linked to the meaning that individuals give to their lives, their spirituality. This moves the focus from the recovery of mental health illness to personal recovery (Lukoff, 2007).

The Care Programme Approach (CPA) has been central to government mental health policy since 1990 (Department of Health, 2008a). The CPA aims to ensure that people with mental health issues who have been in contact with mental health services receive the ongoing care they need through providing:

- Arrangements for holistic assessment
- A care plan documenting agreed mental health goals
- A care co-ordinator who will provide ongoing monitoring and support and co-ordinate care
- Regular review and agreed amendments to the care plan.

Today, the principles of the CPA have a renewed meaning that emphasises the personalisation, promotion of social inclusion, involvement and engagement in individual personal recovery journeys.

Jot This Down

The current unemployment rate in the UK is 4.8% of the economically active population aged over 16 years of age (ONS, 2021b). The unemployment rate of people with a mental health issue is 43% (Health Foundation, 2021b).

Many people who experience long-term mental health issues are unemployed but wish to work. Consider some of the issues facing the person with mental health issues who wishes to enter the labour market.

Drop the Disorder?

There is much debate over definitions of health and disability and what they mean. The World Health Organization (WHO) defines health as 'not merely the absence of disease or infirmity' (WHO, 1946). It further defines mental health as:

'... a state of well-being in which the individual realises his or her own abilities, can cope with the normal stresses of life, can work productively and fruitfully, and is able to make a contribution to his or her community'

(WHO, 2007).

Disability is often understood as a characteristic of individual deficit or personal tragedy, as something arising directly from an impairment; for example, mental health being measured in terms of normality and abnormality. In the International Classification of Functioning, Disability and Health (WHO, 2013), disability retains its character as an unfortunate individual condition:

'Disability is an umbrella term for impairments, activity limitations and participation restrictions. It denotes the negative aspects of the interaction between an individual (with a health condition) and that individual's contextual factors (environmental and personal factors).'

Box 11.2 Guiding Principles for Addressing Stigma and Inequality in Mental Health

- Meaningful engagement with stakeholders
- Genuine partnerships
- Leadership
- Co-production of strategies with people with lived experience of mental health issues

The WHO International Classification of Impairments, Disabilities and Handicaps (1981) encapsulates the core meaning of the biomedical model and its application. The following definitions capture why:

'Impairment: any loss or abnormality of psychological, physiological or anatomical structure or function.'

'Disability: any restriction or lack (resulting from impairment) of ability to perform an activity in the manner or within the range considered normal for a human being'

(WHO, 1976).

Disability, then, is identified as an embodied condition or a physical attribute belonging to an individual. It is seen as a personal flaw and implies a requirement for response in terms of a cure, care or rehabilitation.

There are several models that seek to explain the development of mental health issues. For example, the biomedical model considers mental illness as a product of abnormalities or disease processes within the body. These might include, for example, genetic heritability, dysfunction with neurotransmitters or differences in the structure of the brain among people identified as having mental health illnesses (Kring *et al.*, 2010). The biomedical model also seeks to establish a diagnosis, which forms the basis of clinical decision making with respect to medical care and treatment. Biomedical model thinking has dominated health and social care education and institutional thinking about health in general within the wider society. It is reflected within cultural narratives and the ceaseless recycling of stereotyped representations, portraying disabled people as 'victims' or as 'plucky strugglers' (Cameron, 2014, pp.144–146).

There are two main classification systems used in the field of mental health to inform a diagnosis:

- *International Classification of Diseases*, 11th revision (ICD-11) (WHO, 2021a)
- *Diagnostic and Statistical Manual of Mental Disorders*, 5th edition (DSM-5) (American Psychiatric Association, 2013).

Perceived benefits of a mental health diagnosis include the determination of interventions and treatments, clarity between professionals and access to peer support. A diagnosis may also be considered a comfort to service users (Norman & Ryrie, 2018). However, a diagnosis can be seen as a stigmatising label serving to marginalise or exclude people from communities. Risk exists that a person's lived experience may be lost through diagnosis, as experiences can change over time or symptoms diluted to fit the boxes required. Concerns about the reliability of diagnoses have been debated and are based on subjective observation according to the psychiatrist's personal bias rather than a cataloguing of objective symptoms (De Silva, 2017). These symptoms may be amplified if the person has experienced trauma, neglect or abuse (Bond, 2019). reminding us of the importance of focusing on individual need and enabling people to be active participants in their care (Munro, 2021).

A biomedical lens would perceive a person's behaviour as odd, deviant or objectionable, or not conforming to prevailing 'social norms' and as such they may be considered symptomatic of 'mental illnesses'. It is also important to ensure that cultural differences in communication or behaviour are not misinterpreted. It has often been argued that psychiatric medication can be helpful to individuals in terms of their recovery and medication has been the single most important development in treatment (Krauss & Slavinsky, 1982). However, it must be acknowledged that there are sometimes significant consequences for an individual who has been prescribed medication for mental health issues, including many major side-effects such as toxicity and dependence.

Engel (1977) argued that the biomedical model may restrict our understanding of health and illness and there are other approaches which may offer a fuller explanation of mental distress. The social model is an alternative perspective that was established by the Disabled People's Movement. The social model, developed initially in 1976 by the Union of the Physically Impaired Against Segregation and later by Disabled Peoples' International (DPI), redefines disability as an unequal social relationship within a society that has failed to take account of the needs of people with impairments, or to plan for their inclusion in everyday community life (Cameron & Lingwood, 2020). The social model defines the terms 'impairment' and 'disability' as:

'Impairment: the loss or limitation of physical, mental or sensory function on a long term, or permanent basis.'

'Disability: the loss or limitation of opportunities to take part in the normal life of the community on an equal level with others due to physical and social barriers.'

Whilst policy moves towards addressing discrimination, the attitudes and assumptions relating to mental health issues still require attention (Heaton, 2014, pp.1–3). While the precise causes of mental health issues are unknown, it is believed that social, psychological, biological and environmental factors interact to increase the risk of developing mental issues. Adverse life events and stressors (such as financial troubles, bereavements and unemployment) are often cited, for example, as risk factors for depression. There is growing evidence that the highest rates of depression are to be found in the most deprived neighbourhoods (WHO, 2014).

A person's biology may also be implicated. For example, depression often seems to run in families and those with the most genetic similarity (such as monozygotic twins) seem to have higher concordance rates (Kring *et al.*, 2010). Neurochemical changes in the brain may also play a part in depression (such as decreased levels of the neurotransmitter serotonin) (Cowen & Browning, 2015). There are also higher rates of depression among those who have suffered trauma to their brain (traumatic brain injury) (Brown, 2004). Depression may be associated with lower volumes of grey matter in the prefrontal cortex, the part of the brain which is responsible for speech, decision making and goal-directed behaviour, and people diagnosed with depression show elevated activity in the amygdala (the structure in the brain associated with assessing the emotional importance of a stimulus) (Kring *et al.*, 2010). The impact of adverse socio-economic conditions on people's health, including diet, obesity or risk of trauma, is well known. Experiences of health or ill health are not just 'natural', but rather always experienced within unequal social structures. In addition, poor nutrition and diet have also been linked to mental health problems.

171

Red Flag

Almost 20.6% of adults reported thoughts of suicide and one person in 15 had made a suicide attempt (Adult Psychiatric Morbidity Survey, 2014).

In the UK, there were 5316 suicides in 2020 (ONS, 2021a). Suicide is therefore a serious health issue, with depression being a significant risk factor. It is important that the nurse is vigilant when caring for the person who is depressed and alert to any warning signs that they may be considering taking their lives. Concerns of family members and carers must be listened to and fully acknowledged.

Settings for Mental Healthcare

Mental health service provision in the UK is arranged in a three-tier structure, comprising primary, secondary and tertiary care. Mental health services are commissioned nationally by NHS England, and jointly at a local level by clinical commissioning groups and local authorities.

Primary care mental health support and treatment has historically been predominantly provided by non-specialised professionals such as GPs. GP's and other primary care professionals are generally the first point of contact for anyone experiencing mental health issues, and the response from these professionals will depend on their skills, attitudes and experience. It is therefore imperative that these professionals have the skills to detect mental health issues and can consistently plan for and access the most appropriate, evidence-based approaches to care or refer to specialist services where necessary (PHE, 2017).

In a survey of 1000 GPs, 66% stated that they had experienced an increase in demand for appointments pertaining to mental health issues and that 40% of all appointments made involved mental health (Mind.org, 2018). GPs will usually instigate treatment options based on NICE guidance, including the use of medicines, counselling or talking therapy. The 'Improving Access to Psychological Therapies' (IAPT) programme aimed to reduce waits in the healthcare system through providing increased access to well-being practitioners, trained cognitive behaviour therapists and psychologists (Health Foundation, 2015). Critiques have described IAPT as involving the industrialisation of care. In addition, CBT has faced criticism from person-centred practitioners for its tendency to see the person as the problem (Proctor, 2006).

Integrated primary care services or 'Primary Care Plus' was launched in 2015 to provide specialist mental health liaison services to primary care. Primary Care Plus has four core elements:

- Assessment and referral
- Relapse prevention and shared care
- Health promotion and education
- Training and consultation.

Primary Care Plus has assisted with early intervention to prevent immediate referral to secondary care. It also played a role in the discharge of mental health service users from secondary care back to primary care (NHS London Strategic Clinical Networks, 2014).

Social prescribing, sometimes known as community referral, enables health professionals to refer people to non-clinical services. There are differing models of social prescribing. Most involve a link worker who will holistically support people to improve their own health and well-being. The link worker may be based within a statutory, voluntary, community and social enterprise or charitable organisation. Other models involve health advisors, connectors or navigators (King's Fund, 2020). The role involves supporting someone to consider what is important to them, provide time, signpost or refer the person to the appropriate services. It is hoped that there will be 900 000 referrals to social prescribing by 2023–24, supporting individual care and reducing pressure on the NHS (NHS England, 2019).

Secondary care services are specialist mental health services based in community settings and are part of the national move to reconfigure mental health service provision towards more personalised and cost-effective care (Department of Health, 2010, 2011). It has more recently been recognised that community-based mental health services have been inflexible and disparate, particularly in accessing urgent and emergency assessment and treatment. Out-of-hours crisis care in mental health is not of a standard equal to the care available on weekdays during office hours (Department of Health, 2014a; Care Quality Commission, 2015). This has led to a focus on access to services 24 hours a day, 7 days a week, and implementing urgent care standards aiming towards parity of esteem between physical and mental healthcare (Department of Health, 2013, 2014a).

The remit of secondary care services is to assess and treat people with acute, severe and/or enduring mental health issues. Assessment services and brief treatment services manage referrals for persons over 18 years, excluding those with an organic condition, and provide short-term treatment and follow-up. Community recovery teams such as Assertive Outreach support those with complex presentations, who may not engage, and may present with a co-morbid and dual diagnoses. These teams have now merged with general mental health community teams to drive efficiency savings.

Services also exist for people who are in acute mental health crisis so that they can receive support outside the confines of hospital. These include psychiatric liaison teams, who assess and treat patients in general acute hospitals who may also have mental health and social care needs. Co-morbid mental health and physical health issues can often lengthen a patient's admission to general hospital, and if untreated and unsupported, can lead to a poorer long-term outcome.

Home treatment or crisis resolution teams were implemented nationally as part of the NSF Framework for Mental Health (Department of Health, 1999). Personal benefits to service users include enhanced control over their own mental health and support provided at home by families and friends. Cost benefits exist, with inpatient care being more expensive than community care. The establishment of crisis teams, cafés, safe havens and sanctuaries has been mandated (Department of Health, 2000) and the Crisis Care Concordat pushed for timely access to crisis care (Department of Health, 2014a). In response, crisis and assessment services expanded to provide rapid assessment 24 hours a day, 365 days a year. It is intended that service users will be assessed and treated more rapidly through mobile and home-based interventions as well as 'street triaging' with emergency services, to prevent further deterioration, improve prognosis and reduce crisis presentations to accident and emergency departments (Department of Health, 2014a). In 2020, a measure on waiting times for emergency mental healthcare was established as the first ever of its kind.

Specialist services are in place for older people with organic mental health problems, including cognitive impairment and dementia. Early intervention services exist for young people aged 18–35, presenting with first symptoms of psychosis. Prompt treatment within this group has been shown to improve long-term mental health and reduce suicide rates and hospital admissions (Singh, 2010). Specialist services in perinatal mental health support pregnant and postnatal women and are expanding nationally to support women with mental health problems and their families. Other specialist mental health services include personality disorder services, gender identity clinics, eating disorder services, D/deaf services, police liaison, custody and court diversion services. The voluntary and community sector also plays an important role in supporting and promoting social inclusion relating to mental health issues.

Tertiary care mental health services refer to inpatient care usually provided in hospital-based settings. The main inpatient facilities in the UK are acute services (comprising assessment and recovery wards), psychiatric intensive care and forensic services. As community-based mental health services and a focus on cost efficiency have increased, inpatient facilities have provided shorter care spells to only the most complex service users. Unfortunately, the national reduction in inpatient beds has increased bed occupancy rates, and a greater need to transfer service users to out-of-area hospitals has negatively impacted on care quality, service user experience and safety (King's Fund, 2015).

It has also been identified that the merging of specialist community services and the reduction of inpatient services have led to an increased risk of suicide. This is because high-risk service users are being treated by either generic community services or crisis teams in the community rather than in inpatient settings (Healthcare Quality Improvement Partnership, 2013).

Recovery

Mental health services have often focused on medical symptomatology, and the use of medication. In the words of Murray (2012, p.4), 'in mental health care medication is prioritised at the expense of psychological interventions and social rehabilitation'. 'Recovery' in a biomedical sense may be seen to be achieved if a person is free of symptoms of mental illness or if they have been 'cured' (Matthews, 2008). Many people with mental health issues, in this sense, may not be expected to 'recover' and are therefore perceived to need long-term psychiatric care and medication.

The 'recovery approach' has become increasingly important in mental healthcare, in terms of both policy development and nursing care (Repper & Perkins, 2003). This recovery-focused approach stresses the importance of a hopeful, optimistic, positive approach to the care and treatment of all people who use mental health services (Department of Health, 2001). The recovery approach distinguishes between 'complete recovery' and 'social recovery' (which focuses on supporting the process of recovery, emphasising support for the person to improve their overall quality of life, despite the presence of 'psychiatric symptoms') (Matthews, 2008).

173

The social recovery approach highlights the importance of:

- Working in partnership and shared decision making with service users
- Development of a supportive and empathic professional working alliance
- Approaches that reflect the service user's preference based on an informed discussion
- A recognition of personal strengths, abilities and assets that may be used in the recovery process
- Support to cope with future challenges that mental health issues may bring (Trenoweth & Allymamod, 2010).

Holism

A personal recovery approach requires a holistic focus in the assessment and delivery of nursing care (Sin & Trenoweth, 2010). Holism encompasses the whole of the person, the biological social, psychological and spiritual being.

Spirituality is an aspect of the person often misunderstood and ignored. It is not necessarily the same as religious affiliation, but it may be used to connote belief in a divine power (metaphysical) and as a reference to the philosophies, values and beliefs that help us to make sense of our lives (existential) (Goddard, 1995). There may, of course, be a connection between metaphysical and existential forms of spirituality, but this cannot be assumed or expected. There are also large numbers of people in the UK who have no religious affiliation and it would be incorrect to say that they were not spiritual.

The National Census in 2011 gathered data on religious affiliation; the questions were not mandatory and of those who answered, 25% did not identify with any religion (ONS, 2020a). Listening to the meanings that a mental health service user places on their lives supports understanding of their frame of reference. This requires open-mindedness and effective interpersonal skills, as we encourage people to share with us the issues that matter to them in their lives.

It is recognised that a lack of 'hope' can have a detrimental impact in the trajectory of mental health and the concept of 'hope' is central to an individual's personal recovery (Stickley & Wright, 2011). Hope is:

'a process of anticipation that involves the interaction of thinking, acting, feeling and relating, and is directed toward a future fulfilment that is personally meaningful'

(Stephenson, 1991, p.1459).

174

Caring for Carers

A carer can be defined as someone who helps another person, usually a relative or friend, in their day-to-day life. Each day 6.5 million people have a caring responsibility for another (CarersUK, 2020). Unfortunately, the needs of carers have often been overlooked. It is important to recognise the impact that such caring can have on carers, acknowledging they may require support themselves. In fact, the strains, responsibilities and subsequent emotional and financial implications of caring can lead to carers' own mental health being compromised (Age UK, 2019). **The Care Act** (Department of Health, 2014b) was implemented to strengthen the rights of carers.

Parents may need to take carers' leave from work, which might have career and financial implications for the family. Other family members may be concerned that they may also develop a mental health issue.

Professionals need to signpost carers to support groups and voluntary agencies, provide advice regarding benefit entitlements and information about care and treatment options, and guide carers regarding what to do, and who to contact in the event of a crisis (Department of Health, 2014b). Specialist mental health services have provisions for assessing and responding to the specific needs of carers, aiming to support the balance between the caring role while maintaining their own health and well-being (Department of Health, 2014b).

Comprehensive Assessment in Mental Health

Assessment is considered the foundation on which mental healthcare is based (Coombs *et al.*, 2013). Assessment is therefore a central activity of the mental health nurse. Assessment is a continuous process and is reliant on the therapeutic relationship forged between the service user and mental health nurse. Nurses working in partnership with service users must use appropriate, supportive and empathic communication skills to encourage the individual to share their story (Launer, 2002). Traditional approaches to assessment have focused on problem solving and the pathology of mental health and therefore cannot be seen as comprehensive (Wand *et al.*, 2019).

Supporting recovery is the fundamental goal of mental health nursing. Assessment that uses a strengths-based approach and acknowledges the unique strengths of individuals can aid personal recovery. In addition, the service user is seen as the expert in their care. Assessments must also be culturally sensitive, and the nurse needs to gain the knowledge, skills and values required in understanding and working with diverse communities to enhance the quality of mental health care and assessment (Fogel *et al.*, 2021).

Physical Health

The phrase 'parity of esteem' represents the equal value that should be given to the physical health of people who have mental health issues. More fully, when compared to physical healthcare, it should be characterised by equal access to safe and high-quality care and treatment. Mental health services should be afforded equal efforts to innovate and improve provision, have access to equal educational opportunities and the aspirations of service users should be as high in terms of expectation (Panday, 2016).

'Parity of esteem' hopes to address the inequalities faced and reduce morbidity and mortality. People with long-standing mental health issues are more likely to have an overlap with physical healthcare needs and are less likely to receive preventive or appropriate physical healthcare to meet their needs in comparison to those with no mental health issues. People with mental health issues are at greater risk of premature death and often die 15–20 years earlier than the general population

(Chesney *et al.*, 2014). The stigma attached to mental health is often a barrier to healthcare-seeking behaviour (Clement *et al.*, 2015). This fear is often accompanied by a public fear of mental health (Baker & Gheera, 2020). Other modifiable risk factors include medication side-effects and lifestyle choices (Lawrence & Kisely, 2010). There may be an overemphasis on mental health issues. As such, 'diagnostic overshadowing', where the focus is on a person's primary mental health diagnosis to the exclusion of other health issues, may occur (Dean *et al.*, 2001; Friedli & Dardis, 2002). More worryingly, physical symptoms may be dismissed as being 'all in the person's mind' (Seymour, 2003).

What the Experts Say Physical Health

Our community mental health team runs a monthly 'physical health clinic' for service users less likely to attend their GP surgery or recognise their own physical health issues. Service users often feel more comfortable in familiar, relaxed environments run by healthcare professionals with specialist understanding of mental health issues. Service users are provided an extended appointment which includes measurement of clinical observations, blood sugar levels, body mass index and health promotion assessment and advice. This could include information about smoking cessation, dietary advice and referrals to in-house healthy lifestyles, cooking or sports groups. Reports are then passed on to the service user's GP with recommendations for any follow-up medical care or further investigations. Care co-ordinators are then able to empower and support service users to address any areas that require follow-up and continue with health promoting support.

Community Mental Health Nursing Team member

Red Flag

Never overlook the physical healthcare needs of people with mental health issues. As a nurse, you must ensure that the same advice and support are available to people with long-term mental healthcare needs as the general population. Nurses in all fields must be alert to co-morbid and co-existing health issues, which can affect the holistic well-being of their patients and service users. This may include considering and challenging one's assumptions about the overall healthcare needs of people with mental health issues

(Seymour, 2003).

It is well known that lifestyle factors and the environment influence mental health and are recognised predictors of physical health illness and death (WHO, 2014). Low levels of physical health activity, tobacco and excess alcohol use are more common modifiable lifestyle factors for people who have mental health issues. NHS trusts became smoke free following recommendations to encourage smoking cessation (NICE, 2013) to tackle the impact on health and demands on services.

The Nursing Associate Platform 2 - Promoting Health and Preventing Ill Health

'Nursing associates play a role in supporting people to improve and maintain their mental, physical, behavioural health and wellbeing. They are actively involved in the prevention of and protection against disease and ill health, and engage in public health, community development, and in the reduction of health inequalities' (NMC, 2018).

Case Study

Sarah is 60 years old. She lives alone in an upstairs flat and is not managing the stairs. Sarah is a heavy smoker, she states being alone makes her want to smoke more. She was recently diagnosed with COPD. She is feeling isolated and increasingly depressed. What are the evident holistic needs and how might they be addressed in partnership with Sarah?

175

Risk Assessment and Management

There may be an over-emphasis on the assessment and management of risk in mental health care, influenced by public perception that people with mental health issues are violent (Morgan, 1998). However, most people with mental health issues are not violent. This is not to say that an assessment of the risk of violence or aggression is unwarranted, but nurses need to maintain a sense of perspective. The Royal College of Psychiatrists (2021) provides general principles for assessing risk in the field of mental health. The assessment should take place with informed consent and an understanding of why the assessment is taking place, involve a comprehensive history, include the service user's (and their families/carers) narrative about their own level of risk and consider what the service user feels may reduce risk.

Jot This Down

Why is it, do you think, that there is a perception that people who experience mental health issues are more violent than the general population?

Suicidal behaviours should be met with a mental health suicide prevention strategy. Assessments to identify the risks present are known to often be inaccurate (Carter & Spittal, 2018) and care must be taken to ensure assessment is comprehensive and sensitive in nature. In 2016 rates of suicide were 9.7 per 10 000 people, 2018 saw the highest suicide rate, and in 2019 the suicide rate statistically was 11 deaths per 100,000; in 2020 this fell to 5224 suicides, or 10 deaths per 100,000 people (ONS, 2021a). The reduction is thought to be related to the COVID-19 pandemic and death reporting systems and a reduction in male suicide deaths between 2017 and 2019. Age is an important consideration with the rates increasing in the age group 1–24 years of age and in men 45–64 years of age (ONS, 2020b).

Suicide prevention was a priority of the *NHS Long Term Plan* (Department of Health, 2019), along with bereavement support. Risk assessment should encompass the known risk factors for suicide, as outlined in Box 11.3. Risk assessment must include not only factors relating to a person's previous history and current mental state but also social and environmental factors, which may also increase risk.

Box 11.3 Suicide Risk Factors (National Institute of Mental Health, 2021)

- A history of suicide attempts
- Depression, other mental disorders or substance use disorder
- Chronic pain
- Family history of a mental disorder or substance use
- Family history of suicide
- Exposure to family violence, including physical or sexual abuse
- Presence of guns or other firearms in the home
- Having recently been released from prison
- Exposure, either directly or indirectly, to others' suicidal behaviour, such as that of family members, peers or celebrities

---

What the Experts Say Suicide Risk

One of the questions I am most asked by students is 'How do you know how likely someone is to commit suicide?' I have found that therapeutic relationship and knowledge of individual clients to be one of the most valuable tools in gauging risk. A clinician's instinct or 'gut feeling' is also an important consideration, especially when they know the service user very well. Changes in emotional state, behaviour and social situation can be considered carefully in conjunction with knowledge of the actuarial risk factors. However, we often need to assess individuals we do not know, and it is especially important to try and establish an atmosphere of trust and openness in such situations. It can be challenging asking people sensitive questions, such as their intent to end their lives, and you may find their answers difficult to deal with. Asking key questions sensitively but directly is very important, with the aim of getting honest answers from the individual. Support should always be sought when you do not feel confident in dealing with the level of risk posed.

Mental Health Lecturer

However, people who experience serious, chronic, painful physical illnesses are also at heightened risk of suicide. In a recent study of suicides of people who contacted NHS Direct prior to suicide, over 50% reported physical health problems (Bessant *et al.*, 2008). There have been many strategies over the years to reduce the incidence of suicide. The recent National Suicide Prevention Strategy for England (Department of Health & Social Care, 2021) sets out the plan for a collective approach and a single strategy driving national, local and voluntary sectors to reduce suicide.

People who neglect their own personal health and hygiene are relatively common in mental healthcare. As such, self-neglect is an important risk, which needs to be assessed. The term 'self-neglect' is used to describe a personal lack of self-care to the extent where it threatens the person's health and safety.

Self-neglect may or may not be associated with a mental health issue (Dawson, 2020). On a less severe basis, people may not look after their diet and dental hygiene and not seek medical attention when ill. On the other end of the scale is severe self-neglect, such as a failure to look after physical health issues such as diabetes, the hoarding of rubbish and animals, both alive and dead, the presence of rotting food; poor personal hygiene, which could result in parasitic infestations and other infections; ignoring possible dangers from malfunctioning appliances, and so on (Gibbons *et al.*, 2006). There are many factors which must be taken into consideration when assessing self-neglect. Self-neglect may be associated with deteriorating health in older adults; this is also known as Diogenes syndrome (Box 11.4) (Social Care Institute for Excellence, 2018) and is related to living in squalid conditions, hoarding, social withdrawal, malnutrition (Khan, 2017) and a lack of shame. Self-neglect can also be related to emotional hurt or trauma. It may also result from the use of prescribed medication or be exacerbated by alcohol or drug misuse (Turner, 2019).

Box 11.4 Diogenes of Sinope (412–323 BCE)

Diogenes the Cynic was a philosopher who believed that through abandoning the traditional means of happiness, one could find happiness. He was famous for living in a wine barrel or jar and urinating in public and his rejection of comfort was a choice thought to be politically driven.

Self-neglect may be present among people who have poor social networks and people may have little or no engagement with services, increasing the risk of mortality (Turner, 2019). The Care Act (Department of Health, 2014b) includes self-neglect as a safeguarding issue under the category of abuse. Nurses must be self-aware of their own values and seek always to respect individual choice. Any assessor of self-neglect must consider what they perceive to be socially acceptable standards of cleanliness and hygiene as these are likely to vary between social groups and cultures. It is therefore subjective, and nurses may have different perceptions of what constitutes self-neglect from service users. The Care Act's revised statutory guidance (Department of Health, 2016) adds that: 'Assessment should be made on a case-by-case basis. A decision on whether a response is required under safeguarding will depend on the adult's ability to protect themselves by controlling their own behaviour. There may come a point when they are no longer able to do this, without external support'.

There are many risks associated with mental ill health and any assessment must consider the risks that a person poses to themselves or others. However, the risks to which the person is exposed also need to be considered in any risk assessment, such

Practice Assessment Document

As a student nurse, you are required to provide non-discriminatory, person-centred and sensitive care at all times, reflecting on other people's values and beliefs, diverse backgrounds, cultural characteristics, language requirements, needs and preferences, and taking account of any need for adjustments (PAD 2.5). You could reflect on your personal and professional values and share your reflections with your peers to support you to recognise differences. You could consider the role of clinical supervision and how this will support you with your ongoing professional development.

as the risk of abuse, being a victim of crime, social exclusion, isolation, poverty, poor access to physical healthcare, the risk of relapse, and so on.

The social determinants of health (SDOH) include social, cultural, political, economic, commercial and environmental factors. These factors do not act in isolation; they interconnect. They act together to reduce opportunity for education, work, income, appropriate housing, safety, access to services, health and well-being. They impact on people in differing ways according to a person's age, gender, ethnicity, sexuality and impairment. There is a social gradient that is related to health and illness. The higher the person's socio-economic position, the higher the chances are of good health. The lower people are on the social gradient, the worse the chances are for health. There is also an evident regional gradient in the UK, with the gradient being steeper in the north in comparison to the south (PHE, 2017). Inequalities in disadvantaged groups are likely to lead to certain groups of people having inadequate housing or food, unsafe environments, poorer educational attainment and living standards, and fewer opportunities in terms of employment and healthcare access (WHO, 2021b).

Stigma can result from misconceptions about people with mental health problems and the level of risk that they may be deemed to pose. Discrimination may have significant consequences for the person in terms of their employment prospects. Unemployment can lead to financial problems, thereby exacerbating the feelings of frustration, low self-esteem and entrapment. This, in turn, can increase the potential for suicidal thoughts and behaviour (Mathers & Schofield, 1998). This is recognised in *No Health Without Mental Health* (Department of Health, 2011). The strategy recognises the impact of social injustice and the risks posed by social inequalities, such as those mentioned earlier, which further compounds mental distress.

There is also a potential danger that people with mental health issues may be vulnerable to violence, sexual abuse or exploitation. Individuals, particularly at times of acute emotional or mental distress, may be especially at risk. Here, nurses must be mindful of such risks, particularly when the person has a known history of being physically or sexually abused; when the person appears to lack boundaries in relation to sexual expression or personal space or a lack of awareness, or passivity in the face of, their own risk when exposed to people who may wish to exploit them.

Legal Context

In England and Wales, the Mental Health Act 1983 (amended 2007) is the law which can be used to admit, detain and treat people who are deemed to have a mental health disorder against their wishes in a hospital setting. Imminent changes are expected in the next year. For a person to be detained under the Act, there must be clear grounds that:

- The person is suffering from a mental disorder of a nature or degree which warrants their detention in hospital for assessment and/or to receive treatment
- The person ought to be detained in their interest of their own health and safety with a view to the protection of others.

While a person may be compulsorily detained, the Mental Health Act (MHA) emphasises the need to involve service users in all appropriate aspects of their care and to promote a person's overall health and well-being while supporting their recovery from mental distress (Department of Health, 2008b). The guiding principles of the MHA are highlighted in Box 11.5.

The Mental Capacity Act 2005 (MCA) differs from the MHA, in that its purpose is to ensure that adults (aged 16 or over) who lack the mental capacity to make decisions for themselves are protected under the law. The MCA may apply not only to people with mental health issues, dementia and learning disabilities but also to people who may have a brain injury or are under the influence of substances or sedation.

> **Box 11.5 The Guiding Principles of the Mental Health Act**
>
> The MHA is founded on several important guiding principles, which include:
>
> - Minimum restriction which impacts a person's liberty
> - Respecting a person's views, wishes and feelings as far as possible, recognising an individual's race, religion, culture, gender, age, sexual orientation or impairment
> - The opportunity for service users to participate in their care, including decision making regarding planning and reviewing their care, and the involvement of carers and family members where possible
> - Providing care and treatment, which is effective and efficient in meeting identified healthcare needs.

'The act is intended to assist and support people who may lack capacity and to discourage anyone who is involved in caring for someone who lacks capacity from being overly restrictive or controlling. But the Act also aims to balance an individual's right to make decisions for themselves with their right to be protected from harm if they lack capacity to make decisions to protect themselves'

(Department for Constitutional Affairs, 2007, p.15).

A person may lack capacity if they are unable to:

- Understand information relevant to the decision, or
- Remember the information long enough to make the decision, or
- Weigh up information relevant to the decision, or
- Communicate their decision – by talking, using sign language, or by any other means (Care Quality Commission, 2011, p.5).

There are two stages to making a test of mental capacity. First, consideration must be given to whether there is an impairment

177

or disturbance in the functioning of a person's mind or brain. Then, if there is such impairment, is this sufficient to lead to a lack of capacity to make a particular decision?

The MCA is based on several important key principles: that a person has capacity unless the contrary has been established; people must be helped to make decisions; unwise decisions do not necessarily mean lack of capacity; decisions taken on behalf of the person must be in the person's best interests and must be as least restrictive of freedom as possible (Care Quality Commission, 2011). The MCA also makes it clear that if a person lacks mental capacity to make decisions, this does not imply that they lack capacity to make *any* decisions about their life (Care Quality Commission, 2011). The MCA also provides legal protection for nurses when they offer personal care for a person who lacks capacity (such as washing, dressing or attending to personal hygiene; eating and drinking; walking and assistance with transport), providing they are working within the principles and code of practice of the MCA.

In August 2021, the consultation outcome was published relating the reforms planned for the MHA. The plans for reform were delayed by the COVID-19 pandemic. Four principles, developed by the review and in partnership with people with lived experience, will guide and shape the government approach to reforming legislation, policy and practice. These are:

- Choice and autonomy – ensuring service users' views and choices are respected
- Least restriction – ensuring the Act's powers are used in the least restrictive way
- Therapeutic benefit – ensuring patients are supported to get better, so they can be discharged from the Act
- The person as an individual – ensuring patients are viewed and treated as individuals (Department of Health & Social Care, 2021).

Jot This Down

- What are the key differences between the MHA and the MCA?
- Why do you think the MHA reforms are needed?

Therapeutic Nursing Care

Nursing care is, first and foremost, an interpersonal process and the relationship that nurses establish with service users is crucial to the success of any nursing intervention. Nurses working with people with mental health issues have to be particularly aware of this and need not only to develop excellent social and interpersonal skills, but to be self-aware, open-minded, understanding, accepting, insightful and reflective. Sensitivity, patience, empathy, warmth, and communication and listening skills are also vital qualities that are used consciously and intentionally, in order to make a positive connection with people experiencing mental distress (Heifner, 1993). In so doing, the nurse communicates a genuine concern for and an interest in supporting, understanding and caring for the individual and those who care for them. This is an important part of supporting

individuals on their road to recovery and is known as the 'therapeutic use of self'.

A trusting, safe and supportive relationship helps to build a therapeutic alliance between nurse and service user, within which the person can be supported and possibly helped to address and resolve issues they may be facing. The individual may be experiencing problems with their mood or may have experiences or thoughts which may be overwhelming and distressing. They may feel lonely and isolated. Whatever the symptoms a person may be experiencing, the nursing relationship needs to communicate sensitivity. There also needs to be a readiness and willingness to engage with the person in a positive, sensitive and thoughtful way (Shattell *et al.*, 2006). While this is, of course, the foundation of contemporary professional nursing practice, there is also evidence that therapeutic relationships lead to greater satisfaction with treatment and care, improved attitudes towards medication use and potentially positive clinical outcomes for service users, such as a reduction of symptoms and admission rates and an improved quality of life for service users in the community (Hewitt & Coffey, 2005; Nolan & Badger, 2005).

Often the aspect of mental health nursing care most valued by service users stems from the personal qualities that nurses bring with them. This was recognised by Carl Rogers in the 1950s, whose work on 'client-centred therapy' (Rogers, 1951) has been influential in mental health nursing. Rogers identified three fundamental qualities underpinning a therapeutic relationship.

- Empathy (i.e. listening to, understanding and accepting the service user's frame of reference).
- Non-judgemental warmth or unconditional positive regard (i.e. accepting and valuing the client as a person who is entitled to respect and dignity).
- Genuineness (openness and honesty) (Sin & Trenoweth, 2010).

There have been many studies which have indicated that service users highly rate nurses who are empathic, tolerant and demonstrate personal respect and understanding (Geanellos, 2002; Welch, 2005). For example, Nolan & Badger (2005) identified the following qualities which mental health service users found particularly helpful in their personal recovery.

- Being listened to and understood
- Optimistic attitude from their healthcare workers with reference to treatment options
- Honesty from practitioners in relation to prognosis and outlook
- Practitioners being supportive and nurturing
- Continuity of care
- Specialist knowledge
- Genuine interest and efforts to monitor progress

Empathy is not only a feeling of compassion for another; it is a conscious attempt to understand the frame of reference of the service user and their experiences, perceptions and meanings that they assign to their situation. This will include an awareness of the values and belief systems arising from another's cultural, social and family backgrounds. However, empathy is also the way in which understanding about another is demonstrated and verbalised to them. We should never assume that we fully or truly 'know' another, and we must have humility to recognise that our attempts to understand another person may be limited. We develop our empathy and increase the accuracy of our understanding of another's situation within the therapeutic and trusting relationship where the nurse and service user feel safe to discuss and identify those thoughts, feelings and experiences which seem related to the person's mental health issue.

Empathy begins with understanding our own 'self' – a connectedness to those aspects of our personality which define us as human beings, our values and the way we experience the world (Welch, 2005). An awareness of this helps us to understand how we relate to others, our own attitudes, biases, limitations and strengths and how we are likely to respond to situations and influence our thinking. Such self-awareness helps us to realise that our experiences, like the experiences of others, are subjective, and there are always different interpretations that may be placed on any given situation. Assuming that our viewpoint, and only our viewpoint, is the one which is right or correct and that we have the 'truthful' understanding will not lead to empathic understanding of others. In fact, it may lead to an assumption that our advice is in the service user's best interests. This may be seen as coercion and limiting the service user's choice to live their lives in the way they choose.

Developing our own self-awareness is perhaps one of the most enriching elements of mental health nursing practice – that in the process of helping a person learn about themselves we, in turn and through a process of self-reflection, begin to understand ourselves. This process allows us to become consciously aware of our thoughts, feelings and actions and how they may be interconnected.

Self-disclosure may form an important part of developing a therapeutic relationship with a service user. This may also develop naturally as part of a general social conversation that may develop over time. Indeed, some nurses have consciously used self-disclosure as a therapeutic tool:

'The nurses used their own experiences of living a life to: be seen as ordinary people; be credible; illustrate aspects of being in the world; allow the service users to identify with them; and to normalise the service user's fears and difficulties'

(O'Brien, 2001, p.188).

This, of course, may be perfectly appropriate but needs to be carefully thought through in advance. It is very important to maintain professional boundaries and any aspect of the nurse's personal life must be consciously employed in furtherance of benefiting and supporting the service user as part of a therapeutic relationship and not to use the service user as a sounding board for one's own personal problems. This is reinforced in the NMC Code (NMC, 2018), which requires nurses to maintain clear, professional boundaries by refusing any gifts, which may be seen as leading to preferential treatment, refraining from asking for loans and establishing and maintaining sexual boundaries.

A therapeutic relationship is the foundation for all nursing care, treatment and interventions in mental health nursing. Mental health nurses often use psychosocial interventions (PSI) in their day-to-day practice, which is a collaborative approach using psychological and social principles to support service users and their friends and families (Sin & Scully, 2008). The aim of any PSI approach is to help the person to help themselves (in other words, to optimise their own self-management) by empowering the service user, their families and carers (Repper & Perkins, 2003).

The key features of the PSI approach include the following.

- Structured and systematic assessments undertaken collaboratively with service users (and their families) to explore not only needs but also strengths (such as coping abilities, knowledge, abilities, and so on).
- Educating people about mental health and mental disorders to develop understanding and knowledge and the various treatment options which may be helpful to promote and support recovery (this is often referred to as 'psychoeducation').
- Talking therapies to help the person consider how their thinking patterns may be linked to their feelings and behaviour and helping the person view a situation differently, particularly where the person feels helpless or that there is no way out of their current situation (this is often referred to as 'cognitive therapy').
- Supporting and encouraging the use of medication and optimising the medication regimen and adherence. While medication may be important in supporting and promoting recovery (Bennett, 2008), a PSI approach also seeks to help to psychologically manage symptoms (such as helping people who hear voices to develop control of those voices and to reduce distress, supporting the management of stress by using relaxation techniques, mindfulness and meditation).
- Supporting and working with families and carers to develop their coping abilities and their understanding of mental health problems so that they may be better placed to help and support people who experience mental distress. This may also include 'family therapy' (Sin & Trenoweth, 2010).

Interviews are often used in PSI approaches and mental health nursing as a forum for assessment or counselling. Successful interviewers use the skills mentioned and require skilled and thoughtful interpersonal communication and counselling skills based upon universally agreed approaches. Interviews should be considered a 'purposeful conversation' (Barker, 2004), in which the process (i.e. the way in which the assessment is conducted) is considered as important as the outcome (the assessed information).

A typical interview involves the following aspects.

Establishing Rapport

As Rollnick *et al.* (1999, p.57) suggest, 'If you have a good rapport with someone, you can talk about any subject' and this is an important principle that underpins any interview with a mental health service user. When establishing rapport, a nurse needs to show an interest in the person by using appropriate non-verbal communication (such as eye contact and body language which emphasises calmness and interpersonal warmth, such as appropriate smiling and hand gestures) in an environment which is quiet, safe, private and relaxing.

Understanding the Person's Frame Of Reference

For Nelson-Jones (2003), understanding the person is the basis of being able to offer help most effectively. Here, it is essential to understand the person's frame of reference in an interview by helping the person to talk about their experiences and their thoughts and feelings. This process is facilitated by using verbal and non-verbal prompts. One of the most common ways of

179

doing this is to use open questions (which invite the person to talk freely on a subject, for example, 'How are you feeling?') and closed questions (which invite yes/no or short answers, for example, 'Are you feeling sad today?'). Closed questions should be used sparingly, as they tend to halt conversational flow and if we are interested in developing an understanding of another person, it is important that they are able to do most of the talking and this is best facilitated by open questions.

Other techniques which are important to encourage talk are active listening (i.e. making a conscious effort to hear what the person is saying and demonstrating you are doing this by verbal and non-verbal prompts); reflection (showing that you understand a person's point of view by reflecting back to them what they have said); and summarising (i.e. bringing together all the points that have been discussed as a conclusion to a conversation).

There are times, of course, where an interview may be quite structured, such as when you are conducting assessments to develop a clearer understanding of the nature of the person's issues. At such times, the conversation may centre on the nature of the person's current mental distress and the impact that this has on their life and holistic functioning; the broad context of the current problem, including triggers, which may have precipitated the problem; their past history and factors which may have predisposed the person to mental distress; physical health problems; factors which are helpful and unhelpful in supporting the person; the risks that person may pose to themselves and others; and the strengths and abilities that the person may have which could be marshalled to support their personal recovery. In this way, the nurse can develop an understanding of what the issues might be for the service user and what they would like to do to address their problems. The nurse is therefore able to offer suggestions and develop a care plan in partnership with the service user, ensuring their agreement with their personal goals (Simmons & Griffiths, 2009). This latter point is vital in that a service user is not likely to be willing to work towards addressing such problems if they feel that the action plan has been imposed upon them.

Conclusion

In this chapter, we have explored the fundamental principles of caring for people with mental health issues and the policy context which underpins contemporary mental healthcare. It is important, however, to understand that while the policy context stresses a 'recovery' approach (where emphasis is placed on social recovery and supporting people to achieve quality of life), contemporary mental health services are often primarily medical in nature, where medication is emphasised to the detriment of holistic and psychosocial care. An important aspect of nursing care is being able to promote parity of esteem and respond to the physical healthcare needs of this group. We have explored the settings and contexts for mental healthcare and the principles of nursing care for people experiencing mental distress and their carers, including assessment and treatment options. Finally, we have explored how to provide therapeutic nursing care for this client group.

Key Points

- This chapter has provided you with an overview of the fundamental aspects associated with mental health nursing and the principles of care. The chapter has provided information immersed in the policy context for contemporary mental health nursing care.
- The various approaches to understanding mental health issues have been discussed, and emphasis has been placed on the principles of the personal 'recovery' approach. The values of holism in the delivery of nursing care for people with mental health issues are essential if care is to be person centred.
- The principles of nursing care for people experiencing mental distress and their carers, including assessment, treatment options and therapeutic nursing care, have been discussed with an appreciation of why physical health issues may be elevated in this client group. The chapter has highlighted the need for nurses to be aware of the contexts for mental healthcare, including the various settings for care and the legal contexts.
- Central to the values that underpin effective mental health nursing is the need for all nurses to practise in a holistic, non-judgemental, caring and sensitive manner that avoids assumptions, supports social inclusion, recognises and respects individual choice, and acknowledges diversity. Where necessary, the nurse must challenge inequality, discrimination and exclusion from access to care.
- Emphasis has been placed on the need for all nurses to use therapeutic principles to engage, maintain and, where appropriate, disengage from professional caring relationships, respecting professional boundaries.

References

Adult Psychiatric Morbidity Survey (2014) *Suicidal thoughts, suicide attempts, and self-harm.* https://files.digital.nhs.uk/publicationimport/pub21xxx/pub21748/apms-2014-suicide.pdf (accessed December 2021).

Age UK (2019) *Mental Health (England).* www.ageuk.org.uk/globalassets/age-uk/documents/policy-positions/health-and-wellbeing/ppp_mental_health_england.pdf (accessed December 2021).

American Psychiatric Association (2013) *Diagnostic and Statistical Manual of Mental Disorders* (DSM-5). www.psychiatry.org/psychiatrists/practice/dsm (accessed December 2021).

Anthony, W.A. (2000) Recovery from mental illness: the guiding vision of the mental health system in the 1990's. *Psychosocial Rehabilitation Journal,* 16, 11–23.

Baker, C. & Gheera, M. (2020) *Mental health: achieving 'parity of esteem'.* https://commonslibrary.parliament.uk/mental-health-achieving-parity-of-esteem/ (accessed December 2021).

Barker, P. (2004) *Assessment in Psychiatric and Mental Health Nursing: In Search of the Whole Person,* 2nd edn. Nelson Thornes, Cheltenham.

Bennett, J. (2008) Supporting recovery: medication management in mental health care. In: J. Lynch & S. Trenoweth (eds) *Contemporary Issues in Mental Health Nursing.* John Wiley & Sons Ltd, Chichester.

Bessant, M., King, E. & Peveler, R. (2008) Characteristics of suicides in recent contact with NHS Direct. *Psychiatric Bulletin,* 32(3), 92–95.

Bond, P. (2019) Falling through the net: unrecognised trauma. *Healthcare Counselling and Psychotherapy Journal,* 19(1), 8–13.

Brown, M. (2004) *Coping with Depression after Traumatic Brain Injury.* Brain Injury Association of America. http://nbia.ca/pdfs/coping-with-depression.pdf (accessed December 2021).

Cameron, C. (ed.) (2014) *Disability Studies: A Student's Guide.* Sage, London.

Cameron, C. & Lingwood, L. (2020) What's wrong with seeing the person first? *British Journal of Nursing*, 29(5), 314–317.

Care Quality Commission (2011) *Mental Capacity Act 2005.* www.cqc.org.uk/sites/default/files/Mental%20Capacity%20Act%20Code%20of%20Practice.pdf (accessed December 2021).

Care Quality Commission (2015) *Right Here, Right Now. Help, Care and Support During a Mental Health Crisis.* www.cqc.org.uk/content/new-report-looking-peoples-experience-care-during-mental-health-crisis (accessed December 2021).

CarersUK (2020) *Facts and Figures.* www.carersuk.org/news-and-campaigns/press-releases/facts-and-figures (accessed December 2021).

Carter, G. & Spittal, M.J. (2018) Suicide risk assessment: risk stratification is not accurate enough to be clinically useful and alternative approaches are needed. *Journal of Intervention and Suicide Prevention*, 39(4), 229–234.

Centre for Mental Health (2020) *Call to set budget for wellbeing.* www.centreformentalhealth.org.uk/news/centre-mental-health-calls-government-set-budget-wellbeing-cost-mental-ill-health-england-reaches-ps119-billion (accessed December 2021).

Chesney, E., Goodwin, G.M. & Fazel, S. (2014) Risks of all-cause and suicide mortality in mental health disorders: a meta-review. *World Psychiatry*, 13(2), 153–160.

Clement, S., Schauman, T., Graham, F., *et al.* (2015) What is the impact of mental health-related stigma on help seeking? *Psychosocial Medicine*, 45(1), 11–27.

Coombs, T., Curtis, J. & Crookes, P. (2013) What is the process of a comprehensive mental health assessment? *International Nursing Review*, 60, 96–102.

Cowen, P. & Browning, M. (2015) What has serotonin got to do with depression? *World Psychiatry*, 14(2), 158–160.

Dawson, J. (2020) The conundrum of self-neglect. *British Journal of General Practice*, 70(698), 453.

Dean, C. & Macmillan, C. (2002) *Serving the Children of Parents with a Mental Illness: Barriers, Breakthroughs and Benefits.* Australian Infant, Child, Adolescent and Family Mental Health Association Ltd.

Dean, J., Todd, G., Morrow, H., *et al.* (2001) Mum, I used to be good looking. Look at me now: the physical health needs of adults with mental health problems: the perspectives of users, carers and front-line staff. *International Journal of Mental Health Promotion*, 3(4), 16–24.

Department for Constitutional Affairs (2007) *Mental Capacity Act 2005. Code of Practice.* http://webarchive.nationalarchives.gov.uk/ and http://www.dca.gov.uk/legal-policy/mental-capacity/mca-cp.pdf (accessed December 2021).

Department of Health (1999) *National Service Framework for Mental Health: Modern Standards and Service Models.* Department of Health, London. www.gov.uk/government/publications/quality-standards-for-mental-health-services (accessed December 2021).

Department of Health (2000) *The NHS Plan: a plan for investment, a plan for reform.* https://webarchive.nationalarchives.gov.uk/ukgwa/+/www.dh.gov.uk/en/publicationsandstatistics/publications/publicationspolicyandguidance/dh_4002960 (accessed December 2021).

Department of Health (2001) *The Mental Health Policy Implementation Guide.* Department of Health, London.

Department of Health (2006) *Choosing Health: Supporting the Physical Needs of People with Severe Mental Illness Commissioning Framework.* Department of Health, London.

Department of Health (2008a) *Refocusing the Care Programme Approach.* Department of Health, London. https://webarchive.nationalarchives.gov.uk/ukgwa/20130107105354/http://www.dh.gov.uk/prod_consum_dh/groups/dh_digitalassets/@dh/@en/documents/digitalasset/dh_083649.pdf (accessed December 2021).

Department of Health (2008b) *Code of Practice: Mental Health Act 1983.* Department of Health, London. www.gov.uk/government/publications/code-of-practice-mental-health-act-1983 (accessed December 2021).

Department of Health (2010) *Equity and Excellence: Liberating the NHS.* Department of Health, London. www.dh.gov.uk/en/Publicationsandstatistics/Publications/PublicationsPolicyAndGuidance/DH_117353 (accessed December 2021).

Department of Health (2011) *No Health Without Mental Health.* Department of Health, London. www.gov.uk/government/publications/no-health-without-mental-health-a-cross-government-outcomes-strategy (accessed December 2021).

Department of Health (2013) *A Mandate from the Government to NHS England: April 2014 to March 2015.* www.gov.uk/government/publications/nhs-mandate-2014-to-2015 (accessed December 2021).

Department of Health (2014a) *Mental Health Crisis Care Concordat: Improving Outcomes for People Experiencing Mental Health Crisis.* https://assets.publishing.service.gov.uk/government/uploads/system/uploads/attachment_data/file/281242/36353_Mental_Health_Crisis_accessible.pdf (accessed December 2021).

Department of Health (2014b) *The Care Act.* www.legislation.gov.uk/ukpga/2014/23/contents/enacted (accessed December 2021).

Department of Health (2016) *Care and Support Statutory Guidance Changes in March 2016.* www.gov.uk/government/publications/care-act-2014-part-1-factsheets/care-and-support-statutory-guidance-changes-in-march-2016 (accessed December 2021).

Department of Health (2019) *The NHS Long Term Plan.* www.longtermplan.nhs.uk/ (accessed December 2021).

Department of Health and Social Care (2021) *Preventing Suicide in England: Fifth progress report of the crossgovernment outcomes strategy to save lives.* https://assets.publishing.service.gov.uk/government/uploads/system/uploads/attachment_data/file/973935/fifth-suicide-prevention-strategy-progress-report.pdf (accessed December 2021).

De Silva, P. (2017) How to improve psychiatric services: a perspective from critical psychiatry. *British Journal of Hospital Medicine*, 78(9), 503–507.

Engel, G. (1977) The need for a new medical model. *Science*, 196, 129–136.

Faulkner, A. & Layzell, S. (2000) *Strategies for Living: The Research Report.* Mental Health Foundation, London.

Fogel, A., Nazir, S., Hirapara, K., et al. (2021) *Cultural Assessment and Treatment of Psychiatric Patients.* StatPearls. www.ncbi.nlm.nih.gov/books/NBK482311/ (accessed December 2021).

Friedli, L. & Dardis, C. (2002) Smoke gets in their eyes. *Mental Health Today*, January, 18–21.

Geanellos, R. (2002) Transformative change of self: the unique focus of (adolescent) mental health nursing? *International Journal of Mental Health Nursing*, 11, 174–185.

Gibbons, S., Lauder, W. & Ludwick, R. (2006) Self-neglect: a proposed new NANDA diagnosis. *International Journal of Nursing Terminologies and Classifications*, 17(1), 10–18.

Goddard, N. (1995) Spirituality as integrative energy: a philosophical analysis as requisite precursor to holistic nursing practice. *Journal of Advanced Nursing*, 22(4), 808–815.

Health and Social Care Act (2012) www.legislation.gov.uk/ukpga/2012/7/contents/enacted (accessed December 2021).

Health Care Quality Improvement Partnership (2013) *The National Confidential Inquiry into Suicide and Homicide by People with Mental Illness.* https://documents.manchester.ac.uk/display.aspx?DocID=37595 (accessed December 2021).

Health Foundation (2021) *Latest data highlights a growing mental health crisis in the UK.* www.health.org.uk/news-and-comment/news/latest-data-highlights-a-growing-mental-health-crisis-in-the-uk (accessed December 2021).

181

Health Foundation (2021b) *Unemployment and Mental Health*. www.health.org.uk/publications/long-reads/unemployment-and-mental-health (accessed December 2021).

Heaton, T. (2014) Access. In: Cameron, C. (ed.) *Disability Studies: A Student's Guide*. Sage, London.

Heifner, C. (1993) Positive connectedness in the psychiatric nurse–patient relationship. *Archives of Psychiatric Nursing*, 7(1), 11–15.

Hewitt, J. & Coffey, M. (2005) Therapeutic working relationships with people with schizophrenia: literature review. *Journal of Advanced Nursing*, 52(5), 561–570.

Khan, S. (2017) Diogenes syndrome: a special manifestation of hoarding disorder. *American Journal of Psychiatry Residents' Journal*, August, 9–11.

King's Fund (2015) *Mental health under pressure*. www.kingsfund.org.uk/publications/mental-health-under-pressure (accessed December 2021).

King's Fund (2020) *What is Social Prescribing?* www.kingsfund.org.uk/publications/social-prescribing (accessed December 2021).

Krauss, J. & Slavinsky, A. (1982) *The Chronically Ill Psychiatric Patient and the Community*. Blackwell Scientific Publications, Boston, MA.

Kring, A., Johnson, S., Davison, G. & Neale, J. (2010) *Abnormal Psychology*, 11th edn. John Wiley & Sons, Hoboken, NJ.

Landstedt, E. & Almquist, Y.B. (2019) Intergenerational patterns of mental health problems: the role of childhood peer status position. *BMC Psychiatry*, 19(1), 286.

Launer, J. (2002) *Narrative-based Primary Care: A Practical Guide*. Radcliffe Medical Press, Abingdon.

Lawrence, D. & Kisely, S. (2010) Inequalities in healthcare provision for people with severe mental illness. *Journal of Psychopharmacology*, 24(4), 61–68.

Lukoff, D. (2007) Spirituality in the recovery of persistent mental health disorder. *Southern Medical Journal*, 100, 642–646.

Mathers, C. & Schofield, D. (1998) The health consequences of unemployment: the evidence. *Medical Journal of Australia*, 168(4), 178–182.

Matthews, J. (2008) The meaning of recovery. In: J. Lynch & S. Trenoweth (eds) *Contemporary Issues in Mental Health Nursing*. John Wiley & Sons Ltd, Chichester.

Mental Health Task Force (2016) *Five Year Forward View for Mental Health*. www.england.nhs.uk/wp-content/uploads/2017/03/fyfv-mh-one-year-on.pdf (accessed December 2021).

Morgan, S. (1998) The assessment and management of risk. In: C. Brooker & J. Repper (eds) *Serious Mental Health Problems in the Community: Policy, Practice and Research*. Baillière Tindall, London.

Munro, M. (2021) Mental health diagnosis: looking at a grey area through a critical lens. *Nursing Times*, 117(10), 18–20.

Murray, R. (2012) *The Abandoned Illness: A Report by the Schizophrenia Commission*. www.rethink.org/media/514093/TSC_main_report_14_nov.pdf (accessed December 2017).

National Institute for Health and Care Excellence (2013) *NHS urged to become smoke free*. www.nice.org.uk/news/article/nhs-urged-to-become-smokefree (accessed December 2021).

National Institute for Mental Health (2021) *Suicide Prevention*. www.nimh.nih.gov/health/topics/suicide-prevention (accessed December 2021)

National Mental Health Development Unit (2011) *Improving Access to Psychological Therapies*. NMHDU, England.

Nelson-Jones, R. (2003) *Basic Counselling Skills: A Helpers' Manual*. Sage, London.

NHS (2019) Every Mind Matters. www.nhs.uk/every-mind-matters/mental-wellbeing-tips/your-mind-plan-quiz/?WT.tsrc=Search&WT.mc_id=Brand&gclid=Cj0KCQjww4OMBhCUARIsAILndv7WEJrMUQU4Ca-09ddyS0yVCzNHa1xP3D73DRzYtt4r-PwFVAXlcXsaAiTiEALw_wcB&gclsrc=aw.ds (accessed December 2021).

NHS England (2019) *Social Prescribing*. www.england.nhs.uk/personalisedcare/social-prescribing/ (accessed December 2021).

Nolan, P. & Badger, F. (2005) Aspects of the relationship between doctors and depressed patients that enhance satisfaction with primary care. *Journal of Psychiatric and Mental Health Nursing*, 12, 146–153.

Norman, I. & Ryrie, I. (2018) *The Art and Science of Mental Health Nursing: Principles and Practice*. Open University Press, Maidenhead.

Nursing & Midwifery Council (2018) *The Code: Professional Standards of Practice and Behaviour for Nurses, Midwives and Nursing Associates*. www.nmc.org.uk/standards/code/read-the-code-online/ (accessed December 2021).

O'Brien, A.J. (2001) The therapeutic relationship: historical development and contemporary significance. *Journal of Psychiatric and Mental Health Nursing*, 8(2), 129–137.

Office for National Statistics (2020a) Exploring religion in England and Wales. Available at www.ons.gov.uk/peoplepopulationandcommunity/culturalidentity/religion/articles/exploringreligioninenglandandwales/february2020 (accessed October 2021).

Office for National Statistics (2020b) *Recent Trends in Suicide: death occurrences in England and Wales between 2001 and 2018*. www.ons.gov.uk/peoplepopulationandcommunity/birthsdeathsandmarriages/deaths/articles/recenttrendsinsuicidedeathoccurrencesinenglandandwalesbetween2001and2018/2020-12-08 (accessed December 2021).

Office for National Statistics (2021a) *Deaths caused by Suicide by Quarter in England*. ONS, London.

Office for National Statistics (2021b) *Employment in the UK*. www.ons.gov.uk/employmentandlabourmarket/peopleinwork/employmentandemployeetypes/bulletins/employmentintheuk/october2021 (accessed December 2021).

Panday, S. (2016) *Parity of Esteem Overview and Report*. www.england.nhs.uk/mids-east/wp-content/uploads/sites/7/2018/03/parity-report.pdf (accessed December 2021).

Proctor, G. (2006) Therapy: Opium of the masses or help for those who most need it? In: G. Proctor, M. Cooper, P. Sanders & B. Malcolm (eds) (2006) *Politicising the Person Centred Approach: an agenda for social change*. PCCS, Monmouth.

Public Health England (2017) *Prevention Concordat for Better Mental Health*. https://assets.publishing.service.gov.uk/government/uploads/system/uploads/attachment_data/file/740587/Prevention_Concordat_for_Better_Mental_Health_Prevention_planning.pdf (accessed December 2021).

Repper, J. & Perkins, R. (2003) *Social Inclusion and Recovery: a Model for Mental Health Practice*. Baillière Tindall, Edinburgh.

Rogers, C. (1951) *Client-centred Therapy: Its Current Practice, Implications and Theory*. Houghton Mifflin, Boston, MA.

Rollnick, S., Mason, P. & Butler, C. (1999) *Health Behaviour Change: A Guide for Practitioners*. Churchill Livingstone, Edinburgh.

Royal College of Psychiatrists (2021) *Assessing Risk – Factors to Consider: History, Environment and Mental State*. www.rcpsych.ac.uk/members/supporting-you/assessing-and-managing-risk-of-patients-causing-harm/assessing-risk (accessed December 2021).

Seymour, L. (2003) *Not All in the Mind: The Physical Health of Mental Health Service Users*. Briefing paper 2. Radical Mentalities, London.

Shattell, M.M., McAllister, S., Hogan, B., *et al*. (2006) 'She took the time to make sure she understood': mental health patients' experiences of being understood. *Archives of Psychiatric Nursing*, 20(5), 234–241.

Simmons, J. & Griffiths, R. (2009) *CBT for Beginners*. Sage, London.

Sin, J. & Scully, E. (2008) An evaluation of education and implementation of psychosocial interventions within one UK Mental Healthcare Trust. *Journal of Psychiatric and Mental Health Nursing*, 15, 161–169.

Sin, J. & Trenoweth, S. (2010) Caring for the mind. In: C. Margereson & S. Trenoweth (eds) *Developing Holistic Care for Long Term Conditions*. Routledge, London.

Singh, S. (2010) Early intervention in psychosis. *British Journal of Psychiatry*, 196, 343–345.

Slade, M., Farkas, M., Hamilton, B., *et al.* (2014) Uses and abuses of recovery: implementing recovery-oriented practices in mental health systems. *World Psychiatry*, 13, 12–20.

Social Care Institute for Excellence (2018) *Self-neglect at a Glance*. www.scie.org.uk/self-neglect/at-a-glance (accessed December 2021).

Stephenson, C. (1991) The concept of hope revisited for nursing. *Journal of Advanced Nursing*, 16, 1456–1461.

Stickley, T. & Wright, N. (2011) The British research evidence for recovery, papers published between 2006 and 2009 (inclusive). Part Two: a review of the grey literature including book chapters and policy documents. *Journal of Psychiatric and Mental Health Nursing*, 18, 29–307.

Trenoweth, S. & Allymamod, W. (2010) Mental health. In: C. Margereson & S. Trenoweth (eds) *Developing Holistic Care for Long Term Conditions*. Routledge, London.

Turner, A. (2019) *Safeguarding study reveals knowledge gap in applying MCA to cases of alcohol-based harm. Adults*. www.communitycare.co.uk/2019/07/24/safeguarding-study-reveals-knowledge-gaps-applying-mca-cases-alcohol-based-harm/ (accessed December 2021).

Wand, T., Bechanan-Hagen, S., Derrick, K., *et al.* (2019) Are current mental health assessment formats consistent with contemporary thinking and practice? *International Journal of Mental Health Nursing*, 29(2), 171–176.

Welch, M. (2005) Pivotal moments in the therapeutic relationship. *International Journal of Mental Health Nursing*, 14, 161–165.

Union of the Physically Impaired Against Segregation and the Disability Alliance (1976) *Fundamental Principles of Disability*. UPIAS, London.

World Health Organization (1946) International Health Conference, New York, 19 June to 22 July. *Official Records of the World Health Organization*, 2(100). WHO, Geneva.

World Health Organization (1976) *International Classification of Impairments, Disabilities, and Handicaps*. https://tinyurl.com/wae9mbc (accessed December 2021).

World Health Organization (1981) *International Classification of Impairments, Disabilities and Handicaps*. WHO, Geneva.

World Health Organization (2007) *Mental health: strengthening our response*. Factsheet No. 220. WHO, Geneva.

World Health Organization (2013) *How to Use the ICF. Practical Manual for Using the International Classification of Functioning, Disability and Health (ICF)*. https://tinyurl.com/qqnpo7r (accessed December 2021).

World Health Organization (2014) *Social Determinants of Mental Health*. https://apps.who.int/iris/bitstream/handle/10665/112828/9789241506809_eng.pdf (accessed December 2021).

World Health Organization (2021a) *International Statistical Classification of Diseases and Related Health Problems*, 11th revision (ICD-11). WHO, Geneva.

World Health Organization (2021b) *It's time to build a fairer, healthier world for everyone, everywhere*. https://cdn.who.int/media/docs/default-source/documents/social-determinants-of-health/who-multicountry-special-initiative-sdh-equity.pdf?sfvrsn=dac26a6d_22&download=true (accessed December 2021).

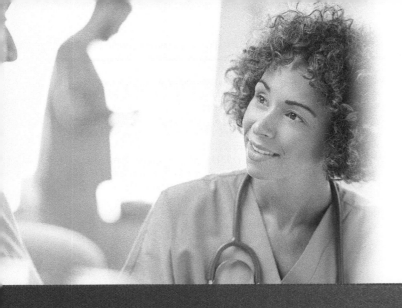

12

The Principles of Maternity Care

Rosemary McCarthy and Jean Mason Mitchell

University of Salford, UK

Learning Outcomes

On completion of this chapter you will be able to:

- **Understand the role of the midwife in maternity care and identify the options available for maternity care and birth**
- **Gain an insight into the physiology of pregnancy**
- **Be aware of screening options offered during pregnancy**
- **Understand the common minor disorders of pregnancy and appropriate management**
- **Understand the care a woman receives in the antenatal, intranatal and postnatal periods and gain insight into the care of the neonate**
- **Identify some of the complications of pregnancy and childbirth**

Proficiencies

NMC Proficiencies and Standards:

- **There are no NMC proficiencies for this chapter. However, the EU Directive states in General nurse training Article 31 of 2005/36/EC, the principle requirements for the training of general nurses (2), that nurses must have theoretical and clinical instruction in maternity care.**

 Visit the companion website at www.wiley.com/go/peate/nursingpractice3e where you can test yourself using flashcards, multiple-choice questions and more.

Nursing Practice: Knowledge and Care, Third Edition. Edited by Ian Peate and Aby Mitchell.
© 2022 John Wiley & Sons Ltd. Published 2022 by John Wiley & Sons Ltd.
Companion website: www.wiley.com/go/peate/nursingpractice3e

Introduction

Nurses will meet pregnant women in a variety of situations and therefore need to have an awareness of pregnancy as a normal physiological event and an understanding of the implications of pregnancy and childbearing on women's health. Registered nurses must:

'support and enable people at all stages of life and in all care settings to make informed choices about how to manage health challenges in order to maximise their quality of life and improve health outcomes. They are actively involved in the prevention of and protection against disease and ill health and engage in public health, community development and global health agendas, and in the reduction of health inequalities'

(NMC, 2018, p.10).

Red Flag

 All health professionals have a responsibility for safeguarding children an sues in any context, including domestic violence. This must include informing the named nurse for safeguarding who will liaise with the midwifery team.

There were 591 759 deliveries during 2019–20 (NHS Digital, 2020). This is a decrease of 2.0% from 2018–19. Most of these births follow healthy, uncomplicated pregnancies that are considered to be low in risk. In low-risk pregnancies the midwife is the lead health professional who delivers and co-ordinates maternity care. The midwife may share this care with other health professionals, depending on the woman's specific and unique needs. If complications or risk factors are identified, midwives refer to obstetricians who manage clinically complex pregnancies.

The Role of the Midwife in Maternity Care

A midwife is a person who has been educated and trained and successfully completed a course of studies in midwifery. The midwife is a healthcare professional who works in partnership with women to give support, care and advice during pregnancy, labour and the postpartum period.

Jot This Down

From your experience, what would you say are the principal roles that the midwife has in pregnancy and aftercare? Consult the link: **www.nmc-uk.org/ Publications/Standards/**

In this exercise, think about the midwife's role in preparing women for motherhood and maintaining safety. Think about opportunities you may have as a nurse to help support mothers as they prepare for their new role. How can you 'Make Every Contact Count'? This might include giving advice or information about diet, exercise, smoking cessation, alcohol, identifying safeguarding issues (adult and child), or other active interventions to improve maternal and family health. You can refer to the 'Making Every Contact Count' (MECC) website for further information at **www.makingeverycontactcount.co.uk**.

The midwife assists the woman birthing and is the lead professional during normal labour and birth and also provides care for the newborn and infant. Midwifery care includes preventive measures, promotion of normal birth, detection of complications in mother and child, accessing of medical care or other appropriate assistance, and carrying out of emergency measures. The midwife also has a vital role in antenatal education, preparation for parenthood, health counselling and education for women and their families (International Confederation of Midwives, 2011).

All midwives in the UK must be registered with the Nursing and Midwifery Council (NMC) which regulates their practice (NMC, 2018).

Overview of the Physiology of Pregnancy

Pregnancy is a normal physiological event and is not pathological; however, pathological processes can occur in pregnancy, as they can in any individual at any time. Thus, nurses need to be aware of the pregnant woman and the potential changes to her physiology and the care she may require.

The duration of pregnancy is 40 weeks or 280 days; this comprises three parts called 'trimesters', each lasting three calendar months. The first trimester is from conception to 12 weeks; the second (mid) trimester is from 12 weeks to 24 weeks; and the third is from 24 weeks to delivery of the fetus. The calculation of the estimated date of delivery (EDD) is described in Box 12.1. Ultrasound scans are commonly used to confirm gestation; the earlier these are undertaken, the more accurate they are.

The signs and symptoms of pregnancy are largely due to hormonal changes and the increasing size of the gravid uterus.

Box 12.1 Example Calculation to Estimate Date of Delivery (Naegele's Rule)

LMP = 8 May 2021
+1 year = 8 May 2022
– 3 months = 8 February 2022
+ 7 days = 15 February 2022 is The estimated delivery date (EDD)

The calculation method does not always result in 280 days because not all calendar months are the same length; it does not account for leap years. Naegele's Rule assumes an average menstrual cycle length of 28 days. In modern practice, calculators, reference cards or sliding wheel calculators are used to add 280 days to LMP.

Calculate the EDD if the LMP is 25 July 2021.

Signs and Symptoms: First Trimester

These are not diagnostic tests and do not confirm pregnancy.

1. Amenorrhoea (absence of menstruation): in women with a previously predictable cycle
2. Positive pregnancy test
3. Breast changes: they may become larger, more tender and veins may appear more prominent and the pigmentation of the areolae may become darker
4. Skin pigmentation
   - *Chloasma*: also known as the 'mask of pregnancy'. This is a brownish pigmentation that appears on the face of approximately 50–70% of women in a butterfly-like pattern. This increases as the pregnancy develops
   - *Linea nigra*: a dark line may be noted on the abdomen between the sternum and the symphysis pubis
   - *Striae gravidarum*: reddish/purple stretch marks that may be noted on the thighs, buttocks, abdomen and breasts
5. Nausea and vomiting (morning sickness) can occur from as early as 2 weeks but usually subsides by 12 weeks
6. Fatigue
7. Frequency of micturition
8. Pica (cravings)

Additional Signs and Symptoms: Second and Third Trimesters

1. Enlargement of the abdomen and the uterus can be felt through the abdominal wall.
2. Fetal movements are felt and heart sounds may be heard from approximately 20–22 weeks in a primigravid woman and 16–18 weeks in a multigravid woman. Many things can affect this, such as the mother's weight, muscle tone and position of the placenta and fetus.
3. Changes may be seen in the cervix and vagina on speculum examination. The colour of the vagina, cervix and labia may appear to be darker purple (Jacquemier's/Chadwick's sign). Stronger pulses may be palpated on vaginal examination (Osiander's sign).
4. Increase in normal vaginal discharge (leucorrhoea).
5. Braxton Hicks contractions: intermittent contractions of the uterus may be felt from the second trimester.

What the Experts Say A Mother to Be

> I think it's [Braxton Hicks contractions] different for everyone, for sure. Mine don't hurt. I can just feel the tightness. It's definitely not comfortable, but not painful at all for me.

(Julie's experience in her first pregnancy)

Diagnostic Tests that Confirm Pregnancy

- Fetal parts palpable abdominally
- Fetal movements felt by examiner
- Fetal heart heard
- Ultrasound scan that confirms the presence of a fetal heart

Overview of Antenatal Care

Pregnancy, birth and motherhood affect women physically, psychologically and socially and the role of the midwife is to support women during this process. Pregnant women often seek out information from a number of sources, including books, websites and health professionals. It is important for nurses to understand the aims of antenatal care, but they should refer to the midwife who is the lead professional in normal childbirth.

Antenatal Appointments

The National Institute for Health and Care Excellence (NICE) (2020) advocates a schedule of antenatal appointments but contact with women during pregnancy should be based on their individual needs. This is commonly ascertained during the booking appointment, which is often the first contact between the mother and maternity services. The appointment is longer than subsequent appointments so that information can be gathered regarding the woman's obstetric, medical, family and social history. The midwife gives the woman information about the pregnancy, screening, options for care and lifestyle choices. This appointment is considered pivotal for assessing risk and identifying the woman's needs.

Care should be sensitive to the needs of the woman and take place at venues that are easily accessible for her; this may be the woman's home or a local medical/family centre. Women with complicated pregnancies or specific medical conditions will be offered consultant-led appointments at the hospital or appointments shared between the consultant and midwife at hospital and community-based venues.

Clinical Care, Assessment and Advice

The clinical care, observations, assessment and advice offered to the woman and her family during the antenatal period are fully explored in NICE's (2019b) *Routine Care for the Healthy Pregnant Woman*.

Abdominal Examination

At each antenatal appointment from the second trimester, the midwife will examine the mother's abdomen to confirm fetal growth and well-being. A full abdominal examination consists of the following.

- *Inspection*: the midwife observes the abdomen for skin changes, scars, shape and size.
- *Palpation*: the midwife palpates the abdomen using the palmar surfaces of the hands. Palpation is divided into three elements.
  - Fundal: the uppermost border of the uterus is palpated. This reflects growth and assists the midwife in determining the presentation of the fetus.
  - Lateral: the sides of the uterus are palpated. This assists the midwife in determining the position of the fetus.
  - Pelvic: the lower aspect of the uterus is palpated to assist the midwife in determining the presentation of the fetus. This is assessed from 36 weeks of gestation, as the presentation will be variable when the fetus is less mature and has more room to move.
- *Auscultation*: the midwife listens to the fetal heart as per NICE intrapartum guidelines (2019a) using a Pinard stethoscope or a hand-held ultrasound device.

Terminology used during the abdominal examination (Figure 12.1)

- *Presentation*: this is the part of the fetus lying lowest in the maternal uterus, i.e. directly above the cervix. Most commonly, this is the head and is called a cephalic or vertex presentation.
- *Position*: this most commonly reflects the position of the head in the maternal pelvis.
- *Lie*: this refers to the long axis of the fetus in relation to the long axis of the maternal uterus, i.e. longitudinal (lengthways), transverse (across), oblique (diagonally).
- *Attitude*: this means the degree to which the fetus has its limbs, body and head flexed. The most common attitude is one of flexion, i.e. the fetal position (curled up).
- *Engagement*: how much of the presenting part, usually the head, has passed through the narrowest part of the maternal pelvis.

The assessment of fetal growth is a vital aspect of the midwife's role as fetal growth correlates with fetal well-being. If growth is less than or more than would be expected for the gestational age of the fetus, the midwife will refer the woman to an obstetrician. Growth is initially assessed by measuring the fundal height of the mother's uterus, as discussed in NICE (2019). Fetal growth is demonstrated pictorially in Figure 12.2. At weeks 1–4, the approximate size is 0.6 cm. By weeks 13–16, the approximate measurement is 18 cm and the uterus containing the pregnancy can be palpated abdominally. The approximate measurement at weeks 26–29 is 32–42 cm and by 36 weeks to the end of pregnancy it is 50 cm.

Antenatal Screening

During the antenatal period, women will be offered a range of screening tests. Tests are usually offered early in pregnancy to check for potential problems. Blood tests and ultrasound scans

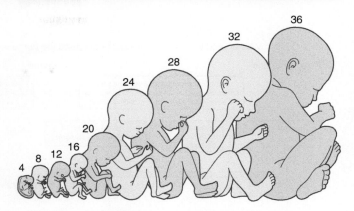

Figure 12.2 Fetal growth from week 4 to week 36.

can be offered to women, who should be given enough information to make an informed choice about the test. You can see the schedule of screening tests for mothers in Figure 12.3.

Common Blood Tests and Investigations
Maternal

- *Haemoglobin (Hb)*: there is an increase in the number of red blood cells in pregnancy but this is not equal to the increase in plasma volume. Consequently, there appears to be a drop in the haemoglobin level; this is called haemodilution of pregnancy. Tests to confirm anaemia may be needed if the haemoglobin level falls significantly.
- *Blood group and antibodies*: these are taken to check for antibodies that may cause a problem in this or subsequent pregnancies.
- *Infection screen*: blood is taken to check for rubella, hepatitis, HIV, syphilis.
- *Haemoglobinopathies* such as sickle cell anaemia and thalassemia are inherited blood disorders.
- *Chlamydia screening* is offered to women under 25 years.

Fetal

- *Early pregnancy ultrasound scan*: confirms the pregnancy and due date and may detect abnormalities.
- *20-week detailed scan*: this does not detect all abnormalities and may also lead to problems being suspected in healthy babies. Subsequent scans may be undertaken to assess fetal growth and well-being.
- *Down syndrome (trisomy 21)*: a chromosomal abnormality detected using a combination of blood tests and sonography at approximately 16 weeks of gestation. An invasive diagnostic test is offered following a positive screening test, e.g. amniocentesis.

Women may feel anxious during pregnancy and need information to reassure them that their pregnancy is progressing normally. This may include information about screening tests and also about the physical changes the woman is experiencing, which can result in minor symptoms of pregnancy. Nurses need to have an awareness of common minor disorders and their treatments but it is important for nurses to refer pregnant women to a midwife for ongoing advice and support. It is important to differentiate between minor symptoms and pathological disorders.

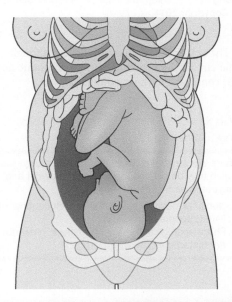

Figure 12.1 Terminology used during abdominal palpation. In this case, the presentation is cephalic. The position is left occipitoanterior (the fetal occiput is anterior and is on the left of the maternal pelvis). The lie is longitudinal. The attitude is one of flexion and the head is not engaged.

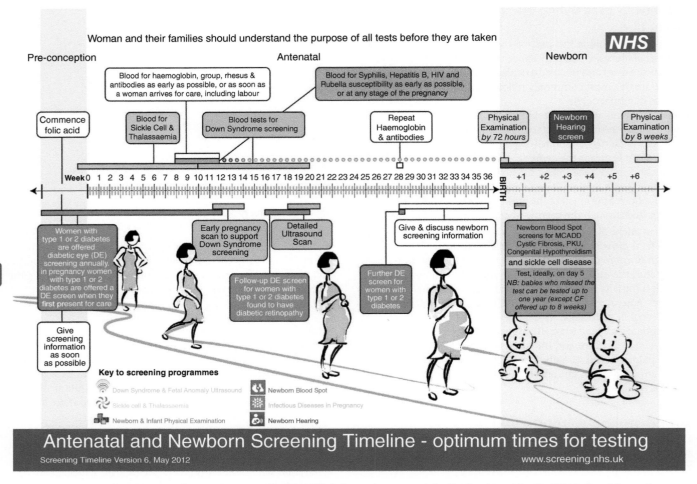

Figure 12.3 **Antenatal and neonatal screening test schedule. This information was originally developed by the UK National Screening Committee/NHS Screening Programmes.** *Source: www.screening.nhs.uk.* © **Crown Copyright 2014.**

Minor Disorders of Pregnancy and Their Management

Nausea and Vomiting

This is very common and affects over 50% of pregnant women. It is usually worse in the first trimester and often occurs in the morning, hence its colloquial name 'morning sickness'. Women should be reassured that this usually resolves by 20 weeks of gestation. The exact cause is unknown but it is thought that high levels of the circulating hormone human chorionic gonadatrophin (hCG) contribute to the condition.

What to Do If. . . A Pregnant Woman Complains of Morning Sickness

There are several ways to manage morning sickness which may be divided into pharmacological and non-pharmacological.

- Non-pharmacological methods include ginger and P6 (wrist) acupressure.
- Pharmacological treatments include prescribed antihistamines.

Red Flag

Women should be referred to a midwife, GP pharmacist or obstetrician for advice on the management of minor disorders of pregnancy, including morning sickness.

Heartburn

Heartburn is also very common in pregnancy. Women complain of retrosternal burning in the chest or discomfort that can be more noticeable when lying down. It is caused by the weight of the pregnant uterus, which affects the emptying of the stomach. Additionally, there is an increase in progesterone that relaxes the cardiac (lower oesophageal) sphincter, leading to gastric reflux. Women who present with symptoms should be advised to eat small frequent meals and avoid fatty foods. An upright position and not lying down after meals may help, and sleeping with extra pillows may alleviate nocturnal heartburn. Antacids may be offered to women whose heartburn remains troublesome.

Constipation

Constipation can occur in pregnancy due to decreased peristalsis in the colon because of the effects of progesterone, which relaxes smooth muscle. This may be exacerbated by oral iron tablets. Women who present with constipation in pregnancy should be advised to take a high-fibre diet with extra fresh fruit, vegetables, bran or wheat fibre. An increase in fluid intake should be encouraged.

Varicosities

Varicosities may develop in pregnancy in the legs, anal area and also the vulva, due to the relaxing effect of progesterone on the vessel walls and the venous stasis caused by the weight of the gravid uterus.

Women should be informed that varicose veins are a common symptom of pregnancy that will not cause harm and that compression stockings can improve the symptoms but will not prevent varicose veins from emerging.

In the absence of evidence of the effectiveness of treatments for haemorrhoids in pregnancy, women should be offered information concerning dietary modification to avoid constipation. If clinical symptoms remain troublesome, standard haemorrhoid creams may be considered.

Women may be distressed or concerned especially about vulval varicosities and should be reassured they will subside after delivery of the baby.

Vaginal Discharge

An increase in vaginal discharge (leucorrhoea) is a common physiological change that occurs during pregnancy. However, women should be advised that if the discharge is associated with itching or soreness, it has an offensive smell or there is pain on passing urine, there may be an infection present and this should be investigated. Common infections can include *Candida albicans* (thrush) and urinary tract infections (UTIs).

Backache

This is caused by softening and relaxation of the ligaments in the pelvis. The gravid uterus results in an exaggerated curvature of the spine that increases back strain and can lead to pain. Exercising in water, massage therapy and back care classes might help to ease the symptoms.

Carpal Tunnel Syndrome

This is caused by soft tissue swelling resulting from increases in the circulating volume that may cause compression of the median nerve in the wrist. The woman may experience weakness and tingling in the thumb and forefinger and pain, particularly at night. The symptoms usually resolve following delivery of the baby. A light splint may support the wrist and alleviate the symptoms along with simple analgesia.

Discussing the physiological changes of pregnancy is an important part of antenatal care. This can take place during antenatal appointments or during sessions delivered by the midwife to help prepare the woman and her partner for birth and parenthood. Antenatal education may also include relaxation techniques, birth choices, infant care and feeding.

Options Available for Birth

Women should have the choice to birth where they feel most comfortable. The birth environment can affect a woman's chances of having a normal birth. Options for birthing currently include home birth, midwifery-led birth centres and obstetric units. Birth centres offer the comforts of a home environment, with a team of midwives available. Birthing in an obstetric unit provides direct access to obstetricians, anaesthetists, neonatologists and other specialist care, including epidural analgesia, and it is important that women are aware of this to enable them to make an informed choice about where they birth their babies (NICE 2019, 2020).

If women give birth at home or in a midwife-led unit, there is a higher likelihood of a normal birth, with less intervention; however, some women require additional care and may be advised to birth in an obstetric unit, for example if the woman has any pre-existing medical conditions, develops complications during the pregnancy or has had a previous complicated birth.

In 2011–2012, over half (51.4%, 299 528) of NHS deliveries took place in designated consultant wards, 35.9% (208 937) in wards associated with a consultant, GP or midwife and 12.3% (71 590) in midwife or other wards. The percentage of deliveries in midwife or non-maternity wards has seen a gradual change to 18.5% in 2019–2020, indicating a trend towards midwifery-led care (NHS Digital, 2020). Although most women in the UK birth their babies in obstetric units, with only 2.1% of births taking place at home (ONS, 2016), this has not always been the case and it is important that women understand all the available options for birth.

Overview of Intranatal Care

Normal birth occurs spontaneously between 37 and 42 completed weeks of a singleton (one fetus) pregnancy, without induction, without the use of instruments and without general, spinal or epidural anaesthetic before or during delivery. It is generally accepted that the head delivers first in normal birth (cephalic).

Giving birth is generally very safe in the UK and over 60% of women will have a normal vaginal birth. This is not the case throughout the rest of the world, particularly in parts of South-East Asia and sub-Saharan Africa, where women birth without professional help. The consequences of this are illustrated in the high maternal mortality rates in those countries.

Labour

Labour is the process by which the fetus, placenta and membranes are born.

The onset of labour is not fully understood but it is thought to be due to a combination of factors, including the influence of maternal and fetal hormones. Labour is confirmed by the presence of regular, rhythmical contractions, which dilate the cervix. Contractions may also be accompanied by a clear or lightly blood-stained plug of mucus per vagina. This is called a 'show'. Rupture of the membranes may or may not accompany labour. Labour is not predictable and is experienced by different women in different ways. Women may also find differences in each of their own pregnancies.

Stages of Labour

Labour is often divided into three stages.

- *First stage*: the onset of labour from the onset of regular rhythmical contractions that result in dilation (opening) and effacement (shortening) of the cervix. The dilation of the cervix is estimated digitally from 1 cm to 10 cm (full dilation), as shown in Figure 12.4.
- *Second stage*: from full dilation of the cervix to the complete expulsion of the fetus. Figure 12.5 demonstrates expulsion of the fetal head during the second stage of labour.
- *Third stage*: from the birth of the baby to the complete expulsion of the placenta and membranes. Figure 12.6 shows the placenta prior to separation after delivery of the baby. This stage of labour also includes the control and management of bleeding.

Normal Labour and Birth

This is considered to occur at term (37–42 weeks); it is spontaneous in onset and the head of the fetus presents. This is called a *cephalic presentation*. The process is completed within 24 hours

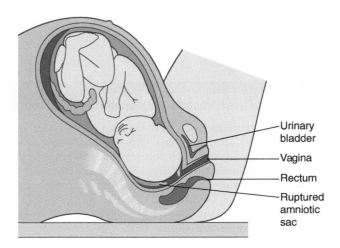

Figure 12.4 **The cervix is effaced and dilated.**

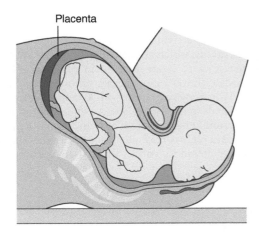

Figure 12.5 **Expulsion of the fetal head during the second stage of labour.**

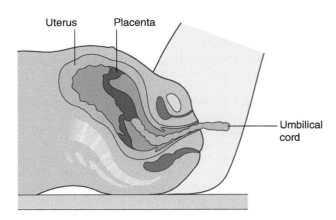

Figure 12.6 **The placenta after delivery of the baby and prior to separation from the wall of the uterus.**

of its onset and there are no complications or interventions (Royal College of Midwives, 2012).

Other Types of Labour and Birth

- *Multiple births*: 1 in 80 births following natural conception in the UK are multiples, i.e. twins, triplets, quadruplets, quintuplets, sextuplets (NICE, 2019c).
- *Induced labour*: this is when the onset of labour is started artificially. Inductions have increased from 29% in 2016–17 to 33% in 2019–20 (NHS Digital, 2020). The method of choice depends on each individual woman and her preferences, as well as the clinical presentation. The cervix may be manually stretched to stimulate labour; this is known as a cervical sweep. Drugs can be administered directly into the vagina or can be given via an intravenous infusion. Finally, a procedure called amniotomy or artificially rupturing the membranes can be undertaken. This is often called 'breaking the waters'.

What To Do If . . .

 You are asked about some old wives' tales and their supposed rationale. Always refer the woman to a midwife for further discussion. Some of these examples may be harmful and professional advice is essential.

Sex: prostaglandins in the semen ripen the cervix and stimulate labour onset.

Castor oil: increases peristaltic action, which can stimulate the uterus to contract.

Walking: upright position and the effects of gravity may help to stimulate the onset of labour.

Raspberry leaf tea: stimulates effective contractions and shorter second stage of labour.

Nipple stimulation: stimulates the release of hormones associated with the onset of labour.

Eating fresh pineapple: meant to help release the enzyme bromelain that in turn softens the cervix.

- *Breech birth*: this happens when the fetus presents by the breech (or buttocks). When this occurs, women are advised to discuss their options with a midwife and obstetrician, as there are concerns about the safety of breech vaginal birth.
- *Caesarean section*: the baby is delivered through an incision made into the abdomen and the uterus. Usually in the UK, this will be a small transverse incision low down on the abdomen and the uterus. Occasionally in an emergency or premature caesarean birth, it is necessary to incise both the abdomen and the uterus lengthways; this is called a classical incision.

Instrumental Deliveries

- *Forceps*: these are spoon-shaped instruments that are applied to the fetal head to allow traction to be applied to aid delivery. This is undertaken by a specially trained practitioner or obstetrician.
- *Ventouse*: this is a suction cup that is applied to the fetal head and allows traction to be applied to aid delivery. This is undertaken by a specially trained practitioner or obstetrician.

Midwifery Care in Normal Labour

The midwife will diagnose the onset and monitor the progress of normal labour, referring to the multidisciplinary team when necessary. During labour, a fundamental role of the midwife is to work with women and their partners to support their choices and facilitate their needs. Evidence has shown that continuous support in labour improves outcomes for mothers in terms of less analgesia, shorter labours, reduced instrumental intervention and fewer caesarean sections (Hodnett *et al.*, 2011; Bohren *et al.*, 2017). The midwife should advise women how to promote normality in birth. This will include advice about positions and movement during labour and hydration and nutrition. Women should consider these things before going into labour and are advised to write a birth plan.

Assessing Progress and Well-being

There are many ways of assessing progress in labour and there are both subtle and obvious changes. These may include changes in the woman's behaviour, such as breathing patterns, movements, mood and the noises she makes. There are also anatomical changes, which the midwife is trained to measure, including the following.

- *Abdominal examination*: the midwife can palpate the strength, length and frequency of the uterine contractions and can assess the descent of the fetus through the maternal pelvis. Contractions need to be strong enough to cause effacement and dilation of the cervix. These are counted over a 10-minute period and up to five contractions in 10 minutes are considered normal. Contractions may last up to 90 seconds. The frequency and length of the contractions may depend on the stage of the labour, with increasing intensity and frequency as labour progresses.
- *Vaginal examination*: this is a procedure during which the midwife feels the dilation and effacement of the cervix. The midwife can also determine the position and descent of the fetal head. This is an extremely intimate examination and women may feel uncomfortable physically and/or psychologically during the procedure. The midwife needs to be sensitive and should explain the procedure fully and gain the woman's consent. It is essential to maintain the woman's privacy and dignity, and at all times the midwife should be aware of the invasive nature of the examination.

The midwife will assess the woman and her unborn baby's well-being throughout the labour. Recordings of blood pressure, temperature, pulse, respiration rate and urinalysis are undertaken and recorded on a labour observation chart called a partogram. This is a graphic record of a woman's well-being and progress in labour and is used by all midwives caring for a labouring woman.

Fetal well-being is also recorded on the partogram and is assessed by regularly listening to the fetal heart (auscultation). If the membranes have ruptured, the colour of the liquor is observed; this should be clear.

Methods of Fetal Heart Rate Auscultation

Intermittent auscultation is when the midwife listens to the fetal heart at intervals during labour, using either of the following.

- *Pinard stethoscope*: this is a simple trumpet-shaped instrument that amplifies fetal heart sounds.
- *Sonicaid Doppler*: this is an electronic hand-held device that amplifies the fetal heart sounds through a speaker so that both mother and midwife can hear.

Continuous electronic fetal heart rate monitoring is sometimes required in more complex labours. This is undertaken using a cardiotocograph (CTG), which is a form of electronic fetal heart rate monitoring that amplifies the heart sounds and makes a recording on graph paper similar to an electrocardiograph (ECG).

Working with Labour Pain

There are two main beliefs about pain in labour: first, that experiencing labour pain is an important part of the labour process and fundamental to normal birth; and second, that pain is unnecessary and can be alleviated. Healthcare professionals should consider how their own values and beliefs inform their attitude to coping with pain in labour and ensure their care supports the woman's choice (NICE, 2019). Women are informed about various options open to them in labour. These can be broadly separated into non-pharmacological and pharmacological methods, as identified in Table 12.1.

Table 12.1 Methods of pain relief in labour.

NON-PHARMACOLOGICAL METHODS	PHARMACOLOGICAL METHODS
Breathing and relaxation techniques	Inhalational analgesia, e.g. Entonox®
Water, e.g. birthing pool/bath	Intramuscular opioids, e.g. pethidine/diamorphine
Massage techniques	Patient-controlled analgesia, i.e. remifentanil
Transcutaneous electrical nerve stimulation (TENS)	Regional analgesia

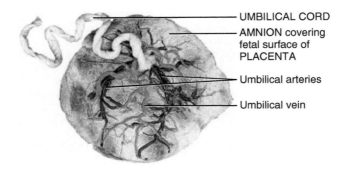

Figure 12.7 **The fetal surface of the placenta. *Source*: Jenkins, G. & Tortora, G.J. (2013) *Anatomy and Physiology: From Science to Life,* 3rd edn. Reproduced with permission of John Wiley & Sons.**

Care Specific to the Second Stage of Labour

During the second stage of labour, uterine contractions may become expulsive and women may feel an urge to bear down and to change to a different position. The midwife continues to monitor maternal and fetal well-being, supports the woman in adopting positions, and encourages behaviours to facilitate a normal delivery, for example encouraging the woman to push when she has the urge to bear down. Women should be encouraged to combine spontaneous pushing with upright positions.

Episiotomy is a surgical incision into the perineum to enlarge the introitus. This should not be carried out routinely during spontaneous vaginal birth.

Care Specific to the Third Stage of Labour

This stage has long been described as the most hazardous for the mother, due to the risk of haemorrhage and other complications (Stables & Rankin, 2017). After the birth, the placenta continues to supply the baby with blood until it separates from the uterine wall or the umbilical cord is clamped and cut by the midwife. Natural separation and birth of the placenta is considered appropriate if the woman has experienced a physiologically normal labour and birth. NICE (2019) states that if a woman at low risk of postpartum haemorrhage requests physiological management of the third stage, she should be supported her in her choice. However, NICE (2019) advocates an active approach involving the use of a drug that stimulates contraction of the uterus. The midwife then clamps and cuts the umbilical cord and delivers the placenta manually. Delayed cord clamping (DCC) is recommended to preserve neonatal iron stores and circulating blood volume (NICE, 2019).

The placenta needs to be examined after birth to check that it is healthy and complete. The maternal surface is dark red in colour. Figure 12.7 demonstrates the appearance of the fetal surface of the placenta.

The midwife may take a sample of blood from the vessels in the umbilical cord to confirm the baby's blood group and Rhesus status. If the maternal and fetal blood group and Rhesus status are not compatible, then there a risk of the mother developing antibodies. This may affect future pregnancies and result in fetal morbidity and mortality.

 Link To/Go To

To understand more about the Rhesus factor and how it affects pregnancy, visit the NHS blood and transplant site: www.blood.co.uk/the-donor/winter2011/am-i-rhesus-positive-or-rhesus-negative.asp

Unexpected and Rapid Deliveries

Occasionally, a woman will deliver her baby unexpectedly or rapidly. If a woman appears to be birthing her baby without a midwife or doctor in attendance, the nurse should proceed as follows.

- Call for help or an ambulance.
- Provide reassurance that help is on the way.
- Consider the woman's privacy and dignity.
- Ensure the area is as warm and draught free as possible.
- Hands off! Let events proceed naturally. Do not cut the cord or attempt to deliver the placenta.
- If the baby delivers, place on mother's abdomen directly on her skin and, if possible, provide a warm cover.
- Do not separate mother and baby.

Initial Care of the Mother and Baby after Birth

This is an important time for the mother and her birth partner to meet the baby and, ideally, the mother and baby should be left undisturbed. It is thought this can help with bonding and breastfeeding. Following delivery, the baby should be dried and placed on the mother's chest. Skin-to-skin contact should be encouraged but it is vital that the baby is not allowed to get cold. The mother's skin temperature will help to keep the baby warm but towels and blankets should cover the baby.

The mother and baby are discreetly observed during this time for signs of normality. The mother will be observed for any signs of bleeding from the genital tract and vital signs will be recorded. Each mother will be assessed individually and will be cared for according to her needs and wishes. It is important to ensure the mother's comfort and dignity during this time.

Table 12.2 Apgar score.

SIGN	SCORE 0	SCORE 1	SCORE 2
Heart rate	Absent	Below 100 beats/minute	Above 100 beats/minute
Respiratory effort	Absent	Weak irregular or gasping	Good, crying
Muscle tone	Flaccid	Some flexion of arms or legs	Well flexed, or active movements of extremities
Reflex irritability	No response	Grimace or weak cry	Good cry
Colour	Blue or pale all over	Body pink, hands and feet blue	Pink all over

Approximately 70% of women will sustain some trauma to the genital tract during birth (NICE, 2019). This can range from minor skin grazes to tears that require suturing. This should be assessed after birth and repairs need to be performed as soon as possible. Urinary incontinence, haematoma, infection and fistulas are rare but possible complications of perineal injury. If these are not identified and treated, they could impact on the quality of the mother's future physical and psychological well-being.

The baby will be assessed at approximately 1 minute after delivery using a scale called the 'Apgar score' (Table 12.2). This score assesses a baby's general well-being at birth and identifies if there is a need for resuscitation. A baby that does not require any intervention will achieve a score of 7 or above.

Overview of Postnatal Care: Mother

The transition to parenthood is one of the most dramatic developmental transitions in the family life cycle. It lays the foundations for the parent–infant relationship, but it can also be a time of increased vulnerability (Wadephul et al., 2019). The postnatal period marks the establishment of a new phase of family life for most women and their partners.

Jot This Down

Consider what 'family' means to you and what it means to other people. How have families changed over the years?
Do most families still consist of mother, father and their children? Think about the needs of different types of families. Will they be the same?

Sadly, some women may experience the loss of their baby or babies may be born with disabilities. Social care services may be involved with support plans or the removal of a child from the mother in extreme circumstances. It is vital that all health professionals caring for these women and their families adopt a sensitive approach to care and incorporate the 6Cs (Care, Compassion, Competence, Communication, Courage and Commitment) of professional practice (Cummings, 2013).

The puerperium or postnatal period lasts between 6 and 8 weeks following birth. During this time, the woman's body reverts to its pre-pregnant state. Ischaemic changes lead to the breakdown of uterine muscle fibres and the uterus returns to its pre-pregnant size, shape and position. This is called *involution*. Lactation will commence and breastfeeding may become established if the mother chooses to breastfeed. Multiple physiological changes to the body that have occurred throughout pregnancy are reversed.

If the woman has birthed at home, then her initial care and ongoing postnatal care will be continued in the home. Women who birth in hospital are generally transferred to a postnatal ward that specialises in the care of new mothers and their babies within a few hours of delivery. The length of the hospital stay will depend on the mother's unique circumstances. However, it is thought to be in the mother and baby's best interests to return home as soon as possible, to establish normal family life and to reduce the risks associated with hospitalisation.

Traditionally, ongoing postnatal care has been offered within the mother's home, but postnatal clinics and telephone support were introduced by some trusts in 2010 (Royal College of Midwives, 2010). The impact of the COVID-19 pandemic has also required a more flexible approach to services. Maternity services currently offer a combination of in-person and remote postnatal follow-up, according to the woman and baby's needs (RCOG, 2020).

Jot This Down

List the advantages and disadvantages of postnatal visiting and newer methods of postnatal support for women.
Which do you think will provide the most effective support?

The midwife's role in the postnatal period is to support the woman and her family, to detect any problems and to refer to an appropriate professional when required. Care should be based on individual circumstances, but the Confidential Enquiry into Maternal Deaths recommended that routine postnatal observations will lead to better recognition and management of potentially life-threatening conditions (Knight et al., 2015).

A range of clinical examinations and observations to assess the mother and confirm normal progress may be undertaken.

- Blood pressure, pulse, temperature and respirations within 6 hours after birth (NICE, 2015).
- *The lochia*: these are the vaginal losses following delivery. They are heavily blood-stained immediately after delivery but become less so as the postnatal period advances.
- *Uterine involution*: abdominal palpation of the uterus is thought to be unnecessary to assess the progress of involution unless the lochia becomes abnormal.
- The midwife should check if the woman has passed urine within 6 hours of birth (NICE, 2015) and assess if micturition continues to be normal.

Following a discussion with the mother, the midwife will determine if additional examinations are necessary, for example if the mother complains of discomfort. The midwife will also ascertain the return of normal bowel function.

It is also important to consider the woman's emotions, as this is a time of immense change. Many women will experience 'baby blues' soon after delivery, usually on the second or third day. Following the initial euphoria after delivery, mothers may feel tired, tearful and low in mood. This is a normal transient occurrence and should resolve spontaneously. It is not fully understood why the baby blues occur, but suggestions include a rapid fall in hormones following delivery and the realisation of the responsibility of motherhood. If the symptoms of baby blues have not resolved within 14 days, the mother should be assessed for postnatal depression (NICE, 2015).

Postnatal depression (PND) is a much more serious mental illness that affects 10–15% of mothers (NICE, 2014). The onset of PND is usually later. If the midwife, mother or her family have concerns about the mother's emotional well-being, the Edinburgh Postnatal Depression Scale can be used to assess for depression. Appropriate referrals must be made to specialist health professionals to ensure the mother receives adequate support and treatment. This is particularly important as recent evidence suggests that in addition to the effect on women and their families, PND can also lead to cognitive and emotional impairment in the baby (NICE, 2014) therefore support and care should be accessed early as this is crucial to achieving optimum health for both the parents and their future children.

> **Jot This Down**
>
> Social isolation is a known risk factor for postnatal depression.
> - What support services are available in your area?
> - Contact local family centres or health visitors for information.
> - How will mothers access these services?

Health and Advice in the Postnatal Period

Mothers will require advice and information about a variety of subjects, depending on their particular circumstances, ranging from baby care to the legal registration of the baby's birth (Box 12.2). The midwife will tailor information to meet the needs

> **Box 12.2 Advice and Guidance for Postnatal Well-being**
>
> - Infant feeding and baby care
> - Sudden infant death syndrome
> - Emotional well-being
> - Contraception and resuming sexual intercourse
> - Diet and exercise
> - Common health problems
> - Life-threatening conditions
> - Breast care
> - Cervical screening
> - Postnatal examination and appointment at 6 weeks
>
> Information about all of these issues can be found at
> **www.nice.org.uk/guidance/cg37**

of the mother, baby and wider family but advice should enable mothers to make choices about their own health and the health and well-being of their babies.

The midwife should ensure that the woman and her family are given information about serious complications that may occur in pregnancy and the postnatal period so they are aware when to access urgent medical attention. Women may present, for example, at GP clinics or emergency departments with complications that may be potentially life-threatening. The signs and symptoms of life-threatening conditions are identified in Table 12.3. Nurses need to be aware of these complications and ensure that women who are pregnant or have recently given birth are identified and receive appropriate and timely treatment.

It is also important that nurses are aware of the potential response to infections during pregnancy, particularly community-acquired Group A *Streptococcus* (GAS). Young children are often carriers of GAS, which is a common causative organism in sore throats. GAS can have devastating effects on pregnant and newly delivered women. This was highlighted back in 2011 by the Centre for Maternal and Child Enquiries when they identified a sudden rise at that time in the number of maternal deaths due to GAS. Nurses should be aware of the need to advise pregnant or newly delivered women about preventing transmission. Women should be advised to wash their hands before and after using the toilet. This is because transmission occurs from contaminated hands to the genital tract when wiping following toilet use. Hands can be easily contaminated when caring for young children. This is an important message health professionals should share during all interactions with pregnant or newly delivered women as this simple advice could save lives.

Urgent liaison with an obstetrician is required if there are any concerns about the health of a pregnant or newly delivered woman.

Postnatal midwifery care continues for as long as the midwife feels it is necessary. Often this will be between 10 and 28 days but will depend on the mother's individual circumstances. Visits should be flexible and arranged to meet the needs of the mother, baby and family. The midwife should liaise with the health visitor and GP to ensure care is provided after discharge from midwifery services.

> **Jot This Down**
>
> The newborn baby can lose heat through four mechanisms:
> *Evaporation, conduction, radiation, convection.*
>
>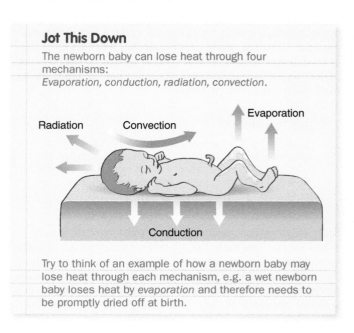
>
> Try to think of an example of how a newborn baby may lose heat through each mechanism, e.g. a wet newborn baby loses heat by *evaporation* and therefore needs to be promptly dried off at birth.

Table 12.3 Signs and symptoms of potentially life-threatening conditions. *Source:* NICE (2015).

POSSIBLE SIGNS AND SYMPTOMS	SIGNS MOTHER NEEDS TO BE AWARE OF	EVALUATE FOR:	ACTION
Sudden or profuse blood loss or blood loss and signs and symptoms of shock, including tachycardia, hypotension, hypoperfusion, change in consciousness	Persistent increased blood loss, faintness, dizziness, palpitations or racing pulse	Postpartum haemorrhage	Emergency action
Offensive excessive vaginal loss, tender abdomen or pyrexia. If no obstetric cause, consider other causes	'Smelly' vaginal loss, abdominal pain, shivering and/or fever	Postpartum haemorrhage, sepsis or other pathology	Urgent action
Pyrexia, shivering, abdominal pain and/or offensive vaginal loss. If temperature exceeds 38 °C, repeat in 4–6 hours. If temperature still high or there are other symptoms and measurable signs, evaluate further	Fever, 'smelly' vaginal loss, abdominal pain and/or shivering	Infection/genital tract sepsis	Emergency action
Severe or persistent headache	Unusual, severe or persistent headache	Pre-eclampsia, eclampsia	Emergency action
Diastolic blood pressure (BP) >90 mmHg accompanied by another sign/symptom of pre-eclampsia, e.g. visual disturbance, oedema, proteinuria, seizures, headache, epigastric pain	Unusual, severe or persistent headache, visual disturbance, excessive swelling, upper abdominal pain, seizures	Pre-eclampsia, eclampsia	Emergency action
Diastolic BP >90 mmHg and no other symptom. Repeat BP within 4 hours. If it remains above 90 mmHg after 4 hours, evaluate	N/A	Pre-eclampsia, eclampsia	Emergency action
Shortness of breath or chest pain	Shortness of breath or chest pain	Pulmonary embolism	Emergency action
Unilateral calf pain, redness or swelling	Calf pain in one leg, redness or swelling	Deep vein thrombosis	Emergency action

195

Care of the Neonate after Birth

The role of the midwife in the early postnatal period is to give the mother the confidence to care for her baby and to confirm normal progress and well-being.

Following birth, the baby should be immediately dried with a warm towel. Parents should be given time to look at and be with their baby soon after birth. Women should be encouraged/offered to have skin-to-skin contact with their baby as soon as possible following birth. Physical contact encourages attachment and initiation of breastfeeding. The baby should be covered with a warm dry towel and a hat applied while maintaining skin-to-skin contact. Initiation of breastfeeding should be encouraged within 1 hour of birth. A woman and her baby should not be separated within the first hour, unless it is necessary for immediate care of the woman or baby. The baby's temperature should be recorded soon after birth, as the effects of cold stress on a newborn baby can include breathing problems and hypoglycaemia. These could result in serious consequences for the baby.

Following the birth of the baby, a thorough examination will be undertaken by the midwife. This examination is to confirm gross normality and to detect any problems that need referral.

An important aspect of this examination is to reassure the parents that their baby appears normal. The baby will be weighed to provide a baseline for future measurement. If birth takes place in a hospital, it is important that name bands and security tags are applied to the baby. Parents should check that the information is correct. Mothers and babies should stay together as one unit throughout their stay in hospital if possible. Vitamin K will be offered to prevent a condition called vitamin K-deficiency bleeding (VKDB).

The examination of the baby in the early postnatal period monitors progress and assesses ongoing well-being. The midwife, in conjunction with feedback from the mother, will confirm that the baby is thriving. Signs of a thriving baby are:

- Alert when awake and asks for feeds
- Good colour (no evidence of grey, blue or ashen tones) and muscle tone
- Calm and relaxed during feeding
- Satisfied after feeds
- Regular wet and soiled nappies
- When feeding established, gaining weight.

The midwife teaches the parents skills, such as bathing, dressing and nappy changing, and by example and discussion will demonstrate good habits such as hand washing. The midwife will teach and advise the parents about how to care for the umbilical cord. The cord will separate by a process of necrosis between day 7 and day 10. Some parents are anxious about care of the umbilical cord but should be advised to keep the cord clean with water and as dry as possible. The midwife will show parents how to put on a nappy leaving the cord exposed. Creams and lotions should not be applied to the cord. Parents should be observant for signs of infection such as redness around the base of the cord, offensive odour or the presence of pus. This should be reported to the GP for appropriate treatment.

A healthy baby should have regular wet and soiled nappies, increasing in frequency. By 7 days, parents should anticipate up to six or more heavy wet nappies with at least two being soiled. Parents should be made aware of the changing stool pattern. The colour and consistency will change from the first stool, which is called *meconium*. This is the sterile content of the baby's bowel and is black and has a sticky tar-like consistency. As the baby starts to breastfeed and milk is absorbed by the bowel, the colour and consistency of the stools change and by 5 days they have a yellow, watery appearance (Figure 12.8). The stools of babies fed artificial milk appear more formed and may also have a seedy appearance.

The midwife also needs to ensure that parents know when to seek advice on other common health problems in babies (Table 12.4).

The early postnatal period is a time for guiding and advising parents and also supporting and encouraging them in their new role. Parents will need information in order to make decisions about neonatal screening tests. (Refer to Figure 12.3 for the antenatal and neonatal screening schedule or visit **www.gov.uk/topic/population-screening-programmes/newborn-blood-spot.**)

Table 12.4 Common health problems in babies. *Source*: NICE (2015).

HEALTH PROBLEM	SIGNS AND SYMPTOMS	ACTION
Jaundice in the first 24 hours	Yellow discoloration of the skin and eyes	Emergency action
Jaundice after the first 24 hours		Monitor overall well-being, hydration and alertness; *refer urgently* if concerned
Jaundice which starts after 7 days and persists after 14 days		Urgent referral
Thrush	Nappy rash and/or white patches on the baby's tongue	Offer information and advice on hygiene; refer for possible antifungal treatment
Nappy rash	Redness, spots, excoriation	Offer information and advice on hygiene; refer for possible treatment
Constipation in formula-fed babies	Reduction in the number of soiled nappies, <1 in 24 hours	Evaluate feed preparation and refer to GP/health visitor
Diarrhoea	Persistent watery stools	Refer to GP
Excessive, persistent crying		Reassure parents and assess the general health of the baby. Refer to health visitor and support groups

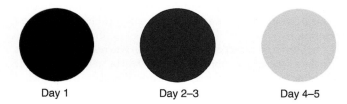

Day 1   Day 2–3   Day 4–5

Figure 12.8 Stool colour chart. Approximate colour guide for the first few days of a baby's life. This should be used as a guide only.

What the Experts Say Caela's Story

Caela's daughter was born with medium-chain acyl-CoA dehydrogenase deficiency (MCADD), which was detected through newborn screening. Caela sits as a parent representative on the MCADD-PKU board, and contributes greatly to the information and resources available for parents.

(Continued)

I have a 5-year-old daughter, J, who was diagnosed with MCADD at 9 days old. I was asked by our clinical nurse specialist if I would become a parent representative on the MCADD board.

The screening for MCADD was initially part of a trial, which we were lucky enough to be a part of, although oblivious of at the time. J's heel-prick test was taken and I vaguely remember being told not to worry as nothing ever shows up.

A few days later, our world was shattered by a phone call from our GP who asked me to call the hospital as something called MCADD had showed up from J's heel-prick test. The next few hours were a whirlwind, as we learned the basics of this condition and prepared to be at the hospital the next morning.

The team that now manage J's MCADD have given us the confidence to meet this condition head on, ensuring J maintains a completely normal life.

We have had our ups and downs with this condition, a few hospital trips with a few days here and there on a glucose drip for J, but it does not consume our lives.

Infant Feeding

There has been a great deal of published research over the last two decades that demonstrates that breastfeeding is a significant factor in improving public health (Brown, 2017; UNICEF, 2010).

Breastfed babies may have better development, cholesterol, blood and dental health. They may also have less cardiovascular disease in later life and a lower incidence of childhood cancers. There is evidence to suggest women who breastfeed are at lower risk of breast and ovarian cancer, hip fractures and poor bone density. Artificially fed babies may be at higher risk of gastrointestinal, respiratory and urinary tract infections, ear infections, eczema, asthma and wheezing, type 1 and type 2 diabetes, obesity, childhood leukaemia and sudden infant death syndrome (UNICEF, 2010).

Infant feeding choices should be made by the parents. It is the midwife's role to give clear, factual information and to support the mother in the feeding method of her choice. Currently in the UK, by the age of 6 weeks, most babies are bottle-fed.

In 2010, the initial breastfeeding rate was 83% and at 6 weeks was 24% in England. The breastfeeding rates were lower in the rest of the UK (Health and Social Care Information Centre, 2012). A systematic review of the Unicef UK Baby Friendly Initiative included papers published between 2002 and 2015. The review demonstrated that the Unicef UK Baby Friendly Initiative increases breastfeeding rates up until the age of 6 weeks and that this is consistent with studies conducted in other resource0rich countries (Fallon *et al.*, 2019).

Mothers who choose to bottle-feed should be shown how to prepare bottles and infant formula, to make sure the principles of hygiene are maintained and ensure the correct nutritional balance of the feed (UNICEF, 2010). It is important to remember that feeding a baby is not just a time for providing nutrients, it is also a time for biological nurturing. Breastfeeding is believed to reduce the risk of sudden infant death syndrome (SIDS). It is important that parents know about the risk of SIDS and all parents should be given advice about safe sleeping. In addition to promoting breastfeeding to reduce risk, other advice includes the following.

- Place your baby on their back to sleep in a cot in a room with you.
- Use a firm waterproof mattress in good condition.
- Never fall asleep with your baby on a sofa or armchair.
- Do not share a bed with your baby if you or your partner:
  – Smoke
  – Have recently drunk any alcohol
  – Have taken legal or illegal medication that could make you sleepy/drowsy.
- Keep your baby smoke free before and after birth.
- Make sure your baby does not get too hot and keep your baby's head uncovered when sleeping.

Conclusion

The role of the midwife in maternity care is to work as part of the larger multidisciplinary team, to provide mothers and babies with high-quality evidence-based care centred around the woman. Much of maternity care is about working in partnership with women to empower them to make decisions about their bodies, their pregnancies and their babies. As nurses, you may come across pregnant women and mothers in a variety of situations. Mothers may ask for your advice and opinions; however, it is your responsibility to refer mothers to the health professional who can provide appropriate care (NMC, 2018).

Key Points

- This chapter has explored the role of the midwife in maternity care and the options available for maternity care and birth.
- It has provided an insight into the physiology of pregnancy and links for further reading.
- There is an overview of the important screening tests offered to women during pregnancy and there are recommended links for further reading.
- There has been discussion of some of the common minor disorders of pregnancy and their appropriate management.
- The importance of the care a woman receives in the antenatal, intranatal and postnatal period and the initial care of the neonate have been emphasised.
- The chapter has highlighted some of the complications of pregnancy and childbirth and the actions required by health professionals.
- There are many opportunities where nurses can impact on maternal and child health to 'Make Every Contact Count'.

References

Bohren, M.A., Hofmeyr, G., Sakala, C., Fukuzawa, R.K., Cuthbert, A. (2017) Continuous support for women during childbirth. *Cochrane Database of Systematic Reviews*, 7, CD003766.

Brown, A. (2017) Breastfeeding as a public health responsibility: a review of the evidence. *Journal of Human Nutrition and Dietetics*, 30(6), 759–770.

Centre for Maternal and Child Enquiries (2011) Saving Mothers' Lives: reviewing maternal deaths to make motherhood safer: 2006–08. The Eighth Report on Confidential Enquiries into Maternal Deaths in the United Kingdom. *BJOG*, 118(Suppl. 1), 1–203.

Cummings, J. (2013) *Compassion In Practice*. Department of Health, London.

Fallon, V.M. Harrold, J.A. & Chisholm, A. (2019) The impact of the UK Baby Friendly Initiative on maternal and infant health outcomes: a mixed-methods systematic review. *Maternal and Child Nutrition*, 15, e12778.

Health and Social Care Information Centre (2012) *Infant Feeding Survey 2010: Summary*. HSCIC, London. http://content.digital.nhs.uk/catalogue/PUB08694/ifs-uk-2010-sum.pdf (accessed December 2021).

Hodnett, E.D., Gates, S., Hofmeyr, G.J. & Sakala, C. (2011) Continuous support for women during childbirth. *Cochrane Database of Systematic Reviews*, 2, CD003766.

International Confederation of Midwives (2011) *ICM international definition of the midwife*. https://internationalmidwives.org/our-work/policy-and-practice/icm-definitions.html (accessed December 2021).

Knight, M., Tuffnell, D., Kenyon, S., Shakespeare, J., Gray, R. & Kurinczuk, J.J. (eds) on behalf of MBRRACE-UK (2015) *Saving Lives, Improving Mothers' Care. Surveillance of Maternal Deaths in the UK 2011–13 and Lessons Learned to Inform Maternity Care from the UK and Ireland Confidential Enquiries into Maternal Deaths and Morbidity 2009–13*. National Perinatal Epidemiology Unit, University of Oxford.

NHS Digital (2020) https://digital.nhs.uk/data-and-information/publications/statistical/nhs-maternity-statistics/2019-20 (accessed December 2021).

NICE (2014) *Antenatal and Postnatal Mental Health: Clinical Management and Service Guidance*. Clinical Guideline No. 45. National Institute for Health and Clinical Excellence, London.

NICE (2015) *Routine Postnatal Care of Women and their Babies*. Clinical Guideline No. 37. National Institute for Health and Clinical Excellence, London.

NICE (2019a) *Intrapartum Care for Healthy Women and Babies*. Clinical Guideline No. 190. National Institute for Health and Clinical Excellence, London.

NICE (2019b) *Routine Care for the Healthy Pregnant Woman*. National Institute for Health and Clinical Excellence, London.

NICE (2019c) *Twin and Triplet Pregnancy*. Clinical Guideline No. 137. National Institute for Health and Clinical Excellence, London.

NICE (2020) *Antenatal Care for Uncomplicated Pregnancies Overview*. Clinical Guideline 62. www.nice.org.uk/guidance/cg62 (accessed December 2021).

Nursing & Midwifery Council (2018) *The Code: Standards of Conduct, Performance and Ethics for Nurses and Midwives*. NMC, London.

Office for National Statistics (2016) *Births in England and Wales: 2016*. www.ons.gov.uk/peoplepopulationandcommunity/birthsdeathsandmarriages/livebirths/bulletins/birthsummarytablesenglandandwales/2019 (accessed December 2021).

Royal College of Midwives (2010) *Audit of Midwifery Practice*. RCM, London.

Royal College of Midwives (2012) *Evidence Based Guidelines for Midwifery-led Care in Labour*. RCM, London.

Royal College of Obstetricians and Gynaecologists (2020) *Guidance for Antenatal and Postnatal Services in the Evolving Coronavirus (COVID-19) Pandemic*. RCOG, London.

Stables, D. & Rankin, J. (2017) *Physiology in Childbearing*. Baillière Tindall, London.

UNICEF (2010) The Baby Friendly Initiative. www.unicef.org.uk/babyfriendly/ (accessed December 2021).

Wadephul, F., Jones, C. & Jomeen, J. (2019) 'Welcome to the World': parents' experiences of an antenatal nurturing programme. *British Journal of Midwifery*, 27, 353–361.

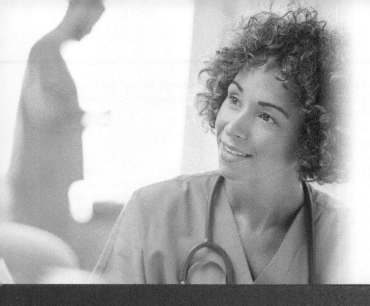

13

The Principles of Caring for People with Long-Term Conditions

Claire Pryor, Annette Hand, Juliana Thompson, Julie Derbyshire, and Sue Tiplady

Northumbria University, UK

Learning Outcomes

On completion of this chapter you will be able to:

- Understand what a long-term condition (LTC) is
- Be able to recognise the impact that LTCs can have on people with LTCs and those around them
- Be able to appreciate the variety of LTC across the lifespan
- Start to consider how communication may support care for people with LTCs

Proficiencies

NMC Proficiencies and Standards:

- Several aspects of the proficiencies equip the newly registered nurse with the underpinning knowledge and skills required for their role in health promotion and protection and prevention of ill health.

Visit the companion website at www.wiley.com/go/peate/nursingpractice3e where you can test yourself using flashcards, multiple-choice questions and more.

Nursing Practice: Knowledge and Care, Third Edition. Edited by Ian Peate and Aby Mitchell.
© 2022 John Wiley & Sons Ltd. Published 2022 by John Wiley & Sons Ltd.
Companion website: www.wiley.com/go/peate/nursingpractice3e

Introduction

Long-term conditions (LTC) are conditions that cannot be cured, but can be controlled with medication and/or the provision of other therapies (Department of Health, 2010). In addition, the World Health Organization (WHO, 2021) describe non-communicable diseases (also known as chronic diseases) as those of long duration which occur due to physiological, environmental, genetic and behavioural components. The most commonly recognised longer conditions are those associated with the cardiovascular system (stroke, myocardial infarction) cancer and respiratory diseases (e.g. asthma), and the ageing population, although LTCs are not exclusive to the older population. The Royal College of General Practitioners (2016) estimates that by 2025 there will be 8.2 million people in the UK living with one or more serious LTC. This represents a significantly increased pressure on health and social care.

The King's Fund (2012) found that in England, over 4 million people who had a physical LTC also had mental health needs. The NHS reports that two-thirds of people with LTCs have co-existing mental health problems, most commonly anxiety and depression. These needs, for many, result in poorer quality of life and health outcomes. The financial cost of this is significant, with the King's Fund (2012) estimating that the NHS spends £8–13 billion pounds a year on LTCs associated with poor mental health. The presence of a co-morbid mental health condition may exacerbate a physical health condition and vice versa. The presence of both is seen to increase the healthcare cost for the individual by more than 45% (King's Fund, 2012).

From this, it is evident that LTCs should not be seen only as involving the physical health of an individual, but also their mental health and well-being and the impact it has on their overall quality of life. The robust link and collaboration between mental health, primary care and chronic disease pathways could significantly enhance the care provided to the individual with LTCs and improve quality of life (King's Fund, 2012).

People of all age ranges are susceptible to the risk factors associated with LTCs, whether that be environmental, poor diet, lack of physical activity, excessive alcohol consumption or exposure to tobacco smoke (WHO, 2021). The WHO (2021) recognises key modifiable and metabolic risk factors for such conditions (Table 13.1). Metabolic risk factors include

Table 13.1 Long-Term Condition Risk Factors.

	RISK FACTOR
Modifiable behaviour	Tobacco use/second-hand smoke
	Excess dietary salt
	Alcohol consumption
	Insufficient physical activity
Metabolic risk	Elevated blood pressure
	Obesity/overweight
	Hyperglycaemia
	Hyperlipidaemia

hypertension (raised blood pressure), being overweight or obese, hyperglycaemia (raised blood glucose levels) and hyperlipidaemia (raised blood fat levels).

Care, dignity and compassion

Conversations about modifiable behaviour and metabolic risk will need a compassionate and empathetic approach. Discussing weight, diet and lifestyle choices needs to be handled sensitively. Respect for the patient is paramount, whilst offering supportive information and any appropriate resources. It is important to ensure the patient feels supported. Non-judgemental and open communication should be maintained.

Practice Assessment Document

Consider how recognition and history taking of environmental, dietary, activity level, substance use and alcohol use may inform your consideration of LTC discussions for your patients. How will you discuss this with your patient and what emotional support may be required?

Nurses/Nursing Students: Review the NMC (2018a) Skills, Annex A
1.5 Use caring conversation techniques
   1.7 Be aware of own unconscious bias in communication encounters
   2.7 Assess motivation and capacity for behaviour change and clearly explain cause and effect relationships related to common health risk behaviours including smoking, obesity, sexual practice, alcohol and substance use
   2.8 Provide information and explanation to people, families and carers and respond to questions about their treatment and care and possible ways of preventing ill health to enhance understanding

Nursing Associates: Review the NMC (2018b) Skills, Annex A
1.6 Use caring conversation techniques
   1.8 Be aware of the possibility of own unconscious bias in communication encounters
   2.9 Engage in difficult conversations with support from others, helping people who are feeling emotionally or physically vulnerable or in distress, conveying compassion and sensitivity

How will you support those you care for when discussing LTCs? What skills and abilities do you need to have to communicate in a caring and compassionate manner whilst potentially discussing sensitive topics (such as lifestyle choices)?

The *Five Year Forward View* (NHS England, 2014) set out the direction and key priorities that the NHS was to take, considering the rapidly evolving health and care needs of the population. This was based on an understanding that people live longer, with more complex health needs, and, may make lifestyle decisions that impact upon future health. Recognising the historical divides between primary, secondary and community-based services, the *Five Year Forward View* aimed to keep LTCs central and encompass the physical, mental and social needs of the population.

The report recognised that people with LTCs may be frequent users of health services, although they actually spend less than 1% of their time with healthcare professionals. The remaining 99% of the time, the person with LTC manages their condition themselves, alongside any family/carers. Thus importance is placed on real person-centred care that aligns to the individual's goal and life. Central to this is the promotion of independence and empowerment. This may be in the form of better access to services, advice and support and taking more control over their care provision. To support empowerment, the NHS focused on key improvements, primarily access to and the type of information provided to people with LTCs. The plan aimed to open health record access to the individuals, and also facilitate sharing of records across health and social care providers. For the patients themselves, increased access to their records, health history and improved clinical information was included.

Following on from this, and supported by improved information provision, the plan aimed to support people to better manage their own health. Self-management courses, peer support groups and education provision were central to this aim with the support of the voluntary sector. The ability for people with LTCs to have choice over service provision location and increase control over the care provided was considered. It was recognised that whilst an option in practice, only half of patients report a choice in location or manner in which they receive care.

The NHS committed to enhancing person-centred care for people with LTCs in 2015 with the production of *Our Declaration: Person-Centred Care for Long Term Conditions* (NHS, 2015). This declaration promised to always hold the individual at the centre of care provision, and to consider their mental and physical well-being together. The declaration covered four key areas.

1. *Person-centred care for all*: this recognised that adults, children and young people may all live with LTCs, and person-centred care is integral to all people. Person-centred care is usually associated with care for frail, vulnerable older people. This declaration placed it at the heart of care for all people with LTCs irrespective of age.

2. *Person-centred care at all stages*: here, a declaration was made to support care that spanned all phases of the individual's life and recognise how these may change over time. Individuals may have no LTCs at one end of the spectrum and engage in proactive lifestyle choices, whilst towards the other end of the spectrum, people may have multiple LTCs and have significantly different needs. As such, the individual's need will change in line with their health.

3. *Collaborative care and support planning as the key to person-centred care*: the introduction of care and support planning as a process is central to allowing professionals and individuals to move towards their specific goals. This approach included not only traditional medical interventions, but wider social participation and strategies.

4. *Person-centred care in the NHS, locally and nationally*: the final declaration seeks to support partnership working with people with LTCs and their carers to co-produce services. This values their experiences and supports professionals to design and deliver services with compassion. In addition, the declaration advocated for the single use of the LTC Framework (The House of Care) to ensure consistent and evidence-led tools uptake across the NHS.

The 2017 review of the *Five Year Forward View* (NHS England, 2017) reported on the 3-year implementation, improvements made and further recommendations for the health and social care service. It found improvements in GP appointment times for people with LTCs through the introduction of streaming patients to facilitate same-day appointments and preserving continuity of care. Improvements have also been seen in integrating community service provision (GP, community nursing, social care, etc.) and increased specialist care provision in the community rather than hospital settings and a move towards better care for older people. This is being achieved through strategies such as Enhanced Health in Care Homes which joins up health and rehabilitations services.

A Framework for LTC Care: The House of Care

Recognising the need for a new way to manage care for people with LTCs, the House of Care model was devised by NHS England (2019) (Figure 13.1). Traditional segregated medical models of care do not represent the current population's needs, and a focus has been placed on patient experiences and the expertise of the person with LTCs. This approach helps support holistic care for the person with an LTC.

The House of Care module has five key elements.

1. Organisational and supporting processes form the roof.
2. Engaged, informed individuals and carers form a wall.
3. Health and care professionals who are committed to partnership working form the second wall.
4. Commissioning forms the floor or foundations of the house.
5. Person-centred co-ordinated care is the centre and heart of the house.

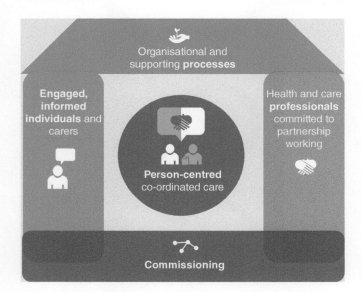

Figure 13.1 **The House of Care model.** *Source:* NHS England (2019).

Care and Support Planning

For healthcare professionals and the people they care for, collaborative Care and Support Planning (CSP) is a way to approach care advocated by the King's Fund (2013a) and the British Heart Foundation (BHF, 2018). Keeping the person at the centre of the process, health professionals work in partnership with the individual with the LTCs to co-ordinate services and support the goals and needs of the individual. The process is dynamic and encompasses a process of disease surveillance, preparation and conversations (BHF, 2018). Throughout the process, the values and experience of the person are paramount. They bring the qualitative experience of the LTC, and the healthcare professional brings clinical expertise. Coming together in a partnership, they hold a conversation about progress, goal setting and forming a care plan (BHF, 2018). A simple version of this is presented in Figure 13.2.

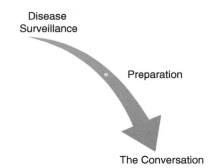

Figure 13.2 **Care and Support Planning process.** *Source:* Modified from BHF (2018).

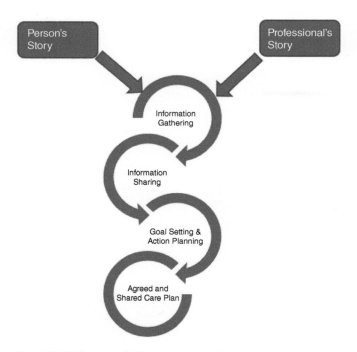

Figure 13.3 **The consultation.** *Source:* Adapted from King's Fund (2013a).

The full process of CSP commences with the recognition that the professional and person both bring their story to the conversation (or consultation). Each will have different experiences or knowledge to share. Health professionals need to recognise that the experience of the person with the LTC and their personal assets are equally as important as the clinical information. Any tests, investigations or health status checks that may be required are carried out. Following this, a preparatory period is undertaken where an agenda for a conversation is set, results from tests are collated and reviewed and a reminder for the conversation appointment is set. At the conversation, an appropriate practitioner and the person with the LTCs will meet as 'equals and experts' to discuss and review progress, visit or revisit goals to highlight what priorities are present, share ideas, discuss and review available options and develop a care plan in partnership. This plan is then agreed and recorded. The King's Fund (2013a) approach to consultation is shown in Figure 13.3.

This collaborative conversation process sits at the very heart of the House of Care.

Cancer and Long-Term Conditions

Cancer is increasingly being seen as a long-term condition as more people are living with a cancer diagnosis, or have other long-term conditions at the same time as cancer. Macmillan (2015) found that 70% of people with cancer also had at least one additional LTC. The addition of LTCs in a person with cancer may impact upon survival rate and increase level of need. The five most common LTCs found in someone with cancer were hypertension, obesity, mental health conditions, chronic heart disease and chronic kidney disease. This has significant parallels with the WHO modifiable and metabolic risk categories (WHO, 2021).

Long-Term Neurological Conditions

Neurological conditions (including Parkinson disease, epilepsy and motor neurone disease) significantly impact on the affected person, their family/loved ones and carers. Whilst some neurological conditions can be intermittent (epilepsy) or stable in presentation (e.g. adults with cerebral palsy), many are progressive (such as Parkinson disease). The care of people with neurological conditions accounts for 14% of the social care budget (NHS England, n.d.). Recognising the significant burden to the person with a neurological condition, the impact on care provision and associated cost, the NHS has placed special focus on neurological conditions as an area for service improvement.

Parkinson Disease

Parkinson disease is a complex neurodegenerative disorder characterised by the gradual depletion of dopamine. Dopamine is a neurotransmitter produced in the substantia nigra, ventral tegmental area and hypothalamus of the brain. Dopamine plays an important role in the brain and body and is required for executive functions, motor control, motivation and reward. The exact cause of Parkinson disease remains unclear but current research suggests that a combination of age, genetic and environmental factors causes the dopamine-producing nerve cells to die (Bloem *et al.*, 2021).

In the UK, due to population growth and an ageing population, the incidence and prevalence of Parkinson disease are increasing. In 2018, there were thought to be 145 519 people with Parkinson disease in the UK, with predictions that the UK Parkinson disease population will have increased to 256 609 people by 2065 (Parkinson's Disease UK, 2018). Currently there is no cure or disease-modifying treatment for Parkinson disease and although it is not life-threatening, it is a life-changing diagnosis. Parkinson disease is an age-related disease, with incidence and prevalence steadily increasing with age (Pringsheim *et al.*, 2014). However, it is not just a disease of older people. The age of onset for almost 25% of affected individuals is younger than 65 years and for 5–10% it is younger than 50 years. Around 1 in 20 people with the condition first experience symptoms when they are under 40 and are often referred to as having young-onset Parkinson disease (Schirinzi *et al.*, 2020).

For many years, Parkinson disease was characterised by its motor features of rest tremor, rigidity, bradykinesia and postural instability but there are over 40 non-motor symptoms which are very common and can include autonomic dysfunction, cognitive dysfunction, neurobehavioural disorders (e.g. depression, apathy, anhedonia), and sensory and sleep abnormalities.

Diagnosis

Parkinson disease remains a clinical diagnosis, meaning there are no tests or scans that can be performed to confirm the diagnosis. Usually individuals will first present to their GP and if they complain of symptoms of tremor, stiffness, slowness, balance problems and/or gait disorder, Parkinson disease should be suspected. Following National Institute of Health and Care Excellence (NICE) guidance (NICE, 2017a), people should be referred quickly and untreated to a specialist in Parkinson disease as there are a number of different diagnoses for this condition. Following the Movement Disorders Society diagnostic criteria (Figure 13.4), specialists will undertake a full patient medical, social and medication history, along with a neurological examination to determine if presenting symptoms could be caused by Parkinson disease.

The diagnosis of Parkinson's disease needs to be reviewed regularly, every 6–12 months, and reconsidered if atypical features develop or if individuals do not respond to Parkinson disease treatment (NICE, 2017a). For patients, this means that it may take several months, or even years, to have a diagnosis of Parkinson disease confirmed.

Everybody reacts to a serious diagnosis, like Parkinson disease, differently. For some individuals, it may be a total shock and very unexpected, for others it may be a relief that they finally have a reason for all their symptoms. It is vital that at this stage people are given the right information and the support they need to help them understand and manage their condition.

Supporting Individuals to Reduce Their Risk of Developing a Long-Term Condition

As with many LTCs, it is important that we understand potential risk factors for developing certain conditions to provide relevant and appropriate health promotion and advice to individuals to reduce the risk of disease development. When examining the causes of Parkinson disease, there are three relevant factors that we need to take into consideration: genetics, environment and the interactions between these. Currently there is a good understanding of the causative genes of Parkinson disease, but this

203

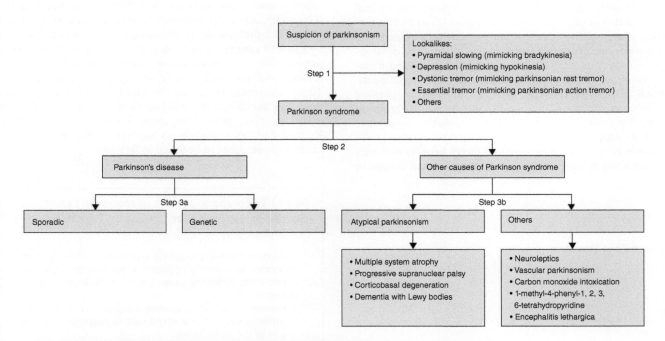

Figure 13.4 The Movement Disorder Society diagnostic criteria for Parkinson disease. *Source:* Bloem et al. (2021).

only accounts for 5–10% of people who develop the disease. Currently genetic screening occurs within specialist centres after careful discussion with individuals or as part of a research study. Until disease-modifying treatments are developed, genetic screening for Parkinson disease in the general population is not recommended.

The assessment of the so-called *environmentome* (i.e. the sum of all potentially causative and protective factors for Parkinson disease that are present in our environment) is not possible at present, but some risk factors have been identified that may inform our practice. One established risk factor for developing Parkinson disease is exposure to environmental toxins such as pesticides, for which there is converging and consistent evidence (Dorsey, 2020). Health and safety regulations regarding the handing of environmental toxins are in place for multiple professions and adherence to these is monitored. Another well-established risk factor is head injury. Research studies and the examination of medical claims databases have shown, for example with former professional soccer players, that traumatic brain injury can be a risk factor for Parkinson disease (Mackay *et al.*, 2019; VanItallie, 2019; Russell *et al.*, 2020). Other sports where traumatic brain injury could occur, such as boxing and rugby, are also under scrutiny due to the potential long-term implications on an individual's physical and mental health.

Negative associations with the risk of developing Parkinson disease have also been identified for smoking, coffee drinking and anti-inflammatory drug use (Noyce *et al.*, 2012). However, you would not recommend people to start smoking, drinking high levels of caffeine or taking regular anti-inflammatory drugs to lower their risk of developing Parkinson disease. These activities in themselves could be very damaging to an individual's health and well-being.

Only by fully understanding the current evidence and being able to discuss this with an individual are you able to promote healthy lifestyle choices. The multiple physical and mental health benefits of physical activity, healthier lifestyles and better fitness are well documented but physical activity may also be an important protective factor for preventing the development of Parkinson disease. In a systematic review and meta-analysis of more than half a million unique participants, physical activity, particularly moderate to vigorous physical activity, was associated with a significant reduction in Parkinson disease risk (Fang *et al.*, 2018). When promoting a healthier lifestyle or supporting an individual to increase activity levels, being able to provide evidence-based direct benefits to health and well-being is important to promote a potential change in lifestyle.

Pharmacological Management of Parkinson Disease

Parkinson disease is treatable, but any treatment strategy must be individualised to meet the specific needs of an individual. There are four main pharmacotherapy treatment strategies used in the management of Parkinson disease and they work by one or more of the following methods.

- Increase the amount of dopamine within the brain (levodopa).
- Act as a dopamine substitute, stimulating the parts of brain where dopamine works (dopamine agonists).
- Block the action of other factors (enzymes) that break down dopamine (monoamine oxidase-B inhibitors and catechol-o-methyl transferase inhibitors).

Prior to the results of a large pragmatic, open-label randomised trial being published by the PD Medication (PD Med) Collaborative Group (2014), any of the treatment strategies could be used from diagnosis. The PD Med trial provided evidence that was incorporated into the Parkinson disease guidance from NICE (2017a) that recommended offering levodopa as the first treatment for those individuals presenting with motor features affecting their quality of life. Ultimately, the decision on when, and which treatment, to start should be made in partnership between the person with Parkinson disease and their specialist following a discussion regarding:

- All available pharmacology choices
- Risk and benefits of treatments
- Expectations from treatment and personal lifestyle choices.

Regardless of which medication is chosen, people with Parkinson disease will be required to maintain strict adherence to an individualised, timed medication regime related to the medication pharmacology. Dosing intervals will also be specific to each individual according to their daily routine. When medications are not administered on time, people with Parkinson disease can experience an immediate increase in symptoms. Delays to medication can result in worsening tremors, increased rigidity, loss of balance, confusion, agitation and difficulty communicating (Grissinger, 2018). If people with Parkinson disease are admitted to hospital, their medicine management is often compromised by a lack of awareness, and a lack of systems and procedures to prevent delayed/missed doses or incorrect prescribing of time-critical Parkinson disease medicines (Oguh & Videnovic, 2012). To try and ensure Parkinson disease medications are given on time, they are classed as critical medicines as an administration delay has the potential to cause harm to the individual. Recommendations for how to support people to have their medication on time can be found in Box 13.1.

Jot This Down

Sam is 54 and has recently been diagnosed with Parkinson disease. Sam is not keen to start medication for Parkinson disease yet but is keen to see if there is any way they can slow the disease down. Sam has seen that smoking may help in Parkinson disease and asks you about using nicotine replacement patches. How would you respond to this?

Box 13.1 How to support a person with Parkinson disease to get their medications on time in a hospital setting

- Parkinson disease medicines should be ordered from the pharmacy as a matter of priority to prevent omission of doses if the individual's own supply of medicine is not available.
- Parkinson's disease medicines are provided as a matter of urgency. Lack of awareness may highlight the learning needs of the wider team.

- Prescribed medicines are administered at the specific times the person with Parkinson disease would normally take them (this may not be the same time as the normal ward drug round).
- People with Parkinson disease are assessed to determine if they can safely self-administer their PD medicines; this should adhere to local policy.

Red Flag

 Individuals with Parkinson disease should not be treated with metoclopramide or prochlorperazine (antiemetics used to treat nausea or vomiting) as they block D2 (dopamine) receptors in the brain, which can worse Parkinson disease symptoms.

Domperidone or ondansetron should be used instead.

Non-pharmacological Management of Parkinson Disease

From the diagnosis of Parkinson disease, a participatory health model should be followed, where health and care professionals not only care for people with Parkinson disease but also encourage individuals to participate in their own care plan. As such, people with Parkinson disease, and their direct family members, should be regarded as members of the multidisciplinary team.

Participatory health also means involving people with Parkinson disease in important medical decisions made on the basis of digestible information tailored to their needs and educational level and combining scientific evidence with the healthcare professionals' experience and the preferences of people with Parkinson disease (van den Heuvel *et al.*, 2020). An example of this could be which medication a person with Parkinson disease should take, and when. This decision should not only be based on evidence-based practice but also on personal preference and lifestyle choice of the individual.

Jot This Down

What is participatory health? Take some time to consider how your practice areas support participatory health.

Participatory health is firmly grounded in patient engagement, shared decision making, patient activation, patient-centred and consumer-directed care.

Practice Assessment Document

 Consider how engaging in participatory healthcare practice may support the NMC Skills Annex A: 1.1, 1.5 and 2.8.

In partnership with your practice supervisor or assessor, take the lead in discussing their proposed care with a patient. Demonstrate active listening skills and appropriate responses to any questions they have.

Remember, it's OK (and very important) to acknowledge when you need to seek information from others.

Reassure the patient and/or carers that their opinions are heard and valued. Using this shared information, discuss the goals or wishes of both the patient and the healthcare team.

Student Nursing Associates

Consider how engaging in participatory healthcare practice may support the achievement of Platform 2: Promoting health and preventing ill health.

Consider platform 2, section 2.2. In discussion with a patient, you may support them by providing information about their condition, and having a caring conversation about the different options they have. This may support their understanding and promote informed decisions.

In order to manage the complex demands of Parkinson disease, there are various models of care provision in the UK. Most people with Parkinson disease are under the care of a specialist service led by a neurologist or a geriatrician with a specialist interest in Parkinson disease. As part of that service, some will also have access to care from a Parkinson disease nurse specialist. A minority of people with Parkinson disease will be managed by their GP alone. The person with Parkinson disease will have a core team of professionals always involved in their care, including their medical specialist, GP and Parkinson disease nurse specialist.

Unfortunately, many features of Parkinson disease do not respond well to optimal pharmacotherapy. The spectrum of motor and non-motor symptoms caused by Parkinson disease, including changes in speech and swallow, impairments in walking, balance and upper limb movement, cannot be effectively managed with pharmacological therapy alone and so many symptoms will also require non-pharmacological interventions. The broader impact that many Parkinson disease symptoms have on activities of daily living requires a multidisciplinary team approach to treatment. For health and care professionals, this means having an awareness of the multisystem nature of the condition and the impact it can have on lifestyle. When assessing people with Parkinson disease, it is important to examine both motor and non-motor symptoms that may be impacting on their quality of life or level of functional ability.

If a problem is identified, and after discussion with the person with Parkinson disease, a prompt referral should be made to the appropriate multidisciplinary team member. Figure 13.5 illustrates the professional disciplines that may be involved in multidisciplinary care for people with Parkinson disease due to disease progression or symptom development. Early referral to physiotherapy is recommended (NICE, 2017a) for assessment, education and advice, including information about physical activity. Aerobic exercise, even when done at home, has been found to be a valuable non-pharmacological treatment for people with Parkinson disease (van der Kolk *et al.*, 2019). There are many ways in which people with Parkinson disease can contribute to their health, including adopting a healthy lifestyle that involves regular exercise and an appropriate diet, but they need information, support and guidance to do so.

Jot This Down

Many people with LTCs are managed by multiple health and care professionals across primary and secondary care. How will you ensure you have the most up-to-date information from their healthcare teams, and how will you ensure effective communication of any care, or changes to care, that you provide?

205

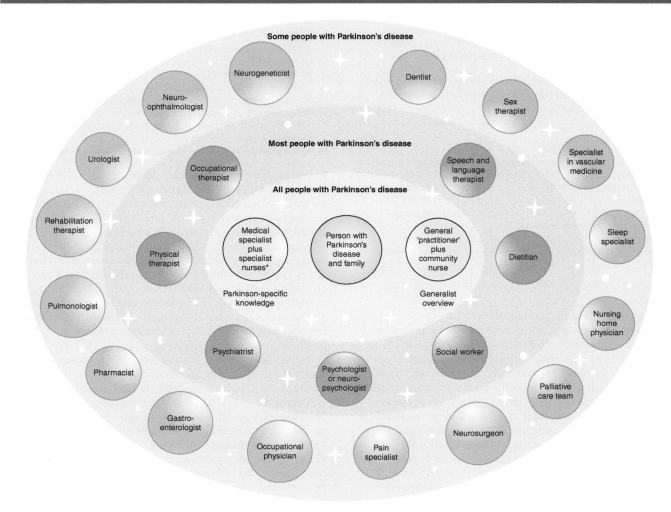

Figure 13.5 Professional disciplines involved in care for people with Parkinson disease. *Source:* Bloem et al. (2021).

Epilepsy

Epilepsy is the most common chronic neurological condition and is characterised by recurrent and unprovoked seizures originating in the brain, with the dysfunction caused by excessive and abnormal neuronal discharge (Hickey, 2017). Epilepsy affects 600 000 or 1 in 103 people in the UK (Epilepsy Action, 2017) and 50 million people worldwide (WHO, 2019). One in 20 people will have a single seizure at some point in their life, but epilepsy is defined as having two or more unprovoked seizures.

Epilepsy varies in its clinical presentation and presents very differently in each person. This can be dependent on the age of the person when the epilepsy develops, and the cause of the epilepsy. The causes of epilepsy can be identified as:

- Structural
- Genetic
- Infectious
- Metabolic
- Immune.

Examples include perinatal trauma, neurological conditions, hereditary susceptibility and metabolic disturbances (WHO, 2019). In many cases a cause for the epilepsy is never identified (Hickey, 2017). It is recommended that patients suspected as having epilepsy be seen by a specialist within 2 weeks to ensure early diagnosis and initiation of therapy as appropriate to their individual needs (NICE, 2012).

A diagnosis of epilepsy has major implications for the person, therefore accurate diagnosis is essential as there is misdiagnosis in 5–20% of cases (NICE, 2012).

Diagnosis

Accurate history and witness description are an essential part of the initial assessment, with a description of events leading up to the seizure being as important as the event itself. Blood tests, electrocardiogram (ECG; to assess for long QT syndrome), electroencephalogram (EEG; to clarify seizure type and syndrome), computed tomography (CT) or magnetic resonance imaging (MRI) and video-telemetry are investigations used to aid the diagnosis, but also to rule out other potential diagnoses (NICE, 2012; Hickey, 2017).

Classification

Seizures have been classified by the International League Against Epilepsy (ILAE), which is a world-wide organisation of epilepsy professionals (Epilepsy Action, 2017). Seizures can vary from the briefest lapses of attention or muscle jerks to severe and prolonged convulsions (WHO, 2019), but are most often categorised into focal and generalised seizures. Table 13.2 details the different types.

Focal seizures present with signs and symptoms depending on the location in the brain where seizure occurs, most often in one hemisphere only. Motor symptoms might include brief irregular jerking movements of limbs, lip smacking and chewing. Non-motor symptoms can include feelings of anxiety, changes to smell, vision or hearing (Epilepsy Action, 2017). Most focal aware seizures are brief, usually lasting between 2 and 3 minutes with full recovery 10 minutes after the seizure (Woodward & Mestecky, 2011), whereas generalised seizures are characterised by more diffuse abnormal electrical activity throughout the whole brain, the most common being a tonic-clonic seizure. These types of seizures often begin with a period of irritability (frequently described as an 'aura') preceding the seizure with a sudden loss of consciousness. Tonic stiff movements of the limbs are followed by a clonic phase which is characterised by rhythm jerking movements of the limbs. Grunting, foaming at the mouth, tongue biting and incontinence can also occur during this type of seizure (Epilepsy Action, 2017). Tonic-clonic seizures can last up to 3 minutes and after the seizure the limbs become limp, breathing is quiet and when the patient awakes, they may be disorientated and often fatigued.

When a tonic-clonic seizure lasts more than 5 minutes, or if the patient experiences three or more seizures in an hour without recovery, it is known as status epilepticus and is considered a medical emergency (NICE, 2012; Hickey, 2017). Immediate care should be focused around maintaining individual safety, with the administration of buccal midazolam. This is particularly seen in the prehospital phase and community setting where access to medical equipment is more limited. Phenytoin is also recommended by NICE (2012) to be given intravenously, prescribed for seizure relapse in hospital, and has to be used with caution due to its action on the heart; thus, cardiac monitoring is required.

Absence seizures are the other main type of generalised seizure, characterised by an abrupt stop to normal activity and short loss of consciousness of 10–30 seconds. The person does not move, their eyes become vacant, and they often stare straight ahead. Absence seizures often go unnoticed because of their short duration but can occur several times a day with a full recovery after the seizure (Epilepsy Action, 2017).

Table 13.2 Classification of seizures. *Source:* Based on Epilepsy Action (2017).

FOCAL SEIZURES	GENERALISED SEIZURES	
Focal aware seizures without impaired conscious level	Absence seizures	
	Myoclonic seizures	
Focal impaired awareness seizures with impaired conscious level	Clonic seizures	
	Tonic seizures	
	Tonic-clonic seizures	
	Atonic seizures	

Treatment

The underlying cause of the seizure will determine treatment interventions, but if there is no underlying condition causing the epilepsy, the mainstay of treatment is directed at management of seizures through medication (Karch, 2017). The drugs that are used to manage seizures are referred to as anticonvulsants or more commonly antiepileptic drugs (AEDs). These drugs aim to control epilepsy in one of three ways.

1. Enhance the activity of the inhibitory neurotransmitter gamma-aminobutyric acid (GABA).
2. Enhance the activity of the excitatory brain neurotransmitter glutamate.
3. Directly block sodium and/or calcium channels in the nerve cell membrane.

Antiepileptic drugs should only be prescribed once an epilepsy diagnosis is confirmed, most often after two unprovoked seizures. The AED strategy for each person should be individualised according to the seizure and epilepsy type, co-morbidity, the person's lifestyle, and the preferences of the person, their family and/or carers as appropriate (NICE, 2018).

The WHO (2019) states that 70% of patients with epilepsy can have seizures reduced or controlled effectively by appropriate use of AEDs. AEDs work by controlling the electrical activity in the brain that causes seizures and are most effective if they are taken regularly, around the same time each day. The aim of AED treatment is to take the lowest dose of the fewest number of AEDs and with the fewest side-effects. They are introduced at a low dose, with gradual increase until seizures are controlled. If seizures are not controlled with a single drug, another drug might be added until optimum management is achieved (Epilepsy Society, 2017).

Table 13.3 lists the different AEDs depending on seizure type used by healthcare teams to guide prescription strategy for patients.

Adults with epilepsy should have an agreed, written epilepsy care plan that includes details about their medication, any preferences and lifestyle issues, which needs to be agreed between the individual with epilepsy and their healthcare team (NICE, 2012).

The role of the nurse in epilepsy is to help people cope better with their epilepsy, which is not limited to management of seizures and medicine optimisation but includes provision of good education for the patient and their family or carers. Information needs are dependent on the patient's gender, age, lifestyle, job and how long they have had epilepsy (Woodward & Mestecky, 2011).

People with epilepsy should be advised to avoid potential triggers for seizures which might include medication non-concordance, lack of sleep, stress, alcohol/recreational drugs, flashing lights, hormonal imbalance and illness (Epilepsy Action, 2017). Health promotion in terms of lifestyle issues is also an important part of patient education, with reviews recommended by epilepsy specialist services if there are any concerns about medication or lifestyle issues (NICE, 2012).

Whilst epilepsy can be a hidden disability, it is a chronic long-term condition which can also have a significant impact on the patient's daily life and well-being, including their mood, relationships, driving and employment. Psychological interventions including talking therapies or cognitive behavioural therapy (CBT) may be used in conjunction with AED therapy, which

Table 13.3 Antiepileptic drugs (AED) by seizure type.
Source: Based on NICE (2018).

SEIZURE TYPE	FIRST-LINE AED	ADJUNCT AED
Focal (partial, complex partial, secondary generalised)	Carbamazepine	Levetiracetam
	Lamotrigine	Clobazam
	Levetiracetam	(and many other AEDs)
	Oxcarbazepine	
	Gabapentin	
	Sodium valproate	
Generalised tonic-clonic	Carbamazepine	Clobazam
	Lamotrigine	Lamotrigine
	Oxcarbazepine	Levetiracetam
	Sodium valproate	Sodium valproate
		Topiramate
Absence	Ethosuximide	Ethosuximide
	Lamotrigine	Lamotrigine
	Sodium valproate	Sodium valproate
		Benzodiazepines
		Levetiracetam
		Topiramate
Myoclonic	Levetiracetam	Levetiracetam
	Sodium valproate	Sodium valproate
	Topiramate	Topiramate
		Levetiracetam
		Clonazepam
		Topiramate

Sudden Unexpected Death in Epileptic People (SUDEP)

Each year in the UK 1200 people die due to epilepsy, and half of those deaths can be attributed to SUDEP, with a lack of awareness amongst those with epilepsy and their relatives. SUDEP is most likely in the 18–24-year-old age group and is defined as when a person with epilepsy dies without warning, most often after nocturnal seizures – at night or during sleep. The risk can be minimised by providing good patient education to people with epilepsy and their families about medicine concordance to optimise seizure control, alongside having an awareness of the dangers of nocturnal seizures (NICE, 2012; Williamson, 2021).

Case Study

Amy is 20 years old and has recently been diagnosed with temporal lobe epilepsy after three unprovoked seizures. Diagnosis was made following EEG and telemetry (this showed simple focal, complex focal and secondary generalised seizures).

Carbamazepine and lamotrigine are both first-line treatments in focal epilepsy. However, Amy is using a combined hormonal contraceptive pill. This may be affected by enzyme-inducing drugs such as carbamazepine, so lamotrigine is prescribed. If she is to consider pregnancy in the future, she is informed that treatment with high-dose folic acid will be needed to reduce the risk of neural tube defects during pregnancy.

The DVLA regulations are discussed with Amy and she is advised that she cannot drive until she has been free of seizures for 1 year. A written treatment plan is provided, and leaflets are given on different aspects of epilepsy diagnosis, medication management and lifestyle issues which may be affected by epilepsy. Amy will be followed up with the practice nurse who will carry out regular reviews.

Red Flag

 Sodium valproate is a common AED but it is not to be used in women or young people of child-bearing age unless a Pregnancy Prevention Programme (PPP) is in place. The risk of birth defects and developmental disorders is significant if pregnancy occurs when taking valproate.

Adapted from NICE (2012), Medicines and Healthcare products Regulatory Agency (2018)

may be associated with improvement in well-being, but there is no evidence to suggest it improves seizure control (NICE, 2012). It is important to signpost the patient and their families to agencies such as the Epilepsy Society and Epilepsy Action for ongoing support and up-to-date information and research on the condition. However, it is the epilepsy nurse specialist who is often the co-ordinator of care and the key point of access on an ongoing basis and the identified expert who conducts the yearly reviews (NICE, 2012).

The prognosis of those with epilepsy is variable, but 70–80% of people who develop epilepsy will at some point be free from seizures with effective treatment, predominantly from medication (Greenstein, 2009). It is important to note that when AEDs are not effective, surgery may be considered for focal seizures where specific areas causing the seizure can be removed in an attempt to prevent further seizures and improve quality of life (Woodward & Mestecky, 2011).

Frailty and Long-Term Conditions

The management of chronic illnesses and LTCs becomes much more complicated due to three primary factors:

1. Frailty
2. Multimorbidity
3. Complex multiple needs.

Frailty is a state of health and is related to the ageing process. Through this process, multiple body systems gradually lose their in-built reserves and ability to fully recover from even minor stressors (British Geriatrics Society, 2014; Skills for Health, NHS England and Health Education England 2018). Frailty may overlap with LTCs and multimorbidity. It is not a term to be used to describe someone who looks old, weak or ill.

Many older people who have frailty may not themselves identify as frail. They may recognise that they have lost some ability or have several conditions that impact on their life but they may not consider themselves frail. This is partly due to the misconception that frailty is associated with vulnerability or dependency. Whilst some frail people may be vulnerable or dependent, others may not (British Geriatric Society, 2014).

Frailty shares common features of other LTCs in that:

- At present there is no cure
- It is progressive in nature and gets worse over time
- It can impact on a person's daily living abilities
- There are episodes of crisis which impact upon recovery
- It is associated with high financial costs to the health and social care economy.

Frailty is a complex presentation due to it being a medical syndrome (a syndrome is a group of symptoms consistently occurring together) rather than a single disease (Harrison *et al.*, 2015; Lyndon, 2015). As such, frailty is a complex LTC in its own right, whilst encompassing potentially several other individually classified LTCs.

Frailty may be identified by considering deficits; these may include disease states, symptoms or signs of frailty, abnormal tests or laboratory values, and disabilities amongst others (Figure 13.6; adapted from Clegg et al. 2016).

As we age, the percentage of people within the population with a frailty presentation increases. Table 13.4 shows the population estimates for people living with frailty by age range.

Often frailty becomes recognised at a time of crisis when a person presents with one or more of the common syndromes of frailty: immobility, falls, susceptibility to side-effects of medication, incontinence, delirium (British Geriatrics Society, 2014).

The consequences of having frailty are profound. Older people living with frailty are at risk of adverse outcomes such as dramatic changes in their physical, cognitive and mental well-being after an apparently minor event which challenges their health, such as an infection or new medication. Because of frailty, full recovery from such events may never occur. Figure 13.7 shows how this works. Initially, the person in this figure has frailty but is just managing to remain functionally independent. When faced with a minor event such as a UTI, a change in medication, catching flu or a fall, the person may become immediately more functionally dependent. They may recover but due to having frailty, a return to their original functional ability is unlikely. In this case, they do not regain independence which has implications for their physical, social, emotional and psychological well-being and care needs.

209

Table 13.4 **Estimated population percentage for frailty.**

AGE	ESTIMATED PERCENTAGE LIVING WITH FRAILTY
65–69	4%
70–74	7%
75–79	9%
80–84	16%
Over 85	26%

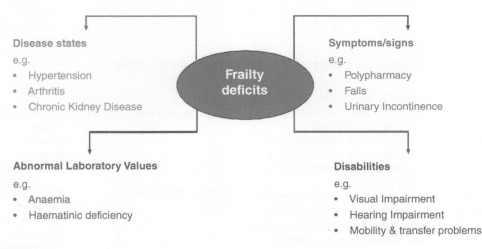

Disease states
e.g.
- Hypertension
- Arthritis
- Chronic Kidney Disease

Symptoms/signs
e.g.
- Polypharmacy
- Falls
- Urinary Incontinence

Frailty deficits

Abnormal Laboratory Values
e.g.
- Anaemia
- Haematinic deficiency

Disabilities
e.g.
- Visual Impairment
- Hearing Impairment
- Mobility & transfer problems

Figure 13.6 **Frailty deficits.**

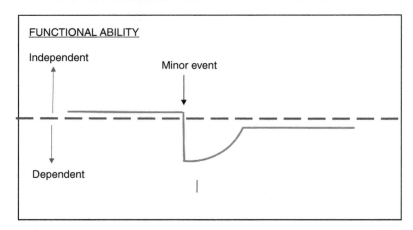

Figure 13.7 Functional ability with frailty and acute illness. *Source: Adapted from Vernon (2018).*

Jot This Down

Frailty syndromes include:

- *Immobility* – the person presents with a change in their mobility, or suddenly becomes immobile
- *Falls* – the person presents following a fall
- *Incontinence* – the person has new or worsening episodes of incontinence
- *Delirium* – the person presents with an acute episode of confusion
- *Susceptibility to medications* – the person presents with signs of medication adverse effects.

How do you bring this information together in practice for your patients? Is there a pathway or document that links these frailty syndromes?

The complexity of the situation of older people with frailty suggests that a comprehensive and integrated approach to assessment and care is needed. Frailty should be clinically identified and assessed and following assessment, appropriate integrated care provision should be planned and provided.

Identification

The BGS recommends four tests to determine if frailty could be present.

1. Consider if the person has displayed any of the common symptoms of frailty (immobility, falls, susceptibility to the side-effects of medication, incontinence or delirium).
2. The gait speed test: you may need to ask for a physiotherapist to complete this for you. The gait speed test would indicate frailty of it takes more than 5 seconds to walk 4 meters (with the person's usual walking aids if appropriate).
3. The timed get up and go test: again, you may need support with this depending on your clinical area and role. Frailty would be indicated if it took more than 10 seconds to get up from a chair, walk 3 metres, turn around, return to the chair and sit down.
4. PRISMA 7 Scale (Raîche *et al.*, 2017).

Assessment

Following the identification of frailty, a Comprehensive Geriatric Assessment (CGA) should be undertaken. Completion of a CGA should be seen as a process, not a single event. It involves multiple professionals from many disciplines assessing and determining medical, physiological, functional, social and environmental impacts and capabilities of an older person (Table 13.5). This is

Table 13.5 Components of the Comprehensive Geriatric Assessment.

COMPONENTS	ELEMENTS TO INCLUDE
Physical assessments	Identified problems Co-morbidities and disease severity Medication review Nutritional status Altered presentation
Assessment of function	Activities of daily living (ADLs) Instrumental ADLs Activity Gait and balance Frailty
Psychological/cognitive assessment	Cognition Mood Anxieties
Social assessment	Informal support Carers Financial Purposeful activity Relationships
Environmental assessment	Home safety Transport Telecare/telehealth/technology Equipment for independence/resilience

used to help plan and co-ordinate an individualised plan of care for that individual.

Following the CGA, the Clinical Frailty Scale (CSF) by Rockwood & Theou (2020) can be used to summarise the overall assessed level of frailty of the individual. This should be undertaken following the CGA process (and not before it). The CFS can be seen in Figure 13.8.

Combined, the CGA and CFS should inform both the level and type of care support needed by the individual. Depending on the identified level of frailty, different approaches to care support should be taken. These range from healthy ageing plans for people who are vulnerable to frailty, supported self-management for those who are mildly frail, through to case management and end-of-life care for people who are severely frail or in receipt of end-of-life care respectively (Table 13.6).

Individuals who are vulnerable to frailty, or have mild frailty, may not need intensive support from the MDT. These individuals may benefit from healthy ageing and supported self-management strategies.

Intensive support is usually required to optimise outcomes for people with higher levels of frailty. Care and support management, and case management will require a Care and Support Plan (CSP). The CSP will depend upon the outcome of the CGA, but all CSPs should include:

- A named key contact who is responsible for co-ordinating care on behalf of the patient and who will be the patient's main point of contact in the community teams

Table 13.6 Levels of frailty care planning.

LEVEL OF FRAILTY	PLAN
Vulnerable	Healthy ageing
Mild frailty	Supported self-management
Moderate frailty	Care and support planning
Severely frail/very severely frail	Case management
End of Life	End-of-life-care

- A health and social care summary which includes symptoms, underlying diagnoses, medications and current social situation
- An optimisation and/or maintenance plan to highlight what the individual's goals are and what actions are going to be taken
- Who is responsible for doing what (including the individual receiving the CGA assessment, any carers, relatives, their doctor and other health professionals – these may include a geriatrician, GP, specialist nurse, old age psychiatrist, older person's mental health team, therapists, dietitian, podiatrist)
- What the timescale is and how and when review will happen
- An escalation plan which describes what the individual or carers may need to look out for in terms of deterioration, who to call if this happens, and an urgent care plan which summarises what the individual wants to happen if a crisis occurs in their

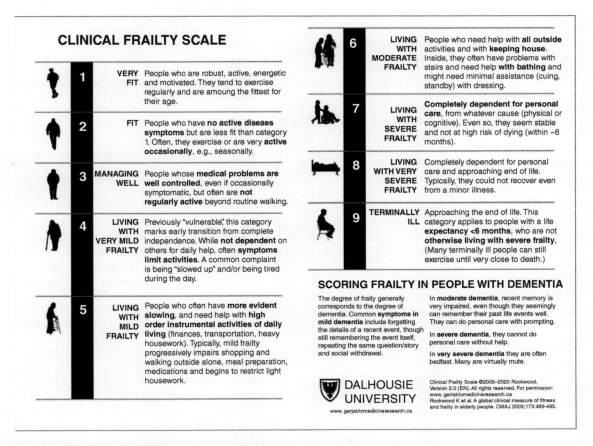

CLINICAL FRAILTY SCALE

1 VERY FIT People who are robust, active, energetic and motivated. They tend to exercise regularly and are among the fittest for their age.

2 FIT People who have **no active diseaes symptoms** but are less fit than category 1. Often, they exercise or are very **active occasionally**, e.g., seasonally.

3 MANAGING WELL People whose **medical problems are well controlled**, even if occasionally symptomatic, but often are **not regularly active** beyond routine walking.

4 LIVING WITH VERY MILD FRAILTY Previously "vulnerable", this category marks early transition from complete independence. While **not dependent** on others for daily help, often **symptoms limit activities**. A common complaint is being "slowed up" and/or being tired during the day.

5 LIVING WITH MILD FRAILTY People who often have **more evident slowing**, and need help with **high order instrumental activities of daily living** (finances, transportation, heavy housework). Typically, mild frailty progressively impairs shopping and walking outside alone, meal preparation, medications and begins to restrict light housework.

6 LIVING WITH MODERATE FRAILTY People who need help with **all outside** activities and with **keeping house**. Inside, they often have problems with stairs and need help **with bathing** and might need minimal assistance (cuing, standby) with dressing.

7 LIVING WITH SEVERE FRAILTY **Completely dependent for personal care**, from whatever cause (physical or cognitive). Even so, they seem stable and not at high risk of dying (within ~6 months).

8 LIVING WITH VERY SEVERE FRAILTY Completely dependent for personal care and approaching end of life. Typically, they could not recover even from a minor illness.

9 TERMINALLY ILL Approaching the end of life. This category applies to people with a life expectancy <6 months, who are not **otherwise living with severe frailty**, (Many terminally ill people can still exercise until very close to death.)

SCORING FRAILTY IN PEOPLE WITH DEMENTIA

The degree of frailty generally corresponds to the degree of dementia. Common **symptoms in mild dementia** include forgetting the details of a recent event, though still remembering the event itself, repeating the same question/story and social withdrawal.

In **moderate dementia**, recent memory is very impaired, even though they seemingly can remember their past life events well. They can do personal care with prompting.

In **severe dementia**, they cannot do personal care without help.

In **very severe dementia** they are often bedfast. Many are virtually mute.

DALHOUSIE UNIVERSITY
www.geriatricmedicineresearch.ca

Clinical Frailty Scale ©2005–2020 Rockwood, Version 2.0 (EN). All rights reserved. For permission: www. geriatricmedicineresearch.ca Rockwood K et al. A global clinical measure of fitness and frailty in elderly people. CMAJ 2005;173:489-495.

Figure 13.8 The Clinical Frailty Scale (CFS). *Source:* Rockwood & Theou (2020).

health (e.g. do they want to go to hospital? Under what circumstances would they want to stay at home? Whether there is a Do Not Attempt Cardiopulmonary Resuscitation [DNACPR] order in place

- An advance care plan or end-of-life care plan (if appropriate) which could describe the individual's wishes with respect to their preferred end-of-life care.

In order to optimise the effectiveness of the CGA and CSP, care models need to go beyond chronic disease monitoring or generic chronic care models. This is because of the complexity involved in caring for older people with frailty, multimorbidity and complex multiple needs. Frailty care should include identification, assessment, appraisal and planning (Box 13.2).

Box 13.2 Frailty care process

Step 1: IDENTIFY: initial frailty assessment including gait speed, timed get up and go test, PRISMA 7 test

Step 2: ASSESS: if frailty is identified, complete a Comprehensive Geriatric Assessment (CGA)

Step 3: APPRAISE: complete a Clinical Frailty Score (CFS) to identify level of frailty

Step 4: PLAN: use the CGA and CFS to determine the type and level of care support required

---

Case Study

Leila Talia is 82 and was admitted to a hospital medical admissions unit via ambulance following a fall at home. Leila's daughter Anita had called to see her mother that morning and found her lying on the kitchen floor. On admission, Leila complained of back, hip and abdominal pain, and appeared confused and agitated. Anita accompanied her mother to the hospital, and brought Leila's medication:

Inhaled tiotropium
Inhaled salbutamol
Theophylline – 200 mg twice daily
Adcal D3 – 1 tablet twice daily
Risedronate – 35 mg weekly
Co-codamol – PRN
Aspirin – 75 mg daily
Atenolol – 100 mg daily
Simvastatin – 20 mg at night
Omeprazole – 20 mg daily
Dipyridamole retard – 100 mg 4 times daily
Bend luazide – 2.5 mg daily

Anita was concerned because she thought her mother may have mixed up her tablets and taken too much theophylline.

Upon examination, Leila was found to be dehydrated and disorientated. She had a reduced range of movement to her left hip, her chest was wheezy, and she had some suprapubic tenderness. A range of diagnostic tests were performed (blood tests, X-rays, CT scans, ECG, urine and sputum cultures), after which Leila was diagnosed with dehydration/renal impairment, theophylline toxicity and urinary tract and chest infections. Luckily, she had no fractures. Antibiotics

and intravenous fluids were commenced, and Leila was transferred to a medical ward. Over the next few days, Leila's condition improved.

Prior to admission, Leila had been experiencing deteriorating mobility and a progressive but slow decline in her mental state (this has occurred over the last 12–18 months). She had a past history of falls, osteoporosis, previous fractured neck of femur, ischaemic heart disease, gastritis, stroke and chronic obstructive pulmonary disease.

Leila had lived on her own in a small bungalow since her husband died 20 years ago. Anita was Leila's only child, and she worked full time as a police officer. She visited her mother every day but felt that Leila was becoming more and more dependent on her. Anita was concerned about her mother's weight loss, her frequent falls, and her reluctance to leave the house. She believed that Leila may have episodes of urinary incontinence but could not get her mother to discuss this issue. Anita also suspected that this may not be the first time that her mother mixed up her medications. Anita had tried to get her mother to agree to a 'home help' but Leila resisted, because she felt that they should 'cope on their own'.

What actions would you take when considering Leila's care planning and how might you support Anita?

Practice Assessment Document

In your clinical area, what frailty pathways of care are available?

Are people screened for frailty?

Is the level of frailty assessed using a clinical frailty scale?

What examples of integrated care have you experienced or seen?

Have you used witnessed the Comprehensive Geriatric Assessment (CGA)?

Multimorbidity and Long-Term Conditions

Often LTCs are observed and planned for in isolation, focusing on a single specified condition at a time. This approach may be detrimental to the overall well-being of the individual, and cause tensions in care as competing recommendations may become confusing for practitioners, the person with LTCs, their carers and family. As we see in frailty, many individuals will have many LTCs or other conditions which need to be factored into the picture and appreciated when planning or providing care.

Multimorbidity is the presence of two or more multiple long-term health conditions in one person (NICE, 2016). It is important to recognise that this does not only include physical health diagnosis but also, and importantly, mental health conditions. In addition, learning disabilities, frailty or other symptom complexes (e.g. chronic pain), sensory impairments and alcohol or substance misuse are included when considering the presence of multimorbidity (NICE, 2016).

The aim of care for people with multimorbidity is to reduce the treatment burden they experience when navigating care and treatment options for the individual conditions present, streamline appointments or provision of care and improve quality of life through informed, shred decision making which holds central the person in receipt of care. Their goals, aims and wishes are of paramount importance.

The complexity of caring for someone with multimorbidity comes in the appreciation that the individual will have many competing recommendations and care regimes. As such, healthcare professionals need to be skilled at working with the individual to best meet their identified needs and goals. It is important that healthcare professionals recognise that treatment recommendations often are formed on the basis of single disease process research. The application of this to people with multimorbidity needs to be balanced and considered in line with the totality of their conditions and presentation.

Multimorbidity approach to care

NICE (2016) recommends an approach to care for people with multimorbidity which places the individual at the centre of their care (Figure 13.9).

Following this approach, care should be assessed, planned and delivered as a partnership with the person with multimorbidity. There should be an understanding of how their conditions impact upon their quality of life, what they wish to happen, their goals and needs, an appraisal of the benefits or risks of using recommendations for single health conditions and how they may impact on their other conditions, review of how any recommendations or treatments may increase or reduce the burden upon the person, how to support them relating to unplanned care episodes, and how to co-ordinate their care across the different services involved.

This is a complex process and may appear overwhelming to both the healthcare professional and person with multimorbidity. Careful and well-timed discussions should be undertaken to agree an individualised plan for their care based on reducing burden and improving quality of life.

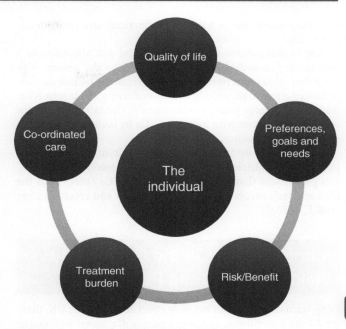

Figure 13.9 An approach to multimorbidity care.

Optimisation and Integrated Care Systems

In order to optimise the effectiveness of the CGA and CSP and to support people with multimorbidity, care models need to go beyond chronic disease monitoring models or generic chronic care models. This is because of the complexity involved in caring for people with frailty, multimorbidity and complex multiple needs. Instead, an integrated care model is required.

The recently published White Paper (Department of Health and Social Care, 2021) recognises the need for integrated care systems (ICS) that place the person at the centre of care design and delivery, seeking to meet individual needs in a co-ordinated and tailored way. The overarching goal should be to improve the quality of care and the person's experience.

Achieving integrated care can be challenging because it requires integration of:

- Primary, secondary and tertiary care
- Health and social care
- Physical and mental health services.

Supporting people with LTCs includes social care and support as well as more traditional physical or mental health support. As healthcare professionals, this is a part of holistic care which needs to be considered, and requires partnership working. NICE (2015a) recommends that consideration should be given to referring older people with LTCs to their local authority. This is to support assessment of needs in relation to their social care or support. This assessment should consider the needs of the person with the LTC, but also involve (if appropriate) any carers they have. It is important that the person with LTCs is involved, and that the appraisal recognises their individual strengths, what they would like to happen (preferences) and their identified needs.

Key to this process is the identification and allocation of a named care co-ordinator (NICE, 2015a). As the person with LTCs may need input from multiple services, the named care co-ordinator is key in organising and co-ordinating the information from an often large team of professionals. The care co-ordinator supports the person with multiple LTCs by being a single point of contact and resource.

The care plan formed by this process is jointly owned by the person with multiple LTCs and the care professionals. As such, it is paramount that the individual with LTCs agrees with the plan and feels involved. They should sign it and receive a copy (NICE, 2015a).

Managing LTCs in the Community: Children and Young People

Long-term conditions do not only affect adults. In the UK, there are 1.7 million children and young people diagnosed with one or more LTCs (NICE, 2021). Similarly to adults, these are most commonly asthma, diabetes and epilepsy (NICE, 2021). In addition, cancer and additional learning needs are considered as key LTC priority areas (Royal College of Paediatric and Child Health, 2020). Cardiovascular conditions are not focused upon in the same manner as LTCs in adults.

For children and young people, the three key LTCs are asthma, diabetes and epilepsy. Children with asthma make up the largest group, with 900 000 children receiving asthma care (NICE, 2021). A key part of LTC care for children with asthma is review of inhaler technique. Proper technique helps control asthma and reduces hospital admissions.

For children with type 1 diabetes, focus has been placed on regular health checks and regular monitoring of blood glucose levels through the HBA1c test. The Royal College of Paediatric and Child Health (2020) identifies that adolescence is a key phase in a person's life and often is associated with suboptimal management of diabetes. Increased focus on this time may support transition to adult diabetes services and improve diabetic control.

In relation to epilepsy, the Royal College of Paediatric and Child Health (2020) emphasises the formation of shared and agreed plans of care (much the same as with older people or those with frailty). At present, one-third of children with epilepsy do not have an agreed individualised care plan. The Royal College of Paediatric and Child Health (2020) recommends that an epilepsy passport is devised for each child to include information on the type of epilepsy they have, their medications, key emergency contacts, any emergency care plans that are in place, and their named healthcare professionals.

Polypharmacy: A Practice Consideration

Polypharmacy is defined as the ongoing use of multiple medicines by one person and is most common in the care of older people (King's Fund, 2013b). Polypharmacy can be clinically justified in some cases but it can also occur due to poor medicines management. This is called inappropriate polypharmacy.

Age UK's (2019) report *More Harm Than Good* identified that inappropriate polypharmacy is a hidden crisis requiring urgent attention, due to the human and financial costs it causes. Results of the report show that:

- More than 1 in 10 people aged over 65 take at least eight different prescribed medications each week. This increases to nearly 1 in 4 people aged over 85
- Around 1 in 5 prescriptions for older people living at home may be inappropriate
- Up to 50% of all medicines for LTCs are not taken as intended.

For many older people living with multiple health conditions or frailty, this could mean taking multiple medicines. Without these medicines, many older people would be living in poorer health. However, we risk undoing the many benefits of medicines and treatments if they are prescribed in excessive numbers (where this is not clinically justified or safe), in unsafe combinations, without the consent and involvement of the older person themselves, or without support to use them properly (NICE, 2017b).

Inappropriate polypharmacy can lead to poor concordance. A report on medicines adherence by PrescQIPP (2017) identified that this is due to patients being confused about when and how to take medications, having difficulty opening containers/packages, or having difficulty swallowing so many medications. If problems with concordance are not recognised by health professionals, higher doses or even more medications may be prescribed (King's Fund, 2013b).

The most significant problem associated with inappropriate polypharmacy is the increased risk of adverse reactions. Physiological changes due to ageing resulting in changes in the metabolism of medications mean that older people are more susceptible to adverse reactions. According to Age UK (2019), 75% of people over 70 years of age will have an adverse drug reaction. The more medicines they take, the more likely they are to experience harmful side-effects. In fact, once a person is taking more than four medicines, the chance of experiencing an adverse drug reaction gets exponentially worse for every new medicine taken.

Common adverse reactions to medication include nausea, dizziness, reduced appetite, low mood, weight loss, muscle weakness, delirium, falls and constipation (Lavan & Gallagher, 2016). The more medications taken, the more likely the patient is to experience multiple types of adverse reaction. This can have a profound impact on quality of life (Age UK, 2019).

Some medications should be prescribed with caution because they increase the risk of falls for older people. NHS Scotland (2020) has produced a guide about medication and falls risk in the older person, and identified 'hot topics' regarding polypharmacy that require particular attention.

- *Anticholinergic burden*: a specific issue for older people is taking too many anticholinergic medicines, leading to anticholinergic burden. Anticholinergic drugs are prescribed for a wide range of conditions, including Parkinson disease, overactive bladder, chronic obstructive pulmonary disease, nausea and vomiting, depression and psychosis. Combining treatments with anticholinergic activity can have harmful cumulative effects and has been associated with impaired cognitive function, increased risk of falls, heart problems, hospitalisation and death.

- *Antipsychotics*: there is currently a move to de-scribe (stop) the use of antipsychotics for people with dementia, as these drugs have limited positive effect and can cause increased risk of falls, stroke and death.
- *Benzodiazepines and z-drugs*: benzodiazepines and the Z-drugs should be avoided in older people, because they are at greater risk of becoming ataxic (abnormal, unco-ordinated movements) and confused, leading to falls and injury.

Medication Review

NHS England recognises the significance of poor medicines management and inappropriate polypharmacy on the health and quality of life of older people. The *NHS Long Term Plan* (NHS England, 2019) made a number of important commitments.

- Patients taking multiple drugs for multimorbidity will receive regular medication reviews.
- Where appropriate, care home residents will receive regular clinical pharmacist-led medication reviews.
- All providers will be required to implement electronic prescribing systems with the aim of reducing medication errors by up to 30%.
- Funding for the new primary care networks will be used to significantly expand the number of clinical pharmacists.
- Where appropriate, social prescribing will be supported as an alternative to medications.

Central to these commitments is medication review, defined as: 'A structured, critical examination of a person's medicines with the objective of reaching an agreement with the person about treatment, optimising the impact of medicines, minimising the number of medication related problems and reducing waste' (NICE, 2015b).

Optimising the benefits of medication and minimising medication-related problems and waste requires effective medication management strategies. A number of medication review tools are available to help clinicians to identify the risks and benefits of medications to individuals. These include the STOPP/START tool (STOPP: Screening Tool of Older People's potentially inappropriate Prescriptions; START: Screening Tool to Alert doctors to Right, i.e. appropriate, indicated Treatments), which is validated for use in the older population and people with multimorbidity; the NO TEARS mnemonic (Box 13.3) prompts the medication review process (**N**eed/indication, **O**pen questions, **T**ests, **E**vidence, **A**dverse effects, **R**isk reduction, **S**implification/switches). The NO TEARS mnemonic is simple and flexible and can be embedded within a routine consultation. In addition, the MAI tool (Medication Appropriateness Index) can be applied to each medication taken by an individual to determine whether it is appropriate. The MAI tool is an effective method of supporting medication reviews in the older population but using it can be a lengthy process.

Box 13.3 NO TEARS mnemonic

Need/indication

Open questions

Tests,

Evidence

Adverse effects

Risk reduction

Simplification/switches

Reducing inappropriate medications (de-scribing) has been shown to reduce adverse medication reactions, promote person-centred medication management, and improve patient–professional relationships and concordance (Woodward, 2003; Le Couteur *et al.*, 2011). An important aspect of medication review is the involvement of patients in the process, as involvement improves the patient's understanding of medications and the professional's understanding of factors influencing the patient's medication concordance decisions (Ostini *et al.*, 2009; Reeve *et al.*, 2013a). Reeve *et al.* (2013b) propose that up to 90% of patients with multimorbidity taking a number of medications would cease a medication if their doctor offered that option. However, many patients are reluctant, or refuse, to stop medications due to a fear that cessation will lead to health deterioration (Williams *et al.*, 2004; Beer *et al.*, 2011).

Conclusion

This chapter has introduced the principles of care for people with LTCs across the lifespan. Specific focus has been placed on key conditions and drivers for contemporary healthcare practice and service provision. By reading and reflecting on this, you will have a better appreciation of the impact that healthcare professionals can make on the lives of those with LTCs.

Key Points

- Long-term conditions (LTC) are conditions that cannot be cured, but can be controlled with medication and/or the provision of other therapies.
- They can be present in people of all ages and stages of life, and may impact on both physical and mental health and well-being.
- Nurses and nursing associates have a responsibility to engage in caring conversations, to support people with LTCs through collaborative working and person-centred care.

References

Age UK (2019) *More Harm Than Good: why more isn't always better with older people's medicines*. Age UK, London.

Beer, C., Loh, P.K., Peng, Y.G., Potter, K. & Millar, A. (2011) A pilot randomized controlled trial of deprescribing. *Therapeutic Advances in Drug Safety*, 2, 37–43.

Bloem, B.R., Okun, M.S. & Klein, C. (2021) Parkinson's disease. *Lancet*, 397, 2284–2303.

British Geriatrics Society (2014) *Introduction to Frailty, Fit for Frailty Part 1*. British Geriatrics Society, London.

British Heart Foundation (2018) *Putting People at the Heart of their Care: The BHF House of Care Programme*. British Heart Foundation, London.

Clegg, A. Bates, C. Young, et al. (2016) Development and Validation of an Electronic Frailty Index using Routine Primary Care Electronic Health Record Data. *Age and Ageing*, 45(3), 353–360.

Department of Health (2010) *Improving the Health and Wellbeing of People with Long Term Conditions*. Department of Health, London

Department of Health and Social Care (2021) *Integration and Innovation: Working Together to Improve Health and Social Care for All.* Department of Health and Social Care, London.

Dorsey, R., Sherer, T., Okun, M.S. & Bloem, B.R. (2020) *Ending Parkinson's Disease: A Prescription for Action.* Public Affairs, New York.

Epilepsy Action (2017) *Seizure classification.* www.epilepsy.org.uk/info/seizure-classification (accessed December 2021).

Epilepsy Society (2017) *About epilepsy.* www.epilepsysociety.org.uk/what-epilepsy#.WgOQ-7p2vIU (accessed December 2021).

Fang, X., Han, D., Cheng, Q., *et al.* (2018) Association of levels of physical activity with risk of Parkinson disease: a systematic review and meta-analysis. *JAMA Network Open,* 1(5), e182421–e182421.

Greenstein, B. (2009) *Clinical Pharmacology for Nurses.* Churchill Livingstone, London.

Grissinger, M. (2018) Delayed administration and contraindicated drugs place hospitalized Parkinson's disease patients at risk. *P & T,* 43(1), 10–39.

Harrison, J.K., Clegg, A., Conroy, S.P. & Young, J. (2015) Managing frailty as a long-term condition. *Age and Ageing,* 44(5), 732–735.

Hickey, J.V. (2017) *The Clinical Practice of Neurological and Neurosurgical Nursing,* 7th edn. Lippincott, Philadelphia, PA.

Karch, A.M. (2017) *Focus on Nursing Pharmacology,* 7th edn. Wolters Kluwer, New York.

King's Fund (2012) *Long-Term Conditions and Mental Health. The Cost of Co-Morbidities.* King's Fund, London.

King's Fund (2013a) *Delivering Better Services for People with Long-Term Conditions: Building the House of Care.* King's Fund, London.

King's Fund (2013b) *Polypharmacy and medicines optimisation: making it safe and sound.* www.kingsfund.org.uk/publications/polypharmacy-and-medicines-optimisation (accessed December 2021).

Lavan, A.H. & Gallagher, P. (2016) Predicting risk of adverse drug reactions in older adults. *Therapeutic Advances in Drug Safety,* 7(1), 11–22.

Le Couteur, D.G., Banks, E., Gnjidic, D. & McLachlan, A. (2011) Deprescribing. *Australian Prescriber,* 34, 182–185.

Lyndon, H. (2015) Reframing frailty as a long-term condition. *Nursing Older People,* 27(8), 32–39.

Mackay, D.F., Russell, E.R., Stewart, K., MacLean, J.A., Pell, J.P. & Stewart, W. (2019) Neurodegenerative disease mortality among former professional soccer players. *New England Journal of Medicine,* 381(19), 1801–1808.

Macmillan Cancer Support (2015) *The Burden of Cancer and Other Long-Term Conditions.* www.macmillan.org.uk/documents/press/cancerandotherlong-termconditions.pdf (accessed December 2021).

Medicines and Healthcare products Regulatory Agency (2018) *Valproate used by Women and Girls: Guidance.* www.gov.uk/guidance/valproate-use-by-women-and-girls (accessed December 2021).

NHS England (n.d.) *Neurological Conditions.* www.england.nhs.uk/ourwork/clinical-policy/ltc/our-work-on-long-term-conditions/neurological/ (accessed January 2022).

NHS England (2014) *Five Year Forward View.* National Health Service, London.

NHS England (2015) *Our Declaration: Person Centred Care for Long Term Conditions.* National Health Service, London.

NHS England (2017) *Next Steps on the NHS Five Year Forward View.* National Health Service, London.

NHS England (2019) *House of Care – A Framework for Long Term Condition Care.* National Health Service, London.

NHS Scotland (2020) *Polypharmacy: Manage Medicines. Hot Topics.* https://managemeds.scot.nhs.uk/for-healthcare-professionals/hot-topics/ (accessed January 2022).

National Institute for Health and Care Excellence (2012) *Epilepsies: Diagnosis and Management.* National Institute for Health and Care Excellence, London.

National Institute for Health and Care Excellence (2015a) *Older People with Social Care Needs and Multiple Long-Term Conditions. NG22.* National Institute for Health and Care Excellence, London.

National Institute for Health and Care Excellence (2015b) *Medicines Optimization: The Safe and Effective Use of Medicines to Enable the Best Possible Outcomes. NG5.* National Institute for Health and Care Excellence, London.

National Institute for Health and Care Excellence (2016) *Multimorbidity: Clinical Assessment and Management. NG56.* National Institute for Health and Care Excellence, London.

National Institute for Health and Care Excellence (2017a) *Parkinson's Disease in Adults: Diagnosis and Management. NG71.* National Institute for Health and Care Excellence, London.

National Institute for Health and Care Excellence (2017b) *Multimorbidity and Polypharmacy. KTT18.* National Institute for Health and Care Excellence, London.

National Institute for Health and Care Excellence (2018) *Epilepsies: Diagnosis and Management. CG137.* National Institute for Health and Care Excellence, London.

National Institute for Health and Care Excellence (2021) *Managing Long-Term Conditions in the Community.* National Institute for Health and Care Excellence, London.

Noyce, A.J., Bestwick, J.P., Silveira-Moriyama, L., *et al.* (2012) Meta-analysis of early nonmotor features and risk factors for Parkinson disease. *Annals of Neurology,* 72(6), 893–901.

Nursing & Midwifery Council (2018a) *Future Nurse: Standards of Proficiency for Registered Nurses.* NMC, London.

Nursing & Midwifery Council (2018b) *Standards of Proficiency for Nursing Associates.* NMC, London.

Oguh, O. & Videnovic, A. (2012) Inpatient management of Parkinson disease: current challenges and future directions. *Neurohospitalist,* 2(1), 28–35.

Ostini, R., Hegney, D., Jackson, C., *et al.* (2009) Systematic review of interventions to improve prescribing. *Annals of Pharmacotherapy,* 43, 502–513.

Parkinson's Disease UK (2018) *The incidence and prevalence of Parkinson's disease in the UK.* www.parkinsons.org.uk/professionals/resources/incidence-and-prevalence-parkinsons-uk-report

PD Med Collaborative Group, Gray, R., Ives, N., Rick, C., Patel, S., Gray, A., Clarke, C.E. (2014) Long-term effectiveness of dopamine agonists and monoamine oxidase B inhibitors compared with levodopa as initial treatment for Parkinson's disease (PD MED): a large, open-label, pragmatic randomised trial. *Lancet,* 384(9949), 1196–1205.

PrescQIPP (2017) *Polypharmacy and deprescribing – medicines adherence.* www.prescqipp.info/umbraco/surface/authorisedmediasurface/index?url=%2fmedia%2f1566%2fb187-polypharmacy-improving-medicines-adherence-20.pdf (accessed December 2021).

Pringsheim, T., Jette, N., Frolkis, A. & Steeves, T.D. (2014) The prevalence of Parkinson's disease: a systematic review and meta-analysis. *Movement Disorders,* 29(13), 1583–1590.

Raîche, M., Hébert, R., Dubois, M.F. and the PRISMA Partners (2017) User guide for the PRISMA-7 questionnaire to identify elderly people with severe loss of autonomy. In: R. Hébert, A. Tourigny & M. Gagnon (eds) *Integrated Service Delivery to Ensure Persons' Functional Autonomy* (pp.147–165). Edisem, Quebec. www2.gov.bc.ca/assets/gov/health/practitioner-pro/bc-guidelines/frailty-prisma7.pdf (accessed December 2021).

Reeve, E., To, J., Hendrix, I., Shakib, S., Roberts, M.S. & Wiese, M. (2013a) Patient barriers to and enablers of deprescribing: a systematic review. *Drugs and Aging,* 30, 793–807.

Reeve, E., Wiese, M.D., Hendrix, I., Roberts, M. & Shakib, S. (2013b) Patient attitudes, beliefs and experiences of polypharmacy and willingness of deprescribing. *Journal of the American Geriatric Society,* 61(9), 1508–1514.

Rockwood, K. & Theou, O. (2020) Using the Clinical Frailty Scale in allocating scarce health care resources. *Canadian Geriatric Journal,* 23, 254–259.

Royal College of General Practitioners (2016) *Responding to the Needs of Patients with Multimorbidity: A Vision for General Practice.* www.rcgp.

org.uk/-/media/Files/Policy/A-Z-policy/RCGP-Responding-to-needs-of-Multimorbitiy-2016.ashx?la=en (accessed December 2021).

Royal College of Paediatrics and Child Health (2020) *Long Term Conditions.* https://stateofchildhealth.rcpch.ac.uk/evidence/long-term-conditions/ (accessed December 2021).

Russell, E.R., McCabe, T., Mackay, D.F., *et al.* (2020) Mental health and suicide in former professional soccer players *Journal of Neurology, Neurosurgery & Psychiatry*, 91, 1256–1260.

Schirinzi, T., Di Lazzaro, G., Sancesario, G.M., *et al.* (2020) Young-onset and late-onset Parkinson's disease exhibit a different profile of fluid biomarkers and clinical features. *Neurobiology of Aging*, 90, 119–124.

Skills for Health, NHS England and Health Education England (2018) *Frailty: A framework of core capabilities.* https://skillsforhealth.org.uk/wp-content/uploads/2021/01/Frailty-framework.pdf (accessed December 2021).

van den Heuvel, L., Dorsey, R.R., Prainsack, B., *et al.* (2020) Quadruple decision making for Parkinson's disease patients: combining expert opinion, patient preferences, scientific evidence, and big data approaches to reach precision medicine. *Journal of Parkinsons Disease*, 10(1), 223–231.

van der Kolk, N.M., de Vries, N.M., Kessels, R.P., *et al.* (2019) Effectiveness of home-based and remotely supervised aerobic exercise in Parkinson's disease: a double-blind, randomised controlled trial. *Lancet Neurology*, 18(11), 998–1008.

VanItallie, T.B. (2019) Traumatic brain injury (TBI) in collision sports: possible mechanisms of transformation into chronic traumatic encephalopathy (CTE). *Metabolism*, 100S, 153943.

Vernon. M (2018) *Ageing Well. Quality Healthcare in Later Life: The Electronic Frailty Index.* http://tvscn.nhs.uk/wp-content/uploads/2018/03/7.-Martin-Vernon.pdf (accessed January 2022).

Williams, M., Pulliam, C., Hunter, R., *et al.* (2004) The short-term effect of interdisciplinary medication review on function and cost in ambulatory elderly people. *Journal of the American Geriatric Society*, 52, 93–98.

Williamson, N. (2021) How can nurses to help reduce the risk of SUDEP in young people. *Emergency Nurse*, 29, 13–14.

Woodward, M. (2003) Deprescribing: achieving better health outcomes for older people through reducing medications. *Journal of Pharmacy Practice and Research*, 33, 323–328.

Woodward, S. & Mestecky, A.M. (2011) *Neurosciences Nursing: Evidence Based Practice.* Wiley, London.

World Health Organization (2019) *Epilepsy.* www.who.int/mental_health/neurology/epilepsy/en/ (accessed December 2021).

World Health Organization (2021) *Noncommunicable Diseases Fact Sheet.* www.who.int/news-room/fact-sheets/detail/noncommunicable-diseases (accessed December 2021).

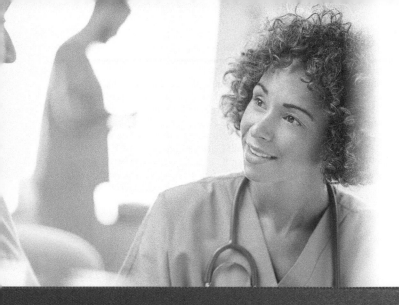

14

The Principles of Surgical Care

Carl Clare

University of Hertfordshire, UK

Learning Outcomes

On completion of this chapter you will be able to:

- Differentiate between the different classifications of surgery
- Discuss the potential reasons for preoperative anxiety and ways of relieving it
- Understand preoperative risks that must be identified on admission
- Understand the American Society of Anesthesiology (ASA) grading system
- Explain the importance of early mobilisation in the postoperative period
- Explore the value of patient-controlled analgesia (PCA) in postoperative pain relief

Proficiencies

NMC Proficiencies and Standards:

- Recognise signs of mental and emotional distress or vulnerability and promote anxiety-reducing techniques
- Promote recovery by teaching postoperative exercises for breathing and circulation
- Carry out a systematic postoperative assessment
- Use aseptic techniques when undertaking wound care, including dressings and suture removal
- Identify, respond to and manage dehydration in the preoperative patient
- Safely discharge the surgical patient, including undertaking an assessment of their ability to self-administer their own medications

 Visit the companion website at www.wiley.com/go/peate/nursingpractice3e where you can test yourself using flashcards, multiple-choice questions and more.

Nursing Practice: Knowledge and Care, Third Edition. Edited by Ian Peate and Aby Mitchell.
© 2022 John Wiley & Sons Ltd. Published 2022 by John Wiley & Sons Ltd.
Companion website: www.wiley.com/go/peate/nursingpractice3e

Introduction

Surgical nursing in the UK is the care of the patient on the ward/unit before and after surgery, as opposed to *theatre* nursing, which is the care of the patient within the operating department. It is the unique role of the surgical nurse to support patients through a procedure that is, for many, a major life event. To the nursing and medical staff, surgery is routine and 'nothing to be scared of'; however, for the patient, the prospect of surgery can be one of the most novel and alien experiences they will ever undergo. Even if the patient has undergone surgery before, any new operation (or repeat procedure) remains an unnerving episode that creates anxiety and stress. The whole process of becoming a patient is debilitating and both the anxiety about the forthcoming surgical procedure and the surgery itself have physical, psychological and social effects. The ongoing care of the patient by the surgical nurse requires that the nurse both recognises and attempts to alleviate or prevent these effects. It is almost unique in the hospital setting that the patient may come into the ward 'well' and then be subjected to procedures that can leave them acutely ill.

Classification of Surgery and Risk

Surgery is primarily classified according to purpose.

- *Diagnostic*: surgery to confirm or establish a diagnosis
- *Palliative*: surgery intended to relieve pain or reduce symptoms of a disease
- *Ablative*: surgery to remove diseased body parts
- *Constructive*: restores function or appearance that has been lost or reduced
- *Transplant*: replaces malfunctioning structures

Jot This Down

Try to place as many surgical procedures as you can think of into the categories defined above. For instance, hip replacement is a form of *transplant* surgery.

Surgery is further classified by the degree of urgency and the degree of risk. The degree of urgency is often defined by the necessity to preserve the patient's life, body part or bodily function. Thus, it is usual to talk of emergency (or immediate) surgery, urgent surgery, expedited surgery and elective surgery.

- *Emergency surgery* is performed immediately to preserve life, limb or function (for instance, to stop bleeding after a trauma).
- *Urgent surgery* is normally carried out within hours of the decision to operate for events that potentially threaten life, limb or function or for the relief of pain (for instance, the fixation of fractures).
- *Expedited surgery* is surgery that is normally carried out within days of the decision to operate and where the condition is not an immediate threat to life, limb or function.
- *Elective surgery* is surgery that is performed when surgery is the preferred treatment to achieve the required outcome for the patient and is planned and booked in advance.

Surgery can also be categorised according to the degree of risk.

- *Major surgery*: involves a high degree of risk in that it may be a complex and/or prolonged operation. Large losses of blood may occur and vital organs may be affected.
- *Minor surgery*: surgery with little risk where few potential complications are expected. Often performed as day surgery or short-stay surgery.

Needless to say, all operations are 'major' to the patient and while these classifications are useful for healthcare staff, there should be consideration of their use around patients and relatives. Furthermore, the degree of risk of surgery is affected by several other factors, independent of the nature of the operation, and these will be discussed later in the chapter (Boxes 14.1 and 14.2).

Box 14.1 Example Surgery Grades

- *Grade 1 (minor)*: excision of lesion of skin; drainage of breast abscess
- *Grade 2 (intermediate)*: primary repair of inguinal hernia; excision of varicose vein(s) of leg; tonsillectomy/adenotonsillectomy; knee arthroscopy
- *Grade 3 (major)*: total abdominal hysterectomy; endoscopic resection of prostate; lumbar discectomy; thyroidectomy
- *Grade 4 (major+)*: total joint replacement; lung operations; colonic resection; radical neck dissection

Source: Modified from NICE (2016).

Box 14.2 Minimally Invasive Surgery

It is worthwhile at this juncture to mention the concept of *minimally invasive surgery* (often referred to as 'keyhole' surgery by patients). It is often associated with a protocol for 'fast-track surgery' or enhanced recovery after surgery (ERAS; Hoffmann & Kettelhack, 2012). Minimally invasive surgery has been used in all surgical specialties (Kehlet & Wilmore, 2008) and its use continues to expand. The use of this technique reduces wound size and thus decreases unwanted inflammatory responses and pain, leading to shortened recovery times and earlier discharge. However, not every patient is suitable for minimally invasive surgery (e.g. obese patients or patients who have undergone previous surgery to the proposed operative site); furthermore, minimally invasive surgery requires specialist expertise and equipment and thus many procedures may not be available outside specialist centres (e.g. minimally invasive cardiac surgery), whereas other procedures (such as arthroscopy) are commonly performed.

Phases of Surgery

Surgery is composed of three distinct phases.

1. *Preoperative*: this phase begins when the patient makes the decision to undergo the recommended surgical procedure and ends when the patient is transferred to the operating theatre.

2. *Intraoperative phase*: begins on admission to the operating theatre and ends on transfer to the recovery area.

3. *Postoperative phase*: begins on admission to the recovery area and ends when healing is complete.

It is the intention of this chapter to discuss the nursing care of the patient on their journey through the preoperative and postoperative phases of their journey. However, as the recovery area is considered to be a critical care area, the postoperative discussion will begin with the transfer of care from the recovery nurse to the collecting (ward) nurse.

Preoperative Surgical Phase

The decision to offer surgery is that of the surgeon but the decision to agree to undergo surgery remains with the patient, unless the patient is deemed not competent to make the decision (see Chapter 2). From that moment on, the patient enters into the preoperative phase of their surgical journey. The effect the decision will have on the patient will vary from individual to individual but in the majority of patients, there will be an element of trepidation and anxiety. While much of the nursing care undertaken during the surgical journey of the patient will be based around physical care (biological care), it is imperative that the nurse does not lose sight of the fact that a major role of the surgical nurse is to educate, reassure and alleviate anxiety.

What the Experts Say

'. . . to understand and respond adequately to patients suffering – and to give them a sense of being understood – clinicians must attend simultaneously to the biological, psychological and social dimensions of illness.'

George Engel (creator of the 'Biopsychosocial model')

It has long been established that patients are anxious about their anaesthetic and surgery and anxiety can focus on many factors (Zemła *et al.*, 2019).

- Fear of the unknown
- Fear of the treatment
- Concerns about pain
- Concerns about safety
- Concerns about recovery and the effect on daily life
- Loss of control
- Fear of death and dying

It is suggested that the patient's experience of anxiety begins at the point that surgery is planned and reaches its peak on the day of the operation. Anxiety causes a wide range of physical responses.

- Tachycardia
- Increased blood pressure
- Increased temperature
- Sweating
- Nausea
- Heightened awareness

In addition, the psychological responses can be varied and include changes in behaviour, such as increased tension, apprehension,

aggression, nervousness and withdrawal. Furthermore, anxiety is a subjective experience and may be affected by factors such as age, gender and previous hospital experiences.

There is a growing body of evidence that addressing the psychological needs of the patient can reduce the risk of complications and improve postoperative outcomes. For instance, anxiety can increase experiences of pain (Ertürk & Ünlü, 2018). The obvious need of the patient is information, and the traditional approach to anxiety reduction is that information giving and allowing the patient to ask questions will reduce preoperative anxiety. However, this is not universally agreed to be the most effective method, as the psychological changes noted earlier may make it more difficult for the patient to attend to information giving and to understand and retain information (Nordfalk *et al.*, 2019). Thus, the suggestion has been made that the use of a validated assessment tool. such as the Amsterdam Preoperative Anxiety and Information Scale (APAIS). to assess anxiety may be valuable in allowing the nurse to stratify the needs of the patient and target anxiety reduction interventions and information (Celik & Edipoglu, 2018).

As well as information giving, it is worthwhile suggesting other anxiety reduction strategies that the patient may wish to try.

- *Medication*: the use of medication in the reduction of preoperative anxiety is gradually decreasing, as it is recognised that it increases postoperative sedation.
- *Distraction techniques*: the use of distraction techniques has long been recommended, including the use of music (Kühlmann *et al.*, 2018).
- *Relaxation techniques*: such as visualisation or deep breathing (Box 14.3).

As noted, for the majority of patients, surgery will be a novel experience and even for those who have undergone surgery before, there may be incomplete memories/recollection. In educating patients, it is always best practice to ascertain what the patient already knows. Even if the patient appears to be reasonably certain

Box 14.3 A Simple Relaxation Technique

Make yourself as comfortable as you can. If you can, loosen any clothes that restrict your breathing.

If you're lying down, place your arms a little bit away from your sides, with the palms up. Let your legs be straight, or bend your knees so your feet are flat on the floor.

If you're sitting, place your arms on the chair arms.

If you're sitting or standing, place both feet flat on the ground. Whatever position you're in, place your feet roughly hip-width apart.

Let your breath flow as deep down into your belly as is comfortable, without forcing it.

Try breathing in through your nose and out through your mouth.

Breathe in gently and regularly. Some people find it helpful to count steadily from 1 to 5. You may not be able to reach 5 at first.

Then, without pausing or holding your breath, let it flow out gently, counting from 1 to 5 again, if you find this helpful.

Keep doing this for 3–5 minutes.

Source: NHS Inform (2018)

of their knowledge, there is always the possibility that they are mistaken in some of their beliefs and thus identifying and rectifying incorrect information may avoid problems for both patient and staff. Increasingly, patients are being given preoperative information leaflets and many are also now asked to watch a video presentation in preadmission clinics (Lin *et al.*, 2016). With the onset of the coronavirus in 2019, there has been an increasing use of telephone and video consultations both in preadmission and postdischarge surgical care (King & Hothi, 2020).

Regardless of the method of information delivery, it is essential that patients and relatives are allowed the time to question staff on matters that have not been addressed or the patient did not understand. Often, information delivery is based on what the staff think the patient should be told, not the patient's priority (Mitchell, 2017), and therefore allowing patients to explore their own information needs ensures that those needs can be addressed.

The information provided to patients preoperatively will vary from institution to institution and according to the surgical procedure to be undertaken. However, as a guide, it can be categorised into five main areas.

- Details of the procedure
- Preoperative preparation
- The theatre environment
- Postoperative expectations (including length of stay)
- Details of the anaesthesia

Other information of value will include visiting times, meal times and, where possible, orientation to the ward environment. It has been a popular model of preadmission care for patients also to be offered a chance to visit the operating theatre or for those who will be admitted electively to a critical care area postoperatively to be able to visit the critical care unit (Van Decar *et al.*, 2019).

The Nursing Associate

Effective information giving is an essential skill before, during and after any intervention (NMC, 2018b). Understanding the processes a client is about to undergo, or has undergone, allows the nursing associate to provide detailed and accurate information to both the client and their family, thus reducing anxiety and promoting care-related behaviours (such as leg exercises).

Jot This Down

Think about the preoperative information needs of different types of clients. How would you tailor the information giving and teaching for:

- Children?
- Clients with learning disabilities?
- Older patients?
- Patients with communication difficulties (such as the deaf patient)?

Preoperative Teaching

Alongside information giving, the preoperative phase is also used for the delivery of teaching to aid the patient with their postoperative recovery, such as deep breathing exercises, leg exercises and splinting/supporting incisions when coughing.

Deep breathing exercises are encouraged, as the postoperative incidence of chest infections is increased when the patient has reduced mobility and thus is not taking breaths deep enough to expand the lungs. Teaching the patient to deep breathe before surgery means they are more likely to undertake the exercise after surgery, encouraging lung expansion and also aiding in the clearance of inhaled anaesthetic gases that may be trapped in the lung bases. An example of a breathing exercise is detailed in Box 14.4.

Teaching patients to splint or support incisions when they are going to cough is important for several types of surgery. Patients who have undergone abdominal or thoracic surgery are less likely to cough after surgery, as they are both frightened that the sudden pressure will 'split the scar' and also because it either will hurt or there is at least a fear that it will hurt. Advise the patient to have a pillow or cushion available when they wish to cough. They can then hold the pillow over the wound site and 'hug it' into the wound just before they cough; this splinting reduces the pain experienced and also reassures patients. Patients who have undergone hernia repair surgery are often taught to support the incision when coughing, as there is the worry that the sudden increase in intra-abdominal pressure may lead to the repair being breached and the hernia reappearing (though this is in fact uncommon).

Leg exercises are taught to patients in an attempt to mitigate the effects of reduced mobility on the circulation. It is preferable for the patient to mobilise as soon as possible after an operation but, depending on the operation the patient has undergone, early mobilisation may not be possible or may only be limited. The reduced mobility leads to pooling of the blood in the veins of the legs (venous stasis) and this in turn can lead to the development of thrombi in the veins (especially the veins in the calf), known as a deep vein thrombosis (DVT). If this thrombus then breaks free and enters the circulation as an embolus, it can travel to the lungs and lead to a pulmonary embolus (PE). It should be noted that both DVT and PE are examples of venous thromboembolism (VTE) and this term is often used when referring to the overall risk (Bircher & Chowdhury, 2020). An example of a passive leg exercise is detailed in Box 14.5 (Figure 14.1).

Box 14.4 Breathing Exercise for Patients

1. Put yourself in a comfortable position, ideally sitting up straight with your back supported.
2. Take a deep breath in and hold your breath for approximately 3 seconds, then breathe out slowly and relax.
3. Repeat step 2.
4. Take a third deep breath in and hold your breath for approximately 3 seconds. Open your mouth wide and force the air out in a short, sharp breath as if you were steaming up a glass window (this is called a huff).
5. Finally, take a deep breath in and perform a strong cough, clearing any secretions/mucus that may be present.

Box 14.5 An Example of a Passive Leg Exercise for Patients

1. With your legs straight, first point your toes, then bring your toes up toward your head. Do this exercise 10 times every hour with one foot and then the other.
2. With your legs straight, rotate your ankles one at a time, as if you were drawing little circles with your toes. Do this exercise 10 times with one foot and then the other.

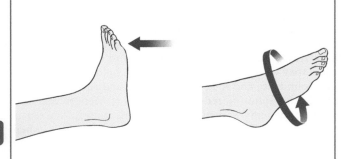

Figure 14.1 **Leg exercises after surgery.**

222

Preadmission Clinics

Patients who are to undergo a planned (elective) surgical procedure are often asked to attend a preadmission clinic, which is often nurse led. A preoperative assessment of the patient is carried out as well as preoperative information giving and teaching.

Suitably educated and trained nurses may carry out a physical assessment, including listening to breath sounds and heart sounds. Depending on local policies, nurses may also carry out or order preoperative tests and investigations if required (otherwise, this will be done by the medical staff).

- *Electrocardiogram (ECG)* to assess the patient for pre-existing cardiac conditions (though it must be noted that a normal ECG does not guarantee the absence of heart disease).
- *Full blood count*: red blood cell count, haemoglobin level and haematocrit are important indicators of the oxygen-carrying capacity of the blood. Reduced capacity will affect recovery postoperatively. Raised white blood cell counts can help to identify infections.
- *Blood grouping and cross-matching*: in case of the need for blood transfusion.
- *Serum electrolytes*: to evaluate fluid and electrolyte status.
- *Fasting blood glucose*: to screen for diabetes mellitus. Diabetes mellitus is a major potential cause of postoperative complications and poor wound healing.
- *Blood urea nitrogen (BUN)*: to evaluate renal function.
- *Alanine aminotransferase (ALT), aspartate aminotransferase (AST) and bilirubin*: to evaluate liver function.
- *Urinalysis*: to assess for potential problems, such as diabetes mellitus, urinary tract infection or renal disease.
- *Chest X-ray (CXR)*: to help evaluate respiratory function and heart size.

- *Methicillin-resistant Staphylococcus aureus (MRSA) screening.*
- *Coronavirus (COVID-19) screening*: though this will usually be done on the day of admission (King & Hothi, 2020).

Risk Assessment

Risk assessment prior to a surgical procedure is a vital element of ensuring patient safety. In general, the degree of risk of an operation begins with a baseline of the grade of the surgery (see Box 14.1). Surgical risk is also increased by the urgency of the operation, in that the more urgent the surgery, the less time there is to both assess the patient and attempt to alleviate any operative risks inherent to the patient. When reviewing patients for surgery, the anaesthetist will usually grade the patient according to the American Society of Anesthesiologists (ASA) grade (Box 14.6). However, the ASA grade is not the only risk factor and must not be taken alone as the sole indicator of risk. Operative risk is a combination of several factors (Mayhew *et al.*, 2019).

- The physical status of the patient.
- The physiological derangement that the operation will cause.
- The skill and experience of the surgeon.
- The skill and experience of the anaesthetist.
- The physiological support service in the perioperative period (including preoperative optimisation and postoperative care).

Optimising the patient's physical condition and health prior to surgery will help to reduce the risk the operation poses to that particular patient. Several factors cannot be altered (such as age) but the control of disease processes and other factors can make a significant difference to operative risk and the speed of recovery.

- *Malnutrition*: can lead to delayed wound healing, increased rates of infection and reduced energy. The body requires a variety of nutrients for recovery, such as protein and vitamins for wound healing and vitamin K for clotting.
- *Obesity*: leads to hypertension, impaired cardiac function and impaired respiratory function. Obese patients are more likely to have impaired wound healing and have an increased risk for wound infections as adipose tissue impedes blood circulation and this reduces the delivery of the nutrients, antibodies and enzymes necessary for wound healing (Frame-Peterson *et al.*, 2017).

Box 14.6 ASA Grades

Though the term 'ASA grade' is in common use, the actual classification system is known as the 'ASA physical status grade' (ASA PS grade) and it is acceptable to use either Roman numerals (I, II, III, etc.) or standard numbers (1, 2, 3, etc.).

ASA Grade Definition

I. Normal healthy individual
II. Mild systemic disease that does not limit activity
III. Severe systemic disease that limits activity but is not incapacitating
IV. Incapacitating systemic disease which is constantly life-threatening
V. Moribund, not expected to survive 24 hours with or without surgery

- *Smoking*: smoking increases the risks of some postoperative complications, such as pulmonary complications, cardiovascular complications and wound-related complications (such as infection). Even a brief period of not smoking may reduce the risk of postoperative complications (Nolan *et al.*, 2017). The use of nicotine replacement therapy (NRT) is certainly recommended in helping patients to stop smoking but there is a theoretical risk of delays in wound healing if this is carried on through the surgical period. It is currently unknown if the use of e-cigarettes ('vaping') is a risk factor for surgical complications though many argue it is no different from NRT (Famiglietti *et al.*, 2021).

Practice Assessment Document

Preoperative smoking cessation, even if only immediately pre and post operation, is an opportunity for the student to show the ability to utilise appropriate opportunities to encourage health behaviours such as smoking cessation in the context of the client's current circumstances (outcome 2.4, NMC 2018a). Discussion can focus on the hospital stay as an opportunity to break the smoking cycle and also information on the immediate benefit of smoking cessation on wound healing may aid the client in their decision making.

Admission to the Ward

On admission to the ward, the patient may understandably feel anxious and disorientated. It is essential for the patient to feel as though they are welcome and expected. There can be little more disturbing to a patient on the day of their operation than to attend the ward only to be ignored or placed in the day room, with little information or even with such phrases as 'We don't know if we have a bed yet'. A welcome from a staff member who is clearly expecting the patient can make all the difference to their early impressions of the hospital and ward. If the patient's bed space is not ready for them to occupy, then the patient should be informed of the delay and reassurance given.

Practice Assessment Document

The standard that requires student nurses to have the skills and abilities to support people at all stages of life who are emotionally or physically vulnerable (NMC, 2018a) can often be a difficult one for student and assessor to measure. What must be remembered is that this is a 'soft' skill that can be evidenced at many points of the client journey and showing an anxious client the care and consideration of greeting them and providing reassurance during the 'limbo' of waiting for a bed on a ward should never be underestimated as an opportunity to evidence this outcome.

Regardless of whether the patient has a bed to go to or is asked to wait in the day room, there should be an immediate orientation to the ward environment (such as the location of the toilets). Once the nurse has been made aware of the presence of the patient, then they should endeavour to at least introduce themselves to the patient and any relatives that may be present. This way, the patient is reassured that they have not been abandoned or forgotten and has the name of a member of staff to whom they can turn if required.

If not already done, a full nursing history should be taken from the patient. Full nursing documentation should be recorded on the relevant paperwork in conjunction with the patient and/or relatives.

- *Breathing*: including baseline respiration rate and smoking status. Any history of respiratory diseases. Take this time to teach, or revise, breathing exercises.
- *Cardiovascular system*: baseline observations. History of cardiac disease, arrhythmias, chest pain or shortness of breath on exertion. Any history of claudication or other peripheral vascular disease: peripheral vascular diseases are linked with an increased risk of deep vein thrombosis (Niu *et al.*, 2021) and any patient with known or suspected peripheral vascular problems should also be considered high risk for pressure sores, including those caused by compression stockings (Hobson *et al.*, 2017; NICE, 2019). A history of hypertension should be recorded, as it is associated with increased risk of cardiovascular complications in surgery and anaesthesia (Aronow, 2017).
- *Maintaining body temperature*: a raised temperature may be an indication of an infection.
- *Hygiene* (*washing and dressing*): building a picture of what the patient was able to do before surgery is a valuable aid to postoperative goal setting ready for discharge and also helps with discharge planning. At the same time, the nurse should be aware of the actual physical state of the patient at the time of admission. Many patients will not be willing to admit that they are struggling with day-to-day tasks or may not be aware of the possibility of aids to washing and dressing or home adaptations. Oral hygiene should be discussed, including the presence of dentures, caps, crowns and loose teeth. A labelled denture pot should be made available where necessary and any loose teeth or implants should be recorded.

Case Study

You are assessing and admitting 80-year-old Mrs Jones to the ward prior to hip replacement surgery. Despite denying any difficulty with washing and dressing at home, Mrs Jones has long dirty toenails, unwashed hair and her clothes are stained and dirty. On inquiring, Mrs Jones states that she lives alone in a flat, she has access to her own washing machine but has to hang her clothes on a line outside. She has a bathroom with a bath but no shower. Mrs Jones was offered home care after her last admission to hospital but refused as she doesn't like 'strangers in her home' and 'anyway it's expensive'.

Take some time to reflect on this case study, look up the discharge advice for a patient post hip replacement and then consider these questions and perhaps discuss them with your colleagues.

1. What do you think may be the reasons for the difference between what Mrs Jones is saying and her physical state?
2. What may be some of the potential reasons for her inability to maintain her own hygiene?

3. How will Mrs Jones manage in the immediate postdischarge period? What could you do to ensure a safe and effective discharge?
4. How can staff encourage the use of home care by Mrs Jones?
5. Where could you refer Mrs Jones to help with the potential cost of home care?

- *Eating and nutrition*: as well as recording patient dietary preferences and normal intake, the nurse should take the time to commence patient education in the benefits of healthy eating and review the patient's normal diet with them. Height and weight should be recorded and body mass index (BMI) calculated. An accurate weight aids the anaesthetist in calculating the correct anaesthetic dose. Enquiring about any significant weight loss in recent times can be a valuable discussion, as if the weight loss was not deliberate it may be an indication of an underlying disease process. Weight loss of greater than 10% in the preceding 6 months is associated with a greater risk of surgical morbidity and mortality and should be addressed with the multidisciplinary team. Fluid intake (including alcohol consumption) should be discussed and recorded.

Red Flag

 Patients who are underweight should have their score calculated on the Malnutrition Universal Screening Tool (MUST) to help direct suitable interventions to improve their nutritional status.
The most recent version of the tool is always available to download from the British Association of Parenteral and Enteral Nutrition website (http://bapen.org.uk).

- *Elimination*: record the patient's normal patterns. Are they often constipated? Do they rely on laxatives? If so, have the patient's normal laxatives been prescribed? Do they have regular bowel movements? A large proportion of patients will find it difficult to have their bowels open during a hospital stay and patients with regular bowel habits should be reassured that this is normal but if they wish, laxatives can be made available. Patterns of micturition should also be recorded. For instance, a patient who routinely wakes in the night to use the toilet may try to get up in the night on a darkened ward and fall. If required, it may be necessary to assess the patient's stool using the Bristol Stool Chart, especially where there is actual or potential constipation.
- *Communication*: note should be made of the patient's native language and any need for a translator. Any difficulties with communication must be noted clearly on patient documentation and handed over effectively to all members of the healthcare team who come into contact with the patient. Hearing aids should be labelled if the patient is going to wear them until the point of anaesthetic, otherwise they should be stored carefully with the patient's belongings. The use of glasses and contact lenses should be noted and storage made available.
- *Mobility*: what is the patient's usual mobility? If the patient has reduced mobility, what is the cause? Being aware of the patient's normal abilities allows for realistic goal setting for postoperative mobilising and also allows the nurse to refer to any appropriate services, such as physiotherapy or occupational therapy for assessment. A 'slips, trips and falls' assessment may be required to help maintain patient safety, as well as a pressure sore risk assessment such as a Waterlow score. Finally, the patient should be assessed for the risk of venous thromboembolism (VTE) using a recognised scoring system (NICE, 2019).
- *Expressing sexuality/gender*: this is a section of the nursing admission that is often ignored but sexuality and gender are important aspects of care delivery. Patients may wish to discuss when they will be able to resume sexual activities and/or if there will be any restrictions. Some patients may have express wishes about wearing make-up until the last possible moment and having make-up available as soon as they are orientated after surgery. Muslim women may have preferences as to who should nurse them and may wish to wear their hijab until they are in the theatre environment. Homosexual patients may be concerned about whether they can record their partner as their next of kin (Fish, 2010). It is important to ask and record patient preference regarding their personal choice of pronouns (Mulkey, 2020). The use of the contraceptive pill should be noted and the date it was stopped checked with the patient, as there may be an increased risk of deep vein thrombosis. The possibility of pregnancy should be considered in all menstruating patients. If, in discussion, they cannot be certain they are not pregnant, then a pregnancy test should be undertaken though some state pregnancy testing should be routine for all women of child-bearing age (Clement *et al.*, 2018).
- *Dying/plans for the future*: it has already been noted that admission to the ward prior to surgery will be a point of great anxiety for the patient. While it may be inappropriate to discuss death and dying with some patients at this point, other patients may wish to address their feelings or to be directed to a place where they can spend some time praying/in contemplation. This is an issue that should be approached with sensitivity and the discussion tailored to the wishes of the patient.
- *Work and leisure*: many patients will wish to know when they can return to work and any limitations on the activities they can undertake at work or for leisure and for how long.
- *Support systems*: will the patient be having visitors? Do they know which ward and what the visiting times are? It is worthwhile allocating one family member who will contact the ward and then update other members of the family. Who is looking after any pets or dependents that are usually reliant on the patient? Who will be available on discharge and what support mechanisms will be available for activities such as shopping? During the current coronavirus pandemic, visiting patients in hospital has stopped to help prevent the spread of the virus. Whilst understandable, this prohibition of visiting adult patients can lead to distress for both the patient and families (Macmillan, 2021); where possible, the use of video calls (patient's own or hospital acquired) may be of value.

Preparation for Surgery

On the day of surgery, the patient will be required to be nil by mouth (NBM). Traditionally, patients have been asked to be NBM from midnight; however, it is now recognised that keeping patients NBM for potentially prolonged periods is not necessary and may even be detrimental. Recent recommendations are that patients can drink clear fluids up to 2 hours prior to surgery and eat food up to 6 hours prior to surgery (King, 2019). However, the nature of surgical theatre lists is such that the patient will often be NBM for longer, due to delays or reorganisation of the running order in theatre (Merchant *et al.*, 2020). Therefore, patients who are NBM are often prescribed intravenous fluids though adherence to preoperative fasting guidelines is considered optimal (Myles *et al.*, 2017); furthermore, mouthcare packs or mouth care should be given to those who cannot perform it themselves. Good communication is necessary between ward and theatres, as when operations are cancelled a patient's NBM status may be prolonged.

Prescribed medication should be reviewed and only those deemed medically necessary should be administered but nurses must be sure that medicines that are critical are administered. Premedication may be prescribed for a variety of reasons and these may be taken with up to 60 mL of water. Care should be taken to ensure that time-critical premedication (such as antibiotics) is given as prescribed.

Unless directed otherwise by the surgeon, the patient should wash or shower the night before surgery using soap and water; antibacterial washes are not considered to be effective (Webster & Osborne, 2015). Nail polish, acrylic nails and make-up should be removed before surgery, as otherwise the effects of cyanosis or shock may not be as evident, as the changes in colour of the nail bed are masked.

If hair removal is required, it should be done on the day of surgery using depilatory cream or electric clippers. If shaving is undertaken, then it should be done in the theatre environment as close to the point in time of surgical skin preparation as possible but outside the theatre itself.

Jewellery should be removed if possible, as rings can harbour bacteria; loose items of jewellery could become snagged while transferring the patient onto and off the operating table; and all metal jewellery increases the risk of burns where diathermy is used during the procedure. Local policy may allow difficult-to-remove rings to be covered with tape. Transdermal patches should also be removed, as they carry a risk of burns or explosion with the use of diathermy or the need for defibrillation if advanced life support is required.

Menstruating patients should be advised of the risk of toxic shock syndrome if they use tampons during the operative period. If a tampon is left in place for more than 6 hours, the risk of toxic shock is increased and therefore patients are best advised to use sanitary towels until after the operation. If a tampon is left in place, then this information must be documented and handed over.

Antiembolic stockings and/or low molecular weight heparin (LMWH) injections may be required. This will depend on surgeon choice, the results of a venous thrombosis risk assessment and the existence of any contraindications to antiembolic stockings. Stockings must be measured and applied appropriately, ensuring a wrinkle-free result to avoid areas of high pressure on the skin. The nurse should ensure that prescribed anticoagulants are administered prior to surgery.

The details on the patient's wristband must be checked with the patient and against the medical notes, X-rays, test results and nursing documentation. Patient allergies should be documented and recorded on a suitable allergy wristband. As well as medication allergies, food allergies should be recorded, as certain food allergies give an indication of the potential for allergies to certain drugs or substances.

The site of the surgery should be marked by the operating surgeon using an indelible marker before the patient receives any medication that may cause drowsiness (Omar *et al.*, 2021).

Red Flag Wrong Site Surgery

 Wrong site surgery is an adverse event in which a surgical procedure is performed on the wrong site (e.g. organ, limb, eye or wrong patient). The effects of wrong site surgery can be devastating to the patient and the use of a preoperative marking checklist is strongly recommended.
Source: NICE (2020a)

The consent form must be placed on the front of the patient's notes (or other prominent place according to local policy) and confirmed with the patient. While a formal written consent is gained for the surgical procedure, note that patients should also be consented for any anaesthetic they are to receive (Yentis *et al.*, 2017), though this is not normally recorded on a formal consent form but in the patient's notes. (For further details of the ethical and legal aspects of consent, please refer to Chapter 2.)

Care, Dignity and Compassion

 Maintaining dignity while wearing a surgical gown is difficult, as they are worn backwards (with the opening to the patient's rear) and patients often complain that the gowns do not keep them covered. Wherever possible, the patient may keep on their underwear until the moment they are to be transferred. Patients who have a dressing gown should be encouraged to wear it; those who do not have a dressing gown with them should be given a second surgical gown to wear in place of a dressing gown.

Waiting on the ward on the day of surgery is the time when the patient's anxiety is most likely to peak and thus the availability of distractions, such as reading materials, televisions or radios, may be useful. Patients with learning disabilities, or children and young adult patients, will benefit from the presence of a family member or familiar carer and this should be encouraged, regardless of standard visiting times.

Surgical Safety Checklist

What the Experts Say

 'The introduction of the WHO Safer Surgery Checklist was a great step forward in the delivery of safer care for patients undergoing operations.'
Dr Mike Durkin, Director of Patient Safety, NHS England

The use of a surgical checklist in the preoperative period is now standard practice in the UK (NICE, 2020a). The checklist is used to ensure that certain mandatory items are not forgotten and gives teams a simple set of checks that have been shown to improve patient safety.

Transfer to Theatre

Once the theatre staff have asked for the patient to be transferred to theatre, the patient should be accompanied by an appropriately qualified member of staff (such as a registered nurse) who remains with the patient until handover to the theatre staff (using the checklist and patient notes) has been completed.

Postoperative Surgical Phase

Collection of the patient from the recovery area must be carried out by a suitably qualified member of staff (such as a registered nurse). The patient is considered safe for discharge from recovery to the ward when:

- They are awake with their eyes open
- They are extubated
- They are maintaining satisfactory blood pressure and pulse
- They are able to lift their head from the pillow on command
- They are not hypoxic
- They are breathing quietly and comfortably
- The are not persistently bleeding from wound sites or into drains
- Appropriate analgesia has been prescribed and is safely established.

Handover from the recovery nurse to the ward nurse must include comprehensive orders for:

- Vital signs
- Pain control
- Rate and type of intravenous fluids
- Urine and gastrointestinal fluid output
- Other medications
- Laboratory investigations.

The handover must incorporate information on:

- The procedure undertaken
- Any complications
- Any changes in treatment from that planned
- A comment on medical and nursing observations.

Red Flag

If the patient is restless, then something is wrong. Look out for:
- · Airway obstruction
- · Hypoxia
- · Uncontrolled pain
- · Shivering/hypothermia
- · Bleeding (external or internal)
- · Vomiting.

If you are unhappy with the state of the patient, then you should refuse to transfer them and request a medical review.

Immediate Postoperative Period

On return to the ward, postoperative patients must be monitored and assessed for any deterioration. Vital signs should be assessed and recorded in line with local policy and guidance and compared with baseline levels (preoperative and immediately postoperatively).

When reviewing vital signs, take into account both the current observations and the trend the vital signs have followed over an appropriate period of time (e.g. the last few hours). Hospital trusts in the UK have adopted the use of early warning scores such as the National Early Warning Score 2 (NEWS 2) (Royal College of Physicians, 2017). The NEWS 2 is an at-risk scoring system that helps in the identification of patients who are clinically deteriorating and measures six parameters.

- Respiratory rate
- Oxygen saturations
- Temperature
- Systolic blood pressure
- Pulse rate
- Level of consciousness or new confusion

While use of the NEWS 2 system has undoubtedly improved clinical recognition of the deteriorating patient, it is preferable that the score is used as part of an ABCDE assessment of the patient, to enable a holistic assessment and gain a complete clinical picture.

When assessing the patient, ensure that you use all the appropriate senses. Touch your patient to feel the skin temperature and assess for clammy skin; listen to the sound of the patient's breathing; look at the colour of the inner eyelid or oral mucosa and be aware of any smells (such as faeces, melaena or acetone breath).

Airway

A disordered airway may be the result of several potential causes.

- Direct trauma to the airway from intubation leading to inflammation and oedema.
- Reduced conscious level leading to a loss of the ability to maintain a patent airway.
- Foreign body aspiration.

Assessing the airway requires the nurse to look, listen and feel. Look at the patient's chest for movement, while at the same time listening and/or feeling for breath being expired from the mouth. Complete airway obstruction will be identified by the lack of air movement from the patient. Partial airway obstruction is often associated with an increased effort to breathe and added noises to the breathing. Listen for:

- Snoring noises
- Crowing noises (stridor)
- Gurgling noises (indicating fluid in the upper airway).

Left untreated, partial airway obstruction will often lead to complete airway obstruction and cardiopulmonary arrest. The treatment of airway obstruction depends on the cause but may include:

- Placing the patient in the recovery position
- The use of suction
- Removal of foreign bodies
- Head tilt-chin lift
- Advanced airway manoeuvres.

For a patient with a disordered airway, constant monitoring is advised until the situation is resolved. In many cases, it is recommended that the nurse asks for an urgent medical review of the patient.

Breathing

Causes of disordered breathing in the surgical patient include:

- Increased bronchial secretions following the use of anaesthetic gases
- Decreased respiratory rate or work of breathing due to opiate analgesia

- Pain
- Pneumothorax
- Respiratory diseases
- Increasing respiratory rates are often the earliest sign of shock.

To assess breathing:

- Look, listen and feel for signs of respiratory distress:
  - Sweating
  - Central cyanosis (inspect the inner eyelid or oral mucosa)
  - The use of the accessory muscles of respiration
- Assess the respiratory rate. A high (or increasing) respiratory rate is a sign that the patient is potentially severely ill and may deteriorate suddenly
- Assess the depth of each breath and whether the chest is expanding equally on both sides
- Note the amount of oxygen being delivered and the oxygen saturation
- Listen for noisy breathing, for example rattling or wheezing.

Red Flag

 When using oxygen saturation monitoring, remember to change the position of the probe regularly to prevent the development of pressure sores.

Treatment of respiratory problems will almost always require medical help to treat the underlying cause but where possible consider:

- Commencing oxygen as prescribed (if not already being administered)
- Positioning the patient in a semi-recumbent position to allow for increased lung expansion.

Circulation

Disturbances of blood pressure and pulse are often late signs of an underlying problem. To assess circulation:

- Look to see if the patient's hands are mottled, pale or blue (or greyish in patients with a darker skin colour)
- Assess the limb temperature by touching the patient's hands
- Measure the capillary refill time
- Monitor the heart rate
- Take a pulse: is it regular or irregular? Weak or strong?
- Take the blood pressure
- Consider the patient's conscious level (poor cerebral perfusion will lead to reduced conscious level)
- Measure and record the hourly urine output (less than 0.5 mL/kg per hour can be a sign of poor renal perfusion due to low blood pressure)
- Measure and record the patient's temperature.

Post anaesthetic, many patients will show a transient drop in blood pressure that will rectify itself quite rapidly. However, patients with a continuing trend of decreasing blood pressure or showing other signs of haemodynamic instability should be assumed to be deteriorating and appropriate help should be sought. In almost all patients with signs of circulatory shock, consider hypovolaemia as the potential cause. Assess the wound site for signs of bleeding and check any drains for output. If the fluid balance is not already being recorded, then this should be commenced.

If haemodynamic compromise is suspected, then consider the following actions.

- Asking for a review by the surgical team.
- Tilting the patient's bed to a head-down position to improve venous return. Be aware that this may be inappropriate in patients with a compromised airway.

Red Flag

 Do not use head-down tilt with patients who have undergone gynaecological surgery, as this can mask vaginal bleeding.

If the patient's temperature is reduced, then consider the use of extra blankets or a warm air blanket. In the event of a raised temperature, consider the potential onset of sepsis. Nursing interventions for pyrexia include prescribed antipyretics and indirect fan therapy. Direct fan therapy and tepid sponging should not be used, as they are fundamentally illogical and based on ritual.

Disability

This part of the assessment is where the patient's conscious level is judged. Measurement using the Glasgow Coma Scale (GCS) is very effective but a quicker method is to use the ACVPU score.

- **A** refers to Alert (a patient who is awake and talking to you).
- **C** refers to a patient with new-onset confusion.
- **V** refers to Voice, i.e. the patient is only responding to voice, such as direct questions or commands.
- **P** refers to Pain, i.e. the patient is only responding to painful stimuli.
- **U** is the Unresponsive patient, who does not even respond to pain.

A patient who scores P or U on the scale is considered to have a GCS score of less than 8 and therefore the airway is in danger – this patient needs to be seen by an anaesthetist as a matter of urgency.

Following on from this, review the patient's drug chart for causes of a change in conscious level (for instance, opiate drugs), check the blood glucose, and consider nursing the patient in the recovery position if appropriate.

Exposure

This refers to exposing the patient in order to carry out a primary survey to assess for bleeding, rashes, early signs of pressure sores, and so forth. Ensure that you expose and assess the whole of the patient from head to toe. Remember to maintain dignity and prevent heat loss at all times. Pay particular attention to wound sites and drains to assess for signs of bleeding.

Depending on the operation, as the patient's blood pressure stabilises they may be able to sit up. The patient may need to be reminded that the operation is over and where they are, as disorientation can occur. Children and young people and patients with learning disabilities will benefit from the presence of a relative or carer at the bedside, while they are recovering from the immediate effects of an anaesthetic.

Case Study Care Post Hemicolectomy

John (he/him) has returned to the ward following a 3-hour operation to remove a section of his large intestine (hemi-colectomy). He was stable in the immediate postoperative period and was deemed safe to return to the ward. You have been charged with the follow-up care on the ward and have been undertaking regular observations and wound checks. In the 2 hours following his return to the ward, John has become increasingly distressed and anxious. His observations are showing an increasing respiratory rate, increasing heart rate and a dropping blood pressure. His hands are cold to the touch and whilst his catheter bag was emptied on his return to the ward, there has been no subsequent urine output noted. The wound site is clean and dry but you do note his abdomen is looking swollen. He has a 1 litre bag of 0.9% saline being administered intravenously over 6 hours. His latest vital signs are as below.

VITAL SIGN	OBSERVATION	NORMAL
Temperature	36.0 °C	36.0–37.9 °C range
Pulse	110 beats per minute	60–100 beats per minute
Respiration	24 breaths per minute	12–20 breaths per minute
Blood pressure	95/50 mmHg	100–139 mmHg (systolic) range
O$_2$ saturations (on air)	92%	94–98%

NEWS 2
John's NEWS 2 score is noted below

PHYSIOLOGICAL PARAMETER	3	2	1	0	1	2	3
Respiration rate							24
Oxygen saturation %		92					
Air or oxygen					Air		
Temperature °C			36.0				
Systolic BP mmHg		95					
Heart rate						110	
Level of consciousness				A			
Score	0	4	1	0	1	2	0
Total	8						

Take time to reflect on this case study and then consider the following.

1. What are your immediate concerns with regard to John's condition?

2. John's heart rate is increasing, and his systolic blood pressure is dropping. What do you think is happening and why?
3. What immediate nursing actions could you take (remember any drugs including oxygen must be prescribed)?
4. Given John's NEWS 2 score of 8, what is the recommended escalation action according to your local policy?

The Nursing Associate

John's case study is directly related to outcomes 3.7 (escalation of care) and 3.11 of the *Standards f Proficiency for the Nursing Associate* (NMC, 2018b). Outcome 3.11 specifically refers to recognising deterioration and escalating as necessary. Using the NEWS 2 scoring system gives the trainee nursing associate a useful tool for recording and reporting patient deterioration.

Complications of Surgery

While each surgical procedure will carry its own potential complications, there are several potential complications that are common to all surgical patients.

Basal Consolidation Leading to Chest Infection

Signs to look for include:

- A raised temperature
- Rapid shallow respirations
- Decreased chest expansion
- Potential chest pain
- A productive cough (though this is less likely in the elderly patient)
- Oxygen saturations may or may not be reduced.

Patients with increased risk of basal consolidation include smokers, patients who have undergone chest or abdominal surgery, and patients who are dehydrated. Prevention requires the encouragement of breathing and coughing exercises, early mobilisation and maintaining appropriate hydration. Patients suspected of basal consolidation should be referred to the physiotherapist and, if possible, a sputum sample should be obtained and sent for microbiological culture and sensitivity testing.

Renal Failure or Urinary Retention

In patients who are not being monitored on a fluid balance chart, this can be missed in the early stages. Patients most at risk of renal failure are those who have had a period of hypovolaemia/hypotension (see Chapter 29 for more details). Renal failure must be distinguished from urinary retention, as renal failure is a medical emergency. Patients with urinary retention will have a full bladder that may also be painful and will be unable to urinate, despite having the urge. It is expected that all patients will pass urine within 24 hours after their operation and when they do, this should be documented in their notes. No patient should be discharged from hospital without documented evidence that they have passed urine. Anaesthesia can affect the bladder, which may make it difficult for the patient to pass urine.

Retention may be prevented by ensuring that the patient is appropriately hydrated, providing privacy and encouraging the patient to sit up to urinate. Where appropriate, male patients can be encouraged to sit on the side of the bed to use the bottle and female patients should be provided with commodes. Until the nurse is confident of patient safety, they should remain with any patient who gets out of bed in case of fainting or collapse. The use of bed pans and urinals in bed should be avoided if at all possible, as the patient will find it difficult and will also not be able to empty their bladder entirely. Mobilising the patient to the toilet once it is safe to do so will often encourage patients to pass urine.

Deep Vein Thrombosis

The most common site for DVT is the calf veins. The cause is often a mix of dehydration, venous stasis and reduced venous return.

Jot This Down

Consider the causes of deep vein thrombosis. How would you help to prevent a DVT occurring in your patient?

The signs and symptoms of DVT are a swollen, painful calf that is hot to the touch. If a DVT is suspected, the medical staff must be informed immediately. Treatment involves bed rest and anti-coagulation. The peak incidence for DVT is 5 days postoperatively, although some patients can be vulnerable up to 12 weeks postoperatively.

Nausea and Vomiting

Postoperative nausea and vomiting (PONV) may be a reaction to opiates, anaesthetics or other drugs. Other potential causes include pain, abdominal distension and electrolyte imbalances in the blood. Those most at risk of PONV are:

- Patients under 3 years or over 70 years of age
- Menstrual age females
- Obese patients
- Patients who were excessively starved preoperatively
- Patients with a history of motion sickness
- Patients with a previous history of PONV
- Patients who are highly anxious (Gan *et al.*, 2019).

The treatment for PONV includes the following.

- If able, find and remove the cause.
- Recovery position for patients at risk of aspiration.
- Suction if required.
- Withhold food and fluids.
- Once the PONV subsides, start the patient on sips of fluids and small amounts of dry solid food (such as biscuits).
- Acupressure wristbands may be of use in some patients.
- If prescribed, antiemetics can be administered.

Haemorrhage

There are three main types of postsurgical haemorrhage.

- *Primary haemorrhage*: occurs at the time of the operation.
- *Reactionary haemorrhage*: occurs within a few hours of surgery and is a reaction to a rising blood pressure.
- *Secondary haemorrhage*: occurs days later, often as a result of infection.

First aid response to haemorrhage is to apply pressure either manually or by applying pads to the dressing. If bleeding persists, then surgical review is required.

Acute Confusion/Delirium

Acute confusion may affect the elderly patient with no previous history of dementia (Helgesen *et al.*, 2021). The key features of acute confusion are:

- Sudden onset
- Impaired attention
- Apathy or hyperactivity
- Thought, perception and short-term memory impairment
- Mood fluctuation, especially at night
- Disorientation in time, place and person
- Disturbed sleep–wake patterns
- Hallucinations and delusions.

Acute confusion tends to last less than a month and is often followed by a full recovery.

Constipation

Often patients reason that, as there has been no food intake, no faeces will be produced and thus tend not to report altered bowel habits to the nurse. Gastrointestinal peristalsis will be decreased for at least 24 hours in patients who have undergone gastrointestinal surgery. Furthermore, immobility, dehydration and opiate analgesia will also contribute to constipation. Nurses must also take into account the psychological effect of using commodes on a busy ward. Where possible, patients should be mobilised to the toilet. Encouraging a high-fibre diet and adequate hydration, as well as encouraging mobility, will help to prevent constipation.

Pressure Injures

Pressure sores can often begin in the operating theatre and it is worth ascertaining the position in which the patient was placed on the operating table, as pressure sores can develop in unusual places. The longer the patient is in the operating theatre, the greater the risk of developing a pressure sore. When assessing patients for pressure sores, the nurse must ensure they inspect areas that are at risk due to equipment use, such as oxygen saturation probes, nasal speculae, the elastic straps from oxygen masks and nasogastric tubes.

Pain

For full details of pain assessment and pain relief, please refer to Chapter 22. One aspect of pain control specific to surgical patients is the use of patient-controlled analgesia (PCA). PCA is any method that allows the patient to control and administer

229

their own pain relief and so can include all methods of drug administration. There are two main systems used for PCA after surgery.

- *Disposable PCA*: this system uses a non-electric pump based on the elastic properties of certain materials, a spring-based mechanism or pressure generated by patient action. Disposable systems have the advantage of not requiring an external power source (useful in transport situations) and eliminating programming errors. However, these systems have been shown to be generally inaccurate, with variations in flow rates being affected by temperature, length of storage, atmospheric pressure and the volume of the remaining solution in the reservoir (Skryabina & Dunn, 2006).
- *Non-disposable PCA*: this is the system most commonly used in the hospital setting. Based on a computerised system with disposable giving sets, these are considered to have much greater accuracy and have the advantage over disposable systems in that they are programmable and thus rates of infusion and delivery can be changed.

Regardless of the choice of delivery system, the principle of intravenous PCA remains the same. Occasionally, the pump device will deliver a preset 'background' infusion rate of analgesia and nurses should be aware of this and be vigilant for the effects of oversedation. Using a hand-held button, the patient can activate the delivery of small doses of bolus analgesia. Once activated, the button is then subject to a timed delay (lock-out), during which the delivery of another bolus dose cannot be activated, thus avoiding potential overdose. The benefits of the patient-controlled system are that the patient can control when analgesia is delivered, thus avoiding waits for nursing staff to be available. Overall, the PCA system has been shown to provide a relatively steady serum concentration of analgesia, avoiding the peaks and troughs of traditional intramuscular regimens (Figure 14.2) and also avoiding excessive pain or sedation.

Not all patients are suitable for PCA, as there is a requirement for baseline levels of dexterity to activate the button and an ability to understand the concept of PCA and its use. If a patient chooses to use PCA, then the preoperative teaching should include the use of PCA, including an opportunity for the patient to handle the device.

Patient-controlled analgesia does not guarantee that the patient will be pain free and thus nurses should be aware of the need to administer further analgesia if required and to refer to the pain control team for the PCA regimen to be altered if it is providing inadequate analgesia for patient comfort.

Further Care of the Surgical Patient

Early Mobilisation
Even short-term immobility and bed rest are associated with:
- Increased risk of DVT
- Muscle wasting
- Decreased pulmonary function and tissue oxygenation
- Increased risk of chest infection
- Loss of appetite
- An inability to effectively empty the bladder, leading to an increased risk of urinary tract infections
- Constipation.

Thus, early mobilisation is a vital part of the recovery of any surgical patient. Walking aids should be available to patients who require them. Depending on the operation performed, there may be particular restrictions on mobility and this should be clearly

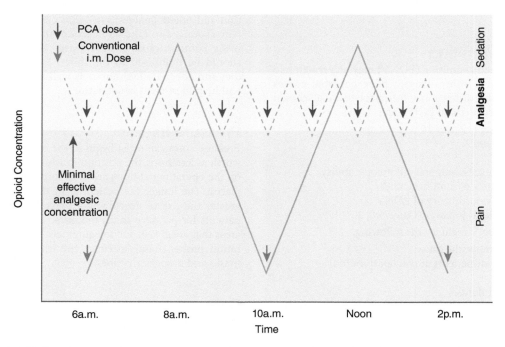

Figure 14.2 **Serum levels of analgesia using PCA and intramuscular regimens.** *Source:* Grass (2005). Reproduced with permission of Wolters Kluwer Health, Inc.

detailed in postoperative plans and the nursing documentation. Patients who cannot mobilise on the day of surgery should be encouraged to perform leg and breathing exercises. On the first day after surgery, the patient should be aiming to spend 2 hours out of bed and on subsequent days the goal should be 6 hours a day up to the day of discharge.

When the patient is to mobilise for the first time, it is essential that the nurse (or other staff member) is present. Have the patient sit on the side of the bed for a few minutes to allow the cardiovascular system to compensate for the effect of any postural hypotension. If the patient does subsequently feel faint, then it is relatively simple for them to lie back onto the bed, thus avoiding a fall. The patient may then stand while the nurse remains in close proximity in order to guide the patient back onto the bed if they feel dizzy. The nurse will then stay with the patient as they attempt to mobilise, to offer support and reassurance until they are sure the patient is safe to mobilise alone.

Patients are often understandably concerned that mobilising will place pressure on their wound and it will then 'split open'. Adequate pain relief and reassurance will be required. The wound will have developed most of its tensile strength immediately after the operation and thus the patient can be reassured that it is safe to mobilise. Mobility can also be restricted by the use of monitoring equipment and intravenous giving sets, and thus it is necessary to ensure that patients are disconnected from any monitoring equipment or intravenous sets as soon as they are no longer required.

Eating and Drinking

As soon as the patient is able, they should be encouraged to take sips of water and the amount taken increased as tolerated. Patients should also be encouraged to eat as they feel able (unless there are medical orders to the contrary). Small, frequent snacks may be better tolerated than full meals in the first days after surgery. In the case of abdominal surgery, appetite may not return for some time and medical orders should be followed as to when eating and drinking may be attempted.

Intravenous Infusions

Many patients return to the ward with an intravenous infusion in progress. The reasons for infusions vary but include the replacement of fluid volume (rehydration), replacement of blood loss (transfusion), or to return serum electrolyte levels to a normal range. Discontinuation of fluids is normally on medical orders. (Further information on intravenous infusions can be found in Chapter 23.)

Surgical Drains

Wound drains are used to remove body fluids and/or air from the area of the operation. Unless removed from the tissues, collections of body fluids can become a focus for infection. A tube is placed in the area where fluid is likely to collect and this tube exits the skin via a puncture wound. The tube is stitched to the skin to prevent it being accidentally dislodged and the exit site is then dressed to prevent infection of the wound. Normally, the drain is attached to a closed system to prevent the entry of pathogens and air into the body via the drainage system.

There are two main types of closed system.

- *Gravity drainage*: a passive collection system that is kept below the level of the wound. If the collection container rises above the level of the wound, then there may be a backflow of fluid into the wound.
- *Suction drainage*: an active collection system that usually uses a vacuum created in the collection container. Occasionally, a vacuum pump may be used. The other form of suction drainage is the underwater seal chest drain (see Chapter 27).

Regardless of the drain type, it is essential that strict aseptic no touch technique (ANTT) is used.

The complications of surgical drain use are:

- Failure to function properly: if the drain has not been placed correctly or has been blocked with tissues or clotted blood, or the vacuum in the container has been released
- Pain
- Inflammatory reaction to the drainage tube
- Accidental disconnection or removal
- Damage to tissues due to excessive suction or movement of the drainage tube.

Patients are often frightened of drains and restrict their movement. Adequate analgesia, education on drain handling and reassurance will help to alleviate this.

Removal of drains is dependent on the decrease in drainage and is often very painful. Removal will almost always require the administration of adequate analgesia, so allow an appropriate amount of time for it to act. Patients often appreciate being given control of the speed of removal of drainage tubes through the use of previously agreed verbal or hand signals.

Wound Care and Surgical Site Infections

The patient will return from theatre with a dressing *in situ* and this should be left in place for at least 48 hours to help reduce the chance of surgical site infection (SSI). The principles of wound healing and wound care are discussed in Chapter 18. An SSI is defined as an infection manifesting within 30 days of a surgical procedure (or within 1 year if a prosthesis is left in place during the procedure) and affecting either the incision or the deep tissue at the operation site (Wong *et al.*, 2019). Symptoms include pus, inflammation, swelling and pain. Fever may or may not be present. The majority of infections will not manifest until after the patient has been discharged from hospital.

The risk of SSI is normally related to the class of surgical procedure undertaken.

- *Clean*: no microbial contamination has been encountered and none of the body spaces are entered.
- *Clean-contaminated*: gastrointestinal, respiratory or urinary tracts are entered under controlled conditions and without contamination occurring.
- *Contaminated*: contamination does occur following entry of the gastrointestinal, respiratory or urinary tract. Recent acute trauma wounds are also classed as contaminated.
- *Dirty*: dead or infected tissue is present at the site of surgery.

Actions to prevent SSIs include the following.

- The administration of prescribed antibiotic prophylaxis in the 60 minutes before surgery starts for patients undergoing high-risk surgery.

- Ensuring the preoperative, perioperative and postoperative core temperature of the patient remains above 36.5°C (NICE, 2020b).
- Leaving the wound covered with an interactive dressing for at least 48 hours postoperatively to ensure the wound seals.
- Ensuring the free drainage of exudates and discharge.
- Removing wound drains at the earliest possible opportunity.
- Dressing changes are undertaken using strict aseptic technique.

Skin Closure Methods

There are two commonly used skin closure methods.

Skin Clips (Staples) These are used when there is little tension on the wound and a good general blood supply. This means they can be removed earlier than sutures (around 4–5 days postoperatively). Each of the different types of clip has an associated removal device, all of which work by deforming the clip, thus freeing the barbs of the clip from the skin. If a clip is proving difficult to remove, it can help to gently rock the clip using the device after the clip has been deformed and then gently pulling the clip away.

Sutures (Stitches) Two commonly used forms of suture are the subcutaneous continuous suture and intermittent skin suture.

- *Subcutaneous continuous sutures* are used to improve the cosmetic end-result of surgery. They can be recognised by the presence at each end of the wound of a retaining bead attached to the end of the suture (Figure 14.3). Removal of the suture is performed by cutting one end of the suture close to the skin (therefore beneath one of the retaining beads) and then applying traction to the opposite end of the suture lateral (along the same axis as) to the wound. The patient will often report that this procedure 'stings' but they should be reassured that the acute sensation will subside quickly to an ache, for which simple analgesics are perfectly suitable.

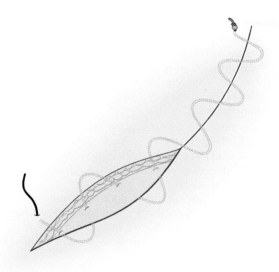

Figure 14.3 Subcutaneous continuous suture showing one of the retaining beads.

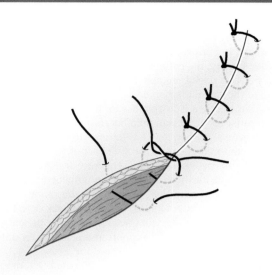

Figure 14.4 Intermittent skin sutures.

- *Intermittent skin sutures* take longer to remove and the patient may wish to have analgesia for this procedure. Each suture will have a knot, which must be identified (Figure 14.4) and lifted slightly away from the skin. Each suture is cut once just below the knot; it is important not to cut both sides of the suture, as otherwise the suture could retract under the skin (the knot will prevent this). The suture is then grasped with forceps under the knot (the knot helps to prevent the suture slipping through the forceps) and traction put on the suture by pulling across the wound to prevent excessive traction on the wound edges.

In many cases, dissolvable sutures may be used, in which case the sutures do not need to be removed but are trimmed close to the skin as the suture under the skin will dissolve over a period of time.

Red Flag

Always be sure of the type of suture you are dealing with. Trimming non-dissolvable sutures on both sides will result in a painful process for the patient when the sutures have to be dug out from under the skin.

Once sutures or clips have been removed, if there is any doubt as to the wound edges (such as the edges gaping open), then adhesive skin closure strips can be applied. Report and document your actions in accordance with local policy and procedure.

Discharge

Wound Infection

Patients should be educated to watch out for:

- Redness and soreness that does not appear to be part of normal wound healing
- Hot and swollen skin around the wound
- Green or yellow discharge (pus) from the wound
- If they feel unwell, feverish or have a temperature.

If any of these symptoms occur, the patient should contact their GP.

Bowels

The patient may find that their bowel habit is altered in the days following surgery. There are several potential reasons for this, including the constipating effects of some analgesics and diarrhoea caused by antibiotic use. Encouraging a healthy balanced diet with plenty of fruit and vegetables and ensuring a good fluid intake will encourage bowel action. It must be stressed to the patient that they should not discontinue the antibiotics except on medical advice.

Dressing and Bathing

The advice given on discharge will depend on the preoperative ability of the patient and the extent to which the operation has affected this ability. Referrals may be made to Social Services (Social Care Services) and occupational therapy, to ensure that the patient has appropriate equipment and support. In the days following surgery (and definitely while clips or sutures are in place), the wound may be exposed to water (such as a shower) but prolonged immersion (such as a bath) should be avoided.

Driving

Generally, patients should not drive for 7–10 days after an operation. While driving is not illegal, the patient's insurance may not be valid and if the patient intends to drive, then they should be encouraged to contact their insurer. After some operations, there may be medical advice not to drive for longer than 10 days; the patient will be advised of this by their surgical team. If the patient still cannot drive 3 months after surgery, then they are required to inform the Driver and Vehicle Licensing Agency (DVLA).

Drugs

The patient must be given verbal and written instructions on any drugs they are to take home. Any changes to the drugs the patient used to take before the operation should be discussed and patient understanding checked.

Exercise

Specific exercises may be prescribed after surgery and these will be taught to the patient by the physiotherapy staff. The patient should be informed that it is essential that they mobilise regularly to avoid complications and aid recovery. Patients can slowly increase daily exercise until they have returned to normal levels.

Rest and Fatigue

The period after surgery often involves episodes of fatigue and this will vary from patient to patient. The patient should be informed that this is normal and that they may need to take afternoon naps for a week or so.

Sexuality

Many patients will wish to know when they can resume sexual activities. It is difficult to give definite timescales and the patient is often the best judge of this. For menstruating patients, there may be the need to discuss appropriate timescales to resume taking the contraceptive pill if this is their choice.

Work

Returning to work will depend on the nature of the surgery and the nature of the work. Patients should be issued with a certificate for the period of their hospital stay and advised to see their GP for a medical note if required.

Wound Care

An appointment must be made to have sutures or clips removed by the community nurses or GP practice nurse.

The appearance of the wound will vary as healing takes place. It will start out red and swollen (densely black in the skin of patients of Afro-Caribbean heritage) and gradually become flat and silvery white (or black). This process may take up to 2 years. Sensations around the wound site will be altered due to the trauma of the incision. Pain and soreness will be related to the incision but also due to bruising and the inflammatory process. Wounds may become itchy but patients should be discouraged from scratching. If the itching must be relieved, then patients are best advised to 'slap' the wound rather than scratch it.

The best results for a scar may be achieved by lightly moisturising the wound but this must not start until 24 hours after any sutures or clips are removed and the wound edges are healed. After a few weeks, thicker creams may be applied and the wound gently massaged to discourage adhesions and to encourage a flatter scar. If the scar is to be exposed to sunlight, then it is best to apply sunblock to the scar for the first year after operation.

Overgrowth of the scar occasionally occurs, which leads to a raised itchy scar (a keloid). The chest and shoulders are the areas that seem to be most at risk of keloid development and they also seem to be more common in patients of Afro-Caribbean heritage. The only treatment option for a keloid scar (if the patient wishes) is referral to a plastic surgeon.

Day-case Surgery

Day-case surgery is becoming increasingly common and the types of operations undertaken as day cases are expanding rapidly. However, the choice of patients for day-case surgery is not just based on the type of operation to be undertaken. Traditionally, only ASA grade I or II patients were considered for day-case surgery but now ASA grade III patients are being treated as day cases so long as their disease processes are well controlled (Solodkyy et al., 2018).

Day-case patients must be able to meet the following social criteria.

- A responsible adult must be available to stay with the patient for 24–48 hours after surgery.
- An escort must be available for the journey home.
- Travel on public transport is not acceptable and so the patient must have access to private transport or a taxi.
- There must be access to a private telephone.
- The journey home must not take more than 1–1.5 hours.

For a patient to be discharged from a day surgery unit, the following criteria must be met.

- Conscious level must be the same as the preoperative level.
- Cardiovascular and respiratory status should be stable.

233

- The patient must have passed urine and be in reasonable fluid balance.
- Pain, nausea and vomiting must be minimal and controlled.
- Bleeding should be minimal.
- Mobility should be at the preoperative level.

Conclusion

This chapter has discussed the role of the surgical nurse in the patient's journey. It has reviewed the preoperative and postoperative periods, discussing the role of the nurse. The primary role of the nurse in a patient's surgical journey is to maintain safety through information giving, appropriate assessment and intervention. While different surgical procedures carry their own individual risks and complications, there are a number of risks and complications common to all operations.

Key Points

- The effect of surgery on patients is not restricted to the physical.
- Preoperative teaching is vital to both patient safety and patient satisfaction.
- Preoperative checklists are an essential tool in ensuring patient safety.
- Collecting patients from the recovery area involves a complete handover and patients should not be transferred unless the nurse is sure it is safe to do so.
- Immediately on return to the ward, the nurse should undertake a complete assessment of the patient including vital signs.
- The trends of vital signs are just as important as any single result and are often more useful to the nurse.
- Mobilising patients early after surgery has the potential to reduce the incidence of several postoperative complications.

References

Aronow, W.S. (2017) Management of hypertension in patients undergoing surgery. *Annals of Translational Medicine*, 5(10), 227.

Bircher, A. & Chowdhury, A. (2020) Current DVT prophylaxis: a review. *Orthopaedics and Trauma*, 34(3), 161–167.

Celik, F. & Edipoglu, I.S. (2018) Evaluation of preoperative anxiety and fear of anesthesia using APAIS score. *European Journal of Medical Research*, 23(1), 1–10.

Clement, K.D., Luhmann, A., Wilson, M.S. & Patil, P. (2018) Current standards for assessing pregnancy status before surgery are subjective and should be replaced with definitive, objective evidence. *Scottish Medical Journal*, 63(2), 60–62.

Ertürk, E.B. & Ünlü, H. (2018) Effects of pre-operative individualized education on anxiety and pain severity in patients following open-heart surgery. *International Journal of Health Sciences*, 12(4), 26.

Famiglietti, A., Memoli, J.W. & Khaitan, P.G. (2021) Are electronic cigarettes and vaping effective tools for smoking cessation? Limited evidence on surgical outcomes: a narrative review. *Journal of Thoracic Disease*, 13(1), 384.

Fish, J. (2010) Promoting equality and valuing diversity for lesbian, gay, bisexual and trans patients. *InnovAiT*, 3(6), 333–338.

Frame-Peterson, L.A., Megill, R.D., Carobrese, S. & Schweitzer, M. (2017) Nutrient deficiencies are common prior to bariatric surgery. *Nutrition in Clinical Practice*, 32(4), 463–469.

Gan, T.J., Belani, K.G., Bergese, S., et al. (2019) Fourth consensus guidelines for the management of postoperative nausea and vomiting. *Anesthesia & Analgesia*, 131(2), 411–448.

Grass, J.A. (2005) Patient-controlled analgesia. *Anesthesia and Analgesia*, 101(55), S44–S61.

Helgesen, A. K., Adan, Y. H., Dybvik Bjørglund, C., et al. (2021) Nurses' experiences of delirium and how to identify delirium – a qualitative study. *Nursing Open*, 8(2), 844–849.

Hobson, D.B., Chang, T.Y., Aboagye, J.K., et al. (2017) Prevalence of graduated compression stocking–associated pressure injuries in surgical intensive care units. *Journal of Critical Care*, 40, 1–6.

Hoffmann, H. & Kettelhack, C. (2012) Fast-track surgery: conditions and challenges in postsurgical treatment. A review of elements of translational research in enhanced recovery after surgery. *European Surgical Research*, 49(1), 24–34.

Kehlet, H. & Wilmore, D.W. (2008) Evidence based surgical care and the evolution of fast track surgery. *Annals of Surgery*, 248(2), 189–198.

King, E. (2019) Preoperative fasting durations for adult elective surgical patients: convenient for the professional, but detrimental to the patient? A narrative review. *Journal of Perioperative Practice*, 29(12), 393–397.

King, L.A. & Hothi, S.S. (2020) Remodelling elective hospital services in the COVID-19 era – designing the new normal. *Future Healthcare Journal*, 7(3), e60.

Kühlmann, A.Y.R., de Rooij, A., Kroese, L.F., van Dijk, M., Hunink, M.G.M. & Jeekel, J. (2018) Meta-analysis evaluating music interventions for anxiety and pain in surgery. *Journal of British Surgery*, 105(7), 773–783.

Lin, S.Y., Huang, H.A., Lin, S.C., Huang, Y.T., Wang, K.Y. & Shi, H.Y. (2016) The effect of an anaesthetic patient information video on perioperative anxiety: a randomised study. *European Journal of Anaesthesiology*, 33(2), 134–139.

Macmillan, P.J. (2021). COVID-19: no visitors. *Journal of Palliative Medicine*, 24, 1404–1405.

Mayhew, D., Mendonca, V. & Murthy, B.V.S. (2019) A review of ASA physical status – historical perspectives and modern developments. *Anaesthesia*, 74(3), 373–379.

Merchant, R.N., Chima, N., Ljungqvist, O. & Kok, J.N.J. (2020) Preoperative fasting practices across three anesthesia societies: survey of practitioners. *JMIR Perioperative Medicine*, 3(1), e15905.

Mitchell, M. (2017) Day surgery nurses' selection of patient preoperative information. *Journal of Clinical Nursing*, 26(1-2), 225–237.

Mulkey, N. (2020). Pronouns and advocacy in medicine. *AMA Journal of Ethics*, 22(3), 255–259.

Myles, P.S., Andrews, S., Nicholson, J., Lobo, D.N. & Mythen, M. (2017) Contemporary approaches to perioperative IV fluid therapy. *World Journal of Surgery*, 41(10), 2457–2463.

NHS Inform (2018) *Breathing exercise for stress*. www.nhs.uk/mental-health/self-help/guides-tools-and-activities/breathing-exercises-for-stress/ (accessed December 2021).

NICE (2016) *Routine preoperative tests for elective surgery*. CG45. National Institute for Care Excellence, London.

NICE (2019) *Venous thromboembolism in over 16s: reducing the risk of hospital-acquired deep vein thrombosis or pulmonary embolism*. CG89. National Institute for Health and Care Excellence, London.

NICE (2020a) *Perioperative care in adults*. CG180. National Institute for Health and Care Excellence, London.

NICE (2020b) *Surgical site infections: prevention and treatment*. CG125. National Institute for Health and Care Excellence, London.

Niu, S., Li, J., Zhao, Y., Ding, D., Jiang, G. & Song, Z. (2021) Preoperative deep venous thrombosis (DVT) after femoral neck fracture in the elderly, the incidence, timing, location and related risk factors. *BMC Musculoskeletal Disorders*, 22(1), 1–9.

Nolan, M.B., Martin, D.P., Thompson, R., Schroeder, D.R., Hanson, A.C. & Warner, D.O. (2017) Association between smoking status, preoperative exhaled carbon monoxide levels, and postoperative surgical site infection in patients undergoing elective surgery. *JAMA Surgery*, 152(5), 476–483.

Nordfalk, J.M., Gulbrandsen, P., Gerwing, J., Nylenna, M. & Menichetti, J. (2019) Development of a measurement system for complex oral information transfer in medical consultations. *BMC Medical Research Methodology*, 19(1), 1–9.

Nursing & Midwifery Council (NMC) (2018a) *Future Nurse: Standards of Proficiency for Future Nurses*. NMC, London.

Nursing & Midwifery Council (NMC) (2018b) *Standards of Proficiency for Nursing Associates*. NMC, London.

Omar, I., Graham, Y., Singhal, R., Wilson, M., Madhok, B. & Mahawar, K.K. (2021) Identification of common themes from never events data published by NHS England. *World Journal of Surgery*, 45(3), 697–704.

Royal College of Physicians (2017) *National Early Warning Score (NEWS) 2: Standardising the Assessment of Acute-illness Severity in the NHS*. Royal College of Physicians, London.

Skryabina, E.A. & Dunn, T.S. (2006) Disposable infusion pumps. *American Journal of Health-System Pharmacy*, 63(13), 1260–1268.

Solodkyy, A., Hakeem, A.R., Oswald, N., di Franco, F., Gergely, S. & Harris, A.M. (2018) 'True day case' laparoscopic cholecystectomy in a high-volume specialist unit and review of factors contributing to unexpected overnight stay. *Minimally Invasive Surgery*, 2018, 1260358.

Van Decar, L., Conover, Z. & Misra, L. (2019) Effective communication in the pre-operative environment. *International Journal of Otolaryngology and Head & Neck Surgery*, 9(01), 1.

Webster, J. & Osborne, S. (2015) Preoperative bathing or showering with skin antiseptics to prevent surgical site infection. *Cochrane Database of Systematic Reviews*, 2, CD004985.

Wong, J.L.C., Ho, C.W.Y., Scott, G., Machin, J.T., Briggs, T.W.R. & National Surgical Site Infection Audit Collaborators (2019) Getting It Right First Time: the national survey of surgical site infection rates in NHS trusts in England. *Annals of the Royal College of Surgeons of England*, 101(7), 463–471.

Yentis, S.M., Hartle, A.J., Barker, I.R., *et al.* (2017) AAGBI: consent for anaesthesia 2017. *Anaesthesia*, 72(1), 93–105.

Zemła, A.J., Nowicka-Sauer, K., Jarmoszewicz, K., Wera, K., Batkiewicz, S. & Pietrzykowska, M. (2019) Measures of preoperative anxiety. *Anaesthesiology Intensive Therapy*, 51(1), 64–69. content, perms

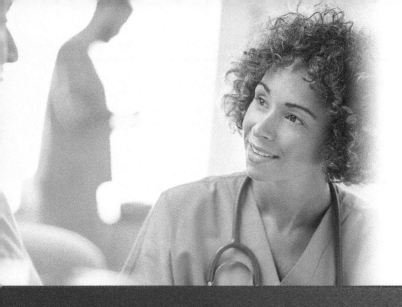

15

The Principles of Cancer Care

Alison Simons and Samantha Toland

Birmingham City University, UK

Learning Outcomes

On completion of this chapter you will be able to:

- **Describe how cancer develops and spreads throughout the body (Platform 1)**
- **Recognise the impact of individual lifestyle choices on the development of cancers (Platforms 1 and 2)**
- **Outline the investigative procedures used to diagnose cancer (Platforms 3–6)**
- **Explain the evidence-based options used to treat cancers, care for a patient living with cancer and end-of life-care (Platforms 3–6)**
- **Explore the holistic support available for people with cancer (Platforms 3–6)**

Proficiencies

NMC Proficiencies and Standards:

- **Evidence-based, best practice approaches to communication for supporting people of all ages, their families and carers in preventing ill health and in managing their care.**
- **Share information and check understanding about the causes, implications and treatment of a range of common health conditions including cancer.**

 Visit the companion website at **www.wiley.com/go/peate/nursingpractice3e** where you can test yourself using flashcards, multiple-choice questions and more.

Nursing Practice: Knowledge and Care, Third Edition. Edited by Ian Peate and Aby Mitchell.
© 2022 John Wiley & Sons Ltd. Published 2022 by John Wiley & Sons Ltd.
Companion website: www.wiley.com/go/peate/nursingpractice3e

Introduction

Cancer is a term used to cover over 200 different diseases. Various cancers have many similarities and evoke similar responses in people, therefore this chapter will take an overview approach to cancer. Cancer is still often perceived as a fatal illness and people dread receiving a cancer diagnosis; however, with the use of combination therapies and newer targeted treatments, and improved survival rates, cancer is increasingly being conceived as a long-term condition, as half of people diagnosed with cancer in the UK live for 10 years or more (Cancer Research UK, 2021a). It is largely a disease of 'older' age; more than a third of all cancers are diagnosed in those 75 years and over (ONS, 2017) and the reasons for this will be explored later. However, younger people can develop cancer: for example, children may develop leukaemia (cancer of the blood cells) and young adults may develop melanoma (skin cancers). However, these age groups only represent 1% of all cancer cases.

Developments in the field are ongoing. As a result of this, the nurse must keep up to date, ensuring that care provision is contemporary and evidence based.

Factors that Increase the Risk of Developing Cancer

Smoking

The link between tobacco and cancer was first made in 1761. The evidence is now indisputable and one in four cancer deaths in the UK occur in smokers. While lung cancer is the most common cancer associated with smoking, people who smoke could develop other cancers such as oral, oesophageal, stomach, pancreatic, liver, kidney, bowel, ovarian, bladder, cervical or leukaemia.

Obesity

Scientists have sought to find a link between what we eat and the potential to develop cancer, obesity being the second highest cause of cancer. Colorectal cancers are associated with a diet lacking in fibre and high in animal fats, red meat and processed meat. Obesity combined with a sedentary lifestyle seems a predictive factor for other cancers such as breast and renal cancers. People keeping a healthy weight could prevent around 22 800 cases of cancer every year in the UK (Cancer Research UK, 2021b).

Case Study

- David is a 35-year-old man.
- He a long-distance lorry driver.
- His BMI is 30 kg/m².
- David enjoys a full English breakfast most mornings.
- He eats take-away food twice a week.
- He doesn't like many different fruits or vegetables.
- He prefers red meat to white.
- David adds salt to most of his food.
- He takes no exercise and his physical activity is minimal.

Consider:
- What type(s) of cancer may he be at risk of developing?
- What diet and lifestyle risk factors does he have?
- What potential changes might you discuss with David?

Alcohol

Drinking alcohol increases the risk of mouth, throat, oesophageal, stomach, liver, bowel and breast cancers. While a small glass of red wine (1.6 units) a day may reduce the incidence of heart disease, it could also pose a risk of developing cancer. Drinking alcohol and being a smoker also further increases the risk of developing this disease.

Infections

Certain infections are associated with a greater risk of developing cancer, including human papillomavirus (HPV), Epstein–Barr virus (EBV) and *Helicobacter pylori*. Strategies are in place to help reduce the risk of infection-linked cancers. For example, as HPV is implicated in cervical cancers, children are now vaccinated at 11–13 years of age to protect them from developing this infection and hence reduce their risk of developing cancers linked to HPV infection such as cervical cancer.

Jot This Down

Can you think of any occupations that could put the person more at risk of developing cancer? What risks do the following workers face that make them potentially liable to develop cancer?
- Builders
- Farmers
- Healthcare workers

Occupational Risks

Some chemical agents have been linked to increasing a person's risk to cancer, for example asbestos, pesticides, diesel engine exhaust, silica, radiation and hazardous drugs. Working in the sun can also increase the risk of skin cancer. Health and safety legislation is in place to protect workers from hazardous substances at work. Employers must prevent or reduce the risk of occupational exposure to these hazardous substances.

Pathophysiology

The cell is the basic unit from which the body develops. The first embryonic cells divide and develop specific functions. They differentiate and become cells of a specific system (e.g. circulatory, nervous, immune). These cells then further differentiate to become specific cell types (e.g. mucosal, myocardial, neuronal). These very specific cells take on different roles within the body, develop at different rates, secrete different enzymes and chemicals, and function in their own unique way.

Cancer starts in a single cell, arising from a mutation that then leads to the development of further cell mutations and overproliferation of cells that form a growth referred to as a tumour or cancer. The many different cancers exist because different cells become cancerous; for example, carcinomas are growths arising from epithelial cells and sarcomas are cancers arising from supporting tissue cells such as bone, muscle and cartilage. Lymphomas are cancers of the lymphocyte cells and leukaemias are cancers of the cells in the blood, usually white blood cells. Cancers are further classified according to the tissue in which they are growing – an osteosarcoma is growing in bone and an adenocarcinoma is growing in a gland.

Cell Division and Replication

Each cell in the body has a determined lifespan. For some cells, such as those that line the mouth, the lifespan is short while others, such as those that make up bone, have a much longer lifespan. Cancers in slow-growing cells develop at a slower rate; however, in a rapidly changing tissue, the cancer may be quite aggressive and this will also affect the rate at which the cancer spreads through the body. Whether the cell is slow growing or fast growing, the cycle through which the cell proceeds remains the same (Figure 15.1).

The starting point is G_0, where the cell is in resting phase, and it is functioning but not dividing. Chemicals signal to the cell nucleus the need to replicate. Under this influence, changes occur within the cell and it moves from the G_0 to the G_1 phase, where the cell prepares for division. There is a checkpoint at the end of the G_1 phase where enzymes, called *kinases*, check that the preparation is in order and, if all is well, the cell proceeds to the next phase, called *S phase*; however, if all is not in order, DNA repair or apoptosis (cell death) is triggered by a protein called p53.

In S phase the cell prepares for replication and DNA in the cell doubles. An enzyme called *helicase* causes the DNA helix to unwind and separate into two strands. This allows the process of DNA replication to take place. The next phase is the final growth and preparation phase called G_2. There is a second checkpoint between the G_2 and M phase, where DNA is checked for damage, repair takes place if required, or if the DNA damage is beyond repair, apoptosis (cell death) is triggered. Again, p53 is involved in this process. The gene that codes for the p53 protein can be mutated or absent in some cancers.

Normal cells replace themselves at regular intervals; once maturity is reached, the cell is instructed to divide; once it has replicated, the old cell is instructed to die.

Cancer cells develop when normal cell growth is unregulated. The reason for this may be unknown, or can be due to the effects of ageing, which is why most cancers develop in older people, or as a result of exposure to agents which cause the cells to mutate. Some agents are initiators, i.e. exposure to them causes cancer, such as some viruses. Other substances are promoters, and prolonged exposure is required before cancer develops, i.e. nicotine and UV light. For example, smoking can cause damage to the squamous epithelial cells lining the bronchus after repeated exposure to cigarette smoke. UV light exposure can cause sunburn and damages cells in the skin, resulting in skin cancers.

Some cancers can be prevented and education of the public to engage in healthier lifestyles could improve health and reduce the risk of developing cancer. The Public Health England Cancer Board (2017–21) published a plan, identifying a work stream on cancer prevention and public health. Its ambition was to significantly reduce the 40% of preventable cancers caused by lifestyle, behavioural, environmental and chemical exposure through increased public awareness, and by providing the evidence to influence policy and support local decision making.

Some of the ways in which it planned to do this was by:

- Reducing smoking
- Addressing obesity
- Promoting the findings of the Alcohol Evidence review (PHE, 2016)
- Continuing to deliver Be Clear on Cancer campaigns
- Rolling out new bowel cancer screening
- Examining inequalities in screening programmes.

In 2018 a report on the PHE's progress towards these objectives was published (PHE, 2018). This update stated that the recommendation requirements were met and further work was continuing. No further review or updates have yet been published.

Some cancers are discovered through screening programmes, where a risk is known and measures can be taken to discover the cancer in its early stages. The UK currently has three national cancer screening programmes (NHS, 2021).

- *Cervical cancer*: women, trans men, trans women and non-binary people registered with their GP as female and aged between 26–49 are invited every 3 years to attend screening, and every 5 years when aged between 50–64. Trans men, trans women and non-binary people registered with their GP as male will not receive automatic invitations but can still have cervical screening on request.
- *Breast cancer*: women, trans men, trans women and non-binary people registered with their GP as female and aged 50–70 are invited every 3 years to attend for breast screening.

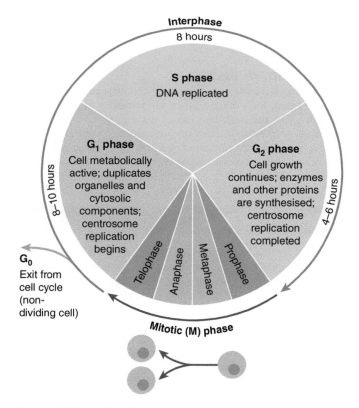

Figure 15.1 The cell cycle.

Trans women, trans men and non-binary people registered with their GP as male can still have breast screening on request. Trials in women aged 47–73 years are currently ongoing.

- *Bowel cancer*: in England people aged 60–74 are offered a home test kit every 2 years.

The Nursing Associate Platform 2 Promoting health and preventing ill health

A Explain why cancer screening is important in terms of promoting health and preventing ill health. Identify those who are eligible for screening and why.

Signs and Symptoms

It is impossible to describe all the signs and symptoms of cancer that people may experience. However, for solid tumors an unexplained lump may be the first indication that something is wrong; for example, if a lump in the breast tissue is discovered this may drive a person to seek medical opinion. People who have an unexplained lump anywhere in the body should seek advice from a healthcare professional.

Changes in bowel habit could indicate colorectal cancers, especially if accompanied by bleeding. Abnormal bleeding and discharge is also an indicator that help should be sought from a healthcare professional as soon as possible.

However, some cancers are difficult to detect until the disease is quite advanced.

Weight Loss

Unexplained weight loss is a key symptom; this may be due to several reasons.

- Lack of appetite
- Nausea
- Difficulty chewing or swallowing
- Tumour mass pressing on stomach or bowel
- Cachexia

Care, Dignity and Compassion

A person may initially welcome a degree of weight loss, but it can soon become apparent that all is not well and that they are looking gaunt. Some people will stop visitors coming to see them and deprive themselves of their company because they do not want to shock friends and family. Helping the person to disguise weight loss by the use of scarves, wearing high-neck clothing and ensuring that their hair is brushed and looking attractive can detract from the gaunt appearance.

Cachexia is the loss of fat and muscle due to the increased demands of the underlying cancer, and develops from altered metabolism within the cells. Cancer cells require amino acids obtained from proteins to grow and develop and obtain these through the breakdown of skeletal muscle. This leads to a raised insulin and sugar level which depresses the appetite.

It is believed that some people may die from muscle wasting as the cachexia depletes muscle from the heart and the intercostal muscles, making respiration difficult.

Various interventions are available to help people eat more, such as promoting a diet with high-protein food and/or nutritional supplements, and the use of anti-inflammatory drugs and appetite stimulants. A holistic approach considering physical, social, cultural and emotional aspects of cachexia should be taken.

Pain

Pain is a feared symptom associated with cancer. However, it is a symptom that may drive people to seek healthcare advice. The heightened stress that accompanies a cancer diagnosis can intensify the pain. Pain also arises physically as the cancer grows and infiltrates nerves or presses on nociceptors (nerve endings that sense pain). Velly (2018) explains that there is a relationship between depression and anxiety and chronic pain. Thus, pain has psychological and physical dimensions.

Cancer pain is complex because it is multidimensional, and cancer treatments can cause pain syndromes (Brant, 2014).

Some people still think of cancer as a fatal illness rather than a chronic illness, so a cancer diagnosis may lead them to question their mortality. This may cause spiritual angst, increasing pain, as spirituality and personal belief can affect perceptions about pain.

Pain is an individual experience that has physical, psychological and spiritual aspects. Therefore, to ensure effective pain management, a holistic approach must be adopted to include these features of pain.

Investigations and Diagnosis

The National Institute for Health and Care Excellence (NICE) (2015) states that over 300 000 new cancer cases are diagnosed each year (NICE have updated this guidance in 2021). The advice to GPs is that if there is a 3–5% chance of the person's symptoms being caused by cancer, they should have urgent direct access to investigations. For most cancers, the person should be seen by a cancer specialist within 2 weeks (NICE, 2015).

The *NHS Long Term Plan* (NHS, 2019) aimed to save thousands more lives each year by dramatically improving how cancer is diagnosed and treated. In terms of diagnostic strategies, this plan stated that:

- The age for bowel screening would be lowered
- New forms of cervical cancer screening and extended lung health checks would be introduced
- Rapid diagnostic centres would be set up across the country so patients displaying symptoms of cancer can be assessed and diagnosed in as little as a day
- Faster diagnosis standards would be introduced, which would ensure that patients receive a definitive diagnosis or ruling out of cancer within 28 days
- Access to more effective tests and treatments, from genomic testing to proton beam therapy, would be improved, to help find more cancers before symptoms appear.

In 2020 the key milestones were summarised (NHS, 2020). Due to the coronavirus pandemic, there was a reduction in the number of people coming forward to have their symptoms checked. However, 95% of those who were urgently referred were seen within 31 days. Working with PHE, subsequent campaigns have been launched to address the barriers deterring patients from accessing the NHS. The spending review has committed £325 million to fund and support diagnostics to help speed up the diagnostic pathway and improve patient outcomes.

The most important part of assessment is the patient history and their reason for seeking medical help. This is followed by a physical examination, as some cancer tumours can be palpated and felt. Cancers can be seen via:

- *Bronchoscopy*: to detect cancer in the lung
- *Cystoscopy*: to detect cancers in the bladder
- *Endoscopy*: to detect cancer in the oesophagus and stomach
- *Sigmoidoscopy*: to detect colorectal cancers.

However, cancers can grow in areas that are difficult to palpate and are not so obvious, necessitating further investigation.

Diagnostic investigations can identify the site and give an indication of the size of the cancer. Depending on the type of cancer suspected, this will include a range of imaging procedures such as:

- Computed tomography (CT)
- Magnetic resonance imaging (MRI)
- Positron emission tomography (PET)
- PET-CT scan
- Ultrasonography
- Bone scan
- Endoscopy
- Colonoscopy
- X-rays.

Biological samples can also assist in the diagnostic work-up.

- *Tissue Biopsy*: tissue samples taken from the suspected tumour and examined using an electron microscope to identify any abnormal cells and the cell of origin that has mutated.
- *Cytological screening*: viewing a sample of cells using an electron microscope which will determine the morphological features of the cells, i.e. their size, shape and degree to which they have changed.
- *Blood samples* can be viewed for the presence of tumour markers; for example, prostate-specific antigen (PSA) levels can be raised in prostate cancer and would need further investigations.

Nursing Care While the Person Is Undergoing Investigations

People undergoing investigations for cancer may be frightened and require psychological support. It is important that they are not given false reassurance, as this can lead to a lack of trust in healthcare staff.

It is not possible to have all the answers and you may not have sufficient knowledge to deal with patient's queries. It is important that this is explained to the patient and referral to others is made to meet the patient's needs.

Treatment of Cancer

There are now numerous options to treat cancer. Surgery, radiotherapy and chemotherapy are the main treatments. More recently, the use of biological and immunotherapy has been introduced. The stage of a cancer will determine the choice of treatment.

Decisions on the Course of Treatment

Staging of solid cancers is most commonly determined using the **TNM** (tumour, node, metastasis) system.

Tumour Size (T)

Primary tumours are graded using the letter T.

- T1, T2, T3, T4: refers to the size and/or extent of the main tumour. The higher the number after the T, the larger the tumour or the more it has grown into nearby tissues. T's may be further divided to provide more detail, such as T3a and T3b.
- Tx: tumour cannot be assessed.
- Tis: carcinoma *in situ*.
- T0: no evidence of tumour.

Node (N)

This refers to the lymph nodes near the site of the cancer. Cancer spreads through the lymphatic and blood system and can seed in adjacent nodes.

- Nx: lymph nodes cannot be assessed.
- N0: no nodal involvement, suggesting the cancer is still relatively new and contained within the tissue where it is found.
- N1: one node near the cancer site has been altered.
- N2: more nodes are involved.
- N3: nodes distant to the tumour are involved.

Metastasis (M)

This refers to the presence and number of different sites to which the cancer has metastasised.

- Mx: metastasis cannot be assessed.
- M0: no distant metastasis.
- M1: metastasis to other parts of the body/organs.

If the person's cancer is graded as T1N0M0, then it is in its early stages and may be easily removed by surgery. Surgery could be followed up with either chemotherapy or radiotherapy, to ensure all the cancer is eradicated. If the person's cancer is graded T3N3M3, it is advanced and may be beyond removal by surgery. In this case, surgery might be used to provide symptom relief by removing obstructions or to insert a stent to keep an opening patent. It may be possible to slow tumour growth using chemotherapy or radiotherapy, but the prospects of curing the person are not realistic. Treatment is 'palliative' and focuses on controlling symptoms and keeping the person comfortable.

Treatment decisions are made at multidisciplinary team (MDT) meetings, where a group of healthcare professionals meet and discuss each individual case.

> **The Nursing Associate** Platform 4 Working in teams
>
> List the healthcare professionals you would expect to attend an MDT meeting for a person with a cancer diagnosis and note their roles and scope of practice. Consider your role within this MDT.

Surgery

Surgical procedures are used to diagnose and stage 90% of all cancers, and to treat 60% of cancers. As a primary treatment, the aim is to remove the whole cancer if possible, with a clear margin of unaffected tissue around it. Adjacent lymph nodes are removed, especially if there is lymph node involvement.

Surgical intervention is not without risk or implications. Surgery results in physical changes to the body; sometimes this is visible, such as removal of a breast or formation of a colostomy/ileostomy. Removal of the lymph nodes may result in the person developing a lymphoedematous limb, which is clearly visible and extremely uncomfortable. Alterations of the body may affect a person's self-image whether or not they are visible.

Nerve plexuses can be damaged, resulting in altered functioning of the body; for example, a man may be left with erectile dysfunction or incontinence following prostatectomy.

Surgical procedures are also used for:

- Bypassing an obstruction
- Reconstructing the body to improve body image, as in breast cancer
- Debulking a tumour so that it does not press on other organs
- Relieving pain
- Palliative measures, as when a stent is inserted to keep the oesophagus open.

Nursing Care for the Person Prior to Having Surgery

Surgery may be the first step of a person's treatment for cancer; they may go on to have radiotherapy and/or systemic anticancer treatments, or they may undergo surgery after radiotherapy and/or systemic anticancer treatment.

Nursing care requires preparing a person for surgery, offering support, advice and information so they know what to expect from the surgery and the care they will have to take following surgery.

Care, Dignity and Compassion

Compassionate care is essential. The person will need to make informed choices at a time when they are feeling vulnerable, and this needs to be respected and time allowed for them to process the information in order to make choices about their care.

Systemic Anticancer Treatment (SACT)

The umbrella term 'systemic anticancer treatment' (SACT) is used to describe all types of pharmacological treatments for cancer, including chemotherapy, biological treatments and immunotherapies. Some of these drugs can be used for non-cancer patients and are effective in treating rheumatoid arthritis, Crohn's disease and renal vasculitis, for example, and some have also been used to terminate ectopic pregnancies. This chapter focuses on the use of these drugs in cancer, where generally much higher doses are used and therefore there is a potential for more severe side-effects.

Chemotherapy

Chemotherapy drugs are usually 'cytotoxic' agents, i.e. they kill cells, attacking both normal and diseased cells – hence the development of significant side-effects. They work by interfering in the process of cell replication, which is why it is important to understand the role of the cell cycle in cancer development. Some agents work in a particular phase of the cell cycle, so are termed 'phase specific', while others act throughout the entire cell cycle of replication and are 'non-phase specific'; however, some cells that are not replicating, including some cancer cells, can be unaffected.

Therefore, to target as many cells as possible, a combination of several chemotherapy agents is used together to obtain the greatest 'cell kill'. However, as the agents target both normal and diseased cells, a balance has to be achieved, so chemotherapy agents are usually given in cycles timed to allow normal cells to recover (about 3 weeks). Cancer cells have a longer recovery time. Chemotherapy is usually used in conjunction with surgery and/or radiotherapy; it is not universally effective against all cancers but can be significantly effective in curing some blood cancers such as leukaemia.

Several cycles are needed, as there is a percentage of cells that escape the effect of the chemotherapy because they were not at the responsive stage in their process of replication.

The cancers that respond best to chemotherapy are:

- Acute lymphoblastic leukaemia (ALL) in children
- Acute myeloid leukaemia (AML)
- Hodgkin lymphoma
- Germ cell testicular cancers
- Choriocarcinoma
- Ovarian cancer
- Wilms tumour
- Embryonal rhabdomyosarcoma
- Ewing sarcoma.

How Chemotherapy Agents Work

Chemotherapy agents (there are over 50 different ones) are grouped together according to their chemical structure or the way that they work. The main groups are as follows.

Alkylating Agents The first chemotherapy agents to be used, alkylating agents were developed from nitrogen mustard. They cause cross-links within DNA molecules, resulting in mutations of the genetic information. This stops the DNA helix unwinding so cell replication cannot take place. They are considered to be non-phase specific as they cause mutation of the DNA and can work during any phase of the cell cycle.

Some examples are:

- Chlorambucil
- Cyclophosphamide
- Melphalan.

These drugs are used mainly for people with leukaemias, lymphomas or solid tumours.

Platinum Agents Platinum agents are very similar to alkylating agents in that they affect the cross-linking of DNA and these two groups of drugs are often linked together into one category. These drugs contain platinum and examples include:

- Carboplatin
- Cisplatin.

Antimetabolites Antimetabolites starve the cell of the building blocks required to manufacture DNA (bases). This ensures that DNA cannot repair itself when damaged and breaks the cross-links in the DNA helix irreversibly – these drugs are considered to be cell cycle phase specific as once a cell has passed through the DNA synthesis phase, they are ineffective. Examples of antimetabolites are:

- Capecitabine
- Gemcitabine
- 5-Fluorouracil (5-FU).

Antimetabolites are used to treat breast, colorectal, haematological (blood) and pancreatic cancers.

Cytotoxic Antibiotics Mainly produced from the *Streptomyces* species of bacteria, these have antibiotic properties but are obviously too toxic to be used as antibacterial drugs. Generally, they bind to DNA, preventing transcription into mRNA, and subsequently prevent replication. Some of these drugs (anthracyclines, e.g. doxorubicin, epirubicin) also inhibit the action of topoisomerase II (an enzyme that helps in the unravelling of the DNA helix and is essential for DNA repair), resulting in cell death (apoptosis). These drugs are considered to be cell cycle nonphase specific.

Examples of cytotoxic antibiotics are:

- Doxorubicin
- Epirubicin
- Bleomycin.

Cytotoxic Plant Alkaloids/Mitotic Inhibitors These drugs are extracted from plant material which now have synthetic derivatives. Mitotic inhibitors affect the microtubules inside the cells; this affects the division of chromosomes, particularly the spindles that pull the chromosomes apart. Mitotic inhibitors infiltrate these tubules, preventing the chromosomes from being drawn to opposite poles of the cell, and thus interrupting mitosis. They are cell cycle phase specific as they only affect cells moving through the mitotic phase of division. Examples include:

- Vinca alkaloids, such as vincristine and vinblastine, from the periwinkle (*Vinca*) plant
- Taxanes, such as paclitaxel and docetaxel, from the bark of the yew
- Camptothecin analogues, such as irinotecan, from the Asian 'happy tree'.

Resistance to Chemotherapy

The tumour can develop resistance to treatment, as it produces cytokines which block the action of the chemotherapy agent; measurement of tumour markers along with scans can indicate whether or not the cancer is responding to the treatment. The solution to the problem of resistance is to use a combination of drugs.

Combination Therapies

Chemotherapy treatment originally used single agents but people can develop resistance to a single agent in a similar way to antibiotic therapy. The only way to achieve a higher rate of tumour cell kill in this case would be to increase the dose and hence increase the risk of greater toxicity/side-effects. However, mixing several agents that work differently allows for more aggressive treatment, which results in a greater 'cell kill', because each can be used to the maximum level without the same toxic effect that occurs if used singly. Cancer cells are less likely to develop resistance to this combined assault. Research has determined which combinations are most effective; the mix includes phase-specific and non-phase-specific agents.

Within the combination, other drugs that are not specifically chemotherapy agents but which improve their action can also be given. Combination therapies are usually known by their acronyms, which usually derive from the first letter of each drug used, for example FEC, which includes fluorouracil, epirubicin and cyclophosphamide to treat breast cancer.

Side-effects of Chemotherapy

As with any drug, allergic reactions can occur both during and after administration. A number of chemotherapy drugs have a higher tendency for this to happen, therefore patients are closely monitored for and informed of any reactions that may take place.

The main side-effects of chemotherapy are associated with the mechanism of action of the drugs, i.e. destruction of replicating cells. Therefore, any cell types that have a fast turnover and replication of cells are most significantly affected – these include mucous membranes, hair follicles and cells involved in blood production within the bone marrow.

Most people know of the side-effects of chemotherapy, sometimes making the treatment quite daunting for patients. Chemotherapy nurses are well placed to provide reassurance that while some side-effects can be challenging, they are almost all temporary and will only last for the duration of treatment. However, some side-effects can be longer lasting and therefore it is essential that intricate assessments are undertaken prior to each cycle of chemotherapy. To mitigate many of the side-effects, routine use of premedication is advocated.

Organ Toxicity Many chemotherapy drugs have dose-limiting organ toxicities; for example, anthracycline agents can cause severe cardiac toxicity and therefore have a lifetime maximum cumulative dose. Most chemotherapy drugs have one or two specific organ toxicity risks – hence the development of combination therapies whereby different drugs tend to be used in combination that have differing toxicities to increase the fraction of cells that are destroyed without reaching any dangerous level of toxicity.

Nausea and Vomiting Chemotherapy-induced nausea and vomiting (CINV) has been described as the most feared side-effect; it can affect up to 90% of patients. Some drugs are more emetogenic (causing nausea and vomiting) than others, cisplatin being one of the worst, and the vinca alkaloids being the least emetogenic. Nausea is sometimes accompanied by vomiting but this is not the most common experience.

Nausea is a subjective individual experience, described as queasiness, unease in the stomach, a feeling of a need to vomit, with or without retching or heaving. CINV may be classified as:

- *Acute*: usually within several hours of chemotherapy administration
- *Delayed*: can be delayed for several days after the treatment
- *Anticipatory*: if nausea and vomiting is not controlled with chemotherapy then the patient may experience a conditioned response of nausea and vomiting before treatment
- *Breakthrough*: if one level of antiemetic fails then the patient should be stepped up to the next level of antiemetic prophylaxis
- *Refractory*: nausea and vomiting occurs despite all levels of antiemetic.

Nausea can be associated with other related symptoms such as fatigue and constipation, anxiety, taste changes in the mouth and heightened perception of smells, thus making it difficult to manage. The person invariably has to cope with this at home because it usually occurs after they have left the hospital; it can be exhausting, disrupts sleep and prolongs the recovery period between treatments.

Thorough assessment is needed before treatment commences to enable tailoring of antiemetic therapy. The person may find keeping a record in a diary is useful, as a pattern usually develops and it may be difficult to remember what has happened between cycles of treatment.

As it is an anticipated side-effect, most people having chemotherapy will be given an antiemetic premedication, usually a $5HT_3$ receptor antagonist (ondansetron) and a steroid (dexamethasone), up to an hour before chemotherapy is given, as it is easier to prevent the symptom than treat it once it has developed. Neurokinin type 1 (NK-1) receptor antagonists such as aprepitant may also be used as antiemetics for drugs with higher rates of emesis; there is now an oral antiemetic available which contains a combination of $5HT_3$ and NK-1 receptor antagonists which is given 1 hour before treatment and then no additional medication other than steroids are required after chemotherapy unless breakthrough CINV occurs. Patients are also given antiemetics to take home in case CINV develops later on; this is usually a combination of a steroid (dexamethasone) and a dopamine receptor antagonist such as metoclopramide.

Antiemetics can cause drowsiness and constipation, which can lead to a requirement for additional medication such as laxatives.

There are non-pharmacological approaches that can be used to control nausea. Progressive muscle relaxation, music therapy, meditation and controlled breathing may be effective and acceptable coping strategies. Guided imagery, where the person focuses on a pleasant scene or an enjoyable calming experience, can be effective because the person has a sense of control over their situation. Some patients may also benefit from the use of ginger, mint or acupressure bands worn on the wrists. The research-based evidence for these interventions is limited but they do have the advantage of being relatively inexpensive and easy to use in practice.

Constipation

Constipation can be as a direct result of the chemotherapy drugs (e.g. plant alkaloids such as vincristine) or can be secondary to other side-effects, such as nausea, where the person has not eaten the right foods or has not felt like drinking enough fluids to remain hydrated. The premedications used to minimise the experience of nausea and analgesics taken to control pain are also constipating because they slow down bowel transit time, resulting in more water being absorbed from the bowel.

Constipation can be a significant problem, requiring assessment to establish the cause. If it is related to a chemotherapy regimen using vinca alkaloids, the problem generally resolves several days after treatment and management may include taking laxatives prophylactically; however, increasing fluids may be sufficient to resolve the problem. If the constipation is secondary to other treatment (iatrogenic), the person needs regular laxative therapy in combination with the analgesics and antiemetics. Bulk-forming laxatives are not generally advised because they require the person to drink plenty of water, which may be difficult when feeling nauseous.

Diarrhoea

Diarrhoea occurs because chemotherapy agents affect rapidly dividing cells, such as those that line the gut. Some of the drugs most likely to cause diarrhoea are:

- Capecitabine
- Cisplatin
- Cyclophosphamide
- Daunorubicin
- 5-Fluorouracil
- Irinotecan.

Episodes of diarrhoea may start within hours of the first treatment and can prove acutely embarrassing. Its severity can result in dehydration, necessitating rapid treatment with drugs such as loperamide or codeine. If the diarrhoea does not subside, it may be necessary to reduce chemotherapy or stop treatment until the person recovers. The compromised immune status may mean the person is more susceptible to developing infections due to *Clostridium difficile*.

Irinotecan can cause an acute cholinergic reaction consisting of severe diarrhoea, abdominal cramping and excessive sweating; this can be life-threatening and subsequent cycles require administration of atropine for prophylaxis.

Hair Loss

Hair loss (alopecia) is a symptom that most people associate with chemotherapy, some saying it is the worst side-effect. However, it does not occur with all agents – some agents cause hair thinning rather than total hair loss. Hair loss occurs because the hair cells replicate quickly, so are very susceptible to the cytotoxic effect of chemotherapy. The hair does regrow once treatment is completed but it may well change in colour and texture. All body hair can be affected, so eyebrows, eyelashes and pubic hair can be lost as well as scalp hair. It is an obviously visible sign that the person is unwell and some people do not wish to disclose their illness and treatment for a variety of reasons, hence assessment and management of this side-effect is an essential part of the chemotherapy nurse's role.

There are several ways to manage this side-effect. The person having chemotherapy can be advised to cut their hair short; as the hair falls out, this tends to be less distressing than when the hair is worn long. Using very mild shampoos, not washing the hair frequently and letting the hair dry naturally also help to preserve hair. A great deal depends on the aggressiveness of the treatment regimen used and the agents involved.

Many people choose to wear some form of head covering to provide warmth and protection of the scalp; there are many varieties of headwear available. Alternatively, they can be provided with a wig; patients are entitled to a synthetic wig free of charge on the NHS (Cancer Research UK, 2014). Remember that men can be as affected by this side-effect as women, so assessment, management and advice should be provided equally.

The loss of eyebrows and eyelashes can be problematic, as these protect the eyes from dust particles, causing discomfort due to dry and sometimes gritty eyes.

Scalp Cooling

Scalp cooling can be used to prevent or minimise hair loss; it works by reducing scalp temperature, causing vasoconstriction and thereby preventing the chemotherapy drugs from affecting the hair follicles. There is mixed evidence for the effectiveness of scalp cooling; it can work very well for some but not for others (particularly those with very thick hair as

243

this can insulate the scalp from the cooler). Chemotherapy suites have scalp cooling machines that keep a cap at a constant temperature. The cap has to fit snugly to the head for the best results, so the right size cap needs to be selected for each person. A poor fit can result in hair loss, which may still occur even with a correct fit. The cap has to be worn for at least 15 minutes before treatment starts and for at least 30 minutes after treatment has stopped. Cool caps lower the person's temperature and they may need extra blankets to keep warm during the process. The caps are heavy as well as cold and some people opt not to continue with the treatment because of the discomfort.

As cooling of the scalp reduces the uptake of chemotherapy agents in the hair follicles, there were some fears that the cancer would metastasise to the scalp as a result but there is currently no research-based evidence to support this claim. However, there are a number of indications for which scalp cooling is not advocated, particularly haematological cancers, and in some chemotherapy regimens scalp cooling is ineffective, particularly those that have a longer half-life.

> ### Jot This Down
> Take some time to think about how hair loss may impact on someone in terms of their psychological, social, sexual and spiritual needs.

Bone Marrow Suppression Blood cell production takes place within the bone marrow (in adults this is mainly within the pelvis, femur and sternum) where rapid replication is required to maintain the cells necessary to combat infection (leucocytes – white blood cells, specifically neutrophils), to maintain oxygenation throughout the body (haemoglobin) and aid clotting (platelet production). Due to the nature of chemotherapy drugs, this production can become suppressed, resulting in anaemia (reduction in haemoglobin), neutropenia (reduction in neutrophils, rendering the person much more susceptible to infections) and thrombocytopenia (reduction in platelets, increasing the risk of bleeding). Patients receiving chemotherapy sometimes require blood and/or platelet transfusions to maintain appropriate levels of haemoglobin and platelets.

Neutropenic Sepsis This is a condition caused by a significant reduction in neutrophils (the main immune cells used to fight infection) whereby infection develops rapidly and requires immediate action, because untreated it can prove fatal. The person receiving chemotherapy is at risk of developing opportunistic infections as they lack the body's first line of defence. The infections may come from the patient themselves; for example, when the oral mucosa is breached, the person can develop ulcers and sores which are a source of infection, or they can develop an infection from a central line if they have one. Infections can also come from any external source, hence people receiving chemotherapy are generally advised to isolate themselves from the general public and avoid crowded places.

A person is classed as being 'neutropenic' when their neutrophil count is lower than 0.5×10^9/L; febrile neutropenia (an indication of neutropenic sepsis) is when the person's temperature is greater than 38°C (NICE, 2012). The optimum timeframe for development of neutropenic sepsis is 7–10 days following immunosuppressive chemotherapy.

A strong indication of neutropenic sepsis is a raised temperature, so the recipient of chemotherapy needs to record their temperature daily. In the event of a raised temperature, the person must contact their healthcare team immediately or report to hospital for a possible emergency admission. Everyone receiving chemotherapy is given a card detailing local arrangements and emergency telephone numbers. Neutropenic sepsis can escalate very quickly and the person can develop overwhelming sepsis, multiple organ failure and die within hours if untreated. Intravenous antibiotics need to be administered within 1 hour of arrival to an emergency department and the neutropenic sepsis protocol needs to be initiated immediately.

What To Do If . . .

A person arrives at the emergency department with a slightly raised temperature of 37.4°C and tells you they had a chemotherapy treatment 7 days previously. The questions you mi ask include:

- Have you got your chemotherapy Alert Card? This will have a record of the treatment and the consultant caring for the person and contact details
- Have you taken any paracetamol? As this can mask a temperature
- Do you have any other signs/symptoms/sources of infection? For example, presence of a central venous catheter.

It is imperative that the person receives treatment quickly and is not made to wait, as they will deteriorate very quickly and reach a point where multiple organ failure and subsequent fatality may result.

A course of granulocyte colony-stimulating factor (G-CSF) may be given to a person at particular risk over a period of 10 days, as this helps the neutrophil levels to recover quickly. G-CSF is also given as a prophylaxis with many chemotherapy regimens with a risk of neutropenia >20%, with the aim of preventing people experiencing this complication.

Some foods could possibly lead to a person developing infection (although there is very little evidence to support this claim), so it is advised that a 'neutropenic or clean diet' is followed, in which uncooked foods such as salads, blue cheeses, unpasteurised milk products and undercooked meats are avoided (Van Dalen *et al.*, 2012).

Fatigue Many people receiving chemotherapy develop quite severe fatigue as a result of treatment (cancer-related fatigue is discussed later). Advice should be given regarding ways to manage this, particularly in relation to energy conservation for the highest priority tasks, exercise, sleep hygiene and other self-management strategies such as meditation, relaxation and yoga. It is important to rule out other causes of fatigue such as anaemia, so bloods are regularly checked to ensure adequate haemoglobin levels are maintained through treatment.

Mucositis As previously mentioned, chemotherapy agents can affect mucous membranes via their impact on replicating cells. This causes erosion of the mucous membranes along the GI tract, leading to a condition known as mucositis, an inflammation of the oral mucosa, which can extend all along the oesophagus and into the gut. Some chemotherapy drugs such as antimetabolites (e.g. fluorouracil, methotrexate) are particularly renowned for causing this side-effect. Advice on prevention can be given, such as maintenance of a basic mouthcare regimen to include regular tooth brushing with a soft toothbrush and regular mouth rinsing with a saline rinse. Treatment includes use of specific mouthwashes and analgesia to enable maintenance of adequate nutrition. Mucositis can also increase the risk of opportunistic infection due to breaches in the mucous membranes whereby micro-organisms are able to enter and colonise, particularly as mucositis tends to be at its peak during the neutropenic phase.

Peripheral Neuropathy Some 30–40% of people are affected by chemotherapy-induced peripheral neuropathies, which occur following treatment with high doses of chemotherapy agents such as the platinum drugs, taxanes and vinca alkaloids. Combination therapies which include these agents can damage the nerves and this is felt in the feet and hands as tingling (paraesthesia) or altered sensations (dysaesthesia), numbness and shooting pain. This condition is painful and can be difficult to manage if the nerve endings are permanently damaged. Reporting this side-effect at once to the healthcare team will result in a reduction of the dose or cessation of treatment for a short while, which reverses the problem; however, it is not always reversible and it can be a major factor in people opting out of further treatment. Supplements such as vitamins E and B may help, but should only be taken following consultation with the medical team.

Neuropathic pain responds better to treatment with analgesics, which are combined with antidepressants or anticonvulsant drugs such as gabapentin, which are more efficient in controlling nerve pain than analgesics alone.

'Chemobrain' and 'Chemofog' Some people observe that during the treatment period they experience memory problems, where they may forget words when they are talking or forget appointments. People receiving chemotherapy treatment can find reliable solutions, such as making lists and keeping a diary. Others report difficulty in concentrating on reading and absorbing information. There may be a variety of reasons for 'chemobrain' and 'chemofog': people may be anxious, have sleep problems and feel fatigued, all of which can affect concentration levels. In general, people report this as a passing problem; either more significant side-effects detract from the focus on concentration or they feel they will adapt to a world of treatment and recovery.

Primary Care

Chemotherapy is usually administered while the person is an outpatient and most of the side-effects can occur once they have returned home, so they may feel vulnerable and alone. Think about what support services might be available in the community, and what support patients may need beyond treatment.

Case Study

- Denise is a 35-year-old woman.
- She has been diagnosed with stage 2 breast cancer – no nodes or metastasis.
- She is currently receiving adjuvant chemotherapy (after surgery) with epirubicin and cyclophosphamide
- She has experienced significant nausea and is having trouble maintaining diet and fluids.
- She has a 2-year-old daughter who is into everything and does not sleep well.
- Her wife has been working away and does not appear to show much interest in Denise when she is home.

Consider:
- How would you assess Denise?
- What treatment and support could you offer?
- What onward referrals might be appropriate in this case?

Nursing Care for the Person Receiving Chemotherapy

Chemotherapy treatment can have a significant impact on a person's well-being, not only physically but also psychologically, socially, sexually and spiritually. Holistic assessments are required throughout treatment, to enable the healthcare team to identify any specific issues and provide tailored support. Every person receiving chemotherapy is given a card that details their local emergency chemotherapy/SACT helpline telephone number which they can contact 24 hours a day, 7 days per week.

Red Flag

 Only nurses who have been assessed annually as competent to do so can administer SACT.
(UK Oncology Nursing Society SACT Passport, 2019)

Before Chemotherapy is Administered

Receiving a diagnosis of cancer can be devastating. During the initial consultation, there is much information that needs to be relayed regarding the diagnosis and treatment options, but often people are in a state of shock, and so they fail to take in much of what is said. For this reason, a period of time is usually given for the person to think about the options, and then return to spend an hour or so with a chemotherapy nurse where they can discuss the treatment plan and are provided with information about the specific SACT regimen and in particular its potential side-effects. This allows for a process of informed consent for the treatment to proceed, as people receiving treatment are better able to focus on the information given. Prechemotherapy consultations are usually conducted by nurses who are trained in giving chemotherapy because they are better placed to deal with any queries. This is also an opportunity to conduct a holistic assessment so that any specific issues can be addressed, and the person can be put at ease regarding any major concerns they may have.

Administering Chemotherapy

Chemotherapy is often given as an intravenous infusion, but there are also a number of oral preparations. Oral drugs have to be capable of withstanding the digestive process, which may alter their effectiveness; in addition, if a person is nauseous and vomits, it is difficult to establish what dosage has been absorbed. Patients often prefer oral medication because this negates the need for frequent hospital visits; however, healthcare professionals are anxious that the regimen may not be strictly adhered to, or conversely that medication continues to be taken even when adverse effects are experienced. As both parties are anxious to maximise the effectiveness of the chemotherapy, intravenous infusions and frequent hospital visits remain the standard pattern for the majority of people.

Medicines Management

 Oral SACTs must never be crushed or broken; they must always be taken whole and all have specific instructions about taking with or without foods as this can affect absorption.

If a patient vomits after taking a dose, they must never take another dose as it is not possible to know how much has been absorbed.

Chemotherapy drugs are usually given in cycles, which are repeated at intervals sufficiently long enough to enable normal cells to recover but short enough to hit cancer cells before they replicate. If the person requires several cycles, a permanent central venous access device (CVAD) such as a Hickman catheter or a portacath can be inserted and this prevents multiple cannulations and venepunctures.

The vast majority of chemotherapy is given in the outpatient setting; people are generally only admitted into hospital for treatment when receiving very high-dose chemotherapy, such as in the case for some blood cancers such as leukaemia, or as pre conditioning for a bone marrow (stem cell) transplant. Otherwise, admission into hospital tends to occur due to severe side-effects or toxicities of treatment. Most people attend specialist chemotherapy suites, which have been designed to be as comfortable as possible, furnished with recliner chairs with environments that are specially designed to enhance a positive atmosphere. The feedback from users indicates that this environment is preferred as it normalises treatment, comparing it with a visit to the hairdressers, where they are hooked up to a giving set instead of a hair dryer.

Before each treatment is commenced, the person must be assessed as fit to receive it, and must have undertaken a blood test to ensure organs are functioning adequately and blood cells are within specific parameters, rendering it safe to proceed with chemotherapy. Box 15.1 outlines the general blood values needed for chemotherapy to proceed – this can vary according to cancer site and treatment regimen.

Nurses need to have additional education and preparation to become competent in administration of chemotherapy due to the complex nature of the treatment and side-effects. The UK Oncology Nursing Society (UKONS) has produced a nationally recognised competency document called the 'SACT Passport' which is now used in most areas. The idea of this is that once a nurse has completed it, the competency can be transferred from hospital to hospital without having to be reassessed in different areas, although reassessment of competency is required annually.

Chemotherapy drugs also pose a health and safety risk to those handling them as many of them are recognised as hazardous drugs and are classed as being mutagenic (can mutate cell DNA), teratogenic (toxic to reproductive organs and fetal development) and carcinogenic (have potential to cause cancer). Part of the additional preparation and education for chemotherapy nurses includes safe handling of these drugs to reduce the risk of occupational exposure. Spillages of chemotherapy in particular need to be handled very carefully, and all units have policies and procedures in place to ensure minimal exposure to staff handling these drugs which all staff in the units need to be familiar with.

Practice Assessment Document

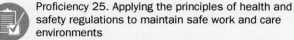 Proficiency 25. Applying the principles of health and safety regulations to maintain safe work and care environments

Considering the above points, think about how you would maintain a safe environment working on a chemotherapy unit. Discuss this with your supervisor and how this can be applied to other healthcare settings – it is not just chemotherapy drugs that can be hazardous!

Extravasation This may be a complication of intravenous administration of SACT whereby the drug leaks out of the vein and infiltrates the surrounding tissues. In some cases, this can lead to significant injury and even necrosis due to the cytotoxic nature of some chemotherapy drugs. People receiving these agents have been known to need extensive skin grafting due to necrotic injuries as a result of extravasation. One class of these drugs, known as 'vesicants', have the greatest risk of causing significant injury if they are extravasated, and chemotherapy nurses are educated in the prevention, recognition and immediate management of this complication. Each unit has policies and guidelines to follow in the management of extravasation as people can have permanent injuries as a result.

Hypersensitivity/anaphylaxis Some SACT agents have a significantly higher risk of causing an allergic or hypersensitivity reaction; this is due to the nature of some SACTs that have molecules that are easily recognisable as 'foreign' by the immune system, initiating an allergic response. Often these reactions are caught in the early stages so are treated as a hypersensitivity reaction with steroids and antihistamines, but some do go on to develop an anaphylactic type reaction which requires treatment according to the UK Resuscitation Council guidelines. Many of these drugs require a premedication to be given (usually an antihistamine with or without a corticosteroid) as prophylaxis of any allergic or hypersensitive reactions.

Where a reaction has occurred, it is possible to try the treatment again, infusing it at a slower rate or lower dose, and it may well be effective once the person has become desensitised.

Box 15.1 General Blood Values Necessary for Chemotherapy to Proceed

Haemoglobin: greater than 100 g/L
Total white cell count: greater than 3.0×10^9/L
Total neutrophil count: greater than 1×10^9/L
Platelets: greater than 80×10^9/L
Creatinine: less than $1.5 \times N$

Biological Therapies and Immunotherapies

These types of therapies are becoming ever more utilised as SACT agents, either alongside traditional chemotherapy drugs or as single agents. Immunotherapy is not a new concept; William Coley, an American surgeon practising in the 1800s, found that one of his patients with a solid tumour went into remission from his cancer following erysipelas (a streptococcal bacterial infection). He experimented by injecting small amounts of streptococcal bacteria into bone tumours in order to stimulate the body's immune system, which targeted the cancer cells, causing them to die, called apoptosis. Other doctors used bacille Calmette–Guérin (BCG) vaccine to treat bladder cancers once it was noted that people with active tuberculosis infections recovered from cancer (Butterfield *et al.*, 2017).

These treatments were used less and less during the 20th century, as radiotherapy and chemotherapy seemed to provide better options. However, they have re-emerged as understanding of malignancy has developed and therefore targeting of specific growth pathways or stimulation of the immune system to combat cancers have become a major part of our current treatment strategies.

Biological Therapies

These agents include monoclonal antibodies, vaccines and antiangiogenesis agents.

Monoclonal Antibodies Monoclonal antibodies recognise and lock onto specific protein receptors excreted by cancer cells, so they are called 'targeted therapies'. They work by either:

- Making the cancer cells responsive to attack from the body's own immune cells which then destroy them, or
- Making the cancer cells resistant to growth factors that would help the cells to replicate.

One example is rituximab, used in the treatment of non-Hodgkin lymphoma; another is trastuzumab (Herceptin®), used in certain types of breast cancer.

Rituximab and trastuzumab are formed from a mixture of murine (mouse) and human antibodies and are used to treat non-Hodgkin lymphoma, a cancer of specific white blood cells (T and B lymphocytes), in conjunction with chemotherapy. Rituximab, when used with the combination chemotherapy of cyclophosphamide, vincristine, doxorubicin and prednisolone (CHOP) as an adjuvant therapy, is almost twice as effective as using CHOP alone. These antibodies target specific antigens (CD20) found on the surface of large B-cell lymphomas. When the two combine, they attract natural killer (NK) cells (lymphocytes in the immune system), which release perforin (a small protein) that enters the targeted cell and causes apoptosis (Graham, 2009).

The person receiving treatment is given a premedication, which consists of an antipyretic (paracetamol) and an antihistamine (usually chlorphenamine) to pre-empt the development of infusion-related reactions. The rate of infusion is important: if given too quickly, it can cause a reaction referred to as 'cytokine release syndrome', which has been described as being similar to the onset of flu with a mild rash. Cytokine release syndrome is more prominent following the first dose, as this is when most cells are targeted and destroyed, reducing the tumour burden. Subsequent treatments affect fewer cells, resulting in fewer cytokines being released. A more severe reaction can occur with breathlessness and hypotension. When a severe reaction occurs, the infusion is stopped immediately and the person is treated with bronchodilators and oxygen therapy.

Once the symptoms abate, the treatment can be recommenced and infused over a longer period. The more severe reactions are similar to a severe allergic reaction, resulting in low blood pressure, breathlessness and bronchospasm, which lead to insufficient oxygen intake and respiratory distress. This reaction usually occurs within minutes of the transfusion starting and affects about 10% of patients, constituting a medical emergency.

Trastuzumab (Herceptin) works by blocking the HER-2 receptor present on breast cancer cells of HER-2 positive breast cancers, preventing the growth factor from landing on its target and subsequently stopping replication of the cancerous cell. This keeps the cancer under control and can do so for many years for some people. There are newer generation HER-2 antibodies available, such as pertuzumab, and a conjugate drug called trastuzumab emtansine, which has a cytotoxic drug attached to the antibody which helps to destroy the targeted HER-2 cancer cells.

There are a number of other monoclonal antibodies available that target specific proteins on cancer cell surfaces. This has been an area of significant development in recent years as new drugs in this category are being developed all the time for different tumour sites.

Immunotherapies

Immunotherapies are a type of monoclonal antibody which targets the cells of the immune system, allowing them to attack cancer cells, by 'unmasking' the cancer cells that have evaded the normal immune response. Drugs such as ipilimumab and nivolumab have revolutionised treatment for some cancers such as malignant melanoma. These therapies are now being used in more tumour sites such as lung, colorectal, head and neck, renal cell and bladder cancers, and are being investigated in many more.

Physiology of the Immune Response The body's immune system differentiates between what is true self and what is foreign, i.e. non-self, which includes cells that have mutated, foreign proteins as in transplanted cells and micro-organisms that have invaded the system. It sets in motion a chain of reactions to rid the body of what is considered harmful and dangerous to the body's continued survival. This means that cancerous cells should be recognised by the immune system and destroyed as they have become mutated cells. However, over time the cancer cells develop mechanisms whereby they can evade destruction by immune cells.

There are three types of lymphocytes: T cells, B cells and natural killer (NK) cells. These cells make up the adaptive immune system whereby the body recognises antigens from previous exposure. B cells produce antibodies to recognise specific antigens and develop memory cells that can initiate an immediate immune response on exposure to the recognised antigen. T cells recognise DNA altered/mutated cells, and those of non-self. The T cells are the target of immunotherapies as these are the immune cells that recognise non-self and cause apoptosis of abnormal cells.

Lymphocytes are produced in the bone marrow and thymus gland; some, like the B cells, stay in lymph tissue until required. The immune system becomes less effective as we age, thus making us more susceptible to the development of cancer.

There are two main types of immunotherapy; one mainly targets specific pathways within T cells that prevent their action on cancer cells and thus stimulates the activation of T cells against cancer cells. The other type of immunotherapy targets cancer cells themselves, effectively unmasking them to allow T-cell destruction. A combination of these two types of immunotherapy has proven extremely effective, particularly in malignant melanoma, although the risk of adverse effects is significantly increased by using this combination.

Side-effects of Immunotherapies As use of these therapies has expanded exponentially in recent years, it is important to recognise that the side-effects of these agents are significantly different from those of traditional types of chemotherapy. As these drugs stimulate the person's immune system, the side-effects are a manifestation of an overactive immune system. Hence they have the potential to create an inflammatory reaction in almost any organ of the body. The most common side-effects are dermatitis, colitis (diarrhoea caused by inflammation of the colon which can be life-threatening) and pneumonitis (inflam-

mation of the lung tissue causing cough and breathlessness – CT scans have a 'ground glass' appearance). Other organs can also be affected; both the kidneys and liver can become inflamed (nephritis and hepatitis respectively) and their function impaired, and there may also be effects on the endocrine system. It is really important that these effects are picked up early as they can be treated very easily with steroids but can be life-threatening if left untreated. Chemotherapy nurses need to incorporate an additional assessment for people receiving these treatments to check for the development of any of these side-effects.

Other Targeted Therapies

Protein Kinase Inhibitors

Protein kinases are enzymes involved in signaling pathways within cells which trigger the cell into replication. Inhibition of these enzymes reduces the signaling within the cell, subsequently stopping the cell from dividing. There are many different types of these drugs on the market; they are all in tablet form which is easier to manage outside the hospital setting, and can be very effective in controlling many cancers, including chronic myeloid leukaemia, a specific type of lung cancer, renal cell cancer, metastatic breast cancer and melanoma. Examples of these include imatinib (the first of its kind), ibrutinib, sorafenib, pazopanib, palbociclib and vemurafenib, to name just a few. Side-effects can include fatigue, nausea, diarrhoea and hypertension.

Antiangiogenesis Agents

Tumours have the ability to grow their own blood vessels to ensure a blood supply which can provide the cancer with the nutrients it requires to grow. Antiangiogenesis agents such as bevacizumab (which is a monoclonal antibody, and is another targeted therapy) inhibits vascular endothelial growth factor (VEGF) from initiating a capillary network in the tumour. VEGF is produced in the growing fetus and in adults is only present when there is a wound, so its effect on other parts of the body is minimal, unlike chemotherapy agents that affect normal and abnormal cells alike. This means that the tumour is prevented from producing any more blood vessels and therefore cannot continue to grow. Bevacizumab is used in combination with taxanes such as paclitaxel and docetaxel to treat breast cancer and also to treat some colorectal cancers.

Bevacizumab can cause hypertension, proteinuria, bleeding in the bladder, epistaxis (nose bleeds) and thromboemboli (blood clots), which can affect the heart, leading to heart failure.

Proteasome Inhibitors

These agents include bortezomib and carfilzomib, used in the treatment of myeloma. They work by inhibiting transcription of genes that produce proteins which promote cell division. This also results in a build-up of proteins which then initiates apoptosis of the cell.

Vaccines

Vaccines, such as the human papillomavirus (HPV) vaccine, are given to prevent the development of cervical cancer. The UK has introduced a vaccination programme for all girls aged over 13 years against HPV types 16 and 18, as these are believed to result in 70% of cervical cancers (Davis, 2008). Paniagua (2006) points out that, unfortunately, the vaccine does not protect against all types of cervical cancers. Cervical cancer represents the second most common cancer affecting women worldwide. While this vaccination programme does not directly target cancer cells, it has a role in the prevention of future cancers.

Personalised Therapy

As our understanding of malignancy develops, it has become clear that each cancer behaves in an individual way, and therefore requires an individualised approach to therapy. Added to that is the fact that many people requiring treatment for cancer are older and have many co-morbidities, so cannot always receive full-dose regimens, and are sometimes unable to tolerate specific drugs due to the inherent risk of toxicity; for example, a person with chronic heart failure would be unable to receive full-dose anthracycline drugs as these are known to carry significant cardiac toxicity risk.

Many of the newer, more targeted therapies also require the presence of specific receptors on cancer cells, or rely on specific pathways within cancer cells to be effective, so additional genomic testing is required for many people to determine the most appropriate types of therapy. SACT has become far more complex in the last few years due to the many significant drug developments made, meaning that nurses providing care for patients receiving SACT need to have extensive knowledge and expertise, as well as being able to show care and compassion for people at very difficult stages of disease and treatment.

Radiotherapy

Radiotherapy can be used as the primary treatment or in conjunction with surgery and SACTs. It may be used before surgery to debulk the tumour, or after surgery to eliminate any remaining cancer cells. It can also be used in palliative disease to manage symptoms.

Examples of what radiotherapy is used to treat:

- Neuroblastomas
- Lymphomas
- Head and neck cancers.

Radiotherapy uses cobalt and caesium; these radioactive agents are delivered by huge machines, which are noisy, and can appear frightening and feel claustrophobic. The person is required to lie very still during treatment.

Radiotherapy is delivered by either teletherapy/external beam radiation or brachytherapy/internal radiotherapy, where the radioactive material is placed close to the tumour. Dosages of radiotherapy are calculated in grays (Gy) and are divided up into units which are delivered at intervals; this is called fractionation. The aim with teletherapy is to ensure that the dose reaches the tumour. To do this, it has to pass through normal tissue and the machines deliver this at different angles into the body – a three-dimensional effect. It is a very precise treatment: the person is measured and the position where the beam needs to enter the body is marked with an indelible pen on the skin.

More recent is the development of cyber/gamma knife machines that deliver radiation in multiple narrow beams which can be more accurate, meaning less surrounding tissue is treated and fewer side-effects experienced.

Skin Care

It is important that the skin through which the radiotherapy beam passes remains dry and the application of creams or ointments must be avoided as these cause skin reactions during treatment. The person is also advised to only wash skin gently with mild soap and water, not to shave or rub the area, or to apply hot or cold packs.

After a few doses of radiotherapy, the skin may become red (erythematous), blanch (look white) or become darker in darker skinned people. The surface layer may peel off, and this may leave dry or wet skin exposed; this reaction is called desquamation.

General Side-effects of Radiotherapy

The side-effects of radiotherapy differ depending on the area of the body being treated. This is because radiotherapy is a local treatment so will affect localised tissues. For example, head and neck cancer treatment may cause mucositis and xerostoma and bowel cancer treatment may result in constipation or diarrhoea.

General side-effects of radiotherapy include:

- Fatigue
- Skin reactions
- Nausea
- Loss of appetite
- Hair loss
- Bone marrow suppression.

Nursing Care for the Person Receiving Radiotherapy

Most people receive radiotherapy as outpatients, so nurses may only be involved if severe side-effects are experienced. For example, if desquamation occurs, the area will require dressing and aseptic wound care.

Since these wounds can be highly visible (as in head and neck cancers) and painful, this can lead to social withdrawal and impact on well-being. A holistic approach to care is imperative.

Common Problems Resulting from All Cancer Therapies

Due to the variety and multimodal approach to treating cancer, and the effect of the disease itself, there are a number of other problems that can arise. These tend to be very specific to the type and site of the cancer and the treatment plan. Some general problems are outlined below.

Weight Loss/Weight Gain

Weight loss, which has been discussed earlier, is often the symptom that triggers a person to seek medical advice. In general, people expect someone with cancer to lose weight, so are not prepared for a person with cancer who gains weight.

Weight gain also occurs in response to pharmacological treatment: steroids may result in weight gain, including cushingoid features (moon face), or hormonal treatments which affect weight management. Other symptoms such as fatigue impact on a person's weight, as they have less impetus to exercise.

Cancer-Related Fatigue (CRF)

Up to 80% of people having cancer treatment experience CRF which affects their quality of life. It is characterised by a subjective feeling of tiredness, weakness or lack of energy, which is not relieved by rest. CRF affects mental and physical processes, making evaluating and planning care of a patient with CRF challenging (Tadman *et al.*, 2019). Often people experiencing CRF fail to report it, believing nothing can be done to improve their quality of life. However, fatigue can be the result of anaemia, increased levels of cytokines (produced by the tumour) and the body's reaction to excretion of the toxins as a result of treatment, all of which are treatable, so should not be ruled out.

Keeping active is advised to boost appetite and improve energy and sleep levels. Exercise offers a distraction, improves mood and outlook, and enhances general feelings of well-being. Cognitive behavioural therapy (CBT) may be beneficial as it helps to reframe the way people view their illness (Mitchell, 2014).

What to Do If. . .

A patient wants advice on how to manage cancer-related fatigue. Some things to consider might be diet and nutrition, keeping a diary, exercise and sleep hygiene. Remember CRF is a multifaceted condition and physical/mechanical/chemical causes must not be overlooked.

Living With and Beyond Cancer

As previously stated, with improved diagnostic strategies, the use of combination therapies and newer targeted treatment, survival rates have improved and cancer is increasingly being conceived as a long-term condition, as half of people diagnosed with cancer in the UK live for 10 years or more (Cancer Research UK, 2021a). The experience of cancer often leaves a physical, mental and emotional legacy for many years afterwards (Macmillan, 2013).

Lynda Thomas (Macmillan Cancer Support) says:

'It is good that we are curing more people of cancer, but we have to recognise that "not dying" is not the same as "being well". No one should face the often severe long-term effects of cancer alone.'

The National Cancer Survivorship Initiative was launched in 2007, and in 2012 the Department of Health undertook a pilot survey using patient-reported outcome measures (PROMS) to assess the quality of life for people following their cancer treatment (Department of Health, 2012; Corner & Wagland, 2013). The main finding of the survey was that overall quality of life was significantly associated with:

- The presence and number of concurrent long-term conditions
- Disease status
- Age
- Physical activity.

'People have feelings of abandonment or isolation once initial treatment has concluded' (Tadman *et al.*, 2019).

Younger people experienced problems when they wished to return to work following treatment. Employers may need to re-evaluate the perceptions of people who have been treated for cancer; many people felt that they were forced to return to work before they were ready and would have benefited from a longer convalescent stage.

The key message is that for effective living with and beyond cancer care, individualised and personalised care is essential. Healthcare professionals have an important role to play in supporting people to have a better quality of life with and beyond cancer, and there have been great strides in developing strategies and interventions such as holistic needs assessments, recovery packages, cancer care reviews and health and well-being education events to enhance the care of people living with and beyond cancer.

The Cancer Quality of Life Survey is a national survey run by NHS England and NHS Improvement and Public Health England. The survey is for people in England who have been diagnosed with cancer. From 2020, people who have had a breast, prostate or colorectal (bowel) cancer diagnosis are being asked to complete the survey around 18 months after diagnosis. The aim of the survey is to find out how quality of life may have changed for people diagnosed with cancer. This will help to improve the way people are supported to live as long and as well as possible.

What the Experts Say

At the Queen Elizabeth Hospital, Birmingham, UK, we have a department called the Patrick Room, which offers cancer information and support to people with cancer and their families. A professional and experienced team, which is supported by trained volunteers, delivers the service, offering telephone helplines, support from health professionals, cancer information materials and access to the internet.
Alison Simons, Senior Lecturer

End-of-Life Care

Cancer is a long-term condition; however, some people present late with an advanced cancer and may be offered palliative care. It can be difficult to have a conversation about end-of-life issues and advance care planning. If the prospect of dying is not discussed initially, the person may never broach the subject again until it is too late to make plans for future care.

Specialist cancer and palliative care nurses are key in their involvement and presence during these initial and consequent consultations. Most specialist cancer nurses have undergone an intensive course to develop their communication skills and are very adept at dealing with these difficult conversations. The best strategy is to:

- Find out why the person is feeling this way. What has been their past experience of people with cancer? Do they know someone who has had cancer?
- Find out what they know about their cancer. Have they looked it up on the internet? What have other healthcare professionals discussed about their cancer with them?
- Find out how they are currently feeling.

Practice Assessment Document

For a variety of reasons, you might not have had the opportunity to demonstrate to your assessor/supervisor how to engage in difficult conversations, including breaking bad news with compassion and sensitivity.

Make an appointment to meet with the palliative care team and ask if you can spend some time with them discussing the interpersonal skills required in this situation. When you have done this, prepare a report for your supervisor/assessor to demonstrate the knowledge you have gained.

Having established the patient's fears and concerns, it helps to know what the next step should be. If you do not have the answers, be honest and say so, but refer the patient on to someone who can give the patient the answers they need.

Professional and Legal Issues

Nursing people with cancer requires skilled care. Most nurses caring for people with cancer have undertaken additional studies at postgraduate level to ensure that they are suitably equipped with knowledge and skills to provide care.

Cancer care is highly charged because people feel pressured to start treatment straight away; the earlier treatment starts, the better the chance of recovery. However, informed consent before treatment commences is vital and people can only give informed consent if they are fully apprised of what the treatment entails.

As we have seen earlier, the side-effects of treatment can lead to death. Side-effects can also be disfiguring and compromise life afterwards, so that life never returns to what it once was.

Conclusion

This chapter has considered and addressed the general approach taken to cancer care. Treatment of cancer is constantly changing and the outcomes for people with cancer continue to improve. However, if the cancer is found in its late stages, the outcomes remain poor.

Cancer is a very personal experience for the person with the diagnosis and their family. It should be remembered that even though patient outcomes have improved, the person still has to come to terms with the devastating impact that the news may have for them. Nursing care demands that we are compassionate and caring and mindful of each individual's needs.

Key Points

- Cancer can develop as a result of lifestyle choices or the cause can be unknown; different cancers require different treatment approaches.
- Cancer is a frightening experience and people need care, compassion and honesty from healthcare professionals and sensitive handling of their issues.

- Cancer is an illness that affects the person with cancer, their families, friends and work colleagues. Nurses and healthcare workers need to consider the impact on the person with cancer and also the people important to them.
- Cancer treatments can be debilitating and perceived as worse than the illness itself, leading to neutropenia and possible death, which requires rapid responses when patients present for emergency care.
- Some people with cancer present too late for curative treatment and palliative care is their only option.
- Cancer is a long-term condition and many people live with and beyond cancer but are in need of support to adjust to life with the long-term effects of treatment or disease.
- Cancer research is at the cutting edge of medical science and to remain proficient in caring for people with cancer, nurses and healthcare workers must ensure their knowledge is current and up to date.

References

Brant, J.M. (2014) cited in Yarbo, C.H., Wujcik, D. & Gobel, B.H. (2014) *Cancer Symptom Management*, 4th edn, p.69. Jones and Bartlett Learning, Burlington, MA.

Butterfield, L.H., Kaufman, H.L. & Marincola, F.M. (2017) *Cancer Immunotherapy: Principles and Practice*. Demos Medical Publishing, New York.

Cancer Research UK (2014) *Wigs*. www.cancerresearchuk.org/about-cancer/coping-with-cancer/coping-physically/changes-to-your-appearance-due-to-cancer/hair-loss/where-to-get-wigs-hats-scarves (accessed December 2021).

Cancer Research UK (2021a) *Cancer Survival*. www.cancerresearchuk.org/health-professional/cancer-statistics-for-the-uk#heading-Two (accessed December 2021).

Cancer Research UK (2021b) *Does Obesity Cause Cancer?* www.cancerresearchuk.org/about-cancer/causes-of-cancer/obesity-weight-and-cancer/does-obesity-cause-cancer (accessed December 2021).

Corner, J. & Wagland, R. (2013) *National Cancer Survivorship Initiative: Text Analysis of Patients' Free Text Comments: Final Report*. University of Southampton, Southampton.

Davis, C. (2008) Stopping cervical cancer in its tracks. *Cancer Nursing Practice*, 7(5), 19–21.

Department of Health (2012) *Quality of Life of Cancer Survivors in England: Report on a Pilot Survey Using Patient Reported Outcome Measures (PROMS)*. Department of Health, London.

Graham, A.H. (2009) Administering rituximab: infusion-related reactions and nursing implications. *Cancer Nursing Practice*, 8(2), 30–35.

Macmillan (2013) *Throwing Light on the Consequences of Cancer*. www.macmillan.org.uk/documents/aboutus/research/researchandevaluationreports/throwinglightontheconsequencesofcanceranditstreatment.pdf (accessed December 2021).

Mitchell, S.A. (2014) cited in Yarbo, C.H., Wujcik, D. & Gobel, B.H. (2014) *Cancer Symptom Management*, 4th edn, p.27. Jones and Bartlett Learning, Burlington, MA.

NHS (2019) *The Long-Term Plan*. www.longtermplan.nhs.uk/wp-content/uploads/2019/08/nhs-long-term-plan-version-1.2.pdf (accessed December 2021).

NHS (2020) *NHS Cancer Programme Quarterly Report: October to December 2020*. www.england.nhs.uk/wp-content/uploads/2019/12/nhs-cancer-programme-update-report-october-to-december-2020.pdf (accessed December 2021).

NHS (2021) *Screening and early diagnosis*. www.england.nhs.uk/cancer/early-diagnosis/screening-and-earlier-diagnosis/ (accessed December 2021).

NICE (2012) *Neutropenic sepsis: prevention and management in people with cancer*. www.nice.org.uk/guidance/cg151/ (accessed December 2021).

NICE (2015) *Suspected cancer: recognition and referral*. https://www.nice.org.uk/guidance/ng12 (accessed December 2021).

Office for National Statistics (2017) *Cancer Registration Statistics, England Statistical Bulletins*. www.cancerresearchuk.org/health-professional/cancer-statistics/incidence/age#ref-1 (accessed December 2021).

Paniagua, H. (2006) Knowledge of cervical cancer and the HPV vaccine. *British Journal of Nursing*, 15(3), 126–127.

Public Health England (2016) *The Public Health Burden of Alcohol: Evidence Review*. www.gov.uk/government/publications/the-public-health-burden-of-alcohol-evidence-review (accessed December 2021).

Public Health England Cancer Board (2017–21) *PHE Cancer Board Plan*. www.gov.uk/government/publications/phe-cancer-board-plan (accessed December 2021).

Public Health England (2018) *PHE progress report on the independent cancer taskforce recommendations*. PHE, London.

Tadman, M., Roberts. D. & Foulkes, M. (2019) *Oxford Handbook of Cancer Nursing*, pp.519–524. Oxford University Press, Oxford.

Van Dalen, E.C., Mank, A., Leclercq, E., *et al.* (2012) Low bacterial diet versus control diet to prevent infection in cancer patients treated with chemotherapy causing episodes of neutropenia. *Cochrane Database of Systematic Reviews*, 9, CD006247.

Velly, A. (2018) Epidemiology of pain and relation to psychiatric disorders. *Progress in Neuro-Psychopharmacology and Biological Psychiatry*, 87, 159–167.

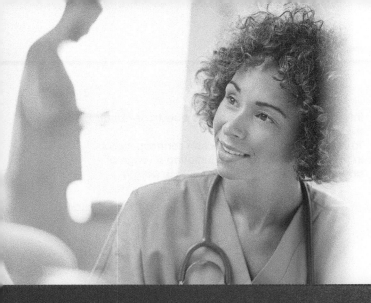

16

The Principles of Infection Prevention and Control (including Pandemics)

Hilarious De Jesus[1] and Nigel Davies[2]

[1]City, University of London, UK
[2]Brunel University, UK

Learning Outcomes

On completion of this chapter you will be able to:

- To follow relevant infection prevention and control legislation, policies, mandatory reporting and risk management duties (outcomes 1.2, 6.1, 6.3, 6.5, 6.6, 7.2)
- To protect health through understanding and applying the principles of infection prevention and control, including communicable disease surveillance and antimicrobial stewardship and resistance (outcome 2.12)
- To use this knowledge in relation to global patterns of health (outcome 2.2) and disease spread (pandemics) and how these relate to health screening programmes (outcome 2.5) and people's choices and motivations about vaccination (outcome 2.11) and behaviour change (Annexe A, 2.7)

Proficiencies

NMC Proficiencies and Standards:

- Use evidence-based, best practice approaches for meeting needs for care and support in the prevention and management of infection, accurately assessing the person's capacity for independence and self-care and initiating appropriate interventions.

Nursing Practice: Knowledge and Care, Third Edition. Edited by Ian Peate and Aby Mitchell.
© 2022 John Wiley & Sons Ltd. Published 2022 by John Wiley & Sons Ltd.
Companion website: www.wiley.com/go/peate/nursingpractice3e

Introduction

The control of infection is essential to the well-being of individuals and society. History teaches us that a lack of understanding of infection prevention and control measures can lead to disease and death sometimes on a large scale, for example, the epidemics of cholera and typhoid in the 19th century and blood-borne viruses such as hepatitis C and HIV towards the end of the 20th century. In the 21st century we have seen the Ebola epidemic in Africa and the global SARS-CoV-2 pandemic caused by a virulent strain of coronavirus in 2020.

In healthcare settings such as hospitals, GP practices and in residential and nursing homes, policies and procedures are often used to guide practitioners treating patients with infections. These polices use the current evidence and research to ensure not only that the patient receives the best treatment for the infection but also to prevent the spread of the infection to others. Sometimes, in diseases that can be particularly serious or transmitted easily to others, the polices are laid down in law and patients are required to follow the treatment regimen, for example, in cases of tuberculosis (TB). These diseases have to be reported to a national database and are known as 'communicable' or 'infectious diseases'. Proportionate to the risk to public health, more restrictive legislation can be imposed such as the national or scaled regional lockdowns imposed to curb the coronavirus transmission in the UK.

It is important for nurses and students working in all healthcare settings to have a good understanding of the principles of infection control, so they can apply the guidelines to prevent further infection and also to explain the reasons for tests and treatment to their patients. Compliance from patients is much greater when the reasons for treatment are understood and this often requires the nurse to interpret the patient's understanding and adapt often complex information in a meaningful way.

This chapter provides an introduction to infection prevention and control to enable you as a nurse to practise confidently and effectively, and to know when to refer to specialist infection control teams for further advice.

Practice Assessment Document

 Identifies potential infection risks and responds appropriately using best practice guidelines
As part of your competencies as a student nurse, knowledge and application of infection

control is crucial. To demonstrate this, you may do case studies of your patients and present them to your practice supervisor. Your case study does not have to be limited to patients with infectious diseases as infection control is applicable in most, if not all, case scenarios.

Development of Infection Control Practices

The science behind infection prevention and control measures has advanced a great deal in the last 150 years. Figure 16.1 outlines some of the milestones which have contributed to the development of infection control. The timeline refers to the revolutionary work of doctors and scientists such as Pasteur, Lister and Koch but also to work specifically related to hygiene by Semmelweis and Florence Nightingale. These discoveries still underpin many of the principles of infection control today such as the importance of hand hygiene. Infection control teams are now common in all hospitals with their evolution traced back to the appointment of infection control officers in the 1920s. However, it was not until the 1950s that the first infection control nurse was appointed and they were not common in all hospitals until the 1980s.

In healthcare settings recently there has been a renewed focus on the control of infections and especially those that are believed to be caused by the treatments people receive (Loveday *et al.*, 2014). These infections are often referred to as healthcare-associated infections (HCAI).

Principles of Microbiology and Virology

This chapter concentrates on the practical aspects of infection control; however, to appreciate your role as a nurse/student nurse in controlling infection, it is important to understand the principles of microbiology and virology. This is so you can discuss the care of patients confidently with colleagues and also explain to patients and relatives the implications of any infection they might have or the potential for cross-infection to and from others. The primary and secondary responses to infection and the associated immune response can be reviewed in an anatomy and physiology textbook (e.g. Peate and Evans, 2020, Chapter 17) and other principles like the classification of bacterial and viruses can be revised in specific infection control texts (e.g. Watson *et al.*, 2016).

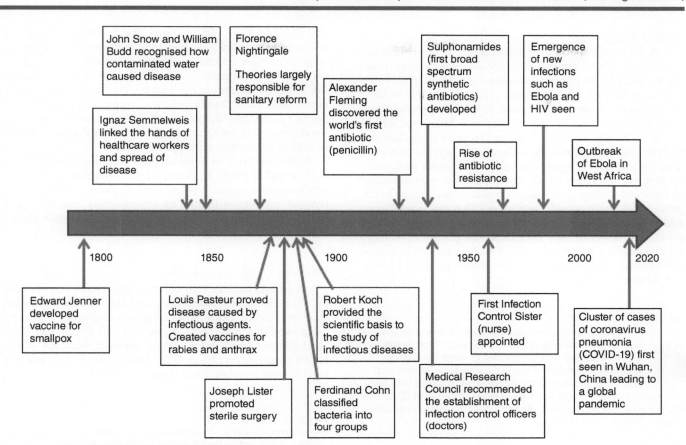

Figure 16.1 Infection control measures – historical timeline.

Jot This Down

Consider whether you can answer these questions.

- How would you describe what bacteria are to a patient?
- Can you explain to a fellow student the difference between a bacterium and a virus?
- Aside from bacteria and viruses, what other infectious organisms do you know of?
- Name three common human diseases caused by viruses.

Preventing the Spread of Infection

Broadly speaking, the spread of infections can be prevented at two levels. First, at the individual level using standard precautions and the isolation of patients. Second, at a population level through public health measures which include surveillance and preventive treatments, principally through social distancing measures and vaccination programmes.

Standard Precautions

Standard precautions (previously called universal precautions) should be applied across all healthcare settings to prevent the transmission of blood-borne and other infections in body substances where potentially infectious materials are present.

These precautions include:

- Routine use of barriers (such as gloves and/or goggles) when anticipating contact with blood or body fluids
- Washing hands and other skin surfaces immediately after contact with blood or body fluids
- Careful handling and disposing of sharp instruments during and after use
- Isolating infected patients
- Respiratory hygiene or cough etiquette.

Monitoring and surveillance are also undertaken to track infections and help prevent the spread of infection (Ruckert *et al.*, 2020).

The Nursing Associate

Part of the required proficiencies of nursing associates (NMC, 2018b, Annexe B, 8.7) is competence related to safe disinfection and effective decontamination.

When disinfecting contaminated surfaces or equipment, it is crucial that appropriate materials are used. Training on disinfection procedures and following the labels are important ways to ensure that disinfection is carried out appropriately. For instance, correct dilution of chlorine-based products is needed to optimise effectiveness. Also, knowledge of different disinfectant wipes is crucial in ensuring effective infection control.

Hand Hygiene

One of the most important aspects of infection prevention and control is good hand hygiene. Although seemingly a simple practice, ensuring health professionals clean their hands effectively is key to preventing cross-infection. The importance of hand hygiene was first noted by Semmelweiss in 1847 when he recognised that fever and subsequent death in large numbers of women following childbirth could be prevented by doctors and midwives washing their hands. Although the importance of good hand hygiene has been generally accepted by health professionals, in recent years there have been campaigns across community and hospital settings to increase compliance and ensure health professionals have greater awareness. This has partly been achieved through the introduction of alcohol hand gels which are used to decontaminate the hands. The gels are often more convenient to use than standard hand washing and can be located at the bedside of all patients. However, alcohol gel is not a substitute for hand washing.

Red Flag

Alcohol gels are only effective on visibly clean hands but are not effective against spores, present for example in *C. difficile*. Therefore if you are caring for a patient with *C. diff* you should ensure you wash your hands with soap and water. In some hospitals, if there is an outbreak of *C. diff* the alcohol gels may be removed. You may need to explain why this is so to patients and relatives.

Cleaning hands in a clinically effective way requires a standard and methodical approach to ensure all the surfaces on the hands are clean. Figure 16.2 describes the process.

It should be noted that the hands need to be wet before the soap is applied and that thorough drying is as important as the process of washing. In healthcare settings, hands should be dried with paper towels as warm air hand dryers can increase the spread of infection.

It is also important that arms are 'bare below the elbows' to ensure effective hand washing. This was recognised by the Department of Health in 2008 in national guidelines for hand hygiene but caused some controversy as it meant some health professionals needed to amend dress codes, for example, doctors no longer wearing long-sleeved white coats. Complying with 'bare below the elbows' policies includes not wearing wrist watches, rings (other than plain wedding bands) or acrylic nails.

Primary Care

Uniforms usually have short sleeves but often in community, social care and nursing home settings, uniform is not always worn and so thought needs to be given in these cases to ensure the 'bare below the elbows' principles can be applied if clinical care of any sort is performed. NICE has produced guidance for primary and community care which includes dress code guidance (NICE, 2017).

The NHS updated its advice in response to concerns that some health professionals wish to keep their arms covered for cultural, religious or other reasons (e.g. extensive tattoos) (NHS England and NHS Improvement, 2020). The Royal College of Nursing (RCN, 2013) has produced general evidence-based guidance for nurses' uniform and work wear and healthcare employers and practice placements will have local uniform policies which you should consult. If there is any doubt then advice should be sought from infection control nurse specialists.

Within the NHS in England, there is now a standard hand hygiene policy (NHS England and NHS Improvement, 2019) which embeds evidence-based hand hygiene in practice and lays out the responsibilities of organisations, managers and staff regarding hand hygiene and personal protective equipment use.

When to Clean Your Hands

It is important to clean your hands at appropriate times to protect the patient and yourself. The situations in which you should clean your hands, either by washing with soap and water or by using hand gels, have been summarised into five moments for hand hygiene which are based on evidence from the World Health Organization (Figure 16.3). They define the key times for hand hygiene in a simple and standardised way.

What To Do If . . .

If you notice that a doctor or other healthcare professional (HCP) has not cleaned their hands when they are about to examine a patient, you should be polite and matter of fact and suggest that they sanitise their hands. You may want to indicate where the alcohol hand rub is by saying something like: 'There's alcohol gel on the table . . .'. Or you may clean your own hands which might prompt your colleague. Remember you need to balance the protection of your patient with ensuring the patient maintains confidence in your colleague and you maintain a good working relationship with them. If a HCP continues to flout good hand hygiene practice, speak to a more senior nurse.

Personal Protective Equipment (PPE)

Gloves, masks, protective eyewear and chin-length plastic face shields are examples of personal protective equipment (PPE). PPE must be provided and worn by staff in all instances where they will or may come into contact with blood or body fluids. This includes, but is not limited to, dentistry, phlebotomy, processing of any bodily fluid specimen and postmortem procedures. See Figure 16.4 for further information.

In addition to knowing the appropriate PPE based on transmission risk, skills in donning and doffing are also crucial. Donning refers to the procedures for putting on the PPE whereas doffing refers to the sequence in removing PPE. Ideally, donning requires supervision by another colleague to ensure that PPE is properly fitted. Consequently, doffing should follow a sequence that starts from the most to the least contaminated part of the PPE.

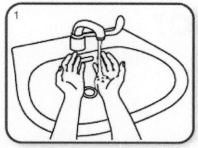

Wet hands with water

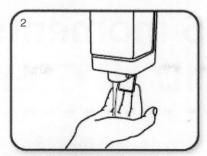

Apply enough soap to cover all hand surfaces

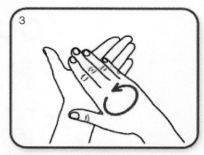

Rub hands palm to palm

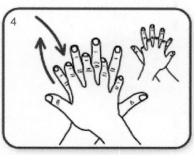

Right palm over the back of the other hand with interlaced fingers and vice versa

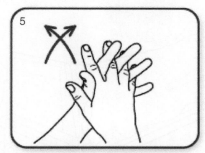

Palm to palm with fingers interlaced

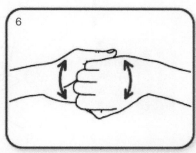

Backs of fingers to opposing palms with fingers interlocked

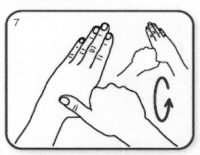

Rotational rubbing of left thumb elasped in right palm and vice versa

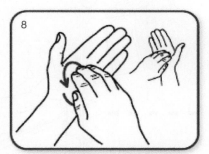

Rotational rubbing, backwards and forwards with clasped fingers of right hand in left palm and vice versa

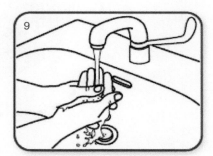

Rinse hands with water

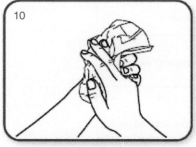

Dry thoroughly with towel

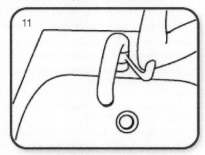

Use elbow to turn off tap

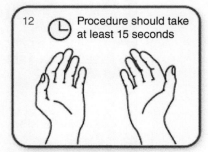

Procedure should take at least 15 seconds

...and your hands are safe

Figure 16.2 Hand washing technique – best practice. *Source:* World Health Organisation.

Your 5 moments for
HAND HYGIENE

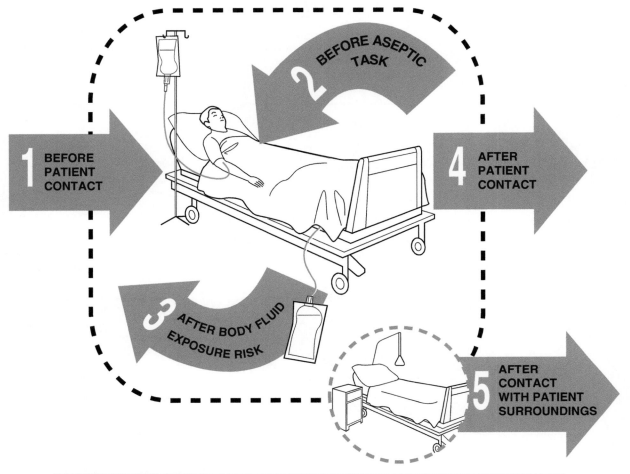

1	**BEFORE PATIENT CONTACT**	WHEN?	Clean your hands before touching a patient when approaching him or her
		WHY?	To protect the patient against harmful germs carried on your hands
2	**BEFORE AN ASEPTIC TASK**	WHEN?	Clean your hands immediately before any aseptic task
		WHY?	To protect the patient against harmful germs, including the patient's own germs, entering his or her body
3	**AFTER BODY FLUID EXPOSURE RISK**	WHEN?	Clean your hands immediately after an exposure risk to body fluids (and after glove removal)
		WHY?	To protect yourself and the health-care environment from harmful patient germs
4	**AFTER PATIENT CONTACT**	WHEN?	Clean your hands after touching a patient and his or her immediate surroundings when leaving
		WHY?	To protect yourself and the health-care environment from harmful patient germs
5	**AFTER CONTACT WITH PATIENT SURROUNDINGS**	WHEN?	Clean your hands after touching any object or furniture in the patient's immediate surroundings, when leaving - even without touching the patient
		WHY?	To protect yourself and the health-care environment from harmful patient germs

Figure 16.3 **Five moments for hand hygiene.**

Gloves

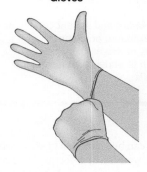

Protective gloves are recommended when dealing with blood or body fluids
- EN374 standard gloves are recommended, rather than latex, to prevent allergy.
- Gloves must be changed after each client.
- Gloves should be worn:
  - When working with blood, blood products, semen, vaginal secretions and any other potentially contaminated body fluids such as cerebrospinal fluid, amniotic fluid and saliva
  - When touching mucous membranes or breaks in the skin
  - When performing or assisting with any invasive procedures, such as venepuncture or surgery
  - When working in situations where hand contamination may occur, such as with an uncooperative patient
  - When the healthcare practitioner has cuts, scratches or other breaks in their own skin

Masks, goggles and visors

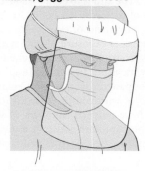

Masks, goggles and/or face shields should be worn
- During aerosol generating procedures
- During all invasive procedures and any procedure in which blood or body fluids may spatter or become airborne, e.g. during endoscopic procedures, during surgery
- During procedures in which heavy bleeding or other extensive fluid loss (such as peritoneal fluid) may occur

259

Gowns and plastic aprons

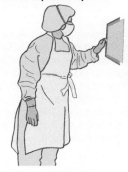

Gowns or aprons should be used when extensive fluid loss may occur
Reusable PPE must be cleaned and decontaminated or laundered by the employer. Lab coats and scrubs are generally considered to be worn as uniforms or personal clothing. When contamination is reasonably likely, protective gowns should be worn. If lab coats or scrubs are worn as PPE, they must be removed as soon as practical and laundered by the employer.

Disposal of equipment

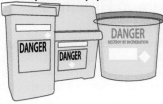

All equipment should be disposed of appropriately to prevent cross contamination
There is now a universal colour-coded system in use across the UK health service.

Needles must not be re-sheathed or re-capped after they are used. Syringes, needles and scalpel blades should be placed immediately in puncture-resistant containers ('sharps-bins'). Whenever possible, small sharps boxes should be taken to the bed side or point of care. (see Chapter 49)

Personal activities

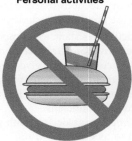

Personal activities
- Eating (including sweets and chocolates), drinking, smoking, applying cosmetics or lip balm and handling contact lenses should be prohibited in work areas that carry the potential for occupational exposure
- Food and drink must not be stored in refrigerators, freezers or cabinets where blood or body fluids are stored or in other areas of possible contamination

Figure 16.4 Protecting yourself and using personal protective equipment (PPE).

Case Study Religion and PPE

Anurag is a third-year nursing student about to go on a placement requiring FFP3 masks to be worn. His religious belief as a Sikh forbids him to shave off his facial hair. However, for the FFP3 masks to fit properly, facial hair should be removed.

To address this, Anurag has a discussion with his university's placement team and the placement trust. Two options were explored: 1. Anurag's placement should be reconsidered to an area or tasks that do not require FFP3 protection, or 2. The trust provides alternative PPE called a powered air purifying respirator, that protects wearers despite having their beards unshaved.

Isolation or Barrier Nursing

Isolating a patient in a single room may take place either to protect others from infection (source isolation) or to protect the patient themselves from infection (protective isolation).

Source isolation is used for patients who are infected with, or colonised by, infectious agents that require additional precautions over and above the standard precautions used with all patients. Common reasons for source isolation include infections that cause diarrhoea and vomiting and infections that are spread through the air. The patient's other nursing and medical needs must always be taken into account and infection control precautions may need to be modified accordingly, for example if a patient needs monitoring in high-dependency or intensive care facilities. Where insufficient single rooms are available for source isolation, they should be allocated to those patients who pose the greatest risk with advice being given by infection control nurse specialists. As a general rule, patients with diarrhoea and vomiting, or serious airborne infections such as tuberculosis, will have the highest priority.

Patients requiring source isolation are normally cared for in a single room, although outbreaks of infection may require affected patients to be nursed in a cohort, that is, isolated as a group. This is sometimes referred to as cohorting. A cohort is a designated group with similar infection or exposure risk. For instance, in large-scale outbreaks such as the coronavirus pandemic, cohorting requires classification based on a screening test. Patients who test positive for the virus will be nursed together as a cohort. Cohorting may also occur among healthcare professionals attending to the patient. Staff exposed to the potential source of infection are limited by breaking the staff group into teams. This may mean that staff may be isolated also in variable periods of time. The duration may vary, being as short as one hospital shift or longer. The needs of both the patients and the staff must be taken into account to ensure sustainable practice and protect well-being.

What to Do If . . .

What would you do if you discovered that you have a tear or a breach of your PPE during care of a patient with a highly infectious condition (e.g. Ebola)?

- Alert a colleague to take over your care responsibilities, leave the work area and proceed immediately to the doffing area.

- Assess the exposure and inform your line manager immediately.
- Depending on the type of exposure and patient condition, administer the relevant postexposure procedures (i.e. blood-borne or respiratory pathogens).
- Report to Occupational Health to undergo postexposure surveillance and/or prophylaxis.
- Document the incident.

Zoning is another practice that can be employed to achieve physical separation from potential sources of infection. Cohorting designates a group of patients, whereas zoning designates physical areas based on exposure risk. The aim is to contain sources of infection and mitigate the risk of exposure. In doing so, traffic flow of people, distancing and movement of equipment can be controlled to further reduce the risk of exposure. Visible signages such as colour-coded prompts, controlled access to entry and exit points and staff training are measures used in zoning.

Protective isolation is used for patients who are particularly at risk of infection, including people with compromised immune systems. These patients often have reduced numbers of white blood cells called neutrophils; this condition is known as neutropenia and people suffering from it are described as neutropenic.

Care, Dignity and Compassion

Being nursed in a single room can literally be very isolating for patients (Barratt et al., 2010). Consider ways in which isolation can be reduced, contact with the patient's wider network maintained and emotional support provided. Chew et al. (2020) reviewed and synthesised several studies concerning patient responses to isolation as a result of infection outbreaks. The authors advocated the use of creative solutions such as technology to provide support to patients while maintaining safety.

Surveillance of Common Healthcare-associated Infections

There are a number of healthcare-associated infections that are monitored nationally (Public Health England, 2018). Every quarter the data collected in the enhanced surveillance are used to produce epidemiological commentaries with the aim of contributing to a better evidence base regarding risk factors for infection. Information is largely collected for the most serious infections which cause bloodstream infections (bacteraemia) or severe illness. The infections that are monitored include:

- *Bacteraemias* including meticillin-resistant *Staphylococcus aureus* (MRSA), meticillin-sensitive *Staphylococcus aureus* (MSSA), *Escherichia coli* (*E.coli*) bacteraemia and glycopeptide-resistant enterococci (GRE) bacteraemia. The latter was previously known as vancomycinresistant enterococci (VRE) and is sometimes still referred to as such by clinicians.
- *Clostridioides difficile* (*C. diff*) *infection* associated with severe diarrhoea (previously referred to as *Clostridium difficile*, the name has been slightly changed recently to reflect better scientific knowledge of the organism).

- *Klebsiella* species and *Pseudomonas aueruginosa*: these two bacteria have been found to be another major cause of blood-stream infections leading to hospitalisation.
- *Surgical site infections*.

Jot This Down

Access the national statistics websites where mandatory surveillance figures and reports are provided (Tip: use a search engine to search for 'HCAI surveillance Country Name', e.g. 'HCAI surveillance Northern Ireland'). Have a look at the data for any infections you have encountered in patients in practice.

- What strikes you about the data on MRSA? Why do you think the number of cases has fallen?
- Look at the data for *C. diff*. Find the data for the hospital or healthcare organisation you are associated with and compare their rates to other trusts.
- Look at the data on surgical site infections and see how wound infections vary between different surgical specialties.

Common Healthcare-associated Infections

Over the last two decades, increased attention has been given to the control of infections that may either be caused by or associated with the treatments people receive. These infections are often referred to as healthcare-associated infections (HCAI) or iatrogenic infections, meaning that they are an adverse effect or complication arising from medical or healthcare treatment. Examples of these infections include meticillin-resistant *Staphylococcus aureus* (MRSA) and *Clostridioides difficile* (*C. diff*). Norovirus can spread quickly between people in close contact, including hospitals, but is also evident in community settings.

Meticillin-resistant *Staphylococcus aureus* (MRSA)

Meticillin-resistant *S. aureus* has been a major infection control challenge in the UK and internationally during the past decade. It has led to public concern about hospital safety and had a major effect on government health policy. Guidelines to reduce the risk of transmission (NICE, 2018; Gould, 2011) emphasise the importance of surveillance, decolonisation strategies, standard infection prevention and control precautions, and antibiotic stewardship.

MRSA – Key Facts

Meticillin-resistant *S. aureus* is a strain of *Staphylococcus aureus* which is resistant to meticillin and other antibiotics. It is an organism that colonises the skin, particularly the nose, skinfolds, hairline, perineum and navel. It commonly survives in these areas without causing infection – a state known as colonisation. A patient becomes clinically infected if the organism invades the skin or deeper tissues and multiplies.

Meticillin-resistant *S. aureus* is prevalent in healthcare environments because individuals tend to be older, sicker and weaker than the general population, which heightens their vulnerability to infection through weakened immunity. In addition, these environments involve a great many people living and working together closely, which provides perfect conditions for transferring MRSA.

The symptoms of a person with MRSA vary depending on what part of the body is infected. Common symptoms include redness, swelling and tenderness at the site of infection. Sometimes, people may carry MRSA without having any symptoms. In order to reduce the spread of MRSA, healthcare staff should ensure that they wash their hands thoroughly between patients (NICE, 2018).

Public Concern about MRSA

During the early 2000s, public concern about the rising numbers of people with MRSA came to the fore. Media campaigns were led by patient groups and the press included stories which led the public to see MRSA as a new 'super-bug'. Although the number of cases of MRSA has now reduced in most hospitals, the myths and stories that were abundant at its height are still remembered by many patients and can cause concern and fear. This needs to be taken into account when patients are screened for MRSA and particularly if patients are colonised or infected.

Nursing Fields Mental Health

Infection prevention and control is an important issue in all settings.

People in mental health facilities will often have more underlying physical health problems than the general population, and because of this they are predisposed to risk factors for HCAIs.

Service users should be offered support and training in order for them to feel able to contribute effectively. The nurse should ensure that service users are treated as equal partners in controlling and preventing HCAIs.

Schweon (2019) discusses some of the challenges to providing infection prevention and control measures within mental health settings. These include the need to prevent items being used for self-harm or as potential weapons. This means:

- PPE (see Figure 16.4) must not be accessible to patients
- Care needs to be taken with placement of hand decontamination items, such as soap dispensers, so they cannot be used as ligature points or alcohol gel ingested
- Secure storage is needed for chemicals used to disinfect body fluid spillages
- The potential for sharps containers to be used for self-harm or as weapons needs to be remembered

Patient Information about MRSA

Because of the public concern about MRSA, most patients have some awareness of the term but often lack detailed knowledge. Hospitals and GP practices have developed patient information leaflets and video presentations to explain what MRSA is, importantly the difference between colonisation and infection, and how it is treated.

Jot This Down

From your own experience personally or from clinical placements, reflect on how you would explain what MRSA is to a patient.

MRSA Screening and Decolonisation

Screening people to detect whether they are carriers of MRSA was introduced in all NHS hospitals for elective admissions in 2009 and for emergency patients in 2011. From 2014, English hospitals require all patients admitted to high-risk units and those with a history of a positive MRSA test to be screened (Department of Health, 2014).

This therefore means that methods of screening and which patients are screened may vary slightly between hospitals and in the community and so reference should be made to local policies. However, typically screening consists of taking swabs (see section later in chapter) from the nose and groin. If the patient has a urinary catheter, intravenous lines or wounds then these are also swabbed. In babies the umbilicus is often swabbed.

If a patient is found to carry MRSA then decolonisation can take place to help prevent infection occurring. Complete eradication of MRSA is not always possible but a decrease in carriage can reduce the risk of transmission to others and the risk of surgical wound infection to the patient themselves (Coia *et al.*, 2006). Decolonisation usually takes the form of two treatments; first, mupirocin or neomycin nasal cream and second, chlorhexidine shower and hair washes (Figure 16.5). Treatment should be prescribed or follow a Patient Group Direction and practitioners should note guidance in the British National Formulary (BNF, 2021).

Clostridioides difficile (C. diff)

Clostridioides (formerly *Clostridium*) *difficile*, commonly referred to as 'C. diff', CDI (*C. diff* infection) or CDAD (*C. diff*-associated diarrhoea), is the leading cause of hospital-acquired diarrhoea. Although it was first described in the mid-1930s, it has come to the fore more in the past three decades. In 1978, *C. difficile* was identified as the primary cause of pseudomembranous colitis and shown to be present in the faeces of patients undergoing antibiotic treatment with clindamycin. Further reports showed a strong correlation between pseudomembranous colitis, antibiotic therapy, *C. difficile* colonisation and toxin production. Collectively, these studies and observations revealed *C. difficile* as an emerging pathogen capable of causing severe gastrointestinal disease in people having antibiotic therapy (Voth and Ballard, 2005; Dingle *et al.*, 2017).

Care, Dignity and Compassion

Any diarrhoea-related care plan should address:
- Elimination needs including safety, dignity and the maintenance of privacy
- Appropriate and effective skin care
- Attention to nutritional needs and hydration.

There are several possible explanations for the increase in *C. difficile* disease during the past three decades.

- Better detection methods which have led to an increase in reported cases of *C. difficile*, including mandatory surveillance and reporting systems (see above).
- The high-frequency use of antibiotics and gastric suppressant medications (e.g. protein pump inhibitors like omeprazole) has increased the likelihood of people acquiring *C. difficile*-associated disease.
- As the frequency of disease has increased, hospitals have become contaminated with spores of *C. difficile*, making infection of susceptible patients more probable.

The government has sought to tackle *C. diff* by addressing these issues (NHS England, 2015) with emphasis on clean hospital campaigns and prudent antibiotic prescribing both in hospitals and by GPs to prevent large outbreaks previously seen in the early 2000s which necessitated ward closures and extensive infection control measures.

Clostridioides difficile is present in the gut of up to 3% of healthy adults and 66% of infants. However, it rarely causes problems in children or healthy adults, as it is kept in check by the normal bacterial population of the intestine (the normal flora). When certain antibiotics disturb the balance of bacteria in the gut, *C. difficile* can multiply rapidly and produce toxins which cause illness.

Clostridioides difficile infection ranges from mild to severe diarrhoea and in some cases severe inflammation of the bowel (pseudomembranous colitis). People at greatest risk are those who have been treated with broad-spectrum antibiotics (those that affect a wide range of bacteria), people with serious underlying illnesses and the elderly; over 80% of *C. difficile* infections reported are in people aged over 65 years.

Preventing Transmission

Clostridioides difficile infection is usually spread on the hands of healthcare staff and other people who come into contact with infected patients or with environmental surfaces (e.g. floors, bedpans, toilets) contaminated with the bacteria or its spores. Spores are produced when *C. difficile* bacteria encounter unfavourable conditions, such as being outside the body. They are very hardy and can survive on clothes and environmental surfaces for long periods. Good hand hygiene is needed (see above) with attention being given to washing hands with soap and water as alcohol gel is not effective against spores.

Norovirus

Norovirus, sometimes referred to as acute non-bacterial gastroenteritis or winter vomiting disease, has increased in incidence in recent years. It is a severe but self-limiting infection causing nausea, forceful vomiting and watery diarrhoea lasting for 1–3 days. Most people recover without treatment but dehydration can cause greater problems in the very young and those vulnerable because of other illnesses (e.g. patients with impaired immune system or the frail elderly). Norovirus can occur at any time of the year but it is much more prevalent during winter months, hence the use of the commonly used alternative name 'winter vomiting bug'.

General guidance	Products
Nasal ointment The ointment should be applied to the anterior nares of both nostrils. A small amount about the size of a match head is applied using a clean cotton bud for each nostril. Squeeze the nose gently after applying to help spread the cream inside the nose. 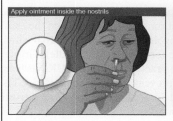 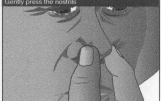	**Mupirocin** (often referred to by its trade name of Bactroban®) Applied 2–3 times daily for 5 days
	Neomycin (often referred to by its trade name of Naseptin®) is used in people who are resistant to mupirocin. It is applied 4 times a day for 10 days.
Body and hair washes The manufacturer's instructions should be followed as they vary slightly between products. Patient should be told to pay particular attention to washing the axillae, groin and skin folds. The lotions are typically applied for 5 days and hair should also be washed with the lotion 2–3 times during this period too.	**Chlorhexidine** (Hibiscrub®) 4% skin wash/shower, daily for 5 days. Skin should be moistened with water before applying the chlorhexidine to reduce the likelihood of reactions. Hair should be washed at least 3 times during the 5 days, if possible. A normal shampoo can be used after the chlorhexidine each time
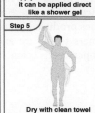 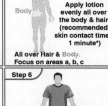	**Octenisan®** is similarly applied in as a lotion. It is also available as hand-mittens/wipes which can be used by patients who are unable to shower/bathe. Hair should be washed twice during the five days.
	Prontoderm foam This is a 'leave on' product. Patients should shower or be assisted to wash as usual paying particular attention to axillae, groin and skin folders and dry with a clean towel. The foam is then applied. It should also be combed through the hair and not washed off. May be an easier option for bedridden elderly patients or patients with sensitive irritated skin.
Treatment should be prescribed or follow a patient group direction, and you should note the most recent guidance in the British National Formulary (BNF 2019). Record in the patient's notes and medicines administration record.	

Figure 16.5 **MRSA suppression**

Care, Dignity and Compassion

When a patient is feeling nauseous or vomiting, the nurse should aim to offer emotional and physical support You could:

- make sure they have a vomit bowl, tissues and water nearby
- try not to move them too quickly, e.g. when sitting up or assisting them to get out of bed
- make sure the patient is positioned comfortably and is not lying flat
- offer cool drinks or flavoured water rather than hot drinks
- suggest eating cold food instead of hot food as strong smells can make people feel sick, and avoid wearing perfume or other strong scents around the patient
- provide a calm and reassuring environment to help patients relax as much as possible and suggest they do breathing exercises when feeling nauseous.

Norovirus is spread easily through airborne droplet contamination, especially if someone has vomited. It is equally spread through contact as the virus can survive on hard surfaces for hours. Prevention through hand washing is vital. This is important for all clinical staff but also for the patient themselves and any visitors. In the past, lack of hand hygiene associated with food preparation has been shown to lead to infection.

In hospitals, a chlorine-based detergent should be used to clean hard surfaces. During outbreaks, this should occur more frequently than standard cleaning. Alcohol gels, while helping to clean hands, are not as effective as hand washing with soap and water (Gould, 2008; Singh *et al.*, 2020).

The incubation period is between 24 and 48 hours. During this time, people can be infectious to others while not yet having symptoms themselves. Therefore, if people are exposed to others with norovirus, e.g. patients in the same hospital bay or passengers on the same cruise ship, care needs to be taken to isolate these patients as well as those with symptoms to prevent spread. In hospital outbreaks, this often means that wards will be 'closed' to admissions, transfers and discharges to isolate both symptomatic patients and those potentially infected from those not affected by norovirus. Hospitals also often impose restricted visiting to reduce the number of people having contact with patients. An escalation approach to closing wards is usually taken, with affected bays being closed first and if necessary, restrictions being placed on the whole ward (Norovirus Working Party, 2012). As well as patients becoming infected, there is also a risk to staff.

Red Flag

 If you suspect that you have norovirus (whether this is confirmed or because you have symptoms of diarrhoea and vomiting), you will need to stay away from the clinical placement while the symptoms are still active and for a further 48 hours after the symptoms subside to ensure you do not pass on the infection to patients or other staff.

Jot This Down

Use the internet to find an example of a norovirus outbreak reported in the media associated with one of the following institutions or environments.

- Hospital
- Nursing or residential care home
- Cruise ship
- School
- Prison
- University hall of residence

Consider the similarities of these cases and how transmission is easier in closely confined environments.

Urinary Tract and Catheter-associated Infections

Urinary tract infections (UTIs) are very common. They can be painful and uncomfortable, but they usually pass within a few days or can be easily treated with a course of antibiotics. UTIs are more common in women than in men, with the main causal agent being *Escherichia coli* (commonly referred to as *E.coli*) bacteria.

It has been estimated that UTIs account for between 20% (Department of Health, 2007) and 40% (IHI, 2013) of all hospital-acquired infections. The majority of hospital-acquired UTIs are attributable to indwelling urinary catheters. It is well established that the duration of catheterisation is directly related to the risk for developing a UTI so regular reassessment of the need for catheterisation is necessary.

Good practice to prevent catheter-associated UTIs falls into two domains; first, actions that must be followed when the catheter is inserted and second, ongoing care (see Figure 16.6 which presents the guidelines in the form of a care bundle). Greater awareness amongst healthcare practitioners in the UK has been promoted in recent years to prevent catheter-associated UTIs, with practice now monitored in acute and community trusts with regular auditing of care bundles.

Antimicrobial Resistance

Antibiotics are needed to treat many infections and have revolutionised healthcare in the last century, reducing mortality markedly. However, they are becoming less effective in some illnesses as bacteria appear to be adapting and finding ways of not responding to the effects of the antibiotic medicines. It's estimated that 25 000 people die each year in Europe because of infections resistant to antibiotics and in the USA the figure is 23 000 people.

The naturally occurring resistance has been further enhanced because of overuse and misuse of medications (Review on Antimicrobial Resistance, 2014). There are therefore campaigns nationally and guidelines produced locally by hospitals and primary care commissioners to ensure antibiotics are used only when needed. This proper use is often referred to as 'antibiotic stewardship'.

Medicines Management

 When helping people with their medicines, it is essential that you provide advice that is accessible and understandable to optimise the therapeutic effects of medicines. People should be reminded that they must complete the full course of antibiotic therapy prescribed, even after feeling well.

Platform 2 – Promoting health and preventing ill health

Antimicrobial stewardship is a required proficiency for all practising nurses in the UK. Nurses are often the final gateway to ensuring that antimicrobial prescriptions are appropriate and follow the established policies. Nurses should challenge inappropriate use and collaboratively work with the healthcare team to improve antimicrobial practice.

Catheter-associated Urinary Tract Infection Care Bundle

Aim: To Reduce the Incidence of Urinary Catheter-associated Infection
Remove catheters as soon as possible
Care for catheters individually

Bundle component	Criteria for compliance with bundle
Check the clinical indication why the urinary catheter is in *situ* – is it still required?	• ALL urinary catheters are indicated. • If there is no clinical indication then the catheter should be removed.
Check the catheter has been continuously connected to the drainage system.	• Urinary catheters must be continuously connected to the drainage bag.
The patient is aware of his/her role in minimising the risk of developing a urinary tract infection or ensure routine daily meatal hygiene is performed.	• Patients are involved in their urinary catheter care and educated as to how they can minimise complications. • Routine daily meatal hygiene is performed.
Regularly empty urinary drainage bags as separate procedures, each into a clean container.	• The urinary catheter bag should be emptied regularly, as a separate procedure, into a clean container. • The use of 'separately' here implies that the same container has not been used to empty more than one catheter bag - without appropriate decontamination of the container, change of personal protective equipment and performing hand hygiene. • If the container is for single use it must not be reused – with or without decontamination.
Perform hand hygiene and wear gloves and apron prior to each catheter care procedure; on procedure completion, remove gloves and apron and perform hand hygiene again.	Decontaminate hands (soap and water or alcohol hand rub/gel). • Before accessing the catheter drainage system. • After glove removal following access to the catheter drainage system. • On removal of gloves.

Figure 16.6 Catheter-associated urinary tract infection care bundle. ***Source:*** **Health Protection Surveillance Centre, Ireland.**

What the Experts Say

'Antimicrobial resistance is a major threat to patient safety and the quality of care. These measures will build on the vital work the NHS is already doing to tackle the overuse and inappropriate prescription of antibiotics, so that in years to come patients can continue to be protected from otherwise lethal infections.'
Sir Simon Stevens, Chief Executive of NHS England

Public Health England (2015) set out different team roles for health professionals to help tackle antibiotic resistance. Nurses should use the principles of 'Making Every Contact Count' to influence public and patient knowledge and expectations of antibiotic prescribing. Nurses have a significant role to play in reducing inappropriate prescribing and can contribute through their roles in:

- Infection prevention and control
- Medicines management
- Immunisation and vaccination programmes
- Promoting health and well-being and immunity.

Care and Treatment for People with Infectious Diseases

Infectious diseases, also known as communicable or transmissible diseases, are illnesses that result from the infection, presence and growth of bacteria or viruses which are pathogenic (i.e. capable of causing disease). Infections may range in severity from asymptomatic to severe and fatal. This section will discuss the principles of prevention, diagnosis and treatment for measles, tuberculosis (TB), human immunodeficiency virus (HIV) and hepatitis C and the global influence of some infectious diseases, such as Ebola.

Measles

Measles is a viral infection spread by droplets passed on through direct contact with someone who is infected. It can be contracted easily by people who have not been vaccinated. People in close proximity are very much at risk which is why outbreaks are often seen in schoolchildren. Measles is a notifiable infection.

The infectious period is from around 4 days before the appearance of the rash to around 4 days after its appearance. It is most infectious before the rash is visible so the virus is often spread before people realise they are infected. Those most at risk of catching measles include babies under 1 year, people whose immune system is suppressed, for example by cancer or HIV, malnourished people, children with vitamin A deficiency and pregnant women – the infection may cause miscarriage or premature delivery. All children who have not been vaccinated are at risk from measles.

The symptoms take about 10–14 days to develop after exposure to the virus (the incubation period). At first people develop symptoms like the common cold. This is followed by tiny white spots on the inside lining of the cheeks. A rash then develops a couple of days later, usually starting on the face and spreading across the body. Abdominal symptoms may occur, including nausea, vomiting and diarrhoea. Symptoms usually last about 2 weeks.

Measles isn't usually serious but there are potential complications that can be fatal, even for otherwise healthy children. These include otitis media, pneumonia, hepatitis, conjunctivitis and encephalitis (inflammation of the brain, which occurs in about one in 5000 cases) (O'Donnell *et al.*, 2019). Although complications involving the nervous system occur in fewer than one in 1000 cases, the long-term effects can be devastating.

> **Nursing Fields** Children
>
> The treatment for most children will be at home with pain and fever-reducing syrups such as paracetamol and they should be encouraged to drink fluids. Hospital treatment, with antiviral drugs, may be needed in more serious cases.

In the UK, measles is now believed to be preventable through the implementation of a long-standing immunisation programme. Children are offered vaccination against measles as part of the MMR vaccine, which is given between 12 and 15 months of age with a later booster dose before the child starts school. However, the uptake of the vaccination in the 1990s and into the 2000s was hampered by now discredited concerns which linked the MMR to autism. The overwhelming body of evidence does not support the concerns and experts are emphatic that the MMR vaccine is safe and effective, preventing illnesses whose real potential to cause damage is greater than many people remember. The lingering fears for some parents continue to mean that vaccination uptake is low in some areas, with large numbers of children not being effectively vaccinated and the potential for outbreaks to occur. This is thought to be the reason for the recent outbreaks (Davies, 2018).

> **What the Experts Say**
>
> Dr Yvonne Doyle, public health director from London, said: 'We are seeing an increase in measles cases across the city, which could be considered an outbreak. The cases are being confirmed mainly in adolescents and young adults – but it's never too late for them to have the vaccine. Those who have not received two doses of the vaccine in the past – or who are unsure – should speak to their GP. There's no harm in receiving an additional dose where there is any uncertainty.'
>
> *Source:* Lydall (2016)

Tuberculosis

Tuberculosis or TB is an infectious disease caused by various strains of mycobacteria, usually *Mycobacterium tuberculosis*, typically attacking the lungs, but can also affect other parts of the body. It is spread through the air when people who have an active infection cough, sneeze or otherwise transmit respiratory fluids. Most infections are asymptomatic and latent but one in 10 latent infections eventually progresses to active disease which, if left untreated, can be fatal in around 50% of those infected.

The typical symptoms of active TB infection are:

- A persistent cough with blood-stained sputum
- Fever
- Night sweats
- Weight loss
- Loss of appetite
- Tiredness and fatigue.

> **The Nursing Associate**
>
> As a nursing associate, part of your competency is proficiency in obtaining vital signs and clinical assessments of your patients. Vital signs are usually an important indicator of a worsening clinical picture. This may include persistent fever, rapid/irregular heart rate and rhythm or out-of-range blood pressure. It is important to work within the limits of your competency and alert the healthcare team to ensure timely escalation and management of care.

Diagnosis of active TB is made following a chest X-ray, as well as microscopic examination and microbiological culture of body fluids. In latent TB, diagnosis can be made using a tuberculin skin test (Mantoux test) and/or blood tests. A blood test known as the interferon-gamma release assay (IGRA) is a more reliable test for latent TB as previous BCG vaccination can affect the accuracy of Mantoux test.

Globally, TB is a very common disease, particularly prevalent in sub-Sarharan Africa and parts of Asia. In the UK, TB is seen more in socioeconomically deprived areas, with cities such as London having the highest rates (Pedrazzoli *et al.*, 2012).

> **Case Study**
>
> **Latent tuberculosis from overseas worker**
>
> Tom, a migrant from South Asia, has been in the UK for 5 years. He has recently been diagnosed with cancer and would need chemotherapy as part of his treatment. During the screening test prior to commencing chemotherapy, he underwent a blood test and was found to have latent TB.
>
> Latent TB occurs when a person is infected with TB bacteria but remains asymptomatic. Treatment choice for latent TB is usually guided by clinical situation. In this case, as Tom's immune system will be weakened by the chemotherapy, his healthcare team advised him to treat the latent TB prior to starting his chemotherapy.

Risk Factors for TB

A number of factors make people more susceptible to TB infections. The most important risk factor is HIV, with 13% of all TB cases associated with the virus. This is particularly the case in sub-Saharan Africa. Tuberculosis is closely linked to overcrowding and malnutrition, making it one of the principal diseases of poverty (Jarvis, 2010).

An understanding of the risk factors helps to explain why different strategies are used to prevent and treat TB. For example, NHS commissioning organisations in some areas of England have targeted immunisation of babies based on the postcode of the parents including those who live in poorer social economic areas as rates of TB in these areas have been increasing. However, universal immunisation of all teenagers, which was the practice between the 1960s and 1990s, no longer takes place as rates are low or non-existent in many areas.

Prevention and Treatment of TB

Tuberculosis prevention primarily relies on vaccination. The only vaccine currently available is the bacillus Calmette–Guérin (BCG). The BCG is effective against disease in childhood but confers inconsistent protection against contracting pulmonary TB and the immunity it produces decreases after about 10 years. It is the most widely used vaccine worldwide, but new vaccines are currently in development.

The treatment and management of TB is with antibiotics. Treatment usually lasts 6 months with combinations of antibiotics. Sometimes people find it difficult to take their medication every day. If this is the case then some patients may be asked to join a programme of 'directly observed therapy'. This can include supervised treatment, involving regular contact between the patient and the treatment team (daily or three times a week) to support and prompt antibiotics administration.

Preventing the Spread of Infection

While patients are contagious, which will usually be for up to 3 weeks into their course of treatment, precautions need to be taken to prevent the spread of TB to others. For most people, the best way to do this is to stay in their normal home environment and not to be admitted to hospital. Patients do not normally need to be isolated during this time, but it is important that they take some basic precautions to stop TB spreading to their family and friends, which include:

- Stay away from work, school or university
- Always cover the mouth when coughing, sneezing or laughing
- Dispose of used tissues carefully in a sealed plastic bag
- Open windows when possible to ensure a good supply of fresh air
- Not sleeping in the same room as other people as coughing or sneezing can occur without realising it.

Unless there is a clear clinical or socioeconomic need, such as homelessness, people with TB should not be admitted to hospital. However, if a patient needs to be admitted then the NICE (2019) and RCN (Story & Cocksedge, 2012) guidelines should be followed. The main component of care for people with TB in hospital is that they should be isolated in a single, ideally negative-pressure room where the air is automatically monitored and vented to the outside (Nursing Times, 2012; NICE, 2019).

Jot This Down

It is important to consider the healthcare advice relating to TB but also not to forget the impact the infection has on patients and carers.

Access both the NICE website to read the TB quality standard produced by UK health professionals, and the 'Truth about TB' website run by patients and carers of people who have contracted TB. Read their stories about diagnosis and care.

www.nice.org.uk/guidance/qs141
www.thetruthabouttb.org/

Using this information, what are your main priorities for care of a patient diagnosed with TB?

What the Experts Say

Tracey, a TB clinical nurse specialist, says:
'I have treated many people with TB; most patients have other needs in addition to their TB treatment as they are vulnerable due to poverty and often don't speak English well. Being a TB nurse specialist allows me to combine the science and art of nursing as I need to understand the pathology of the disease and treatment but the role also requires care, compassion and creativity to tailor a plan of care that will be followed by the patient.'

267

Blood-borne Pathogens

Blood-borne pathogens include any human pathogens present in human blood, but they may also be present in other body fluids. Blood-borne pathogens include HIV, hepatitis B (HBV), hepatitis C (HCV), hepatitis D (HDV), malaria, syphilis, babesiosis, brucellosis, leptospirosis, arboviral infections, relapsing fever, Creutzfeldt–Jakob disease, adult T-cell leukaemia/lymphoma (caused by HTLV-I), HTLV-I-associated myelopathy, diseases associated with HTLV-II and viral haemorrhagic fever.

Human Immunodeficiency Virus/Acquired Immunodeficiency Disease

Many people, including student nurses, have some lay knowledge of HIV and AIDS. This may include knowledge or myths about transmission of the virus as well as out-of-date information about prognosis and treatments. The aim of this section is to concentrate on the infection control principles associated with the transmission and prevention of HIV, especially precautions and procedures for controlling HIV infection amongst healthcare workers. Other specialist texts or articles should be referred to in relation to the care of people living with HIV and treatment of AIDS (e.g. Nursing Times, 2011; Peate, 2019a,b). The British HIV Association has published evidence-based standards of care for people with HIV (BHIVA, 2018). The standards are grouped into 12 themes prioritised as being the most important issues for the care of people with HIV.

HIV Transmission Three factors are needed for HIV to be transmitted (Evans, 2011):

1. An HIV source
2. A sufficient dose of the virus (viral load)
3. Access to the bloodstream of another person.

Different levels and concentrations of HIV have been found in most bodily fluids of infected persons, but only blood, semen, breast milk and vaginal and cervical secretions have been shown to transmit HIV infection.

Transmission occurs mainly through sexual contact with an infected person. The risk of transmission depends on sexual practices, with receptive anal contact without a condom carrying the greatest risk. This is due to the larger surface area of mucous membranes involved. Indeed, receptive partners are at greater risk for transmission of any sexually transmitted infection (STI), including HIV.

Care, Dignity and Compassion

As a nurse, you should remember that sexual identity and gender preference do not always predict behaviour, and that assumptions should not be made about risk of transmission. Safer sex practices should be advocated to all patients and clients.

Professional and Legal Issues: HIV and Equality Act 2010

HIV is one of the few specified disabilities that is cited under the Equality Act of 2010. As such, persons diagnosed with HIV would be protected under the Act from discrimination.

Another common mechanism for transmission of HIV is injection drug use when needles, syringes and other drug use equipment are shared. More rarely, HIV may be transmitted through transfusions of blood or blood products. This is now very uncommon in developed countries as blood is screened for HIV antibodies. HIV can also be transmitted during tattooing or during blood-sharing activities such as 'blood brother' rituals where blood is exchanged or contaminated equipment is shared.

An HIV-positive woman can transmit HIV to her baby during pregnancy, at the time of birth or while breastfeeding. Women newly or recently infected with HIV or those in the later stages of AIDS tend to have higher viral loads and may be more infectious.

Other sexually transmitted infections, such as syphilis, gonorrhoea, genital warts, human papillomavirus (HPV), trichomoniasis, scabies, herpes and chlamydia, can make treatment more complex. Equally, having sores, lesions or inflammation from STIs make the skin or mucous membrane more vulnerable to other infections, including HIV.

HIV Prevention and Risk Reduction HIV/AIDS is preventable. Prevention should be part of a more general sexual health education programme as the prevalence of other preventable STIs has risen. Screening for STIs is recommended since many of those infected do not show symptoms.

The introduction of standard precautions in healthcare has unquestionably prevented thousands of cases of HIV/AIDS, but because the virus is transmitted through behaviours that many people find pleasurable (sexual activity and injection drug use), prevention is more complex. Prevention needs to begin with education and counselling about sexual practices and injection drug use. An unprejudiced approach needs to be adopted with recognition that for many people, 'just saying no' is not a realistic option and therefore there is a need for basic, practical, 'how to' information to reduce risk.

Global Influence of Infectious Disease

Some infectious diseases which previously would not have been considered in the UK or the Western world have recently gained prominence. This is partly due to awareness raised through organisations such as the World Health Organization but also because increasingly greater numbers of people travel and migrate, meaning infections contracted in other parts of the world have significance for healthcare locally.

People travelling to countries where specific infectious diseases are a risk should take advice from their GP or a specialist travel health clinic. Many of these clinics are run by nurse practitioners, with travel nursing being recognised as a public health specialty. You may wish to consider an elective placement or future work in one of these areas if you are interested in this aspect of healthcare.

Prevention is the primary defence and control for many of these infectious diseases. In many cases, this may require people to be vaccinated before travel or to take medications around the time they are at risk.

Platform 2 – Promoting Health and Preventing Ill Health

Part of the proficiency of professional nurses is evidence-based practice around the area of immunisation. Practising nurses should be competent in understanding and translating the best available evidence in counselling patients regarding vaccination. Information should be based on the best available scientific evidence to enable patients to make an informed choice. The Green Book (PHE and Department of Health, 2021) is an excellent resource for information about vaccines for vaccine-preventable diseases in the UK.

Ebola

Ebola is an infectious disease which has become prominent in the media recently. It is a viral haemorrhagic fever (Ward, 2016), first recorded in 1976 and occurring mainly in Africa. The largest outbreak occurred between 2013 and 2016 in west Africa with estimates of around 30 000 people infected and 11 000 deaths. High-profile cases of healthcare workers who became infected while working in Africa have received wide attention in the press.

Signs and symptoms typically start between 2 days and 3 weeks after the virus is contracted and can include fever, sore throat, muscular pain and headaches. This is followed by bleeding into the skin, mucous membranes, organs and gastrointestinal tract with vomiting, diarrhoea, rash and decreased functioning of the liver and kidneys. This leads to low blood pressure from fluid loss, and typically follows 6–16 days after symptoms appear.

Ebola is transmitted in the blood and body fluids. When caring for a patient with Ebola, strict isolation, in the UK in negative-pressure rooms, is needed together with staff wearing PPE that leaves no skin exposed. These measures are recommended for those caring for people with Ebola and also for anyone who may handle objects contaminated by an infected person's body fluids or handling bodies after death. Healthcare personnel need training to put on and remove PPE to ensure that measures adopted remain effective.

You need to be aware of the principles regarding the prevention and treatment of Ebola so you can explain these to concerned patients or service users, especially if they have recently arrived in the UK from Africa. You also need to understand the importance of precautions should you work in an area where Ebola is present. The Public Health England (2019) website contains detailed guidance on the clinical management of Ebola.

Case Study

UK Nurse and Ebola
Pauline Cafferkey, a Scottish nurse, contracted the Ebola virus while working in Sierra Leone in 2014 during an Ebola epidemic. She was successfully treated at the Royal Free Hospital in London in a high-level isolation unit. Nine months after her treatment, she developed some complications from the disease. She has since recovered and was able to give birth to healthy twin boys (BBC News, 2019).

Coronavirus Virus Disease of 2019 (COVID-19)

Key Facts

COVID-19 is a pandemic viral infection first discovered in Wuhan, China, in 2019. Other names associated with this infection are severe acute respiratory syndrome coronavirus 2 (SARS CoV-2), human coronavirus 2019 (hCoV19) and novel coronavirus 2019 (nCoV-19). Coronavirus refers to a family of viruses made up of ribonucleic acid that usually infects mammals and birds. Some coronaviruses may cause mild or no symptoms (the common cold is often caused by a type of coronavirus), whilst others may be severe, such as severe acute respiratory syndrome coronavirus-1 (SARS-CoV-1) in Hong Kong in 2003 and Middle East respiratory syndrome coronavirus (MERS-CoV).

Pandemic

The term 'pandemic' is defined by the WHO as 'the worldwide spread of a new disease'. The definition highlights the potential scale of the infection rather than the severity. In March 2020, the WHO declared that COVID-19 had reached global pandemic status. Although not unique to viral infections, past pandemics typically originated from animal viruses that became infectious to humans, sometimes referred to as zoonotic diseases.

The primary signs and symptoms of the infection include cough, fever and anosmia (loss of sense of smell).

Nursing Fields Children

Symptoms seen in children may vary and in extreme, rare cases may lead to paediatric multisystem inflammatory syndrome (PIMS-TS). Children with this severe condition may present with cardiac, digestive and dermatological symptoms.

Preventing Transmission

COVID-19 is transmitted from person to person through small droplets containing the virus. The main route of entry for the virus is the mucous membranes of the nose, mouth or eyes.

Several prevention strategies have been considered during active transmission of the disease. These include transmission-based precautions, community surveillance and immunisation.

Transmission-based Precautions This preventive strategy is based on understanding of the chain of infection. For COVID-19, this includes social distancing, quarantine and the use of face coverings as public health measures. These are based on the principles of reducing human-to-human contact and limiting the spread of the virus through secretions. Ventilation of spaces is also seen as a significant contributory factor in preventing the spread of the infection.

In high-risk scenarios such as bedside care of confirmed COVID-19 cases, higher levels of PPE that include masks with high filtration standards are warranted. In particular, when performing aerosol-generating procedures (AGP), enhanced levels of PPE protection are required. The Department of Health commissioned an expert panel to produce consensus guidelines on varying levels of PPE (Poller *et al.*, 2018).

Professional and Legal Issues: Fit Test vs Fit Check for Health and Safety

 The coronavirus pandemic has brought into sharp focus the need for hospitals to obtain appropriate respiratory PPE. To ensure that masks provide adequate protection, fit testing and fit checks are essential.

- *Fit test* – is a responsibility of your employer. This is done either qualitatively (i.e. a taste test) or quantitatively (using a special device to measure airflow). Any changes in the masks used by the organisation or the wearer's physical conditions must be taken into account for a retest.
- *Fit check* – is responsibility of the wearer. This is done dependent on the type of respirator or mask. Usually, it can involve ensuring good coverage of the nose and mouth and repeated inhalation-exhalation to ensure there is no air leak.

Community Surveillance Active community surveillance refers to the identification of active cases and isolating these cases until the potential to transmit the infectious disease abates. In COVID-19, and any pandemic, effective systems to identify cases and isolate them from the rest of the population are needed. This can be achieved through effective and efficient screening tests and instituting quarantine measures once cases are identified.

Immunisation During the COVID-19 pandemic, the world has seen the significant impact of vaccines. Through computerised systems, use of artificial intelligence and high-efficiency genomic sequencing, vaccine development has been accelerated and rolled out at an unprecedented rate. With a rapid understanding of the COVID-19 biological mechanism, vaccines that target various parts of the virus were developed. Countries that had an effective rollout of a vaccination programme have seen significant reductions in hospitalisation and death rates within the population.

On the other hand, the issue of vaccine hesitancy emerged as a significant deterrent. This was propagated by public mistrust from sensationalised cases, the spread of 'fake news' and the inadvertent politicisation of vaccines. Consequently, the role of healthcare professionals as advocates of evidence-based practice became more prominent. Government campaigns to address vaccine hesitancy are an important part of public health measures.

Diagnostic Tests and Treatment

There are many diagnostic tests and treatment approaches used by infection control practitioners to identify the cause of infection and determine the best treatment. Diagnostic tests frequently involve a specimen being obtained and then the laboratory performing a series of tests to isolate the organism responsible for the infection and determine which antibiotics the organism is sensitive to. This enables treatment to be well informed and based on evidence about what will be effective. In this section, some common diagnostic tests are explained and the way in which specimens are obtained is discussed as this is frequently either a nursing task or, if the patient is self-caring, requires a nurse to explain how the specimen is obtained. Finally, the section considers the use of technology in infection prevention and control.

Common Laboratory Tests

Microbiology and virology laboratories in hospitals carry out different tests. Increasingly some tests can now be performed outside the laboratory using equipment that enables 'near-patient testing'. This is very helpful in clinical settings such as walk-in centres, emergency departments and sexual health clinics where diagnoses can be made more rapidly and decisions about treatment or whether a patients needs to be isolated can be made. Examples of near-patient testing for infection control can range from a simple urine 'dipstick' test for the presence of protein, suggesting a urinary tract infection, to HIV and CD4 count tests. During the COVID-19 pandemic, the governments in the UK made lateral flow self-testing kits freely available to the public.

Obtaining Specimens

Specimens tend to be obtained most frequently in five ways.
- Blood tests
- Swabs including wound, ear, eye, nose and throat swabs
- Urine samples
- Stool samples
- Sputum samples

Other less common specimens which may be collected include cerebrospinal fluid (CSF) during a lumbar puncture, tissue from biopsies, or bronchial 'washings' in cases of suspected TB.

As with any type of laboratory specimen, there are certain criteria that need to be met for proper collection and transportation of specimens. This will ensure proper stability of the specimen and more accurate test results. Containers need to be clean or in some cases sterile to prevent substances interfering with the analyses. The container needs to have a secure lid and be leak resistant; this is particularly important as other healthcare professionals and ancillary staff should not be exposed to body fluids when handling or transporting the specimens. The local laboratory will issue guidelines and ensure staff know which containers should be used, e.g. specific blood bottles or 24-hour urine collection containers. If in doubt, ring the laboratory or speak to the infection control nurse for advice. In some cases a preservative is added to the container. If this is the case, the guidelines need to be read and followed; for example, it may be necessary to refrigerate the sample or to ensure it is sent to the lab within a specific period of time. Equally, the volume of the specimen needs to be correct otherwise the concentration of the preservative may be too low or too high.

Red Flag

 All specimens should be labelled correctly; this includes the patient's name and identification/hospital number. Care should be taken to ensure that the information on the label and on the requisition form match. Labels should be placed on the container itself, not the lid of the container as this can be removed and mixed up.

All specimens should be labelled correctly. Care should be taken that if a sample is being placed in a fridge, the label is compatible with this, i.e. the ink does not leach. This may be relevant when printed labels are used with some printers.

The collection date and time need to be included on the specimen label. This will confirm that the collection was done correctly. For some timed specimens, e.g. 24-hour urine collection, the start and stop times should be documented.

Blood Tests for Infection

Blood sampling should be performed by a healthcare worker trained and competent in the procedure. In nursing, this is usually a registered nurse, although unregistered practitioners such as phlebotomists can be trained to successfully take blood. As there are many different blood tests, information needs to be obtained about the appropriate laboratory containers (blood bottles) required for specific tests and the amount of blood required. Protective clothing such as gloves and aprons (and facial protection when appropriate) must be used along with an aseptic non-touch technique.

Blood Cultures

Detection of micro-organisms by culture of blood is essential in the diagnosis of bloodstream infections. Accurate positive results provide valuable information to guide antibiotic prescribing which can improve the outcome from blood-borne infections. However, contaminated blood cultures can cause considerable diagnostic confusion and lead to unnecessary antimicrobial therapy so careful collection of the blood using an aseptic non-touch technique is needed.

Swabs

Swabs are used to determine whether there is local infection or colonisation across different parts of the body. Swabs are commonly used to obtain specimens from wounds, ears, eyes, nose and throat (Table 16.1).

Urine Samples

Urine is an important tool for clinical diagnosis (Lee *et al.*, 2021). The clinical information obtained from a urine specimen is influenced by the collection method, timing and handling. A vast assortment of collection and transport containers for urine specimens are available. Determining which urine collection method and container should be used depends on the type of laboratory test ordered. Types of collection range from routine urinalysis completed at ward or department level to complex laboratory

tests. The tests tend to be classified according to the type of collection required.

- *Random specimen*: this is the specimen most commonly sent to the laboratory for analysis, primarily because it is the easiest to obtain and is readily available. Random specimens can sometimes give an inaccurate view of a patient's health if the specimen is too diluted. As the name implies, the random specimen can be collected at any time.
- *Early morning urine (EMU)*: this is the specimen of choice for urinalysis and microscopic analysis, since the urine is generally more concentrated (due to the length of time the urine is allowed to remain in the bladder) and therefore contains relatively higher levels of cellular elements such as protein, if present. The specimen is collected when the patient first wakes in the morning, having emptied the bladder before going to sleep. Proper collection practices and accurate recording of the collection time are important.
- *Midstream specimen of urine (MSU)*: this is the preferred type of specimen for culture and sensitivity testing because of the reduced incidence of contamination. Patients are required to first cleanse the urethral area. The patient should then void the first portion of the urine stream into the toilet. These first steps significantly reduce the opportunities for contaminants

271

Table 16.1 **Swab collection.**

TYPE OF SWAB	PRACTICAL TIPS	TAKE NOTE
Wound swabs	• Obtain the specimen prior to any dressing change or cleaning procedure • Use a sterile swab and gently rotate on the area to collect exudate from the wound • Where there is pus, collect as much as possible in a sterile syringe or sterile container (do not use a swab)	If there are no clinical signs of infection a positive wound swab might just indicate colonisation
Ear swabs	• Antibiotics or other therapeutic agents should not be administered 3 h hours prior to sampling the area • Sample any discharge • Place a sterile swab into the outer ear and gently rotate to collect the secretions	For deeper ear swabbing, a speculum may be used. Only experienced medical staff should undertake this procedure
Eye swabs	• The patient should be asked to look upwards and gently pull the lower lid down or gently part the eyelids • Use a sterile cotton wool swab and gently role the swab over the inside of the lower lid	Hold the swab parallel to the cornea to avoid injury if the patient moves
Nose swabs	• If the nose is dry, moisten the swab in sterile 0.9% saline solution beforehand • Insert the swab into the anterior nares and direct it up into the tip of the nose and gently rotate. • Both nares should be swabbed using the same swab to obtain adequate material	Specify on the lab form if this is a routine admission screen for MRSA or for a suspected infection
Throat swabs	• Place the patient in a good light source to ensure maximum visibility of the tonsillar bed. • Either depress the tongue with a spatula or ask the patient to say 'aahh' • Gently rub the swab over the tonsillar fossa or area where there is exudate or a lesion • Care should be taken not to contaminate the swab by contact with the tongue or oral mucosa on removal	The procedure is likely to cause gagging. It is therefore important to quickly obtain an accurate sample

to enter the urine stream. The urine midstream is then collected into a clean container (any excess urine should be voided into the toilet). This method of collection can be conducted at any time of day or night.

- *24-hour urine collection*: a timed specimen is collected to measure the concentration of substances affected by diurnal variations, over a specified length of time, usually 24 hours. In this collection method, the bladder is emptied prior to beginning the timed collection. Then, for the duration of the designated time period, all urine is collected and pooled into a collection container, with the final collection taking place at the very end of that period. The specimen should be refrigerated during the collection period, unless otherwise requested. Accurate timing is critical to the calculations that are conducted later in the labs.
- *Catheter specimen urine (CSU)*: this method may either be used for a patient with an existing urinary catheter or in some cases a catheter may be inserted specifically to obtain the specimen. Specimens are collected directly from a special port in the catheter tubing via an aseptic sterile technique using a syringe.

Nursing Fields Children's Specimens

For infants and small children, a special urine collection bag is adhered to the skin surrounding the urethral area. Once the collection is completed, the urine is poured into a collection cup or transferred directly into an evacuated tube with a transfer straw. Urine collected from a nappy is not recommended for laboratory testing since contamination from the nappy material may affect test results.

For more information see the Great Ormond Street Hospital for Children's guidelines (GOSH, 2020).

Stool Samples

- The specimen form should state whether the sample is a routine (admission) screening sample or an investigation for suspected intestinal infection.
- If viral gastroenteritis (e.g. Norovirus, Rotavirus) is suspected, the stool specimen should be sent to the virology laboratory. To exclude a bacterial cause, a second stool specimen can be sent to the microbiology laboratory.
- A faecal specimen is more suitable than a rectal swab.
- A specimen can be obtained from a nappy or clean potty.
- Use the scoop attached to the inside of the lid of the specimen container to place faecal material into the container.
- In babies and young children where diarrhoea is present, a small piece of non-absorbent material lining the nappy can be used to prevent material soaking into the nappy.
- Examine the sample for consistency, odour or blood and record observations to monitor changes.
- If segments of tapeworm are seen, send to the laboratory. Tapeworm segments can vary from the size of rice grains to a ribbon shape, 1 inch long.

Sputum

Good-quality sputum samples are essential for accurate microbiological diagnosis of chest infections, pneumonia and bronchitis. Samples contaminated with secretions and saliva are difficult to interpret and can be misleading. The patient should be encouraged to cough, especially after sleep, and expectorate into a container. Physiotherapy may be needed to help facilitate expectoration. You should ensure that the material obtained is sputum and not saliva before sending the sample to the laboratory.

Practice Assessment Document

Use best practice approaches to undertake nasal and oral suctioning techniques

Certain situations such as patients who may be intubated may require suctioning to obtain sputum samples. It is important to use the correct equipment and technique in ensuring a good sample is collected. The use of normal saline prior to suctioning in some cases remains controversial. In your placement areas, ensure that you perform this procedure under expert supervision and follow the local policy regarding the use of saline.

Technology and Infection Control

Technological advances have been used to help prevent and control infection by enabling more rapid diagnoses and faster treatment decisions. Innovations have also been seen in recent years which have helped to develop practice, introduced new medical devices and products, and improved cleaning. Examples include the following.

- Home test kits for HIV and other infections.
- New laboratory tests to enable MRSA screening tests within 1 day rather than 5 days as was previously common thanks to the use of new chromogenic agar.
- Antimicrobial dressings, including those that contain silver, are used to prevent or manage infection in a wide range of wounds with the aim of improving healing (NICE, 2016).
- The use of new products like 'foam' alcohol gel and softer paper hand towels to encourage improved hand hygiene practice.
- Product and furniture design which makes cleaning easier; for example, bed screens made from disposable fabric which can be changed more frequently than traditional fabric curtains have now been adopted almost universally in UK healthcare facilities.
- The wider availability of single-use items which avoid the need for decontamination.
- Rapid genomic sequencing of infectious organisms.
- New vaccine technology such as the mRNA vaccine against COVID-19.

Practice Assessment Document

Utilise aseptic technique when undertaking wound care

Wound care is a skill that you would encounter as a student nurse. Take a proactive approach in observing and developing your skills with your practice supervisor. Pay particular attention to the different dressings used. If you have an opportunity, learn from wound care specialist nurses who are experts in this area.

Kiernan (2009) cautions that while technological advances have resulted in many benefits related to infection prevention and control, advances in some areas have also led to problems. For example, the development of anaesthetic practice and antibiotics has led to more invasive techniques, meaning more people are being treated, with greater survival rates but often subsequent complications. The average age of emergency admissions is rising, and so inpatient populations are increasingly vulnerable. Kiernan (2009) points out that there is also an increasing public expectation that all illnesses are treatable, which may have resulted in a careless attitude towards prevention associated with some infections.

Red Flag Single-use Medical Devices

 You should not reuse medical devices that are labelled with the words 'do not reuse' or display this symbol:

Single-use devices are medical devices that are intended to be used on an individual patient during a single procedure and then disposed of. They must not be decontaminated and reused as this can affect their safety and effectiveness.

Single patient use, in contrast, refers to a device that may be used for more than one episode of use on one patient only, for example a nebuliser.

Conclusion

This chapter has introduced the reader to the principles of infection prevention and control. It is intended that this will enable you to have the knowledge and evidence that underpins this fundamental aspect of nursing care. However, it should be recognised that infection control is a complex and specialised subject and in some cases the information here will not be sufficient and you should refer to a specialist infection control nurse or consultant medical microbiologist for more information and advice.

The chapter has considered why infection control is essential in healthcare settings to prevent disease and promote recovery. The standard approaches to preventing the spread of infection have been described with emphasis given to hand hygiene. The chapter also includes information about the treatment of people with communicable diseases (e.g. tuberculosis and COVID-19) and how their treatment differs from that of people with other infections. The most common healthcare-associated infections that you may come across in practice are discussed, including MRSA, *Clostridioides difficile* and Norovirus, and the common diagnostic tests and treatment approaches used by infection control practitioners are presented. The chapter has included approaches to providing explanations to patients and their families about the prevention and control of infection.

Key Points

- The importance of infection prevention and control has been described, providing the reader with an historical perspective.
- The most common healthcare-associated infections have been discussed.
- The requirement to use a person-centred, evidence-based approach to the treatment of people with communicable diseases has been discussed.
- The unique role and function of the nurse as central in the prevention, monitoring and control of infection has been reiterated.
- The chapter has provided insight and understanding concerning a number of ways of collecting specimens.
- Information giving has been cited as a key factor in the fight against infection prevention and control.

References

Barratt, R., Shaban, R. & Moyle, W. (2010) Behind barriers: patients' perceptions of source isolation for Methicillin-resistant Staphylococcus aureus (MRSA), *Australian Journal of Advanced Nursing*, 28(2), 53–59.

BBC (2019) *BBC News Ebola nurse Pauline Cafferkey gives birth to twin boys*. 14 June 2019. www.bbc.co.uk/news/uk-scotland-glasgow-west-48635678 (accessed December 2021).

BNF (2021) *British National Formulary*. BMJ Publishing Group Ltd and Royal Pharmaceutical Society, London. https://bnf.nice.org.uk/ (accessed December 2021).

British HIV Association (2018) *Standards of care for people living with HIV*. www.guidelines.co.uk/infection/bhiva-standards-of-care-for-people-living-with-hiv/454178 (accessed December 2021).

Chew, Q.H., Wei, K.C., Vasoo, S., Chua, H.C. & Sim, K. (2020) Narrative synthesis of psychological and coping responses towards emerging infectious disease outbreaks in the general population: practical considerations for the COVID-19 pandemic. *Tropical Journal of Pharmaceutical Research*, 61(7), 350–356.

Coia, J.E., Duckworth, G.E., Edwards, D.I., *et al.* (2006) Guidelines for the control and prevention of meticillin resistant Staphylococcus aureus (MRSA) in healthcare facilities. Joint Working Party of the British Society of Antimicrobial Chemotherapy, Hospital Infection Society and Infection Control Nurses Association. *Journal of Hospital Infection*, 63 (suppl 1), S1–44.

Davies, N. (2018) Measles: what you can do, *British Journal of Nursing*, 27(3), 74.

Department of Health (2007) *High Impact Intervention No 6. Urinary Catheter Care Bundle*. Department of Health, London. http://webarchive.nationalarchives.gov.uk/20120118164404/hcai.dh.gov.uk/files/2011/03/Document_-Urinary_Catheter_Care_High_Impact_Intervention_FINAL_100907.pdf (accessed December 2021).

Department of Health (2014) Implementation of modified admission MRSA screening guidance for NHS (2014). https://assets.publishing.service.gov.uk/government/uploads/system/uploads/attachment_data/file/345144/Implementation_of_modified_admission_MRSA_screening_guidance_for_NHS.pdf (accessed December 2021).

Dingle, K.E., Didelot, X., Quan, T.P., *et al.* (2017) Effects of control interventions on Clostridium difficile infection in England: an observational study. *Lancet Infectious Diseases*, 17(4), 411–421.

EAGA (2015) *Updated guidance on occupational HIV post-exposure prophylaxis*. www.gov.uk/government/publications/eaga-guidance-on-hiv-post-exposure-prophylaxis (accessed December 2021).

Evans, N. (2011) *HIV/AIDS Transmission and Infection Control*. www.nursingceu.com/courses/353/index_nceu.html (accessed December 2021).

GOSH (2020) *Collecting a urine sample*. www.gosh.nhs.uk/conditions-and-treatments/procedures-and-treatments/collecting-urine-sample/ (accessed December 2021).

Gould, D. (2008) Management and prevention of norovirus outbreaks in hospitals. *Nursing Standard*, 23(13), 51–56.

Gould, D. (2011) MRSA: implications for hospitals and nursing homes. *Nursing Standard*, 25(18), 47–56.

IHI (2013) *Catheter-Associated Urinary Tract Infections*. Institute for Healthcare Improvement. www.ihi.org/explore/cauti/Pages/default.aspx (accessed December 2021).

Jarvis, M. (2010) Tuberculosis 1: exploring the challenges facing its control and how to reduce its spread. *Nursing Times*, 106, 23–25.

Kiernan, M. (2009) New technology: friend or foe to infection prevention? *Biomedical Scientist*, Dec, 1032–1034.

Lee, H.Y., Wang, J.W., Juan, Y.S., et al. (2021) The impact of urine microbiota in patients with lower urinary tract symptoms. *Annals of Clinical Microbiology and Antimicrobials*, 20(1), 1–12.

Loveday, H.P., Wilson, J.A., Pratt, R.J., et al. (2014) Epic3: national evidence-based guidelines for preventing healthcare-associated infections in NHS hospitals in england *Journal of Hospital Infection*, 86 (Suppl 1), S1–70.

Lydall, R. (2016) Outbreak of measres declared in London after spate of cases. *Evening Standard*. www.standard.co.uk/news/health/outbreak-of-measles-declared-in-london-after-spate-of-cases-a3236556.html (accessed December 2021).

NHS England (2015) *Clostridium difficile infection objectives for NHS organisations in 2015/16 and guidance on sanction implementation*. www.england.nhs.uk/patientsafety/wp-content/uploads/sites/32/2015/02/clostridm-difficile-infect-objct-15-16-guid-feb152.pdf (accessed December 2021).

NHS England (2016) *NHS England launches national programme to combat antibiotic overusage*. www.england.nhs.uk/2016/03/antibiotic-overusage/ (accessed December 2021).

NHS England and NHS Improvement (2019) *Standard infection control precautions: national hand hygiene and personal protective equipment policy*. www.england.nhs.uk/wp-content/uploads/2019/03/national-policy-on-hand-hygiene-and-ppe.pdf (accessed December 2021).

NHS England and NHS Improvement (2020) *Uniforms and workwear guidance for NHS employers*. www.england.nhs.uk/wp-content/uploads/2020/04/Uniforms-and-Workwear-Guidance-2-April-2020.pdf (accessed December 2021).

NICE (2016) *Chronic wounds: advanced wound dressings and antimicrobial dressings*. www.nice.org.uk/advice/esmpb2/chapter/Key-points-from-the-evidence (accessed December 2021).

NICE (2017) *Healthcare-associated infections: prevention and control in primary and community care (CG 139)*. www.nice.org.uk/guidance/CG139 (accessed December 2021).

NICE (2018) *MRSA in primary care*. https://cks.nice.org.uk/topics/mrsa-in-primary-care/ (accessed December 2021).

NICE (2019) *Tuberculosis*. www.nice.org.uk/guidance/ng33/chapter/Update-information (accessed December 2021).

Norovirus Working Party (2012) *Norovirus: managing outbreaks in acute and community health and social care settings*. www.gov.uk/government/publications/norovirus-managing-outbreaks-in-acute-and-community-health-and-social-care-settings (accessed December 2021).

Nursing & Midwifery Council (2018a) *Future Nurse: Standards of Proficiency for Registered Nurses*. www.nmc.org.uk/standards/standards-for-nurses/standards-of-proficiency-for-registered-nurses/ (accessed December 2021).

Nursing & Midwifery Council (2018b) *Standards of Proficiency for Nursing Associates*. www.nmc.org.uk/standards/standards-for-nursing-associates/ (accessed December 2021).

Nursing Times (2011) *HIV Infection – identifying and testing patients*. www.nursingtimes.net/clinical-archive/infection-control/hiv-infection-identifying-and-testing-patients-cpd-unit-03-04-2011/ (accessed December 2021).

Nursing Times (2012) Case management for tuberculosis. Nursing practice guidance in brief. *Nursing Times*, 108(28), 15.

O'Donnell, S., Davies, F., Vardhan, M. & Nee, P. (2019) Could this be measles? *Emergency Medicine Journal*, 36(5), 310–314.

Peate, I. (2019a) Older people with HIV. *British Journal of Healthcare Assistants*, 13(12), 588–591.

Peate, I. (2019b) Human immunodeficiency virus: a review into treatment, *Journal of Prescribing Practice*, 1(12), 596–601.

Peate, I. & Evans, S. (eds) (2020) *Fundamentals of Anatomy and Physiology for Nursing and Healthcare Students*, 3rd edn. Wiley, Oxford.

Pedrazzoli, D., Fulton, N., Anderson, L., Lalor, M., Abubakar, I. & Zenner, D. (2012) *Tuberculosis in the UK: Annual report on tuberculosis surveillance in the UK, 2012*. Health Protection Agency, London.

Poller, B., Tunbridge, A., Hall, S., et al. (2018) A unified personal protective equipment ensemble for clinical response to possible high consequence infectious diseases: a consensus document on behalf of the HCID programme. *Journal of Infection*, 77(6), 496–502.

Public Health England (2015) *Start Smart - Then Focus: Antimicrobial Stewardship Toolkit for English Hospitals*. Public Health England, London.

Public Health England (2018) *Healthcare Associated Infections (HCAI): guidance, data and analysis*. www.gov.uk/government/collections/healthcare-associated-infections-hcai-guidance-data-and-analysis (accessed December 2021).

Public Health England (2019) *Ebola virus disease: clinical management and guidance*. www.gov.uk/government/collections/ebola-virus-disease-clinical-management-and-guidance#history (accessed December 2021).

Public Health England and Department of Health (2021) *Immunisation against infectious disease*. https://assets.publishing.service.gov.uk/government/uploads/system/uploads/attachment_data/file/954759/Greenbook_cover_Jan21.pdf (accessed December 2021).

Review on Antimicrobial Resistance (Chair Jim O'Neill) (2014) *Antimicrobial Resistance: Tackling a Crisis for the Health and Wealth of Nations*. HM Government/Wellcome Trust, London.

Royal College of Nursing (2013) *Wipe It Out: Our chance to get it right: Guidance on uniforms and workwear*, 3rd edn. Royal College of Nursing, London

Ruckert, A., Zinszer, K., Zarowsky, C., Labonté, R. & Carabin, H. (2020) What role for One Health in the COVID-19 pandemic? *Canadian Journal of Public Health*, 111(5), 641–644.

Schween, S.J. (2019) Preventing infection in behavioral health settings. *Nursing2020*, 49(7), 15–17.

Singh, P., Potlia, I., Malhotra, S., Dubey, H. & Chauhan, H. (2020) Hand sanitizer an alternative to hand washing – a review of literature. *Journal of Advanced Oral Research*, 11(2), 137–142.

Story, A. & Cocksedge, M. (2012) *Tuberculosis case management and cohort review – guidance for health professionals*. Royal College of Nursing, London.

Voth, D.E. & Ballard, J.D. (2005) Clostridium difficile toxins: mechanism of action and role in disease. *Clinical Microbiology Reviews*, 18(2), 247–263.

Ward, D. (2016) *Microbiology and Infection Prevention and Control for Nursing Students*. Sage (Learning Matters), London.

Watson, D., Burgess, A. & Roberts, S. (2016) *Infection Prevention and Control at a Glance*. Wiley Blackwell, Oxford. a/w, perms, content

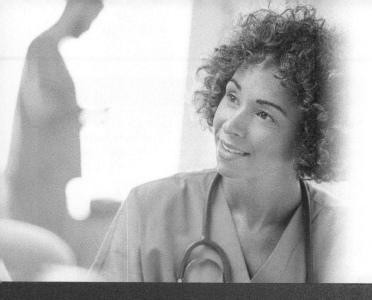

17

The Principles of Nutrition

Pamela Young

University of the West of Scotland, UK

Learning Outcomes

On completion of this chapter you will be able to:

- Identify the components of healthy nutrition
- Recognise factors that lead to malnutrition
- Utilise contemporary nutritional assessment tools
- Identify special group with additional nutritional requirements

Proficiencies

NMC Proficiencies and Standards:

- Observe, assess and optimise nutrition and hydration status and determine the need for intervention and support
- Use contemporary nutritional assessment tools
- Assist with feeding and drinking and use appropriate feeding and drinking aids
- Record fluid intake and output and identify, respond to and manage dehydration or fluid retention
- Identify, respond to and manage nausea and vomiting
- Insert, manage and remove oral/nasal/gastric tubes
- Manage artificial nutrition and hydration using oral, enteral and parenteral routes
- Manage the administration of IV fluids
- Manage fluid and nutritional infusion pumps and devices

 Visit the companion website at www.wiley.com/go/peate/nursingpractice3e where you can test yourself using flashcards, multiple-choice questions and more.

Nursing Practice: Knowledge and Care, Third Edition. Edited by Ian Peate and Aby Mitchell.
© 2022 John Wiley & Sons Ltd. Published 2022 by John Wiley & Sons Ltd.
Companion website: www.wiley.com/go/peate/nursingpractice3e

Introduction

Nutrition is not only vital for health – without food and water, the body cannot function. What we eat reflects both our feelings and our culture.

The food we consume depends on where we live, the availability of food and the means to access it. In 2015, the decline in food poverty reversed and is now steadily increasing. (WHO, 2019a). In the UK, food poverty is increasing. The Trussell Trust has seen an 18% increase in demand from 2019 to 2020, with nearly 1.9 million supplies to an estimated population of 14 million living in poverty (Trussell Trust, 2020).

In contrast, there is an epidemic of obesity in Westernised society. In the UK, nearly one-third of the population is now in the obese category (Baker, 2019). Quite simply, the population's energy expenditure is less than its energy intake, resulting in weight gain. Causes of weight gain are multifactorial and complex but include reduced activity (activity accounts for 5–30% of our energy expenditure), overprocessed food and societal influences (Townsend & Scriven, 2013; Vandevijvere et al., 2019; Sadler et al., 2016; Smith & Toprakkiran, 2019).

Our relationship with food is complex; food is essential for all bodily functions, maintenance and well-being. Proteins are used for tissue building and repair, carbohydrates for energy, fats for insulation and cartilage production, fibre to maintain a healthy gut and get rid of toxins and waste material that accumulates in the body. In the absence of a healthy balanced diet, there is a risk of developing diseases such as:

- Diabetes mellitus
- Hypertension
- Heart disease
- Cerebrovascular disease
- Cancer.

The intake of food and drink is primarily determined by personal preferences but is also significantly influenced by our culture, the society in which we find ourselves and, for some, religious doctrine. Nutrition is more than just 'refuelling the body'; it has psychological, social, spiritual and cultural significance that remains if we are healthy or unwell. For some, mealtimes are a social event when people gather to share part of their day, and special occasions are marked with specific foods, there is feasting after Ramadan, and Christians have special meals for Easter where eggs signify rebirth and a new beginning. We use food to demonstrate affection – special meals are organised to celebrate birthdays, weddings and funerals. Some cultures have stricter rules than others on what should be eaten when we are unwell, and beliefs about the foods consumed to optimise health. There are also culturally determined rituals that need to be observed for food preparation and food eating. If a person cannot wash their hands before eating, they may well decline the food offered, thus compromising their nutritional status.

Before reading the next section, it's important to understand the gastrointestinal tract and digestion physiology. For further details regarding the digestive system, consult McErlean (2020).

The Nutrients

Nutrients are substances in foods required by the body for energy, growth, maintenance and repair. Nutrients can be divided into macronutrients and micronutrients; they can also be organic (i.e. they have a chemical compound that contains carbon, such as carbohydrates, proteins, fats and vitamins) or inorganic (i.e. they do not contain carbon, such as water, minerals and oxygen).

Macronutrients

There are three main categories of macronutrients:

1. Carbohydrates
2. Fats
3. Proteins.

The World Health Organization (WHO, 2021a) suggests that we should limit our macronutrient intake to the following:

- Fats: 15–30% of total energy intake, with saturated fat less than 10%
- Protein: limit to 10–15% of energy intake
- Carbohydrates: 55–75%; limit sugars to less than 10%.

The UK Government developed the Eatwell Guide further to recommendations by the UK Scientific Advisory Committee on Nutrition (SACN, 2015). The guide was developed to ensure the public could comprehend complex information in an easily understandable manner. Figure 17.1 shows the Eatwell Plate guide which underpins all nutritional advice in the UK.

Carbohydrates

Carbohydrates are the primary source of energy. They contain approximately 4 kcal per gram of energy. Patients are often confused when food labels have both carbohydrate and sugar. Patients perceive them as two different nutrients but put simply, carbohydrates and sugar are the same thing but in different forms.

Carbohydrates are formed from three main groups:

1. Monosaccharides
2. Disaccharides
3. Polysaccharides.

Monosaccharides are the most basic form of carbohydrate. They cannot be broken down any further for utilisation by the body. They are highly water soluble so are often known as simple sugars due to the body's ability to use them readily. The most abundant form is glucose which is used in all body tissues for cell energy. All other forms of carbohydrate must be broken down to monosaccharides before they can be used by the body. Other forms of monosaccharides include fructose (found in fruit).

Disaccharides are composed of two monosaccharide molecules and have to be broken down to monosaccharides in the presence of amylase. The most common disaccharides are lactose and sucrose. Lactose is found mainly in milk. Cow's milk contains roughly 4.5–4.8% lactose whereas human milk contains about 7% and represents 40% of the energy provided by breastfeeding mothers to their nursing infants (Shendurse & Khedkar, 2016).

Polysaccharides are made up of multiple monosaccharides and can be made of single or multiple types of sugar. The primary forms of this group are cellulose (From plant based sources) and

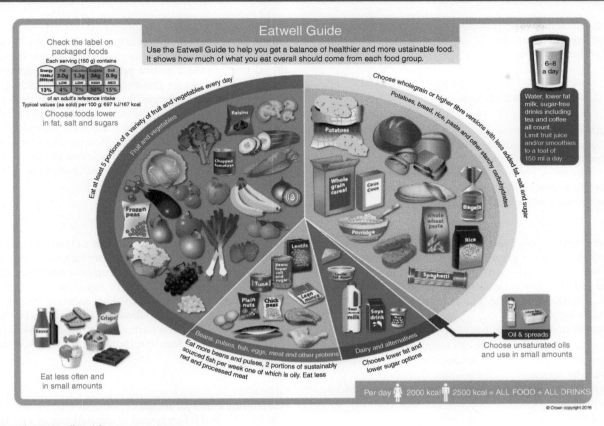

Figure 17.1 The Eatwell Guide. *Source*: © Gov.uk.

glycogen. It is essential to know that excess glucose (a monosaccharide) is not stored by the body in its pure form and instead is stored as glycogen, predominantly in the liver. Access to this store of energy is through the process of gluconeogenesis. The polysaccharides can be described as starchy and non-starchy, starchy being considered the healthier of the two.

Glycaemic Index

Carbohydrates have the most significant impact on raising our blood glucose levels, mainly after we eat (postprandial). How quickly they do this is measured by the Glycaemic Index (GI). Foods that are more readily made available for energy, such as glucose, will have a higher glycaemic index, whereby carbohydrates that are more complex, such as the starchy carbohydrates, must be broken down in the gastrointestinal (GI) tract, so their glycaemic affect is lower but will be prolonged (Figure 17.2).

The British Dietitians Association provide more information on low GI, which can be found at the following website: **www.bda.uk.com/resource/glycaemic-index.html**

There is lots of discussion around the impact of low-GI diets but more recent evidence suggests that low-GI eating reduces obesity and the risk of type 2 diabetes and cardiovascular disease (Peacock et al 2010; Schwingshackl *et al*., 2015).

Simple carbohydrates such as glucose are high GI. The fast release of energy from food sources with a high GI forms the basis of using foods to treat low glucose levels such as in hypoglycaemia or for high-impact activities where fast energy is required.

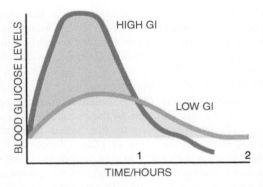

Figure 17.2 The Glycaemic Index. *Source*: © www.glycemicindex.com

Food and fluids such as full sugar drinks, gel sweets or even jam or honey are often used for this purpose.

Complex carbohydrates such as the starchy carbohydrates are more often used where energy release needs to be over a prolonged period. Foods in this group include bread with wholegrains, oats, wholemeal pastas, brown rice and leafy vegetables which contain cellulose which is harder for the GI tract to break down. These form the basis of the lower GI foods and are used to lose weight, and where energy may be required over a prolonged activity such as endurance sports (porridge is a staple for many endurance athletes). Furthermore, foods that have a higher GI rating can have their glycaemic load reduced by combining them with foods that are predominantly fat, as fat slows digestion. One example of this would be:

$$\text{Mashed potato}\left(\text{higher GI}\right)+\text{grated cheese}\left(\text{fat}\right)$$
$$=\text{lower GI mashed potato}$$

It is worth noting that food labels are particularly confusing when it comes to carbohydrates. The public are often confused by the labelling of both sugar and carbohydrate content and perceive this to be two separate items. This is particularly confusing when offering patients dietary advice and requires explanation and support from knowledgeable staff.

Fats

Fats are the most energy dense of all the macronutrients, being approximately 9 kcal per gram. The Eatwell Plate recommendations are that 20–35% of our energy should be from fats.

Fats are described as either *saturated*, those found in animal products, or *unsaturated*, those found in plants, as in seeds, nuts and vegetable oils.

Fats are required in the diet because:
- They are the building blocks for cell membranes
- They are in the form of triglycerides, the primary source of energy in the muscle
- They are needed for the absorption and metabolism of fat-soluble vitamins
- They are necessary to produce bile salts
- In the form of adipose tissue, they protect organs in the body and provide a layer of insulation under the skin, which keeps us from feeling the cold.

The WHO recommends that less than 10% of our fat intake should be from saturated fat (WHO, 2019b). We know that saturated fats, such as those from animal products, significantly contribute to the formation of 'bad' cholesterol, i.e. low-density lipoproteins (LDLs).

There are two types of lipoproteins.

- *Low-density lipoproteins (LDLs)*: cholesterol formation is initially caused by inflammation on the endothelial wall of the artery. LDL fats contribute to that initial inflammatory response, ultimately resulting in plaque formation. These plaques can grow sufficiently large to occlude the blood vessel or break off, leading to myocardial infarction/cerebrovascular accidents or, in diabetes, lower limb ischaemia.
- *High-density lipoproteins (HDLs)*: known as the 'good' cholesterol as they have a protective effect. They remove cholesterol from the arteries and transport it to the liver for excretion. HDLs are found in coldwater fish, such as tuna, salmon and mackerel, and we should consume at least three portions of fish a week to maintain a healthy balance in the body.

When a blood sample is obtained, the total cholesterol is broken down into total cholesterol, LDL, HDL and LDL:HDL ratio. When appraising the results, both the National Institute for Clinical Excellence (NICE, 2014a) and the Scottish Intercollegiate Guidelines Network (SIGN, 2010) recommend both the HDL and total cholesterol should be considered when assessing a patient's cardiovascular risk. This will indicate the proportion of good fat to bad fat and is an indicator of the types of fats the patient is consuming.

Protein

Protein has similar energy density to that of carbohydrate, but its function is much more than just providing energy. Proteins are altered through the digestive process to become amino acids, which the body uses for growth and repair, the building of cells and development of enzymes. Sources of proteins include meat, fish, eggs and dairy products, which are complete proteins. Other sources, such as are found in legumes, nuts, grains, cereals and vegetables, are referred to as incomplete proteins; the process of altering these proteins into amino acids in the body is a little more complex but, while not considered the optimum source of protein, they are perfectly adequate.

Micronutrients

Micronutrients are commonly known as vitamins and minerals. They are available from the food we eat and are essential for normal body function, fetal development and prevention of disease. If we lack any of them in significant quantity, it can lead to conditions such as pernicious anaemia (vitamin B12), rickets (calcium) and night blindness (vitamin A) or affect the body's ability to function normally, e.g. normal blood clotting (vitamin K), cardiac function (potassium) or thyroid function (iodine).

Vitamins

Vitamins are either *fat soluble* or *water soluble*. Fat-soluble vitamins (A, D, E and K) are bound to ingested fats, so a fat-free diet would eliminate these vitamins and result in illnesses. Vitamins C and B complex are water soluble and these vitamins, usually found in green leafy vegetables, tomatoes and fruit, can leach out during a long cooking process and deteriorate during a long period of storage. These vitamins are absorbed in the GI tract; excess amounts are excreted in the urine. Vitamin B12 needs special mention as it requires the presence of intrinsic factor (a substance secreted by the gastric mucous membrane) before it can be absorbed. Absence of this leads to the person developing anaemia.

Due to poverty, malnutrition diseases that were once disappearing are now re-emerging. In the USA and UK, the incidence of rickets was 0 per 100 000 in children under 3 years of age in the 1970s but by the 2000s this had risen to 7.5 per 100 000 in children under 5 years of age in the UK (Carpenter *et al.*, 2017). Table 17.1 highlights the most common vitamins, and the effect of deficiency.

Minerals

Essential minerals are:
- Calcium
- Iron
- Magnesium
- Phosphorus
- Potassium
- Sodium
- Sulphur.

Minerals are required by the body and are found in food. Some manufacturers add extra minerals, such as sodium (salt), in their products, so we may unwittingly consume more than is necessary, which can have implications for health.

Table 17.1 **The most common types of vitamin deficiencies.**

VITAMIN	SOURCES	DEFICIENCY EFFECTS
A (retinol)	Cheese, eggs, oily fish, liver, fortified cereals, cantaloupe melon	Poor night vision, thickened cornea, growth retardation
B (thiamine)	Wholegrains, meat, fish	Beri beri, Wernicke encephalopathy (often seen in alcoholism)
B12 (cyanocobalamin)	Leafy green vegetables	Tingling in nerves, pernicious anaemia
Folic acid (folate)	Broccoli, Brussels sprouts, chickpeas	Neural tube defects (early pregnancy)
C (ascorbic acid)	Citrus fruit, peppers, broccoli	Scurvy, poor wound healing
D (calcium)	Oily fish, eggs, fortified cereals	Rickets, muscle weakness, fatigue

Minerals are essential for:

- Maintaining fluid balance in the cells and interstitial spaces
- Building and maintaining bones and healthy teeth
- Metabolising food and converting it to energy.

Minerals are found in all types of food: meat, fish, dairy, vegetables, fruit and nuts.

Jot this Down

Consider the components of a healthy diet. What do you think may be some of the barriers to accessing a healthy diet?

Malnutrition

The WHO (2020a) defines malnutrition as 'deficiencies, excesses, or imbalances in a person's intake of energy and/or nutrients'. Malnutrition is perceived as limited access to food but it also covers imbalances in nutrition relating to both undernutrition and overweight/obesity.

Undernutrition is commonly associated with countries where access to food is limited but affluent countries have significant rates of poverty which invariably leads to food hunger. Additionally, our family dynamics have changed over many decades. The decrease in extended families, who often looked after their most vulnerable members, has resulted in state responsibility for care. This has seen a rise in vulnerable patients being at risk of malnutrition even in the institutions we once considered safe, such as the NHS.

The British Association for Parenteral and Enteral Nutrition (BAPEN) national survey on malnutrition and nutritional care in 2019 showed a 42% level of malnutrition in England, with 29% being in hospital care (BAPEN, 2019).

Malnutrition impairs the body's ability to respond to disease, repair and grow. The groups most at risk of undernutrition are:

- The elderly
- Children
- Pregnant women
- Those with chronic disease.

Elderly patients are particularly prone to undernutrition as they face issues associated with ageing and reduced mobility such as:

- Reduced ability to go out shopping
- Reduced appetite
- Reduced physical ability, e.g. stroke
- Cognitive impairment, e.g. dementia
- Reduced income
- Low mood due to contributing factors, e.g. depression/isolation
- Bereavement.

In addition:

- 24–35% of older people admitted to hospital are at risk of malnutrition
- They are more likely to have a longer stay in hospital, require more support on discharge and be in need of more care
- 70% of patients weigh less on discharge from hospital than their admission weight (Malnutrition Task Force, 2020).

Pregnancy requires increased calorie intake as well as holistic nutrition to form a healthy fetus. Lack of adequate vitamins and minerals can lead to stunted growth or fetal abnormality due to the following:

- Neural tube defects due to inadequate folic acid
- Iron deficiency leading to low birth weight
- Alcohol intake leading to fetal alcohol syndrome
- Iron and calcium deficiency leading to maternal death (Black et al., 2013).

Children are particularly vulnerable to undernutrition. They require a healthy diet to ensure growth and repair. Undernutrition in children leads to:

- Failure to thrive
- Prevalence of disease
- Stunting of height
- Physical impairment
- Loss of cognitive development.

Screening Tools

The Malnutrition Universal Screening Tool (MUST) is the most commonly used tool in the NHS and is widely used across both hospital and community care. BAPEN provides guidance regarding the MUST tool which you can use to help you understand

and apply this in practice. The tool can be found at the following website: **www.bapen.org.uk/pdfs/must/must_full.pdf**

The screening tool is based on calculating the person's body mass index (BMI), by dividing the person's weight by their height squared (kg/m²).

However, screening requires a holistic perspective and should also include assessment of the following.

- Physical assessment
  - History of recent weight loss
  - Whether the person has dentures and if these fit
  - The person's ability to prepare food or feed themselves
- Social assessment
  - Does the person live at home or are they in residential care?
  - Does the person live alone?
  - Can the person shop for food?
- Psychological assessment
  - Has the person recently experienced a bereavement?
  - Is the person depressed?
  - Is there any cognitive impairment?
- Clinical assessment
  - What is their medical status?
  - Does this affect the person's ability to feed themselves?
  - Does it affect their ability to eat?
  - Does it affect their ability to digest food?

While nurses can undertake screening, a complete nutritional assessment involving biochemical and anthropometric measurements in addition to the data collected above is predominantly done by dietitians or nurses who have undergone additional training.

To complement the MUST tool, and to meet the needs of carers in the community setting, the Patients Association (2018) has produced a Nutrition Checklist which is simple to use and provides patients and carers with practical advice on how to increase weight. Information on the Patients Association Nutrition Checklist can be found at the following website: **www. patients-association.org.uk**

What the Experts Say

The Malnutrition Task Force (2021) provides tips on supporting eating in hospitals and care homes. These include:
- Telling staff of the person's food preferences
- Letting staff know the patient's preferred meal times
- Encourage relatives to bring in preferred foods
- Caregivers should ensure packaging is easy to open
- Food to meet religious or cultural and specialist diets
- Support with eating should be dignified but enjoyable.

Nutritional Support

It is better to keep a person eating before resorting to invasive measures, such as enteral or parenteral feeding. There are many reasons why someone is unable to meet their nutritional demands, ranging from mechanical inability to swallow, such as in a stroke to having poorly fitting dentures that make eating difficult.

Food can be fortified by adding extra proteins such as adding cheese to mashed potatoes or eggs to sauces; extra carbohydrates can be added using cream; extra fats can be added by using butter.

Nutritional supplements often come as prepacked branded formulas; some people tolerate them well but others find the taste, smell and texture difficult. Some taste better at room temperature, while some patients prefer them to be very cold or even frozen and served as ice-cream.

There are three levels of nutritional support.
1. Oral supplements to supplement dietary intake
2. Enteral feeding
3. Parenteral feeding

Supplementary Feeding

Patients who are undernourished and deemed 'high risk' on nutritional screening will need their normal dietary intake to be supplemented to achieve weight gain. To put it simply, their nutritional intake must outweigh their nutritional requirements. To achieve this, patients can have their meals supplemented with high-calorie, high energy-dense foods. The simplest way to do this is to fortify the normal dietary intake. Some examples of this include:

- Swapping to full-cream milk
- Adding full-cream milk to puddings/soups
- Adding in snacks after the evening meal before going to bed
- Exchanging snacks to calorie-rich foods such as scones/ biscuits
- Supplementing the normal dietary intake with oral nutritional supplements such as high-calorie drinks/soups/puddings.

Despite trying the above measures, some patients may not be able to supplement their oral intake. This can be due to many factors such as diseases that impair the swallowing reflex, e.g. stroke/ motor neurone disease, or their nutritional requirements are high due to inability to absorb nutrients in the normal way, e.g. cystic fibrosis, or exceptionally high due to severe illness, e.g. sepsis. The European Society of Parenteral and Enteral Nutrition guidelines recommend that critically unwell patients should receive 80–100% of their energy expenditure (ESPEN, 2016) but this is difficult to estimate so patients should receive a daily calorie intake based on the following equation: 20–25 kcal/kg/day (Singer et al., 2019).

Patients unable to tolerate oral intake may be fed via two routes.

- Enteral (via a functioning gastrointestinal tract) or
- Parenteral (via an intravenous route).

Enteral Feeding

There are various types of tube used to administer feed via the enteral route. Table 17.2 highlights common feeding tubes and some advantages and disadvantages of using each tube.

Inserting a Nasogastric Tube

There are many risks with inserting a nasogastric tube, including migration into the lungs, causing hypoxia and potentially an aspiration pneumonia. Additionally, nasogastric tubes are contraindicated in basal skull fractures. The procedure can be distressing for patients so it is important to provide reassurance and support during the procedure.

Table 17.2 **Advantages and disadvantages of common feeding tubes.**

TYPE OF TUBE	ADVANTAGES	DISADVANTAGES
Nasogastric	· Inserted by nurse/doctor · Can be aspirated (suitable postoperatively) · Can be used for up to 30 days · Tube obstruction less likely · Bedside tube placement with pH strips · Suitable to deliver drugs	· Uncomfortable · Easily pulled out · Easily displaced from stomach
Fine-bore feeding tube	· Inserted by nurse/doctor · Better patient tolerance · Can be used for up to 30 days	· More prone to blocking, especially drugs · Cannot be aspirated (unsuitable postoperatively) · Bypass more readily · Easily dislodged
Nasojejenal tube	· Can feed even when stomach not functioning · Feed directed to jejunum · Feeding not disrupted if need to aspirate	· Must be passed with an endoscope · Tube can kink · Position difficult to establish if it slips · Can be challenging to deliver some drugs
Gastrostomy	· For longer term feeding, more than 30 days · Less likely to block due to large bore	· Surgical/endoscope insertion · Needs regular stoma care/hygiene · Feed can bypass tube and irritate skin · Can affect the patient's body image

281

Information on how to insert a nasogastric tube can be found by accessing *The Royal Marsden Manual of Clinical Nursing Procedures* (Lister *et al.*, 2020).

What to Do If. . .

You Suspect the Tube Has Moved
1. Reassure the patient and explain what you are doing
2. Stop any feed that may be infusing
3. Obtain baseline patient vital signs to exclude respiratory distress
4. Aspirate the tube to obtain gastric fluid to test the pH is still acidic
5. If in any doubt about the position, call for senior nurse/doctor review

The NHS has produced a short film about the risks of nasogastric tube misplacement. The film can be found at the following website: **https://youtu.be/7dSEKQLMa18**

Once the tube position is confirmed by a chest X-ray, feeding is commenced. Patient feeding depends on individual requirements but is usually worked out by a dietitian considering the following.

- Age/weight/height.
- Disease process/route of administration.
- 24-hour nutritional requirement.
- Does the patient need a nutritional rest period, e.g. to get drugs?
- Does the patient need a pause to eat (some patients supplement eating with NG feed through the night)?
- Does the patient need to have bolus feeding to match insulin dosing?

Medicines Management

Feeding tubes are susceptible to damage from many drugs if they are not properly 'flushed' through the tube. This can result in a patient requiring a change of tube which can be distressful for the patient. Always follow your local protocols for flushing tubes in between drug administrations.

Psychosocial Impact of Enteral Feeding

Long-term feeding can result in diarrhoea, constipation, bloating and nausea. This can significantly affect a person's quality of life.

The person being fed in this manner may experience feelings of frustration, loss of control and anger at the perceived alterations to their body image. They may interpret being fed as a return to their childhood and these feelings may impinge on the way they react socially, resulting in isolating themselves from others (Holmes, 2010).

The Nursing Associate

The role of the nursing associate in enteral feeding is to:

· Administer the artificial feed as prescribed
· Document the feed and fluid balance in the appropriate feeding charts
· Identify when there is suspected tube slippage/blockage
· Stop the feed if tube slippage is suspected
· Support the comfort of a patient with a feeding tube placement.

Practice Assessment Document

Students may find that there is no-one in their placement area with a feeding tube. To gain experience caring for patients with feeding tubes, the following advice may be helpful.

- Ask your practice assessor/supervisor to identify key areas where patients may have a feeding tube, e.g. stroke care, critical care.
- Ask to spend time with key staff who would see patients with feeding tubes placed, e.g. gastrointestinal specialist nurses, stroke care specialist nurses.
- Contact the dietitian team to spend some time with them. They see all patients with feeding tubes.
- Gather the documentation required for caring for a patient with a feeding tube and discuss this with your practice assessor/supervisor.

Parenteral Feeding

Parenteral feeding is introduced when a person's gastrointestinal tract is not functioning or accessible for feeding by other methods. Parenteral feeding is inserting nutrients directly into the bloodstream. The solutions infused usually contain amino acids, glucose, fats, electrolytes, vitamins and minerals. Some commercial preparations do not contain all the minerals and vitamins, but these can be supplemented according to individual need. Due to the significant risk of introducing infection, any nutrients added to the individualised feed are introduced under aseptic pharmaceutical controlled conditions.

Red Flag

If an invasive line delivering parenteral nutrition becomes red and inflamed, it may be a sign of line sepsis and must be immediately reported to senior medical/nursing staff.

Parenteral nutrition can be administered through a peripheral cannula or a peripherally inserted central catheter line in the short term, but if the person requires longer-term therapy, a Hickman line or central line is inserted into the subclavian or internal jugular vein, providing central venous access. These lines/devices are inserted in theatre, X-ray environments or under guidance with bedside ultrasound such as in critical care units. Their position is always confirmed by X-ray to verify the line is in position before feeding commences. Feeding via the intravenous (IV) route is high risk for the following reasons.

- Potential for introducing infection
- Risk of line misplacement
- Potential for line sepsis leading to systemic sepsis
- Staff training is required to competently manage the lines

Any patient who has been undernourished who commences feeding via the enteral or parenteral route needs monitoring of blood results for a phenomenon known as refeeding syndrome. This is where significant abnormalities of electrolytes can happen when the patient is renourished.

Weight Loss and Cancer

Approximately 80% of people developing cancer notice weight loss as the first symptom that all is not well; this and pain is what prompts patients to seek medical advice. The weight loss is termed cancer 'cachexia' because the triggers and responses are different from weight loss due to starvation. In cancer, the tumour produces cytokines (chemical messengers) that alter cellular metabolism, so that the tumour has the requisite nutrients to grow and develop. The changes affect the liver's ability to convert stored glucose and promote resistance to insulin; consequently, the person has a raised basal metabolic rate (BMR) and a higher blood glucose level, which depresses the appetite. The cytokines can also alter the motility of the digestive tract, so food takes longer to process, which also affects a person's appetite; they still feel full from the previous meal.

Cancer treatments can also affect a person's nutritional status. Chemotherapy regimens lead to:

- Feeling nauseous
- Dysgeusia (altered taste)
- Xerostomia (dry mouth; as discussed, saliva is needed to commence digestion of food in the mouth)
- Mucositis (inflammation, possibly with infection, of the mucosa from the mouth to the bottom of the oesophagus, which is very painful)
- Dysphagia (difficulty in swallowing)
- Hyperosmia (altered sense of smell, which can affect the desire to eat).

Loss of more than one-fifth of the person's body weight means patients have a poor prognosis and are much less likely to respond to treatment. Approximately one in five people with cancer dies because of malnutrition, rather than the cancer itself.

More information on supporting a person with cancer can be found in Chapter 15 of this text.

Obesity

Obesity now affects nearly 1.9 billion people worldwide. Overweight and obesity are defined as 'abnormal or excessive fat accumulation that may impair health' (WHO, 2020b). Obesity can lead to:

- Type 2 diabetes
- Cardiovascular disease
- Cancer
- Fatty liver disease
- Mobility problems
- Mental health issues
- Fertility problems.

The cost of treating obesity-related diseases such as hypertension and diabetes is having a significant impact on services. The cost to the NHS of treating these diseases is expected to increase to £9.7 billion by 2050 (Public Health England, 2017).

Obesity is classified into distinct categories with the adverse impact on health being greater with each increase in category. Table 17.3 outlines the classification of obesity.

It is worth noting that BMI is based on research from pre-world war adult body types, and it is now recognised that it has

Table 17.3 Classification of Obesity. *Source*: Adapted from SIGN (2010).

CLASSIFICATION	BODY MASS INDEX (BMI)
Overweight	25–29.9
Obesity I	30–34.9
Obesity II	35–39.9
Obesity III	>40

Table 17.4 Body fat types and their function.

TYPE OF FAT	FUNCTION
Essential fat	· Temperature regulation · Nerve conduction · Drug metabolism · Formation of bone marrow
Subcutaneous fat	· Temperature regulation
Visceral fat	· Protection of organs

limitations such as in individuals who have a muscular build, Asian populations with a higher percentage of body fat at a lower weight or even in those with amputations. A valid tool to assess weight-related cardiovascular risk is the waist-to-height ratio.

To weight to height chart can be accessed on the following webpage: **www.ashwell.uk.com/shapechart.pdf**

Jot This Down

What is the impact of your weight on your long-term health? Using the Ashwell chart, assess your own BMI and obtain your waist-to-height ratio. What does this tell you about how healthy you are?

Types of Body Fat

Body fat is essential for normal body function. Table 17.4 highlights the different types of body fat and their function in the body.

Increases in visceral fat have a significant detrimental impact on health. For every 1 kg/m increase in BMI, there is an increased risk of adverse health outcomes of 6–13% (Hingorani *et al.*, 2020).

Causes of Obesity

The causes of obesity are complex and not easily identifiable. Meldrum *et al.* (2017) state that obesity is mostly caused by the 'obesogenic environment'. That is, society now consumes more sugar/processed food in an environment that is becoming increasingly automated, thus calorie intake exceeds calorie requirements. The control of appetite (satiety) is multifactorial but mediated by the hypothalamus via a set of inhibitory and stimulatory peptides.

Obesity in Pregnancy

Women who are overweight are known to be at higher risk of adverse outcomes (Davies & O'Mahony, 2015). Complications can include:

- Spontaneous abortion/stillbirth
- Maternal hypertension
- Gestational diabetes
- Shoulder dystocia
- Increased risk of thromboembolism.

Overweight mothers can affect the future health of their unborn child. A study by Lindell *et al.* (2018) found that overweight mothers were more likely to have offspring who developed type 1 diabetes. Kislal *et al.* (2020) suggested that offspring were at increased risk of cardiovascular disorders including hypertension, insulin resistance and central adiposity.

Tackling Obesity

In the UK there are clear guidelines to manage obesity (NICE, 2014b; SIGN, 2010). Both guidelines have common themes on managing obesity ranging from lifestyle interventions to extensive surgery.

Lifestyle Interventions

These are interventions that can be acted upon by the individual or the community they live in.

- Healthy eating (using the Eatwell Plate model)
- Increased activity
- Goal setting
- Psychosocial interventions
- Behaviour change

Structural-based Interventions

These are interventions that require support from healthcare professionals to achieve shared goals.

- Community interventions to encourage healthy behaviors
- Healthcare staff training
- School years education
- Signposting to community-based support programmes
- Healthy school meals

Advanced Obesity Management

This area will always be managed by specialist teams. Some of their interventions will include:

- Specialist dietitian input
- Cognitive behavioural therapy
- Liquid-based diets
- Pharmacotherapy
- Bariatric surgery.

What to Do If . . .

Consider how you would support a patient who is significantly overweight but needs to lose weight to gain a new hip. What strategies could you employ to support them?

Hydration

A chapter on the principles of nutrition is incomplete without mention of fluid intake. In addition to nutrients, a person requires 1.5–2 L of fluid a day. Women need slightly less than men although will require 300–700 mL more fluid when pregnant or breastfeeding (BDA, 2020).

Dehydration

Dehydration occurs when there is a net loss of fluid from the body, i.e. output is greater than intake. We can become dehydrated due to lack of intake, sweat (insensible loss), urine and faeces. However, older people 65 years and over are particularly susceptible to dehydration as their body water content is reduced (Morley, 2015).

Dehydration can lead to:

- Headaches
- Cognitive impairment
- Renal calculi
- Urinary tract infections
- Delirium
- Lethargy
- Hallucinations.

The kidneys are particularly prone to dehydration as they require an adequate blood supply to ensure renal function is maintained. In severe dehydration, urine output decreases, causing inadequate excretion of waste products. This in turn can eventually lead to acute kidney injury if not treated. Signs of dehydration include:

- Tachycardia
- Thirst
- Reduced skin turgor (less predictive in the elderly)
- Reduced urine output (normally 0.5 mL/kg per hour)
- Hypotension.

It can be particularly challenging to manage dehydration in the community setting as patients find it difficult to communicate particularly if they have cognitive impairment. NHS Inform (2020) recently produced a colour-coded chart which is easy for patients to interpret to assess their level of hydration. Figure 17.3 shows the 1–8 Must Hydrate campaign poster.

You can access the chart on the following website: www.nhsinform.scot/campaigns/hydration

As with food, it is particularly important to monitor fluid intake in vulnerable patients as many are unable to express that they feel dehydrated or how much they have had to drink. Family and carers can support monitoring of fluid intake using pictorial charts representing common fluids, thus facilitating more accurate fluid recording.

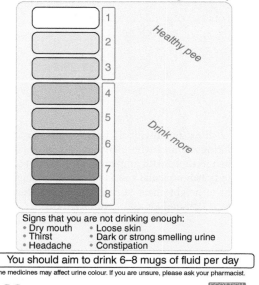

Figure 17.3 **1–8 Must Hydrate.** *Source*: © NHS (2017).

Vulnerable patients in the hospital setting will require monitoring of fluid intake via the hospital fluid balance chart. This can be a challenge in a busy ward setting and may include many forms of fluid intake including oral and intravenous. It is important to ensure fluid balance charts are kept accurate in this setting. Hydration is a key component of patient safety and is currently poorly administered. In a study of a rural hospital's fluid balance charts, 68% of charts were found to be clinically inaccurate (Cole & White, 2020).

If a patient is unable to drink for a substantive period, then intravenous fluids may need to be administered.

The Nursing Associate

The role of the nursing associate in caring for people receiving IV fluids is to:

- Identify signs of dehydration
- Accurately complete the fluid balance chart identifying fluid intake and output
- Identify when IV infusions are not delivering as prescribed
- Accurately document the patient's condition in relation to their hydration status.

What the Experts Say

Cook *et al.* (2019) offered some approaches to improving fluid intake in care homes, including:
- Encourage drinking through social interaction
- Provide prompts to drink
- Offer additional fluids with social activities
- Use adapted/modified larger drinking vessels
- Create a drinking-conducive environment.

Practice Assessment Document

Students often ask how they can evidence their competence in recording fluid intake and output in the community setting, especially when on community placements. Here are some options for the student to consider.

1. If you visit the patient regularly, start a fluid chart. It doesn't need to be complicated. A simple diary for 24–48 hours would do.

2. If possible, involve the patient in this aspect of care. Ask them to help you fill in the chart,
3. Discuss with the patient their common drinks. Using the measuring jug, measure the volume of each drink and write it down to assist the patient in recording their fluid intake.
4. Where possible, use pictorial charts to assist in fluid intake.
5. Enlist the support of family and carers to monitor fluids.
6. If possible, ask the patient to measure their urine in a dedicated measuring jug and record this for 24-48 hours in their fluid diary.
7. Ask the patient for signs of dehydration such as dry mouth, thirst and dark urine (the 1–8 Must Hydrate fluid chart can be left in the house). Even patients with significant cognitive/learning impairments find these symptoms easy to communicate to their carers.

Nutrition in Cardiovascular Disease

Cardiovascular disease remains the biggest cause of premature death in the UK although deaths are declining (Bhatnagar *et al.*, 2016).There are many dietary contributors to poor cardiac health including high-fat/low-fibre diets, processed food high in saturated fat and salt, and excess alcohol intake. Poor food choices can result in:

- Hypercholesterolaemia
- Hypertension
- Weight gain
- Long-term poor health.

In the past decade, UK health policies have provided funding to improve the cardiovascular health of the nation, supporting strategies that encourage healthy behaviours. The Eatwell Plate is based around this model. It is known that cardiovascular health begins in childhood. We know that children who live at a socio-economic disadvantage will not have equitable access to healthy diets and are more likely to have a higher BMI (Zilanawala *et al.*, 2015). This can affect their long-term health outcomes.

It is recognised that the most successful healthy eating plan for cardiovascular health is based on the Mediterranean diet.

- Vegetables
- Wholegrains
- Fruits
- Healthy oils such as olive oil
- Beans, nuts, and seeds
- Minimal red meat
- Low to moderate intake of fish, poultry and dairy

A meta-analysis by Rosato *et al.* (2019) found that those with the highest adherence to the Mediterranean diet reduced their risk of a heart attack/stroke by 20–25%. However, this type of healthy eating is criticised for being unobtainable by those on a low income as it is expensive to buy fresh fruit and vegetables.

In addition to a Mediterranean diet, salt intake should be reduced to as low as possible due to its effect on blood pressure. All recommendations agree that salt intake should be reduced to less than 6 g per day. Studies agree that this has a positive effect on reducing blood pressure and potentially

more so in patients with Black and Asian heritage (Graudal *et al.*, 2020). However, many foods, particularly processed foods, have high levels of salt that patients are often unaware of. Patients should be given advice on how to check food labels. Key points to advise patients on when selecting processed food are:

- Foods with less than 3% fat are considered low fat
- Look at the label to establish if the food contains salt
- Look at the type of fat; is it saturated?
- Are the calories high?

Food labelling is improving, with newer labels being traffic light coded, i.e. green is lowest, red is highest. Patients should be advised to predominantly purchase foods in the green. In the UK, food labelling is a legal requirement but this can be challenging to apply with imported foods or those that are bought loose.

Alcohol intake should be reduced to avoid additional calories and those who drink alcohol should be advised to drink within moderation which is 14 units per week for both men and women (Gov.uk. 2016).

Diabetes and Nutrition

It is estimated that 5.3 million people will have diabetes in the UK by 2053; 50% of those will die prematurely (Diabetes UK, 2021).

Type 1 diabetes occurs when there is autoimmune destruction of the insulin-producing cells in the pancreas. Insulin is a hormone that facilitates the utilisation of glucose by the cells for energy. In the absence of insulin, blood glucose levels rise which results in high levels of circulating blood glucose, causing both short-term and long-term complications if left untreated (Bilous and Donnelly, 2010).

Type 2 diabetes is a more complex disease caused by many factors, including being overweight, having a family member with diabetes (any type) or being from African-Caribbean, Black African or South Asian heritage (Holt *et al.*, 2017). Patients with type 1 diabetes must be managed with injectable insulin to survive. Patients with type 2 diabetes can be managed on diet alone, pharmacotherapy or injectable therapies such as glucagon-like peptide 1 or insulin.

Nutrition is the foundation for managing both types of diabetes. Diabetic diets are no longer advocated in favour of healthy eating, but any person with diabetes needs to be aware of the effect different types of foods have on their blood glucose. The main food group to affect blood glucose levels is carbohydrates. Other groups do affect blood glucose levels, but their effect is much slower and there is still debate on how this can be meaningfully calculated.

The first step for patients is to recognise which foods contain carbohydrates. The next step for some patients who use insulin is to commence carbohydrate counting. Carbohydrate counting enables a person with diabetes to match their insulin to the carbohydrate content in any given food, essentially matching what would be physiological normal. For example, 10 g of carbohydrate is matched to 1 unit of insulin; this is known as a 1:1 ratio. Patients then learn to match and adjust ratios to individualise their insulin requirements to their dietary intake and effect on their blood glucose. For example:

BREAKFAST	
1 slice of toast	15g carbohydrate
1 banana	20g carbohydrate
Butter	Not counted (fat)
Cup of tea	Not counted (tea has no carbohydrate)
Milk (splash)	Not counted unless more than 10g
Result	35g total carbohydrate
Insulin Requirement	3.5 units of quick acting insulin = 1:1 ratio

Ratios are increased in ½ units so if blood sugar control is inadequate on a 1:1 ratio, the ratio is increased to 1.5:1, i.e. 1.5 units for every 10g, and so on. Patients with type 2 diabetes require larger ratios as they need to overcome insulin resistance to achieve the same effect.

Carbs and Cals© (www.carbsandcals.com/) is a pictorial representation of many foods and fluids. It has significantly simplified carbohydrate and calorie counting for patients with diabetes and is now widely used as a tool to enable patients to learn carbohydrate counting.

Foods that are high GI, i.e. release their energy quickly, are used to treat hypoglycaemia (a blood glucose of less than 4 mmol/L). Treating hypoglycaemia requires 15–20g of fast-acting carbohydrate such as:

- 100–120 mL of full-sugar cola/lemonade
- 5 jelly babies
- 4–6 glucose tablets (may vary depending on brand)
- 150 mL of fruit juice.

Once the hypoglycaemic event has been treated with fast-acting carbohydrate, longer acting carbohydrate is given to prevent an immediate recurrence of the low blood glucose. Examples of longer acting carbohydrate snacks include:

- Bread/toast
- Bananas
- Large glass of milk
- Dark chocolate is acceptable as it has less sugar.

Case Study

Muna: Diabetes during Ramadan

Muna is 42 and has type 2 diabetes. She recently commenced insulin therapy, as her oral medications were not controlling her diabetes. She remained symptomatic with polyuria and polydipsia.

Muna is concerned about how she will fast for Ramadan as all Muslims must fast from sunrise to sunset. She attended her diabetes nurse for advice. Her diabetes nurse advised her that permission can be obtained from her Imam not to fast. Diabetes is included under the exemptions for fasting. Her Imam can recommend to her that missed fasting days can be made up before the next Ramadan.

Muslim patients with diabetes during Ramadan are at risk of hypoglycaemia due to lack of carbohydrate or ketone formation due to fasting. Muna needs to take her insulin to alleviate her symptoms; therefore, working together, Muna and her nurse composed a plan to help her manage her diabetes during Ramadan. This included:

- Testing her blood sugars more frequently during fasting
- Consider reducing her insulin doses if hypoglycaemia becomes an issue
- Consider a change of insulin. Basal-bolus regimes are best for fasting
- Consider eating before sunrise
- Ensure she drinks lots of fluids when fast breaks at sunset.

Once Muna eats in the evening, she chooses healthy but low GI foods to ensure there are no significant peaks in her blood sugar.

Muna felt reassured that she could maintain both her faith and her health during the month of Ramadan.

Nutrition and Renal Disease

Approximately 3 million people in the UK have chronic kidney disease (Kidneycare.uk, 2020).

One of the key wastes excreted in the urine is potassium. High potassium levels can be extremely dangerous, leading to cardiac arrhythmias and potentially death. In addition, patients are often on restricted fluid intake to avoid excess extravascular fluid accumulation which can lead to peripheral and, in severe cases, pulmonary oedema.

Red Flag

 Patients on renal replacement therapy can find fluid restrictions challenging. If a patient on dialysis accumulates a significant amount of weight in a short period, it could be related to fluid accumulation and may lead to further complications such as pulmonary oedema.

The Renal Association has published practice guidelines for managing nutrition in chronic kidney disease. Key recommendations from the guidelines include:

- Daily energy intake of 30–40 kcal/kg
- Protein intake of 0.8–1.2 kg/day depending on treatment type
- Water-soluble vitamins for patients on dialysis
- Regular nutrition screening (Wright *et al.*, 2019).

In addition, there is consensual agreement that dietary potassium intake should be no more than 50–70 mmol per day. Renal diets are based on the following factors.

- Low-potassium foods
- Iron supplementation to reduce anaemia
- Salt restriction
- Fluid restriction

Patients with renal disease can often become demoralised by the continual dietary restrictions, so it is important to remember to be supportive and empathetic. Referral to a specialist renal dietitian can help patients explore alternatives that may lift mood and well-being.

Nutrition and Mental Health Issues

People experiencing mental health issues are more likely to die 20 years early, partially because of the effect of weight gain due to medication (Teasdale *et al.*, 2017). When our mental health is affected, our attachment to food can result in resulting in disordered eating. It has long been thought that poor nutrition can lead to poor mental health such as depression, but a longitudinal study of a large UK cohort found that there was no correlation between poor diet and depression (Northstone *et al.*, 2018).

When mental health deteriorates, normal eating can be affected. Common patterns include:

- Depression: loss of interest in food/weight loss
- Bipolar disease: loss of interest in food/binge eating; forget to eat as thoughts/behaviour become more manic
- Disordered eating: bulimia/anorexia
- Hallucinations: believing food is poisoned.

Caring for patients who have altered eating whilst ill can be challenging. Food choices may not follow traditional eating patterns; however, the primary concern should always be maintenance of calories irrespective of choice of food.

Nutritional support for patients with mental health disease focuses on maintenance of healthy nutrition but if this is not possible then maintenance of calorie intake. There are some simple effective measures that can be taken, including:

- Lots of snacks for patients in hypermanic states (to maintain calorie intake)
- Dietitian support to encourage weight gain in hypomania
- Identifying food preferences
- Supplementary foods to support/maintain weight
- Medication that stimulates appetite
- Psychological support to discuss disordered relationships with food.

Alcohol is best avoided in low mood states due to its depressant effect; however, alcohol consumption tends to increase when a person is feeling depressed. Its diuretic effect leads to dehydration, which increases irritability and low mood. In addition, alcohol contains calories but has no nutritional affect.

Patients with schizophrenia have been known to consume increased quantities of caffeine which can lead to increased anxiety and agitation (Teasdale *et al.*, 2017); caffeine-free drinks may be suitable alternatives.

To conclude, managing nutrition in patients with mental ill health can be challenging. The goal of treatment should be nutritional interventions that support the holistic well-being of the person whilst experiencing ill health and not necessarily the healthiest diet. However, long-term health considerations should be appraised when planning nutritional interventions.

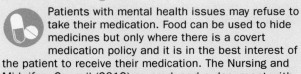
Nutrition in Dementia

Dementia is a term used to describe diseases that affect memory, speech and thought, the most common of which are Alzheimer disease, vascular dementia, dementia with Lewy bodies and frontotemporal dementia (Alzheimer's Research UK, 2021). People with dementia exhibit:

- Amnesia, where they fail to remember names, where they are, what they were about to do
- Agnosia, where they fail to recognise familiar people and objects
- Aphasia, where they fail to recognise words or find words to express themselves
- Apraxia, where they can no longer co-ordinate movement
- Associated psychological and social behavioral symptoms of distress.

All the above can affect patients' nutritional status, as they may forget to eat, forget what to use in the way of cutlery, fail to perceive what is presented as food, and fail to feed themselves because of lack of co-ordination. The dementia may cause changes to the sense of smell and taste, so the person does not recognise the food they are being given. Adding sugar or honey to sweeten food may make it more appetising but the extra calories do not make a significant impact.

People with dementia may also have a greater need for more calories than an older person might require. Increased energy is expended through constant walking and agitated behaviours and a raised BMR, and potentially patients may exhibit aggressive behaviour when hungry and in pain. Night hunger is common, which can be mitigated with fortified warm drinks at bedtime to sustain them through the night. Mealtimes should be regular and adhere to a similar ritual or pattern. Finger food is easier to manage than cutlery.

What the Experts Say

The European Society for Clinical Nutrition and Metabolism (ESPEN, 2016) guidelines recommend the following for nutrition in dementia.

- Every person with dementia should be screened for malnutrition.
- Bodyweight should be regularly monitored in all patients with dementia.
- Meals should be provided in a pleasant home-like atmosphere.
- Food should be provided according to individual preferences and beliefs.
- Adequate food intake should be encouraged as well as adequate support to eat.

As the disease progresses, patients may develop dysphagia (difficulty in swallowing) and will require a speech and language therapist (SALT) assessment. Refusal to eat is extremely distressing for families. This is usually a sign that patients are now in an advanced stage of dementia; however, it is difficult to predict if they have reached the terminal phase of their illness which makes decisions about nutritional support difficult and challenging.

Case Study

John: Nutrition in Advanced Dementia
John is 83 years old. He lives in a care home and is now in the advanced stages of dementia. The carers noticed that John appeared to be losing weight and leaving his food. His clothes seemed loose fitting. When they weighed him, he had lost 7 lb in the previous 3 months. His MUST score was 1. His care team decided to compose a plan of care to ensure his weight loss was reversed and he would gain weight. His plan of care included the following.

- A weekly goal of 1 lb weight gain (it is good to have a clear goal to aim for).
- Commence a food diary to establish his current food intake.
- Speak to John to find out his food preferences/dislikes.
- Ensure John's food preferences are clearly communicated in his nursing documentation.
- Speak to John's family to support his nutritional intake (patients will often eat family-cooked food as this is a pleasant memory).
- Provide John with snacks in between meals if necessary.
- Swap his milk to full cream from semi-skimmed.

Nutrition and Wound Healing

For more information on the wound healing process, please refer to Chapter 18 of this text.

Wounds are significantly more difficult to heal if the person is malnourished, and the cost of this to the NHS is estimated to be over £7000 per patient per annum (Phillips *et al.*, 2020).

It also affects a person's quality of life, as they will experience pain and loss of physical ability, which has repercussions for their social life (Medlin, 2012).

It is estimated that a person's normal protein needs are 1–1.4 g/kg ideal body weight; for wound healing, this rises to 2 g/kg ideal body weight in cases of severe wounds. Wounds that have high exudate losses will require 3 g/kg ideal body weight of protein. The person also requires 100–200 mg/day of vitamin C, which is available if they can eat at least five portions of fruit and vegetables (excluding potatoes) a day. This diet would also give the person sufficient zinc, iron and copper to facilitate wound healing.

In addition to proteins, a person requires an adequate carbohydrate intake, as the body's cells will use protein for energy if there is insufficient carbohydrate, thus depleting the reserves of protein for wound healing to take place.

If a person cannot manage this diet, then the nutrients need to be gained from food supplements. There are many commercially prepared nutritious drinks that are either milk or fruit based, which contain all the essential amino acids.

Nutrition for the Person Who Is Dying

People who are dying have more than medical issues requiring medical solutions; they and their families require evidence-based, person-centred nursing and caring interventions, which includes nutritional care.

While nutrition does not prolong life, it does:

- Give the person strength and time to meet their goals and objectives they have set
- Allow death with dignity and not from starvation
- Give the person control over their disease process; dehydration can cause pain as the inactive metabolites of morphine are not flushed out of the body, thus blocking active metabolites from linking to the pain receptors and suppressing the painful stimuli.

As a person reaches the end of their life and their condition is deemed terminal, whatever their disease, their nutritional status may alter in the following ways.

- Bodily functions slow down: this includes gastric emptying and absorption of nutrients, so there is less need for food and drink
- Medication used, such as analgesics and sedatives, alter the person's sense of taste and desire for food
- Fatigue and lack of energy also depress the appetite
- Psychologically, the person just does not feel like eating; it ceases to be important to them.

This can cause great distress, particularly to those (family and friends) who care deeply and would like to see the person make every effort to stay alive. However, the dying person has personal preferences and where possible these should be respected. It should also be recognised that these preferences and priorities can and do change over time.

There is some debate as to whether tube feeding is a medical treatment or not. It raises several ethical questions.

- Should people die because of lack of nourishment?
- Should nutritional support be withdrawn, knowing it will lead to death?
- Will the withdrawal of nutritional support cause suffering rather than offer relief of suffering?

The aim of end-of-life care is to:

- Provide relief of physical symptoms, such as pain, breathlessness, terminal agitation
- Provide social, psychological and spiritual support to the person and those closest to them
- Allow the person to live until they die and maintain their 'quality of life'
- Not artificially hasten death but allow death with dignity.

Exemplary palliative care shifts the focus from the disease to the person, enabling them to live until they die, and participate in making choices as to how their symptoms are managed and supporting them in their choices where it is possible to do so. This includes respecting their wishes regarding their diet and fluid intake.

Nutritional Nursing Care for the Person at the End of Life

Nursing care commences with assessment (the MUST tool has already been outlined). In addition, the nurse needs to establish:

- How the person views their nutritional status: what are their priorities?
- How those closest to the person view nutrition: how realistic are their expectations for the person at the end of their life? Aggressive persuasion to eat results in conflict and distress for all involved
- What the person would like – taste changes.

The goal of care should be to make mealtimes an enjoyable experience and at the end of life, it is important that memories are created that are pleasant and worthy of keeping. Nurses can help create a caring atmosphere by ensuring:

- Bedpans and vomit bowls are cleared away and the environment smells clean
- The person is positioned so that they can eat with ease
- The food tray or table is set attractively; disposable tray clothes and china crockery all help to create a special atmosphere
- Food portions are small and set attractively on the plate; using smaller plates helps with this
- Use of cutlery and china as opposed to disposable paper and plastic utensils.

The dying person has little time left, while we have all the time in the world, and therefore we should make every effort to deliver compassionate care.

Care, Dignity and Compassion

When patients are nearing the end of their life, small things such as a preferred drink or a favourite food can bring immense satisfaction. Facilitating patients' food choices respects their individual needs and brings comfort to families who can get involved in this aspect of care.

Dehydration at the End of Life

While people can accept that a dying person may not require nutrition at the end of life, it is more difficult to accept the reduced need for fluids, especially if the dying person has a dry mouth and cracked lips. The research-based evidence for providing

What the Experts Say

The Specialist Palliative Care Audit and Guidelines Group (SPAG, 2017) provide guidelines on the administration of subcutaneous hydration. The guidelines recommend the following.

- Maximum continuous infusion rate of 100 mL/h
- Maximum infusion volume of 1.5–2 L in 24 hours in any one site
- Maximum bolus of 500 mL in 1 hour
- The fluid of choice should be sodium chloride 0.9% or dextrose 4% and sodium chloride 0.18%

Chapter 20 of this text discusses end-of-life care in more detail.

medical hydration, either by intravenous or subcutaneous infusion, at this stage is very mixed and studies are flawed for various reasons (e.g. sample sizes too small, parameters for measurement too vague or subjective).

Some people want and need to be more aware, so they can say 'goodbye' and respond to people they love and care for. This level of hydration may not assuage their feelings of thirst because the sensation of thirst is associated with a dry mouth. The best way to deal with this symptom is to provide meticulous mouthcare.

However, maintaining hydration artificially does mean the person has invasive tubes, which they may find distressing. This is perceived by some as the 'medicalisation' of the natural process of dying. Excess fluids retained in the body can add to the symptom burden: it may increase breathlessness and bubbly noisy breathing, which is very distressing for the person and their family. It may increase oedema, which can also be uncomfortable. The decision to commence subcutaneous hydration is always taken based on individual patient needs.

Families and those close to the person who is dying may perceive the withdrawal of nutrition and fluids as abandonment of the person – the giving up of hope by the healthcare professionals – and interpret it as a lack of care. Families and staff may require support at this difficult time and reassurance that withdrawal of nutrition and fluids does not increase suffering. Replacing feeding the person with regular mouthcare reassures everyone that the healthcare professionals are maintaining vigilant care at the end of life.

Nutrition in COVID-19

In March 2020 the UK went into a national lockdown due to a global pandemic caused by a coronavirus labelled COVID-19. In the first few weeks of lockdown, food shortages emerged due to panic buying, resulting in restrictions being imposed by all major supermarkets.

COVID-19 is a respiratory disease that is diagnosed with signs of fever, persistent cough, loss of sense of taste (ageusia) and loss of smell (anosmia) (Gov.uk. 2021); 85–90% of COVID-19 cases have anosmia and ageusia which can have a severe impact on the pleasure gained from food and pose a risk of malnutrition (Meunier *et al.*, 2020). A study of patient self-reported symptoms by Sudre et al. (2021) identified six clusters of symptoms; in the cohort with mild symptoms, skipping meals was frequent, in another cohort gastrointestinal symptoms such as vomiting and diarrhoea were common in addition to skipping meals. Anker *et al.* (2020) found that nutritional impacts of COVID-19 included reduction in food intake, weight loss, malnutrition, cachexia and appetite loss.

Populations affected with the most serious disease are the elderly and the clinically vulnerable (WHO, 2021b). Li *et al.* (2020) found that 42% of elderly patients were at risk of malnutrition due to cachexia and catabolic overdrive.

This chapter has highlighted nutritional requirements in vulnerable groups; therefore, the same principles apply for COVID-19. However, patients with COVID-19 have unique problems due to some advanced respiratory requirements such as continuous positive airway pressure (CPAP) masks which have to be kept on continuously or the use of high-flow oxygen. This remains an area where evidence is still emerging but there are some general considerations such as:

- Nutritional scoring is essential to identify those at risk
- Supplementary and enteral nutrition may be required to ensure adequate calories are maintained when oxygen requirements are high.
- Patients with COVID-19 have high metabolic demands due to, for example, pyrexia, cough, sepsis
- Critically unwell patients with COVID-19 may require parenteral nutrition
- Hydration needs to be closely monitored due to the increased risk of blood clots
- Patients with diabetes need to be closely monitored for ketone formation due to anorexia and metabolic nutritional demands.

Conclusion

Nursing has advanced in complexity and technicality over the years and nurses have developed skills that once were the remit of medical practitioners; yet 'to nurse' is inherently to nourish and sustain a person, especially when they are ill.

Nutrition is pivotal to the well-being of a person. It is needed to sustain life, it is needed to recover from illness, and it is needed when a person is dying.

This is a field of care where nurses can make a significant impact and reap rich rewards from the satisfaction of seeing people recover more quickly from illness and disease or gain comfort at the end of life. Nutrition should be considered equally important as oxygen and water. It is something we gain enjoyment from and it forms part of our identity. Our mental health is inextricably linked with what we eat. Our relationship with food starts at birth and continues until we die. As nurses, we must never underestimate that relationship and should do all we can to ensure that it is maintained during both health and disease.

Key Points

- Food poverty is now steadily rising.
- Food is essential for physical, emotional and psychosocial well-being.
- Nutrition support is an essential care activity enabling us to bond with patients.
- Patients' nutrition should be person centred and individualised to their specific care needs.

References

Alzheimer's Research UK (2021) *A quick guide to dementia.* www.alzheimersresearchuk.org/dementia-information/quick-guide-dementia/ (accessed December 2021).

Anker, M.S., Landmesser, U., Haehling, S., Butler, J., Coats, A.J.S. & Anker, S.D. (2021) Weight loss, malnutrition, and cachexia in COVID-19: facts and numbers. *Journal of Cachexia, Sarcopenia and Muscle*, 12(1), 9–13.

Baker, C. (2019) *Obesity Statistics.* https://researchbriefings.files.parliament.uk/documents/SN03336/SN03336.pdf (accessed December 2021).

BAPEN (2019) *National survey on malnutrition and nutritional care in adults.* www.bapen.org.uk/pdfs/reports/mag/national-survey-of-malnutrition-and-nutritional-care-2019.pdf (accessed December 2021).

BDA (2020) *Fluid.* www.bda.uk.com/uploads/assets/337cfde9-13c5-4685-a484a38fbc3e187b/Fluidfood-fact-sheet.pdf (accessed December 2021).

Bhatnagar, P., Wickramasinghe, K., Wilkins, E. & Townsend, N. (2016) Trends in the epidemiology of cardiovascular disease in the UK. *Heart*, 102(24), 1945–1952.

Bilous, R. & Donnelly, R. (2010) *Handbook of Diabetes*, 4th edn. John Wiley & Sons, Hoboken, NJ.

Black, R.E., Victora, C.G., Walker, S. P., *et al.* (2013) Maternal and child undernutrition and overweight in low-income and middle-income countries. *Lancet*, 382(9890), 427–451.

Carpenter, T.O., Shaw, N.J., Portale, A.A., Ward, L.M., Abrams, S.A. & Pettifor, J.M. (2017) Rickets. *Nature Reviews. Disease Primers*, 3(1), 17101–17101.

Cole, O. & White, G. (2020) Fluid balance chart audit in a rural district general hospital. *Future Healthcare Journal*, 7(Suppl 1), s82.

Cook, G., Hodgson, P., Hope, C., Thompson, J. & Shaw, L. (2019) Hydration practices in residential and nursing care homes for older people. *Journal of Clinical Nursing*, 28(7-8), 1205–1215.

Davies, E.A. & O'Mahony, M.S. (2015) Adverse drug reactions in special populations – the elderly. *British Journal of Clinical Pharmacology*, 80(4), 796–807.

Diabetes UK (2021) *Diabetes Statistics.* www.diabetes.org.uk/professionals/position-statements-reports/statistics (accessed December 2021).

ESPEN (2016) *Guidelines on nutrition in dementia.* www.espen.org/guidelines-home/espen-guidelines (accessed December 2021).

Gov.uk (2016) *Alcohol guidelines review.* https://assets.publishing.service.gov.uk/government/uploads/system/uploads/attachment_data/file/489795/summary.pdf (accessed December 2021).

Gov.uk (2021) *Main symptoms of coronavirus COVID-19.* www.nhs.uk/conditions/coronavirus-covid-19/symptoms/main-symptoms/ (accessed December 2021).

Graudal, N.A., Hubeck-Graudal, T. & Jurgens, G. (2020) Effects of low sodium diet versus high sodium diet on blood pressure, renin, aldosterone, catecholamines, cholesterol, and triglyceride. *Cochrane Database of Systematic Reviews*, 12, CD004022.

Hingorani, A.D., Finan, C. & Schmidt, A.F. (2020) Obesity causes cardiovascular diseases: adding to the weight of evidence. *European Heart Journal*, 41(2), 227–230.

Holmes, S.(2010) Nutrition in the palliative care of chronic and life threatening conditions. *British Journal of Nursing*, 15, S24–S30.

Holt, R.I.G., Cockram, C., Flyvbjerg, A. & Goldstein, B.J. (2017) *Textbook of Diabetes.* John Wiley & Sons, Hoboken, NJ.

Kidneycare.uk (2020) *Facts and stats.* www.kidneycareuk.org/news-and-campaigns/facts-and-stats/ (accessed December 2021).

Kislal, S., Shook, L.L. & Edlow, A.G. (2020) Perinatal exposure to maternal obesity: lasting cardiometabolic impact on offspring. *Prenatal Diagnosis*, 40(9), 1109–1125.

Li, T., Zhang, Y., Gong, C., *et al.* (2020) Prevalence of malnutrition and analysis of related factors in elderly patients with COVID-19 in Wuhan, China. *European Journal of clinical Nutrition*, 74(6), 871–875.

Lindell, N., Carlsson, A., Josefsson, A. & Samuelsson, U. (2018) Maternal obesity as a risk factor for early childhood type 1 diabetes: a nationwide, prospective, population-based case–control study. *Diabetologia*, 61(1), 130–137.

Lister, S.E., Hofland, J., Grafton, H. (eds) (2020) *The Royal Marsden Hospital Manual of Clinical Nursing* Procedures, 10th edn. Wiley-Blackwell, Oxford.

Malnutrition Task Force (2020) *Signs of Malnutrition*. www.malnutritiontaskforce.org.uk/professionals/signs-malnutrition (accessed December 2021).

Malnutrition Task Force (2021) *Eating and drinking well in later life*. www.malnutritiontaskforce.org.uk/eating-well-tips-everybody/eating-while-hospital-care-homes-or-if-you-rely-someone-else-your-meals (accessed December 2021).

McErlean, L. (2020) The digestive system. In: I. Peate & S. Evans (eds) *The Fundamentals of Anatomy and Physiology for Nursing and Health Care Students*, 3rd edn. Wiley, Oxford.

Medlin, S. (2012) Nutrition for wound healing. *British Journal of Nursing*, 21(Suppl. 12), S11–S15.

Meldrum, D., Morris, M. & Gambone, J. (2017) Obesity pandemic: causes, consequences, and solutions – but do we have the will? *Fertility and Sterility*, 107(4), 833–839.

Meunier, N., Briand, L., Jacquin-Piques, A., Brondel, L. & Pénicaud, L. (2020) COVID 19-induced smell and taste impairments: putative impact on physiology. *Frontiers in Physiology*, 11, 625110.

Morley, J. (2015) Dehydration, hypernatremia, and hyponatremia. *Clinics in Geriatric Medicine*, 31(3), 389–399.

National Institute for Health and Care Excellence (2014a) *CG181. Cardiovascular disease: risk assessment and reduction including lipid modification*. www.nice.org.uk/guidance/cg181/resources/cardiovascular-disease-risk-assessment-and-reduction-including-lipid-modification-pdf-35109807660997 (accessed December 2021).

National Institute for Health and Care Excellence (2014b) *CG 189. Obesity: identification, assessment and management*. www.nice.org.uk/guidance/cg189/resources/obesity-identification-assessment-and-management-pdf-35109821097925 (accessed December 2021).

NHS Inform (2021) *Hydration*. www.nhsinform.scot/campaigns/hydration (accessed December 2021).

Northstone, K., Joinson, C. & Emmett, P. (2018) Dietary patterns and depressive symptoms in a UK cohort of men and women: a longitudinal study. *Public Health Nutrition*, 21(5), 831–837.

Nursing & Midwifery Council (2019) *Professional Guidance on the Administration of Medicines in Healthcare Settings*. www.rpharms.com/Portals/0/RPS%20document%20library/Open%20access/Professional%20standards/SSHM%20and%20Admin/Admin%20of%20Meds%20prof%20guidance.pdf?ver=2019-01-23-145026-567 (accessed December 2021).

Patients Association (2018) *Nutrition Checklist*. www.patients-association.org.uk/patients-association-nutrition-checklist-toolkit (accessed December 2021).

Phillips, C.J., Humphreys, I., Thayer, D., *et al.* (2020) Cost of managing patients with venous leg ulcers. *International Wound Journal*, 17(4), 1074–1082.

Public Health England (2017) *Health matters, obesity and the environment*. www.gov.uk/government/publications/health-matters-obesity-and-the-food-environment/health-matters-obesity-and-the-food-environment--2 (accessed December 2021).

Rosato, V., Temple, N.J., La Vecchia, C., Castellan, G., Tavani, A. & Guercio, V. (2019) Mediterranean diet and cardiovascular disease: a systematic review and meta-analysis of observational studies. *European Journal of Nutrition*, 58(1), 173–191.

SACN (2015) *Carbohydrates and Health*. https://assets.publishing.service.gov.uk/government/uploads/system/uploads/attachment_data/file/445503/SACN_Carbohydrates_and_Health.pdf (accessed December 2021).

Sadler, M., Ashwell, M., Buttriss, J., *et al.* (2016) Developments in nutrition: 20 years back, 20 years forward. *Nutrition Bulletin*, 41(2), 180–187.

Schwingshackl, L., Hobl, L.P. & Hoffmann, G. (2015) Effects of low glycaemic index/low glycaemic load vs. high glycaemic index/high glycaemic load diets on overweight/obesity and associated risk factors in children and adolescents: a systematic review and meta-analysis. *Nutrition Journal*, 14(1), 87.

Shendurse, A.M. & Khedkar, C.D. (2016) Lactose. In: B. Caballero, P. Finglas & F. Toldrá (eds) *Encyclopedia of Food and Health*, pp.509–516. Academic Press, New York.

SIGN (2010) *Management of Obesity*. www.sign.ac.uk/assets/qrg115.pdf (accessed December 2021).

Singer, P., Blaser, A.R., Berger, M.M., *et al.* (2019) ESPEN guideline on clinical nutrition in the intensive care unit. *Clinical Nutrition*, 38(1), 48–79.

Smith, M. & Toprakkiran, N. (2019) Behavioural insights, nudge and the choice environment in obesity policy. *Policy Studies*, 40(2), 173–187.

SPAG (2017) *Guideline for the use of subcutaneous hydration in palliative care*. www.palliativedrugs.com/download/180214_Subcutaneous_hydration_in_palliative_care_v2.4_Final.pdf (accessed December 2021).

Sudre, C.H., Lee, K.A., Lochlainn, M.N., *et al.* (2021) Symptom clusters in COVID-19: a potential clinical prediction tool from the COVID Symptom Study app. *Science Advances*, 7(12), eabd4177.

Teasdale, S.B., Samaras, K., Wade, T., Jarman, R. & Ward, P.B. (2017) A review of the nutritional challenges experienced by people living with severe mental illness: a role for dietitians in addressing physical health gaps. *Journal of Human Nutrition and Dietetics*, 30(5), 545–553.

Townsend, N. & Scriven, A. (2013) *Obesity*. Public Health Mini Guide, Elsevier Ltd.

Trussell Trust (2020) *What we do*. www.trusselltrust.org/what-we-do/ (accessed December 2021).

Vandevijvere, S., de Ridder, K., Fiolet, T., Bel, S. & Tafforeau, J. (2019) Consumption of ultra-processed food products and diet quality among children, adolescents and adults in Belgium. *European Journal of Nutrition*, 58(8), 3267–3278.

World Health Organization (2019a) *Nutrition and Food Security*. www.who.int/foodsafety/areas_work/nutrition/en/ (accessed December 2021).

World Health Organization (2019b) *Draft guidelines on saturated fatty acid and trans-fatty acid intake for adults and children*. https://extranet.who.int/dataform/upload/surveys/666752/files/Draft%20WHO%20SFA-TFA%20guidelines_04052018%20Public%20Consultation(1).pdf (accessed December 2021).

World Health Organization (2020a) *Malnutrition*. www.who.int/health-topics/malnutrition#tab=tab_1 (accessed December 2021).

World Health Organization (2020b) *Obesity*. www.who.int/health-topics/obesity#tab=tab_1 (accessed December 2021).

World Health Organization (2021a) *Healthy Diet*. www.who.int/news-room/fact-sheets/detail/healthy-diet (accessed December 2021).

World Health Organization (2021b) *Coronavirus*. www.who.int/health-topics/coronavirus#tab=tab_1 (accessed December 2021).

Wright, M., Southcott, E., MacLaughlin, H. & Wineberg, S. (2019) Clinical practice guideline on undernutrition in chronic kidney disease. *BMC Nephrology*, 20(1), 370.

Zilanawala, A., Davis-Kean, P., Nazroo, J., Sacker, A., Simonton, S. & Kelly, Y. (2015) Race/ethnic disparities in early childhood BMI, obesity and overweight in the United Kingdom and United States. *International Journal of Obesity*, 39(3), 520–529.

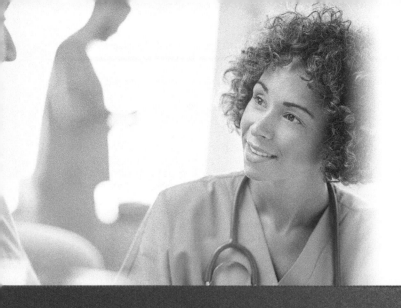

18

The Principles of Skin Integrity

Melanie Stephens

University of Salford, UK

Learning Outcomes

On completion of this chapter you will be able to:

- **Identify and describe the structures of the skin, hair and nails, explaining the processes involved in wound healing**
- **Explain the functions of the skin**
- **Review the psycho-socioeconomic aspects of wound care**
- **Categorise the factors that affect skin integrity and breakdown and how these impact on wound-healing processes**
- **Recognise and review common wounds, including the assessment of wounds, their clinical management and the involvement of the interdisciplinary team**

Proficiencies

NMC Proficiencies and Standards:

- **Use evidence-based, best practice approaches for meeting the needs for care and support with hygiene and the maintenance of skin integrity, accurately assessing the person's capacity for independence and self-care and initiating appropriate interventions**
  - **Observe, assess and optimise skin and hygiene status and determine the need for support and intervention**
  - **Use contemporary approaches to the assessment of skin integrity and use appropriate products to prevent or manage skin breakdown**

 Visit the companion website at www.wiley.com/go/peate/nursingpractice3e where you can test yourself using flashcards, multiple-choice questions and more.

Nursing Practice: Knowledge and Care, Third Edition. Edited by Ian Peate and Aby Mitchell.
© 2022 John Wiley & Sons Ltd. Published 2022 by John Wiley & Sons Ltd.
Companion website: www.wiley.com/go/peate/nursingpractice3e

Introduction

Nurses who are aware of the changes in skin integrity through the lifespan and the phases of healing are more likely to take an active role in the prevention and management of wounds of the patients for whom they care. Although the largest organ of the body, the skin is often the first organ to be ignored when patients are acutely ill or experiencing an exacerbation of their chronic illness. The multifaceted factors that can lead to skin breakdown make the challenge of prevention and management of the skin a testing but rewarding specialism of nursing.

Anatomy and Physiology of the Skin

The integumentary system is made up of the hair, nails and skin, which provides the body with an external cover, acting as a divider between the organs of the body and the external environment. It is the largest organ of the body, weighing 2.7–3.6 kg and with an average surface area of 1.9 m². It has many functions related to the structures that make up the layers of the skin.

The Hair

A hair bulb, with a root enclosed in a hair follicle, produces hair. It is situated in the dermis of the skin; however, in the scalp this is below the dermis. Visible hair, named the 'shaft', is mainly made up of dead cells. Only the palms of the hands, soles of the feet, nails, parts of the external genitals, lips and nipples do not have hair. The function of hair is protection and many factors influence its growth, including nutrition, genetics and hormones. The role of hair is to protect the scalp in particular from ultraviolet rays, heat loss and injury. Eyebrows and lashes stop foreign bodies from entering the eye, as do hair in the nostrils and ears. Hairs, through touch receptors in the hair root, sense light touch.

The Nails

Dead cells arising from the stratum germinativum of the epidermis make up the keratinised plates called nails. The cells form clear, solid coverings to the dorsal and distal section of fingers and toes. The role of nails is to aid the development of fine motor skills such as grasping, scratching and manipulation. A nail also provides protection against trauma to the fingers and toes.

A nail has three segments: body, free edge and root (Figure 18.1). The body is the visible portion of the nail and often looks pinkish in colour due to the flow of blood in the underlying capillary network. The free edge is the part of the nail that may extend past the end of a finger or toe. The nail root is that aspect of the nail that is buried in the fold of the skin.

There is also the cuticle, a thin strip of epidermis that stretches over the nail margin; the matrix, the proximal portion of epithelium deep to the nail root; and the lunula, the whitish crescent-shaped end of the nail.

The Skin (Figure 18.2)

The Epidermis

The outermost layer of the skin is composed of epithelial cells and is slightly acidic (pH 4.5–6). These cells are normally 4–5 layers thick, with most layers being present on the palms of the hands and soles of the feet. The epithelium is made up of the stratum corneum, stratum granulosum, stratum lucidum, stratum spinosum and stratum basale (Figure 18.3).

The *stratum corneum* consists of 20–30 sheets of keratin fragment-filled dead cells arranged in what is termed 'shingles', which flake off as dry skin. It makes up 75% of the epidermis total thickness.

The *stratum granulosum* helps reduce loss of water from the epidermis as it contains a glycolipid. Keratinisation, a process by which the cells' plasma membranes thicken, also begins in this layer. In areas of thick skin, flattened dead keratinocytes are present and this is known as the *stratum lucidum*.

The innermost layer of the epidermis is where keratin and melanin are produced by melanocytes. The role of melanin is to shield the skin from the harmful effects of ultraviolet light, protecting the underlying keratinocytes and nerve endings. Melanocyte activity possibly explains the variation in skin colour in humans. The protective quality of the epidermis is due to the fibrous and water-repellent nature of the protein keratin. Keratinocytes move up through the layers of the epidermis as they mature, eventually becoming the dead cells that flake off as dry skin. Flaking of cells occurs daily when rubbing of the skin takes place, for example when drying with a towel or removing a piece of clothing. As flaking occurs, so does the production of replacement cells in the stratum spinosum, which is 8–10 cells thick. In this layer mitosis occurs, although not as abundantly as in the stratum basale, and cells that began in the bone marrow migrate to the epidermis.

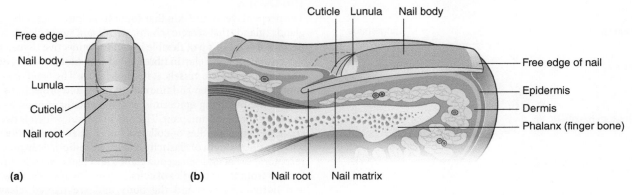

Figure 18.1 **Structure of the fingernail.**

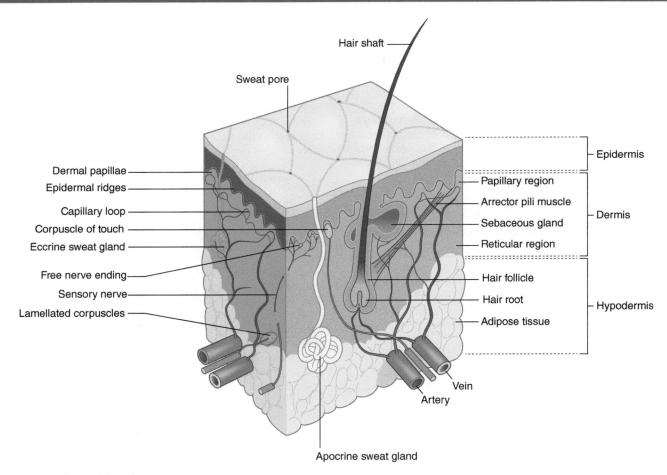

Figure 18.2 **Cross-section of the skin.**

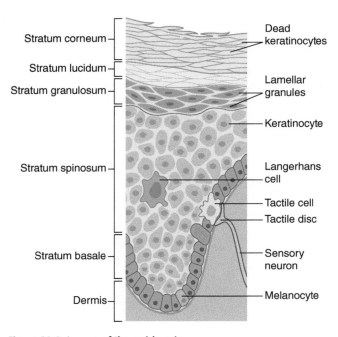

Figure 18.3 **Layers of the epidermis.**

Other cells found in the epidermis include Langerhans cells (found in the stratum spinosum) and tactile cells. Langerhans cells help other immune system cells to detect an infecting micro-organism and destroy it. Tactile cells contain a disc that detects touch and are in the deepest part of the epidermis. They are numerous around areas such as the fingertips, armpits, genital region and soles of the feet and are found in the stratum basale.

The Dermis

The deeper layer of the skin that contains hair follicles, sebaceous glands (glands that secrete sebum, an oil) and sweat glands is the dermis. It is made up of flexible irregular connective tissue, from woven collagen and elastin fibres, filled with blood vessels, nerve fibres and lymphatic vessels. It has two layers. The *papillary* layer contains thin collagen and fine elastin fibres and projections that serrate the overlying epidermis. It also contains capillaries and receptors for touch and pain. The *reticular* layer, which is deeper, contains dense bundles of collagen fibres (that provide the skin with tensile strength of elasticity and extensibility), deep pressure receptors, sweat and sebaceous glands and blood vessels. Ridges formed from these bundles of collagen run downwards, forwards and horizontally around the body and are named 'cleavage lines' and are genetically determined and unique for each person.

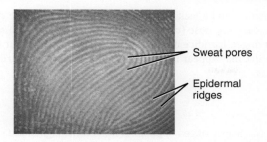

Figure 18.4 Epidermal ridges and sweat pores. *Source:* Jenkins, G. & Tortora, G.J. (2013) *Anatomy and Physiology: From Science to Life,* 3rd edn. Reproduced with permission of John Wiley & Sons Ltd.

Any surgical incision should run parallel to the cleavage lines in order to promote healing with less scarring. Macrophages, known as 'wandering cells', are contained within the reticular region (Figure 18.4).

Hair Follicles

A hair follicle, composed of stem cells, produces hair in three cycles. *Growth* is when cells of the hair matrix divide, adding new cells to the hair root, and this is when hair grows fast, around 1 cm every 28 days; scalp hair in particular stays in this phase for 2–7 years. *Cessation* occurs at the end of the growth stage and the stimulus for this is unknown. This is a short phase of 2–3 weeks and the blood supply to the hair is cut off and the hair becomes fully keratinised; the hair becomes a 'club hair' and enters the final stage. The *rest* phase is when the hair begins to fall out and can prematurely enter this phase in periods of extreme stress. This stage can last up to 3 months; 50–100 club hairs are shed daily from the scalp.

The structure of a hair follicle comprises a papilla, matrix, root sheath, hair fibre and bulge (Figure 18.5). The *papilla* is a large structure at the base of the follicle made up of connective tissue. The *matrix* is a collection of epithelial cells scattered with melanocytes and is where the hair *sheath* and *fibre*, made of

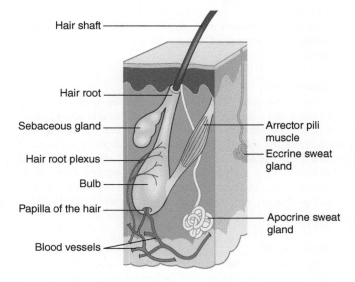

Figure 18.5 Structure of the hair.

keratin, are formed through cell division; this is the fastest growing cell population in the human body (but can be affected by radiotherapy and chemotherapy). The *bulge* accommodates stem cells, providing the hair follicle with new cells for growth and, if needed, also takes part in wound healing.

Attached to the hair follicle is the arrector pili muscle, which when stimulated allows the hair to stand perpendicular to the skin and protrude slightly to create goose bumps. Sebum and sweat are secreted by the sebaceous glands and apocrine glands on to the hair follicle for protection, lubrication and pliability.

Hair Follicle Pigmentation

Hair colour is affected by the amount of melanin in the cells. Various forms of melanin produce a range of hair colours: dark hair contains true melanin; blonde and red hair contain variants of melanin; and grey hair contains less melanin due to a decline in its production. White hair is due to air bubbles in the hair shaft and a lack of melanin.

Blood Vessels

Blood vessels contained within the skin include arterioles, capillary networks and venules. Flow of blood through the capillaries is controlled by hormones and the nervous system. Blood vessels in the skin transport and distribute oxygen, nutrients and hormones and remove waste products.

Nerve Fibres

The dermis contains both sensory and motor nerves. Sensory nerve endings are sensitive to touch, or initiate signals that produce sensations of warmth, coolness, pain, pressure, vibration, tickling and itching. The sensory receptors are found throughout the skin and include tactile discs in the epidermis, corpuscles of touch in the dermis and hair root plexuses around hair follicles. Motor nerves aid the vasodilation and vasoconstriction of blood vessels and glands and the contraction and relaxation of muscle tissues, i.e. the arrector pili.

Lymphatic Vessels

The lymphatic system parallels the blood vessel supply and function, but as its permeability is greater than that of the capillaries, it frequently absorbs proteins, lipids and interstitial fluid, which often occurs when pressure is greater in the interstitial fluid (which surrounds cells of the body tissues) than in the lymph. The role of the lymphatic system is to transport lymphatic fluid, aid in circulating body fluids and help guard against disease-triggering agents.

Subcutaneous Tissue

Primarily adipose tissue (fat) lies under the dermis and helps the skin adhere to underlying structures.

Glands of the Skin

There are many glands of the skin and each has its own function.

Cerumen is the yellow-brown waxy secretion of ceruminous glands, which are in the external auditory canals. Their role, along with hair follicles, is to prevent entry of foreign substances.

Cerumen also waterproofs the canal and prevents bacteria and fungi from entering the cells.

Sebaceous glands are located all over the body except for the palms and soles and are mostly connected to hair follicles. The glands are stimulated by androgens (sex hormones). Their role is to secrete an oily substance called sebum, a mixture of triglycerides, cholesterol, proteins and salts, which lubricates and softens the skin and hair and lessens water evaporation in low humidity. Sebum also destroys bacteria, protecting the skin from infection. Related medical conditions include sebaceous cysts and acne vulgaris.

Sudoriferous glands are small tubular structures that produce perspiration. There are two types. The forehead, soles and palms contain a higher number of *eccrine* glands, which are situated in the dermis and have a duct that opens in a pore at the surface of the epidermis. The sweat produced by the eccrine glands is mainly composed of water, but also contains antibodies, sodium, chloride, urea, uric acid, ammonia, amino acids, glucose and minute amounts of vitamin C and lactic acid. A person may sweat in response to their emotional state, for example when anxious, or to maintain homeostasis through the regulation of body temperature via perspiration. This is all regulated by the sympathetic nervous system. *Apocrine* sweat glands are located in the armpits (axillary), anal and genital area and are considered remnants of mammalian sexual scent glands. The sweat produced in these areas varies slightly, as fatty acids and proteins are also secreted, but is odourless; however, when bacteria on the skin metabolise, the sweat produced from these glands has a musky unpleasant odour.

Skin Pigmentation

Pigmentation levels affect the colour of the skin a human is born with; skin colour can vary from black and brown to pinkish white. The pigments that affect skin colour are haemoglobin, carotene and melanin. Those born with a golden skin tone, such as persons of Asian ancestry, have large amounts of carotene (a yellow-orange pigment) and melanin (a yellow-brown pigment). However, in all persons, carotene is found where the stratum corneum is thickest. Those born with brown or black skin have greater levels of melanin; however, lengthened exposure to the sun can cause an accumulation of melanin, resulting in darkening or tanning of the skin. A pink skin tone, conversely, is due to lack of melanin, which allows red blood cells carrying haemoglobin in the blood vessels of the skin to show through the almost translucent epidermis of Caucasians. Regardless of a person's racial origin, all scar tissue heals pink.

Jot This Down

Take some time and think of the different illnesses and emotions that can affect skin colour.

What could make the skin change to the following colours: red, bluish, paleness, yellow to orange, black hard leather appearance?

In this exercise, you might have thought about reddening of the skin due to embarrassment, fever, hypertension or inflammation. Other causes are a drug reaction, sunburn or rosacea. Poor

oxygenation and a lack of haemoglobin may give a blue colour to lips, ears and nose (cyanosis). Pallor may appear with shock, fear or anger. Jaundice may give a yellow to orange colour of the skin. Pink may appear in the healing of skin in Afro-Caribbean patients.

Care, Dignity and Compassion

Skin changes in patients with darker pigmented skin or neonates with jaundice may present differently. It is important that nurses are culturally aware of these differences in skin tone when they assess patients. Three classification systems for objectively assessing human skin colour include the Munsell skin tone chart (Konishi et al., 2007), which can assist with predicting pressure ulcer risk, the 6 Fitzpatrick (1988) skin types for assessing risk of damage from ultraviolet light and the neonatal skin colour scale (Maya-Enero et al., 2020).

Function of the Skin

The skin, hair and nails each have many functions which are categorised in Box 18.1.

Box 18.1 Function of the Nails, Hair and Skin

Protection
Sensation
Synthesis of vitamin D
Excretion
Absorption
A storage reservoir
Regulation of body temperature

Wound Healing (Figure 18.6)

When there is loss of integrity of the skin, a chain of events is initiated in order to return the skin to near-normal structure and function. The process of wound healing includes four main phases.

Haemostasis

The initial reaction of the skin to injury is bleeding, saturating the wound bed with blood. The purpose of this is to release platelets to the injured area so that they will adhere to the exposed collagen of the damaged vessel(s). The platelets then become sticky, fibrin connects with the platelets and any circulating red blood cells form a plug and haemostasis occurs. Fibrinolysis (breaking down of the clot) then occurs and other cells, such as macrophages and new platelets, arrive at the wound bed and the next phase of healing commences.

Inflammation

The inflammatory stage requires the release of many cells, substances, hormones and growth factors to aid wound healing. During this stage, the wound is cleansed and bacteria, debris and

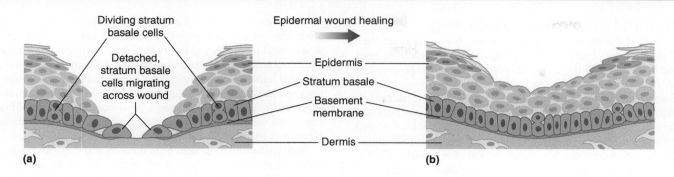

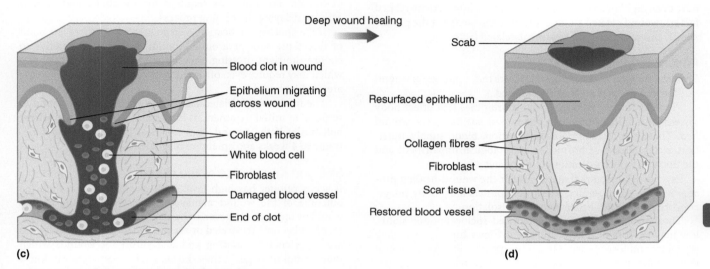

Figure 18.6 **Healing of epidermal and deep wounds.**

devitalised tissue are removed. Often, during this stage of wound healing the patient complains of pain, heat, swelling and redness at the wound bed.

Proliferation

Growth factors released by macrophages stimulate angiogenesis and cell migration to aid the formation of granulation tissue during this phase. Tissue made from collagen, fibrin, fibronectin, proteoglycans, glycosaminoglycans and glycoproteins develops. The function is to provide shape and offer metabolic and structural support to the surrounding cells. The wound bed is often seen as red and granular in all skin tones and wound edges start to close together, as muscle fibres are contracting. Pink epithelial sites are noted, as basal cells have travelled from the stem cells of the hair bulge across the moist wound bed, stopping only when they meet another basal cell (contact inhibition).

Maturation

Cell migration, cell growth and collagen deposition occur during maturation, increasing the tensile strength of the wound. Blood supply and cellular activity are reduced and the outcome for some wounds is scar formation. However, some patients who are younger than 30 years and have darker pigmented skin have abnormal repair such as keloid and hypertrophic scarring.

Case study

Marland is a 27 year old who was admitted for biopsy of an unusual lesion to the right knee. Marland stated that the lesion had increased in size over the last 2 years after the initial trauma from a fall. The lesion presented as pink in colour and 10 × 5 cm in size. Histology of the biopsy showed features of hypertrophic scar with no neoplasia. The wound was diagnosed as a keloid scar. Marland was advised that treatment for the scar would include surgery, silicone sheeting and corticosteroid injections. However, Marland was informed of the high recurrence risk of hypertrophic and keloid scarring due to genetics.

Psycho-Socioeconomic Aspects of Wound Care

Many factors can affect the healing or non-healing of any wound. The factors are classified as wound complexity and healing (Vowden et al., 2008), psychosocial factors and wound healing (Moffatt et al., 2008) and the economic burden of hard-to-heal wounds (Guest et al., 2020).

Wound Complexity and Healing

Predicting the likely healing time of any wound is often very difficult. Usual methods include regular wound measurement and assessment. This informs the practitioner of the progression of the wound as the radius and wound edges decrease. The Commissioning for Quality and Innovation (CQUIN) framework introduced by the Department of Health (2010) requires nurses to improve the assessment of wounds to aid prediction of wound healing. Performance targets and standards were set to reduce the number of wounds that have failed to heal after 4 weeks of treatment, by focusing on wound assessment and documentation.

To improve holistic assessment of wounds, four main factors have been highlighted as affecting wound healing: patient-related factors, wound-related factors, skill and knowledge of the professional, and resources and treatment-related factors.

Patient-related Factors

Physical, social and psychological factors may impinge on wound healing and should be regularly assessed.

Physical factors include any co-morbidities that affect body systems that in turn influence the rate of healing at the wound bed. These can include poor oxygenation, blood supply, nutrition, sleep, release of hormones, neurological impairment and the impact of any medication, to name but a few.

Psychosocial factors that can impair the wound-healing process include pain, gender, stress, economic status, body image, concordance, health beliefs and social isolation.

These problems can lead to reduced socioeconomic status, low income, loss of relationships and friendships, poor coping strategies and loss of meaning and purpose in life. As a result of their wound, these individuals suffer from restricted lives, experiencing further social isolation, being discredited and burdening others (Charmaz, 1983).

What the Experts Say

"Whenever I carry out a full assessment of a patient with a wound, in particular ones that are on visible parts of the body, I ask the patient to complete the Wound Quality of Life Assessment Scale. I do this as often those with the smallest of wounds suffer the most emotional stress and those with larger wounds have better coping mechanisms. The score helps provide objective data to the subjective data I have been assessing and collecting and then I can speak with the patient and their GP to consider other therapies such as counselling, occupational therapy, psychotherapy and medication for depression.

Ashanti, community nurse

Wound-related Factors

Many wound characteristics affect the rate of healing, including wound duration and wound senescence.

The chronicity of a wound often correlates with the number of senescent cells that develop, i.e. the number of cells in a wound bed that are unable to replicate.

The size and depth of wound can affect the healing process and due to the biological nature of wound healing, large deep-cavity wounds will take longer to heal than smaller superficial wounds. However, fistulas or sinuses are often small but deep.

The presence of necrotic and sloughy tissue can not only affect the correct assessment of a wound but also delay the wound-healing process, as this type of tissue requires assessment and consideration of the implications of debridement.

Many hard-to-heal wounds have high bacterial counts, more than one bacterium infiltrating the wound bed and/or the presence of a biofilm can fuel a chronic inflammatory response. This can cause inhibition of cell growth and angiogenesis and an increase in tissue degradation.

Poor perfusion of the skin from diseases and surgical complications such as atherosclerosis, atheroma, thrombus, calcification, dehydration and hypothermia can deprive the wound bed of oxygen and nutrients required for metabolic and cellular activity, delaying the healing process.

If the anatomical location is in an area where there is a point of direct pressure or around a joint, then it is imperative to choose the right dressing, secured with the right material and which may require even off-loading or having the pressure to the area redistributed.

The final wound-related factor is the ability of the wound to respond to initial treatment. It is essential to reassess the patient holistically if the wound does not heal in the accepted timeframe of 4 weeks and amend management accordingly.

Skill and Knowledge of the Nurse

If a practitioner has high-level skills and knowledge, then the outcome of the wound management received by the patient would be optimal. However, in hard-to-heal wounds, professionals often become frustrated or are overwhelmed by patients who are experiencing suffering and discomfort for wounds which they cannot manage. In these instances, it is imperative to know one's limitations and seek further support, as advocated by the NMC (2018a).

Resource and Treatment-related Factors

Wound management products and services have developed rapidly, in both number and design. Practitioners' knowledge of these advances varies, and patients can receive either appropriate, timely, evidence-based interventions or ritualistic traditional practice based on habit. Wound care resources in relation to guidelines, formularies and access to equipment and staff have created an 'atlas of variation' across the UK and therefore where a patient lives will affect the wound management they receive.

The Quality Agenda and Wound Management

Evidence from a retrospective cohort analysis indicated unnecessary variation in UK wound care services, insufficient delivery of evidence-based practice and an excess of ineffective practices (Guest et al., 2017).

In 2018 NHS England and NHS Improvement commissioned the development of a National Wound Care Strategy Programme (NWCSP) to improve the prevention and care of people with pressure ulcers, lower limb ulcers and surgical wounds. Their mission is to implement a consistently high standard of wound care across England by reducing unnecessary variation, improving safety and optimising patient experience and outcomes.

Interdisciplinary Care

Wound management is complex, and an interdisciplinary approach is vital to aid prevention and management. Professions who work together optimise patient well-being, but also ensure the delivery of seamless service (Bellingham & Stephens, 1999). Not only does interprofessional working put the patient at the centre of their care, it also enables best practice that is cost-effective and efficient (Barr *et al.*, 2002).

Patients

Enabling people to be more in control of their own care leads to better and often more cost-effective outcomes. This is particularly true for those with long-term conditions or people who need to use services more intensively (Care Quality Commission, 2016). During the COVID-19 pandemic, the NWCSP produced a document to help health professionals assess whether patients can manage their own wounds.

Nurse Specialists/Nurse Consultants in Tissue Viability/Leg Ulcer/Lymphoedema

The nurse specialist/consultant role is a lead position in wound prevention and management, undertaking the four key roles of working alongside other members of staff and acting as consultant, researcher, educator and manager. Duties include developing policy and guidance; educating staff; reviewing chronic and hard-to-heal wounds; appraising and carrying out research and managing budgets; writing bids and monitoring expenditure for the benefit of patient care.

Directors, Leads and General Managers

Final accountability for the implementation and management of patient care lies with professional leads, managers and directors, the provision of which is directed through the allocation of resources and education of staff.

Medical Staff

Doctors have overall responsibility for patient care and therefore must work with others to address the potential and actual complications of acute and chronic illness that may impede skin breakdown or wound healing.

Registered Nurses

Nurses are in the ideal position to offer holistic care that addresses the needs of the patient, be that in hospital, the home, hospice or nursing and residential home. Utilising the Nursing Process, the nurse can assess, plan, implement and evaluate the care delivered to patients and their significant others.

Nursing Associates

Nurse associates will assist the registered nurse in the monitoring of people with wounds, providing care and supporting the maintenance of skin integrity.

Support Workers, Trainee Assistant Practitioners, Healthcare Assistants

Support workers, trainee assistant practitioners and healthcare assistants assist and support registered nurses in the delivery of care. It is essential that they do not accept duties that are beyond their roles and responsibilities or have them delegated to them within the field of wound management.

Podiatrists

The role of the podiatrist is essential in the prevention and management of wounds in the foot. They provide advice, support and treatment for many patients and should be the first point of call for any diabetic patients for full examination of the foot.

Dietitians

The role of the dietitian is to provide detailed advice and support to the patient, their family and other members of the interprofessional team on nutrition and hydration.

Occupational Therapists

The role of the occupational therapist is to assess and maximise function and independence, promoting meaning and purpose of the activities of daily living a patient may undertake in their normal day-to-day routine, including recommendations for equipment with regular follow-up.

Physiotherapists

Physiotherapists promote independence and movement, offering advice on repositioning, correct body alignment and posture. They can provide equipment to aid independence.

Prosthetists and Orthotists

A prosthetist will ensure the patient is fitted with the most appropriate artificial limb. An orthotist will provide equipment such as splints, braces and casts to aid movement, resolve alignment and relieve pressure.

Radiographers

Radiographers provide a service in which the underlying pathology of wounds can be explored through X-rays, scans and imaging.

Healthcare Scientists

There are three broad areas of healthcare science.

- *Life sciences*: investigating the causes of illness and how it progresses using blood diagnostics, infection services, tissue and cellular science and genetics.
- *Physiological sciences*: investigating the functioning of organ/body systems to diagnose abnormalities and find ways to restore function and/or reduce disabling consequences to the patient.
- *Clinical engineering and medical physics*: developing methods of measuring what is happening in the body, devising new ways of diagnosing and treating disease and ensuring that equipment is functioning safely and effectively.

Bioengineers and Estates

Bioengineers and estates ensure the equipment used for patients is cleaned, serviced and maintained, complying with the Medical Devices Agency regulations. However, some trusts have outsourced this service to suppliers. All staff have a duty to report faulty equipment, replace it and remove it from the workplace until reviewed by these members of staff.

Wound Care and Management

There are many ways in which to classify a wound, including by aetiology, morphology and tissue colour, to name but a few.

299

Table 18.1 Classification of wound types.

CLASSIFICATION OF WOUND	TYPES OF WOUND
Acute	Surgical incisions, traumatic injuries: lacerations, bites, abrasions, burns and avulsions
Chronic	Pressure ulcers, leg ulcers, burns, dehisced surgical wounds, diabetic foot ulcers
Palliative	Malignant lesions of the skin, epidermolysis bullosa and progressive arterial disease

Wounds can be classified by the process by which they are healing. *Primary intention* occurs in surgical or traumatic wounds where there is no tissue loss and the edges of the wound are brought together for suturing, gluing or taping. *Secondary intention* is when the edges of the wound are too far apart and, because of the degree of tissue loss, the wound needs to fill with granulation tissue before epithelialisation occurs. *Tertiary intention* is when the wound is primarily left open for up to 5 days before closing with sutures or staples, allowing the drainage of exudate or infected pus.

Classification can be based upon the severity and depth of tissue damage and can be 'superficial', partial thickness' and 'full thickness', involving respectively the epidermis or tissue destruction occurring right through the epidermis and dermis to underlying structures, exposing bone and body tissues.

Wounds can also be classified by the length of time they have been present, often referred to as acute or chronic. Wounds that result in timely restoration of anatomical and functional integrity without complication are considered *acute* wounds. *Chronic* wounds are those that last longer than 4–6 weeks, take longer to heal than normally expected and may not provide full restoration in anatomical and functional integrity. One type of wound that cannot be classified as acute or chronic is a *palliative* wound, which is when wound healing is unattainable and care is based on symptom management rather than common management, such as moist wound healing and wound bed preparation. Table 18.1 provides a list of wounds that can be attributed to the terms 'acute', 'chronic' or 'palliative'.

Wound Assessment

Holistic wound assessment includes the gathering and analysis of data used to diagnose the underlying cause of the wound and aid decision making relating to implementing (and monitoring) patient and wound management (Benbow, 2016). The assessment should include the fundamentals of the generic wound assessment minimum dataset developed by Coleman *et al.* (2017) which includes general health information, wound baseline information, wound assessment parameters, wound symptoms and specialists the patient will be referred to for further investigation. It is, however, important that the patient is not seen in isolation and the impact of the family, work life, social life, etc. is taken into consideration.

Cause of the Wound

It is important to identify the cause of the wound. Alongside the cause, the clinician should ask how long the wound has been present (acute, chronic or palliative) and what previous interventions have been used. Inappropriate assessment of the cause will lead to poor management in the future.

Wound Size

No method of wound measurement is 100% accurate; however, all wounds should be measured for length, width and depth at each dressing change as an initial baseline for assessment and for further wound progression. The three most common guides are the linear measurement or clockface, the greatest width times greatest length and wound tracing.

- The *clockface* measures the wound by carrying out the following actions: when measuring length, the head is at 12 o'clock and the feet at 6 o'clock. Tunnelling would be measured by using the clockface for direction, i.e. the tunnelling occurs at 4 o'clock and is 3 cm in depth from the epidermis to the end of the tunnel.
- *Greatest width × greatest length* measures the wound lengthways (from head to toe) and widthways (perpendicular to this). The measurements are then multiplied to give the surface area of the wound.
- The third method is to complete an acetate grid *wound tracing* and count up the squares in the outline of the wound.

Photographs and wound management digital systems (WMDS) are now being used to record wound assessments. Consent to capture images for use within the patient record must be recorded in accordance with the Data Protection Act 1998. A WMDS enables wound photography and wound measurement (using a semi-automated wound measuring tool) and for each tissue type. It also allows the recording of co-morbidities and medication. An advantage is that every clinician can access the graphical representation of the patient's wound healing. The photo needs to be clear, have the relevant identifying data and be respectful of patients' personal dignity.

What to Do If . . .

 . . . you want to photograph a wound and your patient lacks capacity to consent due to mental health or learning disabilities.

Where capacity is assessed as lacking, the practitioner can consider making a 'best interests' decision following Mental Capacity Act 2005 guidance.

Ask yourself whether the photograph of the wound is in the patient's best interests and seek authorisation from the appropriate senior professional.

Only use the photographs for clinical purposes.

Wound Site

The wound site can assist in the identification of any co-morbidities or processes that could be connected with the occurrence of the wound. For example, a diabetic foot ulcer occurs on the foot, usually where there has been uneven pressure distribution, while a venous ulcer is common in the gaiter region. Naming and documenting the site of the wound is vital, specifically if there is more than one area of loss of skin integrity.

Colour and Type of Tissue at the Wound Bed

The colour and type of tissue at the wound bed can often indicate the stage of wound healing or the presence of a complication. Those wounds healing by secondary intention can be classified as necrotic, infected, sloughy, granulating and epithelialising.

Wounds can contain more than one tissue type and colour and present as a mixed wound, but prior to assessment of colour and tissue type, the old dressing should be removed and the wound should be cleansed.

- *Necrotic* tissue is where ischaemia has occurred and the tissue has died, forming an eschar or scab, presenting as hardened black or brown coloured tissue. Other necrotic tissue can present as thick layers of slough and can be grey, brown, off-white or dark purple. It is necessary to remember that the wound underneath the eschar may be more extensive than is visible as the scab masks the actual size of the wound. Often after debridement (if advocated), the true extent of damage is seen and can be shocking to both staff and patient.
- *Infected* wounds normally produce a purulent discharge and, in most cases, a host reaction. The type of bacteria causing the infection can affect the colour of the exudate, which can be yellow, green or fluorescent in colour and may even contain old or new blood. In many instances, a wound swab may be taken, but this is not to prove an infection is present, as assessment has demonstrated this, but to aid identification of the bacteria present. The discharge from an infected wound may also be extensive and have an offensive odour. Granulation tissue in an infected wound may be a darker red colour and the peri-wound area may show signs of infection; however, in neuropathic diabetics or immunocompromised patients, the natural immune response may not be visible.
- *Sloughy* tissue is characteristically yellow-white in colour; however, a note of caution here as tendons and ligaments are a shiny, creamy white and should not be classified as slough. Slough is the collection of dead cells collected in the exudate and is related to the endstage of the inflammatory phase of healing. It can easily be removed by macrophages and disappears as the wound heals.
- *Granulation* tissue is red and granular in appearance. This is the tops of the capillary loops that develop during the proliferation phase of wound healing. This tissue is often friable and can bleed easily if touched. If granulation tissue is dark red, this could signify an infection or poor tissue perfusion.
- *Epithelialising* tissue is pinky white in colour and is seen as the wound margins start to contract and island sites are visible on the surface of the wound bed. All scars heal pink and careful care of the scar is needed and involvement of other services depending on the patient's natural skin tone and the site of the scar itself.

Suitable dressings for different wound types are shown in Figure 18.7.

Level of Exudate

Exudate is assessed by reviewing the colour, consistency, odour and amount. It is normally clear, amber coloured and has no odour. An easier method to assess amount is to look at the interaction with the dressing after use: is the removed dressing dry, moist, wet, saturated or leaking (WUWHS, 2007)? This can help with assessing whether exudate levels have increased, decreased or not changed.

The level of exudate can impede the wound-healing process as too little leads to the wound drying out and too much causes maceration or excoriation of the peri-wound area.

Signs and Symptoms of Infection

During wound assessment, clinicians should determine if the wound bed is contaminated, colonised or infected, and this should also be differentiated from the inflammatory response of wound healing. Prompt diagnosis of infection aids treatment and requires clinical assessment and diagnostic testing.

There are classic signs of infection, such as pyrexia, oedema, pain, inflammation and an increase in exudate production. Additional signs include delayed healing, increased watery exudate rather than pus, pocketing at the wound base, bridging, increased pain, malodour, friability of tissues, a change in the colour of granulation tissue and wound breakdown. However, some patients with diabetes may fail to present with any symptoms apart from closer observation of a delay in wound healing (Patel, 2010).

A routine method of diagnosing the offending bacteria is via a wound swab but the reliability of this depends on the method used. Deep tissue biopsy is considered the most reliable method of diagnosing wound infection, but its use in day-to-day wound care is restricted due to the trauma to the patient and by the choice of professional allowed to take the biopsy, limited only to doctors and podiatrists.

Practice Assessment Document

If a PAD requires the assessment of performance of wound care skills and as a student, you are on a placement where there aren't any patients or clients currently with a wound, you can ask to 'spoke out' to a placement where patients are frequently assessed and managed by nurses such as a surgical ward, accident and emergency, the community or a wound care clinic to develop your competence and confidence.

You could also ask your practice supervisor to simulate a wound care scenario that would be seen in that specialty with help from the practice education facilitator (many have simulation suites and manikins).

You could also ask to spoke out to the tissue viability or leg ulcer service.

Pain at the Wound Bed

Pain at the wound bed can be due to a variety of causes, such as neuropathy in the patient with diabetes, anticipatory as the patient waits for the dressing to be removed, and iatrogenic due to self-harm. A full pain assessment includes visual analogue score, history, body map and location/site of the pain. This can aid appropriate dressing selection and pain management approaches (WUWHS, 2008). Regular reassessment is imperative to review strategies and progress. Pain does not always correlate with the size and depth of wound and the cause of the pain

Wound type		Characteristics	Examples of suitable dressings
Epithelialising	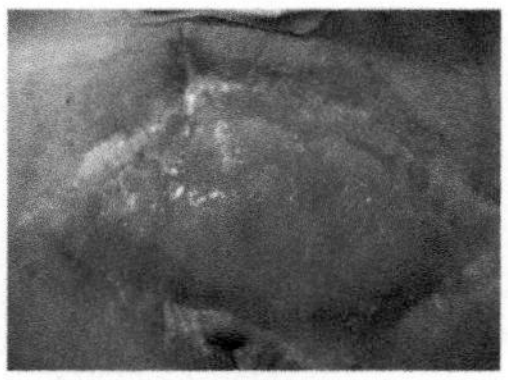	Clean, superficial, low to medium exudate, pink in colour	Low and non-adherent dressings, knitted viscose, paraffin gauze, film dressings
Granulating	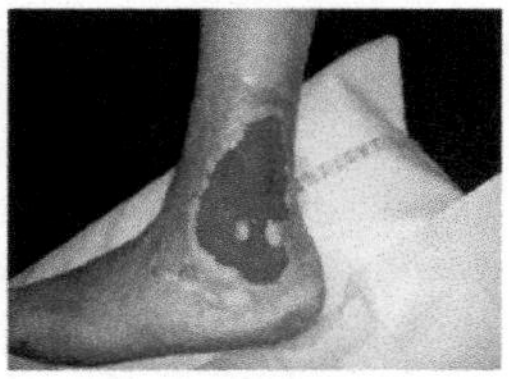	Clean, low to medium exudate, red in colour with granular appearance	Alginates, hydrocolloids, foams
Sloughy	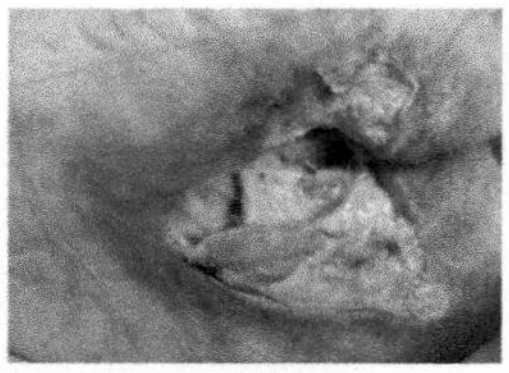	Medium to high exudate, yellowish-grey in colour, partially or completely covered in slough	Hydrogels, alginates, spun hydrocolloids
Necrotic wounds	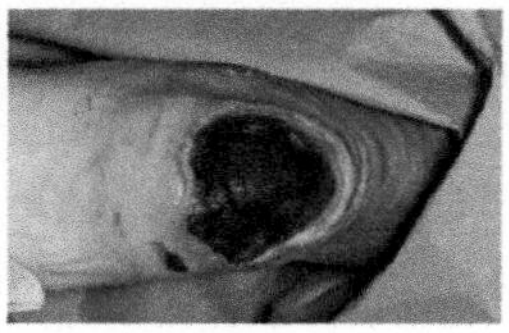	Black, dry, eschar devitalised tissue	Hydrogels, hydrocolloids
Infected wounds	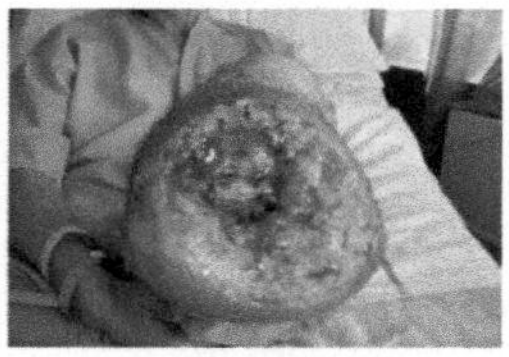	Painful, moderate to high exudate, malodorous, crusting	Silver-impregnated dressings, hydrogels, spun hydrocolloids
Blistering	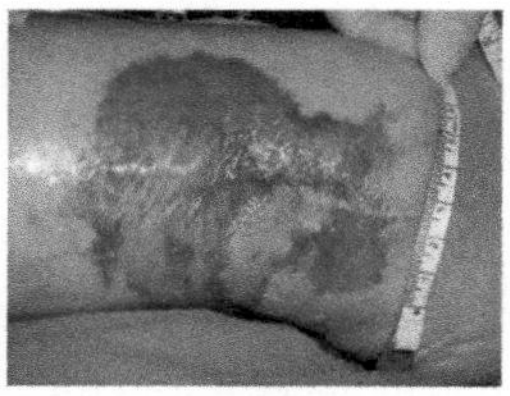	Clean, superficial, low to medium exudate	Non-adherent dressings

Figure 18.7 **Suitable dressings for different wound types.** *Source*: Buxton & Morris-Jones (2013). Reproduced with permission of John Wiley & Sons Ltd.

can often be psychological rather than physical; both pharmacological and non-pharmacological approaches should be explored to aid wound healing.

Surrounding Skin

The margins of the wound will change as the wound progresses through the phases of wound healing. Changes in colour and appearance can indicate healing or wound breakdown, for example redness may indicate infection. The peri-wound area can become macerated or excoriated if the wound produces too

much exudate for the dressing to handle and the clinician then needs to explore the use of more absorbent dressings, more frequent dressing changes and protective barrier skin products for the peri-wound area (Figure 18.8).

Other Clinical Data

A clinician may also record the type of wound, the phase of wound healing, any grading, staging or classification for that particular type of wound, factors affecting wound healing, diagnostic tests and any current management.

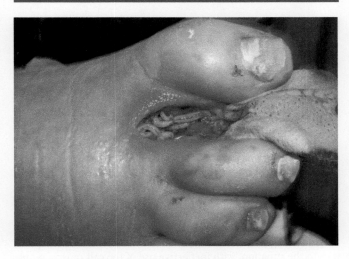

Figure 18.8 Using larvae to clean a peri-wound area.
Source: Buxton & Morris-Jones (2013). Reproduced with permission of John Wiley & Sons Ltd.

Types of Wound

Minor Injuries
Many wounds are trivial in nature such as wounds seen in minor injury units, walk-in centres, practice nurse clinics and accident and emergency. These wounds are classified as follows.

- *Avulsions*: these occur when the skin has been pulled off with or without the involvement of bone by doors and machinery. This usuall affects digits, but can occur in the legs and arms of patients who have previously had steroidal treatment, as their skin is friable and easily avulsed.
- *Contusions*: these are bruises that occur from trauma to the skin and bleeding arises in the tissue spaces. Bruising can be graded from 0 to 5, with 5 being a critical bruise from bleeding into the brain or compartment of a muscle and 0 being a light bruise with very little damage. Underlying medical conditions can cause bruising, such as leukaemia, coagulation problems and infection. Carry out a full assessment to exclude these and explore other factors such as physical abuse.
- *Cuts*: these are wounds with well-defined edges, little bruising and usually straight in alignment. They usually occur due to sharp implements and are easily repaired with sutures, staples, glue or Steri-Strips.

- *Abrasions*: scrapes to the knee when falling on gravel, for example, are brought about by the action of friction and shear between a blunt item and the skin. These types of wounds often dry out, scab over and heal without scarring; however, if gravel is embedded in the skin, it should be removed to prevent permanent tattooing of the skin.
- *Bites*: human or animal bites can cause heavily contaminated wounds, which require thorough assessment for the type of toxins and bacteria present, so correct antibiotics can be prescribed. These types of wounds are healed through tertiary wound healing.
- *Skin tears*: shear and friction forces that separate the epidermis from the dermis or dermis from the subcutaneous layers lead to skin tears. They mainly occur in the elderly, because of the fragility of the skin from medication, age and altered skin function. Healing may be lengthened due to co-morbidities; treatment can vary from dressings and compression bandaging to surgery. Skin tears can be classified (see later). Steri-Strips are no longer advocated for skin tears in older adults.
- *Lacerations*: falls, blows to the skin and crushing injuries from blunt instruments cause a break in the skin with an irregular wound edge, which heals by secondary intention.

Surgical Wounds
Postsurgery wounds can be classified as clean, clean contaminated, contaminated and dirty or infected (NICE, 2008, p.9). The descriptions are given in Table 18.2.

Table 18.2 Types of surgical wound.

TYPE OF SURGICAL WOUND	DESCRIPTION
Clean	An incision in which no inflammation is encountered in a surgical procedure, without a break in sterile technique and during which the respiratory, alimentary or genitourinary tracts are not entered
Clean contaminated	An incision through which the respiratory, alimentary or genitourinary tract is entered under controlled conditions but with no contamination encountered
Contaminated	An incision in which there is a major break in sterile technique or gross spillage from the gastrointestinal tract, or an incision in which acute, non-purulent inflammation is encountered as well as open traumatic wounds that are more than 12–24 hours old
Dirty or infected	An incision in which the viscera (internal organs) are perforated or when acute inflammation with pus is encountered (e.g. emergency surgery for faecal peritonitis) and for traumatic wounds where treatment is delayed, there is faecal contamination or devitalised tissue

Classification of Surgical Wound Complications

Fistulas can occur when patients have a malignancy and inflammatory bowel disease; however, others have no one cause. A passage is formed between two organs, for example bowel and vagina (recto-vaginal), and faeces from the bowel will pass out of the vagina. Common fistulas occur between the bowel and skin (enterocutaneous).

A cavity or bursa that leads from the outside of the body inside is known as a sinus. It is lined with epithelial cells and is caused by infection, a foreign body or breakdown of dead tissue. Patients with sinuses often have surgical intervention, as recurrence rate is high. Factors that increase the vulnerability of a sinus include recent blunt trauma and haematoma formation, immobility, sedentary job and lifestyle, previous abscess formation and surgery at the site.

Dehiscence, or the unplanned opening of a wound post surgery, is often triggered by poor surgical technique, haematoma formation, insufficient number of sutures, infection, age, diabetes and trauma to the wound. Wound healing is often by secondary or tertiary intention and grafts made of Teflon® are used to add strength to the peritoneal lining.

Evisceration is a very frightening experience for both patient and clinician. It occurs in 30% of all surgical wounds and is when the gastrointestinal tract protrudes through the wound opening (Figure 18.9). The patient should be observed for signs of shock, the open wound and bowel covered with moist sterile dressings, the person let down with the foot of the bed elevated 20° and medical attention sought immediately. Again, as in a dehisced wound, a return to theatre and the use of Teflon grafts is often advocated.

Factitious/Iatrogenic/Self-harm Wounds

Wounds caused by self-harm are routinely peculiar, with sharp geometric margins surrounded by normal-looking skin (Gupta *et al.*, 1987). How these wounds present on assessment depends on the cause, for example burn, tourniquet, excoriation or chemical injury, and can present as blisters, purpura, ulcers, erythema, oedema, sinuses or nodules. At times, skin loss can be so significant that the person requires plastic surgery. Timely identification is vital to avert unnecessary surgery and morbidity (Tantam & Huband, 2009). The wounds tend to occur in areas that are easily accessible, i.e. the opposite arm to the dominant writing hand, the abdomen or legs. They are often asymmetrical and appear quickly, with no previous history of injury or disease. Patients are often those with dermatological conditions (Harth *et al.*, 2010) and may have no suicidal intent. NICE (2011) guidance is provided for clinicians who care for patients who have wounds due to self-harm. Self-harm wounds are categorised into two types: pathological and non-pathological.

Leg Ulcers

Leg ulcers affect 1% of the population at any particular time and can be defined as an open lesion between the knee and the ankle joint that occurs in the presence of venous disease and takes more than 2 weeks to heal (NICE, 2013).

Venous Leg Ulcers

The major cause of leg ulceration (60–80%) is venous hypertension and is treatable. Valves in the superficial, deep and perforator veins become damaged and impair the flow of blood returning to the heart, initiating a backflow. This backflow leads to varicosities, venous stasis, lower leg oedema and a change in the colour and integrity of the skin. The tissue becomes fibrous and woody in nature and brown staining appears (lipodermatosclerosis). Many patients complain of itchiness, pain and tenderness, especially when walking. This creates immobility and adds further complexities to the situation, with ineffective use of the calf muscle pump to aid venous return. Ankle flare (dilation of the superficial veins of the leg near the ankle) and atrophie blanche (white/paler plaque spots near the ankle) can often be visible on examination.

The ulcer is usually shallow and flat, located on the medial malleolus and gaiter region of the leg; pain is dull, aching and relieved by elevation (Figure 18.10). Oedema reduces with management and elevation. High levels of exudate are common; there is often wet or dry eczema in the peri-wound area. Ankle brachial indices would be between 0.8 and 1.3 (NICE, 2021).

Susceptibility to venous leg ulceration includes family history, a sedentary job and lifestyle, gender (women more than men), pregnancy, diet, obesity, reduced mobility, malnutrition and intravenous drug use.

Arterial Leg Ulcers

Arterial disease affects 22% of those who have a leg ulcer and is attributed to smoking, a history or family history of cardiovascular problems, high cholesterol, high alcohol intake, diabetes, age over 50, sedentary lifestyle and male gender. Arterial disease is caused by hardening and narrowing of the arteries due to the deposition of fat (atheroma and atherosclerosis). A cascade effect occurs, where lack of oxygen and nutrients to the leg occurs, causing ischaemia and cell death, or total occlusion of a blood vessel and thrombosis, which leads to gangrene and mummification of the toes.

Classic signs and symptoms when detecting arterial disease include a punched-out ulcer anywhere on the foot, a history of

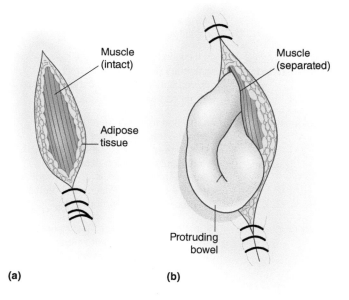

(a) Muscle (intact), Adipose tissue

(b) Muscle (separated), Protruding bowel

Figure 18.9 **Evisceration of a wound can be frightening for the patient.**

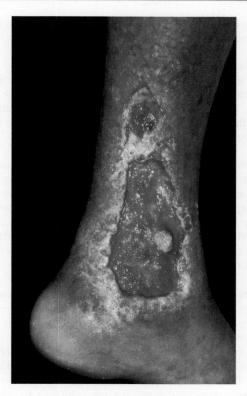

Figure 18.10 **Venous leg ulcer.** *Source:* Buxton & Morris-Jones (2013). Reproduced with permission of John Wiley & Sons Ltd.

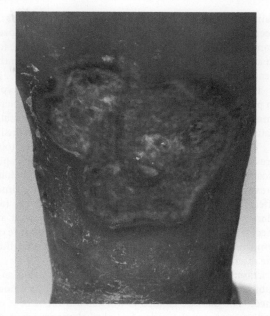

Figure 18.11 **Arterial leg ulcer.** *Source:* Buxton & Morris-Jones (2013). Reproduced with permission of John Wiley & Sons Ltd.

rest pain (pain experienced at night when lying in bed with elevated legs, relieved by dangling legs out of bed or sitting in a chair). Intermittent claudication, triggered on exercise, with cramping pain in the hips, thighs, buttocks and calf muscles, is due to inadequate supply of oxygenated blood. There is absence of foot pulses, poor capillary refill, coldness, hairless, mottled appearance of the skin (bluish-red in Caucasians, purple bluish-black in Black people and ashen grey-yellow in Asians), brittle toenails, breaks that do not heal and sunset rubra (skin turns red/purple hue on dependence). The person may also complain of numbness and tingling in the toe, foot or leg (Figure 18.11). Ankle brachial indices would be below 0.8. Often referral to a vascular surgeon is necessary or indeed urgent.

Rheumatoid Arthritis and Systemic Vasculitis

Nine percent of leg ulcers occur in patients with rheumatoid arthritis and include other underlying components, such as an arterial, venous or vasculitic component.

Diabetic Ulcers

Five percent of leg ulcers are diabetic, usually have multiple aetiology and result from a combination of diabetes and venous disease or diabetes and arterial disease.

Iatrogenic Leg Ulcers

Leg ulcers can be classified as a hard-to-heal wound where there is no significant reason for non-healing; however, it may be that the patient is removing the dressing, picking at the wound or causing other wounds (self-harming) due to a lack of company in

their life. Referral to social and local services such as a 'leg club' is necessary to increase contact with others in their local community and promote healing.

Pressure Ulcers

According to NHS Improvement (2018, p.7) a pressure ulcer is defined as '. . . localised damage to the skin and/or underlying tissue, usually over a bony prominence (or related to a medical or other device), resulting from sustained pressure (including pressure associated with shear). The damage can be present as intact skin or an open ulcer and may be painful'. A number of contributing or confounding factors are also associated with pressure ulcers; the significance of these factors is yet to be clarified.

Causes of Pressure Ulcers

The causes of pressure ulcers are either direct or indirect forces.

- *Indirect forces* include those that affect the physical, social and mental well-being of a patient and can include nutrition, body temperature, dehydration, age, medication, immobility, sleeping, elimination, anxiety and depression (this list is not exhaustive).
- *Direct forces* include the impact of pressure, friction and shear.
  - *Pressure*: when the skin is compressed between a hard surface and a bony prominence, either from a high pressure for a short period of time or a low pressure for a long period of time, pressure damage can occur. This often leaves a wound that is circular in shape and can often affect the epidermis, dermis and underlying structures and bone. A cascade effect takes place when the pressure impedes the flow of blood in the underlying layers of the skin. Initial tissue hypoxia occurs, which if unrelieved becomes ischaemia and then cell death occurs. Initial damage may often not be visible, as the damage occurs at the bony prominence. Days later, a large necrotic wound appears and the extent of the

damage is now visible. In instances where patients have been admitted to hospital after being found collapsed at home, it is imperative to ask which position they were found in and for how long they had been in that position; therapeutic interventions should be commenced.

In health, a person will reposition themselves in response to pressure exerted on the skin; however, in the vulnerable, immobile, frail, elderly and acutely sick or chronically ill patient the risk of skin damage from pressure is intensified.

Tissue tolerance, i.e. the ability of the skin to tolerate pressure without adverse problems, depends upon capillary closing pressures. Healthy individuals can normally tolerate pressure exerted on the capillaries without detrimental effect, i.e. blood flow being disturbed and harm taking place. However, this does not take into account other mechanical and indirect forces or the closing pressure of the lymphatic system, whose role is to drain away excess fluid in the interstitial spaces.

- *Friction*: abrasions or blisters occur when the skin surface rubs across another surface, such as a heel along a hospital sheet. The damage created is worsened if the skin is moist and exacerbates the risk of further damage, when other mechanical forces are involved.
- *Shear*: the repositioning of patients can greatly increase the risk of wounds from shearing forces. During moving and handling, the surface of the skin can become fixed while the rest of the body tries to move, causing underlying structures to be stretched, distorted and torn. This can often be seen as puckering of the skin and occurs when sliding patients up the bed incorrectly or from patients sliding down the bed. The wound is often tear shaped and has a deep cavity.

Risk Assessment

According to NICE (2014) guidance, all patients should have initial and ongoing assessment of their risk of developing pressure ulcers. There are many risk assessment tools to choose from, but local policy will dictate which tool is used and how. Most important for clinicians is that they use their clinical judgement

alongside the assessment, as many tools have limitations in relation to over- or underprediction.

Classification of Pressure Ulcers

In order to provide consensus across the world in the care and management of pressure ulcers, the National Pressure Injury Advisory Panel, European Pressure Ulcer Advisory Panel and Pan Pacific Pressure Injury Alliance (PPPIA) developed a common classification system.

Category/Stage I: Non-blanchable Erythema Intact skin with non-blanchable redness of a localised area usually over a bony prominence. Darkly pigmented skin may not have visible blanching; its colour may differ from the surrounding area. The area may be painful, firm, soft, warmer or cooler, when compared with adjacent tissue. Category/stage I may be difficult to detect in individuals with dark skin tones. May indicate 'at risk' persons (a heralding sign of risk).

Category/Stage II: Partial Thickness Partial thickness is loss of dermis presenting as a shallow open ulcer with a red-pink wound bed, without slough. May also present as an intact or open/ruptured serum-filled or serosanguineous filled blister. Presents as a shiny or dry shallow ulcer without slough or bruising (bruising indicates deep tissue injury) (Figure 18.12). This category should not be used to describe skin tears, tape burns, incontinence-associated dermatitis, maceration or excoriation.

Category/Stage III: Full-thickness Skin Loss Subcutaneous fat may be visible but bone, tendon or muscles are *not* exposed. Slough may be present but does not obscure the depth of tissue loss. *May* include undermining and tunnelling. The depth of a category/stage III pressure ulcer varies by anatomical location. The bridge of the nose, ear, occiput and malleolus do not have (adipose) subcutaneous tissue and category/stage III ulcers can be shallow. In contrast, areas of significant adiposity can develop extremely deep category/stage III pressure ulcers. Bone/tendon is not visible or directly palpable.

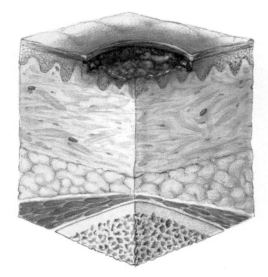
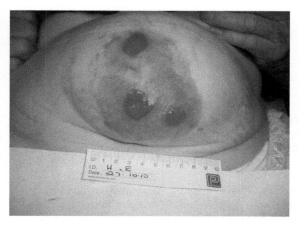

Figure 18.12 **Category/Stage II pressure ulcer.** *Source:* Flanagan (2013). Reproduced with permission of John Wiley & Sons Ltd.

Category/Stage IV: Full-thickness Tissue Loss Full-thickness tissue loss with exposed bone, tendon or muscle. Slough or eschar may be present. Often includes undermining and tunnelling. The depth of a category/stage IV pressure ulcer varies by anatomical location. The bridge of the nose, ear, occiput and malleolus do not have (adipose) subcutaneous tissue and these ulcers can be shallow. Category/stage IV ulcers can extend into muscle and/or supporting structures (e.g. fascia, tendon or joint capsule), making osteomyelitis or osteitis likely to occur. Exposed bone/muscle is visible or directly palpable.

Unstageable/Unclassified: Full-thickness Skin or Tissue Loss – Depth Unknown Full-thickness tissue loss in which actual depth of the ulcer is completely obscured by slough (yellow, tan, grey, green or brown) and/or eschar (tan, brown or black) in the wound bed. Until enough slough and/or eschar are removed to expose the base of the wound, the true depth cannot be determined but it will be either a category/stage III or IV. Stable (dry, adherent, intact without erythema or fluctuance) eschar on the heels serves as the body's natural (biological) cover and should not be removed.

Suspected Deep Tissue Injury – Depth Unknown Purple or maroon localised area of discolored intact skin or blood-filled blister due to damage of underlying soft tissue from pressure and/or shear. This may be preceded by tissue that is painful, firm, mushy, boggy, warmer or cooler, when compared with adjacent tissue. Deep tissue injury may be difficult to detect in individuals with dark skin tones. Evolution may include a thin blister over a dark wound bed. The wound may further evolve and become covered by thin eschar. Evolution may be rapid, exposing additional layers of tissue, even with optimal treatment.

Pressure Ulcer or Moisture Lesion?

Recently some pressure ulcers have been misdiagnosed and were in fact moisture lesions. In order to identify whether a wound to the skin is a pressure ulcer or moisture lesion, the EPUAP, NPUAP & PPPIA (2014) published a position statement which asks the clinician to consider a list of questions; if the answer is yes to all of them, the wound is to be considered a moisture lesion. The questions focus on moisture being present, the skin presenting as shiny and wet, incontinence, location of the lesion, exclusion of shear and friction, shape of the lesion, copy lesions in other clefts, depth, presence of maceration and whether the lesion improves with use of barrier products.

Reactive Hyperaemia

The characteristic bright red flush of skin in a patient with white/pink skin that occurs when pressure is released from the skin is reactive hyperaemia. It can be assessed by applying light fingertip pressure to the area affected for 10 seconds and then observing the reaction. The skin initially should be white, which should then turn to its original colour, demonstrating that the skin is healthy and has a good blood supply. If the skin does not react and retains the same bright red flush, this is indicative of a stage I pressure ulcer and a revised approach to care should be taken.

Reactive hyperaemia is difficult to distinguish in patients with black or brown skin; pressure ulcer development will be indicated instead by areas where there is localised heat that does not dissipate, or where there is damage, coolness, purple-black discoloration, localised swelling (oedema) or tissue hardness (induration).

Medical Device-related Pressure Ulcer

Medical device-related pressure ulcers (MDRPU) are those 'that result from the use of devices designed and applied for diagnostic or therapeutic purposes. The resultant pressure ulcer generally closely conforms to the pattern or shape of the device' (EPUAP, NPUAP & PPPIA, 2014, p.119). This can be from a cannula, plaster of Paris cast, oxygen tubing, mask or catheter, to name but a few. Best practice is to assess the cause of pressure and reduce the risk. However, in some cases the medical device is needed and therefore cannot be removed. It is therefore important to ensure that when using medical devices, one is not creating an avoidable pressure ulcer.

Burns

A burn is an injury to the skin caused by heat, electricity, chemicals, radiation or friction (Table 18.3). Over 250 000 people each year suffer a burn injury and 330 of these people die (Edwards, 2012). Most are accidental in nature and many involve children, the elderly and adults who are obese or have cardiovascular and neurological conditions.

Table 18.3 **Burn injuries.**

TYPE OF BURN	INJURIES SUSTAINED	SYMPTOMS
Radiation from sunburn, radiotherapy and radiation	Affect the epidermis and dermis, mainly superficial in nature	Headache, chills, local discomfort, nausea and vomiting. Reddened blistered skin
Electrical from high voltage of electricity	Entry and exit wounds which are small and mask the true extent of damage	Tissue necrosis, gangrene, cardiac monitoring for ventricular fibrillation and cardiac arrest
Thermal from fire, combustible products, fireworks, excessive heat, steam, cold, liquid and surfaces	Can be superficial epidermis to deep wounds down to bone and underlying structures	Charring of the skin, blood vessels, muscle tissue, nervous tissue and bone
Chemical from corrosive substances (acid and alkali)	Can be superficial to deep wounds	Depend on the agent and the mechanism of action, duration of contact and body surface exposed

Table 18.4 Classification of burns.

CLASSIFICATION OF BURN	APPEARANCE	PAIN	HEALING TECHNIQUES AND TIMES
Full thickness	Pale, waxy, yellow, brown, mottled, charred or non-blanching red. Surface is dry, leathery and firm to touch, thrombosed blood vessels are visible	No sensation of pain or light touch	Require excision and skin grafting and are hard to heal. Often require initial fasciotomy and escharotomy. Often have contractures and hypertrophic scarring
Deep partial thickness	Pale and waxy, moist or dry, ruptured blister may occur that appears as tissue paper	Less pain than superficial thickness as areas of decreased sensation	Excision and grafting. More than 21 days' healing time often with contractures and hypertrophic scarring
Superficial partial thickness	Bright red, moist glistening appearance with blisters. Blanches on pressure	Pain is severe in response to air and temperature. Pain and touch response intact	Dressing products and skin substitutes. Healing within 21 days with minimal or no scar formation
Superficial	Pink to bright red in colour	Stinging sensation	Water-soluble lotions and dressings. Healing in 3–6 days; no scar

Classification

The classification of burns is in accordance with the depth of tissue damage (see Table 18.4 for appearance and estimated healing times).

Burns Assessment

Alongside a comprehensive wound assessment, pertinent information particular to burns includes history of the burn, time of injury, causative agent, early treatment, age and body weight. Most questions should be asked quickly, as initially on arrival burns patients are awake, but conscious states can alter quickly in a major burn injury.

The extent of damage of a burn in a child is assessed through use of the Lund and Browder tool. Damage to the surface area is measured by body parts affected (Figure 18.13). In adults, the Rule of Nines is used, by division of the body into five surface areas (see Figure 18.13); only partial- or full-thickness burns are included in the estimation.

Any patient with a burn who meets any of the following criteria should be transferred to a specialist burns unit for further management (National Network for Burn Care, 2012): burns to the face, hands or feet, to a person aged 5 years and under and 60 years and over, circumferential to a joint, chemical and electrical burns, inhalation injuries, more than 5% total body surface in children, more than 10% body surface in an adult, or burn not healed in 14 days.

The Diabetic Foot

Over 4 million people in the UK have diabetes, 7000 people with diabetes have leg, foot or toe amputations each year in England and up to 80% of people die within 5 years of having an amputation (Kerr, 2017).

Box 18.2 Signs and Symptoms of Diabetic Foot Ulcer

- *Loss of sensation*: might not feel heat, cold, pressure, friction or shear
- *Dry skin*: from autonomic neuropathy, which leads to cracks, fissures and callus formation
- *Infection and osteomyelitis*: may not be visible but can be seen as mummification of toes and gangrene in the foot
- *Foot deformities*: Charcot's foot, claw toes, prominent metatarsal heads, altered gait and muscle atrophy

---

A diabetic foot ulcer is defined as 'a full-thickness lesion of the skin, i.e. a wound penetrating through the dermis; lesions, such as blisters or skin mycosis (infection) are not included' (International Working Group on the Diabetic Foot, 2003). This type of foot contains not just an ulcer but an assortment of pathological changes, such as loss of sensation (neuropathy), reduced blood flow (ischaemia and calcification), deformities of the foot (Charcot) and uneven distribution of pressure. Signs and symptoms are shown in Box 18.2.

Diabetic Foot Assessment

Interprofessional working is the key to effective diabetic foot ulcer assessment and management. Diabetic patients should have regular assessment of their feet which includes the examination of the foot based on the IWGDF (2003) Pedis system. This takes into consideration perfusion of the foot, extent and size of ulcer/damage, depth of tissue loss, infection and sensation. Podiatrists who usually carry out this assessment

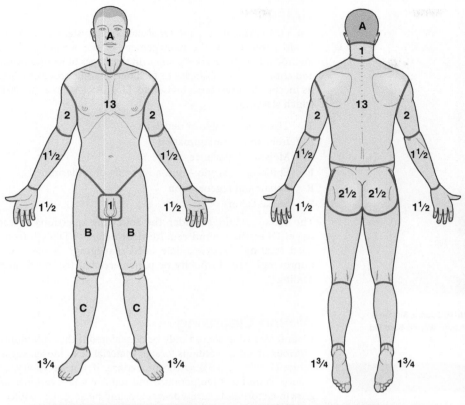

Region	%	
	PTL	FTL
Head		
Neck		
Ant. trunk		
Post. trunk		
Right arm		
Left arm		
Buttocks		
Genitalia		
Right leg		
Left leg		
Total burn		

Area	Age 0	1	5	10	15	Adult
A = ½ of head	9½	8½	6½	5½	4½	3½
B = ½ of one thigh	2¾	3¼	4	4½	4¼	4¾
C = ½ of one lower leg	2½	2½	2¾	3	3¼	3½

Figure 18.13 **Lund and Browder tool.**

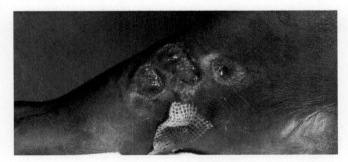

Figure 18.14 **The diabetic foot.** *Source:* Buxton & Morris-Jones (2013). Reproduced with permission of John Wiley & Sons Ltd.

investigate the patient's gait, mobility, posture, balance, reflexes, sensory function (vibration perception, protective pain sensation and neuropathy), foot pulses, Doppler and toe pressures (Figure 18.14).

Malignant and Fungating Wounds

Malignant wounds are frequently found in head and neck and breast cancers; however, they can also occur in the skin. They develop at the primary site of the cancer or at lymph nodes, for example the groin or axillae.

A fungating wound occurs when the tumour has invaded the epithelial layer of the skin and breaks through the surface, forming an ulcerative area (crater) or proliferative area (cauliflower-like nodules) (Dealey, 2005). It is imperative to assess if the ulcer is malignant, especially as management would be focused on symptoms rather than healing. In leg ulcers, it is recommended that if an ulcer fails to improve within a 12-week period, then a biopsy for malignancy should be taken, as often the ulcer is cancerous and not a typical venous one (Scottish Intercollegiate Guidelines for Nurses, 2010). Some patients are offered radiotherapy, chemotherapy or surgery for short-term symptom relief; however, because cancer cells continue to grow, the wound will not disappear and will regress at a later stage (Figure 18.15).

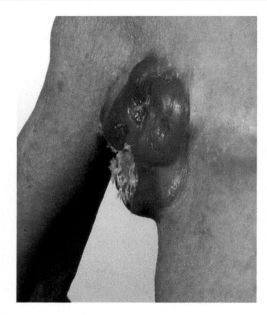

Figure 18.15 Malignant and fungating wound. *Source:* Buxton & Morris-Jones (2013). Reproduced with permission of John Wiley & Sons Ltd.

Nursing Management

After a thorough holistic patient and wound assessment, it is imperative for the clinician to plan, implement and evaluate the care provided. If after the initial assessment the patient requires more advanced care than the clinician can provide, referrals for advice, support and guidance must be sought immediately and if necessary, a transfer of care.

Moist Wound Healing

From 1962 onwards, the principles of moist wound healing challenged previous presumptions of leaving a wound to dry out and scab over. George Winter (1962) in his study on pigs highlighted that if wounds were kept moist and the scab removed, cell migration is encouraged. His work has been repeated and is the basis of treatment for most wounds, as the advantages of moist wound healing include reduction in infection, less injury to the wound bed, less pain, assisting debridement and cost-effective treatment.

Wound Bed Preparation

In order to optimise wound healing and ensure the dressings and equipment function at their best, it is imperative that the practitioner manages and prepares the wound bed. Wound bed preparation, according to Falanga (2000, p.1), is 'the management of a wound in order to accelerate endogenous healing or to facilitate the effectiveness of other therapeutic measures'. Falanga suggests that effective wound bed preparation is achieved through the following actions: restoration of bacterial balance; management of necrosis; management of exudate; correction of cellular dysfunction; and restoration of biochemical balance.

TIMERS

The TIME principle (Schultz *et al.*, 2003) is a systematic approach to aid clinicians in the management of the wound bed. The method allows the nurse to focus on the stages of wound healing and eliminate any obstacles to facilitate healing processes. Since its inception, it has been revised to TIMERS (Atkin *et al.*, 2019) which stands for:

T   Tissue non-viable or deficient
I   Infection or inflammation
M   Moisture imbalance
E   Epidermal margin – non-advancing or undermined
R   Repair and regeneration
S   Social factors

The nurse should consider the following questions at each stage: Does the wound require debridement? Does infection need treating? Does exudate need managing? Is the wound improving? Are chronicity or patient-related factors delaying healing?

Wound Cleansing

Wound cleansing should only be considered if the wound has a previous dressing, contains foreign material or to loosen surface debris (Dealey, 2005), as the procedure, if not necessary, can reduce wound bed temperature and remove vital cytokines and growth factors and cause a delay in wound healing. The choice of method for cleaning a wound should be based on a full assessment and no-touch technique. Some wounds are suitable for cleaning with warm tap water, in the shower, bath or a bowl, while others require 0.9% saline solution.

Dressing Selection

The sheer number of dressings available in order to create prompt and cosmetically acceptable healing can often be baffling and lead to the wrong type of dressing being chosen and a delay in the healing process. However, understanding the category in which the dressing is classified can aid appropriate dressing choice.

The selection will be based on a full patient and wound assessment, the goals of the wound intervention, knowledge of the dressing to be used, its uses, side-effects and contraindications, the evidence base, the clinician's personal choice, the patient's concordance with treatment, known allergies and cost. Most organisations have developed wound care formularies and guides to aid prescribing and selection; manufacturer's guidelines should be followed regarding application, wear time and removal. A guide to actions and dressings for consideration is given in Table 18.5.

Not only must the clinician choose the correct dressing for the type of wound and appropriate wound bed management, they must also address other factors that are affecting wound healing, for example nutrition, pressure relief, repositioning, lack of sleep and pain. There should be consideration of other members of the MDT aiding diagnosis and management, use of specialist equipment and adjuvant therapies such as hyperbaric oxygen, medication, pressure-relieving and-reducing devices and cosmetic camouflage.

Medicines Management

Reporting of adverse reactions from wound care products
Adverse incidents from wound care products should be reported to the appropriate monitoring body to enable a clear examination of the safety and efficacy of wound dressings/products.

Actions that monitoring bodies may take after assessment of the situation can include withdrawing a dressing or product from use. There are two methods of reporting adverse reactions.

Those with a product licence (PL).

- Inspect the packaging for a number preceded by the letters PL.
- Fill in the Yellow Card (in the back of any British National Formulary, MIMS or from a pharmacy).
- Ask the doctor or pharmacist to sign the card before sending to the Committee on Safety of Medicines (CSM); nurses at present are not recognised reporters of the scheme.
- Send a copy to the CSM.

Those without a product licence.

- Fill in a Medical Device Agency form.
- Send to MDA adverse incident centre.
- Anyone can fill in these forms and send them to the MDA. A counter signature is not needed.

Multiple Pathology and Wound Care

Care of the Older Person's Skin

Common skin conditions that affect the elderly include eczema, psoriasis, infections, infestations and pruritus (Davies, 2008); however, skin tears, pressure ulcers and incontinence-related damage can also occur (Figure 18.16, Table 18.6). Skin conditions,

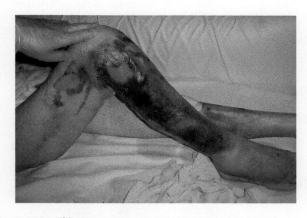

Figure 18.16 Skin tear. *Source:* Flanagan (2013). Reproduced with permission of John Wiley & Sons Ltd.

Table 18.5 Dressings.

CLINICAL OBSERVATION	ACTION TO ACHIEVE WOUND BED PREPARATION	TYPE OF DRESSINGS	OTHER ACTIONS FOR CONSIDERATION
Tissue non-viable or deficient	Debridement of necrosis or slough	Consider debridement via autolytic, sharp surgical, enzymatic, mechanical or biological methods	Seek further advice before intervening on foot ulcers for patients who present with impaired vascular flow, diabetes and neuropathy. Consider surgical and vascular opinion. Utilise podiatry
Infection or inflammation	Remove infection or biofilm	Topical antimicrobials, antibacterials, antiinflammatories, protease inhibitors. Charcoal dressings to manage malodour	As above and ensure diagnosis of infection is correct. Try a 2-week antimicrobial challenge
Moisture imbalance	Moisten dry wounds or remove excess exudate	Moisture rebalancing Dry wounds: use films, hydrocolloids, hydrogels and foams Heavily exuding wounds: compression therapy, foams, alginates, hydrofibres, wound managers, topical negative pressure	Consider skin protection to the peri-wound area in heavily exuding wounds
Edge of wound: non-advancing or undermined	Reassess cause and consider debridement, advanced therapies or surgical intervention	Debridement skin grafts Biological agents	Consider biopsy if non-healing. Utilise adjuvant therapies such as hyperbaric oxygen, referral to other members of the MDT. Consider palliative wound and symptom management. Consider peri-wound area: is it viable, does it require management/ protection, is it suitable for adhesive dressings or tapeless/non-adhesive ones?

Table 18.6 Classification of skin tears. *Source:* **Based on Carville *et al.* (2007).**

SKIN TEAR CLASSIFICATION (STAR)	SKIN DAMAGE
Category 1a	A skin tear where the edges can be realigned to the normal anatomical position (without undue stretching) and the skin or flap colour is not pale, dusky or darkened
Category 1b	A skin tear where the edges can be realigned to the normal anatomical position (without undue stretching) and the skin or flap colour is pale, dusky or darkened
Category 2a	A skin tear where the edges cannot be realigned to the normal anatomical position and the skin or flap colour is not pale, dusky or darkened
Category 2b	A skin tear where the edges cannot be realigned to the normal anatomical position and the skin or flap colour is pale, dusky or darkened
Category 3	A skin tear where the skin flap is completely absent

like general health issues, often go under-reported in the elderly as they may feel defeatist with regard to health and well-being issues or prefer to be stoical. It is therefore important on admission and at regular intervals to assess the skin of the older person and also regularly enquire for further problems that may be considered trivial, as often the skin problem is a sign or symptom of an underlying condition, for example diabetes, renal failure, thyroid dysfunction or iron deficiency anaemia.

In 2008, a best practice statement was developed by a team of specialists on behalf of Wounds UK; this was updated in 2012 and advocates holistic assessment, exploration of underlying conditions, twice per day emollient application, keeping nails short, early detection of areas of excess moisture, good continence care, assessment of the risk of skin tears and good end-of-life care.

Neuroischaemic Diabetic Foot Ulcer

Sixty percent of diabetic foot ulcers are neuroischaemic in nature (Gershater *et al.*, 2009). Patients present late and often have gangrene. The focus of their care should be on revascularisation but because of the gangrene, patients are often considered unsuitable and tend not to be listed for surgery but for amputation instead. Early vascular assessment of diabetic patients with neuropathy is essential in prevention of ulcers and gangrene (IWGDF, 2007). Assessment of toe pressures and ankle pressures can guide early treatment options such as reconstruction, vascular surgery or pharmacology (Apelqvist, 2010). Debridement of neuroischaemic wounds may be initially delayed due to the risk of trauma.

If the gangrene is dry and mummified, the practitioner may leave the wound alone and seek an urgent vascular opinion (Wounds International, 2013).

Conclusion

The prevention and management of wounds have progressed over the last 30 years from a simple wound assessment to the biological, psychological and economic impact of the wound on the patient, carers, clinicians and healthcare providers. Practitioners more than ever need to acquire the necessary knowledge, skills and attitudes in order to assess, plan, implement and evaluate the care delivered for this group of patients. As technology moves forward, so does the need to critically appraise the evidence provided within the realms of cost-effectiveness and efficiency. The quality agenda will promote the collection of outcomes measures and metrics, in order for clinicians to quantify their decisions to ensure the right treatment for the right patient at the right time.

References

Atkin, L., Bućko, Z., Montero, E. C., *et al.* (2019). Implementing TIMERS: the race against hard-to-heal wounds. *Journal of Wound Care*, 28(Suppl.3a), 1–50.

Apelqvist, J. (2010) A paradigm shift is needed in diabetic foot care. www.woundsinternational.com/resources/details/a-paradigm-shift-is-needed-in-diabetic-foot-care (accessed December 2021).

Barr, H., Freeth, D., Hammick, M., Koppel, I. & Reeves, S. (2002) A *Critical Review of Evaluations of Interprofessional Education*. HEA, London.

Bellingham, J. & Stephens, M. (1999) Bridging the hospital/community gap. *Community Nurse*, 5(8), 51–52.

Benbow, M. (2016). Best practice in wound assessment. *Nursing Standard*, 30(27), 40–47.

Buxton, P.K. & Morris-Jones, R. (2013) *ABC Dermatology*, 5th edn. John Wiley & Sons Ltd, Chichester.

Care Quality Commission (2016) *Better care in my hands*. www.cqc.org.uk/sites/default/files/20160519_Better_care_in_my_hands_FINAL.pdf (accessed December 2021).

Carville, K., Lewin, G., Newall, N. *et al.* (2007) STAR: a consensus for skin tear classification. *Primary Intention*, 15(1), 18–28.

Charmaz, K. (1983) Loss of self: a fundamental form of suffering in the chronically ill. *Sociology of Health and Illness*, 5(2), 168–195.

Coleman, S., Nelson, E. A., Vowden, P., *et al.* (2017) Development of a generic wound care assessment minimum data set. *Journal of Tissue Viability*, 26(4), 226–240.

Davies, A. (2008) Management of dry skin conditions in older people. *British Journal of Community Nursing*, 13(6), 250–257.

Dealey, C. (2005) *The Care of Wounds*. Wiley Blackwell, Oxford.

Department of Health (2010) *Using the Commissioning for Quality and Innovation (CQUIN) payment framework – a summary guide*. Department of Health, London.

Edwards, J. (2012) Burn wound and scar management. *Nursing in Practice*, 9, 41–44.

EPUAP, NPUAP & PPPIA (2014) *Prevention and Treatment of Pressure Ulcers: Quick Reference Guide*. www.epuap.org/wp-content/uploads/2010/10/Quick-Reference-Guide-DIGITAL-NPUAP-EPUAP-PPPIA-16Oct2014.pdf (accessed December 2021).

Falanga, V. (2000) Classifications for wound bed preparation and stimulation of chronic wounds. *Wound Repair Regeneration*, 8, 347–352.

Fitzpatrick, T.B. (1988) The validity and practicality of sun-reactive skin types through VI. *Archives of Dermatology*, 124, 869–871.

Flanagan, M. (2013) *Wound Healing and Skin Integrity. Principles and Practice*. John Wiley & Sons, Chichester.

Gershater, M.A., Löndahl, M., Nyberg, P. et al. (2009) Complexity of factors related to outcome of neuropathic and neuroischaemic/ischaemic diabetic foot ulcers: a cohort study. *Diabetologia*, 52(3), 398–407.

Guest, J.F., Ayoub, N., McIlwraith, T., et al. (2017) Health economic burden that wounds impose on the National Health Service in the UK. *International Wound Journal*, 14, 322–330.

Guest, J.F., Fuller, G.W. & Vowden, P. (2020) Cohort study evaluating the burden of wounds to the UK's National Health Service in 2017/2018: update from 2012/2013. *BMJ Open*, 10(12), e045253.

Gupta, M., Gupta, A. & Haberman, H. (1987) The self-inflicted dermatoses: a critical review. *General Hospital Psychiatry*, 9(1), 45–52.

Harth, W., Taube, K.M. & Gieler, U. (2010) Factitious disorders in dermatology. *Journal der Deutschen Dermatologischen Gesellschaft*, 8(5), 361–373.

International Working Group on the Diabetic Foot (2003) *Definitions and criteria for diabetic foot disease*. https://iwgdfguidelines.org/wp-content/uploads/2019/05/definitions-and-criteria-final.pdf (accessed December 2021).

International Working Group on the Diabetic Foot (2007) *Peripheral arterial disease and diabetes: international consensus*. https://iwgdfguidelines.org/ (accessed December 2021).

Kerr, M. (2017) *Diabetic foot care in England: an economic study*. https://diabetes-resources-production.s3-eu-west-1.amazonaws.com/diabetes-storage/migration/pdf/Diabetic%2520footcare%2520in%2520England%2C%2520An%2520economic%2520case%2520study%2520%28January%25202017%29.pdf (accessed December 2021).

Konishi, N., Kawada, A., Morimoto, Y. et al.(2007) New approach to the evaluation of skin color of pigmentary lesions using Skin Tone Color Scale. *Journal of Dermatology*, 34(7), 441–446.

Maya-Enero, S., Candel-Pau, J., Garcia-Garcia, J., Giménez-Arnau, A.M., & López-Vílchez, M. Á. (2020) Validation of a neonatal skin color scale. *European Journal of Pediatrics*, 179(2).

Moffatt, C., Vowden, K., Price, P. & Vowden, P. (2008) Psychosocial factors and wound healing. In: *Hard to Heal Wounds: A Holistic Approach*, pp. 10–14. European Wound Management Association, Frederiksberg, Denmark.

National Health Service Improvement (2018) *Pressure ulcers: revised definition and measurement framework*. www.england.nhs.uk/pressure-ulcers-revised-definition-and-measurement-framework/ (accessed December 2021).

National Institute for Health and Care Excellence (2008) *Prevention and Treatment of Surgical Site Infections. CG74*. NICE, London.

National Institute for Health and Care Excellence (2011) *Self-harm in over 8s: long-term management*. NICE, London.

National Institute for Health and Care Excellence (2013) *Clinical knowledge summaries: Leg ulcer – venous*. https://cks.nice.org.uk/topics/leg-ulcer-venous/ (accessed December 2021).

National Institute for Health and Care Excellence (2014) *Pressure Ulcers: Prevention and Management*. www.nice.org.uk/guidance/cg179 (accessed December 2021).

National Institute for Health and Care Excellence (2021) *How should I interpret ankle brachial pressure index (ABPI) results?* https://cks.nice.org.uk/topics/leg-ulcer-venous/diagnosis/interpretation-of-abpi/ (accessed December 2021).

National Network for Burn Care (2012) *National Burn Care Referral Guidance*. www.britishburnassociation.org/wp-content/uploads/2018/02/National-Burn-Care-Referral-Guidance-2012.pdf

Nursing & Midwifery Council (2018a) *The Code*. NMC, London.

Nursing & Midwifery Council (2018b) *Future Nurse Standards*. NMC, London.

Patel, S. (2010) Investigating wound infection. *Wound Essentials*, 5, 40–47.

Schultz, G., Sibbald, G., Falanga, V. et al. (2003) Wound bed preparation: a systematic approach to wound management. *Wound Repair Regeneration*, 11, 1–28.

Scottish Intercollegiate Guidelines for Nurses (2010) *Management of Chronic Venous Leg Ulcers*. SIGN Guideline 120. SIGN, Edinburgh.

Tantam, D. & Huband, N. (2009) *Understanding Repeated Self-injury: A Multidisciplinary Approach*. Palgrave Macmillan, Basingstoke.

Vowden, P., Apelqvist, J. & Moffatt, C. (2008) Wound complexity and healing. In: *Hard to Heal Wounds: A Holistic Approach*, pp. 2–9. European Wound Management Association, Frederiksberg, Denmark.

Winter, G.D. (1962) Formation of the scab and the rate of epithelization of superficial wounds in the skin of the young domestic pig. *Nature*, 193, 293–294.

World Union of Wound Healing Societies (2007) *Wound Exudate and the Role of Dressings. A Consensus Document*. WUWHS, London.

World Union of Wound Healing Societies (2008) *Wound Infection in Clinical Practice. A Consensus Document*. WUWHS, London.

Wounds International (2013) *Best Practice Guidelines: Wound Management in Diabetic Foot Ulcers*. www.woundsinternational.com/uploads/resources/33c16c714942cc022a74420bfdb5f3fd.pdf (accessed December 2021).

Wounds UK (2012) *Best Practice Statement: Care of the Older Person's Skin*, 2nd edn. Wounds UK, London.

313

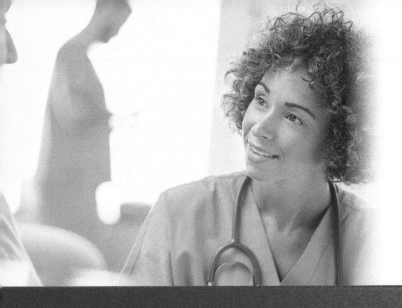

19

The Principles of Medicine Administration and Pharmacology

Barry Hill

Northumbria University, UK

Learning Outcomes

On completion of this chapter you will be able to:

- Define the term 'pharmacology'
- Differentiate between the terms 'pharmacokinetics' and 'pharmacodynamics'
- Evaluate up-to-date information on medicine management and work within national and local policies
- Administer medicines safely in a timely manner, including controlled drugs
- Discuss the advantages and disadvantages of various routes of drug administration
- Keep and maintain records within a multidisciplinary framework and as part of a team

Proficiencies

NMC Proficiencies and Standards:

- Demonstrate an understanding of professional, legal and ethical frameworks relating to safe administration of medicines in practice
- Work within the professional, ethical and legal framework that underpins safe and effective medicine administration and management
- Demonstrate an ability to safely store and dispose of medicines
- Ensure safe administration of medications and maintain accurate records of the procedure
- Use knowledge of commonly administered medicines to act promptly in cases where side-effects and adverse reactions occur
- Work in partnership with other healthcare teams

 Visit the companion website at www.wiley.com/go/peate/nursingpractice3e where you can test yourself using flashcards, multiple-choice questions and more.

Nursing Practice: Knowledge and Care, Third Edition. Edited by Ian Peate and Aby Mitchell.
© 2022 John Wiley & Sons Ltd. Published 2022 by John Wiley & Sons Ltd.
Companion website: www.wiley.com/go/peate/nursingpractice3e

Introduction

Administering drugs means more than just giving a medicine to a patient; the process must involve the patient, their relatives and other healthcare practitioners but primarily it must be safe. Nurses must adhere to national, local and professional guidelines so the administration process meets professional, legal and ethical requirements. Nurses care for patients who are better informed, in part due to access to the internet, and are involved in preparing patients for safe discharge back to the community as well as having an understanding of differing health contexts, such as an ageing population. An important requisite is that nurses should have a sound knowledge base that includes pharmacology, as this will help to inform clinical decision making. Knowledge of pharmacology, encompassing nomenclature (what drugs are called), pharmacokinetics (how the body deals with drugs) and pharmacodynamics (how a particular drug works in the body), is essential.

In 2016, the National Institute for Health and Care Excellence (NICE) published a quality standard entitled *Medicines Optimisation*, covering the safe and effective use of medicines (NICE, 2016a); all nurses should familiarise themselves with this standard. Additionally, due to changes to the Nursing and Midwifery Council's (NMC) standards of education, nurses now use the Professional Guidance on the Administration of Medicines in Healthcare Settings (Royal Pharmaceutical Society (RPS) and Royal College of Nursing (RCN), 2019).

The Nursing Associate (NMC, 2018a)

3.15 must understand the principles of safe and effective administration and optimisation of medicines in accordance with local and national policies.

As a valued member of the health and care team, the nursing associate, at the point of registration, must understand the key principles associated with the safe and effective administration of medications along with medicine optimisation. At all times local policy and procedure is to be followed.

A starting point must be a consideration of definitions within the legal framework. Some sections of the Medicines Act 1968 and the Misuse of Drugs Act 1971 have been incorporated into the newest regulations, the Human Medicines Regulations 2012 (SI 2012/1916), known as HMR 2012. The Commission on Human Medicine's functions are set out in regulation 10, and it must advise ministers on the safety, efficacy and quality of medicinal products. The regulations define medicinal products as being:

'any substance or combination of substances that may be used by or administered to human beings with a view to restoring, correcting, or modifying a physiological function by exerting a pharmacological, immunological or metabolic action, or making a medical diagnosis'.

The Medicines Act 1968, section 2(7) requires market authorisation before any medicine can be used for humans. A drug has been defined as a substance which exerts a pharmacological, immunological or metabolic action (EU Directive 2001/83), so a drug is the chemical substance – the active ingredient in a medicine – but often the terms are used interchangeably.

In terms of ethical practice, Beauchamp and Childress's (2013) four principles (autonomy, non-maleficence, beneficence and justice) will be considered throughout the chapter. You should consider patient autonomy – the right to self-determination – to help patients make decisions in relation to medicines. Beneficence is about promoting benefit for the patient, non-maleficence about not doing harm, and justice is about fairness and access to treatment options.

Pharmacology

Pharmacology is defined by the RPS and RCN as the science or practice of the preparation and dispensing of medicinal drugs (RPS and RCN, 2019). Pharmacology encompasses pharmacokinetics, pharmacodynamics, therapeutics and toxicology. While there are many pharmacology textbooks written for nurses, no single source covers all medications prescribed but one resource that is updated regularly is the *British National Formulary* (BNF, 2020a).

Most drugs are used to treat disease such as diabetes and coronary heart disease, but some are taken for recreational purposes, such as body builders' use of anabolic steroids and illicit use of cannabis/marijuana.

Pharmacokinetics

This is the study of what the body does to a drug as when it enters, moves through and exits the body. Nurses therefore require knowledge of absorption, distribution, metabolism and excretion. For example, the choice of administration route will affect the speed at which drug action occurs. Pharmacokinetics is also dependent on patient-related factors such as renal function, age and sex.

Absorption

This needs to take place before the drug reaches the cell. Drugs are administered via different routes of absorption, including:

- Injections, i.e. intramuscular (IM), intravenous (IV), subcutaneous (SC)
- Vaginal
- Buccal
- Aural (ear)
- Sublingual
- Oral
- Rectal
- Inhalational
- Intrathecal.

The Nursing Associate (NMC, 2018a)

3.17 must recognise the different ways by which medicines can be prescribed.

The role of the nursing associate demands that you can provide care that is safe and effective. Recognising the various ways in which medications can be prescribed can help with this.

Jot This Down

These routes of absorption can be divided into subgroups: enteral, parenteral and topical. Can you order them according to the fastest route for drug absorption?

For an oral drug, absorption takes place through the intestinal wall and into the plasma before it reaches the site of action. Any drug given via the oral route is absorbed from the gastrointestinal (GI) tract and is transported to the liver via the portal circulation (hepatic portal vein) (Figure 19.1).

In the liver, the drug is metabolised by the hepatic enzymes before it is returned to the general circulation. One of the liver's functions is to detoxify the drug, which may reduce its effect; this is called 'first-pass metabolism' or 'first-pass system' (Figure 19.2). The amount of drug that returns into general circulation after it has passed through the liver is now available for therapeutic use. Not all drugs are available for action, particularly if they have undergone protein binding (see later). Some drugs pass through the liver without any biotransformation, the process whereby the parent compound is metabolised; it may be increased or decreased or not change at all. Barber & Robertson (2020) give the example of codeine, which is metabolised to morphine, a much stronger opiate.

Drugs administered by other routes, such as by injection, will bypass the first-pass metabolism. Drugs given using these routes enter the bloodstream directly so their bioavailability is much higher compared with medications taken orally.

If there is food in the GI tract at the time a medication is taken, this can affect the absorption of the drug. This is because digested food particles compete with drug molecules at the same absorption site, resulting in low plasma concentration and causing delayed action of the drug. Unless the medication should be taken with food, drugs should be administered an hour before eating.

Jot This Down

Think about conditions or surgery that a person may have had that can affect absorption of drugs from the GI tract and what could be the consequences for the patient.

Absorption is facilitated by certain transport systems in the body.

- *Active transport system (Figure 19.3)*: requires cellular energy to move drugs from an area of low concentration to an area of high concentration.
- *Passive transport system (Figure 19.4)*: does not require cellular energy. Drugs move from an area of high concentration to an area of low concentration.
- *Facilitated diffusion (Figure 19.5)*: drugs are transported into the cells by carrier proteins found on the surface of the cells.

Distribution

This is the movement of a drug to and from the blood and various tissues of the body (e.g. fat, muscle, brain tissue) and the relative proportions of drug in the tissues. After a drug is absorbed into the bloodstream, it rapidly circulates throughout the body. As blood circulates, the drug moves from the bloodstream into the body's tissues. Drugs pass more readily between the intravascular and interstitial compartments than between other compartments,

316

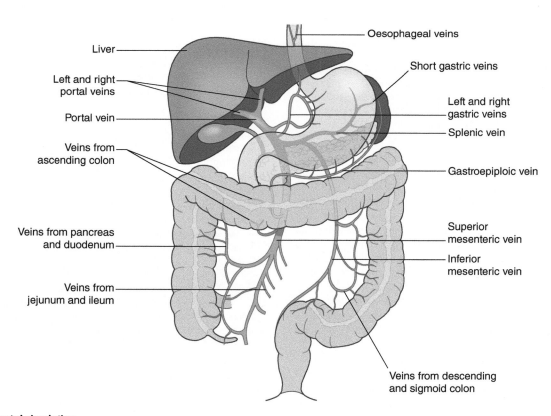

Figure 19.1 Portal circulation.

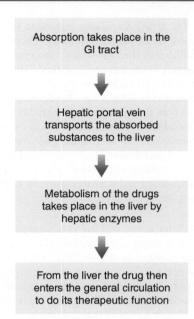

Absorption takes place in the GI tract

↓

Hepatic portal vein transports the absorbed substances to the liver

↓

Metabolism of the drugs takes place in the liver by hepatic enzymes

↓

From the liver the drug then enters the general circulation to do its therapeutic function

Figure 19.2 **First-pass metabolism.**

for example the central nervous system (CNS). Many factors affect drug distribution in the body, including:

- *Lipid solubility*: the greater the lipid solubility, the greater the distribution
- *Drug molecule size*: smaller molecules are distributed more extensively throughout the body than larger molecules
- *Cellular binding*: drugs may exist in free or bound form. Bound forms of drugs exist as reservoirs. The free and bound forms co-exist in equilibrium. Cellular binding depends on the plasma-binding proteins
- *Plasma protein binding*: the level of plasma proteins affects distribution. The most important and abundant plasma protein is albumin. Others include globulins, glycoproteins and lipoproteins.

Once the drug reaches the general circulation after passing through the liver, drug molecules are distributed mainly by four methods:

- Blood flow
- Plasma protein binding
- Solubility of the drug
- Storage sites.

Blood Flow Drugs are distributed to many or all parts of the body by the circulation. The distribution of drugs is dependent on vascular permeability, blood flow, tissue uptake of the drug and plasma protein binding. Organs that are highly vascular, such as the heart, liver and kidneys, will rapidly acquire a drug because of the rich blood supply. However, the levels of a drug in bone, fat, muscle and skin may take some time to rise due to reduced vascularity and perfusion. The person's level of physical activity and local tissue temperature may also affect drug distribution to the skin and muscle. Other factors affecting drug distribution include heart disease, blood pressure and blood volume.

Jot This Down

Think about any other conditions that may affect drug distribution by increased or decreased blood flow.

Plasma Protein Binding In the circulation, a drug is either bound to circulating plasma proteins or is 'free' in an unbound state. The plasma protein usually involved in binding a drug is albumin. If a drug is bound, then it is said to be inactive and cannot have a pharmacological effect. Only the free drug molecules can cause an effect. As free molecules leave the circulation, drug molecules are released from plasma protein to re-establish the ratio between the bound and the free molecules. Certain drugs compete with other drugs for drug-binding sites on albumin.

317

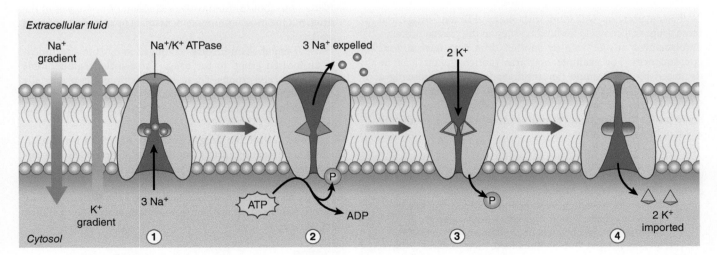

Figure 19.3 **Active transport system.**

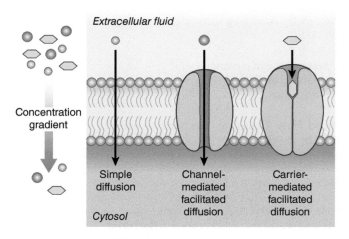

Figure 19.4 Passive transport system.

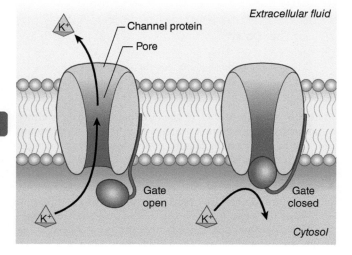

Figure 19.5 Facilitated diffusion.

Plasma proteins will bind with many different drugs and these drugs will compete for binding sites on the plasma proteins. Displacement of one drug by another drug may have serious consequences. For example, warfarin (anticoagulant) can be displaced by tolbutamide (an antidiabetic drug), producing a risk of haemorrhage as the level of warfarin in plasma increases, while tolbutamide can be displaced by salicylates (used as an analgesic for the treatment of mild-to-moderate pain), producing a risk of hypoglycaemia.

Red Flag

Certain diseases, such as nephrotic syndrome, severe burns and malnutrition, can affect the availability of plasma protein-binding sites. In these conditions, the level of plasma protein is reduced, thus increasing the plasma concentration of a drug and leading to a greater effect on the body systems.

Solubility of the Drug Capillaries supplying the CNS differ from those in most other parts of the body. They lack channels between endothelial cells through which substances in the blood normally gain access to the extracellular fluid. This barrier constrains the passage of substances from the blood to the brain and cerebrospinal fluid and is termed the blood–brain barrier. Lipid-soluble drugs, such as diazepam, will pass readily into the CNS, whereas lipid-insoluble drugs will not. This is because the cell membrane is composed of lipid (Figure 19.6) and lipid-soluble drugs cross the cell membrane much more readily than water-soluble drugs. This explains why certain fat-soluble drugs, such as barbiturates, tranquillisers and cannabis, can have lingering effects hours or days after initial use.

Storage Sites Fatty tissue will act as a storage site for lipid-soluble drugs, for example anticoagulants. Drugs accumulating in the fatty tissue may not be released until after administration of the drug has ceased. Calcium-containing structures such as bone and teeth can accumulate drugs that are bound to calcium, such as tetracycline (antibiotic). Drugs that accumulate in fatty tissues leave the tissues so slowly that they circulate in the bloodstream for days after a person has stopped taking the drug.

Distribution of a given drug may vary from person to person. Obese people may store large amounts of fat-soluble drugs, whereas very thin people may store relatively little. Older people, even when thin, may store large amounts of fat-soluble drugs, because the proportion of body fat increases with ageing.

Metabolism

Metabolism is the transformation of drugs in preparation for excretion from the body. This is mainly carried out in the liver by the hepatic enzymes and, to some extent, in other areas such as the intestines, lungs and plasma (Peate & Hill, 2021). Enzymes responsible for the biotransformation of drugs belong to the group of cytochromes P450 that are found in the smooth endoplasmic reticulum of a cell. The products of drug metabolism are called metabolites. Inactive metabolites are excreted from the body; if they are not excreted, they can become toxic. Metabolism occurs in two phases: I and II.

- *Phase I* metabolism can involve reduction or hydrolysis of the drug, but the most common biochemical process that occurs is oxidation.
- *Phase II* metabolism involves conjugation, i.e. the attachment of an ionised group to the drug. These include glutathione, methyl or acetyl groups. These metabolic processes principally occur in the hepatocyte cytoplasm. Other sites of drug metabolism include epithelial cells of the GI tract, lungs, kidneys and skin.

To reiterate, fat-soluble drugs could take longer to metabolise, whereas water-soluble drugs are different. The opiate diamorphine, also known as heroin, is water soluble; it is not stored in the body and is metabolised quickly, so illicit users must readminister the drug every 4–5 hours to maintain a 'high'. For patients, a more slowly metabolised opiate like slow-release morphine would be more suitable.

Excretion

Excretion is the removal of a drug from the body; the organs of excretion include the kidneys, GI tract and skin through sweat (e.g.

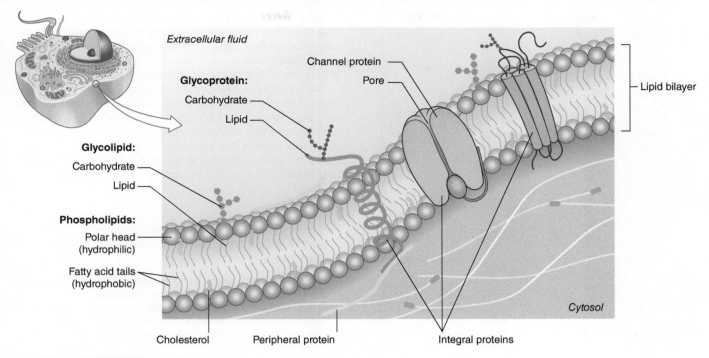

Figure 19.6 Cell membrane.

vitamin B), the breast and lungs. The rate of excretion depends on the physical status of the person. If the person has renal or heart failure, the drug may stay in the system longer, resulting in drug toxicity. The lungs are the main route of excretion for anaesthetic gases and, to some extent, alcohol. The kidneys are the principal organs of excretion for drugs. Most water-soluble drugs are excreted by the kidneys, while fat-soluble drugs are excreted in the faeces.

Jot This Down

Can you name any conditions that may affect drug excretion?

Half-life

Half-life is the amount of time required for the concentration of drug in the body to be reduced by half; sometimes the symbol $t\frac{1}{2}$ is used. Understanding half-life is important when calculating the dosage and frequency of a drug as it may interact to enhance or decrease physiological response.

Pharmacodynamics

This is the study of drug action at the biochemical and pharmacological level and the effect of drugs on the body. By acting on receptors (proteins) on a cell, a drug can either change the environment of a cell or alter the rate of cell function; drugs can either increase or decrease certain physiological functions. Metformin increases receptor sensitivity to insulin in patients with type 2 diabetes whilst tamoxifen can block normal cell function and activity, thus reducing the proliferation of tumour cells. When a drug enhances the physiological action of another drug, it is called an agonist. One that decreases the physiological function of another drug is called an antagonist.

Drug Interactions

Drug interactions may be beneficial or detrimental to the person. The interaction may take place during absorption, distribution, metabolism or excretion. The interaction can occur between drugs or between drugs and chemicals in food (Barber & Robertson, 2020). A comprehensive account of drug interactions, for example drug–food interactions, can be found in a specific chapter within the BNF.

Receptors

Receptors are protein molecules embedded in the cell membrane, organelles in the cytoplasm (e.g. mitochondria, Golgi complex) and the nucleus of a cell (Figure 19.7). They transport drug molecules into the cell. There are different types of receptors.

The Role of the Nurse in Pharmacology

The nurse's role involves promoting the responsible use of chemicals to enhance health and minimise side-effects. This requires knowledge and understanding not only of the physical and social sciences but also the legal and ethical issues pertaining to nursing care. In carrying out drug administration, nurses must be skilled in the procedure required to interpret prescriptions, and handle, control and administer drugs using invasive and non-invasive techniques safely. Nurses need to fulfil their record-keeping obligations in line with professional guidance and be able to defend their acts or omissions in line with professional accountability. The person and their family should be part of the decision-making process.

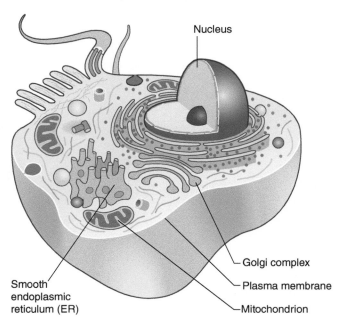

Figure 19.7 **Anatomy of a cell.**

Labels in figure: Nucleus, Golgi complex, Plasma membrane, Mitochondrion, Smooth endoplasmic reticulum (ER)

Methods

Registrants must only supply and administer medicinal products in accordance with several specific processes.

- Patient-specific direction (PSD)
- Patient medicines administration chart (may be called medicines administration record, MAR)
- Patient group direction (PGD)
- Medicines Act exemption
- Standing order
- Homely remedy protocol
- Prescription forms

What the Experts Say

'If a person with Parkinson's disease does not get their medication on time all of the time, it can lead to them becoming immobile and extending any hospital stay, as it can take weeks to get the therapeutic effect of the medicine back to where it should be, hence the Parkinson's UK campaign 'Get it on Time' (Parkinson's UK, 2019).'

Sarah, Neurology Nurse Specialist

The nurse is responsible for knowing about anything that affects nursing care in relation to drug use, such as timing of doses, special techniques for administration, precautions to take before administering a drug, assessment of the toxicity, drug interactions and side-effects.

Jot This Down

Consider the implications for a patient who is having enteral feeding via a nasogastric tube over 20 hours per day. How would they get their prescribed analgesia?

Side-effects are undesirable physiological effects exerted by the drug other than the intended therapeutic effect, more commonly referred to as adverse drug incidents. Some drugs have a multitude of side-effects, such as suppression of respiration and retention of urine, in the case of opioid drugs, and nausea and vomiting.

Nurses must be aware of the contraindications and precautions of the drugs they are administering. Contraindications are symptoms that alert healthcare professionals to the potential dangers where a drug should be avoided if the person has the condition mentioned; for example, glaucoma is a contraindication for anticholinergic drugs as these drugs may increase intraocular pressure and precipitate or aggravate glaucoma (Box 19.1).

Box 19.1 Outline of the Nurse's Role in Medicine Management

Refer to the BNF if unsure of the therapeutic use, side-effects and contraindications of the drug you are giving.

- *Awareness of the person's care plan.* Check the care plan to make sure the person's care has not changed because of the drug or the person has developed any adverse reactions
- *Consent from the person that it is acceptable to administer the medication.* The person may refuse to take the medication they are prescribed
- *Check the identity of the person.* A hospital number is unique to every person. Check against their identity bracelet and treatment chart, adhere to local policy and procedures
- *Check the orientation level of the person* (ask for name and date of birth). This ensures the correct person is receiving the medication but also might help in considering the capacity of the patient
- *Check the prescription chart.* To ensure the correct treatment chart corresponds to the correct person
- *The prescription must be clearly written and legible.* It is a requirement for the prescriber to prescribe all medications legibly using capital letters; the nurse can query and refuse to give the medication until it is legibly written
- *Double-check the medication has not been administered at an earlier time.* Check the signature box for the corresponding time and date
- *Check allergies.* Check with the person and their medical notes to ensure the person is not allergic to the medication. Any allergies should be notified immediately to the prescriber and documented in the person's notes. It is common for a patient to wear an identity bracelet that alerts others that the patient has an allergy
- *Clear prescription label* on the medicine to be administered
- *Check expiry date* of the medicine being administered
- *Consider dosage* in line with weight, method of administration, route and timing
- *Administer/withhold* depending on the person's condition
- *If medication has been administered orally*, ensure all medication has been taken by the person
- *Observe for effects/side-effects* and report accordingly
- *Clear, accurate and immediate record* of:
  - Medicines administered
  - Medicines withheld (giving rationale)
  - Medicines refused
  - Delegation of the task.

The Nursing Associate (NMC, 2018a)

3.16 Must demonstrate the ability to recognise the effects of medicines, allergies, drug sensitivity, side-effects, contraindications and adverse reactions.

Caring in a holistic manner requires you to be aware of and alert to the effects (positive and negative) of the medicines people are taking. You must also report and document any concerns you may have.

The *Professional Guidance on the Administration of Medicines in Healthcare Settings* (RPS and RCN, 2019) details certain criteria that must be fulfilled with regard to medicines.

- *Administration of medicines*: medicines are administered in accordance with a prescription, patient specific direction, patient group direction or other relevant specified exemption.
- *Covert administration*: medicines are administered covertly only to people who actively refuse their medication and who are considered to lack mental capacity in accordance with an agreed management plan.
- *Transcribing*: 'the act of making an exact copy, usually in writing. In the context of this guidance, transcribing is the copying of previously prescribed medicines details to enable their administration in line with legislation (i.e. in accordance with the instructions of a prescriber)' (RPS and RCN, 2019, p.6).

Red Flag

Healthcare organisations must have a policy for self-administration of medicines. Patients maintain responsibility for the administration of some or all of their medicines during a stay in the healthcare setting, unless a risk assessment indicates otherwise (RPS and RCN, 2019, p.3).

What the Experts Say

It is easy to neglect communication about medicines when you have only a few minutes with each patient, so attitudes need to change to recognise that taking the time to discuss medicines now will help to prevent errors and worsening health – saving more time in the long run. There needs to be a cultural change across the healthcare professions to raise awareness.

Nurse consultant in thrombosis and anticoagulation

Primary Care

Advise the patient on the following.
- Learn the names of medications being taking and why they are taken. Know unwanted effects of drugs prescribed.
- Keep all medication in a cupboard and out of reach of children.
- Always check the medication label to ensure they are taking the correct medication at the correct time.
- If unsure of any medication, check with the local pharmacist.
- Check for the expiry date of the drug, dispose of any unwanted medicines in a safe manner, return unwanted drugs to the chemist or pharmacy department.

- If a patient misses a dose, do not double the dose for the next intake. Always seek advice from the prescriber, pharmacist or practice nurse.
- Never stop prescribed medications unless advised to do so.
- Do not crush or open capsules without checking with the pharmacist or prescriber.
- Take the medications as directed by the prescriber.
- Order repeat medication in good time before the medication runs out.
- Always check with the pharmacist when taking non-prescription medications with prescribed medications, for drug interactions.
- Make sure the patient is aware of the shelf-life of the medicines.

Source: Adapted from Berman et al. (2015).

Patient Group Directions

Patient group directions (PGDs) constitute a legal framework allowing certain registered healthcare professionals to supply and administer medicines to groups of patients who fit the criteria laid out in the PGD (NICE, 2017). A PGD is defined in the Health Service Circular (HSC2000/026) as 'Written instructions for the supply or administration of medicines to groups of patients who may not be individually identified before presentation for treatment'. It is a written direction that allows the supply and/or administration of a specified medicine or medicines, by named authorised health professionals, to a well-defined group of patients requiring treatment of a specific condition (RPS and RCN, 2019).

Patient-specific directions (PSDs) differ from PGDs in that there are written instructions signed by a doctor or non-medical prescriber for a medicine to be supplied and/or administered to a named patient. An example could be a vaccination clinic where the nurse would have a list of named patients, so the nurse can administer the prescribed vaccine to those on the list.

Nurse Prescribing

The role of the nurse is varied and ever changing; this is also true of the role of the nurse in relation to prescribing medication. While non-registered practitioners (including students) are not permitted to prescribe medications, the notion of limited prescribing is something the registered graduate nurse may encounter due to new higher education (HE) curricula that teach pharmacology and prescribing theory and offer supervised 'prescriber ready' practice (NMC, 2018b).

Proficiency

Prior to undertaking limited prescribing at the point of registration, students must demonstrate proficiency regarding a list of outcome-based standards, including being prescriber ready (NMC, 2018b). The proficiencies describe the roles, responsibilities and accountabilities for all registered nurses, including prescribing.

Generic and Brand Names

Licensed medicines have three names: a chemical name, a generic name and one or more brand names. The generic name is a drug's common scientific name, sometimes referred to as non-proprietary. A brand or proprietary named drug is a medicine discovered, developed and marketed by a pharmaceutical company. An example of a generic drug, one used for diabetes, is metformin hydrochloride; the brand name is Glucophage®. Another generic drug, used for hypertension, is metoprolol, whose brand name is Lopressor®. Medicines sold under generic names are usually cheaper because the research and development costs are lower. However, they contain the same active ingredient as the equivalent branded medicines.

The brand name is clearly given on any packaging and the generic name appears on the packet in small print. Prescribers are encouraged to prescribe using the generic name.

Legislation and Policies Governing Drug Administration

One of the main Acts governing medicine administration is the Medicines Act 1968, partially subsumed into the Human Medicines Regulations 2012, but there are many other pieces of legislation or policy governing day-to-day practice.

Jot This Down

During clinical placement, have you witnessed any situation where professionals did not exercise their professional judgement when giving out medicines to patients?

When administering medications, it is important to understand relevant legislation and policies. The legislation relates to the prescribing, supply, storage and administration of medicines. Classification of medicinal products is outlined in HMR 2012, Part 1 (5).

- *General sales list* (GSL): do not need a prescription, sold in a general store and direct pharmaceutical supervision is not required.
- *Pharmacy only medicines* (P): sold only under control of a pharmacist.
- *Prescription only medicines* (POMs): supplied or administered to a person under the direction of a UK registered doctor, dentist or non-medical prescriber. A person may not administer a POM unless he or she is a practitioner or acting in accordance with the direction of a practitioner.

Misuse of Drugs Act 1971

This Act controls the import, export, production, supply, possession and manufacture of controlled drugs to prevent abuse. There are five schedules within the Act. Schedule 1 names drugs considered to have little or no therapeutic value and are subjected to the most restrictive control. Schedule 3 are those drugs which can be held legally by someone with a prescription, for example a patient who requires morphine for analgesia. Schedule 5 includes those drugs with a therapeutic value and which are

readily available as over-the-counter medicines. The Act is also designed to promote research and education relating to drug dependence (Dougherty *et al.*, 2015). The level of control depends on the potential for abuse or misuse. This framework allows criminal penalties to be set when a drug is used illegally.

The drugs subject to control are termed 'controlled drugs'. They are classified into three groups.

- *Class A (Part I)*: examples are Ecstasy, LSD, heroin, cocaine, crack, magic mushrooms, amphetamines (if prepared for injection).
- *Class B (Part II)*: examples are amphetamines, cannabis, methylphenidate (Ritalin®), pholcodine.
- *Class C (Part III)*: examples are tranquillisers, some painkillers, gamma-hydroxybutyrate (GHB), ketamine.

The classification system is reviewed regularly. Safe custody of drugs was governed by Misuse of Drugs and Misuse of Drugs (Safe Custody) (Amendment) Regulations 2007 and this was revoked when the Controlled Drugs (Supervision of Management and Use) Regulations 2013 came into force.

Large organisations such as NHS trusts, hospices and care homes have to appoint a Controlled Drug Accountable Officer (CDAO) whose duties include compliance with the Misuse of Drugs legislation, having in place a system for reporting and recording concerns or untoward incidents about controlled drug use, and the development of standard operating procedures related to controlled drugs (NICE, 2015a).

With the exceptions of drugs in Schedules 4 and 5, controlled drugs must be kept in a locked cupboard and the keys kept by the person in charge of the ward or their deputy (Table 19.1). All drugs administered are recorded in a controlled drugs register. Every drug must have its own page with the drug's name as the heading, the date and time of administration, name of the person, signatures of the nurse administering the drug and the witness. The number of ampoules or tablets or the amount of elixir before and after is recorded. No cancellation or deletion must be made, and all entries must be in ink. The register itself must be kept for 2 years from the date of the last entry.

In 2016, NICE produced new guidance on the safe management of controlled drugs after a 7-year review of incidents related to controlled drug use (NICE 2016b).

Cold Chain

A cold chain is continuous maintenance of low temperature required for biologicals from the point of manufacture, during transportation and storage prior to administration; vaccines are an example, as is blood for transfusion. The storage temperature needs to be monitored regularly, alarm systems checked and fridges maintained, all part of the nurse's role.

Preparation of Drugs

Drugs come in many forms: tablets, liquids, suppositories, ointments, patches and creams. Tablets are sugar-coated, starch-based or film-coated, produced in this format because they are broken down in either the stomach or the intestine. Sugar coatings are used to improve appearance and palatability. In all starch-based

Table 19.1 A schedule table with examples of drugs within the schedules.

SCHEDULE 1	SCHEDULE 2	SCHEDULE 3	SCHEDULE 4	SCHEDULE 5
Cannabis, raw opium	Most opiates commonly used, such as diamorphine, morphine, fentanyl, pethidine	Minor stimulant drugs and barbiturates, pentazocine, temazepam	Benzodiazepines, such as diazepam, anabolic and androgenic steroids	Minimal risk of abuse. Drugs such as low-strength morphine, cocaine, morphine
Must be kept in a locked cupboard where access is restricted	Must be kept in a locked cupboard where access is restricted	Varies: some drugs are required to be kept in a locked cupboard, such as buprenorphine	No requirement	No requirement
Controlled drug register must be used	Controlled drug register must be used	No requirement	No requirement	No requirement

tablets, the breakdown of the starch coating takes place in the mouth by the salivary enzyme amylase. Tablets must disintegrate in the GI tract before they can be broken down and absorbed. Tablets may be formulated to achieve controlled release as they pass through the GI tract.

Enteric-coated Tablets

Coated with a hard shell so that breakdown of these tablets takes place in the intestine where the pH is alkaline and not in the stomach where it is acidic, known as enteric-coated tablets. Some of the drugs in enteric-coated tablets are gastric irritants and should be taken with food or after a meal. Enteric-coated medications should never be crushed as this may render the drug ineffective (Gracia-Vásquez *et al.*, 2017).

Red Flag

 Do not crush enteric-coated tables; doing so will render the drug ineffective.

Capsules

Some drugs are prepared in a capsule so they are easy to swallow. The capsule is made of gelatin and the contents may be a powder, solid, liquid or even paste. If the capsule is difficult for the person to swallow, the capsule should not be removed and the contents sprinkled on food to give to patients (Dougherty *et al.*, 2015). Breaking the capsule could render the drug ineffective. Masking the drug with food before feeding elderly or confused patients is then causing harm to the patient. Patients have the right to know what they are taking and the effects it may have on them. For

Medicines Management

 In exceptional circumstances, where a change or addition to the administration details is required and a delay in administering a medicine (other than a Schedule 2 CD) would compromise patient care, verbal orders are used. The process is underpinned by risk assessments and organisational policy and/or procedures (RPS and RCN, 2019, p.5).

those patients whose belief or faith bars them from using animal-based gelatin, some capsules are produced in a vegetable-based gelatin.

If a drug is eliminated rapidly, the plasma concentration will fall rapidly and the person may have to take the drug more frequently. This is avoided by giving the person medications in a slow-release preparation. Tablets such as aspirin and omeprazole are available in this format (Barber & Robertson, 2020). Crushing these tablets will render the drug ineffective.

Liquid Preparations

Some people find it difficult to swallow tablets because of their unpleasant taste. Many drugs, especially antibiotics, are prepared in liquid format. These preparations may use certain flavourings and sugar to make them more palatable. However, some medications, such as penicillin, are unstable in solution and are therefore prepared in a powder format and water is added to the powder to make a suspension.

Creams and Ointments

The preparation of creams and ointments is different, in that creams are water based while ointments are oil based. Some of the water within the drug molecule in a cream gets absorbed via the aqueous pores. However, ointments are lipid based and absorption can be significant, depending on the application. If a dressing is applied over the ointment, the absorption is better as the skin under the dressing becomes soft and the drug penetrates the skin much more quickly. Nurses should always wear gloves to administer creams and ointments.

Sublingual and Buccal Drugs

Although the mucous membrane of the mouth is not highly vascular, certain drugs, such as glyceryl trinitrate (vasodilator given to treat angina and heart failure), are administered using the sublingual route (Figure 19.8). The drug is absorbed quickly and is available for action within a short time. The other important factor is that drugs given via this route bypass the first-pass metabolism. Moreover, gastric enzymes and juices are avoided as they may interfere with drug metabolism and absorption.

Some drugs are administered by the buccal route (Figure 19.9).

323

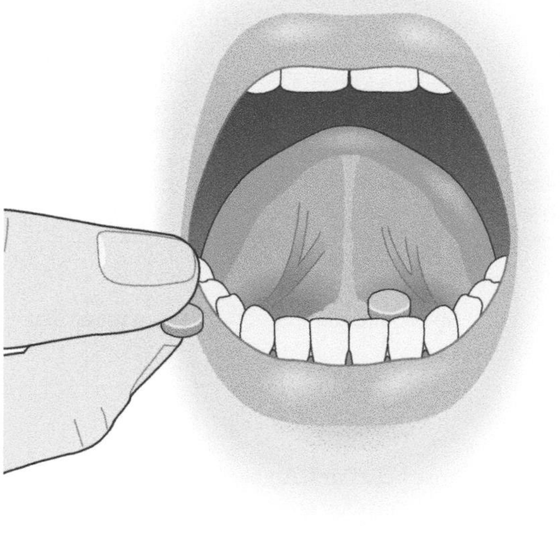

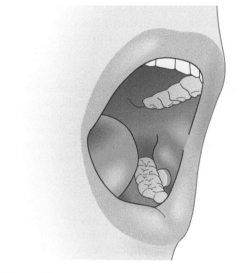

Figure 19.8 **Sublingual route.**

Figure 19.9 **Buccal route.**

Rectal Route

Many drugs can be administered rectally, including non-steroidal anti-inflammatory drugs (NSAIDs) such as diclofenac, mild tranquillisers such as diazepam, glycerol suppositories (for treating constipation) and many others. There are advantages and disadvantages to using this route, as detailed in Table 19.2.

Jot This Down

A medication given rectally may work better than one given orally. Why is this? Think about the anatomy of the rectum (Figure 19.10).

Retention enemas as bowel evacuants and in some cases medications such as diazepam are administered via this route (Dougherty *et al.*, 2015). The advantages of this route include

Table 19.2 Advantages and disadvantages of using the rectal route.

Advantages
- Bypasses first-pass metabolism
- If a person is unconscious, this route can be used to administer drugs when other routes such as IV, IM are not easily accessible
- If the person is vomiting, then the oral route will be a problem, so the rectal route could be used
- Some patients may have difficulty in swallowing, in which case the rectal route is available

Disadvantages
- Constant use of the rectal route may cause anal trauma and even perforation
- The person may find it uncomfortable
- Patient co-operation is needed to retain the suppository
- The procedure can be painful for the person if they suffer from anal stricture or have haemorrhoids, in which case some bleeding may take place

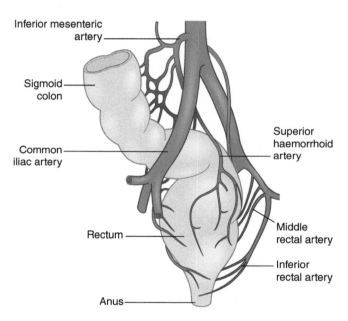

Figure 19.10 **Rectal anatomy.**

bypassing first-pass metabolism, avoiding gastric irritation as seen with some medications, and the abundant supply of blood vessels (see Figure 19.10). Enemas for bowel movement are hypertonic. An enema causes water to move from the body into the rectum, aiding defaecation.

When inserting suppositories or an enema, the nurse must instruct the patient to:

- Lie on the left side with their knees brought right up to the chest. This facilitates insertion of the suppositories or an enema, which should be at room temperature
- Retain the suppository or the enema for approximately 15 minutes before opening their bowels.

Some patients may find the rectal route unacceptable and expel the suppository or the enema before it has had a chance to work.

What To Do If . . .

. . . the person refuses to have an enema or a suppository? How might you deal with this situation? Some nursing actions you may consider include:

· Discussing with the patient their anxieties and worries
· Discussing the benefits of taking the prescribed bowel laxatives
· Ensuring privacy and dignity.

Jot This Down

A person has had an abdominoperineal (AP) resection and formation of a colostomy for rectal cancer. Theya re prescribed metronidazole (antibiotic) suppositories as a prophylactic treatment for infection. What will you do?

Vaginal Administration

This route may be used for the treatment of vaginal infection with antibiotics such as metronidazole. The suppository or pessaries are inserted high up in the vagina and therefore manufacturers often supply an applicator in the package. Women should be advised to wear a small pad or panty liners so their clothing will not be soiled as the medication may leak out as it dissolves.

Intramuscular/Intravenous Routes

Many medications are administered using these routes. When a person is unable to take oral medication because of nausea and vomiting or they are nil by mouth, drugs may be administered using one of these routes. Intramuscular (IM) injections are given using the dense muscles – the gluteus medius in the buttocks (Figure 19.11), the deltoid muscle of the upper arm (Figure 19.12) and the rectus femoris and vastus lateralis (Figure 19.13) of the thigh. Nurses need to adhere to local policies when giving IM injections. The advantage of using this route is that it bypasses the first-pass metabolism. The disadvantage is that IM injections can be painful, depending on the drug.

Medicines Management

The prescribing and dispensing/supply and/or administration of medicines should normally remain separate functions performed by separate healthcare professionals to protect patient safety.
RPS and RCN (2019)

Professional and Legal Issues

Pre-registration education for nurses and midwives has dramatically changed a student's role and their participation within the intravenous (IV) medication process. For example, the NMC (2018b) Skills Annex B includes information regarding IV drugs.

With direct and constant supervision throughout the procedure by a practice supervisor (PS) or practice assessor (PA) competent in the skill, students may:

· Draw up and prepare intravenous medication
· Administer intravenous medication according to accepted protocol within the clinical placement area, for example, via bolus push or additive to a bag of fluid.

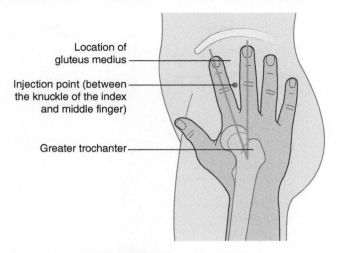

Figure 19.11 **Location of the gluteus medius muscle.**

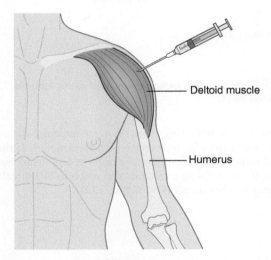

Figure 19.12 **Location of the deltoid muscle.**

The PS/PA will ensure the medication is checked by themselves and another registered member of staff as per local protocol and policy.

Intravenous injections are given by doctors and registered nurses who have had instruction in their administration. When giving medication through this route, the drug is given straight into the bloodstream and therefore its bioavailability is 100%. The first-pass metabolism is avoided, resulting in very fast action of the drug. The IV route is also used to administer chemotherapy drugs, antibiotics and others when quick action is needed.

At all times nurses must adhere to the RPS and RCN (2019) guidelines in the safe preparation and administration of injections.

Subcutaneous Injections

The subcutaneous (SC) route is used to administer a small amount of drug into the subcutaneous tissue for slow absorption. This method is used to give drugs that otherwise cannot be given orally, such as insulin, which is rendered ineffective by gastric juices. Another drug commonly given subcutaneously and postoperatively to prevent complications such as deep vein thrombosis is enoxaparin (Clexane×), which is an anticoagulant. See Figure 19.14 for the recommended sites.

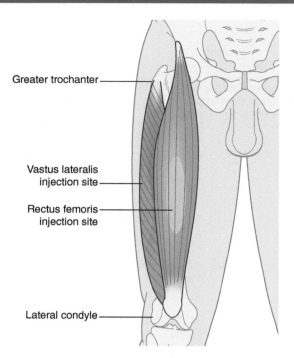

Figure 19.13 Location of the rectus femoris and vastus lateralis muscles of the thigh.

Whatever the method of injection, the nurse must also ensure safe disposal of sharps in accordance with local policy. If the patient has an intravenous cannula, the nurse is responsible for assessment of the site using a vein infusion phlebitis (VIP) scale and for changing the cannula (Lister *et al.*, 2020).

Inhalers

Some drugs, such as salbutamol inhaler and oxygen, are administered via the respiratory tract by inhalation via the oral or nasal route. This method is preferred when quick local action is required. Salbutamol works by acting on beta-2 receptors in the lungs. Drugs can be inhaled via other devices, such as spacers and metered-dose inhalers, and nurses should be aware of the differences in action. Inhaled medication allows rapid action but poor inhaler technique means therapeutic effect may not be optimal so patient education is imperative to improve the safe administration and compliance of inhaled medicines (Peate & Hill, 2021).

> **Care, Dignity and Compassion**
>
> Many people with learning disabilities, mental health and physical dexterity problems may require more support with inhaler administration and use of spacers. Remember to always respect their needs and utilise both the art and science of nursing.

Aural Route

Used to administer medications such as eardrops to treat ear infection or soften ear wax.

Transdermal Route

Used for drugs which usually have a delayed release, such as nicotine patches for smoking cessation and estradiol patches for postmenopausal symptom management.

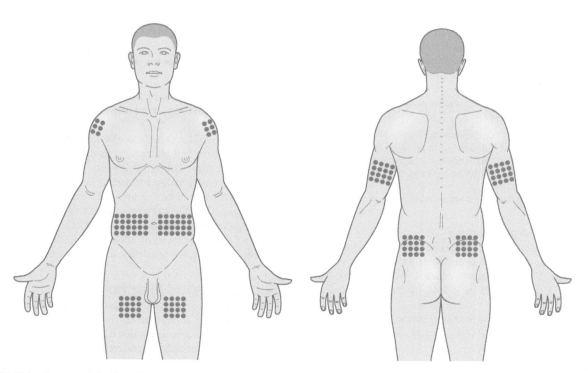

Figure 19.14 Subcutaneous injection sites.

326

Medical Abbreviations

In practice, you will come across standard abbreviations used by prescribers when prescribing medications. At all times adhere to local policy and practice so as to ensure safe practice.

Compliance, Concordance and Adherence

Medicines adherence is about the patient's action matching the agreed recommendation and thus taking a medicine as prescribed. Non-adherence can be intentional or non-intentional. Factors affecting adherence can be divided into different categories.

- *Patient:* age, cost of prescription, cognitive ability/difficulty.
- *Nurse–patient:* lack of confidence in the nurse who cannot allay the patient's fears; a misunderstanding of instructions.
- *Disease process:* a patient may not be able to visualise the benefit, for example where treatment might be lengthy and improvement is not quick.
- *The medicines themselves:* patients taking several medicines at the same time (polypharmacy) may find it difficult to adhere to timings as they impinge on day-to-day activities or they simply do not like the formulations (Peate & Hill, 2021).

NICE (2009) *Medicines Adherence: Involving Patients in Decisions about Prescribed Medicines and Supporting Adherence* is a guide that nurses should be familiar with.

Jot This Down
How can you as the nurse promote adherence?

Pharmacovigilance

The term 'pharmacovigilance' comes from the Greek *pharmakon* meaning 'drug' and *vigilar* meaning 'to keep alert'. HMR 2012 implemented European directive 2010/84/EU, which introduced new pharmacovigilance requirements that defined roles and responsibilities as well as a greater involvement of patients and healthcare professionals in reporting safety issues. The Medicines and Healthcare products Regulatory Agency (MHRA) published *Good Pharmacovigilance Practice for Medicines* in 2014; its aim is to monitor adverse drug reactions (ADRs). In Peate & Hill (2021) there is further discussion regarding adverse drug reactions (ADR) that may help you gain further insight and understanding.

Another cause of ADRs is when a drug error has occurred, so that the wrong drug is given to the wrong patient. It is vital that nurses remember their responsibilities in line with the Duty of Candour (NMC/GMC, 2015) – a duty to inform patients when things go wrong, giving an apology and working towards a remedy. Risks must be discussed before treatment commences.

Some Common Drugs Used in Practice and Their Action

Antibiotics

What are Antibiotics?
The word 'antibiotic' comes from the Greek *anti* meaning 'against' and *bios* meaning 'life' – life of the bacteria. Antibiotics are also known as antibacterials, and they are used to treat infections caused by bacteria.

Today most antibiotics are synthesised in medical laboratories. Antibiotics may be classed as 'broad spectrum', which means they can affect a wide range of different bacteria, examples being amoxicillin and cefotaxime. Other antibiotics only work against specific types of bacteria and are known as 'narrow-spectrum' antibiotics; these include vancomycin and teicoplanin.

Although there are several different types of antibiotic, they all work in one of two ways.

- A 'bactericidal' antibiotic kills the bacteria. Penicillin is bactericidal. A bactericidal usually interferes with the formation of the bacterium's cell wall or its cell contents.
- A 'bacteriostatic' stops a bacterium from multiplying. This group of antibiotics works with the host's immune system to get rid of the organisms that are in the body.

How Do Antibiotics Work?
Antibiotics work by interfering with the growth of bacteria through:

- Inhibiting cell wall formation
- Blocking protein synthesis
- Disrupting cell membranes
- Interfering with nucleic acid synthesis
- Preventing synthesis of folic acid.

The issue of antibiotics can be complex; in Peate & Hill (2021) antibiotics are discussed in more detail.

Jot This Down
What do you understand by the terms broad-spectrum and narrow-spectrum antibiotics?

Side-effects
All antibiotics have adverse effects, which vary from drug to drug. Some can be very severe and can cause severe toxic effects resulting in anaphylactic shock. The drugs may damage body tissue or organs and interfere with body function. In some cases, they destroy the normal flora of the body, resulting in an increase of bacteria that cause illness. Apart from the common side-effects, such as nausea and vomiting, diarrhoea and upset stomach, the person may develop symptoms such as allergy, drug toxicity, meticillin (methicillin)-resistant *Staphylococcus aureus* (MRSA) and antibiotic-related colitis.

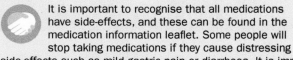

Care, Dignity and Compassion

It is important to recognise that all medications have side-effects, and these can be found in the medication information leaflet. Some people will stop taking medications if they cause distressing side-effects such as mild gastric pain or diarrhoea. It is important to be supportive and understanding when answering any health-related queries, and to encourage a person to complete their course of antibiotics to gain maximum benefit from the medication.

Allergy One of the most common side-effects of any antibiotic is an allergic reaction, which may be minor or severe. In some patients, a small allergic reaction such as diarrhoea is not uncommon. Patients who have never had any drug therapy may develop allergic reactions when they are treated with antibiotics. This may be due to a variety of factors, for example the body's reaction to foreign chemicals or contamination of the drug by environmental factors. If the reactions are severe, where a patient develops respiratory and/or cardiac problems, then the treatment should be discontinued immediately and documented in the person's notes. The person should also be informed of their allergic reaction so they are aware of their allergy and can inform healthcare practitioners in the future.

Jot This Down

Can you think of any other allergic reactions that the person may have because of antibiotics?

What To Do If . . .

What should you do if the person develops an anaphylactic reaction during antibiotic therapy?
· Call for help.
· Stop the antibiotic therapy immediately.
· Report the patient's condition to the person in charge.
· Stay with your patient and assess their airway, breathing, circulation and vital signs; use the National Early Warning Score 2 (NEWS2) assessment tool.
· Document all outcomes in the patient's care plan.

Drug Toxicity

Apart from fighting infection, antibiotics can also damage the body as a result of toxic effects, including kidney failure, liver failure, bone marrow defects and nerve damage. Other less severe symptoms include diarrhoea, nausea and vomiting. Drugs such as the sulphonamides can cause renal problems when they crystallise in the kidneys and form kidney stones. Some drug combinations involving diuretics, for example gentamicin (an antibiotic) and furosemide (a diuretic), can be nephrotoxic if they are not regulated and monitored correctly. Liver problems can develop as a result of drug toxicity. Diseases such as liver cirrhosis may occur, thus affecting liver function, which can be fatal.

Some drug toxicity may affect the CNS, resulting in the person developing convulsions, ataxia, nervousness, insomnia and temporary blindness. The most common symptom is acoustic nerve damage, resulting in tinnitus and deafness.

Antibiotic Resistance

Bacteria are termed drug resistant when they are no longer inhibited by an antibiotic to which they were previously sensitive. The spread of antibacterial-resistant bacteria has continued to grow, due to both the overuse and misuse of antibiotics. Treating a patient with antibiotics causes the microbes to adapt or die, a process known as 'selective pressure'. If a strain of bacterial species acquires resistance to an antibiotic, it will survive the treatment. Antibiotics can destroy many of the harmless strains of bacteria that live in and on the body. This allows resistant bacteria to multiply quickly and replace them. Consult NICE (2015b) for further details on effective antimicrobial medicine use.

MRSA

Meticillin-resistant *Staphylococcus aureus* is sometimes known as a superbug. There are various subtypes (strains) of *S. aureus* and some strains are classed as MRSA. MRSA strains are very similar to any other strain of *S. aureus*. That is, some healthy people are carriers, and some people develop MRSA infections. *Staphylococcus aureus* is a bacterium (germ). It is often abbreviated to 'S. aureus' or 'Staph'. *Staphylococcus aureus* bacteria are often found on the skin and in the nose of healthy people. These people are called *S. aureus* carriers. In healthy people who are carriers, *S. aureus* is usually harmless (Department of Health, 2014).

However, *S. aureus* bacteria sometimes invade the skin to cause infection. This is more likely if the person has a cut or graze, allowing bacteria to get under the surface of the skin. Sometimes, these bacteria move into the bloodstream and can cause septicaemia, pneumonia and endocarditis

Antibiotic-related Colitis

The normal flora of the gut protects the lining of the GI tract. Uncontrolled use of antibiotics may destroy the normal flora; this is more evident in persons treated with oral antibiotics. One of the most widely discussed infections in hospital is caused by a bacterium called *Clostridium (Clostridioides) difficile* (C. difficile or C. diff). This is a normal bacterium in the gut, which protects the lining of the GI tract. However, due to misuse of some antibiotics, these bacteria multiply in great numbers and produce toxins, resulting in the person developing severe diarrhoea and fever (Peate & Hill, 2021).

Anticoagulants

Blood clotting is the mechanism by which blood sticks together to form small solid clots. It is a natural and vital function of the body, without which a person would bleed to death after an injury. The blood has a complex system that regulates when or how clots form. Blood clotting is triggered by small blood cells called *platelets*. The clotting blood goes through a series of chemical reactions before clots are formed.

Anticoagulants are prescribed for patients who experience clotting disorders, postoperatively and after a myocardial infarct (MI).

Aspirin, warfarin and heparin (dalteparin) are currently the drugs of choice for oral anticoagulant therapy. Anticoagulant medicines reduce the ability of the blood to clot. This is necessary if the blood clots too quickly, as these clots can block blood vessels and lead to conditions such as a stroke or an MI. Some conditions in which anticoagulants are used include:

- *Deep vein thrombosis (DVT)*: blood clot in the veins resulting from poor circulation, for example in patients who are on prolonged bedrest after major surgery
- *Pulmonary embolism (PE)*: blood clot in the lungs
- *Atrial fibrillation (AF)*: irregular heartbeat. AF increases the risk of stroke.

For further discussion of anticoagulants, the reader is directed to Peate & Hill (2021). Detailed information regarding anticoagulant therapy is provided there, enhancing learning and understanding.

Analgesia

Strategies for coping with pain vary from person to person. Coping methods that were perceived as helpful in the past are often used by the person and may become habitual. It should be remembered that pain is a personal experience and is unique to the individual. There are different pain assessment tools used in clinical practice to assess the level of pain. If pain is not assessed properly and appropriate analgesia administered as prescribed, the patient will remain in pain and their progress will be affected (Peate & Hill, 2021). There are different types of analgesics.

- Non-opioid analgesics such as paracetamol, used to treat mild to moderate pain.
- NSAIDs such as aspirin, which act on the peripheral nerve endings, inhibiting prostaglandin synthesis.
- Opioids such as morphine, used to treat severe pain.
- Synthetic opioids such as codeine, tramadol and fentanyl.

The World Health Organization developed a three-step 'ladder' (Figure 19.15) for cancer pain relief in 1986 and it continues to be used today. If pain occurs, there should be prompt oral administration of drugs in the following order: non-opioids (aspirin and paracetamol); then, as necessary, mild opioids (codeine); then strong opioids, such as morphine, until the person is free of pain.

Opioids

Opioid drugs exert their action by stimulating receptors in the CNS. These receptors are opioid agonist, which means they will allow opioids to attach to them and produce a response. The three main CNS receptors for opioid analgesia are the mu, kappa and delta receptors.

Side-effects

Some common side-effects of opioid analgesia include:

- Constipation
- Retention of urine
- Suppression of respiration
- Drowsiness
- Pupil constriction (miosis)
- Dry mouth
- Nausea and vomiting
- Cough suppression.

Jot This Down

In hospital, can patients receiving opioid analgesia be addicted to the drug? Is there a difference between dependency and addiction?

NSAIDs

These drugs, such as aspirin, paracetamol, ibuprofen, diclofenac and indometacin, are given for mild to moderate pain and have an analgesic and anti-inflammatory effect. They inhibit prostaglandin synthesis. Prostaglandins are mediators of the inflammatory response and are involved in the production of pain and fever. When tissues are damaged, white blood cells flood to the site to try to minimise tissue destruction. Prostaglandins are produced as a result, which then cause pain at the site of injury. There is further discussion of NSAIDs in Peate & Hill (2021).

Side-effects The side-effects of NSAIDs include:

- Abdominal pain
- GI bleeding
- Melaena
- Kidney damage
- Hypotension
- Fluid retention.

Case Study

Sunita Garcia is a 38-year-old female who works as a registered nurse and has been experiencing lower back pain for 3 weeks. She has been reviewed by the practice nurse and has been prescribed oral tablets of ibuprofen and paracetamol. She has been taking this medication as prescribed but her pain in the lower back remains. Sunita's pain score has elevated by 2 points up to 8/10. She is barely able to mobilise.

- As a nurse or healthcare professional, how are you able to support Sunita?
- What suggestions or recommendations could you make to Sunita's practice nurse?
- Are there any other more suitable formulations and routes of administration for these medicines and if so, what are they?
- What other analgesia could be considered in this circumstance, and why?

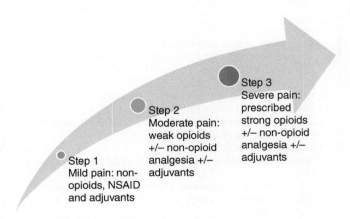

Step 3
Severe pain: prescribed strong opioids +/– non-opioid analgesia +/– adjuvants

Step 2
Moderate pain: weak opioids +/– non-opioid analgesia +/– adjuvants

Step 1
Mild pain: non-opioids, NSAID and adjuvants

Figure 19.15 Analgesic steps.

329

Non-pharmacological Therapies

There are many complementary therapies available instead of using drugs. Non-pharmacological interventions for pain management include the following.

- *Transcutaneous electrical nerve stimulation (TENS):* a pair of electrodes is applied to the skin and the area is stimulated by a small electric current.
- *Acupuncture*: needle insertion into acupuncture points of the body.
- *Massage:* manual stimulation of muscles is used as pain relief.
- *Yoga:* a meditative technique; breathing and posture are used as a healing process.
- *Aromatherapy*, the use of essential oils on the body through gentle massage technique.

Other techniques include:

- Herbal medicine
- Music therapy
- Reflexology
- Homeopathy.

Herbal medicines are also regulated under the HMR 2012 and can cause interactions with other drugs. For example, garlic increases the potency of insulin and warfarin; St John's wort has many interactions as it is an inhibitor of the cytochrome P450 system; valerian, often used as an aid for sleeping, increases the effect of sedatives.

Bronchodilators

In chronic obstructive pulmonary disease (COPD), the constriction of airway smooth muscle gives rise to symptoms such as chest tightness, wheezing and breathlessness (NICE, 2019). Patients are administered bronchodilators to relieve these symptoms.

Drugs administered as gases, such as sprays and aerosols, penetrate the cell linings of the respiratory tract easily and rapidly. They are absorbed almost as fast as they are inhaled, because the blood and the lung membrane are in close proximity. Drugs given in this form are bronchodilators, such as salbutamol.

Patients with COPD include those who have:

- Asthma (extrinsic and intrinsic)
- Chronic bronchitis
- Emphysema
- Cystic fibrosis.

Bronchodilator medicines are available in short-acting and long-acting varieties. The three most widely used bronchodilators are:

- Beta-2 agonists
- Anticholinergics
- Theophyllines.

The pharmacology associated with bronchodilators requires the nurse to demonstrate insight and understanding so as to ensure care provision is safe and effective. In Peate & Hill (2021), there is further discussion of bronchodilators.

Case Study

Princess Adeyayo is a 42-year-old female living in Edinburgh. During the winter months, Princess has been experiencing chest tightness and has an audible wheeze. She has been prescribed a salbutamol inhaler, but is reluctant to take it

---

as she says 'it makes her heart race out of her chest' and 'makes her very hot and sweaty'.

- What are the side-effects of beta-2 agonists such as salbutamol?
- What does an audible wheeze tell the healthcare professional?
- What is the nurse's role in this case scenario?

Cardiac Glycosides

Cardiac glycosides are termed *inotropic* agents. Inotropic drugs can have either positive or negative properties.

Positive inotropic drugs improve contraction force of the heart muscle, thus increasing cardiac output. They are used in the treatment of heart failure with AF. One of the common drugs used in practice to treat heart failure is digoxin. Digitalis is a generic term for all 'cardiac glycosides'. Digoxin acts on the autonomic nervous system to slow the heart rate and on the atrioventricular node of the heart to slow the conduction of the ventricles.

Negative inotropic drugs decrease myocardial contractility and are used to decrease cardiac workload in conditions such as angina. Examples of drugs that have a negative inotropic effect include beta-blockers such as metoprolol and calcium channel blockers such as nifedipine. Metoprolol is a beta-adrenergic receptor blocker. It blocks the beta version of epinephrine (adrenaline) from attaching and sending signals to the cardiac tissue, thus lowering pulse rate, stroke volume and cardiac output. The action of negative inotropic drugs also results in a decrease in the electrical activity in the heart. Calcium channel blockers inhibit inward movement of calcium ions through the slow channels of active membranes, thus reducing the afterload of the heart.

Side-effects As the margin between the therapeutic and toxic levels of cardiac glycosides is so narrow, nurses need to be cautious when administering these drugs. Side-effects include:

- Nausea and vomiting
- Visual disturbance
- Headache
- Confusion
- Diarrhoea
- Bradycardia (slow heart rate, below 60 beats/minute)
- ECG changes, for example prolonged PR interval and shortened QT complex.

Care, Dignity and Compassion

Older people, especially the very old, require special care and consideration from prescribers (BNF 2020b; see https://bnf.nice.org.uk/guidance/prescribing-in-the-elderly.html).

Healthcare professionals must avoid excessive, inappropriate consumption of medicines by older people.

- Before administering the medication, consider whether the person needs the drug.
- Limit the range of drugs.
- Prescribe lower dosage of drugs than would be used for a younger adult.
- Review medications regularly. Discontinue if not needed.
- Write down precise instructions on how and when to take the medications.
- Advise the person on the proper disposal of unwanted drugs.

Drug Calculations

Nurses must use mathematical calculations to administer medications to patients, and some of these calculations may be required during an emergency. Calculations made for tablets and fluids involve converting larger units to smaller units and smaller to larger units. To convert larger units to smaller, the larger is multiplied, for example:

- kilograms (kg) to grams (g) = kg × 1000
- litres (L) to millilitres (mL) = L × 1000
- milligrams to micrograms (mcg or μg) = mg × 1000.

To convert smaller units to larger, the smaller is divided, for example:

- grams to kilograms = g/1000
- millilitres to litres = mL/1000
- micrograms (mcg or μg) to milligrams = mcg/1000.

By definition, 1 gram = 1000 milligrams and 1 milligram = 1000 micrograms.

SI Units

Some examples of conversions:

- 200 mg = 0.2 g; 0.6 g = 600 mg; 600 mcg (or μg) = 0.6 mg
- 2000 mL = 2 L; 0.030 m = 30 mm; 0.03 mg = 30 mcg (or μg).

In practice, most of the drugs supplied from pharmacy will have already been adjusted by the pharmacist, and nurses must ensure that they administer the medication correctly, adhering to local and national policies. However, there are times when nurses may need to calculate the dosage of a drug before dispensing, especially when administering IV fluids to patients. This is when nurses need to use their calculating skills to obtain the correct dosage for the person.

Jot This Down Exercise 1

1. Convert 550 mg to g
2. Convert 0.1 g to mg
3. Convert 50 mcg (or μg) to mg
4. Convert 100 mL to litres
5. Convert 0.125 g to mg
   Answers: **1.** 0.55 g; **2.** 100 mg; **3.** 0.5 mg; **4.** 0.1 L; **5.** 125 mg

Jot This Down Exercise 2

A person is prescribed 120 mg of verapamil but the tablets are available as 40 mg each. How many tablets are required? The answer involves finding how many 40s are in 120, in other words, 120 divided by 40.
Always remember this formula for calculating tablets:
Number of tablets = what you want/what you have
So in the above example, 120/40 = 3

Jot This Down Exercise 3

1. 600 mg is prescribed, tablets are 300 mg each: how many tablets will you give?
2. 50 mg is prescribed, tablets are 12.5 mg each: how many tablets will you give?
3. 1 mg prescribed, tablets are 500 micrograms: how many tablets will you give?
4. 625 mg prescribed, tablets are 1.25 g each: how many tablets will you give?
5. 3 tablets each contain 250 mg. What is the total dose in milligrams?
   Answers: **1.** 2 tablets; **2.** 4 tablets; **3.** 2 tablets; **4.** ½ tablet; **5.** 750 mg.

Liquid Medications

When a medication is in liquid form, you should consider the concentration of the drug in that liquid. For example, pethidine hydrochloride is available as 50 mg/mL. This means that 50 milligrams of pethidine hydrochloride are dissolved in every millilitre of liquid. In this case, it is the volume you need to consider.

For example, a drug is available as 25 mg/mL and 75 mg is required. What volume will be given in mL?

Formula: volume of the drug = amount prescribed/amount per measure

So in the above example: 75/25 = 3 mL.

Another example: A child is prescribed amoxicillin 250 mg every 6 hours. The liquid medicine dispensed is 125 mg in 5 mL. What volume of medicine should be dispensed?

Using the above formula: 250/125 × 5 mL = 2/1 × 10 mL

331

Jot This Down Exercise 4

1. Drug available as 10 mg/mL, prescription is for 20 mg: how many mL will be given?
2. Drug available as 10 mg/2 mL, prescription is for 5 mg: how many mL will be given?
3. Drug available as 20 mg/5 mL, prescription is for 40 mg: how many mL will be given?
4. Drug available as 10 mg/mL: how many mg will there be in 3 mL?
5. Drug available as 20 mg/5 mL: how many mg will be in 7.5 mL?
   Answers: **1.** 2 mL; **2.** 1 mL; **3.** 10 mL; **4.** 30 mg; **5.** 30 mg.

Intravenous Infusions

Sometimes patients are administered medication via the parenteral route because either the person cannot swallow any tablets or the drug may be destroyed by chemicals in the stomach. Intravenous infusions are administered to patients, and nurses are required to ensure the infusion runs on time. One needs to bear in mind that the drops per minute will vary between an adult and a child. It is estimated there are 20 drops per mL for the adult IV administration tubes. However, this is slightly less for blood.

In the case of blood, it is calculated that there are 15 drops in 1 mL of blood. If in any doubt, check the packaging which will indicate the drops per mL. One reason for this is that blood is thicker than clear fluid and therefore there are slightly fewer drops in 1 mL. To calculate the flow rate, you can use the following formula to calculate drops per minute.

$$\text{Drops per minute} = (\text{volume} \times 20 \text{ drops}) / (\text{times} \times 60 \text{ minutes})$$

Example: The person is prescribed 1 litre of normal saline over 4 hours. How many drops per minute should the drip rate be? The drip factor is 20 drops per mL.

Using the formula above:

$$\text{Drops per minute} = (1000 \times 20) / (4 \times 60) = 2000 / 24$$
$$= 83 \text{ drops} / \text{minute}$$

You can round the figure to a whole number.

Jot This Down Exercise 5

Using the formula above, calculate the drip rate for the following examples.

1. The person is prescribed 500 mL of normal saline over 6 hours: what is the drop rate?
2. If a person requires 1000 mL in 6 hours, what is the rate?
3. If a person is to be given 500 mL by IV infusion using a controller with a drip factor of 20 drops/mL over 6 hours, what would you set the drip rate to?
4. If a person is to be given 750 mL by IV infusion using a controller with a drip factor of 20 drops/mL over 12 hours, what would you set the drip rate to?
5. The person is written up for 1 unit (475 mL) of blood over 3 hours through an adult blood administration set. What is the drip rate?

Answers: **1.** 28 drops; **2.** 56 drops; **3.** 28 drops; **4.** 21 drops; **5.** 40 drops.

Practice Assessment Document

Whilst working to achieve proficiency in medicine administration, you are required to demonstrate that you can manage:

- The administration of IV fluids
- Fluid and nutrition infusion pumps and devices
- Inhalation, humidifier and nebuliser devices.

Demonstrating proficiency in medicine administration can be daunting, so do not worry if you feel a little intimated. As this chapter has demonstrated, there are so many skills you need to hone and fine tune that have to be underpinned by a solid evidence base.

Think about this; on each practice learning experience you attend, make it a point to learn about three commonly used medications in that area; ask your practice supervisor if they

think the medications you have chosen are appropriate. Learn as much as you can about the medicine, for example, generic and brand names, usual doses, possible routes of administration, whether the medication is a GSL, POM, P or CD product, what the side-effects are, what information you need to give to the patient regarding the medication. You can discuss this at your initial or midpoint interview; you could even have the list prepared prior to placement as you prepare for practice. Make this a learning outcome, one that is specific, measurable, achievable, relevant and time bound (SMART). Try and engage with medicine administration rounds, think about the ways in which medicine are administered in settings other than the hospital setting, and what the challenges are. Practise drug calculations as often as you can, remembering that practice makes perfect. Your university will have numeracy resources available to you, for example SN@P; make use of these as they will help you perfect your skills as you grow into becoming a proficient and confident practitioner.

Conclusion

This chapter has explored some aspects of drug administration, including reference to policies and legislation governing drug administration. Nurses should always adhere to the local, professional and national policies in the safe administration of medicine. The nurse's role involves more direct care compared with other healthcare professionals and therefore nurses need to ensure a high standard of nursing care with respect to drug administration.

Key Points

- All drugs produced have a generic and one or more brand names. The generic name is a drug's common scientific name. The brand name drug is a medicine that is discovered, developed and marketed by a pharmaceutical company.
- Drug administration does not just involve giving out medication to patients; it involves working with the person, their relatives and other healthcare professionals in the safe administration of medicines. Nurses also must follow the local, national and their professional guidelines to ensure that they carry out their duties confidently and professionally.
- The chemical nature of the drug determines how and where absorption takes place. Absorption takes place through the intestinal wall and into the plasma before it reaches the site of action.
- Drugs administered orally have a major hurdle to overcome before they reach the general circulation. This is called first-pass metabolism.
- Some enteric-coated tablets are gastric irritants and therefore should be taken with food or after a meal. Thus, nurses should never crush enteric-coated medications as this may render the drug ineffective.
- Anticoagulant medicines reduce the ability of the blood to clot. If the patient is overdosed with an anticoagulant, prompt action is needed to reverse the action of the drug. Some of the serious side-effects include bleeding from the GI tract, haematuria, bleeding from the gums and epistaxis.

References

Barber, P. & Robertson, D. (2020) *Essentials of Pharmacology for Nurses*, 4th edn. McGraw Hill Education, Maidenhead.

Beauchamp, T.L. & Childress, J.F. (2013) *Principles of Biomedical Ethics*, 7th edn. Oxford University Press, Oxford.

Berman, A., Snyder, S. & Frandsen, G. (2015) *Kozier & Erb's Fundamentals of Nursing: Concepts, Process and Practice*. Prentice Hall, Harlow.

BNF (2020a) *British National Formulary*. https://bnf.nice.org.uk/ (accessed December 2021).

BNF (2020b) *Prescribing in the Elderly*. https://bnf.nice.org.uk/guidance/prescribing-in-the-elderly.html (accessed December 2021).

Department of Health (2014) *Who to screen for MRSA*. www.gov.uk/government/publications/how-to-approach-mrsa-screening (accessed December 2021).

Dougherty, L., Lister, S. & West-Oram, A. (eds) (2015) *The Royal Marsden Hospital Manual of Clinical Nursing Procedures*, 9th edn. Wiley Blackwell, Chichester.

Gracia-Vásquez, P. González-Barranco, I.A. Camacho-Mora, O. & González-Santiago, S.A. (2017) Medications that should not be crushed. *Medicina Universitaria*, 19, 50–63.

Home Office (2014) *A Change to the Misuse of Drugs Act 1971: control of NBOMe and benzofuran compounds, lisdexamphetamine, zopiclone, zaleplon, tramadol and reclassification of ketamine*. Home Office Circular 008/2014.

Lister, S., Hofland, J. & Grafton, H. (2020) *The Royal Marsden Hospital Manual of Clinical Nursing Procedures*, 10th edn. Wiley Blackwell, Chichester.

Medicines and Healthcare products Regulatory Agency (2014) *Good Pharmacovigilance Practice for Medicines*. www.gov.uk/guidance/good-pharmacovigilance-practice-gpvp (accessed December 2021).

National Institute for Health and Care Excellence (2009) *Medicines Adherence: Involving Patients in Decisions about Prescribed Medicines and Supporting Adherence. CG76*. (accessed December 2021).

National Institute for Health and Care Excellence (2015a) *Medicines Management in Care Homes. QS85*. www.nice.org.uk/guidance/qs85 (accessed December 2021).

National Institute for Health and Care Excellence (2015b) *Antimicrobial Stewardship: Systems and Processes for Effective Antimicrobial Medicine Use. NICE Guideline 15*. www.nice.org.uk/guidance/ng15 (accessed December 2021).

National Institute for Health and Care Excellence (2016a) *Medicines Optimisation. QS120*. www.nice.org.uk/guidance/qs120 (accessed December 2021).

National Institute for Health and Care Excellence (2016b) *Controlled Drugs: Safe Use and Management. NICE Guideline 46*. www.nice.org.uk/guidance/ng46 (accessed December 2021).

National Institute for Health and Care Excellence (2017) *Patient Group Directions. Medicines Practice MPG2*. www.nice.org.uk/guidance/mpg2 (accessed December 2021).

National Institute for Health and Care Excellence (2019) *Chronic Obstructive Pulmonary Disease in Over 16s: Diagnosis and Management. NG115*. www.nice.org.uk/guidance/ng115 (accessed December 2021).

Nursing & Midwifery Council (2018a) *Standards of proficiency for nursing associates*. www.nmc.org.uk/globalassets/sitedocuments/education-standards/nursing-associates-proficiency-standards.pdf (accessed December 2021).

Nursing & Midwifery Council (2018b) *Standards of proficiency for registered nurses*. www.nmc.org.uk/globalassets/sitedocuments/education-standards/future-nurse-proficiencies.pdf (accessed December 2021).

Nursing & Midwifery Council/General Medical Council (2015) *Openness and honesty when things go wrong: the professional duty of candour*. NMC, London.

Parkinson's UK (2019) *Get it on time*. www.parkinsons.org.uk/sites/default/files/2019-10/CS3380%20Get%20it%20on%20Time%20Report%20A4%20final%2026.09.2019-compressed%20%281%29.pdf (accessed December 2021).

Peate, I. & Hill, B. (2021) *Fundamentals of Pharmacology*. Wiley, Chichester.

Royal Pharmaceutical Society and Royal College of Nursing (2019) *Professional Guidance on the Administration of Medicines in Healthcare Settings*. www.rpharms.com/Portals/0/RPS%20document%20library/Open%20access/Professional%20standards/SSHM%20and%20Admin/Admin%20of%20Meds%20prof%20guidance.pdf?ver=2019-01-23-145026-567 (accessed December 2021).

World Health Organization (1986) *Cancer Pain Relief*. WHO, Geneva.

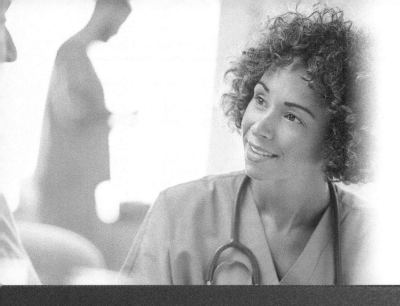

20

The Principles of End-of-Life Care

Aby Mitchell[1] and Scott Elbourne[2]

[1] University of West London, UK
[2] Berkshire Healthcare NHS Foundation Trust, UK

Learning Outcomes

On completion of this chapter, you will be able to:

- Identify the role of the nurse in supporting dying patients and their families
- Demonstrate the core skills of:
  - Communication
  - Assessment
  - Symptom control
  - Advance care planning
- Apply the principles of ethics to end-of-life (EoL) care nursing practice
- Demonstrate insight into the application of models of care delivery in promoting effective EoL nursing care
- Describe the main principles of loss, grief and bereavement

Proficiencies

NMC Proficiencies and Standards:

- Treat people with kindess, respect and compassion
  - communicate effectively using a range of skills and strategies with colleagues and people at all stages of life and with a range of mental, physical, cognitive and behavioural health challenges
  - demonstrate the skills and abilities required to support people at all stages of life who are emotionally or physically vulnerable
- Identify and assess the needs of people and families for care at the end of life, including requirements for palliative care and decision making related to their treatment and care preferences

(Continued)

Nursing Practice: Knowledge and Care, Third Edition. Edited by Ian Peate and Aby Mitchell.
© 2022 John Wiley & Sons Ltd. Published 2022 by John Wiley & Sons Ltd.
Companion website: www.wiley.com/go/peate/nursingpractice3e

Proficiencies *(Continued)*

- **Work in partnership with people to encourage shared decision making in order to support individuals, their families and carers to manage their own care when appropriate**
- **Demonstrate the knowledge and skills required to prioritise what is important to people and their families when providing evidence-based person-centred nursing care at end of life including the care**

- of people who are dying, families, the deceased and the bereaved
- **Understand the principles of safe and effective administration and optimisation of medicines in accordance with local and national policies and demonstrate proficiency and accuracy when calculating dosages of prescribed medicines**

 Visit the companion website at www.wiley.com/go/peate/nursingpractice3e where you can test yourself using flashcards, multiple-choice questions and more.

Introduction

This chapter will explore the principles of care at the end of life for those facing death and their families and loved ones. It will examine the historical context of death and dying and look at the sociological development of its current place in contemporary society. It will investigate the wider philosophical and psychosocial context surrounding death, dying and bereavement as well as the principles and practice of its effective delivery. The complex area of grief, loss and bereavement and the conceptual models that underpin modern grief theory will be explored along with their implications for healthcare today.

Palliative and end-of-life care is an important aspect of nursing. Around 500 000 people die in England every year and it is expected that, by 2040, this will rise to 590 000 (Dying Matters, 2020). The main aetiology of death is stroke and heart failure; however, one in four people in the UK will die of cancer (Office for National Statistics (ONS), 2020). It should also be borne in mind that due to an increasing and ageing population, a significant proportion of older adults will be living with co-morbidity and therefore an increase in deaths due to co-morbidity and frailty will probably occur as a leading course of mortality in the coming years (National Institute for Health and Care Excellence (NICE), 2016). In response to this, nurses need to manage and deliver services that can identify and care for people who require palliative care and are likely to be approaching the end of their lives (NICE, 2019; Mitchell & Elbourne, 2020).

Palliative and End-of-Life Care

The terms 'palliative care' and 'end-of-life care' are often used interchangeably but they are not the same. This may seem confusing, and it is often difficult for nurses and other health professionals to agree on what the term 'end-of-life care' means, whether end of life means the final, terminal stages of a person's illness or a broader view of the care required at the latter part of their life. The terms may be even more unclear for patients and families

and it could be argued that such discussion about definitions is meaningless and what is important is access to the right support, at the right time according to their needs.

Palliative care is an area of healthcare that encourages nurses and others to view death and dying as a normal and natural process rather than from an overtly medical model perspective. It should focus on a person's quality of life, not necessarily the quantity, and should try to address their holistic needs and not just their physical symptoms.

The term 'palliative' is derived from the Latin word *pallium* meaning 'to cloak'. It aims to express the notion that palliative care perhaps protects and shields the individual. However, another perspective is that the term can mask the true nature of the disease.

The World Health Organization (2015) provided what is often referred to as the definitive explanation of the meaning of palliative care.

'Palliative care is an approach that improves the quality of life of patients and their families facing the problems associated with life-threatening illness, through the prevention and relief of suffering by means of early identification and impeccable assessment and treatment of pain and other problems, physical, psychosocial and spiritual.'

End-of-life care is commonly referred to as care that is required during the last 6–12 months of life, regardless of the individual's diagnosis (General Medical Council (GMC), 2010). Traditionally, palliative care has been more clearly aligned to those with a cancer diagnosis; however, it is becoming increasingly recognised that other diseases such as organ failure, cardiovascular disease and dementia dominate the main causes of death in the UK (ONS, 2020; NICE, 2015). End-of-life care helps people live as well as possible until they die, focusing on dignity and support for family or carers.

'End of Life Care is care that helps all those with advanced, progressive incurable illness to live as well as possible until they die. It enables the supportive and palliative care needs of both patient and family to be identified and met throughout the last phase of life and into bereavement. It includes management of pain and other symptoms and provision of psychological, social, spiritual and practical support'. (National Council for Palliative Care, 2010; Department of Health, 2008)

Marie Curie (2018) also explains the difference and similarities between the two terms: palliative care and end-of-life care. Palliative care is treatment, care and support for people with a life-limiting illness. The aim of palliative care is to support the patient to have a good quality of life, which includes being as well and active as possible for the time the person has left. This can involve:

- Planning for future care with a detailed advance care plan that expresses the person's individual needs and wishes
- Controlling physical symptoms, such as pain
- Emotional, spiritual and psychological support needs
- Social care needs, including assistance with washing, dressing or eating
- Support for the person's carers, family and friends.

Similarly, end-of life care also focuses on treatment, care and support of patients, but is for those who are thought to be in the last year of their life. This includes people with:

- Advanced, progressive, incurable conditions
- Frailty and co-morbidity that place them at increased risk of dying within the next 12 months
- Existing conditions whereby they are at risk of dying suddenly from acute crisis (NICE, 2019)
- Life-threatening acute conditions caused by sudden catastrophic events (GMC, 2010).

It may be best to view EoL care as an overarching term that encompasses all care that is focused on improving quality of life and planning for a peaceful dignified death, over the last 6–12 months of life. Palliative care can therefore be viewed as a key component within such an approach – both terms are mutually inclusive and share the same ethos and principles.

Jot This Down Activity

- Think about the end-of-life patients you may have cared for in the past. What prompted you to think they were at the end of their life?
- Can you recall any conversations that took place between nurses, other professionals and the patient and family around EoL care?
- Who was involved in their care and how effective was the communication between them?

Approaches to Delivery of End-of-Life and Palliative Care

A clear, well-disseminated plan helps nurses and other health and social care professionals to co-ordinate their input to deliver care that is patient and family focused and facilitates robust communication across various services 24 hours a day, 7 days a week. The key elements of providing the right care at the right time for patients at the end of life is early identification of the patient and their needs and effective communication between all involved. To this end, many organisations are developing, or already have in place, systems that allow providers and commissioners of care to more clearly and systematically identify those individuals who may be entering into the last 6–12 months of life and ensure their needs are met.

Communication

Communication underpins virtually all nurse–patient interactions and is the bedrock of any therapeutic relationship. It perhaps comes into even sharper focus when dealing with the challenges of such an emotionally charged situation as caring for a dying patient and their family. Effective care at the end of life depends heavily on the ability of the individual practitioner to develop a trusting relationship with patients and those close to them. Patient- and family-centred communication that is honest and sensitive is therefore essential.

What the Experts Say

I had a handover and found out that in the bay where I was working was Vijay, a 45-year-old man who was diagnosed with a malignant brain tumour 18 months ago. He had been admitted to our medical ward as he had deteriorated rapidly overnight and was now thought to be dying. Vijay had an end-of-life care plan in place and his wife Michaela was with him. I really didn't know what to say so I just asked her if she was comfortable or needed anything. She said she was fine but just as I was about to leave, she asked me if I thought Vijay was looking better.

Anna, second-year student nurse

Jot This Down

- Have you ever not known what to say? How did this feel?
- How might you have answered Michaela's question?
- What do you think are the skills required to communicate effectively with Michaela?

Core Conditions

Effective communication is based on what are known as the core conditions – congruence, empathy and respect (Rogers, 1951). These are the foundations of a therapeutic encounter and it is suggested that without these, it is difficult to have a full and open relationship which may lead to a closing off and a creation of barriers between people.

- *Congruence*: genuineness, honesty with the patient or family member.
- *Empathy*: the ability to understand and appreciate what the other person is feeling and to convey this understanding in a relationship.
- *Respect*: acceptance, unconditional positive regard towards the other person.

Communication Skills

Whilst it is essential to have the core conditions in place, there are a number of practical skills and approaches to both verbal and non-verbal communication that can positively enhance communication with patients and family members.

Picking Up on Cues

A cue is a verbal or non-verbal hint that there is something more to be explored. It could take the form of a direct question, a comment or body language or facial expression. Picking up on cues is important – the patient or family member will be reluctant to offer further cues if their initial ones are not picked up. Linking an open question to a cue is much more likely to promote further disclosure than when not linked to a cue, as it is not focusing on the main concern of the patient or relative.

> **Michaela:** *Do you think he's looking better?*
> **Anna:** *What do you mean by better?*

Here the cue is the word 'better'. It suggests to Anna that Michaela is unsure about the situation and that to explore more about what she understands would be the best way to go. As the conversation continues, Anna will use more skills to respond to Michaela's concerns and facilitate further discussion.

Reflective Responding/Paraphrasing

Reflecting back the words used by a patient or relative can suggest that you have been listening carefully. It can be presented in the form of a question seeking more clarity or merely as an acknowledgement and indication of your attention and engagement. It allows the other person to hear their own words and that you are focused on what they are saying.

> **Michaela:** *His colour seems better so I'm kind of hoping he's coming round.*
> **Anna:** *Coming round?*

Here Anna may begin to understand what Michaela's perception of the situation is. Is she unaware and lacking information or is she struggling to accept the emerging reality that Vijay is now thought to be entering the last few hours or days of life?

Paraphrasing is similar to reflective responding but instead of using the other person's words, you reflect back what they have said using your own. This demonstrates that you have heard what has been said and that you have thought about it and communicated that understanding.

Summarising is an important skill to help the professional to take stock of where a conversation is going, what has been discussed and how to proceed. It also demonstrates that you have been listening carefully and by summarising the points discussed so far and checking that you have understood them correctly, you are both clear about what is the issue or difficulty.

> **Anna:** *I can see you're tired, and it must be hard to take in everything that's happening, but it seems to me that you're not sure what is happening regarding Vijay's care at the moment.*

Open Discussion and Information Giving

Facilitating an open discussion may help to clarify views in the situation by picking up on cues and other information. If, given her responses, Anna thinks Michaela is unclear about what is happening about Vijay and his condition, she may present this as a question.

> **Anna:** *I'm getting the feeling, Michaela, that you're a bit unsure as to what's going on regarding Vijay's condition, is that right?*
> **Michaela:** *Well, when we arrived last night he seemed really poorly, fitting and everything, and it all happened really fast and now he seems much more better than when we arrived.*

Information gathered from verbal and non-verbal cues in open discussions demonstrates a wish to understand and be clear about the person's concerns. Once the person's/family's concerns have been established and information needs have been identified, it is important that information is tailored to the individual at the right amount and the right pace. Communication is not a one-way process and it is important to ensure that the information is received and understood. Discussing with patients and families their main concerns can help them make sense of difficult situations.

> **Anna:** *What's the most difficult part of all of this, Michaela?*
> **Michaela:** *I'm not ready for this* [Michaela becomes upset]. *I wasn't expecting this when we came in! How am I going to tell the children? Do I need to make some calls?*
> **Anna:** *I'm sorry this has been such a difficult conversation and it wasn't the news you were hoping for* [pause]. *I can see you're very upset* [pause]. *If you like we could talk about where we can go from here.*

Empathic Response

An empathic response is one which demonstrates that you have some insight into the feelings being experienced by another. Having broken the news to Michaela that Vijay is dying, it is important that her feelings and emotions are acknowledged.

> **Michaela:** *I just don't know what to think. It's all too much to take in.*
> **Anna:** *This must be a very confusing time for you, it must seem overwhelming.* [Anna lightly touches Michaela's shoulder]

By acknowledging how someone is feeling and communicating this to them, you are demonstrating empathy, one of the core conditions. Touch, be it holding a hand or a hand on the shoulder, if done within the context of the core conditions, can be a powerful conveyor of empathy, concern and compassion.

Patient-centred Care – Holistic Assessment

There is a plethora of health and social care guidelines, policy and law related to care provision for patients who require palliative care or EoL care, but before we review this, it is vital to appraise and understand the needs of the person through a detailed holistic assessment.

Patient-centred care is a core component of good palliative care. It promotes the importance of viewing each individual holistically and acknowledges the impact of a person's illness on their psychological, emotional, social and spiritual well-being. It includes the giving of bad news, respecting and developing coping strategies, and acknowledging fears and maintaining hope. It plays an important role in determining how patients and families respond to the impact of the illness and aids in coping with the experiences of loss and change as well as in expanding the sense of what is possible.

Effective biopsychosocial care is dependent on an approach to assessment that identifies these issues and acknowledges them

---

Box 20.1 Common Holistic Assessment Tool

Domain 1: Background information and assessment preferences

- Demographic and contact details, history of illness, treatment plan, professional involved, next of kin.
- Consent to assessment, previous assessments undertaken, preferences for setting of assessment and family involvement.

Domain 2: Physical well-being

- Impact of illness on physical well-being, symptoms such as pain, nausea and breathlessness, effect on sleep, energy levels, nutrition, weight loss.

Domain 3: Social and occupational well-being

- Type of accommodation, who the patient lives with, level of dependency and sources of help with shopping, meal preparation and so forth.
- Work and financial issues, family and close relationships, needs related to children (talking to them about death).

Domain 4: Psychological well-being

- Mood, anxiety, adjustment to worsening illness or treatment, knowledge/understanding of disease/treatment, sources of emotional support, unresolved concerns, coping strategies and strengths, perception of the future.

Domain 5: Spiritual well-being and life goals

- Identification of views on faith or belief, impact of illness on faith/belief, practical support or other needs related to religion or spiritual matters (contact with faith leader, opportunity/space to pray).
- Discussion of important life goals or exploring what endows life with meaning and purpose.

---

equally alongside the medical, symptom and treatment-related aspects of care (Engel, 1977). According to the National End of Life Care Programme (2010), holistic assessment is vital in order to identify where a person's needs are currently not being addressed and indicates where other health and social care professionals could be involved to address this. Individual preferences and wishes can also be highlighted, enabling the person to be more in control of what is happening and promote dignity and choice (National Palliative and End of Life Care Partnership, 2015). The Common Holistic Assessment Tool (Box 20.1) provides guidance for holistic assessment of the supportive and palliative care needs of adults. All people who are approaching the end of their life should be offered this type of biopsychosocial assessment (National End of Life Care Programme, 2010).

There are milestones within a person's EoL care journey that may indicate when an assessment may be appropriate. A structured approach to holistic assessment is valuable at key points in a person's care pathway, such as at diagnosis when the person is identified as approaching the end of life or when the individual is thought to be entering into the dying phase (actively dying) or at any other time that a patient, family member or professional carer may deem necessary. The following holistic assessment can be carried out by any professional who knows the person, their condition and its management and has the appropriate skills to ensure each person is seen as an individual (Department of Health, 2008; National End of Life Care Programme, 2010; National Palliative and End of Life Care Partnership, 2015).

The Common Holistic Assessment is divided into five 'domains'. Each time an assessment is carried out, each domain

should be reviewed with the patient. As the patient progresses through their EoL care trajectory, the depth to which each domain is covered will depend on the individual needs of the patient and should be 'concerns led'; for example, a patient with a newly diagnosed illness may not wish to engage in advance planning discussions, therefore the first domain might be a short discussion, in comparison with a patient who is further along in their disease trajectory (National End of Life Care Programme, 2010).

The order in which the domains are asssed in each discussion with a patient is important. Some domains, such as psychological well-being and spiritual well-being, do require a degree of trust and understanding between the assessor and individual and therefore muiltiple assessments will allow for therapeutic relationships to develop. Patients may also have concerns that are relevant to more than one domain, e.g. physical problems such as pain may raise psychological needs such as depression and/or anxiety. In this guidance, items for discussion are listed only once. The assessor should use their professional judgement if they need to appraise several domains to avoid repetition as this can be a source of frustration for patients. A good example could be when assessing nutrition, you might find you need to assess physical, psychological, social and spiritual domains to fully appraise the concerns of the patient. The assessment should follow a conversational style and it is imperative to support the individual to identify and articulate their own needs.

Psychosocial Assessment at the End of Life: Points to Remember

- Assessment should be led by patient concerns.
- It should be carried out *with* patients and families, not *on* them.
- It should be done in a conversational style rather than viewed as a series of boxes that must be ticked.
- Helping patients to assess their own needs should be central to the process.
- Patient consent is necessary to the assessment process.
- Professionals undertaking assessment should have reached an agreed level of competency in key aspects of assessment.
- Patient preference for communicating with professionals, their family and friends should be considered (National End of Life Care Programme, 2010).

A comprehensive holistic assessment affords health and social care professionals the opportunity to understand the needs of the patient and their families/carers. In doing so, we can support the notion of providing EoL care that promotes a 'good death'.

What Do We Mean By a Good Death?

Jot This Down Activity

- What would be your idea of a good death?
- What could you do to ensure you achieved your 'good death'?
- What have been your experiences of a good death?
- Have you witnessed what you felt to be a bad death?

The concept of a 'good death' may seem strange to many but how and where people die is often very important to individuals and their families. Within contemporary society, the idea of what constitutes a good death might vary according to one's cultural group and the view of death that comes from either a religious or non-religious view (O'Gorman, 1998).

Traditionally, religion gave a structure to the preparation for death but within an increasingly secular society, a more individual response to the understanding of the meaning of death appears to be emerging. In individualistic societies in the 'modern West', a 'bad death' is perhaps seen as that of the person with no autonomy, for instance the patient with a stroke or Alzheimer disease, who cannot communicate their wishes. Our society's concept of a 'good death' is perhaps therefore one characterised by choice and control – a death that occurs where one would choose it, in one's own home with loved ones around, one that was free of pain or anguish and fear – a death that was anticipated but not one that came after a protracted time of disability and increasing weakness, confusion or dependence.

The London End of Life Clinical Network (2015) promotes the following attributes as necessary for any service providing EoL care.

- Access to psychological and spiritual support.
- Tailored pain management.
- Timely assessment and provision of bereavement services.
- Care which is competent, confident, compassionate and personalised.
- Joined-up, co-ordinated services and pathways which are easy to access and navigate.
- A supportive culture that fosters excellence, confidence, innovation and education in all staff.

We will now explore the following points in more detail through the appraisal of guidelines, policy and law that supports patients, their families/carers and health professionals to offer care provisions that support a 'good death'.

End-of-Life Care Strategy

'How we care for the dying is an indicator of how we care for all sick and vulnerable people'

(Department of Health, 2008)

With an ageing population and an unprecedented number of people living with advanced progressive diseases, increasing attention is being paid to how we should care for those who are dying. The hospice movement set the standard regarding how palliative care could be delivered, yet there were many inequalities in care across disease and demographic groups and EoL care was a low priority compared to other health issues. In 2008, the *End-of-Life Care Strategy* (Department of Health, 2008) was the first systematic review of how people died in the UK and provided a quality framework for how they and their families should be cared for. It is subject to annual reviews of progress against its stated aims to improve EoL care for everyone.

The strategy highlighted that there was a lack of public discussion around death and even clinicians had difficulty in initiating EoL discussions and struggled to identify people approaching the end of life. There was a distinct lack of patient and carer satisfaction in the quality of EoL care, with 54% of complaints in acute hospitals related to care of the dying/bereavement care (Healthcare Commission, 2008). The strategy placed a strong emphasis on improving education and training around EoL care for all practitioners in order to achieve the aim of allowing more people to die in the place of their choice. Research

highlighted by Dying Matters (Shucksmith *et al.*, 2013) showed disparity between where people would wish to die and their preferred place of care, and the actual place of death. This research found that around 70% of people would choose to die at home but 50% of people were dying in hospital. However, there appears to be a downward trend in patients dying in hospital. According to Public Health England (2016), in 2004 57.9% of patients died in hospital, whereas in 2016 this number had fallen to 46.9%, with more people dying at home (23.5%) or in their preferred place of care, i.e. a nursing home (21.8%) or hospice (5.7%). However, there was significant variation across the country by district and local authority, with the proportions of deaths in hospital ranging from 34.2% to 63.1% (ONS, 2020).

Jot This Down Activity

- Why do you think more people are dying in their preferred place of care?
- Why do you think that people rate hospice care so highly?
- What are the challenges of providing EoL care in a hospital setting?

Ambitions for Palliative and End-of-Life Care

'The essential challenge is to learn how to work together, collectively and differently to achieve these ambitions and the standard set out in the NICE Quality Standard for End-of-Life Care (2011)'

(National Palliative and End-of-Life Care Partnership, 2015–2020)

In 2015, the Ambitions for Palliative and End-of-Life Care were introduced, not to replace the End-of-Life Care Strategy and the improvements that followed but to build upon its commitment to improving EoL care through national partnership. The National Palliative and End-of-Life Care Network (2015) proposes six ambitions for improving palliative and EoL care as a framework for local implementation, whereby individuals and organisations can lay these foundations on their own or collectively.

1. Each person is seen as an individual.
2. Each person gets fair access to care.
3. Maximising comfort and well-being.
4. Care is co-ordinated.
5. All staff are prepared to care.
6. Each community is prepared to help.

Full details of the ambitions are available at: **https://acpopc. csp.org.uk/system/files/documents/2021-05/FINAL_ Ambitions-for-Palliative-and-End-of-Life-Care_2nd_ edition.pdf**

Each of the six ambitions is accompanied with a statement to give focus to the ambition in practice from the viewpoint of the person nearing the end of life. The attention is on the experience of the dying person, but each of the ambitions should also be viewed as an ambition for carers, families and, where appropriate, for people who have been bereaved. The impetus is for open and honest conversation and the importance of integrated care delivered by compassionate, caring and competent health and care staff (National Palliative and End-of-Life Care Partnership, 2015).

Gold Standards Framework

The End-of-Life Care Strategy states that all organisations providing EoL care are expected to implement a systematic approach to care and encourage the use of evidence-based, quality-assured tools to promote effective EoL care. One such tool is the Gold Standards Framework (2021) (GSF). The GSF aims to improve palliative care provided by the whole primary care team and enables those approaching the end of life to be identified, their care needs assessed, and a plan of care involving all relevant agencies created and put in place. The framework focuses on optimising continuity of care, teamwork, advanced planning (including out of hours), symptom control and patient, carer and staff support. The GSF provides practitioners with various prompts and tools to help them identify when someone may be entering the dying phase.

Prognostic Indicator Guidance

There are a number of indicators that suggest someone may be entering the last 6–12 months of life. These range from quite general indicators to much more specific ones relating to specific conditions and the physical changes that occur as it progresses.

Triggers That Suggest That Patients are Nearing the End of Life

The Surprise Question: would you be surprised if this patient were to die in the next 6–12 months? This is an intuitive question and encourages the practitioner to think about how an individual is coping day to day with an advancing disease, by looking at the context of:

- *Patient choice*: the patient with advanced disease makes a choice for comfort care only
- *Patient need*: the patient is in special need of supportive or palliative care
- *Clinical indicators*: general predicators of end-stage illness and cancer-specific indicators (any patient whose cancer is metastatic or inoperable) (Gold Standards Framework Prognostic Indicator Guidance, 2021).

General Predictors of End-stage Illness

- Multiple co-morbidities
- Weight loss: greater than 10% weight loss over 6 months
- General physical decline
- Reducing performance status
- Dependence in most activities of living (ALs)
- Repeated unplanned/crisis admissions

Specific Clinical Indicators

As well as general indicators of end-stage illness, more specific markers exist that help clinicians to arrive at a more accurate prognosis. These are more specific to individual diseases such as cancer, chronic obstructive pulmonary disease (COPD), heart failure, renal disease, neurological disease (motor neurone and Parkinson disease, multiple sclerosis), dementia, general frailty and stroke. Using more disease-specific measurements about the particular disease and its progression may allow a more evidence-based and accurate prognosis.

Dying Trajectories

Different diseases progress at different rates and have different patterns of periods of stability punctuated by exacerbations and stages where the patient's condition will deteriorate. Malignant diseases such as cancer often follow a predictable trajectory of deterioration, which therefore makes care planning easier to anticipate. However, some illnesses can be problematic in predicting timeframes of mortality, particularly for those patients who have non-malignant life-limiting illnesses. As an example, in chronic obstructive pulmonary disease, it can be challenging to determine if the patient is having an acute exacerbation or if they are at the end of life (Cohen-Mansfield *et al.*, 2018). Similarly, a person with dementia may have a longer and slower trajectory, with often almost imperceptible changes that over time mean that they will become weaker, more dependent and more prone to opportunistic infections or other problems such as difficulty swallowing, poor nutritional intake and mobility problems.

Therefore, it is important to understand that some people might only receive EoL care in their last weeks, days or hours. Every effort should be made to ensure that wishes and preferences, such as the person's preferred place of care or advance decisions to refuse treatment, are sensitively discussed and documented in advance care plans as early as possible with patients and family members (National Palliative and End of Life Care Partnership, 2015; Mitchell & Elbourne, 2020).

Despite the different patterns of progression, all patients with advanced progressive disease will at some point experience a deterioration in their condition that will necessitate EoL care. The challenge for health professionals is to identify the triggers, such as recurrent exacerbations requiring repeated hospitalisations, deterioration in general condition, weight loss, increasing lethargy and dependence. It is important to develop an attitude of proactive planning and anticipation rather than waiting for an event and then reacting to it. This can be facilitated with advance care planning.

Advance Care Planning

Advance care planning is a voluntary process of discussion about future care between an individual and their care providers irrespective of discipline. It is the process of identifying how an individual wishes to be cared for before they lose capacity and can inform such things as where a person may wish to die, what their view regarding certain treatments or interventions may be, who they want to be present, and perhaps what may be important to them to maintain their dignity (Mitchell & Elbourne, 2020).

Jot This Down Activity

- How would you feel about exploring advance care planning with a patient you were caring for?
- What skills or approaches would you use to help the discussion take place?
- When would be the best time to have these discussions?

Red Flag

It is important to remember that not all patients will wish to enter into such discussions and many may prefer not to talk about such things and should not be pressed to do so. However, for some it will be very important and a way of maintaining autonomy and control over their care.

An advance care plan (ACP) can take many forms – it could be a verbal discussion or documenting wishes in a person's healthcare records; however, the more clearly and explicitly documented and the more members of the caregiving team across the different organisations who are aware of the ACP, the more likely it is that an individual's wishes will be realised (Marie Curie, 2020a). If the individual wishes, family and friends can be involved but it may be important to point out that if the person's wishes for EoL care involve, or are in some way dependent on, other members of the family, opening up discussion around this is very important. For example, if a person wishes to die at home but this makes other members of the family anxious about their ability to cope with caring for them, it is important to identify this early and discuss this difficulty and any possible solutions to it.

The value of an ACP is that it opens up a dialogue between the patient, their family and the professionals involved in their care; without this, preferences are unknown and families and professionals are left to try to guess what a person may have wanted. As a person's illness progresses, so may their views on the type of care they may want or need; this is why it is important to regularly review ACPs to ensure that they remain in line with what the person is thinking and feeling at the time (Thomson *et al.*, 2016).

Advance care planning promotes patient-centred care as it tailors the patient's wishes and preferences to their care. It also opens up the possibility of discussion around prognosis ('How long have I got?') and also possibly what the immediate and longer-term future may hold ('What is going to happen to me?') and also helps them plan and predict what they feel they may need ('What support will I need, who will be able to look after me and my family?'). It can help the professional to anticipate what resources may be needed and promotes a dialogue between patients, family and carers, addressing any fears or concerns early in the process.

By asking people what they want, we can continue to put their wishes at the heart of the plan of care, ensuring that they remain in control even when they become too ill to tell us what they want. By dealing with these issues, an ACP can provide people with hope that at least their views and wishes are recognised as important and will be respected.

The Nursing Associate Student

According to the NMC (2018) standards of proficiency, nursing associates will work with registered nurses to provide care and support patients to plan for their end of life, giving information to patients, their families and the bereaved and providing care to the deceased. It is important that you are familiar with advanced care planning and have practised the appropriate communication skills to develop the ability to act autonomously in the delivery of this care. The nursing associate is a valued member of the care team and has much to offer in the provision of high-quality patient-centred end-of-life care.

Ethics and Decision Making at the End of Life

The very nature of EoL care and the profound ethical questions it raises for health and social care practitioners demand an understanding of the underpinning ethical theories and the part they play in clinical decision making. A common framework often applied in nursing and healthcare fields is the 'four principles' approach (Beauchamp & Childress, 2019). These reflect four core moral principles (Box 20.2) which should be acknowledged and evaluated in relation to each other and their importance to the ethical challenge in question.

Mental Capacity

The Mental Capacity Act came into force in 2005 and became fully effective in 2007. It aims to empower and protect people who lack capacity and to ensure that the decision-making process remains focused on their best interests and that their wishes and preferences remain at the centre of the process. It allows people to plan ahead for the eventuality that they may lose capacity in the future and clarifies who should be involved in decision making and what the process should entail (Figure 20.1).

The Mental Capacity Act 2005 is underpinned by five key principles.

1. A person must be assumed to have capacity unless it is established that they lack capacity.
2. A person is not to be treated as unable to make a decision unless all practicable steps to help them to do so have been taken without success.
3. A person is not to be treated as unable to make a decision merely because they make an unwise decision.
4. An act done, or decision made, under this Act for or on behalf of a person who lacks capacity must be done, or made, in their best interests.
5. Before the act is done, or the decision is made, regard must be had to whether the purpose for which it is needed can be as effectively achieved in a way that is less restrictive of the person's rights and freedom of action.

The application of the Mental Capacity Act to EoL care is clearly apparent. The progressive nature of a terminal illness will

---

Box 20.2 Four Principles of Biomedical Ethics

Autonomy: Concerned with the ability of the individual to act freely and to not be constrained or restricted. It relates to the right of the individual to self-determination. Respect for autonomy is fundamental for informed consent and advance directives

Beneficence: To do good, to act in such a way that promotes the best interests and well-being of others. This is a fundamental aspect of our caregiving role

Non-maleficence: To do no harm, to ensure that no action or omission of action is detrimental to the health and well-being of the patient

Justice: Fairness, to ensure that people are treated without prejudice and are seen as equal. It also relates to the allocation and distribution of resources

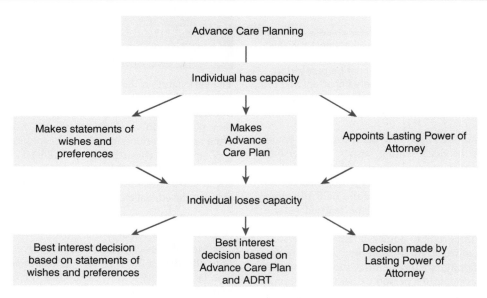

Figure 20.1 Relationship between advance care planning, best interest decision making, Advance Decision to Refuse Treatment (ADRT) and Lasting Power of Attorney.

undoubtedly lead to a person losing capacity to make decisions at some point.

Best Interest Decision Making

When a person loses capacity and their wishes are not clearly known, there is an expectation that health professionals, guided by the views of the family, should make a decision that is in the individual's best interests. The Mental Capacity Act 2005 clearly states that any previously stated views and preferences must be taken into account when making such a decision but, ultimately, following a discussion with all the key people involved, including a relative (or appointed representative if there is no family), it would fall to an individual who is in the best position to understand the implications of various courses of action and can see the overall picture.

What the Experts Say

> Andrea had lived at Ford House for about 5 years. He was 50 and had lifelong severe learning disabilities. He loved being in the house with the other tenants. But I had seen Andrea getting worse, as his breathing worsened due to his heart condition. He was struggling to manage diet and fluids as he kept coughing and the nurses were worried that dust was entering his lungs and that this was why he kept getting chest infections. When he was admitted to hospital, I went with him and after a couple of days the nurses and doctors called a meeting. Myself and Andrea's mum and dad were there, and the nurses and doctors wanted to know how we felt about Andrea's worsening condition and what Andrea would most likely want to happen if he could tell us. The nurses and doctors felt that if Andrea's heart were to stop beating then it would not be appropriate to try to resuscitate him. Both Andrea's parents and I felt that given how poorly Andrea was, he would want to be kept comfortable and not be kept alive by tubes and machines if he wasn't going to get back to how he was. So, we all agreed this was for the best and Andrea died peacefully a few days later.
>
> Jana, learning disability domiciliary care manager

In the preceding example, a capacity assessment had been made and found that Andrea lacked capacity due to his learning disability and physical condition. He was unable to understand, retain and weigh information material to the decisions and any alternatives. Andrea was also unable to communicate a decision, therefore a 'best interests' decision meeting was held with the key people involved: the nurses and other members of the healthcare team looking after him, his parents and his care manager. The meeting looked at Andrea's condition, his prognosis and options for care. The outcome was that, given Andrea's deteriorating condition and poor prognosis and the views of his family regarding what he would wish if he were able to choose himself, he should be kept comfortable and to attempt cardiopulmonary resuscitation would be futile and not in his best interests.

Red Flag

 It should not be assumed that a person with learning disabilities lacks capacity. Capacity must always be assessed using the Mental Capacity Act.

Lasting Power of Attorney

If an individual wants to ensure that their wishes are unequivocally stated and that someone they identify is able to make decisions on their behalf, then they can choose to appoint another person as their Lasting Power of Attorney (LPA) (Marie Curie, 2020a). Previously, this role was concerned solely with financial affairs and arrangements, but since 2007 an individual can be appointed as an LPA (through officially being recorded as such with the Office of the Public Guardian) in order to make proxy decisions concerning a person's care and medical treatment. It is important to identify if an LPA has been appointed and, if so, that this decision was made in accordance with the LPA process, superseding any other previously recorded wishes or views, for example in an ACP or an advance decision to refuse treatment.

If a person has no one who can act as an advocate on their behalf if they lose capacity, an independent mental capacity advocate (IMCA) may be appointed. IMCAs are independent of the NHS and local authority bodies and can represent a person who has lost capacity (MCA, 2005; Social Care Institute for Excellence, 2010).

Preferred Priorities for Care

The Preferred Priorities for Care (PPC) document is one way of identifying and recording a patient's wishes. It comprises a patient-held record, which records the patient's wishes, the socioeconomic circumstances of the family, the services being accessed, reasons for change in their care and a needs assessment that documents care on an ongoing basis. It has been used in the domiciliary setting and also in care and residential homes and is becoming more commonplace in hospitals.

Advance Decisions to Refuse Treatment

An Advance Decision to Refuse Treatment (ADRT) replaces previously used terms such as 'living wills' and 'advance directives'. It is a clearly documented statement of wishes and preferences regarding the withholding and withdrawing of treatment. It comes into effect if an individual loses capacity to make such decisions; until this time, the normal process of consent applies. An ADRT forms part of an ACP in that it identifies individual wishes and preferences regarding treatment and can be used to open discussions with health and social care professionals about how best to plan for the future. Examples of ARDTs include Do Not Attempt Resuscitation (DNAR) and the refusal of artificial feeding or hydration (Macmillan, 2019).

reSPECT Forms

Patients can also complete a reSPECT form with a clinician. These forms are not legally binding like ADRTs, but their aim is to develop a shared understanding between the healthcare professional and the patient of their condition, the outcomes the patient values and those they fear and then how treatments and interventions, such as cardiopulmonary resuscitation (CPR), fit into this. It supports the important principle of personalised care (Resuscitation Council UK, 2019).

What the Experts Say

When Adam was brought in, the first thing his husband told us was that he had an ADRT. Adam had been admitted a couple of times previously with worsening symptoms due to his heart failure and been treated with diuretics and other medication. Adam was too ill to discuss this, but we sat down with his husband and he told us about Adam's wishes and what he had written on his ARDT. He showed us the document and it clearly stated that if Adam had a cardiac arrest due to his heart failure, he did not want anyone to attempt cardiopulmonary resuscitation. We discussed it as a team, and we were happy to respect it. Adam died peacefully a couple of days later with his husband by his side.

Yukiko, cardiac consultant nurse

What Adam's story tells us is that as nurses, we must be sure that what is written in an ADRT form meets several essential criteria that reinforce its validity.

- *Has the person lost capacity?* All efforts must be made to maximise a person's ability to make an informed decision but in the event that capacity has clearly been lost, then discussion must take place with family and/or LPA.
- *Is the decision valid?* Is the situation in keeping with what the person was anticipating, have they changed their mind or done or said anything that might be inconsistent with the ADRT? Have they appointed an LPA since the ADRT was written?
- *Is the advance decision applicable?* Does the ADRT specify which treatment the person wishes to refuse?
- *Does the decision refer to life-sustaining treatment?* Does the ADRT clearly refer to a decision by the patient to refuse life-sustaining treatment? Is it signed by the person and by a witness?

Care in the Last few Days of Life

Diagnosing Dying: Signs and Symptoms of Approaching Death

Understanding the clinical indications of the dying process is an important skill if nurses are to support patients and family members effectively. Communicating honestly and appropriately at this time is important if families are to have important conversations or act on a patient's preference about how and where they die. Predicting when a patient might die is difficult (Mitchell & Elbourne, 2020): some patients survive for a long period despite a poor initial prognosis, while others may deteriorate rapidly and unexpectedly. Families often seek some indication from professionals about 'how long?' It is prudent to avoid guessing or to be pressured to be too exact. It is best to support the family with the uncertainty of the situation and talk in terms of 'days', 'weeks' or 'months' accordingly, perhaps focusing on the immediate present and what might be done to improve the patient's comfort and dignity.

However, there are common signs and symptoms that signify that a patient is approaching the terminal stages of their illness and that death is imminent.

- Profound tiredness and weakness
  - Reduced interest in getting out of bed
  - Needing assistance with all care
  - Less interest in things happening around them
- Diminished intake of food and fluids
- Drowsy or reduced cognition
  - May be disorientated in time or place
  - Difficulty concentrating
  - Scarcely able to co-operate and converse with carers
- Gaunt appearance
- Difficulty swallowing medicine (Marie Curie, 2020b)

Other signs of active dying may include:

- Decreasing blood perfusion
- Neurological dysfunction
- Decreasing level of consciousness
- Decreased ability to move

343

- Joint position fatigue
- Increased need for care
- Tachycardia, hypotension
- Peripheral cooling, cyanosis of extremities
- Mottling of skin
- Loss of ability to swallow, sphincter control
- Diminished urine output
- Terminal delirium
- Changes in respiration
- Weak/no radial pulse (Kennedy *et al.*, 2014; Farrell & Paice, 2019).

Common signs and symptoms in the last 48 hours of life include:

- Pain
- Restlessness/agitation
- Upper airway secretions
- Nausea and vomiting (Mitchell & Elbourne, 2020).

Symptom Control at the End of Life

Pain

It is important to ensure that these common symptoms are anticipated and addressed proactively. When a person is unable to communicate their pain verbally due to their condition, staff must observe for non-verbal signs such as facial expressions (grimacing), groaning or moans. The patient's relatives may communicate that they feel the patient is in pain – they know the person better than the nurses do and we must address their concerns and administer prescribed analgesia appropriately. However, it is essential to be aware that terminal agitation and restlessness may also be present and not to confuse the two symptoms as they require different approaches to management. Chapter 22 of this text discusses pain in more detail.

Restlessness/Agitation

Restlessness and agitation are recognised symptoms of the terminal phase and will require management through the use of prescribed sedative and anxiolytic medication. However, it is imperative to exclude or address all possible causes of restlessness and agitation before administering sedative and anxiolytic medication. The following are common causes of restlessness and agitation in EoL patients.

- Pain
- Urinary retention
- Full rectum
- Nausea
- Cerebral irritation
- Anxiety and fear
- Side-effects of medication
- Poor positioning (Farrell & Paice, 2019)

Upper Airway Secretions

Profound weakness at the end of life can lead to accumulation of upper airway secretions that the patient is too weak to expectorate and this results in moist, noisy breathing. This is often referred to as the 'death rattle' and occurs in 50% of patients (Marie Curie, 2020b). The noise can be distressing for those witnessing it and often family members will feel the patient is choking or cannot breathe, though if deeply unconscious the patient may be unaware. It is best to try to avoid this symptom occurring in the first place if possible, as once established, secretions are more difficult to remove than to prevent. Repositioning can help but if treatment is required, antimuscarinic drugs such as hyoscine butylbromide or glycopyrronium can be given subcutaneously to prevent further secretions (Joint Formulary Committee, 2020; NHS Scotland, 2020).

Nausea and Vomiting

There are many causes of nausea and vomiting in advanced disease, such as gastric stasis/obstruction, drug induced and metabolic (i.e. hypercalcaemia/renal failure). However, in the final stages of life it is sometimes not possible or appropriate to identify a specific cause and broad-spectrum antiemetics to cover the main possible causes may be the most prudent approach. Drugs such as cyclizine and levomepromazine are commonly administered continually via a syringe driver and as required via subcutaneous injection (Joint Formulary Committee, 2020; NHS Scotland, 2020).

Ethical Challenges at the End of Life

Artificial Hydration and Nutrition

> **Case Study**
>
> Mrs Patel has just been told that her husband is dying, and the main treatment aim is to keep him comfortable. Mrs Patel is confused and questions the nurse attending to his care why he doesn't have a drip as he is not drinking, and he is likely to die of thirst.
>
> - What would you say to Mrs Patel?
> - How will you manage her distress?
> - *Autonomy*: how could you ensure that you act in accordance with Mr Patels' views, wishes and preferences?
> - *Beneficence*: what is in Mr Patel's 'best interests'? Would artificial fluids make him more comfortable?
> - *Non-maleficence*: would withholding or commencing artificial fluids at this point do harm to Mr Patel?
> - *Justice*: should all patients in this situation be treated exactly the same? Should we give equal weight to all of Mrs Patel's concerns?

Evidence suggests that giving artificial hydration at the very end of life when someone is unable to tolerate oral fluids affects neither the length of remaining life nor the patient's comfort (NICE, 2015) and current literature suggests that the benefits of providing artificial hydration are limited and do not clearly outweigh the burdens (Raijmakers *et al.*, 2011). Therefore, not commencing them would be doing good and minimising harm. Administering artificial fluids may lessen Mrs Patel's immediate distress, but the reality remains that her husband is dying. It is possible to give mixed messages to relatives about the goals of care at this point and this can lead to inconsistencies in approaches to Mr Patel's care by different members of the team, and perhaps facilitate false hope, thus doing more harm. It may be best to make an evidence-based decision as to the benefits of hydration for Mr Patel as this will be in his best interests. It would not be ethically justifiable to treat Mr Patel in order to minimise distress to Mrs Patel but it would be important to sensitively discuss this with Mrs Patel and explore her understanding and feelings around this and allay any fears she may have.

Red Flag

 A blanket policy approach of either always initiating or always withholding or withdrawing artificial fluids for people in this situation is ethically indefensible. Each situation must be looked at individually and the benefits and burdens of such treatment weighed against the needs of the individual.

Nursing Fields of Practice

How would these issues relate to other people who had impaired capacity, such as:
- People with dementia or mental health problems?
- Individuals with learning disabilities?
- Young children and babies?

Syringe Drivers

A syringe driver is useful for symptom control when oral administration is not possible and repeated subcutaneous injections or administration of medication by other routes are inappropriate, ineffective or impractical. Although syringe drivers are primarily used in EoL care, they may also be appropriate for patients who are not imminently dying. Consider using medication via a syringe driver for the following.

- Persistent vomiting
- Reduced consciousness
- Dysphagia
- Weakness
- Bowel obstruction or malabsorption
- Significant tablet burden
- Unwilling to take tablets by mouth
- Unable to absorb oral medications
- For patients who have head and neck lesions or surgery
- Terminal respiratory secretions in unconscious patient
- Poor symptom control with oral drugs
- Improve patient comfort (O'Brien, 2012; NHS Scotland, 2014; Dougherty & Lister, 2020)

The goals for administering medication using a syringe driver should be discussed with the patient and any concerns addressed. It is important to explain to patients and family members that although the syringe driver may allow symptoms associated with the dying process to be helped, it will not expedite the dying process. Patients and family members should be assured that the decision to start a syringe driver is not irrevocable and if the patient's symptoms improve, this may be stopped (Thomas & Barclay, 2015). See Table 20.1 for advantages and disadvantages of using syringe drivers in EoL care.

The most common portable syringe driver nurses will encounter in the UK in homes and care settings requires refilling every 24 hours and administers consistent therapeutic drug levels, set in milliliters (mL) per hour. Safety features include a mechanism to stop the infusion if the syringe is not properly and securely fitted, alarms that activate if the syringe is removed before the infusion is stopped, and an internal log to record pump activity.

Medications Suitable for Syringe Drivers An understanding of the drugs that can be used in syringe drivers and the therapeutic effects is an essential component of end-of-life care

Table 20.1 Advantages and disadvantages of syringe drivers in end-of-life care.

ADVANTAGES	DISADVANTAGES
• Repeated injections are not required • Symptom control with a combination of drugs • 24-hour symptom control and comfort without peaks and troughs • Only needs reloading once every 24 hours • Patients can remain ambulant	• Staff training required • Possible inflammation and pain at infusion sites and increased risk of infection • Skin site availability may become a problem in emaciated patients • Requires daily visits from district nurses and other health professionals and 4-hourly ward checks • Not all drugs can be used with this system

(Table 20.2). Nurses must safeguard the interest of patients at all times by accepting responsibility only for duties in which they are competent and able to practise safely without supervision (NMC, 2018). It is suggested that theoretical knowledge alone is insufficient, and nurses must be deemed competent through locally agreed competency frameworks that incorporate best practice and requirements for continuous training (O'Brien, 2012).

Medications are mixed with water for injection (sterile water) or normal saline (NaCl 0.9%). Sterile water is compatible with most medicines except levomepromazine, ondasetron, hyoscine butylbromide and octreotide, which should be diluted with normal saline. One of the advantages of syringe drivers is that two or more drugs (occasionally up to four) can be mixed together and infused. Knowledge of drug compatibility is therefore essential (Table 20.3) and observation of physical compatibility such as precipitation, discolouration or cloudiness of the infusion mixture (Thomas & Barclay, 2015). Seek pharmacy advice for three or more drugs and follow local procedure guidelines.

Setting Up a Syringe Driver

Equipment
- Syringe driver
- Luer Lock syringes – manufacturers recommend the size of syringe that should be used with their devices. Syringe drivers are calibrated in mL per hour. It is important to establish the final volume required before choosing the size
- Drug label
- Butterfly needle or infusion set cannula
- Transparent surgical dressing
- Syringe driver case and battery
- Subcutaneous infusion set
- Water for injection or normal saline
- Medicines
- Sharps box
- Prescription and monitoring chart
- Non-sterile gloves
- Skin cleansing agent

Table 20.2 Common medicines used in syringe drivers and indications. *Source:* Joint Formulary Committee (2020), NHS Scotland (2020).

DRUG	INDICATIONS	DOSE
Opioids for pain relief		
Diamorphine 5 mg, 10 mg, 30 mg, 100 mg, 500 mg powder ampoules	Opioid-responsive pain, breathlessness	5–10 mg/24 hours, if no opioid before Can be diluted in a small volume Preferred for high opioid doses
Morphine sulfate 10 mg, 30 mg in 1 mL, 60 mg in 2 mL	Opioid-responsive pain, breathlessness	5–10 mg/24 hours, if no opioid before First-line opioid analgesic
Oxycodone	Opioid-responsive pain, breathlessness	2–5 mg/24 hours, if no opioid before Second-line opioid analgesic if morphine/diamorphine not tolerated
Antiemetics		
Cyclizine 50 mg in 1 mL	Nausea and vomiting due to mechanical bowel obstruction, raised intracranial pressure and motion sickness	50–150 mg/24 hours Can cause redness, irritation at the site Incompatible with normal saline, always use water for injection
Haloperidol 5 mg in 1 mL, 10 mg in 2 mL	Opioid for metabolic-induced nausea, delirium	2–10 mg/24 hours
Levomepromazine 25 mg in 1 mL	Complex nausea, terminal delirium/agitation	5–25 mg/24 hours as antiemetic 100 mg/24 hours as sedative Initially 12.5–50 mg/24 hours, titrated according to response (doses above 25 mg should be given under specialist supervision) Second-line sedative if midazolam ineffective If purple or yellow discolouration, discard – this can be caused by light exposure
Metoclopramide 10 mg in 2 mL	Nausea and vomiting (peristaltic failure, gastric stasis/outlet obstruction)	30–100 mg/24 hours
Anticholinergics		
Glycopyrronium bromide 200 mcg in 1 mL, 600 mcg in 3 mL	Chest secretions or colic	0.6–1.2 mg/24 hours for bowel colic and excessive secretions Second-line; non-sedative Longer-duration action than hyoscine
Hyoscine butylbromide (Buscopan®) 20 mg in 1 mL	Chest secretions, bowel obstruction (colic, vomiting)	60–300 mg/24 hours for bowel colic 20–120 mg/24 hours for excessive respiratory secretions First-line; non-sedative
Hyoscine hydrobromide 400 mcg in 1 mL, 600 mcg in 1 mL	Chest secretions	1.2–2 mg/24 hours for bowel colic and excessive secretions Third-line; sedative Can precipitate delirium
Sedatives		
Midazolam 10 mg in 2 mL	Myoclonus, seizures, terminal delirium/agitation	Initially 10–20 mg/24 hours, adjusted according to response; usual dose 20–60 mg/24 hours 20–40 mg/24 hours for convulsions in palliative care
Steroids		
Dexamethasone 3.3 mg in 1 mL	Brain metastases, nausea and vomiting, anorexia, bowel obstructive symptoms, emergency management of suspected superior vena cava obstruction (SVCO) or malignant spinal cord compression (MSCC)	Dose depending on indication, ranges from 2 mg to 16 mg for emergency management of SVCO or MSCC. Contact specialist palliative care team for advice

Table 20.3 Drug compatibility.

NAME OF DRUG	MORPHINE SULFATE	DIAMORPHINE	OXYCODONE
Cyclizine[a]	✓	✓	✓
Haloperidol	✓	✓	✓
Glycopyrronium	✓	✓	✓
Hyoscine butylbromide	✓	✓	✓
Hyoscine hydrobromide	✓	✓	✓
Levomepromazine	✓	✓	✓
Metoclopramide	✓	✓	✓
Midazolam	✓	✓	✓

[a] Use water for injection as diluent for cyclizine.

Procedure Explain the rationale for setting up the syringe driver and the procedure to the patient and relatives.

- Obtain consent.
- Wash hands.
- Check patient name and ID number.
- Ask the patient (or carers/family) if they have any known allergies.
- Check the battery for the syringe driver. If the battery is below 40% at the start of the infusion, discard the old battery and use a new one.
- Set the rate: this is the rate at which the syringe plunger will be moved forward by the motor in mL/hour (McKinley T34 syringe driver model). Special attention should be paid to the rate if the machine has returned from servicing.
- Test the start button: this must be tested before administering the infusion. Press the start/test button and hold it down. Releasing the button starts the syringe driver. If the alarm does not sound, the system is not safe to use (O'Brien, 2012).
- Establish the final volume required in the syringe. It is considered good practice to make the solution as dilute as possible to reduce the likelihood of problems with drug compatibility and to minimise site irritation. Check with the drug compatibility tables and pharmacist if advice is needed (NHS Highland and NHS Greater Glasgow and Clyde, 2007).
- Select syringe size. Make sure that the syringe is a good quality and Luer Lock type (attached by twisting action) to avoid disconnection (O'Brien, 2012). The dimensions of syringes will vary depending on the manufacturer.
- Draw up the medication: make sure to check which diluent to use and drug compatibility.
- Write the medication on the label along with date, time and signature of nurse.
- Prime the line and extension set. This must be primed to the tip of the needle (O'Brien, 2012). This needs to be done manually and prior to needle/cannula insertion. Measure the volume prior to priming the set. This will ensure that correct concentration levels are administered as prescribed. If replenishing the driver, the infusion will finish early the following day. If the prescription is changed, the line needs to be reprimed (NHS Highland and NHS Greater Glasgow and Clyde, 2007).
- Re-explain procedure and check that the patient is in a comfortable position.
- Wash hands and put on gloves.
- Use skin cleansing agent to decontaminate the skin around insertion site (Gabriel, 2015) and allow 30 seconds to dry (see Box 20.3 for unsuitable infusion sites).
- Gently pull the protective sheath away from the stylet.
- Keep the skin taut over the insertions site and insert at a 45° angle.
- Insert the needle/cannula into subcutaneous fat to enhance absorption of medication.
- Remove stylet and dispose of immediately in a sharps container.
- Connect primed infusion set and start infusion.
- Cover cannula with a transparent surgical dressing.
- Ensure that the device is not placed too far above the level of the infusion site. This will increase the risk of a bolus delivery (O'Brien, 2012).
- Place the syringe driver into a locked box to avoid the pump being tampered with or damaged during infusion.
- Dispose of equipment as per organisational policy.
- Remove gloves and wash hands.
- Ensure that the patient is comfortable.
- Check the last service date of the syringe driver. Record the serial number of the syringe driver, record the syringe make and size. Document the flow rate in mL per hour, battery percentage, diluent name and batch number. Record the drug name and batch number, total volume in the syringe (mL) of drugs and diluent. Document the site used and appearance, syringe and signature of persons preparing and checking the syringe driver (NHS Highland and NHS Greater Glasgow and Clyde, 2007).
- The pump should be checked at each visit in the community and primary care settings and every 4 hours in hospital and hospice settings. Record the time and date of check.
- Check the infusion site for redness, swelling, discomfort/ pain, leakage of fluid.
- Report and record any findings. It may be necessary to resite the cannula if the infusion site has been compromised.

347

Box 20.3 Unsuitable infusion sites

· Skinfolds – the infusion site cannot be easily observed, and the device cannot be safely secured. There is also a potential risk of impaired absorption
· Limb oedema/lymphoedema – this is an infection risk and can impair absorption
· Previously irradiated skin – impaired blood supply could reduce absorption and increase infection risk and damage to dry/delicate skin
· Bony prominences – reduced subcutaneous tissue, impaired absorption, and device difficult to secure safely
· Near joints/areas of flexion – uncomfortable for the patient and a greater potential for the device to become dislodged
· Dry skin areas – increased potential for skin breakdown and risk of infection
· Infected/broken skin – increased risk of infection

Practice Assessment Document

In your PAD, you are required to observe and assess the need for intervention for patients, families and carers, identify, assess and respond to uncontrolled symptoms and manage and monitor effective relief medication, infusion pumps and other devices. You can ask to 'spoke out' to a placement where patients are frequently assessed and managed by nurses such as a hospice or community to develop your competence and confidence.

You could also ask your practice supervisor to simulate an end-of-life care scenario and speak with specialist nurses such as Macmillan and hospice staff.

Summary

· Palliative and end-of-life care are an essential part of nursing care. With more people choosing to die at home, it is important that nurses are competent in managing this process.
· End-of-life care should always be patient centred and include advance care planning when considering treatment.
· Syringe drivers are useful when the oral route of administration is not possible or absorption of medication is not optimal.
· It is important that discussions about medication management occur throughout the dying process and are tailored to meet individual needs.

Grief, Loss and Bereavement

The process of dying often involves a series of losses and emotional reactions to those losses. This often affects all those involved, from the individual themselves to family and friends and often the professional caregiver. This section discusses the nature of such loss and possible grief reactions and the theoretical and practical issues that often arise.

There has been a clear and dramatic change in the way that society reacts to death and bereavement in the UK over the past 100 years (Klass *et al.*, 1996). Living in a more secular society has reduced the importance of communal rituals and beliefs in favour of more individualistic ones.

Definitions

· *Loss* is the state of being deprived of, or being without, something one has had and the death of a loved one is perhaps the most traumatic loss of all (Murray Parkes, 2010).
· *Grief* is the multifaceted psychological response of pain and suffering experienced after loss (Walter & McCoyd, 2009).
· *Bereavement* is the process of losing a close relationship and mourning is the period during which signs of grief are made visible in the form of depression (Buglass, 2010).

Models of Loss and Grief

Numerous models have been developed that seek to help us understand the complexity of thoughts and emotions often experienced when we are bereaved. Elisabeth Kübler-Ross developed one of the most influential conceptual models of loss and grief, the five stages of grief model (Kübler-Ross, 1969). This model proposes that there are several stages that bereaved people and those facing loss through the diagnosis of a terminal illness experience and has influenced contemporary thinking and education around the subject for many years.

The five stages of grief model proposed that people experience progressive stages of:

1. Denial
2. Anger
3. Bargaining
4. Depression
5. Acceptance.

Other proponents of the stage or phase theory of grief include John Bowlby and his four stages of grief model (Bowlby, 1961) and Colin Murray Parkes' phases of grief theory (Murray Parkes, 2010).

Worden (1991) suggested that the bereaved need to complete certain tasks, namely to accept the reality of the loss, experience the pain of grief, adjust to an environment with the deceased missing, and to withdraw emotional energy and reinvest it into other relationships. This 'task' model described the importance of individuals 'working through' their grief to find a place of resolution and acceptance and the expression of grief was seen to be central to this.

There have been some attempts to question the validity of the models for grief. Grief is a very individual process and does not always follow a linear process, Stroebe and Schut's (1995) dual process model (Figure 20.2) builds on the stage theory of grief but adds a degree of dynamism to explain how a grieving individual may move back and forth between grief-oriented and restorative-oriented states. Some commentators contend that grief, like depression, has become a medical 'problem' to be diagnosed and treated rather than a natural human response to challenging life events (Illich, 1975; Parker, 2007). However, it is clear that sometimes the traumatic experience of losing a loved one or the realisation that one's own life may be coming to an end can cause serious clinical problems, such as anxiety and depression, and that a distinction should be made between normal and complicated grief reactions. This 'complex grief' can cause severe psychological reactions, can be associated with adverse health outcomes and should be treated medically (Hawton, 2007).

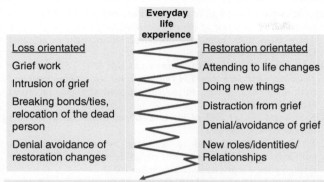

Figure 20.2 **Stroebe and Schut's dual process model.** *Source:* Modified from Stroebe & Schut (1999).

Jot This Down

Think of a time when you lost something (this does not have to be about bereavement – something as simple and everyday as losing your keys or purse will be fine).

· *How did it make you feel?* What emotions did it create? What physical feelings did it create?
· *What did it make you think?* What were the thoughts going around in your head?
· *What did it make you do?* How did the loss make you act? What behaviours did it encourage?

Think about these for a while and then imagine how someone faced with the loss of a loved one may feel about such a loss or the reality of such a loss in the near future.

Conclusion

This chapter has highlighted how the pattern and trajectory of death and dying have changed significantly over the past few generations. Some say that death has become medicalised, professionalised and institutionalised and therefore hidden from society; others have suggested that we are becoming reacquainted with death and dying, which is becoming less of a taboo subject.

The hospice and palliative care movement has done much to improve the care of people who are dying, providing a clear evidence base for many of its approaches, and the End-of-Life Care Strategy has highlighted how all individuals with progressive diseases can have access to the right kind of care at the end of life irrespective of what condition they have.

Nurses and other health and social care providers require a good knowledge base not just of the physical and symptom control needs of patients who are dying but also the psychosocial and spiritual healthcare needs as well as the underpinning issues related to loss, grief and bereavement. A clear understanding of the legal, ethical and professional issues that can arise when caring for dying patients and their families is also a prerequisite to effective care.

Through advance care planning and a systematic approach to co-ordinating care for patients at the end of life, more people can

have a peaceful dignified death in the place of their choosing. Sensitive honest communication at the end of life will ensure that more people will have not just their physical care needs addressed but also their emotional, psychological and spiritual needs.

Practising in this particular field of care can demand a degree of emotional commitment on the part of nurses and it is essential for them to understand the importance of ensuring their own psychological health through the development of appropriate support strategies.

Key Points

· The concept of a 'good death' may seem strange to many, but how and where people die is often very important to individuals and their families.
· Promoting comfort is the main aim of any management at the end of life and a holistic approach must be taken that acknowledges the inter-relationship between the emotional, psychological, spiritual and physical.
· It can often be difficult to truly hear what another is saying. Actively listening and helping the other person stay focused on their concerns can be difficult and it is all too easy to move the focus of the conversation to one which we assume is more relevant or that makes us feel more comfortable.
· The very nature of end-of-life care and the profound ethical questions it raises for health and social care practitioners demands an understanding of the underpinning ethical theories and the part they play in clinical decision making.
· As nurses, when patients are dying, our natural sense of accomplishment from helping someone to return to independence or to heal from an episode of injury or illness is missing.
· Numerous models have been developed that seek to help us understand the complexity of thoughts and emotions that are often experienced when we are bereaved.
· Nurses are repeatedly faced with loss and grief and caring for dying patients for a sustained period of time can provoke intense feelings of grief.

References

Beauchamp, T. & Childress, J. (2019) *Principles of Biomedical Ethics*, 8th edn. Oxford University Press, New York.

Bowlby, J. (1961) Processes of mourning. *International Journal of Psychoanalysis*, 42, 317–339.

Buglass. E (2010) Grief and bereavement theories. *Nursing Standard*, 24, 44–47.

Cohen-Mansfield, J., Skornick-Bouchbinder, M. & Brill, S. (2018) Trajectories of end of life: a systematic review. *Journal of Gerontology B: Psychological Sciences and Social Sciences*, 73(4), 564–572.

Department of Health (2008) *End of Life Care Strategy: Promoting High Quality Care for Adults at the End of their Life*. Department of Health, London.

Dougherty, L. & Lister, S. (2020) Patient comfort and end-of-life care. In: *Royal Marsden Hospital Manual of Clinical Nursing Procedures*, 9th edn. Wiley-Blackwell, Chichester.

Dying Matters (2020) *Frequently asked questions about the Dying Matters coalition*. www.dyingmatters.org/page/frequently-asked-questions (accessed December 2021).

Engel, G. (1977) The need for a new medical model: a challenge for biomedical science. *Science*, 196, 126–129.

Farrell, B. & Paice, J. (2019) *Oxford Textbook of Palliative Nursing*, 5th edn. Oxford University Press, Oxford.

Gabriel, J. (2015) Syringe drivers: their key safety features. *International Journal of Palliative Nursing*, 21(7), 328–330.

General Medical Council (2010) *Treatment and care towards the end of life: decision making*. www.gmc-uk.org/ethical-guidance/ethical-guidance-for-doctors/treatment-and-care-towards-the-end-of-life (accessed December 2021).

Gold Standards Framework (2021) *Proactive Identification Guidance*. https://goldstandardsframework.org.uk/pig (accessed December 2021).

Hawton, K. (2007) Complicated grief after bereavement. *British Medical Journal*, 334(7601), 962–963.

Healthcare Commission (2008) *Spotlight on Complaints. A Report on Second-stage Complaints about the NHS in England*. Healthcare Commission, London.

Illich, I. (1975) The medicalization of life. *Journal of Medical Ethics*, 1, 73–77.

Joint Formulary Committee (2020) *British National Formulary*. https://bnf.nice.org.uk (accessed December 2021).

Kennedy, C., Brooks-Young, P., Brunton Grey, C., *et al.* (2014) Diagnosing dying: an intergrative literature review. *British Medical Journal Supportive and Palliative Care*, 4, 263–270.

Klass, D., Silvermann, P.R. & Nickman, S. (eds) (1996) *Continuing Bonds. New Understandings in Grief*. Routledge, New York.

Kübler-Ross, E. (1969) *On Death and Dying*. Tavistock, London.

London End of life Clinical Network (2015) *What is a good death?* www.londonscn.nhs.uk/publication/what-is-a-good-death (accessed December 2021).

Macmillan (2019) *Advanced decision to refuse treatment*. www.macmillan.org.uk/cancer-information-and-support/treatment/if-you-have-an-advanced-cancer/advance-care-planning/advance-decision-to-refuse-treatment (accessed December 2021).

Marie Curie (2018) *What are palliative care and end of life care?* www.mariecurie.org.uk/help/support/diagnosed/recent-diagnosis/palliative-care- end-of-life-care (accessed December 2021).

Marie Curie (2020a) *Planning your care in advance*. www.mariecurie.org.uk/help/support/terminal-illness/planning-ahead/advance-care-planning (accessed December 2021).

Marie Curie (2020b) Signs that your loved one might be dying. www.mariecurie.org.uk/help/support/being-there/end-of-life-preparation/signs-of-dying (accessed December 2021).

Mental Capacity Act (2005) *Code of Practice (2007)*. TSO, London.

Mitchell, A. & Elbourne, S. (2020) *Advance Care Planning and Syringe Drivers*. British Journal of Nursing. (29)17, pp. 1010–1015.

Murray Parkes, C. (2010) *Bereavement: Studies of Grief in Adult Life*, 4th edn. Penguin, London.

National Council for Palliative Care (2010) *Changing Gear: Guidelines for Managing the Last Days of Life in Adults*. NCPC, London.

National End of Life Care Programme (2010) *Holistic Common Assessment of Supportive and Palliative Care Needs for Adults Requiring End of Life Care*. http://webarchive.nationalarchives.gov.uk/20130718122921/http://www.endoflifecare.nhs.uk/care-pathway/step-2-assessment,-care-planning-and-review/holistic-common-assessment.aspx (accessed December 2021).

National Institute for Health and Care Excellence (2015) *Care of dying adults in the last days of life*. NG13. National Institute for Health and Care Excellence, London.

National Institute for Health and Care Excellence (2016) *Multimorbidity: clinical assessment and management*. NG46. www. nice.org.uk/guidance/ng56 (accessed December 2021).

National Institute for Health and Care Excellence (2019) *End of life care for adults: service delivery*. NG142. www.nice.org.uk/guidance/ng142/chapter/Recommendations (accessed December 2021).

National Palliative and End of Life Care Partnership (2015) *Ambitions for palliative and end of life care: a national framework for local action 2015-2020*. http://endoflifecareambitions.org.uk/ (accessed December 2021).

NHS Highland, NHS Greater Glasgow and Clyde (2007) *Syringe pump guidelines CME McKinley T34 (ml/hour): For use within Argyll and Bute CHP and Clyde*. https://tinyurl.com/y6bptgxh (accessed December 2021).

NHS Scotland (2014) *End of life care*. https://tinyurl.com/y4w7u8rs (accessed December 2021).

NHS Scotland (2020) *End of life care: syringe pumps*. www.palliativecareguidelines.scot.nhs.uk/guidelines/end-of-life-care/syringe-pumps.aspx (accessed December 2021).

Nursing & Midwifery Council (2018) *The code: professional standards of practice and behaviour for nurses, midwives and nursing associates*. https://tinyurl.com/zy7syuo (accessed December 2021).

O'Brien, L. (ed.) (2012) Syringe driver/pump management and symptom control in palliative care. In: *District Nursing Manual of Clinical Procedures*. John Wiley & Sons, Chichester.

Office for National Statistics (2020) *Leading causes of death, UK: 2001-2018. Registered leading causes of death by age, sex and country*. https://tinyurl.com/yxc5unu4 (accessed December 2021).

O'Gorman, S.M. (1998) Death and dying in contemporary society: an evaluation of current attitudes and the rituals associated with death and dying and their relevance to recent understandings of health and healing. *Journal of Advanced Nursing*, 27, 1127–1135.

Parker, G. (2007) Is depression overdiagnosed? Yes. *British Medical Journal*, 335(7615), 328–329.

Public Health England (2016) *Recent trends in place of death in England*. Health and Social Care Information Centre, London.

Raijmakers, N., van Zuylen, L., Costantini, M., *et al.* (2011) Artificial nutrition and hydration in the last week of life in cancer patients. A systematic literature review of practices and effects. *Annals of Oncology*, 22, 1478–1486.

Resuscitation Council UK (2019) *Resuscitation Council UK introduces version 3 of ReSPECT form*. www.resus.org.uk/about-us/news-and-events/resuscitation-council-uk-introduces-version-3-respect-form (accessed December 2021).

Rogers, C. (1951) *Client-Centered Therapy*. Riverside Press, Cambridge, MA.

Shucksmith, J., Carlebach, S., Whittaker, V., for NatCen Social Research (2013) *Dying: Discussing and planning for end of life*. www.bsa.natcen.ac.uk/media/38850/bsa_30_dying.pdf (accessed December 2021).

Social Care Institute for Excellence (2016) *MCA Lead Toolkit*. www.scie.org.uk/mca/directory/pan-london-commissioner-toolkit (accessed December 2021).

Stroebe, M. & Schut, H. (1995) *The dual process model of coping with loss*. Paper presented at the International Workshop on Death, Dying and Bereavement, Oxford.

Thomas, K., Armstrong-Wilson, F. & Tanner, T. (2016) Evidence that use of GSF helps improve advance care planning discussions. www.goldstandardsframework.org.uk/cd-content/uploads/files/2%20%20%203%20Evidence%20that%20use%20of%20GSF%20Improves%20ACP%20n%20different%20settings%20vs%203%20(002)%20JAW%20(002)%20(1).pdf (accessed December 2021).

Thomas, T. & Barclay, S. (2015) Continuous subcutaneous infusion in palliative care: a review of current practice. *International Journal of Palliative Nursing*, 21(2), 60–64.

Walter, C.A. & McCoyd, J.L.M. (2009) *Grief and Loss Across the Lifespan: A Biopsychosocial Perspective*. Springer, New York.

Walters, T. (1994) *The Revival of Death*. Routledge, Abingdon.

Worden, J.W. (1991) *Grief Counselling and Grief Therapy*, 2nd edn. Routledge, London.

World Health Organization (2015) *WHO definition of palliative care*. Factsheet No. 402. WHO, Geneva.

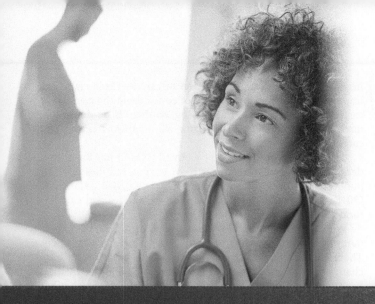

21

The Principles of Supporting Families and Carers in Practice

Mary E. Braine

University of Salford, UK

Learning Outcomes

On completion of this chapter you will be able to:

- Provide an introduction to the context of supporting families and carers in the practice setting
- Understand the knowledge, skills, attitudes and behaviours necessary to form appropriate professional relationships with families and other carers
- Identify and discuss the issues relating to appropriate involvement of families and other carers in the assessment, planning, delivery and evaluation of care
- Analyse the impact of caring on family and other carers across care settings
- Explore the relationship between formal/professional caregiving and informal caregiving by families and other caregivers

Proficiencies

NMC Proficiencies and Standards:

- Evidence-based, best practice approaches to communication for supporting people of all ages, their families and carers in preventing ill health and in managing their care.
- Understand the principles and processes involved in supporting people and families with a range of care needs to maintain optimal independence and avoid unnecessary interventions and disruptions to their lives

Visit the companion website at **www.wiley.com/go/peate/nursingpractice3e** where you can test yourself using flashcards, multiple-choice questions and more.

Nursing Practice: Knowledge and Care, Third Edition. Edited by Ian Peate and Aby Mitchell.
© 2022 John Wiley & Sons Ltd. Published 2022 by John Wiley & Sons Ltd.
Companion website: www.wiley.com/go/peate/nursingpractice3e

Introduction

Nurses are crucial to ensuring that carers and families are fully included in nursing care across all fields of practice. It is fundamental to nursing that opportunities to be collaborative and inclusive with carers and families take place and genuinely happen.

Opportunities are plentiful for nurses to identify and engage with families and carers in practice. We all have a responsibility to take a moment to think about the potential and real long-term gains from good assessments and discharge planning, compliance with care and treatments, with rather than on or for caregivers and patients (Braine & Wray, 2016). By practising in this context, it is likely that you will be promoting *salutogenesis*, which focuses on factors that support human health and wellbeing, an important goal for all nurses.

Carers

Context of Carers

The generic term 'carer', now well accepted throughout the UK, means family, relatives and friends who take on an informal unpaid caring role of a loved one or someone they take responsibility to care for. Specifically, an 'informal' carer is someone of any age or ethnicity, including children, young people and adults, without whose help the family member, partner or friend would be unable to manage alone (Box 21.1). However, carers are not a homogeneous group and each circumstance is unique. The common attribute is that they all care for someone who needs help and assistance and that becoming a carer can occur to anyone at any time whatever their status.

Typically, people do not expect or plan to be carers – 'it just happens' – and can happen suddenly or gradually. Through the collection of data from the UK census (Office for National Statistics 2001, 2011; White 2013), we now have a better understanding of the prevalence, impact and experiences of carers, although the census data offer only best estimates; however, what is evident is that these figures are huge and rising.

Caring can become a way of life but being aware of the carer's existence and respecting them is important, as their 'job' (role) can be a long, lonely and hard one with limited support (Braine & Wray, 2016). Within the UK from April 2015, the Care Act 2014 and the Children and Families Act 2014 sought to

improve the rights and recognition of carers. These rights are important for nurses to be aware of considering the number of carers is around 6 million and rising, so there is no doubt that nurses will be meeting and engaging with family caregivers and carers frequently in practice.

The Nursing and Midwifery Council (NMC) has for several decades made explicit reference to carers and families in all its publications for guiding nursing practice. NMC standards (2018a, 2018b) are clear that inclusion of families and carers is fundamental to nursing practice.

With advanced technology in modern medicine, life expectancy has improved dramatically for many people in our society. Therefore, diversity in caregiving and patterns of carers have changed with these advances in modern medicine and medical health research so that now there is an emergence of what has been termed a 'new survivors' generation. In addition to this medical progress and new survivor generation, we are also seeing what has been termed 'career carers' (Aneshensel *et al.*, 1995); in other words, relating caring to a career, with carers experiencing transitions, key events and role changes over time as in any career. Montgomery & Kosloski (2000) suggest that 'caring is like a career with a beginning, discernible temporal direction and end'. Of note, in England alone 10 million people have two or more long-term conditions (NHS, 2021). Given this context, it is imperative to understand the contextual factors regarding the type of caregiving and the temporal nature of caring, regardless of whether it is in the short or long term.

Jot This Down

Take some time to think whether you have met informal carers.

- Have you included them in the care you have been giving?
- If not, why not?
- If you did, what did you learn?
- Perhaps you could write a reflective account of your experiences with families and carers (this could be useful for your NMC revalidation in the future).

Types of Carers

Regardless of carer type, a significant number of carers do not consciously recognise themselves as carers. Instead, they see themselves as a husband, wife, daughter, son, relative or friend and are often described as 'hidden carers'. The term 'carer' is not their word and, if questioned, many would not proclaim to be a carer. Society's attitudes towards family responsibilities and the availability of services to support both carers and people with health limitations vary widely across countries, thus influencing the pattern and declaration of informal caring. Perhaps this perspective contributes to the notion of 'hidden patients' (Fengler & Goodrich, 1979) or 'secondary patients' as the caregivers' psychological, physical and emotional stresses often go unnoticed due to the primary focus being on the needs of the person cared for.

Becoming a carer can happen at any time in a person's life; however, different terms are useful in understanding the

---

Box 21.1 Defining Carers

There are varying definitions of carers within the literature depending on the care activities and the identity of the care recipient, but what they all agree on is that a carer is unpaid and, in most cases, untrained. The definition most often adopted is:

Anyone who cares, unpaid, for a friend or family member who due to illness, disability, a mental health problem, or an addiction cannot cope without their support

(Carers Trust, 2021).

Table 21.1 Examples of other terms used for different types of carers as seen in the literature. *Source*: Adapted from Braine & Wray (2016).

TERM	MEANING
Career carer	Likening caring to a career, with carers experiencing transitions, key events and role changes over time, as in a more formal career
Compound carer	Compound caregivers are those parents who are already providing considerable caregiving responsibilities to their child with intellectual disabilities, who subsequently becomes a caregiver for an additional family member (Perkins & Haley, 2010)
Distance carer	People who provide any kind of meaningful support to a relative but do so from a distance (Carers UK, 2011)
Expert carer	Carers who are established, in that they have been caring for a family member or significant other for some time
Grandparent carers	An emerging group of carers: grandparents raising their grandchildren
Primary carer	Primary carer is the family member deemed to bear the most responsibility in caring for the patient (mainly mothers and wives) (Perlesz et al., 2000)
Sandwich carer	Providing simultaneous care to their young or adolescent children and at the same time to an older family member or friend
Secondary carer	Secondary carers are those who are next in line to take on most responsibility (mostly fathers and eldest siblings) (Perlesz et al., 2000)
Tertiary carer	Tertiary carers follow on from secondary carers in being the next most responsible (mainly siblings) (Perlesz et al., 2000)

different types of carers (Table 21.1). This table does not provide an exhaustive list but can alert nurses to the carers they will meet in different practice settings.

Number of Carers

Changes in population, longer life expectancy, increases in the numbers of people living with long-term conditions, family structures and employment are likely to increase the future numbers of carers and the patterns of care that they provide. For example, the increasing ageing population (World Health Organization, 2020), together with the phenomenon of older parents of young children, has seen an increase in the number of sandwich-generation carers. Consequently, it is even more critical that nurses recognise and work alongside carers as key partners in the provision of care. Evidence to support the numbers of

Table 21.2 Estimated numbers of carers in the UK.

SOURCE AND DATE	NUMBER OF CARERS	DEFINITION OF CARER USED IN THE DATA
Family Resources Survey: financial year 2019 to 2020 (Department for Work and Pensions, 2021b)	4.5 million 33% of all adult carers were still in full-time employment	A person who gives help on an informal basis (that is, where caring is not a paid job). Examples of care may include helping with shopping, preparing meals and feeding, and household chores
Census 2011	6.5 million	A person who provides unpaid help or support to someone due to long-term physical or mental ill health or disability, or problems related to old age

informal carers in the UK is variable according to the data sources, partly because not all carers will identify themselves as carers, and thus these figures are likely to be an underestimation (Table 21.2).

The 2011 census indicates that around 1 in 10 in England and Wales is an unpaid carer, supporting a friend or family member (White, 2013). Caregiving tends to decrease at older ages, due to health limitations. On average, unpaid carers are more likely to care for a close relative, such as their parents or spouse. Regarding gender, there are some differences across all age groups in both England and Wales: women account for 58% of unpaid carers and men 42%. Again, the 2011 census data (White, 2013) highlights that unpaid care provision by gender is as follows.

- Unpaid care is highest for both men and women in the 50–64 age range.
- Women provide a higher share across ages 0–64, but men aged 50–64 do provide a higher percentage of unpaid care than women aged 25–49.

Until the release of the 2021 census, data from other sources indicate the continued upward trend in the number of carers in the UK. Figures from Carers UK (2020a) reveal 17% of adults are providing unpaid care i.e. 1 in 6, with an additional 9% of adults providing unpaid care since the COVID-19 pandemic. Thus, overall 26% of adults provide care: this is 1:4 adults and up to 13.6 million people providing unpaid care in the UK.

Traditionally, women can be socialised into the 'ethic of care' – our moral responsiveness to the nature of caring, social justice and empathy – and consequently the caring role has

353

tended to be adopted routinely by women. This trend is changing, with more men undertaking caregiving in the UK (White, 2013) and increases in male caregivers have been noted in other countries. As nurses, we need to be aware that more men are likely to take on caregiving roles in the future. Although men may approach caring differently and engage in different tasks from those of women – typically, indirect tasks – the responsibilities can impact similarly on men and women. Regardless, such a variable and often unpredictable workload can evolve into a balancing act between caregiving and other activities such as work, family and leisure activities. Whether this is as a family unit, with several family members working together, or caring alone, the demands can be physically, socially and psychologically huge.

It is estimated that over one-third of carers provide 20 hours or more of care a week and nearly 48% of carers provide care for 35 hours per week, whereas the number of people caring for 50 hours or more a week has increased by 25% (Carers UK, 2015). Notably, in the report *Valuing Carers 2015*, which looked at carers' support of the UK economy, it was found that unpaid carers save the UK £132 billion a year; in other words, the cost of a second NHS. Carers providing at least 35 hours of care may be entitled to the main carer's benefit, the Carer's Allowance, although only 1.3 million carers claimed payment in 2020 (Department for Work and Pensions, 2021a).

Caregiving is associated with a reduction in employment and working hours; as the demands of caring increase, participation in paid employment suffers. In some cases, the carer may change to lower-paid jobs or occupations that may provide a better balance between work and family obligations. Coupled with this is a higher risk of poverty and higher prevalence of mental health problems than among non-carers (Colombo *et al.*, 2011).

Nursing Fields Children and Young People

The Carers Trust (https://carers.org) definition of a 'young carer' includes someone under 18 years old who helps look after someone in their family, or a friend who is ill, disabled, has a mental health condition or misuses drugs or alcohol. It also defined a 'young adult carer', as young people aged 16–25 who care, unpaid, for a family member or friend.

There are at least 800 000 young adult carers in the UK (Children's Society, 2021). The 2011 census identifies 166 363 young carers aged under 18 years old in England.

Helping to care for a family member is something that many young people are happy and proud to do. It can help them develop a sense of responsibility and skills they will use later in life. However, young carers are more likely to need long-term interventions and specialist support to enable them to have the same life opportunities as their non-carer peers. Young carers are more prone to being hidden or ignored within UK society and caring for adults with mental health issues.

There may be more than one young carer in the family and the caring role may include not just caring for a family member with an illness or disability, but also taking siblings to school, looking after their needs and practical tasks in the home. Often, the care that these young people are providing can be age inappropriate and can have a significant negative impact on their

lives. A lack of engagement with positive activities outside the home, including school attendance, and ensuring children are safe is important in seeking to both identify young carers and ensuring that they have appropriate support. Carers charities all agree that:

- We need to identify young carers early
- Support needs to identify causes of inappropriate caring roles
- All forms of support have to be presented sensitively and appropriately for children and young people
- The support provided for the family's needs to be personalised, integrated and holistic.

Jot This Down

Watch this film: *We're Not Different, We Just Do Different Things* (2012)
www.youtube.com/watch?v=aHO8iRSuxyc
Make a note of what you consider to be the issues raised in this film.
- How might this family be helped?
- Who could have helped them?
- Do you think stigma was an issue for the children?
- How might this be managed?

Identifying Carers

Several policy initiatives (Department of Health, 1999, 2010) and nursing organisations such as the Royal College of Nursing (RCN) and the Queen's Nursing Institute (QNI) have made concerted efforts to raise awareness of carers and facilitate early identification of them. Alongside the Carers' Strategy published in 2008 (Department of Health, 2008) and updated in 2010, priority was given to supporting early recognition and self-identification so that carers are fully supported as expert care partners. Further support is offered by the UK Carers Act 2014 and the Children and Families Act 2014, which entitles carers and the people they care for to a clear assessment of their needs irrespective of their finances or level of need (Box 21.2). The nature of caring may mean that, for some, being a carer is an unexpected or unplanned event, while for others it may feel like a 'natural course' (Given & Given, 1991).

Aneshensel *et al.*'s (1995) conceptualisation of the 'carer career' to describe the various phases of caregiving can provide

Box 21.2 Carer's Assessment

A carer's assessment is for carers over 18 years old who are looking after another adult over 18 years who is disabled, ill or elderly. It is an opportunity to record the impact caring has on their lives and what support or services they may need and whether they are able or willing to carry on caring (Carers UK, 2020b).

For young carers under 18 years, their rights for an assessment fall under the Children Act (2004) and Children and Families Act (2014).

Under the Carers (Scotland) Act 2016, young carers in Scotland have the right to a Young Carer Statement which specifies that certain things must included in support planning for carers.

insights into the type of help and support that might be needed, and when. The three broad phases are:

- Preparation for, and acquisition of, the caregiving role
- Enactment of caregiving
- Disengagement from caregiving.

Regardless of context, by identifying carers nurses can provide a fundamental opportunity to signpost them to information about their rights and circumstances.

Red Flag

Think Carer for every contact with a patient or relative.
- Ask the question: 'Do you look after someone?'.
- If so, ask: 'Who will be looking after them?', 'Do they live with you or close by?', 'Have you been offered an assessment of your needs?'.

You may well need to ask the same question more than once (NMC, 2018a).

Often the notion of being a carer has connotations of 'low status' and stigma in society and even within families. Such perceptions may be attributed to the nature of the caring role and the tasks that carers undertake (Box 21.3). Because of the perceived low status of caring, in particular direct physical tasks, carers may avoid identifying themselves or be reluctant to accept the word 'carer'. Losing control over their lives and dealing with increasing levels of dependency and uncertainty can add to notions of low status and sigma perceptions (Braine & Wray, 2016). Understanding these perceptions and respecting carers' dynamic roles are fundamental for all practitioners and staff within the healthcare system.

Think Carer

- Carers have a key part to play in supporting the care provided by health and social care services.
- Carers can help nurses to understand the needs of the people that they are caring for.
- Carers can be an invaluable source of information and knowledge about their loved one, for example, medical history, preferences and well-being.

Box 21.3 Direct and Indirect Caring Experiences

Direct care: physical or practical tasks
- Support in activities of daily living (ADL), for example, washing and dressing, feeding, toileting and managing incontinence, preparing meals, ensuring that medications are taken on time
- Household activities, for example, housework, preparing meals and shopping, help with household maintenance such as repairs, gardening

Indirect care: psychosocial or emotional tasks
- Managing financial issues, for example paying bills, online shopping
- Emotional support, i.e. keeping company and sharing mutually enjoyable activities
- Monitoring care, which includes ensuring that the care recipient's needs are being met and that services provided are of an appropriate standard

---

- Involving carers can improve the patient's experience.
- Enhanced feelings of safety by the patient when the carer is present.
- Can reduce the assumptions about carers (who is doing what, when and how).
- Help to identify health needs of the carers themselves.
- Can reduce hospital admissions and readmissions rates.

Families

Definition

Historically, a family was defined as 'married partners and children residing in a household'. However, in contemporary society, this definition does not encompass the current nature of families, such as single parents, individuals unmarried but co-habiting, blended families, or gay and lesbian couples. Murray & Barnes (2012, p.533) present a more representative perspective, stating that 'a family is a specific blend of social relations that have been constructed and reconstructed in many different forms throughout history'. From a nursing perspective, Hanson (2005, p.5) refers to the family as 'two or more individuals who depend on one another for emotional, physical and economical support'.

Families come in many different sizes depending on the number of children, stepchildren, parents and other people not unrelated by birth or marriage who may be living in the family, for example foster children. Families also change over time. In general, families are getting smaller, with increasing geographical distances between family members, and increased divorce rates and falling marriage rates have raised the number of single-person households across Europe. This trend in smaller families may result in carers providing a larger proportion of care needs. Blended families, which include children from two or more previous relationships, are becoming increasingly common, but even this term is changing. Traditionally, parents of a blended family would be married but more and more parents of blended families are not married. Thus, when considering family members, it is important to consider the nature and diversity of families.

Each family is also highly influenced by their cultural background – their values, opinions, attitudes and behaviours. Culture is influenced by several factors, such as language, age, gender, education, race, ethnicity, geography, religion/spirituality and experiences. In essence, the cultural influences within the family are both dynamic and continually changing and are also personally and contextually determined.

Family Systems

Despite the varying definitions, nurses need to be aware that each family is unique and characterised by the dynamic interactions, relationships and experiences of the individual members. For example, a family with several children is different from a single-parent family. To understand how and why these complex interactions shape families, along with individual family members' behaviours and actions, an understanding of the family systems framework is necessary.

Viewing family as a system has become a commonly held perspective among psychiatrists, family sociologists, family

355

therapists and researchers and offers an insight into how families function. Systems thinking is based on the simple idea that what makes a system is the relationships between its parts and not the parts themselves and seeks to explain the behaviours of complex organised systems, from micro-organisms to families.

By considering the family as a system, the inter-relationships among family members, rather than the individual family member, are central to our understanding of the uniqueness of each family. In other words, whatever happens to one of the family members happens to all of them. The systems theory helps to explain family functioning, family communication and interactions such as conflict, cohesion, integration and adaptation to change. Thus, the family strives to achieve a balance in relationships and function or homeostasis (Steinglass, 1987).

What the Experts Say

'' Virginia Satir, a highly influential family therapist, used the metaphor of a hanging mobile to describe the family system perspective. She explains that:
'In the mobile all the pieces, [family members] no matter what size or shape, can be grouped together and balanced by shortening or lengthening the strings attached or rearranging the distance between the pieces. So it is with a family. None of the family members are identical to any other; they are all different and at different levels of growth. As in a mobile, you can't arrange one without thinking of the other . . .'

Source: Satir (1972, pp.119–120)

Thus, as in the mobile, all the pieces are connected, but each shape (family member) is different. Considering the situation when a family member becomes acutely ill and is hospitalised, we then need to consider all the other family members, i.e. how the family (mobile) functions together to maintain a balance.

Family systems theory views a family as having two dimensions.

1. *Structure*: who makes up the family, i.e. family members and the way the family organises itself through its own unique rules.
2. *Tasks*: the responsibilities of the family members.

Another important component in family systems theory is that boundaries exist between family members and that boundaries result from the interaction of family members with each other and the interaction of the family with outside influences. For example, some families may be more open to healthcare support and advice than others.

Think Family

Understanding how family members interact with each other is vital if nurses are to provide support that targets the family carer, most importantly the relationship between family members, for example, the carer and the person they are caring for and the relationship between the family and the healthcare provider. Regardless of frameworks and models regarding families, we need to remind ourselves that to care and understand the patient, we need to also understand their family, their values and goals. Respecting these factors will result in better healthcare, safety and patient satisfaction.

Building on family systems theory, family nursing science is based on the idea that illness of an individual equally influences the health and well-being of their family. The family-centred approach to nursing, a distinct theoretical framework conceptualised by Wright & Leahey (1990), focuses on the whole family as the unit of care. In this context, nurses are not just caring for the patient but the family as a patient. This requires nurses to shift their way of thinking from focusing only on the patient to including the family, recognising the relationship between the family carer and their loved one. Of critical importance is the relationship that the nurse establishes with each unique family.

Jot This Down Think Family

Think about a patient you have cared for.
- Did you consider who in the patient's family was involved in their care?
- Was the family involved in the care and decision making?
- Were they given the opportunity to tell their story?
- Were their concerns listened to?
- Were their expectations and needs assessed and addressed?

Challenging Families and Carers

Sometimes one family can be more difficult to work with than others. When a patient is admitted to hospital, it is not uncommon that some family members find it difficult to deal with the patient's illness and the associated uncertainty. Equally, caring for families and patients during difficult times, for example, end-of-life care or discussion of treatment options that are risky or uncertain, can result in unsettled emotions. The unpreparedness of family carers to deal with the situation adds to their worries, tensions, frustrations and anxieties, which may, in turn, result in hostile, overbearing or demanding behaviours that can lead to family members being pigeon-holed as 'difficult' or 'challenging'. When care intensity is moderated or lessened, carers or families may feel increasingly anxious about such changes in care provision, for example moving care from a ward environment to a nursing home (Box 21.4).

The nurse needs to verify the family's feelings, let them know you are listening to them, and that you understand their concerns. Sensitively establishing what their understanding of the situation is, what they have been told and what their expectations are may help. In addition, provide families with objective information and encourage them to talk about their differences. However, the overarching premise is that we need to set acceptable boundaries with families so we can provide a quiet, healing environment for the patient. For some family members, visiting is too difficult and can result in them abstaining from visiting or disengaging. We need to be mindful of these variations and not judge that person in terms of notions of caring. Understanding how the family functions provides the tools to interact with 'difficult' families professionally for the best interests of our patients.

After a loved one moves into a nursing home, families often suffer from overwhelming guilt and a sense of loss. The family caregivers often feel that they have failed or let their loved one down by not being able to care for them in their own home. Other family members and friends may even be critical of their decision, adding to their feelings of guilt. Information that

Box 21.4 Family Case Study

Mrs Gupta is a pleasant and co-operative 75-year-old widow who has suffered a stroke and recently been transferred from hospital to a nursing home for her ongoing care needs. Her extensive family seem angry at the nursing home. They are frequently rude and inappropriate, using up large amounts of nursing staff time with numerous telephone calls, requests, demands and complaints. Mrs Gupta appears to be embarrassed by the members of her family and frequently apologises for their behaviour. Understanding the family situation and not making assumptions may help to allay the family's fears and anxieties. The cause of these behaviours may be attributed to:

· Unrealistic expectations and perceptions about the care in the home
· Concerns about a 'stranger' caring for their loved one
· Underlying disputes/issues within the family may have been compounded by the situation
· The family may have past histories of things going wrong on previous hospital visits
· Misunderstandings or interpretations of information provided to them
· Genuine fear of nursing homes, hospitals and healthcare professionals
· Feelings of guilt
· Access to visit their loved ones may be restricted.

By providing opportunities to empathically listen and acknowledge the family's concerns, the nurse can start to build a trusting relationship with the family. By encouraging the family to ask questions, they may feel more valued and respected. Answering questions and explaining procedures can help to alleviate some of their fears and anxieties.

highlights the necessity and appropriateness of the need to reside in a nursing home may help to alleviate their anguish and concerns. By discussing with the family that continuity of communication can help, say for example by appointing a primary carer by name or a designated spokesperson for all the family, ensures that information given is consistent, and reduces the risks of misinformation and misunderstandings.

Some family caregivers may feel it necessary to be present and participate in care as a way of trusting staff and ensuring quality care for their family member. This may occur when a patient who has been cared for by a family member at home is readmitted to hospital, and the responsibility for care shifts back to the hospital; equally, when a family member is transferred to a care home from the home environment. In these circumstances, carers try to balance their shifting role as they hand over control and power to the healthcare professionals with the desire for involvement in the decision making. However, their expertise and knowledge about the patient may not always be recognised or acknowledged and thus can be a source of anger, uncertainty, frustration and exclusion.

What the Experts Say

 Researchers have found that giving families opportunities to engage in meaningful caregiving in unfamiliar institutional settings can provide a sense of hope and positive reward and foster feelings of

being part of the nursing home community, along with helping to come to terms with the change in relationship with their relative (Kellett, 2007).

Research by Agard *et al.* (2015) found that when patients are readmitted to hospital and the care responsibility shifts back to the hospital, caregivers tend to 'watch over' the care. This process requires sensitivity and negotiation that respects this handing back of care to professionals and being aware that the notion of carers 'watching over' is partly a coping mechanism.

Opportunities for Family and Carer Involvement

The following sections provide information that aligns to everyday practices that nurses will be involved in as leaders or key participants. These topics have been chosen as examples of typical opportunities for engaging with families and carers. In all cases, an underpinning principle offered by Dalton (2003), called a 'triad' relationship between client, caregiver and nurse, is useful. Dalton's (2003) theory promotes decision making in nursing practice triads, through increased interactions and collaboration with caregivers, whereby goals can be mutually agreed between patients, family caregivers and professionals. This triad partnership can influence feelings of control, well-being, confidence and compliance with treatments.

In 2010 the Princess Royal Trust for Carers (now known as the Carers Trust) and the National Mental Health Development Unit launched a collaborative model (triad) termed the Triangle of Care. The core principle of the triangle (Figure 21.1) is that 'carers, people who use services and professionals should work in equal partnership to promote safety, support recovery and sustain well-being' (Carers Trust, 2020, p.5). This triangle has also been adapted to meet the needs of carers of people with dementia (Carers Trust, 2016). Seizing opportunities to work collaboratively with carers and families to improve the care of patients rather than fragmenting care or being partial in care provision is vital across all care settings.

357

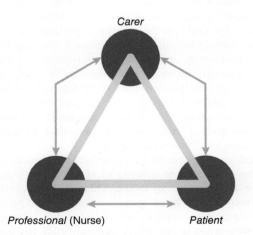

Figure 21.1 **Triangle of Care.** *Source:* Adapted from Carers Trust (2013).

The support and reassurance carers and families can offer during clinical procedures should not be underestimated or discounted. Traditional practices of totally excluding a family carer can prevail in some care settings and, we would argue, need to be questioned and thought through for their value and relevance. As nurses, we have a responsibility to consider this dimension in our care of all patients and their families and carers. Their knowledge base and skills in supporting their loved ones can enhance the care offered by nurses and other healthcare practitioners. For example, in children's services, parents have become successful partners in providing care or involving the family in calming the child/patient. While age is not the main factor for involving carers in care, such involvement does need to be negotiated and considered in all care settings. The benefits of the calming influence of the family/friend or carer during clinical encounters, even during an invasive procedure, should be considered.

Practice Assessment Document

Receiving feedback in each placement from someone whom you have directly cared for and or their carers can help with your learning. By reflecting on this feedback and discussing the outcomes with your assessor, any change in practice can be actioned.

Protected Mealtimes

The Protected Mealtimes Initiative (PMI) was introduced in 2006 as a UK policy directive for patients in hospital (National Patient Safety Agency, 2007). It has also been implemented in other countries around the world. In brief, the PMI was designed to enhance the quality of the mealtime experience and maximise nutritional intake for patients in hospitals. A core element was to reduce unnecessary and needless interruptions, providing an improved mealtime environment conducive to eating, and helping staff to provide patients/clients with support and assistance with meals. However, this initiative has had varied effects with only minor improvements in nutritional intake (Hickson *et al.*, 2011) and research indicates insufficient data for widespread implementation (Porter *et al.*, 2017).

Practice settings can be busy and there are pressures in finding time to encourage patients to eat well and consistently improve their nutritional intake. There is no doubt that the involvement of a family caregiver in helping to feed patients and improving mealtime experiences can be beneficial. The nature of such involvement at mealtimes connects with family-centred care and can provide opportunities for interactions and

discussions. Indeed, it can be during mealtimes that revelations may arise about a caregiver's knowledge of food/nutrients (or lack of) and, as such, learning and educational opportunities could unfold in partnership with carers and families. Clearly, there is potential for family carers to play a vital role during mealtimes but careful consideration of the logistics needs to be thought through.

Jot This Down

- In what contexts might carers or families be excluded from the PMI?
- Have you encountered inclusion of carers and families at mealtimes?
- What are the benefits?
  At mealtimes *Think Carer, Think Family*.

Visiting

Visiting arrangements in hospitals, homes and community facilities have stimulated much debate for many decades irrespective of nursing field. Overwhelmingly, research has shown that isolating patients at the most vulnerable times from the people who know them best places them at risk for medical error, emotional harm, inconsistencies in care and costly unnecessary care. Furthermore, requesting visiting outside visiting hours can result in friction and anxiety for both carers and patients.

In some care settings, particularly dementia care, there is recognition that a flexible approach to visiting practices is needed. The 'Carer Passport' scheme aims to improve and embed identification, recognition and support for carers in the day-to-day life of an organisation or community (Carer Passport, 2021). The *NHS Long-Term Plan* (2019) sets out an ambition for 'national adoption of carer's passports'. The passport acts like an access card/badge that allows a named carer to identify themselves to staff and leads to the provision of support, services and other benefits. Other schemes that identify carers also exist, for example John's Campaign for those caring for someone with dementia and the Butterfly scheme.

The meanings and constructions that people attach to visiting hospitals can inform both their behaviours and actions. Place of care matters and care environments, by their nature of being an institution, have 'rules' and this impacts on those working and residing in a shared space, for example hospital wards (Braine & Wray, 2016). Clarifying our values about the contribution and involvement of patients' families or relatives can go some way to informing visiting practices. Inflexibility can lead to potential communication breakdown and unnecessary negative behaviours and attitudes. Pragmatic visiting practices can have their place in some care settings, such as critical care or high-risk areas that aim to preserve cleanliness and limit risks of hospital-acquired infections (e.g. COVID-19 and MRSA), or times in the day to ensure rest and quiet times for enhancing recovery and recuperation. Visiting arrangements in hospitals need to be geared towards meaning and purpose for both the patient and their family.

You are likely to experience different visiting arrangements across all fields of practice and often throughout the same hospital. Opportunities exist for carer and family involvement in caregiving activities to enhance their skills, competencies and roles in preparation for transfer of care to the home. Reflecting on the purpose and benefits of visiting arrangements and the role of the nurse during visiting are important considerations in enhancing a holistic recovery.

Jot This Down
- What do you routinely do during visiting times?
- Do you talk to visitors? If not, why not?
- How would you know if someone had limited family support?

Patient Hotels

'Patient hotels' originated in Scandinavia and have seen huge benefits in terms of patient and family experience, reduced hospital admissions and readmissions. In the UK, this concept is growing, and several NHS trusts and health charities have opened patient hotels, offering accommodation for patients and their relatives, and children and young people and their families. Within the patient hotel, the family, as primary carers, play a pivotal role in caregiving (Agard & Lomborg, 2010) and opportunities to involve carers and families are plentiful. One criterion for residing in a patient hotel is a relative (primary carer) taking care of the patient as part of the ongoing care trajectory, in preparation for the patient going home. In essence, patient hotels are designed to relieve busy wards and support patients who could go home but feel uncertain or unwell or lacking in confidence; thus, it is a place of transition and helps reduce potential readmission. It is expected that the actual care is provided by carers or families but in the knowledge that nursing and medical staff are available should they be required. The concept is essentially halfway between going home and staying in hospital, with the expectation that self-care is achieved and supported by carers who are themselves supported to partake in all interventions as if they were at home.

Enhanced Recovery Programmes

Enhanced recovery programmes (ERPs) are a growing movement in the NHS to help people get better sooner following major surgery. Arguably, a driving force embedded within ERP connects with a sense of well-being throughout and is aligned to the theory of salutogenesis. With its origins in surgical care, ERP is a structured approach to the whole patient pathway from preoperative to postdischarge care and returning to normal function. An underpinning ethos is to involve both patients and their carers/family so that together they understand the benefits of ERP in its entirety. ERP relies on good-quality communication and information that is explained clearly at every stage of the process.

Enhanced recovery programmes are mentioned here in the context of supporting families and carers, as their involvement from the very outset facilitates reduced psychological factors, most notably stress, in both themselves and their loved ones (patients). With shortened hospital stays and rapid discharge processes, having families and carers well informed and prepared is very important. Opportunities for nurses to engage in dialogue and information sharing need to be embraced with carers and families.

Living Well with Cancer (Health and Well-being Clinics)

National cancer follow-up programme initiatives that promote health and well-being in living with and beyond cancer are increasing. Carers are included in activities ranging from preparation for end of cancer treatment to care and support after treatment. The effects of cancer treatment can be long-lasting and impact both families and patients but in different ways. For instance, families and carers often defer their needs until treatments have ceased as they prioritise their loved one. Cancer follow-up programme initiatives involving family caregivers afford perfect opportunities for family-centred nursing approaches and holistic nursing.

Transition Back Home after Hospitalisation

Among the most significant encounters for family caregivers in hospital settings is the interaction with practitioners regarding discharge, either back home or to other care settings such as nursing homes. UK government policies have consistently highlighted the need to inform and involve families and carers fully in the hospital discharge process (Department of Health, 1999, 2004; NHS, 2020). Yet there is growing evidence indicating that breakdowns in care during the transition from hospital to home result in negative outcomes, such as lack of access to vital community-based services, poor patient satisfaction, breakdown of home care and high readmission rates to hospital.

Discharge from hospital is a process that ideally starts at the admission stage. Yet too often family and caregiver involvement begins at the point of discharge.

Omission of carers from the discharge process often results in care planning provision needing to be revised or delayed and carers feeling uninvolved, unsupported and in turmoil due to being undervalued and discounted in the communication processes. Therefore, nurses must identify, assess and support carers as expert partners in the entire hospital discharge process. Importantly, it is key to consider carers' views and wishes as to whether they have the ability or willingness to continue care and in what ways. Box 21.5 identifies the main principles of carers as partners in the discharge planning process.

Box 21.5 Principle of Carers as Partners in the Discharge Planning Process

- Identify carers as early as possible, being aware that family members may not view themselves as carers.
- Provide information, seeking permission to share information related to the patient, such as the illness and its consequences, as well as information concerning the patient's condition, financial cost of caring, follow-up care, sources of help and support.
- *Assessment*: inform the carer that they have a right to an assessment.
- *Planning for discharge*: fully involve carers at all stages of the discharge planning process, viewing carers as partners in the process and acknowledging their individual needs, considering cultural difference, age, gender, race, religious backgrounds and disability.

(Continued)

- *Provide support*: offer training to care safely, for example moving and handling and the use of equipment, and providing services that meet the needs of the carer, and who to contact if necessary.

Source: Based on Carers UK (2016)

We all have a responsibility to stop and think about the potential and real long-term gains from good assessments and discharge planning, compliance with care and treatments, and more involved caregivers and patients (Braine & Wray, 2016). A systematic assessment of the carer's needs concerning discharge from hospital of the care recipient is essential. Ewing *et al.* (2018) identified the Carer Support Needs Assessment Tool (CSNAT), as an intervention in supporting carers in the transition of a loved one from hospital to home.

Care, Dignity and Compassion

Notions of privacy/confidentiality must not be used *per se* to exclude families and carers. The interests and wishes of both the patient and the carer require a balanced dialogue and approach in the context of discharge processes. Unless there are over-riding reasons, an inclusive and open dialogue between care recipient and carer must be respected. However, carers may be reluctant to contradict what the patient is saying for fear of betraying or offending them. So, it may be important to make time to hear what the carer has to say in private.

The Nursing Associate

At the point of registration, the nursing associate will be able to: demonstrate the knowledge, communication and relationship management skills required to provide people, families and carers with accurate information that meets their needs before, during and after a range of interventions (Platform 3) (NMC, 2018b).

Sharing Information

Nurses are in key positions to explain to the patient the advantage of sharing information with carers, such as access to the right level of information that can help support the care recipient/patient and aid in the recovery process. However, in some cases the patient may lack capacity to consent to information sharing, and in such cases the Mental Capacity Act 2005 Code of Practice sets out the legal position. In summary, it states that information may be shared in such circumstances if it is in the best interests of the person who lacks capacity. Sharing knowledge may require sharing some hard truths about the family situation, which may be difficult and cause tensions within the family, and some may view this is as an intrusion. However, addressing information sharing may mean better services (e.g. financial). How this is handled depends on the nurse's skills and relationship with the family.

Adaptability and Coping

Being a carer can be demanding, difficult and stressful and the process of coping can be complex, dynamic and multidimensional. While coping defines the process of planned and learnt responses to solving problems and situations to reduce stress, coping strategies refers to the actions or practices that individuals use to lessen and manage the stressful situation. Understanding how family carers cope with the challenges they face is important for informing relevant support and intervention strategies. Much has been written about coping and coping with caregiving, and three key theoretical frameworks that have emerged in the literature explain how families and carers deal with their situations.

- The stimulus response model originally developed by Selye (1956), in which stress is caused by the non-specific response to any demand.
- Stress and life events in which stress results from an accumulation of demands or 'pile-up' (Hill, 1958), and whether these demands overwhelm the family system ability to cope with stress.
- The transactional model views stress as a dynamic and interactive process in which it is carers' subjective appraisal of their situation or event that is important in determining whether the situation or event is stressful or not.

The transactional model, originally developed by Lazarus & Folkman (1984), has undergone several modifications over the years but is widely used to explain the carer's situation. This framework acknowledges that each carer may appraise the situation they face differently; for some, the situation or event may be viewed as stressful but for others, it is not.

The outcome of family coping and adaptation depends on the relationship with several factors, such as pre-existing, and subsequent new, resources and the perceptions held by the family/carer about the situation. Several factors have been found to influence their perceptions, including the carer's individual values and beliefs, personal characteristics such as personality and levels of motivation, gender, ethnicity, culture and socioeconomic and marital status. Critically, the cause of stress and the way individuals and families adjust and adapt to stressors invariably differ considerably according to their caregiving situations. When a family member can cope and adapt, the whole family system benefits and likely achieves a balance (homeostasis) that then contributes to positive adjustment.

Coping Strategies

Coping strategies can be broadly divided into two main categories: problem-focused coping (aimed at modifying the sources of the stressor/problem) and emotion-focused coping (aimed at reducing the emotional effect of the stress or problem) (Lazarus & Folkman, 1984). It is important here to recognise that coping strategies can lead to a positive (adaptive) outcome (i.e. effective in helping to cope with the situation) or a negative (maladaptive) outcome (i.e. non-effective). For example, problem-focused strategies may be effective in reducing the burden of caring, while an emotion-focused strategy may help to reduce psychological stress. However, a problem-solving approach is not helpful when a problem or situation cannot be resolved. Equally, an emotion-focused approach can result in burnout and disengagement.

Table 21.3 Coping strategies that families and caregivers may use. *Source:* Adapted from Braine & Wray (2016).

PROBLEM-FOCUSED COPING (INFORMATION SEEKING)	EMOTION-FOCUSED COPING
Adaptive (positive) · Seeking advice and information to help understand the situation and empower themselves · Aiming to become competent in caregiving tasks · Identifying and prioritising problems that can be solved · Planning (setting goals) and evaluating solutions to the situation · Focusing on the situation · Identifying tasks that other family members or friends can do to help **Maladaptive (negative)** · Trivialising the issues or situation · Avoiding information that may cause them distress	**Adaptive (positive)** · Seeking emotional support from others by talking about their feelings · Seeking support from others · Attending a self-help group · Accepting and positively viewing the situation or problem **Maladaptive (negative)** · Denial · Negative thoughts · Unrealistic hopes and expectations · The use of alcohol, tobacco or other substances to try to cheer themselves up · Keeping feelings and thoughts to themselves

Families and carers often use a combination of strategies to cope with the problems they face and these may also change over time. Nurses need to be aware of family caregiver strategies and seek to support coping patterns if appropriate. Table 21.3 provides some examples of the behaviours that family carers may deploy.

In supporting families and carers, we should not assume that carers are motivated to actively seek information. Indeed, some carers do not want, need or use information and will avoid information if it causes them discomfort. On the other hand, others seek knowledge and information to reduce uncertainty, to make sense of or give meaning to the challenges that they face. Thus, it is important to understand that new information may increase or decrease anxiety and uncertainty in carers.

Red Flag

 Many signs may indicate that the caregiver is not coping and may need support.
· Short-tempered and feeling angry and resentful towards other family members
· Emotional outbursts, for example, crying unexpectedly and feeling emotionally fragile
· Changes in sleep patterns, for example, trouble getting off to sleep
· Weight gain and weight loss
· Physical symptoms, for example, headaches, frequent colds and muscular pains
· Loss of motivation and energy

The Impact of Caregiving

Caregiving activities can take their toll and the welfare of family caregivers is an increasing concern. It is important to note here that the effects of caregiving are multidimensional and often change during the carer's career. The impact of being a carer can have serious physical, emotional, psychological, social and financial consequences and can go unnoticed in the context of treating carers as the 'hidden patient'. While serious illness can strengthen, renew and deepen relationships within a family, it can also cause relationships to become conflicted, troubled and fragmented. Ultimately, the extent to which the care recipient and the caregiver can cope effectively with the situation they face contributes to the health and well-being (salutogenesis) of both individuals.

Evidence demonstrates that the caregiving journey is often perceived by the caregiver as a negative experience: difficult, burdensome, stressful and time-consuming. It is well documented that carers often suffer from high levels of stress and anxiety and show higher levels of depression than the general population. Family caregivers who suffer from debilitating stress can jeopardise their health and well-being, thus impacting the quality of care and the relationship with the person they are caring for. In addition, unrelenting periods of caregiving have the potential to create chronic stress, which in turn further affects family relationships and functioning. The detrimental physical effects of caregiving are in general less severe than the psychological effects.

However, the caregiving experience may also be appraised as a positive and enriching experience. The extent to which a carer perceives their experiences as positive or negative depends on several factors, including the nature and extent of the caring responsibility, the relationship between the caregiver and care recipient, caregiver age and the extent to which the caregiver is willing to provide informal care.

To fully understand the impact of caregiving, both the negative and positive dimensions of caregiving need to be considered by nurses.

Caregiver Burden

Burden is one of the most frequently investigated caregiving outcomes and can be defined as the overall consequences associated with a demanding and stressful caregiver situation. Notions of burden can be endured by a primary carer or distributed among several family members and friends. Much research on burden indicates that levels vary, and some caregivers are at increased risk of burden, for example women, children and young caregivers. In essence, burden can be viewed as the caregiver's perception that their situation exceeds their available resources to cope. According to Hoenig & Hamilton (1966), caregiver burden has two distinct components.

1. *Objective burden of care*: the actual physical or instrumental provision of care to the recipient. The burden is quantifiable and can thus be measured by various burden scales.
2. *Subjective burden*: the caregiver's appraisal of the situation and the extent to which a caregiver perceives the burden of care.

Burden is conceptualised as a primary source of caregiver stress and one that is influenced by the caregiver's background and the caregiving context (Pearlin *et al.*, 1990). Gender is frequently cited as being a major influencing factor, with women overall suffering more burden than men. This may be attributed to the more direct care activities that women tend to engage in during their caring role (see Box 21.3). Although burden is unique to each carer, other notable influencing factors increase the predictions of caregiving burden, including being a primary carer and/or a spouse, culture, lack of available supporting resources, and the primary disease of the care recipient (e.g. long-term physical diseases). Recognising these factors can help to predict caregiver burden and influence nursing care.

Change in Roles

Being a carer can mean a loss of other roles in life, loss of identity and loss of relationships. Most family caregivers are untrained and feel ill prepared to take on the caregiving role. Within the family, roles are constantly changing, whereby people may relinquish a role and assume another. For example, taking on the role of a carer can mean drastic changes to their role within the family, in their social role and social networks. A useful theory that emerged in the social science literature during the 1920s and 1930s was 'role theory'; it has been applied to healthcare to understand the demands that caregivers face as they perform their caring role. In general, a role is defined as an expected pattern or set of behaviours associated with a particular position or status in society. The notion of role theory, Goode (1960) argues, is that individuals have limited personal resources, such as time and energy, to fulfil their various roles.

Often carers assume a combination of roles, and this has the potential for introducing role conflict. Biddle (1986) states that role conflict occurs when the expectations of the various roles an individual hold become incompatible. This may lead to role overload or strain. The family system is then thrown into disarray and roles need to be renegotiated as family members decide what needs to be done by whom to enable the family to cope effectively.

By using role theory, nurses can help to develop coping strategies for individual family members through identifying role demands, negotiating new roles and identifying resources to support the new roles, along with any barriers to meeting their caregiving demands.

Physical Health

Caregivers are also physically less healthy than non-caregivers and have more chronic illnesses, such as heart disease, diabetes and arthritis, than non-caregivers (Pinquart & Sörensen, 2007). They may also suffer from poorer immune function and fatigue, muscular injuries and exhaustion along with sleep problems and gastric disturbances. Poor physical health not only puts caregivers at risk of illness and harm but has the potential for negative effects on the person they are caring for; difficulty in performing their role may result in ineffective care (unintentional) and place their loved one at an increased risk of harm. Because of the demands of caring, caregivers may even neglect their own care needs. Nurses need to be alerted to, and intervene with, those carers who neglect their own healthcare appointments and who change their health-related activities, such as diet and exercise regimes, to prevent the onset of adverse healthcare problems.

Psychological Distress: Depression

Depression among caregivers is well documented, with consistently high levels of depressive symptoms reported compared with the general population (Braine & Wray, 2016).

As the care recipient's condition worsens and the intensity of the caregiving increases, so does the caregiver's level of depressive symptoms (Denno *et al.*, 2013). Much research has focused on the link between caregiver burden and depression and indicates that there are several predictors of depression in caregivers, including:

- A decline in caregiver physical health
- Perceiving their caregiving activities as a restriction on their routine activities
- Increase in problematic behaviours evidenced by the care recipient
- Female carers are more likely to suffer depression than non-carers and male carers
- Maternal depression symptoms are high among caregivers of children with chronic conditions.

By being aware of these predictors, nurses can help identify those who are at greater risk due to caregiver circumstances.

Loss

Studies of grief and loss are normally associated with death, but loss and grief are constant insidious companions for caregivers. The losses that caregivers experience in their caregiving journey are multifaceted and often more severe than the grief experienced in death. Illness and disease bring a loss of normal expectations and create uncertainty for the future of carers. For many carers, loss and grief can be significant in their caregiving journey and can make coping difficult. Each family caregiver's losses are unique and may include several losses at any one time.

The losses that caregivers may experience often go unnoticed by both the caregiver and healthcare professionals, with the caregiver suffering in silence without support. Doka (1989) explains this hidden grief as being outside the 'grieving rules' and uses the term *disenfranchised grief* to describe it. Doka (1989, p.4) defines disenfranchised grief as the person's experience when they 'incur a loss that is not or cannot be openly acknowledged, mourned or socially supported'.

It is important that nurses differentiate between the variations of loss and their associated meaning so that appropriate support can be offered. Loss without death has been the subject of research, and several theories and concepts have evolved to explain the phenomenon. Of note are the concepts of ambiguous loss (Boss, 1999, 2016), predeath grief, anticipatory grief (Rando, 2000), non-finite loss (Bruce & Schultz, 2001) and chronic sorrow (Olshansky, 1962). Although this is not an exhaustive list, all highlight the multiple realities of the continuing presence of indefinite loss of a loved one experienced by families and caregivers.

Loss of Couplehood

With a growing interest in dementia care, a more holistic, broader view of the burden of carers has unfolded. This emerging view has resulted in researchers exploring the unique relationship between the caregiving spouse and the person with dementia and the significant losses in their couple relationship. Ade-Ridder & Kaplan (1993, p.20) describe this relationship as 'couplehood', meaning the extent to which there is still a sense of 'we' in the relationship. Couplehood is best understood as the extent to which individuals have feelings of 'we'-ness (strong couplehood), rather than being an 'I' (no couplehood). Although this area of research has been focused on dementia care, the concept has implications for many other long-term degenerative diseases, such as Parkinson disease, multiple sclerosis and mental illnesses.

Through partnership working (see Figure 21.1 and Dalton's 2003 triad theory), nurses can understand the quality of past relationships in couples and gain an insight into their perceived couplehood and how this may affect the caregiving relationship when they are living together and when living apart as a non-homogeneous group. For those couples who were not so close before illness, this may affect the caregiver's willingness to undertake caregiving responsibilities and may require alternative care arrangements, such as institutional care, to be made. In couples who strive to maintain their sense of couplehood, separation (e.g. when a spouse with dementia is placed in a long-term facility) poses significant challenges to their sense of belonging. Førsund *et al.* (2014) found that this can create a strong sense of being alone and loss of couplehood for the caregiver and highlights the vulnerability of the spouse in this situation. Nurses, especially those working in the community, can help to facilitate couplehood by identifying services that accommodate and support the concept of couplehood.

Caregiver Neglect/Abuse

Caregivers may be emotionally, verbally and occasionally physically neglected or abused by the care recipient. Common causes of emotional abuse towards caregivers include changing behaviours due to the nature of the illness, such as dementia and acquired brain injury and/or frustration at the disability or disease progression. Caregivers can also experience emotional neglect or abuse by their family members, who expect the individual to provide all the care to the care recipient, regardless of desire or ability to do so. If caregiver abuse is suspected, a caregiver assessment and raising awareness is an immediate action. If the abuse is extreme, the process of safeguarding actions needs to be employed. Statutory arrangements should be made for additional relief help from other family members, or even paid assistance, to lessen the caregiving demands. In addition, encouraging and helping the caregiver to attend support groups or educational sessions to learn beneficial coping skills may help them be more prepared to deal with their situation.

Caregivers may be embarrassed to reveal their neglect or abuse, in part due to a sense of feeling 'it's in the line of duty' for their loved one. Thus, it is not always apparent to caregivers how they are being affected by their responsibilities or their loved one's changing condition. Consideration needs to be given to the prior relationships between the caregiver and care recipient.

Red Flag

 Caregiver neglect or abuse can cause emotional and/or physical distress to the caregiver. The carer's voice needs to be heard when they feel abused by the person they are caring for. Signs of caregiver abuse may include:
· Fear that the person they are caring for will become violent
· Feeling controlled

· Suffering from low self-esteem
· Viewing caregiving as lonesome and a burden.
Recognise that carers who are neglected or abused are vulnerable people and need support and protection. Asking the carer questions, alone without their loved ones present and without suggesting abuse, may help them to feel safe and secure enough to be able to share any abusive experiences. Record and report accurately any findings following legislation (NMC, 2018a).

Carers can, in some circumstances, become the abuser themselves. By assessing both the patient and their carers in their home environment, carer abuse may be identified and prevented. Regular assessment of high-quality respectful care, which is responsive to individual patient preferences, needs and values over time, is critical as a decline in respect may serve as an early warning signal that the caregiving situation is deteriorating toward abusive behaviour. This may require separate conversations with the patient and the caregiver, to identify these misguided practices or tasks and prevent abuse and neglect. Furthermore, a holistic assessment involving the home environment may help to identify risk factors for unintentional harm and neglect and thus inform prevention processes to help reduce such harms (Braine & Wray, 2016). For further information about safeguarding the vulnerable person, see Chapter 8.

Positive Outcomes of Caregiving

So far, some of the negative impacts of caregiving have been considered, but some carers achieve long-term benefits from their role as carer. There is mounting evidence that the caregiving journey can be uplifting and contribute to positive health outcomes for the carer. This effect can be attributed to the individual's appraisal of their situation as highlighted in Lazarus & Folkman's (1984) transactional model of stress. It is important not to assume that all caregivers are consumed by negative experiences and although not all can experience positive benefits, for some carers both negative and positive consequences of providing care may exist simultaneously. The positive experiences reported by caregivers include:

- Personal reward and satisfaction
- Gaining a more meaningful relationship with their loved one through their caregiving
- Self-worth benefits from supporting a friend or relative
- Discovery of personal strengths and feelings of accomplishment and competence
- Enabling new skills to be learnt and mastering the complexity of caregiving.

In their interactions with caregivers, nurses should focus on both the strengths and weaknesses of the carers; if we view caregiving only as a negative experience, we limit our ability to help and support positive factors that can improve the caregiving experience.

Interventions to Support Families and Carers

By identifying the positive aspects of the caregiving experience, nurses can enhance their relationship with family caregivers. Through positive reinforcement, nurses can help family members to endure their caregiving work during difficult times; it may also help foster motivation and manage their situation. However, the positive impact of caring should not be viewed as a reason to keep a care recipient at home when it may not be safe or appropriate to do so. It is also important to consider that some carers may overplay their positive experiences to give the impression that they can cope. Nurses also need, through careful questioning, to explore the carer's situation and experiences, focusing on the strengths and resources of the caregiver rather than limiting the assessment to problems and deficits.

Given that caregivers face difficult and demanding issues and carry a significant burden, they need effective resources and support. If we are to support and engage with the wider family, this requires an understanding of:

- family dynamics/issues
- how to signpost to where support is available from other services to target appropriate referrals.

One perspective that is useful in supporting families and carers is a strengths-based approach to care. This is concerned with drawing on an individual's strengths, hopes, aspirations and capabilities and in doing so helping the individual to deal with their challenges and meet their needs. While negative experiences are not ignored in a strengths-based approach, they are acknowledged and used to focus on the individual's strengths. Indeed, in the Care Act (2014) local authorities must consider a person's strengths and capabilities and maximise those strengths to enable them to achieve their desired outcomes. Strengths-based approaches in nursing can be useful for focusing on possibilities and opportunities, enabling and empowering families to deal with their caring role.

Importance of Signposting

Nurses have a crucial and unique role to play in providing families and carers with good-quality information and other services to facilitate and influence health and well-being (i.e. salutogenesis). Knowledge of local services in order to signpost families and carers in an appropriate and timely manner is critical. The application of the Triangle of Care or Dalton's (2003) triad comes into play once again and emphasises the importance of partnership working (see Figure 21.1).

The charity sector, along with local authorities, can provide respite opportunities. Carers' charities have much experience in being innovative and resourceful regarding respite, and signposting to these charities is well worth the effort. Respite comes in many guises, ranging from actual rest and time off from caring duties to one-off offers of help or resources that enable relaxation and 'switching off'.

Medicines Management

Many carers help with medicines and this is an integral part of the caring role. However, it is often an issue of concern for many carers, especially when caring for the older person, who often has several co-morbidities. Carers may be involved in a variety of medication-related tasks, ranging from collecting prescriptions to administering several drugs via a variety of routes. Although medicines can legally be administered by anyone, provided it has been prescribed by an appropriate practitioner, administration of a medicine can be challenging for the carer and has the potential to harm the patient. Not only do the nurse and the carer need to appreciate their loved one's right to confidentiality, but some carers may perceive the management of medicines as demanding and burdensome and in some cases may provoke anxiety and stress. Nurses need to explore skills in administering medicines and not assume that the carer or family member is skilled or competent.

Nurses have a central role in providing support, information and advice about medications to family carers, especially before the patient is discharged to the community. This may include:

- Information about the medication, i.e. effectiveness and potential side-effects
- Advice on the use of blister packs/dosage boxes, alarms or telephone calls as reminders to take medicines
- Information about repeat prescriptions may involve medication that is packaged differently or has a different name due to a different brand of the same generic drug
- Medication should be reviewed once a year
- Safely store and dispose of medication according to manufacturer instructions
- If a young carer is helping to administer medications to a relative who cannot do so themselves, then this needs to be performed safely. If they need to pick up the medication from the pharmacist, this will require some special arrangement with the pharmacist.

Primary Care

Community nurses are in a unique position to know the whole family and their dynamics. Community nurses liaise between the hospital and the community and are in a prime position to use their negotiation skills to challenge health partners that they can do better. There may be an issue with the carer's capacity to cope, and community nurses should use their knowledge to decide the limits of this capacity. The well-being of everyone in the family matters, so it is important that community nurses navigate support before carers reach crisis burnout and thus enable carers to feel that their health and well-being are as important as those of the patient. A recurring problem for carers is meeting new people and having to tell their story over and over again to different community nurses and healthcare practitioners. Therefore, wherever possible, community nurses need to keep accurate detailed records and show sensitivity towards carers and their plight. In doing so, nurses can mitigate fragmentation of information and support for carers. Community nurses, with their knowledge of the family, can help to provide the right support at the right time and can monitor the quality of life.

Box 21.6 describes a carer's story that illustrates the unique opportunities nurses have to gently enquire and encourage a carer to recognise their role and the need for self-care. Such conversations need not be onerous but can be hugely valuable, as they can lead to better support for the carer as well as the

Box 21.6 Carer's Case Study

Frank and June

Frank, who is aged 66 years, cares for his wife, June, who has several chronic health conditions. As well as helping June to wash, dress and go to the toilet, Frank takes care of the household chores, and accompanies June to all her GP and hospital appointments. It was during a visit to their GP practice, while June was seeing her doctor, that the practice nurse noticed that Frank was looking very tired. When she asked Frank how he was, he reluctantly confessed to being exhausted as he never had a 'proper night's sleep'; that he 'shouldn't complain', as June was the one who was ill, not him.

The nurse decided to ask Frank a few more questions. With gentle encouragement, Frank revealed that his inability to get a good night's sleep stemmed from the fact that June suffers from severe pain and wears a morphine patch during the night. Unfortunately, the patches make June feel very dizzy and so, whenever she wakes up to go the bathroom (which happens at least three times a night), Frank must accompany her to make sure she doesn't fall. Even when June is asleep, Frank always has 'one ear open, just in case'. It soon became clear that Frank had been giving very little thought to his own health and well-being. 'Morning, noon and night, it's June I'm focused on', he explained. 'How is she feeling? Will she be OK if I go to the shops? How will she cope with the next operation?' He couldn't remember the last time he'd had his blood pressure taken or stepped on his bathroom scales to check his weight.

Even though Frank's conversation with the practice nurse was brief, it proved to be cathartic. Through being given an informal, non-threatening opportunity to 'offload' in private, Frank was able to recognise that he was now June's carer, as well as her husband, that his caring role was becoming more and more demanding and that it was vitally important to look after himself as well as June.

cared-for. It also touches on a subject that is less often discussed: the impact on the carer of the care recipient's medications, and highlights potential issues and opportunities.

Conclusion

This chapter has provided an overview of the context of carers and their importance in nursing practice across care settings and fields of practice. Some of the common issues that nurses face in working with carers and families have been highlighted. It has been emphasised that building therapeutic relationships and trust is the basis for holistic care for patients, carers and their loved ones. Suggestions to advance your knowledge base and inform your practice are offered in a genuine desire to facilitate triad partnership working and we must support, include and respect carers. Small things matter, such as acknowledging their existence, involving them in decision making and working together in meaningful ways to implement actions that can help. Remember that we can all make a difference and we all have a responsibility – it is a collective endeavour supporting family carers (Braine & Wray, 2016).

Key Points

- Nursing practices in whatever field should be rooted in building mutual respect and trust with families and carers.
- Whatever the practice setting, being mindful and aware of the existence of carers and families in the lives of patients they are caring for is vital.
- Globally, caregivers play an increasingly important and ever-expanding role in supporting the care provided by nurses and other healthcare professionals.
- It is important for nurses to both recognise and understand the carers as 'hidden patients' and know how to support this valuable and sometimes vulnerable group.
- The caregiving journey can be a negative or burdensome experience, but it also has positive and rewarding benefits.
- Insights into what it is like to be a family caregiver matter to a family. Empathy matters, listening matters – we can't always do something, but being there and offering understanding can truly help and nurses should not underestimate that.
- Understanding and sensitivity are required concerning the practice of 'watching over', particularly the ethics of care and the division of labour and roles between carers and nurses.
- Support and interventions need to be individualised for the family.

References

Ade-Ridder, L. & Kaplan, L. (1993) Marriage spousal caregiving and a husband's move to a nursing home: a changing role for the wife? *Journal of Gerontological Nursing*, 19, 13–23.

Agard, A.S. & Lomborg, K. (2010) Flexible family visitation in the intensive care unit: nurses' decision-making. *Journal of Clinical Nursing*, 20, 1106–1114.

Agard, A.S., Egerod, I., Tonnesen, E. & Lomborg, K. (2015) From spouse to caregiver and back: a grounded theory study of post-intensive care unit spousal caregiving. *Journal of Advanced Nursing*, 71(8), 1892–1903.

Aneshensel, C.S., Pearlin, L.I., Mullan, J., Zarit, S.H. & Whitlatch, C.J. (1995) *Profiles in Caregiving: The Unexpected Career*. Academic Press, San Diego, CA.

Biddle, B. (1986) Recent developments in role theory. *Annual Review of Sociology*, 12, 67–92.

Boss, P. (1999) *Ambiguous Loss*. Harvard University Press, Cambridge, MA.

Boss, P. (2016) The context and process of theory development: the story of ambiguous loss. *Journal of Family Theory and Review*, 8(3), 269–286.

Braine, M.E. & Wray, J. (2016) *Supporting Families and Carers: A Nursing Perspective*. CRC Press, Boca Raton, FL.

Bruce, E.J. & Schultz, C.L. (2001) *Nonfinite Loss and Grief*. Paul H. Brooke Publishing, Sydney.

Care Act (2014) www.legislation.gov.uk/ukpga/2014/23/contents (accessed December 2021).

Carer Passport (2021) *What is a Carer Passport scheme?* https://carerspassports.uk/about-carer-passport-schemes (assessed December 2021).

Carers Trust (2013) *The Triangle of Care, Carers Included: A Guide to Best Practice for Dementia Care (England)*. carers.org/resources/all-resources/67-the-triangle-of-care-carers-included-a-guide-to-best-practice-for-dementia-care-england#:~:text=In%202013%2C%

365

20Carers%20Trust%20worked%20with%20the%20Royal,cared% 20for%20was%20adapted%20to%20a%20general%20hospital

Carers Trust (2016) *The Triangle of Care, Carers Included: A Guide to Best Practice for Dementia Care.* https://carers.org/resources/all-resources/67-the-triangle-of-care-carers-included-a-guide-to-best-practice-for-dementia-care-england (accessed December 2021).

Carers Trust (2020) *The Triangle of Care for Children and Young People's Mental Health Services. A Guide for Mental Health Professionals.* https://carers.org/resources/all-resources/66-the-triangle-of-care-for-children-and-young-peopleas-mental-health-services-a-guide-for-mental-health-professionals- (accessed December 2021).

Carers Trust (2021) *About caring.* https://carers.org/about-caring/about-caring (accessed December 2021).

Carers UK (2011) *Caring at a Distance: Bridging the Gap.* www.carersuk.org/news-and-campaigns/press-releases/caring-at-a-distance-bridging-the-gap (accessed December 2021).

Carers UK (2015) *Valuing Carers 2015: The Rising Value of Carers' Support.* www.carersuk.org/news-and-campaigns/news/unpaid-carers-save-the-uk-132-billion-a-year-the-cost-of-a-second-nhs (accessed December 2021).

Carers UK (2016) *Coming out of hospital.* www.carersuk.org/help-and-advice/practical-support/coming-out-of-hospital (accessed December 2021).

Carers UK (2020a) *Carers Week Research Report The rise in the number of unpaid carers during the coronavirus (COVID-19) outbreak.* www.carersuk.org/images/CarersWeek2020/CW_2020_Research_Report_WEB.pdf (accessed December 2021).

Carers UK (2020b) *Assessments. Your guide to getting help and support in England.* Factsheet E1020-1118. Carers UK, London.

Children Act (2004) www.legislation.gov.uk/ukpga/2004/31/contents (accessed December 2021).

Children and Families Act (2014) www.legislation.gov.uk/ukpga/2014/6/contents (accessed December 2021).

Children's Society (2021) *Supporting Young Carers.* www.childrenssociety.org.uk/what-we-do/our-work/supporting-young-carers (accessed December 2021).

Colombo, F., Llena Nozal, A., Mercier, J. & Tjadens, F. (2011) *Help wanted? Providing and paying for long-term care.* OECD, Paris. www.oecd.org/els/health-systems/47903344.pdf (accessed December 2021).

Dalton, J.M. (2003) Development and testing of the theory of collaborative decision-making in nursing practice for triads. *Journal of Advanced Nursing*, 41(1), 22–33.

Denno, M.S., Gillard, P.J., Graham, G.D., *et al.* (2013) Anxiety and depression associated with caregiver burden in caregivers of stroke survivors with spasticity. *Archives of Physical Medicine and Rehabilitation*, 94(9), 1731–1736.

Department of Health (1999) *Caring About Carers: A National Strategy for Carers.* Department of Health, London.

Department of Health (2004) *Quality and Outcomes Framework Guidance.* Department of Health, London.

Department of Health (2008) *Carers at the Heart of 21st Century Families and Communities: Improving support for carers.* Department of Health, London.

Department of Health (2010) Annex A: Response to the call for views on priorities. In: *Recognised, Valued and Supported: Next steps for the Carers Strategy.* Department of Health, London.

Department for Work and Pensions (2021a) *National Statistics DWP benefits statistics: February 2021.* www.gov.uk/government/statistics/dwp-benefits-statistics-february-2021/dwp-benefits-statistics-february-2021 (accessed December 2021).

Department for Work and Pensions (2021b) *Family Resources Survey financial year 2019 to 2020.* www.gov.uk/government/statistics/family-resources-survey-financial-year-2019-to-2020/family-resources-survey-financial-year-2019-to-2020#disability-1 (accessed December 2021).

Doka, K. (1989) *Disenfranchised Grief: Recognizing Hidden Sorrow.* Lexington Books, Lexington, MA.

Ewing, G., Austin, L., Jones, D. & Grande, G. (2018) Who cares for the carers at hospital discharge at the end of life? A qualitative study of current practice in discharge planning and the potential value of using The Carer Support Needs Assessment Tool (CSNAT) Approach. *Palliative Medicine*, 32(5), 939–949.

Fengler, A.P. & Goodrich, N. (1979) Wives of elderly disabled men: the hidden patients. *Gerontologist*, 19(2), 175–183.

Førsund, L.H., Skovdahl, K., Kiik, R. & Ytrehu, S.W. (2014) The loss of a shared lifetime: a qualitative study exploring spouses' experiences of losing couplehood with their partner with dementia living in institutional care. *Journal of Clinical Nursing*, 24, 121–130.

Given, B.A. & Given, C.W. (1991) Family caregiving for the elderly. *Annual Review of Nursing Research*, 9, 77–101.

Goode, W. (1960) Theory of role strain. *American Sociological Review*, 25, 483–496.

Hanson, S.M. (2005) Family health nursing: an introduction. In: S.M. Hanson (ed.) *Family Health Care Nursing: Theory, Practice and Research*, 2nd edn, pp. 3–33. F.A. Davies, Philadelphia, PA.

Hickson, M., Connolly, A. & Whelan, K. (2011) Impact of protected mealtimes on ward mealtime environment, patient experience and nutrient intake in hospitalised patients. *Journal of Human Nutrition and Dietetics*, 24(4), 370–374.

Hill, R. (1958) Social stress and the family: 1. Generic features of families under stress. *Social Casework*, 49, 139–150.

Hoenig, J. & Hamilton, M.W. (1966) The schizophrenic patient in the community and the effect on the household. *International Journal of Social Psychiatry*, 12, 165–176.

Kellett, U. (2007) Seizing possibilities for positive family caregiving in nursing homes. *Journal of Clinical Nursing*, 16(8), 1479–1487.

Lazarus, R.S. & Folkman, S. (1984) *Stress Appraisal and Coping.* Springer, New York.

Mental Capacity Act (2005) www.legislation.gov.uk/ukpga/2005/9/contents (accessed December 2021).

Montgomery, R.J.V. & Kosloski, K.D. (2000) Family caregiving: change, continuity and diversity. In: M.P. Lawton & R.L. Rubestein (eds) *Interventions in Dementia Care: Towards Improving Quality of Life.* Springer, New York.

Murray, L. & Barnes, M. (2012) Have families been rethought? Ethics of care, family and 'whole family' approaches. *Social Policy and Society*, 9(4), 533–544.

National Health Service (2019) *The NHS Long-term Plan.* www.longtermplan.nhs.uk/ (accessed December 2021).

National Health Service (2020) *Hospital Discharge Service: Policy and Operating Model.* https://assets.publishing.service.gov.uk/government/uploads/system/uploads/attachment_data/file/962885/Hospital_Discharge_Policy_1.pdf www.longtermplan.nhs.uk/ (accessed December 2021).

National Health Service (2021) *Enhancing the quality of life for people living with long term conditions.* www.england.nhs.uk/wp-content/uploads/2014/09/ltc-infographic.pdf (accessed December 2021).

National Patient Safety Agency (2007) *Protected Mealtimes Review: Findings and Recommendations Report.* https://webarchive.nationalarchives.gov.uk/20170906201728/http://www.nrls.npsa.nhs.uk/resources/search-by-audience/hospital-nurse/?entryid45=59806&cord=DESC&p=11&char=0-9 (accessed December 2021)

Nursing & Midwifery Council (2018a) *Future Nurse: Standards for proficiency for registered nurses.* NMC, London.

Nursing & Midwifery Council (2018b) *Standards for proficiency for nursing associates.* NMC, London.

Office for National Statistics (2001) *2001 Census and earlier.* www.ons.gov.uk/ons/guide-method/census/census-2001/index.html (accessed December 2021).

Office for National Statistics (2011) *Census data.* www.ons.gov.uk/census/2011census (accessed December 2021).

Olshansky, S. (1962) Chronic sorrow: a response to having a mentally defective child. *Social Casework*, 43, 190–193.

Pearlin, L.I., Mullan, J.T., Semple, S.J. & Skaff, M.M. (1990) Caregiving and the stress process: an overview of concepts and their measures. *Gerontologist*, 30(5), 583–594.

Perkins, E.A. & Haley, W.E. (2010) Compound caregiving: when lifelong caregivers undertake additional caregiving role. *Rehabilitation Psychology*, 55(4), 409–417.

Perlesz, A., Kinsella, G. & Crowe, S. (2000) Psychological distress and family satisfaction following traumatic brain injury: injured individuals and their primary, secondary and tertiary carers. *Journal of Head Trauma Rehabilitation*, 15(3), 909–929.

Pinquart, M. & Sörensen, S. (2007) Correlates of physical health of informal caregivers: a meta-analysis. *Journal of Gerontology B: Psychological Sciences and Social Sciences*, 62(2), 126–137.

Porter, J., Ottrey, E. & Huggins, C.E. (2017) Protected Mealtimes in hospitals and nutritional intake: systematic review and meta-analyses. *International Journal of Nursing Studies*, 65, 62–69.

Princess Royal Trust for Carers (2010) *The Triangle of Care: Carers Included: A Guide to Best Practice in Acute Mental Health Care*. Princess Royal Trust for Carers, Woodford Green, Essex.

Rando, T.A. (2000) *Clinical Dimensions of Anticipatory Mourning: Theory Practice in Working with the Dying, Their Loved Ones and Their Caregivers*. Lexington Books, Champaign, IL.

Satir, V. (1972) *Peoplemaking*. Science and Behavior Books, Palo Alto, CA.

Scottish Government (2018) *Carers (Scotland) Act 2016 Statutory Guidance*. Edinburgh, Scotland.

Selye, H. (1956) *The Stress of Life*. McGraw Hill, New York.

Steinglass, P. (1987) *The Alcoholic Family*. Basic Books, New York.

White, C. (2013) *2011 Census Analysis: Unpaid Care in England and Wales, 2011 and Comparison with 2001*. www.ons.gov.uk/people populationandcommunity/healthandsocialcare/healthcaresystem/articles/2011censusanalysisisunpaidcareinenglandandwales2011and comparisonwith2001/2013-02-15 (accessed December 2021).

World Health Organization (2020) *Decade of Healthy Ageing: Baseline Report*. World Health Organization, Geneva.

Wright, L.M. & Leahey, M. (1990) Trends in nursing of families. *Journal of Advanced Nursing*, 15, 148–154.

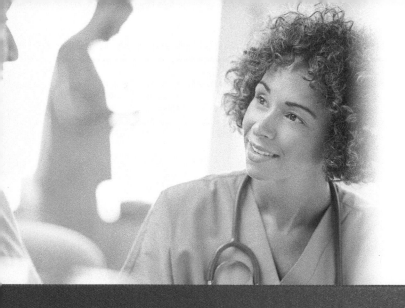

22

The Principles of Pain Management

Anthony Wheeldon

University of Hertfordshire, UK

Learning Outcomes

On completion of this chapter you will be able to:

- Recognise the importance of pain recognition as part of a comprehensive patient assessment
- Demonstrate the ability to perform a comprehensive assessment of an individual's pain
- Recognise the cardinal signs and symptoms of acute pain
- Plan effective pain management, which incorporates both pharmacological and non-pharmacological methods of pain control
- Work collaboratively with other members of the multidisciplinary team to ensure that patients receive care interventions that are based on the best available evidence
- Promote self-management strategies in individuals living with chronic pain

Proficiencies

NMC Proficiencies and Standards:

- Demonstrate the knowledge and skills required to identify and initiate appropriate interventions to support people with commonly encountered symptoms including pain.
- Observe, and assess the need for intervention for people, families and carers, identify, assess and respond appropriately to uncontrolled symptoms and signs of distress including pain.

Visit the companion website at www.wiley.com/go/peate/nursingpractice3e where you can test yourself using flashcards, multiple-choice questions and more.

Nursing Practice: Knowledge and Care, Third Edition. Edited by Ian Peate and Aby Mitchell.
© 2022 John Wiley & Sons Ltd. Published 2022 by John Wiley & Sons Ltd.
Companion website: www.wiley.com/go/peate/nursingpractice3e

Introduction

Everyone throughout their lifetime will experience pain at various times to varying degrees. In all care settings, the nurse will encounter individuals experiencing and living with pain. Yet despite being ubiquitous, it remains a complex phenomenon that can be difficult to conceptualise.

Pain is often defined as an unpleasant or uncomfortable sensation that acts as a warning of tissue damage, which occurs as a result of injury, strain or disease, for example. However, there are times when pain lacks such a useful purpose and continues long after healing is completed. Pain is a common factor shared by all human beings but it should be treated as a personal and individual experience. This is because it is widely recognised that the way individuals express and cope with their pain is influenced by a multitude of determining factors, which may include culture, life experiences and personality but could equally be difficult to determine or characterise. Pain can also be an emotional experience unrelated to tissue damage. Pain is often used to describe feelings of loss, grief and even unrequited love.

Whatever the cause or nature of pain, it is vital that nurses recognise that, if inadequately controlled, pain can be detrimental to the individual's physiological and psychological well-being. Although pain management is often associated with the use of analgesia, there are a number of non-pharmacological methods of pain management that can help patients live with and cope with their pain. Successful assessment and control of pain is, therefore, reliant upon an individualised holistic plan of care that utilises a range of treatments.

The Physiology of Pain

Pain physiology encompasses both physiological and psychological concepts, some of which are not fully understood. As a result, pain physiology is a complex and intricate phenomenon. The transmission and sensation of pain follow very distinct processes. First, tissue damage is detected by the peripheral nervous system by specialised nerve cells called nociceptors. Peripheral sensory neurones are then innervated, and nerve signals are sent towards the central nervous system, where the meaning and location of the pain are determined (Figure 22.1). For a more detailed breakdown of the pathophysiology of pain, please refer to Wheeldon (2021).

Classification of Pain

Pain is classified according to its duration and is categorised as being:

- Transient
- Acute
- Chronic.

Transient pain is a short episode of pain that occurs as a result of minor injury. Although the pain could be intense and even cause the individual to become momentarily upset, it will be eventually be considered to be pain of no significance. Transient pain is short-lived, and the individual is unlikely to seek medical attention. *Acute and chronic* pain are the major reasons for individuals

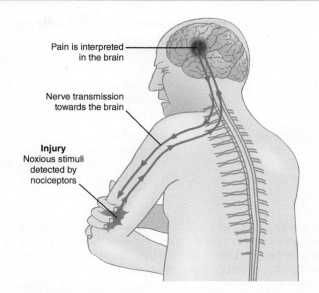

Figure 22.1 Pain pathway of transmission and interpretation.

Pain is interpreted in the brain

Nerve transmission towards the brain

Injury Noxious stimuli detected by nociceptors

seeking medical attention. There are distinct differences between acute and chronic pain, and it is essential that the nurse recognises and fully understands the major differences between these two pain states if they are to provide holistic care to their patients with pain (Table 22.1).

Acute Pain

Acute pain is associated with a severe sudden onset of intense localised or generalised pain that continues until healing begins. Its purpose is to indicate tissue damage. Acute pain is intense and can be an intolerable experience and in response individuals experience an autonomic stress response that manifests as hypertension, tachycardia, diaphoresis, tachypnoea and increased muscle tension. Patients in acute pain may also feel cool and clammy to touch and may complain of nausea and vomiting. Acute pain is also associated with a strong emotional response, which may present with altered facial expressions, verbal expression, guarding and high levels of anxiety.

Chronic Pain

The term 'chronic pain' is used to describe pain that continues even though healing is complete. Acute pain is a symptom of an associated medical condition or injury whereas chronic pain exists after the injury has healed or the disease has ceased. For this reason, chronic pain is often considered as a syndrome – a medical condition in its own right (Melzack & Wall, 1988). Chronic pain is more likely to be perceived as generalised by the patient, which means that they will often find it difficult to inform practitioners of the exact location of their pain.

Due to its long-term nature, chronic pain is usually more difficult manage than acute pain. Stress responses are difficult to maintain over sustained periods of time and therefore despite experiencing pain that may remain as intense as acute pain, there is often little or no autonomic stress response. This could result in patients in tremendous pain presenting without any of

Table 22.1 **Differences between acute and chronic pain.** *Source*: Adapted from Hubert & VanMeter (2018).

TYPE OF PAIN	DESCRIPTION	NEURONES RESPONSIBLE	NATURE OF PAIN
Acute pain	Fast, intense, localised	Fast, wide diameter myelinated Aδ fibres	Sudden, short term Present until healing starts Associated with a stress response
Chronic pain	Slow, diffuse, prolonged	Slow, thin diameter, non-myelinated C-fibres	Long term, disabling Associated with fatigue, irritability and loss of hope Difficult to manage

the cardinal signs of pain, i.e. tachycardia, hypertension and diaphoresis. Often chronic pain does not have a specific or apparent cause, which results in a long-term debilitating experience that has a number of psychological and physical side-effects. Patients with chronic pain complain of a range of psychosocial disorders such as disturbed sleep, reduced appetite, reduced libido, social isolation, depression and a loss of hope.

Care, Dignity and Compassion

Patients with chronic pain may present with no visible symptoms of pain (tachycardia, hypertension or diaphoresis, for example). However, the intensity of their pain may be as severe as an episode of acute pain. In such circumstances, individuals will require the same level of comfort and reassurance as those in acute pain. Remember 'Pain is what the patient says it is'.

Superficial and Deep Pain

Pain can be classified according to its location. Pain is often described as being either *deep* or *superficial*. Superficial pain occurs in tissue situated towards the surface of the body, whereas deep pain comes from tissue deep within the body. Deep pain can be either *somatic* or *visceral*. Visceral pain is caused by the stimulation of nociceptors in organs, kidneys, stomach, gall bladder and intestines. Somatic pain arises from structures such as bones, muscles, joints and tendons. Superficial pain is often described as a sharp, pricking sensation, whereas deep pain is described as a duller and more prolonged ache.

Understanding the nature of deep and superficial pain aids pain assessment. Although nociceptors are present in almost all body tissues (except for the brain), they are more abundant in tissue in the outer regions of the body. In deep tissue, such as the organs within the abdomen, nociceptors are fewer in number and are spaced farther apart. As a result, the brain finds it harder to pinpoint the precise location of pain in deep tissue. Injuries that occur closer to the surface of the skin are often more easily located and therefore more readily diagnosed. People experiencing pain that emanates from deep tissue, such as the abdomen, often find it very difficult to describe its exact location. Given the number of organs and structures within the abdomen, it can therefore be difficult for practitioners to make a diagnosis when assessing a patient with acute abdominal pain (Daniels *et al.*, 2020).

Jot This Down

Make a list of all the organs and structures that are found in the abdomen and pelvic regions of the body. Then take some time to think about all the possible conditions that could cause acute abdominal pain.

While pain is an integral part of life, pain expression will differ from individual to individual. This is because pain expression is dependent on a multitude of influencing factors. It is vital that nurses appreciate that pain is an individual and personal experience that will be influenced by life history, culture and psychosocial circumstances. In addition, each individual will ascribe meaning to their pain that is often influenced by circumstances rather than intensity. A broken arm, for instance, may be excruciating but may be less worrying than sudden unexplained intense abdominal pain. The deep somatic pain from the injured bone will cause intense pain. However, while the sudden unexplained abdominal pain may be less intense, the affected individual's pain experience may be exacerbated due to anxiety generated by there being no discernible cause. Pain could also have a positive meaning for some individuals. Postoperative pain, for example, may be considered to be part of the healing process and as healing is a positive and temporary phenomenon, patients may feel more able to cope with and tolerate the pain associated with their surgery. Past pain experience can also be a contributing factor. Patients who have been exposed to severe pain during a prior medical procedure may become anxious about future treatments and ultimately sense greater levels of pain. An individual's circumstances can also influence the pain expression; sports people have been known to 'play' through intense pain and individuals can dismiss pain when dealing with particularly stressful situations, escaping from violent conflict, for instance. People also learn how to express and react to pain by observing those around them. A patient's attitude towards their pain may be influenced by their environment, socio-economic status or ethnicity and culture (Mackintosh-Franklin, 2021).

We should conclude therefore that the management of pain is a significant nursing challenge and that nurses must accept that the pain experience is subjective and requires a holistic and individualised plan of care. It is perhaps for this reason that the most noteworthy explanation of pain is McCaffery's definition, which states that, 'Pain is whatever the experiencing patient says it is, existing when he says it does' (McCaffery, 1979, p.11).

The Nursing Associate

Being an accountable professional
Nursing associates act in the best interests of people in pain, putting them first and providing nursing care that is person centred, safe and compassionate.

This is of particular relevance to Platform 1 – Being an accountable professional. Specifically:

1.4 demonstrate an understanding of, and the ability to, challenge or report discriminatory behaviour

1.11 provide, promote, and where appropriate advocate for, non-discriminatory, person-centred, and sensitive care at all times. Reflect on people's values and beliefs, diverse backgrounds, cultural characteristics, language requirements, needs and preferences, taking account of any need for adjustments

1.12 recognise and report any factors that may adversely impact safe and effective care provision.

NMC (2018b)

Professional and Legal Issues

Comprehensive pain assessment is closely aligned to many of the key aspects of the NMC Code (NMC, 2018a).

Prioritise people
Pain control is a basic human right
Patients need to be involved in decisions about their pain and its control and management
Pain is a psychological as well as physiological experience
Ensure your patient understands any pain assessment and any pain management intervention and why you recommend its use
If a pain control intervention does not work or is inappropriate, try another one

Practise effectively
Nurses should only recommend or implement pain control interventions that are based on the best available evidence
It is vital that all members of the multidisciplinary team are aware of patient preferences and successful pain interventions

Preserve safety
You must continue to assess and re-evaluate individuals with pain
Ensure you are adequately knowledgeable to undertake a pain assessment. If you are not, seek guidance from a more experienced member of staff
Nurses must act if they feel a patient's pain is not being adequately assessed or dealt with
Analgesia, including controlled drugs, must be administered safely and nurses must keep an accurate record of all drugs administered

Promote professionalism and trust
Ensure that the well-being of patients with pain is protected
Nurses must work at all times to ensure that patients requiring assistance with pain control have a positive experience

Influence of Emotion

The limbic system in the brain processes our emotional response to pain. Pain expression is therefore influenced by our personality and state of mind. The limbic system interacts closely with the frontal lobes of the cerebral cortex, which are responsible for cognitive thought. This explains why people may at times act and behave irrationally when in pain. Conversely, individuals are often able to control their emotions when pain occurs, when it is socially unacceptable to cry out or complain. An individual's state of mind has a significant influence on pain intensity and the pain experience. Anxiety and stress can all increase pain intensity, whereas a relaxed or distracted frame of mind can reduce pain sensation (Marieb & Hoehn, 2019).

The Meaning of Pain

Individuals ascribe meaning to their pain experience. This perceived meaning or reason for pain determines its level and intensity. For example, patients recovering from surgery may report less pain than people who have suffered sudden traumatic accidents. The patient recovering from surgery may view their pain as a symptom of surgery and therefore possibly something positive. Their postsurgical pain could be intense, but they may require less analgesia and be more able to cope because, from their perspective, their pain means 'healing' or 'getting better' and possibly relief. In situations when it is difficult to explain why pain has occurred, anxiety and stress can increase and heighten and pain sensation. The individual with sudden acute abdominal pain, for example, may not be able to explain the cause. From the individual's perspective, their pain means 'something is seriously wrong'. Circumstances and outside influences may alter the individual's pain perception and change the meaning of their pain. For instance, slight abdominal pain may be dismissed as a mild 'tummy bug' until the individual discovers that it may be something serious, in which case the pain may become severe and intense. Similarly, pain levels may reduce when the patient learns that the cause of their pain is trivial and/or easily resolved.

Pain Threshold

Care, Dignity and Compassion

Acute pain can be very distressing, and patients may describe their pain as intolerable. Pain relief should be prioritised, and patients will require constant comfort and reassurance.

The term 'pain threshold' is often used to describe an individual's ability to cope with pain; for example, it is not uncommon for people to be described as possessing a 'high or low' pain threshold. Often, social stereotypes and popular culture reinforce this theory, a good example being the popular misconception that women possess higher pain thresholds than men. This interpretation of pain threshold is misleading and unhelpful for nurses aiming to provide optimum care for the patient living with pain.

The pain threshold is the point at which an individual will report pain and it is generally accepted that all humans have a similar pain threshold. Where individuals differ is in the manner in which they express their pain. Nurses should bear in mind that the expression of pain is influenced by emotional state, personality, life experience, culture, social status and current circumstances, rather than a personal pain threshold that is determined by sex or social stereotypes (Coll & Jones, 2020).

Practice Assessment Document

Respects different cultural beliefs and traditions. Is non-judgemental in their approach to care.
By employing a holistic, open-minded approach to pain management, you can demonstrate that you are non-judgemental. When discussing respect for difference with your practice assessor, demonstrating an appreciation for the need for care planning that is individual and not based on preconceptions or stereotypes associated with pain will enable them to gauge your ability to achieve assessments that centre around respect, dignity and holism.

Pain Theory

The nature of pain is a complex and intricate phenomenon, which involves both physiological and psychological changes. Many pain theories have been developed, all of which attempt to conceptualise the influence of both mind and body on the pain experience. Commonly utilised pain theories include the following.

- The *specificity theory*, which hypothesises that pain is sensed when specific neurones are stimulated. Pain sensation is then transmitted to a specific pain centre within the brain. However, rather than the brain interpreting pain, it is the characteristics of the original stimulus that determine the intensity of the pain.
- The *pattern theory* postulates that there is no separate system dedicated to pain transmission and sensation, but rather pain is sensed and interpreted by the brain when intense peripheral nerve stimulation occurs.
- The *gate control theory* proposes that pain messages must pass through a theoretical 'gate' situated at the dorsal horn of the spinal cord. The wider the opening of the gate, the greater the level of pain experienced. Noxious substances force the gate open, whereas positive descending brain activity seeks to close the gate. Levels of pain are therefore determined by the balance of injury and an individual's psychological response to their pain.

For a more detailed breakdown of the gate control theory of pain, please refer to Wheeldon (2021).

Pain Assessment

Pain is a complex multifaceted phenomenon, and its assessment poses a significant nursing challenge. Nevertheless, effective pain management is essential if the nurse is to plan and implement an appropriate range of both pharmacological and non-pharmacological interventions. The pain experience involves four interlinked dimensions (Figure 22.2). Nursing assessment must pay attention to physiological, psychological, emotional and social aspects of pain, if effective holistic care is to be achieved. Accurate nursing assessment can also be hampered by the subjective nature of the pain experience. Nurses must often rely upon the patient's description of their pain. Many patients, however, are unable to verbalise or describe their pain and in such instances, nurses must look for visual non-verbal cues.

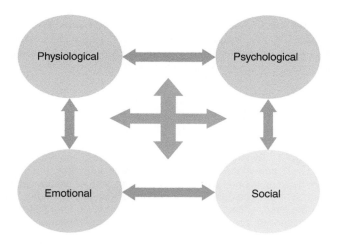

Figure 22.2 The four dimensions of the pain experience.

However, a description of pain is rarely enough to determine appropriate treatment. Further information on the location, duration and onset of pain can assist nurses and other healthcare professionals when establishing the extent, nature and impact of an individual's pain. Every pain assessment must include the following.

- The location of the pain – where is the pain, does it move or radiate elsewhere?
- The duration of the pain – how long has the patient been in pain?
- Onset – when did the pain start and what was the patient doing at the time?
- Frequency – is the pain constant or spasmodic; if spasmodic, how often does the pain occur and for how long does it last?
- Intensity – how painful is it, does the level of pain ever change?
- Aggravating factors – does anything make the pain worse?
- Relieving factors – does anything make the pain feel better?
- Sleep – does the pain disturb sleep; does it keep the patient awake at night?
- Other symptoms – does the pain cause other associated symptoms, i.e. dizziness, nausea, vomiting, shortness of breath, loss of appetite, diaphoresis (adapted from Mackintosh-Franklin, 2021 and Ford, 2019).

Pain assessment must also address the patient's psychological and emotional response to their pain. Therefore, every pain assessment must gather information on the following.

- The individual's expectations of any potential treatments.
- The individual's concerns about the cause of their pain.
- Does the individual have any personal or spiritual beliefs?
- What level of pain would the individual find acceptable?
- What level of pain would allow the individual to return to work?
- Does the individual have any feelings of stress of anxiety?
- Does the individual use any coping strategies?
- What are the individual's preferences regarding treatment options? (Adapted from Ingadottir & Zoega, 2017 and Quinn, 2020).

Acute pain will produce an autonomic response and often, patients will present with the signs and symptoms of stress. Therefore the following would also need to be recorded.

- Blood pressure – many patients in pain can experience hypertension.
- Pulse – to check for tachycardia.
- Respiratory rate – pain often produces changes in respiratory rate. Tachypnoea may suggest stress. Shallow respiratory effort is indicative of thoracic pain. Patients in acute pain may also periodically hold their breath.

Pain Assessment Tools

Formal structured pain assessment tools can facilitate and enhance the nurse's pain assessment. There are a wide variety of pain assessment tools at the nurse's disposal, ranging from simple single-dimension scales to comprehensive pain questionnaires. The verbal rating scale, the visual analogue rating scale and the numerical rating scale are the three most commonly used single-dimension scales. The verbal rating scale (Figure 22.3) asks the patient to select an adjective, from a predetermined list, which best describes their pain. The verbal analogue scale uses a numerical scale, 0–10 or 0–3 for example, from which the patient selects the number that most accurately represents their pain. Numbers at the lower end of the scale signify low or no pain, whereas the higher numbers represent intolerable or worst pain imaginable (Figure 22.4). The visual analogue scale has a more basic format. It consists simply of a rudimentary continuum, which runs from no pain to the worst pain imaginable. The patient can point or state where on the continuum their pain is (Figure 22.5).

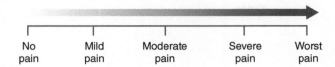

Figure 22.3 **The verbal rating scale.**

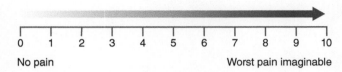

Figure 22.4 **The verbal analogue scale.**

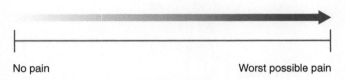

Figure 22.5 **The visual analogue scale.**

The main advantage of simple scales such as these is their ease of use. They can be utilised swiftly and do not overburden an individual in acute pain. However, it should be remembered that these scales only assess one aspect of pain, its intensity, and there is an assumption that the patient will be literate.

A common example of a multidimensional pain assessment tool is the McGill Pain Questionnaire (Figure 22.6). The McGill Pain Questionnaire is a comprehensive assessment tool that comprises a series of descriptive terms from which the patient selects the most appropriate to describe their pain. The adjectives are separated into the three classes: sensory, affective and evaluative. The assessment tool also utilises a simple rating scale, which runs from 0 (no pain) to 5 (excruciating). The assessment of pain is based on three separate measures: the pain rating index (PRI), which is based on numerical values assigned to each number, the number of words selected and the rating scale or present pain index (PPI). The McGill Pain Questionnaire also utilises line drawings of the human body that can facilitate the identification of the location of the pain.

In order to simplify pain assessment, tools that utilise mnemonics are popular among nurses and can ensure a comprehensive and holistic approach. Two good examples are OPQRST and SOCRATES, with each mnemonic listing important areas that the nurse must explore with their patient if they are to execute a thorough assessment of the pain experience. OPQRST, for example, stands for *onset, provokes, quality, radiates, severity* and *time* whereas SOCRATES stands for *site, onset, character, radiates, associations, timing, exacerbating factors* and *severity* (Ford, 2019).

What to Do If . . .

 . . . my patient doesn't speak English
Most pain assessment tools rely on self-reporting. Therefore, if your patient does not speak English or they

have difficulty communicating, you should observe for the visual signs of pain. People in pain often display visible symptoms of discomfort, such as grimacing, guarding and sweating. Their demeanour may also suggest they are in pain, for example, they may be irritable, angry, upset or very still and quiet. You may also wish to explore the use of visual rating scales that use faces as indicators of discomfort. The Wong-Baker FACES tool (Figure 22.7), originally devised for children, has been used to good effect in adults too (Kettyle, 2018).

Platform 3 – Assessing needs and planning care
Registered nurses prioritise the needs of people when assessing and reviewing their pain.
Specifically:
- 3.2 demonstrate and apply knowledge of body systems and homeostasis, human anatomy and physiology, biology, genomics, pharmacology, and social and behavioural sciences when undertaking full and accurate person-centred nursing assessments and developing appropriate care plans
- 3.4 understand and apply a person-centred approach to nursing care, demonstrating shared assessment, planning, decision making and goal setting when working with people, their families, communities, and populations of all ages
- 3.15 demonstrate the ability to work in partnership with people, families, and carers to continuously monitor, evaluate and reassess the effectiveness of all agreed nursing care plans and care, sharing decision making and readjusting agreed goals, documenting progress and decisions made
- 3.16 demonstrate knowledge of when and how to refer people safely to other professionals or services for clinical intervention or support.

Pain Management

Pain management is associated with the use of pain-relieving medications. However, there are also a number of non-pharmacological pain management interventions. As the name suggests, 'non-pharmacological pain management' does not involve any drugs. As pain is a total experience, effective pain control is often achieved through a combination of both approaches.

Pharmacological Interventions

Pharmacological preparations administered for the relief of pain are referred to as *analgesia* or *analgesics*. There are two main types of analgesia:

- Opioids (or opiates)
- Non-opioids.

Opioids (Opiates)

Opioids should be prescribed for moderate-to-severe pain. Opioids mimic the body's own endogenous opiates (endorphins, enkephalins and dynorphins) and bind to opiate receptors within the central nervous system. Opiate receptors such as mu (μ),

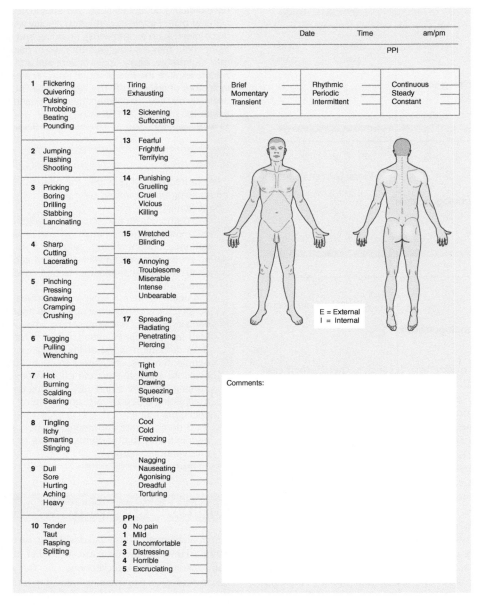

Figure 22.6 The McGill Pain Questionnaire.

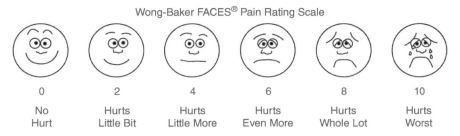

Figure 22.7 The Wong-Baker FACES Pain Rating Scale. *Source:* © 1983 Wong-Baker FACES Foundation. www.WongBakerFACES.org, used with permission.

374

kappa (κ), sigma (σ) and delta (δ), if stimulated, block the action of substance P, the neurotransmitter responsible for the transmission of pain. However, opioids differ from endogenous opiates in that they are not rapidly broken down by the body. As a result, their analgesic properties are powerful and long-lasting (MacIntyre & Schug, 2021).

Stimulation of the central nervous system's opiate receptors not only produces pain relief; it can also produce other, often unwanted, side-effects (Table 22.2).

Jot This Down

Have a look at the list of side-effects in Table 22.2 and take some time to think about the effects opiates may have on those who are addicted to their use.

Red Flag Side-effects of opiate analgesia

 Opiate analgesia has many unwanted side-effects (see Table 22.2). Nurses should continually assess for the presence of side-effects as left untreated, they could be detrimental to the patient's well-being. Important side-effects to look out for are:
- Respiratory depression
- Nausea and vomiting
- Constipation
- Bradycardia and hypotension.

The administration of opioids is governed by the Misuse of Drugs Act 1971and is therefore subject to strict regulation.

Table 22.2 Actions of opiate receptors.

RECEPTOR	PHYSIOLOGICAL EFFECTS
Mu (μ)	Analgesia Euphoria Respiratory depression Bradycardia Nausea and vomiting Inhibition of gut motility Miosis Pruritus Smooth muscle spasm Physical dependence
Kappa (κ)	Analgesia Sedation Dysphoria Respiratory depression Physical dependence
Delta (δ)	Analgesia Euphoria Respiratory depression Miosis Inhibition of gut motility Smooth muscle spasm Physical dependence

Opioids are classified as either weak or strong. Despite their name, weak opioids are very strong analgesic agents. Strong opioids commonly used include:
- Buprenorphine – Temgesic®, Transtec®, Butrans®, Subutex®
- Diamorphine
- Dipipanone – Diconal®
- Fentanyl – Durogesic®, Matrifen®, Effentora®, Abstral®
- Hydromorphone – Palladone®
- Methadone
- Morphine – Oromorph®, Sevredol®, morphine sulfate tablets, Zomorph®
- Oxycodone – Oxynorm®, Oxycontin®
- Pentacozine
- Pethidine
- Tramadol – Zydol®, Zamadol®.

Weak opioids commonly prescribed include:
- Codeine
- Dextropropoxyphene
- Dihydrocodeine – DF118®
- Meptazinol – Meptid®.

Practice Assessment Document

 Applies knowledge of basic pharmacology and how medicines interact with body systems.
Knowing how analgesics work and their major side-effects is a vital if patient safety is to be maintained. Demonstrating an understanding of the differences between opioid and non-opioid analgesics and their major side-effects may enable your practice assessor to establish your safety in the administration of medicines. When looking to achieve skills associated with pharmacology, explaining the impact analgesia has on people is a good way of demonstrating knowledge.

Patient-controlled Analgesia

In many instances, after surgery for example, patients can administer their own opioid pain relief via a system known as patient-controlled analgesia (PCA). A small syringe that contains the prescribed opioid drug is attached to the patient via a small subcutaneous needle. The syringe is operated by a button, which when pressed by the patient delivers a set dosage. After each dose, the syringe driver locks for a short time to ensure that no drug can be delivered even if the button is pressed, therefore protecting the individual against overdose (for a more detailed exploration of patient-controlled analgesia, see Chapter 20).

Red Flag A patient with no visible signs of pain requests opiate analgesia

One concern in situations such as these is that the request is due to dependence rather than analgesia. Nurses must remember that pain is what the patient says it is and it would be unethical to leave a patient in pain. However, under the Misuse of Drugs Act 1971, prescribers should not prescribe diamorphine to an addict or suspected addict without a special Home Office licence. In such situations, it will be the prescriber's decision, but the nurse must act as the patient's advocate and act in their best interests.

Non-opioid Drugs

Non-opioid analgesia drugs are prescribed for mild-to-moderate pain. As such, they are rarely effective in acute or postoperative pain control. They are mainly associated with transient pain, such as muscle strains or headaches. In the main, non-opioid analgesic medications are either:

- Non-steroidal anti-inflammatory drugs (NSAIDs), or
- Paracetamol (acetaminophen).

Paracetamol (acetaminophen) is the most common non-opioid drug. Its precise pharmacological action remains controversial but it is widely accepted that it suppresses the production of prostaglandins. Prostaglandins are hormone-like substances that stimulate and maintain inflammatory processes. They also chemically stimulate nociceptors, which in turn innervate first-order neurones and send pain signals towards the central nervous system and promote pain sensation. Despite being an effective analgesic, paracetamol rarely maintains its analgesic effects for longer than 4 hours and as a result, may not be appropriate for prolonged pain. Although considered a relatively safe pharmacological preparation, paracetamol can cause liver failure, even in small doses (McFadden, 2019).

Medicines Management

 Paracetamol if used correctly can be an effective and safe analgesia. However, liver failure can occur even in small overdoses. Care should be taken to ensure that the drug is administered as prescribed and its use in patients with liver disease should be avoided.

Non-steroidal anti-inflammatory drugs (NSAIDs) also suppress prostaglandin production. Prostaglandins are derived from arachidonic acid, which is released from damaged cells (as a result of trauma, inflammation and so forth). The production of prostaglandins from arachidonic acid is accelerated by the actions of an enzyme called cyclo-oxygenase 2 (COX-2) (Figure 22.8). NSAIDs inhibit the actions of COX-2 and therefore the production of prostaglandins is severely reduced. As a result, inflammation is condensed, and pain signals are diminished. In addition to the suppression of COX-2, NSAIDs may also suppress a similar enzyme called cyclo-oxygenase 1 (COX-1). Unlike COX-2, COX-1 promotes prostaglandin production in the stomach, where it plays an important role in the protection of the stomach wall from erosion by gastric acid. A major side-effect of NSAIDs therefore is the development of gastric irritation and ulcers. Care should also be taken in patients with respiratory disease as NSAIDs are also associated with hypersensitive reactions in people with asthma (McFadden, 2019).

There are many different NSAIDs used within the UK (Box 22.1). However, the major drugs used include:

- Aspirin
- Ibuprofen
- Diclofenac – Volterol®
- Indomethacin
- Naproxen.

Medicines Management

 One of the most likely side-effects of NSAIDs is gastric irritation and drugs such as ibuprofen, diclofenac, indomethacin and naproxen should be administered either with or just after food to minimise the risk.

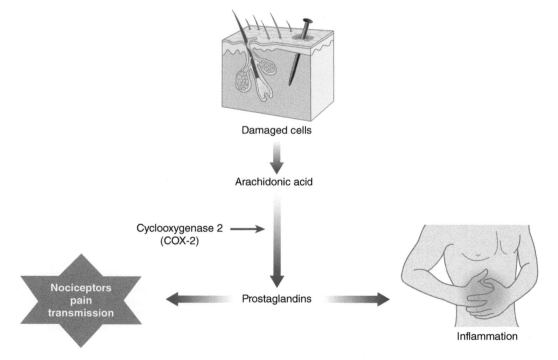

Damaged cells

Arachidonic acid

Cyclooxygenase 2 (COX-2)

Nociceptors pain transmission

Prostaglandins

Inflammation

Figure 22.8 **The action of cyclo-oxygenase-2 (COX-2) in enhancing prostaglandin action.**

Box 22.1 Common NSAIDs, with trade names in brackets

Aceclofenac (Preservex®)
Etoricoxib (Arcoxia®)
Mefenamic acid (Ponstan®)
Acemetacin (Emflex®)
Fenbufen (Fenbufen®)
Meloxican (Mobic®)
Aspirin (Caprin®)
Fenoprofen (Fenopron®)
Nabumetone (Relifex®)
Azapropazone (Rheumox®)
Flurbiprofen (Froben®)
Naproxen (Arthroxen®)
Celecoxib (Celebrex®)
Ibuprofen (Brufen®)
Piroxicam (Brexidol®)
Dexibuprofen (Seractil®)
Indometacin (Rimacid®)
Sulindac (Clinoril®)
Dexketoprofen (Keral®)
Ketoprofen (Orudis®)
Tenoxicam (Mobiflex®)
Diclofenac (Volterol®)
Tiaprofenic acid (Surgam®)
Etodolac

In addition to analgesia, non-opioid drugs have other potentially therapeutic effects, i.e. temperature control and prophylaxis of heart disease. Because prostaglandins promote pyrexia in addition to inflammation, NSAIDs and paracetamol may reduce core body temperature and are often prescribed solely to counteract pyrexia. Aspirin, in addition to analgesia, has antiplatelet properties. When used in small doses, it has been shown to reduce the risk of cardiovascular disease; it is also used in large doses in patients with a suspected myocardial infarction (MI) (McFadden, 2019).

Opioid and Non-opioid Combinations

Some opioids are combined pharmacologically with non-opioid analgesic drugs, such as paracetamol and aspirin. A combination of opioid and non-opioid drugs can reduce opioid usage by 20–40% (Macintyre & Schug, 2021). Such combinations are often prescription-only medications, rather than controlled drugs (HMSO, 1968).

Examples of common, weak opioid and non-opioid analgesic combinations are:

- Co-codamol – codeine phosphate combined with paracetamol
- Co-codaprin – codeine phosphate combined with aspirin
- Co-dydramol – dihydrocodeine combined with paracetamol
- Tramacet – tramadol combined with paracetamol.

The Analgesic Ladder

The analgesic ladder was first produced by the World Health Organization (WHO) in 1986. It postulates that there are three rungs or levels of treatment. On each rung, there is a recommended level of pharmacological treatment (Figure 22.9). The aim is for the patient to be on the lowest point on the ladder that keeps them pain free. Treatment therefore should start on the lowest rung of the ladder and if unsuccessful, it should be escalated to the

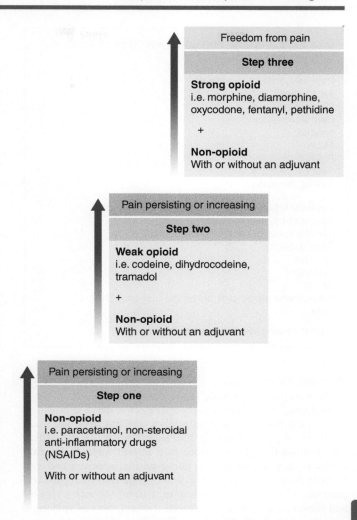

Freedom from pain

Step three

Strong opioid
i.e. morphine, diamorphine, oxycodone, fentanyl, pethidine

+

Non-opioid
With or without an adjuvant

Pain persisting or increasing

Step two

Weak opioid
i.e. codeine, dihydrocodeine, tramadol

+

Non-opioid
With or without an adjuvant

Pain persisting or increasing

Step one

Non-opioid
i.e. paracetamol, non-steroidal anti-inflammatory drugs (NSAIDs)

With or without an adjuvant

Figure 22.9 The WHO analgesic ladder (WHO, 1986).

next step. Step one involves the use of non-opioid drugs, step two recommends a weak opioid, and the final stage advocates the use of strong opioids. Each rung of the ladder also suggests the use of an adjuvant. Adjuvants are a range of drugs that are normally prescribed for non-pain-related conditions, but if used in conjunction with analgesia, can enhance their painkiller effect. Antidepressants, anticonvulsants, muscle relaxants, steroids and local anaesthetics have all been shown to reduce pain when used in conjunction with opioid and non-opioid drugs.

The WHO analgesic ladder has been used for simple and valuable pain-relieving guidance in pharmaceutical pain management for many years. However, with the development of medical history, notions about pain physiology and pain management, it needs to be used with caution and adapted to meet pain-relieving needs.

Non-pharmacological Pain Management

A wide variety of non-pharmacological pain management interventions are widely available (Box 22.2). They are divided into two distinct categories:

- Physical interventions – i.e. TENS machines, massage and acupuncture
- Psychological interventions – i.e. talking therapies.

Box 22.2 Popular non-pharmacological methods of pain management

Psychological interventions
Art therapy
Distraction
Herbal remedies
Imagery
Music
Relaxation
Rest
Talking therapies

Physical interventions
Acupuncture/acupressure
Application of hot and cold substances
Body position
Exercise
Massage
Tai chi
Transcutaneous electric nerve stimulation (TENS)
Yoga

Source: Adapted from Cunningham (2017).

Physical Interventions

Many non-pharmacological pain control techniques have a physiological basis. A transcutaneous electric nerve stimulation (TENS) machine, for example, sends a constant stream of small electrical impulses through the skin (Figure 22.10). These impulses are thought to reduce pain in two ways. In the first instance, they are thought to stimulate the neurones that can transfer messages of touch, heat and cold quicker than pain and therefore interrupt the pain impulses travelling along smaller and slower neurones, in very much the same way as rubbing a mild injury can alleviate discomfort. Second, the continuous electrical stimulation could increase circulating levels of endogenous opiates, such as endorphins within the central nervous system (MacIntyre & Schug, 2018). TENS machines are widely

used for the treatment of acute and chronic pain, phantom limb pain and lower back pain. Despite this wide use and positive patient feedback, evidence of its effectiveness remains inconclusive (Gibson *et al.*, 2019).

Acupuncture entails the insertion of fine needles at a multitude of strategic anatomical points around the human body to alleviate pain (Appleyard, 2018). Acupuncture is widely used throughout the world and is accepted as an effective analgesia in many countries and research into its use for cancer pain, fibromyalgia, headaches, chronic back pain has demonstrated that people find it beneficial (Linde *et al.*, 2016; Mu *et al.*, 2020).

Psychological Interventions

Given that pain is an individual, personal and holistic experience, the psychological aspects are an integral element of the pain experience. Any psychological intervention that aims to alleviate anxiety or stress or is able to help the individual to cope with their pain could be beneficial.

There are many psychological pain control interventions at the nurse's disposal (see Box 22.2). The most commonly used psychological non-pharmacological approaches to pain management are talking therapies, such as cognitive behavioural therapy (CBT) and dialectic behavioural therapy (DLT). Both have been shown to help people live with chronic pain (Williams *et al.*, 2020; Barret *et al.*, 2021). The National Institute for Health and Care Excellence (NICE) also recommends talking therapies such as CBT and Acceptance and Commitment Therapy (ACT) to enable people over the age of 16 to cope with chronic pain (NICE, 2021).

The Nursing Associate

A **Provide and monitor care**
Nursing associates must provide compassionate, safe and effective support to people living with and experiencing pain.
This is of particular relevance to Platform 3 – Provide and Monitor Care. Specifically:
3.2 demonstrate and apply knowledge of body systems and homeostasis, human anatomy and physiology, biology, genomics, pharmacology, social and behavioural sciences when delivering care
3.8 demonstrate and apply an understanding of how people's needs for safety, dignity, privacy, comfort and sleep can be met
3.12 demonstrate the knowledge and skills required to support people with commonly encountered symptoms including anxiety, confusion, discomfort and pain
3.16 demonstrate the ability to recognise the effects of medicines, allergies, drug sensitivity, side effects, contraindications and adverse reactions.

Source: NMC (2018b)

Platform 4 - Providing and evaluating care

Registered nurses take the lead in providing evidence-based, compassionate and safe nursing interventions when caring for an individual in pain.
Specifically:
4.1 demonstrate and apply an understanding of what is important to people and how to use this knowledge to ensure their needs for safety, dignity, privacy, comfort

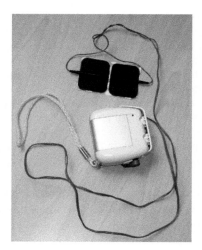

Figure 22.10 Transcutaneous electrical nerve stimulation (TENS) machine. *Source:* Nair, M. & Peate, I. (eds) (2013) *Fundamentals of Applied Physiology.* Reproduced with permission of John Wiley & Sons Ltd.

and sleep can be met, acting as a role model for others in providing evidence-based person-centred care

4.5 demonstrate the knowledge and skills required to support people with commonly encountered physical health conditions, their medication usage and treatments, and act as a role model for others in providing high quality nursing interventions when meeting people's needs

4.8 demonstrate the knowledge and skills required to identify and initiate appropriate interventions to support people with commonly encountered symptoms including anxiety, confusion, discomfort, and pain

4.14 understand the principles of safe and effective administration and optimisation of medicines in accordance with local and national policies and demonstrate proficiency and accuracy when calculating dosages of prescribed medicines

Nursing Management of Acute Pain

Acute pain is an indicator of tissue damage. It is associated with a sudden onset and is often described in terms such as 'excruciating', 'unbearable' and 'intolerable'. Despite causing discomfort, acute pain has a limited lifespan and reduces as healing progresses. Acute pain is not a diagnosis; it is a symptom and nurses should tailor their assessments and interventions to suit the nature or cause of their patient's acute pain, be it postoperative, abdominal pain, chest pain, burns or musculoskeletal.

Signs and Symptoms

Acute pain is associated with an autonomic nervous system response and individuals may present with signs and symptoms of stress. Acute pain is an emotional as well as physical experience and individuals may also verbalise their pain and may visually project their suffering. The major signs and symptoms of acute pain are:

- Tachycardia
- Hypertension
- Diaphoresis
- Altered respiratory rate
- Increased muscle tension
- Cool and clammy skin and peripheries
- Reduced peripheral blood flow
- Vomiting
- Anxiety, fear
- Altered facial expression, i.e. grimace
- Verbalisation of pain
- Agitation, restlessness, anger, irritability
- Guarding.

Investigations and Diagnosis

- Pain assessment
- Remember pain is what the patient says it is

Nursing Care and Management

The main nursing aims for the patient in acute postoperative pain are to reduce discomfort and promote healing and recovery and the main nursing objectives are:

- An accurate pain assessment (see Pain Assessment section) – in order to best establish choice of interventions
- Safe administration of prescribed analgesia (see Opioid and Non-opioid analgesia section)
- Monitor for evidence of the main side-effects of opioid therapy (Box 22.3)
- Use of psychological interventions such as relaxation, distraction and imagery to complement pharmacological interventions
- Monitor patient for signs and symptoms of stress – to evaluate success of nursing strategies
- Regularly reassess pain intensity – to evaluate success of pharmacological and psychological interventions.

Consequences of Unresolved Acute Pain

Prolonged acute pain can result in pathophysiological changes that can have further detrimental effects on well-being. The individual facing unresolved acute pain may also experience symptoms associated with respiration, cardiovascular function, mobility and gastrointestinal problems.

Acute Pain and Respiration

Pain in the thoracic region may result in an involuntary reduction in muscle contraction in the chest and abdominal area. Clinicians often refer to this phenomenon as 'muscle splinting', which means that muscles contract on either side of the injury in order to 'splint' the area and prevent movement. Closure of the glottis can also occur, and individuals can present with a 'grunting' breathing sound. This response is a natural defence mechanism, which facilitates along with muscle spasms an increased intra-abdominal and intrathoracic pressure that braces against an impending injury.

Respiratory changes if left untreated will lead to reduced respiratory function and in turn regional atelectasis. The development of atelectasis results in reduced gaseous exchange and the development of hypoxaemia and hypoxia. Splinting can also result in an inability to cough and clear chest secretions, increasing the likelihood of chest infections.

Acute Pain and Cardiovascular Function

The stress response associated with the acute pain experience increases cardiovascular workload. Stress responses increase heart rate, peripheral resistance, blood pressure and cardiac heart rate. The resultant escalation in cardiac effort will increase myocardial oxygen consumption. Simultaneously, intensification of heart rate also reduces diastolic filling time and oxygen delivery to the myocardium. In the patient with acute pain, there is the potential for a mismatch between myocardial oxygen demand and myocardial oxygen delivery and the potential for myocardial ischaemia and chest pain. Patients with pre-existing cardiac disease are at greater risk of such an event. Unresolved acute pain and prolonged autonomic stress responses are also associated with reduced arterial flow and reduced venous emptying.

> **Box 22.3 Major Side-effects of Opioid Therapy**
>
> - Respiratory depression
> - Bradycardia
> - Nausea and vomiting
> - Drowsiness
> - Hypotension

379

Acute Pain and Mobility

Acute muscular pain promotes muscle spasm and increased pain on movement. As a result, the patient becomes locked in a vicious circle of increased anxiety, increased pain and lack of mobility. A reduction of mobility is associated with reduced muscle metabolism, atrophy and a delayed return to normal muscle function.

Acute Pain and Gastrointestinal Function

The stress response associated with acute pain increases intestinal secretions and smooth muscle sphincter tone but slows down intestinal motility. Gastric stasis and paralytic ileus may also occur. The reduced intestinal motility may be detrimental to the patient's nutritional status.

Postoperative Pain

Pain after surgery remains a significant healthcare quality issue. Worldwide, 65–90% of patients report pain in the aftermath of surgery, with 30% reporting severe pain (Ingadottir & Zoega, 2017). A significant contributory factor to postoperative pain is anxiety, which can increase pain intensity. Anxiety and depression prior to surgery lead to high levels of anxiety postoperatively. In order to reduce postoperative pain, nurses and allied health professionals should select appropriate preoperative care interventions that counteract the impact of preoperative anxiety, including patient education (Powell et al., 2016). Nurses are ideally placed to minimise postoperative pain as they are responsible for the administration and evaluation of prescribed analgesics.

The main nursing objective for the patient in acute pain post surgery is the minimisation of the impact of their pain. This is because unresolved pain leads to a complicated postsurgical recovery. Pain in the chest or abdomen, for example, can affect respiration. The resultant tendency to breathe shallowly and avoid coughing can cause retention of secretions and possibly chest infection. Painful movement can also render patients reluctant to mobilise, which when coupled with reduced arterial inflow and venous emptying leads to an increased risk of venous thromboembolism and pulmonary emptying. Acute postoperative pain can reduce gastric emptying and intestinal motility. The resultant decreased nutrition will reduce healing and lead to prolonged recovery.

Protracted acute pain also increases anxiety, which can have a severe detrimental effect on the patient's postoperative recovery. Prolonged anxiety will lead to a stress response as the body attempts to maintain homeostasis. During stress, numerous hormones released by the neuroendocrine system increase blood pressure and myocardial oxygen consumption. Metabolism, wound healing and respiration are also adversely affected, and patients can also be at risk of venous thromboembolism, urinary retention and muscle wasting (Macintyre & Schug, 2021).

Case Study

Ikram Mahmood

Ikram is a 56-year-old social worker who has undergone a right nephrectomy to remove a tumour. Twenty-four hours after their surgery, Ikram is still experiencing severe pain. On assessment, Ikram's wound is clean and dry and their vital signs are within normal ranges. However, Ikram informs the nurse that the pain is debilitating and does

not wish to be moved or disturbed. They describe the pain as being intense and 9 out of 10. When trying to move, Ikram winces and grimaces, and clearly looks upset and in some discomfort. The nurse asks if Ikram has any concerns of anxieties and they state that the pain is worse than anticipated and is concerned that it means that something is wrong.

The nurse talks to Ikram about their surgery and that everyone's pain is different. They administer prescribed analgesia and help Ikram into a position that is more comfortable. The nurse also encourages Ikram to read the books their partner had left for them. When the nurse assesses Ikram later that morning, they note that Ikram is experiencing less pain and feels less anxious.

Jot This Down

Unresolved postoperative pain can prolong recovery and lead to postoperative complications. Make a list of all the potential complications that could occur if postoperative pain is not effectively managed.

Acute Abdominal Pain

Abdominal pain is a very common symptom that occurs in all age groups. In many cases, abdominal pain has no apparent physical cause and symptoms subside spontaneously. Nevertheless, acute abdominal pain has several causes and diagnosis and determination of the cause of pain can be problematic. To aid diagnosis, the abdomen is divided into quadrants and the location of the pain informs clinicians on the most likely cause (Box 22.4).

Box 22.4 Common Causes of Acute Abdominal Pain

Left upper quadrant	Right upper quadrant
Perisplenitis	Acute cholecystitis
Splenic infarct	Biliary colic
	Acute hepatic distension or inflammation
	Perforated duodenal ulcer

Left lower quadrant	Right lower quadrant
Acute diverticulitis	Acute appendicitis
Pyogenic sacroiliitis	Mesenteric lymphadenitis
	Infective distal ileitis
	Crohn's disease
	Acute pyelonephritis
	Acute cholecystitis
	Acute rheumatic fever
	Ectopic pregnancy
	Ruptured ovarian cyst

Central abdominal pain

Gastroenteritis
Small intestinal colic
Acute pancreatitis

Case Study

Lisa Boakye

Lisa is a 28-year-old teacher who was brought into the emergency department by their partner after complaining of severe abdominal pain for the past 2 hours. On examination, Lisa is cold and clammy to touch. Lisa tells the nurse that the pain started in the middle of the tummy but has now moved to the lower right-hand side of the abdomen. Lisa also feels nauseous but has not vomited. The nurse administers a prescribed opioid analgesia and explains that Lisa will need to undergo an ultrasound scan to establish the cause of the pain. On their return from the scan, Lisa tells the nurse that although they remain anxious their pain is less intense and they are more comfortable.

Jot This Down

Acute abdominal pain can cause anxiety and distress. How might you assess the impact of an individual experiencing sudden and severe pain?

Chest Pain

Acute onset of chest pain is a common presentation in many emergency departments. Chest pain is normally associated with myocardial pathology but there are many other causes of chest pain which relate to other parts of the body, most notably the respiratory system (Table 22.3). For a more detailed description of the treatment of chest pain, see the appropriate chapter in this book. However, it is noteworthy that the first-line treatment for myocardial chest pain is opioid analgesia, which is used for both pain relief and reduction of anxiety and therefore a reduced cardiac workload.

Burns

Pain control for burns victims presents a significant nursing challenge. This is due to a variety of different components that contribute to the severe pain people with burns experience. These multiple components ensure that there is constant changing

Table 22.3 Main Causes of Chest Pain.

CAUSE	
Cardiovascular	Myocardial infarction
	Unstable angina
Pulmonary	Pleurisy
	Pulmonary embolism
	Pneumothorax
	Pneumonia
Musculoskeletal	Costocondritis
	Trauma
Gastrointestinal	Reflux
	Gastric ulcers
	Gallstones
	Pancreatitis
Psychological	Anxiety

pattern to the patient's pain, resulting in complex analgesic prescription issues. It is vital that nurses caring for burns victims fully appreciate and recognise the factors that contribute to their pain experience. The contributing factors can be categorised as:

- Background pain
- Breakthrough pain
- Procedural pain
- Pain associated with tissue regeneration.

Background pain is the pain that emanates from the burn wound sites and the surrounding areas. Pain may also be present in areas of normal skin that have been harvested for skin grafts (donor sites). This pain will be constant and at times excruciating. Movement, such as walking, changing position or in some instances breathing, can cause *breakthrough pain*, which will exacerbate the patient's background pain. *Procedural pain* is caused by the numerous necessary procedures carried out by nurses and other healthcare workers, which form part of their therapeutic treatments, such as wound cleansing, dressing changes and physiotherapy. Finally, *pain associated with tissue regeneration* concerns the pain associated with the healing process and the regeneration of nerve tissue. Patients often describe the pain of regeneration as being an itching or intense tingling sensation.

What the Experts Say Pain associated with re-dressing burns

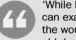

'While burns themselves can cause intense pain, we can exacerbate this pain when we re-dress or debride the wound. Pain can also result from the removal of old dressings. We need to take extra care when cleaning and re-dressing wounds caused by burns to ensure we don't cause any extra or unnecessary pain. Take extra care when re-dressing burns and be judicious in your choice of dressing. Always seek expert help when dealing with wounds, especially when frequent dressing changes are required.'

Alvin Salvador, senior emergency nurse

Nursing Management of Chronic Pain

Chronic pain is a pain sensation that occurs in the absence of any obvious biological cause. In many instances, individuals develop chronic pain over time and it is associated with unresolved prolonged acute pain, which leaves the sufferer in chronic pain even though the injured tissue has fully healed. It is often classified as a psychological phenomenon and often described as 'pain syndrome', suggesting that the pain sensation is a maladaptive psychological response to a protracted pain response. There are, however, a number of chronic health conditions that are associated with chronic pain, Chronic musculoskeletal disorders such as back pain, neuropathies, arthritis and cancer pain are common examples of chronic conditions that cause chronic pain, but cardiovascular disease, gastrointestinal disease, diabetes, stroke and multiple sclerosis are also associated with chronic pain.

Signs and Symptoms

The stress responses associated with acute pain are difficult to maintain over sustained periods of time. People living with chronic pain therefore may not present with the some of the cardinal signs of pain, i.e. tachycardia, hypertension and diaphoresis. Chronic pain often results in long-term debilitating psychological effects and those experiencing chronic pain may measure their pain by reporting the impact it has on their life. Factors the nurse must consider include:

- Sleep patterns – does the pain keep the patient awake?
- Appetite – does the patient have reduced appetite?
- Libido – does the patient's pain have a negative impact on their sex life?
- Social isolation – is the patient able to maintain social activities?
- Depression.

Investigations and Diagnosis
- Pain assessment.
- Remember pain is what the patient says it is.

Nursing Care and Management
The main nursing aim for the individual living with chronic pain is to reduce the impact of chronic pain on quality of life. The major nursing objectives are:

- An accurate pain assessment (see Pain Assessment section) – in order to best establish choice of interventions
- Safe administration of prescribed analgesia (see Opioid and Non-opioid analgesia section)
- Monitor for evidence of the main side-effects of opioid therapy (see Box 22.3)
- Use of psychological interventions such as relaxation, distraction and imagery
- Consider talking therapies
- Establish a pain management plan
- Monitor the individual's quality of care
- Refer to chronic pain services (Box 22.5).

Box 22.5 Functions of Pain Management Services
- Introduction of pain policies, protocols and guidelines
- Education of staff and patients
- Audit and evaluation of services
- Alleviation of pain
- Reduction of disability and restoration of function
- Rationalisation of medication
- Rationalisation of use of all health services
- Attention to social, family and occupational issues
- Ensuring a multidisciplinary approach to chronic pain

Case Study

Luke Stokes
Luke is a 48-year-old delivery driver who has been suffering from lower back pain for the past 6 months. The intensity of the pain has increased gradually over the past couple of days, and as a result Luke has not been able to go to work. Luke has a very physical job, working for a removals firm, and believes continual lifting is the source of the pain. The pain is such that sleep is difficult and sitting is uncomfortable. Today, Luke has visited the general practice (GP) for more advice. Luke is recovering from a traumatic relationship breakdown and has recently moved away, to start a new life.

Luke feels lonely and low and informs the nurse that finding new friends has been difficult. The nurse refers Luke to the local pain management service, where nurses help them to explore the impact of their work and social issues on pain. In the weeks that follow, Luke feels their pain is more manageable and is sleeping better. They also feel more able to socialise and enjoy their work.

Jot This Down
How does mental health exacerbate the pain experience? Explore how mental health impacts on chronic pain and how pain management services can enable people to live with their pain.

Arthritis
Arthritis encompasses over 100 conditions, with rheumatoid arthritis and osteoarthritis being the two most predominant. The pain of arthritis can be caused by inflammation in the synovial membrane, tendons and ligaments, and muscle strain. Many of the different forms of arthritis cause chronic pain, which could range from mild to severe and can last for weeks, months or even years. Pain due to arthritic inflammation is unpredictable, rendering pain management complex and challenging. The treatment of arthritis should include:

- Education – to enhance the individual's understanding of their condition
- Disease-modifying antirheumatic drugs (DMARDs) for rheumatoid arthritis, such as methotrexate, leflunomide or sulfasalazine
- Non-steroidal inflammatory drugs for moderate-to-severe pain with a proton pump inhibitor, such as omeprazole, to protect the gastrointestinal tract
- Physiotherapy
- Occupational therapy – to enable people to cope with their everyday activities
- Promotion of ideal body weight
- Psychological interventions such as relaxation, stress management or cognitive coping skills (NICE, 2018).

Chronic Back Pain
Lower back pain is one of the most common reasons for individuals to seek medical attention for pain. Back pain can be classified as follows:

- Transient back pain
- Acute back pain
- Persistent back pain.

Transient back pain tends have a short lifespan and does not normally require medical attention, with the patient treating themselves. Often the cause of pain is unknown and does not have any long-term issues or any lasting significance to the patient. *Acute low back pain* is a long-term manifestation of pain, which can be of a few days to a few months in duration. Treatments include analgesia and bedrest and surgery if associated with spinal injury/inflammation. *Persistent low back pain* is back pain that persists for more than 6 months. Those with this type of pain may become preoccupied with the pain and depression and anxiety may occur.

Almost every drug used in psychiatry can also serve as a pain medication. Relieving anxiety, fatigue, depression or insomnia with mood stabilisers, benzodiazepines or anticonvulsants will also ease any related pain. The most versatile of all psychiatric drugs, the antidepressants have an analgesic effect that may be at least partly independent of their effect on depression since it seems to occur at a lower dose.

The two major types of antidepressants, tricyclics and selective serotonin reuptake inhibitors (SSRIs), may have different roles in the treatment of pain. Amitriptyline (Elavil®), a tricyclic, is one of the antidepressants most often recommended as an analgesic, partly because its sedative qualities can be helpful for people in pain. SSRIs such as fluoxetine (Prozac®) and sertraline (Zoloft®) may not be quite as effective as pain relievers, but their side-effects are usually better tolerated, and they are less risky than tricyclic drugs. Some physicians prescribe an SSRI during the day and amitriptyline at bedtime for pain patients.

Neuropathy

Neuropathic pain arises from damaged nociceptors and neurones. Patients with neuropathies describe their pain as being a burning, electric or tingling sensation that can be continuous or spasmodic. The nervous tissue in ascending pain pathways is described as plastic as it changes in response to different psychological and physical stimuli. Such changes include altered sensitivity of nociceptors, which then begin to generate pain impulses in response to ordinary feelings of touch. The patient may also complain of pain in response to slight pressure exerted on the site of injury, even after healing has occurred – a phenomenon called *allodynia*. Damaged nervous tissue also produces increased sensitivity to painful stimuli and often individuals with neuropathy will verbalise pain that is out of proportion to the level of tissue damage. This increase in pain sensitivity is referred to as *hyperalgesia*.

Neuropathic pain can be classified as being central, peripheral or mixed, depending on whether the pain stems from the central or peripheral nervous system. Table 22.4 lists examples of central, peripheral and mixed neuropathy.

Cancer Pain

Cancer pain has numerous causes, but the most likely contributing factor is bone metastases. Cancer pain can be classified as being either nociceptive or neuropathic. Table 22.5 summarises the main causes and descriptions of cancer pain. The aim of palliative care is to minimise pain and its associated distressing symptoms (NICE, 2019). Cancer pain is therefore classified according to when it occurs or if it becomes more intense and unmanageable. The three main classifications of cancer pain are:

- Breakthrough pain
- Incident pain
- End of dose failure pain.

Breakthrough pain occurs in addition to the underlying cancer pain. It is more intense than the patient's normal pain levels. *Incident pain* is caused by incidental activities, i.e. walking, lifting, climbing stairs, washing and dressing. *End of dose failure pain*

Table 22.4 Examples of Neuropathic Pain.

CLASSIFICATION	EXAMPLES
Central	Post-stroke pain
	Spinal pain (i.e. infarction, syringomyelia)
	Multiple sclerosis
	Phantom limb pain
	Parkinson disease
	Fibromyalgia
Peripheral	Postherptic neuralgia
	Postamputation pain
	Chronic pelvic pain
	Entrapment neuropathies
	Neuromas
	Radiculopathies
	Diabetes
	Diseases that suppress immunity (i.e. HIV)
Mixed	Spinal stenosis
	Hereditary neuropathy disease, i.e. Charcot–Marie–Tooth disease
	Cancer pain
	Complex regional pain syndrome

Source: Kandil & Perret (2019).

occurs if the therapeutic effects of the patient's prescribed analgesia subside before the next dose is due. Breakthrough and incident pain are common even in patients whose pain is well controlled. End of dose pain, however, is an indicator that the patient's current pain control may need reviewing (Lister *et al.*, 2019).

What the Experts Say Pain Relief in Cancer Pain

'Morphine is the most researched and most widely used opioid and is therefore the analgesia of choice for the patient in severe cancer pain. Morphine is a safe drug when used properly – the simplest method of dose titration is four-hourly, with the same dose used for breakthrough pain. The total dose of morphine should then be reviewed daily, and the regular dose then adjusted accordingly.'

Deborah, palliative care nurse specialist

Referred and Phantom Limb Pain

Referred pain occurs when tissue damage in one area of the body manifests as pain elsewhere, for example pain as a result of angina that can be felt in the left arm. Although tissue damage occurs in the coronary arteries, pain is also felt radiating down the left arm and despite the intense pain present in the left arm, the tissue there remains perfectly healthy. Referred pain occurs because the damaged or inflamed organ and the area where the referred pain is felt are served by neurones from the same segment of the spinal cord. Another example is pain due to liver or gallbladder inflammation leading to intense pain in the right shoulder. Figure 22.11 highlights the main instances of referred pain.

Phantom limb pain occurs when amputees verbalise pain sensed in the area where their removed limb once was. It is estimated to

Table 22.5 Types of cancer pain, their source, causes and descriptions. Note: Listed in order of prevalence. Most patients have a combination of somatic and visceral nociceptor pain. *Source:* Adapted from Kochhar (2002).

TYPE OF PAIN	STRUCTURES AFFECTED	CAUSES	PATIENT DESCRIPTION
Somatic nociceptor	Muscle and bone	Bone metastases Surgical incisions	Aching, sharp, gnawing or dull easily located
Neuropathic	Nerves	Chemotherapy Tumour	Burning, itching, numbness, tingling, shooting
Visceral nociceptor	Organs of the abdomen, pelvis and thorax	Tumour	Crampy, colicky, aching, deep, squeezing, dull
			Less easily located

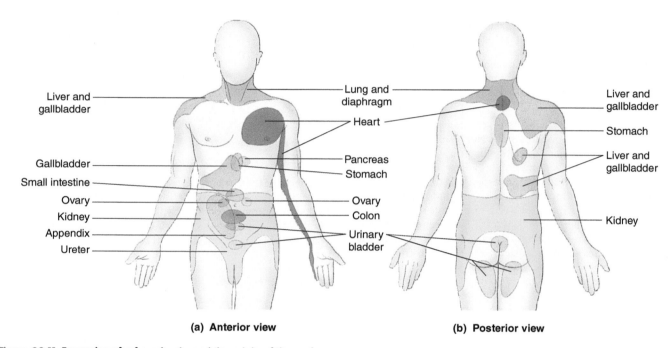

(a) Anterior view   **(b) Posterior view**

Figure 22.11 **Examples of referred pain and the origin of tissue damage.**

occur in up to 50% of people who have had amputations. The precise pathophysiology remains unexplained, but the two most plausible explanations relate to brain interpretation. For instance, when the brain interprets pain impulses from damaged fibres in and around the site of amputation (the stump), it processes the pain signals for the whole (now non-existent) limb. Another theory suggests that the brain contains neurones that provide awareness of body shape and that the neurones that processed information relating to the removed limb remain and continue to be active (Colquhoun *et al.*, 2019).

Conclusion

Pain is an integral part of life. We will all experience pain from time to time. The pathophysiology of pain is complex and should be viewed as a physiological and psychological phenomenon. Pain is a personal and subjective experience and all pain care

should be individualised, encompassing both physical damage and psychosocial circumstances. It is the nurse's aim that patients remain pain free or able to live with and cope with their pain. While the main treatment options are analgesic in nature, many non-pharmacological interventions are at the nurse's disposal.

Key Points

- Pain is a universal phenomenon – everyone experiences pain at some point in their life.
- Nurses must always be non-judgemental in their assessment of the individual with pain – remember pain is what the patient says it is.
- Pain can be acute (short term) or chronic (pain which continues after healing is complete).
- Acute pain is often accompanied by visible and recordable symptoms, whereas chronic pain may not present with symptoms.

- Pain is both a physical and emotional experience and nurses need to pay equal attention to both if they are to provide effective holistic care.
- Unresolved pain has many unwanted physiological consequences which can exacerbate the patient's condition and affect well-being.
- Nurses must carry out a comprehensive pain assessment for all patients experiencing pain.
- Nurses must be able to explain, select and administer a range of both pharmacological and non-pharmacological pain control interventions.

References

Appleyard, I. (2018) Use of acupuncture in the management of pain. *Nursing Standard*, 33, 24–29.

Barret, D., Brintz, C.E., Zaski, A.M. & Edlund, M.J. (2021) Dialectical pain management: feasibility of a third-wave cognitive behavioural therapy approach for adults receiving opioids for chronic pain. *Pain Medicine*, 22(5), 1080–1094.

Coll, A. & Jones, R. (2020) Role of the nurse in the assessment and management of post-operative pain. *Nursing Standard*, 35, 53–58.

Colquhoun, L., Shepherd, V. & Neil, M. (2019) Pain management in new amputees: a nursing perspective. *British Journal of Nursing*, 28(10), 638–646.

Cunningham, S. (2017) Pain assessment and management. In: T. Moore & S. Cunningham (eds) *Clinical Skills for Nursing Practice*, pp.104–131. Routledge, Abingdon.

Daniels, J., Griffiths, M. & Fisher, E. (2020) Assessment and management of recurrent abdominal pain in the emergency department. *Emergency Medical Journal*, 57, 515–521.

Ford, C. (2019) Adult pain assessment and management. *British Journal of Nursing*, 28(7), 421–423.

Gibson, W., Wand, B.M., Meads, C., Catley, M.J. & O'Connell, N.E. (2019) Transcutaneous electrical nerve stimulation (TENS) for chronic pain – an overview of Cochrane reviews. *Cochrane Database of Systematic Reviews*, 4, CD011890.

HMSO (1968) *The Medicines Act*. Her Majesty's Stationery Office, London.

HMSO (1971) *The Misuse of Drugs Act*. Her Majesty's Stationery Office, London.

Hubert, R.J. & VanMeter, K.C. (2018) *Gould's Pathophysiology for the Health Professions*, 6th edn. Elsevier, St Louis, MO.

Ingadottir, B. & Zoega, S. (2017) Role of patient education in postoperative pain management. *Nursing Standard*, 32(2), 50–61.

Kandil, A. & Perret, D. (2019) Classification of neuropathic pain. In: J. Cheng (ed.) *Neuropathic Pain: A Case Based Approach to Practical Management*. Oxford University Press, New York.

Kettyle, A. (2018) Pain management. In: C. Delves-Yates (ed.) *Essentials of Nursing Practice*, 2nd edn. Sage, London.

Kochhar, S.C. (2002) Cancer pain. In: C.A. Warfield & H.J. Fausett (eds) *Manual of Pain Management*, 2nd edn. Lippincott Williams & Wilkins, Philadelphia, PA.

Linde, K., Allais, G., Brinkhaus, B., *et al.* (2016) Acupuncture for the prevention of tension-type headache. *Cochrane Database of Systematic Reviews*, 4, CD007587.

Lister, S., Dougherty, L. & McNamara, L. (2019) *The Royal Marsden Manual of Cancer Nursing Procedures*. Wiley-Blackwell, Chichester.

Mackintosh-Franklin, C. (2021) Recognising and assessing acute pain. *Nursing Standard*, 36, 61–66.

MacIntyre, P.E. & Schug, S.A (2021) *Acute Pain Management: A Practical Guide*, 5th edn. CRC Press, Boca Raton, FL.

Marieb, E. & Hoehn, K. (2019) *Human Anatomy and Physiology*, 11th edn. Pearson, San Francisco, CA.

McCaffery, M. (1979) *Nursing Management of the Patient with Pain*, 2nd edn. J.B. Lippincott, New York.

McFadden, R. (2019) *Introducing Pharmacology for Nursing and Healthcare*, 3rd edn. Routledge, Abingdon.

Melzack, R. & Wall, P. (1988) *The Challenge of Pain*, 2nd edn. Penguin, London.

Mu, J., Furlan, A.D., Lam, W.Y., Hsu, M.Y., Ning, Z. & Lao, L. (2020) Acupuncture for chronic nonspecific low back pain. *Cochrane Database of Systematic Reviews*, 12, CD013814.

National Institute for Health and Care Excellence (2018) *Rheumatoid arthritis in adults: management*. www.nice.org.uk/guidance/ng100/resources/rheumatoid-arthritis-in-adults-management-pdf-66141531233989 (accessed July 2021)

National Institute for Health and Care Excellence (2019) *End of life care: service delivery*. www.nice.org.uk/guidance/ng142/resources/end-of-life-care-for-adults-service-delivery-pdf-66141776457925 (accessed July 2021).

National Institute for Health and Care Excellence (2021) *Chronic pain (primary and secondary) in over 16s: assessment of all chronic pain and management of chronic primary pain*. www.nice.org.uk/guidance/ng193/resources/chronic-pain-primary-and-secondary-in-over-16s-assessment-of-all-chronic-pain-and-management-of-chronic-primary-pain-pdf-66142080468421 (accessed June 2021).

Nursing & Midwifery Council (2018a) *The Code. Professional standards of practice and behaviour for nurses, midwives and nursing associates*. NMC, London.

Nursing & Midwifery Council (2018b) *Standards of proficiency for nursing associates*. NMC, London.

Powell, R., Scott, N.W., Manyande, A., *et al.* (2016) Psychological preparation and post-operative outcomes for adults undergoing surgery under general anaesthesia. *Cochrane Database of Systematic Reviews*, 5, CD008646.

Quinn, B.G. (2020) Responding to people who are experiencing spiritual pain. *Nursing Standard*, 35, 59–65.

Wheeldon, A. (2021) Pain and pain management. In: I. Peate (ed.) *Fundamentals of Applied Pathophysiology: An Essential Guide For Nursing and Healthcare Students*, 4th edn. Wiley-Blackwell, Chichester.

Williams, A.C. de C., Fisher, E., Hearn, L. & Eccleston, C. (2020) Psychological therapies for the management of chronic pain (excluding headache) in adults. *Cochrane Database of Systematic Reviews*, 11, CD007407.

World Health Organization (1986) *Cancer Pain Relief*. WHO, Geneva.

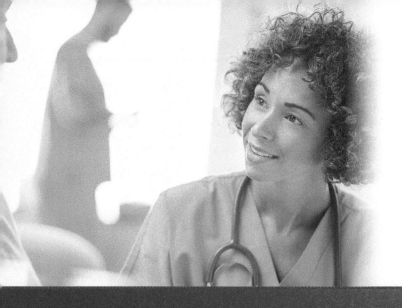

23

The Principles of Fluid and Electrolyte Imbalance and Shock

Noleen P. Jones

School of Health Studies, Gibraltar

Learning Outcomes

On completion of this chapter you will be able to:

- Discuss the fluid compartments of the body
- Compare and contrast the causes, effects and care of the patient with fluid and electrolyte imbalance
- Discuss the risk factors, aetiologies and pathophysiologies of hypovolaemic, cardiogenic, obstructive and distributive shock
- Recognise and report reasons for poor fluid intake and output

Proficiencies

NMC Proficiencies and Standards:

- All nurses must be able to assess and monitor fluid and electrolyte balance, prioritising nursing care based on assessment data.
- The nurse must be able to assess symptoms of physical deterioration and improvement as well as effectively evaluating the care of patients with fluid and electrolyte imbalance.
- The Standards of Proficiency reflect what the NMC expects a newly registered nurse to know and be capable of doing safely and proficiently at the start of their career.
- These two proficiencies are related to fluid intake:
  - record fluid intake and output and identify, respond to and manage dehydration or fluid retention
  - manage the administration of IV fluids

 Visit the companion website at **www.wiley.com/go/peate/nursingpractice3e** where you can test yourself using flashcards, multiple-choice questions and more.

Nursing Practice: Knowledge and Care, Third Edition. Edited by Ian Peate and Aby Mitchell.
© 2022 John Wiley & Sons Ltd. Published 2022 by John Wiley & Sons Ltd.
Companion website: www.wiley.com/go/peate/nursingpractice3e

Introduction

In health, fluid intake and output are equally balanced by the body. Fluid and electrolytes are essential for homeostasis, and the body is usually able to compensate for environmental changes through the constant movement of fluid and electrolytes between intracellular and extracellular compartments. Movement of fluid and electrolytes ensures that cells are continuously supplied with electrolytes such as sodium, chloride, potassium, magnesium, phosphates, bicarbonate and calcium, necessary for cellular function. Even subtle changes in fluid and electrolyte balance can lead to death in patients unable to maintain homeostasis due to illness. Fluid loss via the skin and lungs will increase with fever, burns and severe injuries. Nurses must consequently have a good understanding of fluid and electrolyte balance to observe for and anticipate any changes which may harm patients. This chapter considers fluid and electrolyte balance and looks at some diseases resulting from fluid and electrolyte imbalance.

Body Fluid Compartments

Water is distributed between two major sections within the body, medically termed the intracellular and extracellular compartments. The intracellular compartment, the space inside a cell, contains intracellular fluid (ICF). The extracellular compartment and fluid outside the cell is called extracellular fluid (ECF) (Peate & Evans, 2020). The extracellular compartment is further divided into the extravascular (interstitial) compartment, intravascular compartment (plasma) (Figure 23.1), lymph and transcellular fluid (e.g. saliva, cerebrospinal, ocular and synovial fluid). Two-thirds of body fluid, approximately 40% of total body weight, is found inside the cell. One-third of the fluid is outside the cell and accounts for 20% of total body weight. Eighty percent of ECF is in the interstitial compartment and 20% in the intravascular compartment as plasma (see Figure 23.1).

Movement of fluid between compartments is primarily controlled by two forces:

- *Hydrostatic pressure*: pressure exerted by the fluid
- *Osmotic pressure*: pressure exerted on a solution to prevent the passage of water through a selective permeable membrane.

Function of Water

Body fluid is composed of water, electrolytes (e.g. sodium and potassium), gases (e.g. oxygen and carbon dioxide), nutrients, enzymes and hormones. Water is essential for the body as it:

- Lubricates, facilitating swallowing and joint movement
- Is a major component of the body's transport system for various substances: nutrients, gases, hormones, waste products of metabolism and electrolytes
- Regulates body temperature
- Provides an optimal environment for cellular function and chemical reactions
- Helps to process food in the gastrointestinal tract.

Fluid Balance

Fluid balance concerns the maintenance of the correct amount of fluid in the body. This varies with disease and illness. Individual fluid composition depends on the patient's physical condition, their exercise and the environment. Normally, water intake is balanced by water loss and so body fluid remains constant. Most water is obtained through drinking, some from food and some from cellular metabolism. The kidneys are the major organs responsible for maintenance of fluid balance, excreting excess water in urine. Other organs, for example the lungs, remove water through respiration. The skin eliminates water through sweat and the intestines through faeces. See Table 23.1 for a guide to fluid intake and output.

Osmosis

Osmosis is the net movement of water across a selectively permeable membrane, driven by a difference in solute concentrations on the two sides of the membrane. A selectively permeable membrane is one that allows unrestricted passage of water but not of solute molecules or ions. Thus water flows from the solution with the lower solute concentration into the solution with the higher solute concentration (Figure 23.2). The number of particles dissolved in a unit of water determines concentration, expressed as osmolality or osmolarity. Osmolality refers to the number of osmoles per kilogram of water while osmolarity refers to the number of osmoles per litre of solution. When referring to body fluid, the correct term to use is osmolality.

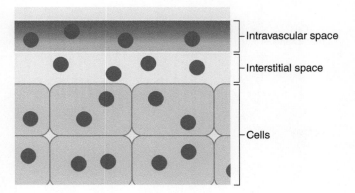

Figure 23.1 Body fluid compartments.

- Intravascular space
- Interstitial space
- Cells

Table 23.1 **Fluid intake and output.** *Source*: **Peate et al. (2012).**

INTAKE		OUTPUT	
Drinking	1500–2000 mL	Urine	1500–2000 mL
Water from food	700–1000 mL	Faeces	100 mL
Cellular metabolism	300–400 mL	Expiration	600–800 mL
		Skin	300–600 mL
Total balance	2500–3400 mL		2500–3400 mL

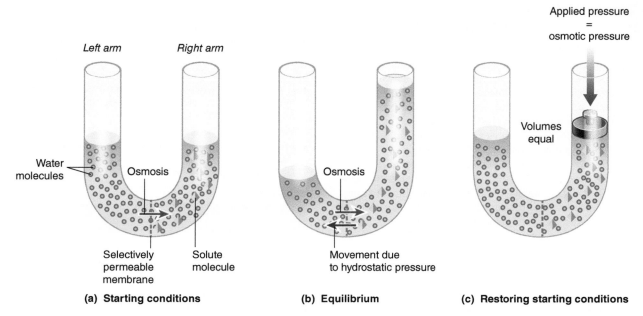

Figure 23.2 **Osmosis.**

Jot This Down

The term 'tonicity' is sometimes used instead of osmolality. Solutions are termed isotonic, hypotonic and hypertonic. Think about the intravenous fluids you have encountered in practice. Can you give one example that falls into each of these groups?

Simple Diffusion

Diffusion describes the movement of solutes such as sodium, potassium and urea from areas of higher concentration to areas of lower concentration (Figure 23.3). Diffusion is further subdivided into simple and facilitated diffusion.

Soluble molecules and gases move by a process of simple diffusion through a concentration gradient, while larger molecules such as glucose and amino acids are transported across the cell membrane by facilitated diffusion (Figure 23.4). An example of

simple diffusion is the exchange of oxygen and carbon dioxide between the alveoli and lung capillaries. The rate of diffusion depends on several factors:

- Gases diffuse much more rapidly than liquids
- Environmental temperature
- Molecular size – smaller molecules diffuse faster than larger ones
- Concentration gradient.

Electrolytes

Electrolytes are ions (charged atoms or molecules) in solution with the capacity to conduct electricity. Electrolytes are positively (cations) or negatively (anions) charged, and carry electrical impulses through nerves for certain physiological functions.

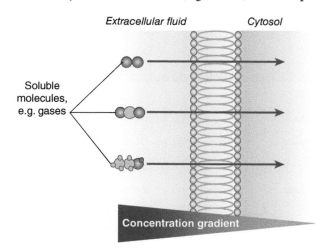

Figure 23.3 **Simple diffusion.**

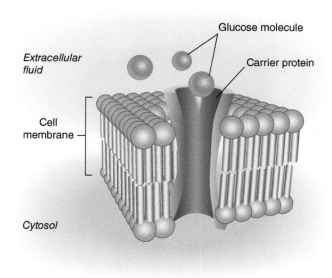

Figure 23.4 **Facilitated diffusion.**

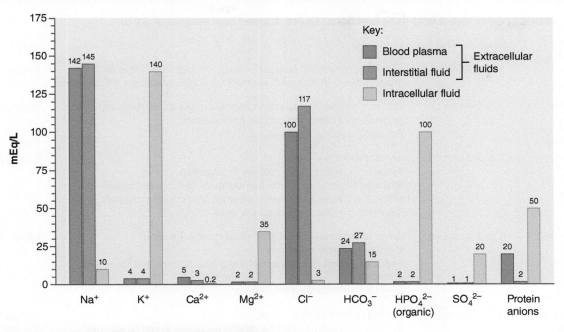

Figure 23.5 **Electrolytes of intracellular and extracellular compartments.**

They also maintain the fluid and acid–base balance of the body. The balance of electrolytes such as potassium (K^+), sodium (Na^+), chloride (Cl^-), magnesium (Mg^{2+}) and phosphate (HPO_4^{2-}) is essential for normal cell and organ function. The composition of electrolytes differs between the intracellular and extracellular compartments (Figure 23.5).

Functions of Electrolytes

Electrolytes are important for:

- Regulating fluid movement between compartments, thus ensuring balanced fluid levels inside and outside cells
- Regulating blood pH levels
- Carrying electrical impulses across the cell and to neighbouring cells, promoting muscle contractions and nerve impulses
- Enzyme reactions.

Table 23.2 gives a summary of the principal electrolytes and their functions.

Practice Assessment Document

By the time they register, nurses are expected to recognise and respond to potential hazards that may affect a patient's safety (NMC, 2018a–c), for example, their altered fluid status. They need to be able to identify the clinical indicators for fluid interventions, and to report these for attention.

You may show your supervisor your knowledge and understanding of intravenous fluids, for instance, by discussing the differences between hypotonic, isotonic and hypertonic fluid, or show your ability to evaluate treatment by discussing the effectiveness of a patient's response to them.

You could also demonstrate the application of your knowledge on a patient's fluid status by competently maintaining and recording a fluid balance chart, identifying issues of concern and escalating these promptly and appropriately.

Acid–Base Balance

Optimal cellular function requires the maintenance of hydrogen ion (H^+) concentration within a relatively narrow range in body fluids. Hydrogen ions determine the relative acidity of body fluids. Acids release hydrogen ions in solution; bases (alkalis) accept hydrogen ions in solution. The acidity or alkalinity of a fluid is measured as pH. A pH of 7 is neutral. The relationship between hydrogen ion concentration and pH is inverse, i.e. as hydrogen ion concentration increases, the pH falls below 7, and the solution becomes more acidic. Fluid alkalinity (pH above 7) depends on hydrogen ion concentration falling.

Not all parts of the body operate within the same pH range because body organs function at different levels of acidity and alkalinity. Chemical and enzyme reactions are continuously occurring around the body. A narrow pH range is necessary for many of these reactions to be performed. Small changes in pH levels can therefore profoundly affect the body's overall function. Urine, for example, is usually acidic and saliva mostly neutral. The pH of blood is slightly alkaline, with a pH ranging from 7.35 to 7.45. A pH outside this range, below 7.35 or above 7.45, can cause life-threatening problems. See Figure 23.6 for the pH scale.

Most acids and bases in the body are weak, i.e. they neither release nor accept significant amounts of hydrogen ions (Hamilton *et al.*, 2017). A number of mechanisms work together to maintain the pH system within acceptable ranges.

Metabolic processes in the body continuously produce acids, categorised as being volatile and non-volatile. Volatile acids are eliminated from the body as carbonic acid (H_2CO_3). It dissociates (separates) into carbon dioxide (CO_2) and water (H_2O) and is eliminated through the lungs. All other acids produced in the body are non-volatile acids, metabolised or excreted from the body in fluid. Examples of non-volatile acids are lactic acid, hydrochloric acid and phosphoric acid.

389

Table 23.2 Principal electrolytes and their functions. *Source:* Adapted from Peate *et al.* (2012).

ELECTROLYTE	NORMAL VALUE	FUNCTION	MAINLY FOUND
Sodium (Na^+)	135–145 mmol/L	Transmits nerve impulses and muscle contractions. Plays an important role in fluid and electrolyte balance. Maintains blood volume	Extracellular fluid
Potassium (K^+)	3.5–5 mmol/L	Transmits nerve impulses and muscle contractions. Regulates pH balance, maintains intracellular fluid volume Regulates cardiac impulses	Intracellular fluid
Calcium (Ca^{2+})	2.1–2.6 mmol/L	Important clotting factor Assists neurotransmitter release in neurones Maintains muscle tone and excitability of nervous and muscle tissue Maintains cardiac pacemaker automaticity Activates enzymes (pancreatic lipase and phospholipase)	Extracellular fluid
Magnesium (Mg^{2+})	0.5–1.0 mmol/L	Helps to maintain normal nerve and muscle function Maintains regular heart rate Regulates blood glucose and blood pressure Essential for protein synthesis Operates sodium–potassium pump	Intracellular fluid
Chloride (Cl^-)	98–117 mmol/L	Regulates acid–base balance Buffer for oxygen and carbon dioxide exchange in red blood cells Regulates extracellular fluid volume	Extracellular fluid
Bicarbonate (HCO_3^-)	22–30 mmol/L	Main buffer of hydrogen ions in plasma Maintains a balance between cations and anions of intracellular and extracellular fluids	Extracellular fluid
Phosphate (PO_4^-)	0.8–1.1 mmol/L	Essential for the digestion of proteins, carbohydrates and fats and absorption of calcium Essential for bone formation Regulates pH balance	Intracellular fluid

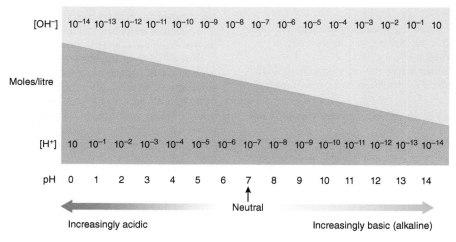

Figure 23.6 **The pH scale.**

Investigations and Diagnosis

In practice, analysis of arterial blood gases provides the following information.

- *pH*: determines overall blood acidosis or alkalosis.
- *Carbon dioxide (CO_2) partial pressure (Paco$_2$)*: respiratory acidosis/alkalosis disorders are identified by increased or decreased CO_2.

- *Standard bicarbonate*: analysis of blood gases provides a bicarbonate level, calculated from the Paco$_2$ using the Henderson–Hasselbalch equation.
- Bicarbonate (HCO_3^-) is increased in metabolic alkalosis and decreased in metabolic acidosis. Otherwise, the change is compensatory (i.e. normal or raised in respiratory acidosis; normal or decreased in respiratory alkalosis).

Buffer Systems

Buffers are substances that prevent major changes in pH by removing or releasing hydrogen ions. When excess acid is present in body fluid, buffers bind with hydrogen ions to minimise changes in pH. If body fluids become too basic (alkaline), buffers release hydrogen ions, restoring the pH. Although buffers act within a fraction of a second, their capacity to maintain pH is limited (Hamilton *et al.*, 2017). For example, in the respiratory and renal systems, chemical buffers such as bicarbonate–carbonic acid, catalysed by the enzyme carbonic anhydrase (Figure 23.7), phosphate buffer systems and protein buffers help to maintain pH balance in the body.

The lungs regulate acid–base balance by eliminating or retaining carbon dioxide. Increases in either carbon dioxide or hydrogen ions in the blood stimulate the respiratory centre in the brain so that the rate and depth of respiration increase and carbon dioxide is exhaled. The levels of carbon dioxide in the blood are measured as P_{CO_2}. Pv_{CO_2} measures the pressure of carbon dioxide of venous blood, whereas Pa_{CO_2} measures the pressure of carbon dioxide in arterial blood The normal Pa_{CO_2} is between 4.6 and 5.6 kPa (35–42 mmHg), while the partial pressure of arterial oxygen (Pa_{O_2}) is between 11.3 and 14 kPa. Note that Pa_{CO2} measures alveolar mean pressures of carbon dioxide (Messina & Patrick, 2021).

The renal system is responsible for long-term regulation of acid–base balance in the body. Unlike the respiratory system, the kidneys are slower to respond to changes, requiring hours to days to correct imbalances. Excess non-volatile acids produced during metabolism are normally eliminated by the kidneys. The kidneys also regulate bicarbonate levels in extracellular fluid by regenerating bicarbonate ions, as well as reabsorbing them in the renal tubules. When excess hydrogen ion is present in blood and the pH falls (acidosis), the kidneys reabsorb and regenerate bicarbonate ions. Conversely, the kidneys will excrete bicarbonate ions and retain hydrogen ions in alkalosis.

Acidosis and Alkalosis

Acidosis and alkalosis are terms used to describe abnormal conditions when a patient's blood pH may not fall within the range 7.35–7.45. Disorders of acid–base balance are primarily either respiratory or metabolic. Acidosis occurs when there is a high level of hydrogen ions, resulting in a pH of below 7.35. Respiratory acidosis is caused by a build-up of carbon dioxide from disorders of the respiratory tract. Other conditions affecting the respiratory centre, such as exacerbation of chronic obstructive pulmonary disease (COPD), muscular dystrophy, hypoventilation

syndrome (Pickwickian syndrome), neuromuscular disorders and drugs that suppress breathing (e.g. narcotics), especially when combined with alcohol, may also result in respiratory impairment. Respiratory alkalosis (pH above 7.45) oppositely occurs from hyperventilation, for example, due to anxiety, stroke or liver impairment.

Metabolic acidosis is the result of low pH and low levels of bicarbonate ions because of shock, hypoxia, diabetes and renal failure, among other conditions. Metabolic alkalosis occurs because of an excess of bicarbonate ions, for example, in burns, vomiting and hypokalaemia. The management of these conditions depends on identifying and treating the underlying cause.

Antacids (alkaline) are prescribed for patients with gastric problems that include acid reflux. Most antacids contain aluminium, magnesium hydroxides or derivatives of carbonates. Overuse could cause metabolic alkalosis.

All the organs of the body are affected when there is severe loss of fluid and electrolytes. The heart is unable to pump enough blood to the organs, leading to inadequate tissue perfusion which causes multiple organ dysfunction.

Fluid Volume Deficit

Fluid volume deficit (FVD) develops when water loss exceeds water intake. Examples include:

- Excessive fluid losses from the gastrointestinal tract, e.g. diarrhoea and vomiting; profuse sweating
- Dehydration
- Failure of regulatory mechanisms
- Diseases including renal failure, diabetes, diabetes insipidus
- Trauma, surgery, haemorrhage
- Medications, e.g. diuretics or laxatives
- Pyrexia resulting in severe sweating
- Fluid loss into the third space.

Fluid volume deficit is a relatively common problem, existing alone or in combination with other electrolyte or acid–base imbalances. The term 'dehydration' refers exclusively to loss of water, although it is often used interchangeably with FVD.

Red Flag

Small water losses of 1–2% can impair mental and physical performance. Loss of as little as 7% of body fluid can lead to circulatory collapse. Nurses should report and document any changes, however minimal, in the patient's vital signs, especially low blood pressure, tachycardia and low urine output.

Pathophysiology

Fluid volume deficit may result from lack of fluid intake, inability to request or drink fluids, oral infection, diarrhoea or conditions such as diabetes mellitus or diabetes insipidus. Elderly people are at particular risk for FVD (Picetti *et al.*, 2017). FVD can develop slowly or rapidly, depending on the type of fluid loss. Electrolytes can also be lost along with fluid. When both water and electrolytes are lost, the serum sodium level remains normal, although levels of other electrolytes such as potassium may fall. Fluid is drawn into the vascular compartment from the interstitial spaces as the body attempts to maintain tissue

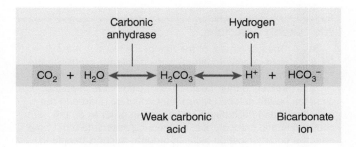

Figure 23.7 Bicarbonate–carbonic acid buffer reversible reaction.

perfusion. However, fluid loss from the interstitial space also results in fluid moving out from the intracellular compartment, depleting intracellular volume.

Third Fluid Space Infection or burns may cause movement of fluid into what is medically known as the third space. Fluid from the vascular space shifts into an area, e.g. the pleura, peritoneum, joint and pericardial cavities, where the trapped fluid is not available for physiological function.

Signs and Symptoms
- Dry mucosa
- Weight loss
- Poor skin turgor (elasticity)
- Hypotension
- Flat neck veins, decreased central venous pressure
- Tachycardia
- Pallor
- Oliguria (scanty urine output)
- Sunken eyeballs

> **Jot This Down**
>
> Think about fluid compartments and fluid movement between compartments. Is a patient overhydrated or dehydrated if large volumes of fluid are trapped in the third space?

Care, Dignity and Compassion

Mouth care is often overlooked in acute hospitals (Davis *et al.*, 2019). However, evidence shows that good oral health improves patient recovery and is related to general health and well-being (Health Education England, 2016).

Dehydration will normally cause the mouth to dry. Absence of saliva can lead to cracked lips, a fissured tongue and fungal infections. Implementing a tool like the Challacombe Scale (King's College London, 2011) will help the nurse to identify early problems and treatment options.

Along with the nurse's obligation to monitor for signs of oral problems (NMC, 2018a,b), there are other ways in which patient comfort can be promoted. For instance, for the patient who is nauseated, small sips of cold water or sucking on ice chips may help to provide relief as well as hydration.

Nursing Care and Management
Nurses have a responsibility to identify patients at risk for FVD (NMC, 2018a, b), carrying out measures to prevent and treat it, as well as monitoring the effects of therapy. The aim is to identify the cause of FVD and replace fluid loss. However, in order to achieve full fluid replacement with crystalloids, the volume infused must be three times the volume of fluid lost (Pierce *et al.*, 2016). Nurses need to monitor the patient closely and:

- Weigh and record the patient's weight daily. This should be done at the same time every day, when possible. *Weight helps to assess fluid loss or gain.*
- Maintain strict input and output records. *Accurate records importantly assess ongoing fluid balance.*

- Check the patient's prescription medications regularly. *Diuretics or antihypertensive medications may cause excessive fluid losses.*
- Regularly monitor vital signs. *Vital sign changes, e.g. increased heart rate, decreased blood pressure, may indicate hypovolaemia. Observations are also good indicators of the patient's response to treatment.*
- Administer prescribed fluids. *To ensure that the patient is getting the correct amount of fluid.*
- Provide frequent oral hygiene. *Oral mucosa becomes dry because of a loss of interstitial fluid loss.*
- Check pressure areas every 4 hours to ensure skin integrity. *Patients with poor skin turgor are at risk of developing pressure sores.*
- Assist with mobility if the patient is unsteady when walking. *Lower blood pressure may result in mobile instability.*

> **Jot This Down**
>
> During treatment, what do you think might be happening with the patient if they respond to your questions inappropriately/appear confused?

What To Do If . . .

If a patient with FVD on intravenous therapy complains of breathlessness and has difficulty in breathing, your actions should include:

- Reporting this immediately
- Taking and recording vital signs
- Stopping the infusion until the patient is reviewed by a doctor
- Documenting actions and outcomes.

Health Promotion and Discharge
- Patients should be made aware of the importance of sufficient fluid and salt intake, particularly when exercising, if they have diarrhoea and vomiting or have a fever.
- Inform patients of the signs and symptoms of dehydration.
- Advise patients of adequate intake (no less than 1.5 L/day).
- Advise weekly weight monitoring to monitor for weight loss.
- Patients should seek advice from their practice nurse if they are concerned.

The Nursing Associate

One key aspect of the role of the Nursing Associate is to be able to clearly and confidently explain to the individual and family how their lifestyle choices may influence their health. This includes the impact of common health risk behaviours that could be related to the individual's diet (including fluid intake). In order to do this with confidence and competence, the nursing associate must have effective communication skills in order to support people to prevent ill health and to manage their health challenges.

Primary Care

Before discharging the patient, nurses need to ensure that the patient is well informed about their condition and the care they will need in place when discharged home. Discuss the increased risk for FVD with adults, providing information about prevention and maintenance of adequate fluid intake, particularly when exercising and during hot weather. Advise the patient (or their caregivers) that thirst decreases with ageing and that regardless of thirst, they should maintain a regular fluid intake of about 1500 mL per day.

Care, Dignity and Compassion

Encouraging people to eat and drink is an important part of the nurse's role. Fear of incontinence resulting in the loss of dignity may lead to some patients denying themselves adequate fluid or nutritional intake. Nurses need to be sensitive and compassionate in the delivery of care to older people.

Find out more about the guidelines of the Social Care Institute of Excellence at the link below: www.scie.org.uk/dignity/care. These guidelines include the following points.

- Encourage people to drink regularly throughout the day. The Food Standards Agency recommends a daily intake of 6–8 glasses of water or other fluids. However, warn of the dehydrating effects of alcohol.
- Provide education, training and information about the benefits of good hydration to staff, carers and people who use services, and encourage peer-to-peer learning.
- Provide promotional materials to remind service users, staff and carers of the importance of hydration.
- Ensure there is access to clean drinking water 24 hours a day.
- If people are reluctant to drink water, think of other ways of increasing their fluid intake, for example with alternative drinks and foods that have a higher fluid content (e.g. milky breakfast cereals, soup, fruit and vegetables).
- If people show reluctance to drink because they are worried about incontinence, reassure them that help will be provided with going to the toilet.

Fluid Volume Excess

Fluid volume excess (FVE) is the abnormal retention of fluid and sodium in the extracellular space which leads to tissue swelling (oedema). This could occur if a patient is overinfused with intravenous normal saline, or eats foods containing high amounts of sodium.

Pathophysiology

Fluid volume excess usually results from conditions that cause retention of both sodium and water. The risk of fluid overload is higher in elderly patients, especially if there is cardiac or renal impairment, sepsis, major injury or major surgery (Ko *et al.*, 2019). As individuals age, natural decline in physiological functioning makes the elderly vulnerable to health-related illnesses that include fluid retention and electrolyte imbalance.

Retention of water and sodium could originate from:

- Drinking large amounts of hypotonic fluid, e.g. water. Water moves from the intravascular space, resulting in tissue oedema
- Administration of excessive amounts of saline infusions
- Excess intake of dietary salt
- Diseases such as liver cirrhosis, renal failure, congestive heart failure
- Administration of drugs that cause sodium retention, blood transfusion, plasma volume expanders.

Investigations and Diagnosis

Initial investigations which will assist a diagnosis include:

- *Electrocardiogram (ECG)*: detects cardiac arrhythmia, infarction or hypertrophy
- *Chest X-ray*: identifies pulmonary oedema and other chest pathology, e.g. pneumonia
- *Serum urea, creatinine and electrolytes*: examines renal function and electrolyte contributions to problems
- *Full blood count*: for anaemia and features of infection
- *Liver function tests*: albumin and protein levels.

Symptoms

Fluid volume excess causes symptoms such as:

- Distended neck and peripheral veins
- Cough, dyspnoea
- Orthopnoea
- Moist crackles in the lungs
- Pulmonary oedema
- Polyuria with normal renal function
- Ascites/weight gain
- Peripheral oedema
- Possible cerebral oedema
- Confusion/headache/seizures/coma
- Full bounding pulse/hypertension.

Nursing Care and Management

Nursing of the patient with FVE includes interventions such as the administration of diuretics, maintaining sodium and fluid restriction as well as monitoring the status and effects of the excess fluid volume, particularly critical in the elderly because of the age-related decline in cardiac and renal functions. In its report following a dignity and nutrition inspection programme in 2012, the Care Quality Commission found that staff were inaccurately monitoring patients' food and fluid balance at 34 of the 50 hospitals visited. Its recommendations therefore included improving the standards of record keeping at these facilities. Nurses must remain ever aware of the role of hydration in maintaining health and promoting recovery, ensuring that they observe for and track signs of ill health.

- Assessment of vital signs and heart sounds is imperative because hypervolaemia can cause hypertension and tachycardia. Patients should be assessed for peripheral oedema, particularly in the lower extremities, the back and sacral region. With pulmonary oedema, gas exchange may be impaired by fluid in the alveolar sac. *Assessment of vital signs is important to detect signs of deterioration.*
- Administer oxygen as prescribed and monitor its effect on the patient's respiratory status. *Supplementary oxygen improves tissue oxygenation by promoting gas exchange across the alveolar-capillary membrane.*
- Weigh the patient daily and record the result. *Acute weight gain or loss represents fluid gain or loss. A weight gain of 1 kg is equivalent to 1 L of fluid gain.*
- Advise the patient and their relatives on the necessity of fluid regulation.

Table 23.3 Three major group of diuretics and their site of action.

DRUG	GROUP	TARGET SITE IN THE KIDNEY
Furosemide	Loop diuretic	Thick ascending loop of Henle
Chlorothiazide	Thiazide-type	Distal tubule and collecting ducts
Amiloride	Potassium-sparing diuretic	Cortical collecting ducts

- All fluid intakes must be calculated. *Accurate fluid measurement is important to ensure that the patient is not in positive balance and developing complications of fluid retention.*
- Provide oral hygiene 2 hourly. *Oral hygiene may help prevent oral infections and also promotes patient comfort.*
- Advise the patient about sodium-restricted diets. Check food content if brought in from home. *Excess sodium promotes water retention, so a sodium-restricted diet is advised to reduce water retention.*
- Monitor the patient's urine output hourly if indicated, maintaining a strict input and output chart. *Fluid volume excreted is a good indicator of the patient's response to treatment.*
- Monitor the effects of prescribed diuretics on urine output and serum electrolytes. Furosemide, chlorothiazide and amiloride are some of the diuretics that may be used to treat FVE (Table 23.3). *Diuretics can have undesirable side-effects such as excess fluid loss and loss of sodium and potassium chloride.*
- Check the patient's skin regularly for ruptures caused by oedema. Problems can occur if the volume of interstitial fluid in the limbs exceeds its capacity to retain it (Bradford & Rossiter, 2020), causing blistering and leakage of interstitial fluid onto skin and potentiating infection. *Skin breaks down rapidly in pressure areas as a result of oedema.*

Medicines Management

Postural hypotension is common in elderly patients taking both thiazides and loop diuretics. Advise the patient to stand up slowly and in stages. Compression support stockings may help venous return and prevent this problem.

Medicines Management

- Advise your patient to avoid foods high in potassium while taking potassium-sparing diuretics.
- Advise patients to check with their practice nurse, doctor or pharmacist before taking herbal remedies at the same time as a diuretic (or other medications) as they may provoke adverse drug reactions.

Red Flag

Do not use adhesive dressings on grossly oedematous legs because they may cause pain and tear the very fragile, taut skin in these areas.

Jot This Down

Following fluid therapy, the patient's circulation is in danger of becoming overloaded. Why might this occur?

Health Promotion and Discharge

- Patients should be informed of the risk of fluid retention and high intake of sodium. Salt helps to retain fluid in the body, resulting in fluid overload.
- Patients who have heart or kidney diseases should be advised on fluid and electrolyte balance and referred to a dietitian for information on food containing high amounts of salt.
- Encourage the patient to weigh themselves weekly and to inform the practice nurse of any gain in weight.
- Advise the patient and their relatives to read food labels properly for salt additives in the food.

Primary Care

Prior to discharge, the nurse should offer health promotion advice related to fluid volume excess focused on teaching preventive measures to patients who are at risk (e.g. those who have heart or kidney failure). Discuss the relationship between sodium intake and water retention. Provide guidelines for a low-sodium diet, and educate the patient to carefully read food labels to identify 'hidden' sodium. Advise the patient to weigh themselves daily, using the same scale and wearing the same clothing. Inform the practice nurse if they gain more than 2 kg in a day. Encourage the patient to monitor their urine output.

Electrolyte Imbalance

Levels of electrolytes in the body can become too low or too high. This can happen with fluctuating water changes in the body. For example, when sweating as a result of exercise, hot weather or illness, the levels of some electrolytes such as sodium and potassium may be lowered. Vomiting and diarrhoea may also cause electrolyte imbalances because of excessive fluid loss.

Where there is an imbalance in electrolytes, the aim is to restore normal levels as soon as possible otherwise it could prove a serious health risk for the patient. See Table 23.4 for a summary of electrolytes: causes, signs and symptoms and nursing interventions.

Sodium Imbalance (Hyponatraemia)

Sodium is the most abundant cation in the ECF, with normal serum sodium levels ranging from 135 to 145 mmol/L. Hyponatraemia refers to a lower than normal level of sodium (below 135 mmol/L) in the blood. Sodium is the primary regulator of volume, blood pressure and osmolality of ECF. More than 95% of body sodium is in the ECF. The level of sodium is regulated by the renin–angiotensin–aldosterone systems. The adrenal gland secretes aldosterone which stimulates the kidney to retain sodium from urine. Addison disease, which damages the adrenal gland, can therefore lead to low levels of sodium in the body.

Sodium is important for maintaining neuromuscular activity. About 40% of the body's sodium is contained in bone, some is

Table 23.4 Summary of electrolytes: causes, signs and symptoms, and nursing interventions. *Source*: Adapted from Kozier *et al.* (2012) *Fundamentals of Nursing: Concepts, Process and Practice.* Pearson Education, Harlow.

ELECTROLYTE	CAUSES	SIGNS AND SYMPTOMS	NURSING INTERVENTIONS
Sodium (hyponatraemia), serum sodium below 135 mmol/L	Excessive sweating, diarrhoea and vomiting. Excessive consumption and infusion of hypotonic fluids, diuretics. Inappropriate secretion of ADH and aldosterone Liver, kidney and heart diseases	Confusion, irritability, abdominal cramps, muscle twitching, personality changes, coma and convulsion if sodium level is very low Depression Headaches	Monitor fluid intake Maintain strict input and output chart Monitor and record vital signs If permitted, encourage high salt intake until level is within normal range Monitor effects of diuretics if prescribed
Sodium (hypernatraemia), serum sodium above 145 mmol/L	Diarrhoea Excessive infusion of hypertonic fluids Excessive intake of salt in diet Hyperventilation Fever	Feeling thirsty, dry mucous membranes, fatigue, seizures, coma, death	Monitor fluid intake Maintain input and output chart Obtain and record vital signs Advise on restricted salt intake in diet
Potassium (hypokalaemia), serum potassium below 3.5 mmol/L	Diarrhoea and vomiting Non-potassium-sparing diuretics Excessive sweating	Muscle weakness, feeling tired, cardiac dysrhythmias (atrial and ventricular), poor tendon reflexes Alkalosis, T-wave flattening and ST-segment depression	Obtain and record vital signs Administer potassium in IV infusion Advise patient to eat food containing potassium, such as bananas
Potassium (hyperkalaemia), serum potassium above 5 mmol/L	Renal failure Excessive intake of salt with potassium Undersecretion of aldosterone Potassium-sparing diuretics	Confusion, cerebral agitation, cardiac arrest, muscle weakness	Obtain and record vital signs, especially heart rate Administer non-potassium-sparing diuretics and monitor the effects Advise patient to avoid potassium-containing salts
Calcium (hypocalcaemia), serum calcium below 4.5 mmol/L	Hypoparathyroidism resulting from surgery Alkalosis Acute pancreatitis	Tetany Painful muscle spasm of hands Painful muscle spasm of feet Facial muscle spasms Facial grimacing Lip paraesthesias (tingling, pricking or numbness of the lip) Tongue, finger, foot paraesthesias	Monitor and record vital signs, especially respiration and pulse rates Encourage diet rich in calcium Administer calcium supplement tablets
Calcium (hypercalcaemia), serum calcium above 5.5 mmol/L	Prolonged bedrest Hyperparathyroidism Sarcoma of the bones Excessive intake of calcium-rich food such as cheese and milk Paget's disease Calcium supplement	Urinary calculi, weakness, polyuria, heart block, flank pain, nausea and vomiting	Encourage mobility Advise patient to take diet with less calcium Encourage fluid intake to flush kidneys Advise patient on the signs and symptoms of osteoporosis

ADH, antidiuretic hormone.

found within organs and cells, and the remaining 55% is in blood plasma and other fluids outside the cell.

Sodium is essential for:

- Regulating blood pressure
- Regulating blood volume
- Function of nerves and muscles.

Pathophysiology

Exercise, sweating, vomiting, diarrhoea and excessive hypotonic fluid intake can cause extra sodium loss. Renal disease and the loss of skin from extensive burns can also result in hyponatraemia. Other reasons for hyponatraemia include:

- Systemic diseases such as congestive heart failure, renal failure or cirrhosis of the liver

- Syndrome of inappropriate secretion of antidiuretic hormone (SIADH), in which water excretion is impaired
- Excessive administration of hypotonic intravenous fluids
- Severe malnutrition
- Aldosterone deficiency
- Overhydration
- Compulsive water drinking.

> **Nursing Fields** Mental Health: Hyponatraemia
> Excessive water intake may be an issue in some people with mental health problems. The syndrome is referred to as 'compulsive water drinking' in those with obsessive-compulsive disorder or delusional psychosis. Nurses caring for patients with these conditions need to be aware of hyponatraemia.

Investigations and Diagnosis

- Serum sodium level.
- Serum potassium; if raised, consider Addison disease.
- Urine sodium level; if >20 mmol/L, a renal function test is carried out to exclude renal disease.
- Serum thyroid-stimulating hormone and free thyroxine level are checked to exclude hypothyroidism.
- Random serum cortisol levels or adrenocorticotropic hormone (ACTH) tests are carried out in patients with suspected adrenal suppression (e.g. those who have recently taken oral steroids).
- Further investigations may be indicated in some clinical situations, e.g. a chest X-ray in suspected congestive cardiac failure or a CT brain scan in patients with confusion or altered consciousness.

Symptoms

- Nausea and vomiting
- Abdominal cramps
- Anorexia
- Diarrhoea

As sodium levels continue to decrease, the brain and nervous system are affected by cellular oedema which can lead to:

- Headache
- Depression
- Personality changes
- Irritability
- Lethargy
- Hyper-reflexia
- Muscle twitching
- Tremors.

Convulsions and coma are likely to occur if serum sodium falls dangerously low.

Nursing Care and Management

Care of the patient with hyponatraemia focuses on identifying those at risk and treating the underlying cause.

Fluid and Dietary Management In mild hyponatraemia, increasing the intake of foods high in sodium, e.g. meats, and adding salt to the patient's diet may be sufficient. Fluids are often restricted to help reduce ECF volume and correct low sodium levels. However, nurses need to ensure that the patient does not become dehydrated as a result of fluid restriction.

- When both sodium and water have been lost (hyponatraemia with hypovolaemia), sodium-containing fluids are administered to replace both fluid and sodium. These fluids may be given orally, subcutaneously or intravenously. Isotonic solutions such as normal saline (0.9% NaCl) may be administered to replace fluid and sodium (Guest, 2020).
- Loop diuretics are administered to patients who have hyponatraemia with normal or excess ECF volume. Loop diuretics promote an isotonic diuresis and fluid volume loss without hyponatraemia; however, thiazide diuretics are avoided because they cause a relatively greater sodium loss in relation to water loss.
- Monitor urine output strictly in input and output charts.
- Check with the patient regularly for symptoms such as stomach cramps or feelings of nausea, which are early signs of hyponatraemia.

- Check serum sodium levels daily to ensure that treatments are effective and to ensure a safe rate of correction (NICE, 2015).
- Provide support in maintaining personal hygiene.
- Monitor and record any central nervous system (CNS) changes such as muscle twitching, confusion and restlessness, signs of cerebral oedema, and increasing pressure within the brain.
- Assess muscle strength and tone, and deep tendon reflexes. Increasing muscle weakness and decreased deep tendon reflexes are symptoms of increasing hyponatraemia.

The Nursing Associate

It is essential that fluid balance charts are accurately completed in order to determine a patient's fluid input and output and identify any potential fluid loss or gain that may be detrimental, requiring escalation of care.

Fluid input/output charts in hospital inpatients are an invaluable source of information for healthcare practitioners when reviewing intravenous fluid prescription, but they can be incomplete and inaccurate.

The concept of a fluid balance chart seems simple but in practice it can be difficult to maintain and many issues with the recording process have been identified. The nursing associate is ideally placed to increase awareness of the importance of fluid balance and the significance of monitoring amongst staff and patients.

Health Promotion and Discharge

- Hyponatraemia can result from excessive sweating, vomiting and diarrhoea. Nurses should advise the patient to replace the fluid loss. They should also be informed that drinking excessive amounts of water could result in hyponatraemia.
- Advise the patient and their relatives of signs and symptoms, for example, abdominal cramps, irritability and muscle weakness, and to seek advice from their GP or practice nurse if they are concerned.
- Encourage the patient to drink varied types of fluid, not just water, when feeling thirsty.
- Encourage the patient to take fluid containing electrolytes when exercising.
- Advise on salt supplement when cooking or eating food low in sodium.

Primary Care

Before discharging patients, nurses should offer information about:

- The causes of hyponatraemia
- The signs and symptoms of hyponatraemia
- The types of food and fluid that are rich in sodium content
- The importance of patients monitoring their urine output
- The importance of maintaining hydration during exercise and in hot weather
- Checking with the practice nurse if diarrhoea and vomiting persists for more than a day
- The importance of drinking oral fluid to balance fluid loss if diuretics are being taken.

Hypernatraemia

Hypernatraemia is defined as a serum sodium concentration exceeding 145 mmol/L. Serum sodium concentration, and hence osmolality, is normally kept from rising significantly by the release of antidiuretic hormone (ADH) which regulates water losses, and by the stimulation of thirst, which increases water intake.

Pathophysiology

The fundamental problem in hypernatraemia is hyperosmolality, an overall deficit of total body water. It may be a consequence of insufficient water intake due to severe nausea/vomiting or poor health, or secondary to renal diseases. Hypernatraemia causes cellular dehydration by direct extraction of water by the osmotic load of sodium, or by the body's free water deficit. The result is that cells shrink and transport electrolytes across the cell membrane to compensate for the osmotic force. Intracellular organic solutes are generated in an effort to restore cell volume and avoid structural damage.

Investigations and Diagnosis

- Serum urea and electrolyte check for sodium, potassium, urea, creatinine, calcium and plasma glucose.
- Urine and serum osmolality if diabetes insipidus is suspected; there would be a high serum osmolality (>300 mOsmol/kg) combined with an inappropriately dilute urine (less than serum osmolality).

Signs and Symptoms

- Polydipsia and polyuria.
- Hyperosmolality of extracellular fluid.
- Water is drawn out of cells, leading to cellular dehydration. The most serious effects of cellular dehydration are seen in the brain. Neurological manifestations develop as brain cells contract. The brain shrinks, causing mechanical traction on cerebral vessels.
- Altered neurological function, such as lethargy, weakness and irritability, can progress to seizures, coma and death in severe hypernatraemia.
- Orthostatic hypotension.
- Tachycardia.

Nursing Care and Management

- Treat underlying disorders. If diabetes insipidus or any other disease is present, this should be addressed and appropriate treatment provided.
- Correct dehydration by replacing free water losses.
- Correct hypovolaemia by giving electrolytes in addition to free water.

Risk for Injury

As a result of hypernatraemia, the patient may present with central nervous system-related symptoms that could lead to harm.

A full risk assessment of the patient and preventive measures are required.

- Administer any intravenous fluid as prescribed and monitor the outcome. Ensure that serum sodium levels and osmolality are checked daily and report rapid changes immediately. Rapid water replacement or rapid changes in serum sodium or osmolality can cause fluid shifts within the brain, increasing the risk of cerebral oedema.
- Record neurological observations hourly and check with the patient if they have headaches or are feeling nauseous. Careful monitoring of the patient is vital to detect changes in mental status that may indicate cerebral oedema.
- Monitor vital signs such as heart rate, blood pressure and respiration rate and report any changes immediately.
- Administer medications prescribed, if any, and note the effects and report any side-effects immediately.
- Maintain a strict input and output chart.
- Weigh the patient daily to detect any rapid gain or loss in weight.
- Document interventions and outcomes.

Health Promotion and Discharge

- Elderly patients are at risk of developing hypernatraemia as a result of dehydration or other illnesses. Advise the patient and their relatives of the importance of adequate fluid intake at regular intervals.
- Advise the importance of restricting salt intake in their diet.
- Advise the patient and their relatives about the signs and symptoms of hypernatraemia.
- Advise them to see their GP or practice nurse if symptoms of hypernatraemia persist.

Primary Care

- Advise the patient and their relatives of the importance of an adequate fluid and normal sodium intake.
- Discuss foods that are appropriate for a low-sodium diet, if indicated.
- Advise the patient and their relatives to avoid over-the-counter medications that are high in sodium.
- Educate the patient about the early signs of hypernatraemia, such as polyuria, nausea, vomiting and orthostatic hypotension, and advise relatives to observe the patient's mental status. Encourage the patient and their relatives to see their GP or practice nurse if any of these signs and symptoms occur.

Hypokalaemia

Hypokalaemia is a lower than normal level of potassium in the blood. It is probably the most common electrolyte abnormality affecting hospitalised patients. Most cases are mild, with a serum potassium in the range 3.0–3.5 mmol/L, but in 5% of cases it is below 3.0 mmol/L, and in 0.03% of cases less than 2.5 mmol/L. Even mild hypokalaemia can increase the incidence of cardiac arrhythmias.

Pathophysiology

Hypokalaemia can result from the use of diuretics or occur via the gastrointestinal tract as a result of nausea and vomiting. Large amounts of potassium could be lost through inappropriate use of non-potassium-sparing diuretics or corticosteroids. Another cause is excessive secretion of aldosterone, a hormone that regulates electrolyte balance.

Patients who suffer from diabetes mellitus are also at risk of developing hypokalaemia, as large amounts of potassium could be lost through glycosuria and osmotic diuresis. Hospitalised patients are at risk, especially those on extended parenteral fluid therapy with solutions that do not contain potassium. Poor dietary intake of potassium is also a factor.

Investigations and Diagnosis

- *Blood test*: urea and electrolytes.
- *ECG*: all patients with moderate or severe hypokalaemia need an ECG to determine whether the hypokalaemia is affecting cardiac function. Typical ECG findings with potassium lower than 3.0 mmol/L are:
  - Flat T waves
  - ST depression
  - Prominent U waves (Figure 23.8).
- *Urine test*: low urinary potassium may suggest poor intake, shift into the intracellular space or gastrointestinal loss. High levels indicate increased output. Low urinary sodium combined with high urinary potassium suggests secondary hypoaldosteronism.

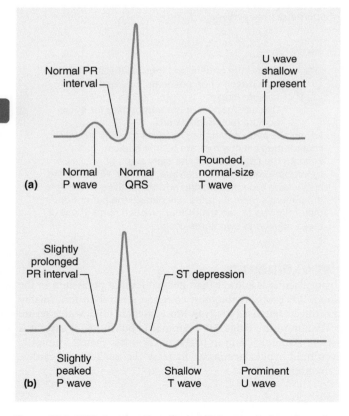

(a)
- Normal PR interval
- Normal P wave
- Normal QRS
- Rounded, normal-size T wave
- U wave shallow if present

(b)
- Slightly prolonged PR interval
- Slightly peaked P wave
- ST depression
- Shallow T wave
- Prominent U wave

Figure 23.8 ECG showing the effects of (a) normokalaemia and (b) hypokalaemia.

Signs and Symptoms

- Characteristic ECG changes of hypokalaemia: flattened or inverted T waves and a depressed ST segment. The most serious cardiac effect is an increased risk of atrial and ventricular dysrhythmias.
- General malaise/muscle pain/constipation.
- In severe cases, the patient may have advanced muscle weakness and paralysis (beginning in the lower extremities, progressing to the upper extremities and torso).
- Respiratory failure (due to involvement of respiratory muscles).
- Paralytic ileus (due to involvement of gastrointestinal muscles).
- Paraesthesia.
- Tetany.

Red Flag Potassium Chloride

 Potassium chloride must never be administered in a bolus as it can cause severe cardiac problems and lead to death. If the patient is to have intravenous potassium, it must be mixed in intravenous fluid and given slowly via a volumetric infusion pump. Where possible, use a ready-mixed solution rather than adding potassium to an infusion bag. If this is necessary, make sure that you mix (invert) the fluid bag thoroughly to disperse contents before administering it as potassium has a higher density than water and therefore settles to the bottom of the bag.

The concentration of potassium for peripheral intravenous administration should not exceed 40 mmol/L, as higher strengths can cause line phlebitis and pain. This can be avoided further by ensuring that the cannula is only available for potassium infusions and labelled to indicate that it should not be used for other drugs.

The infusion site must be checked prior to use for signs of inflammation and every 2–4 hours. Check with the patient that they are not in any pain as a result of the infusion.

Nursing Care and Management

As hypokalaemia can be life-threatening, it is important to recognise early signs and take necessary measures to protect the patient. Any loss of potassium through diarrhoea and vomiting should be replaced quickly. Monitor vital signs, including blood pressure and peripheral pulses. Tachypnoea, dyspnoea, tachycardia and/or a change in blood pressure may indicate decreasing ability to tolerate activities.

If the hypokalaemia is caused by diuretic or laxative abuse, advise the patient on the importance of maintaining adequate levels of potassium. Encourage diet and drinks high in potassium such as spinach, raw carrots, pork, beef, banana, orange juice and cod.

If the patient is to have intravenous potassium, great care needs to be taken in the safe administration of potassium. Closely monitor intravenous flow rate and response to potassium replacement therapy. Nurses need to be aware that rapid potassium infusion is dangerous and can lead to cardiac arrest.

While the patient is receiving an intravenous infusion of potassium, monitor vital signs hourly and report changes immediately. Check infusion sites for inflammation and ask the patient if the site of infusion feels uncomfortable.

Muscle cramps and weakness are early signs of hypokalaemia. Advise the patient to take periods of rest during exercise and to keep well hydrated.

Health Promotion and Discharge

- Identify patients who are risk of developing hypokalaemia.
- Discuss the importance of a good intake of potassium with patients at risk.
- If the patient is on a non-potassium-sparing diuretic, stress the importance of a potassium supplement in their diet.
- Advise the patient to seek advice from their GP or practice nurse if signs and symptoms of hypokalaemia are evident.
- Advise the patient that intense exercise and sweating can lower serum potassium and therefore advise caution in undertaking strenuous activities.
- Encourage intake of fluids rich in potassium, such as orange juice, when excess fluid is lost through sweating, vomiting or diarrhoea.

> **Primary Care**
>
> Before discharge into the community, the patient and their relatives will need health promotion advice regarding the maintenance of adequate potassium levels.
>
> - Advise on the importance of taking any prescribed medications, including potassium supplements, and their unwanted effects.
> - Recommend diet and drinks rich in potassium like carrots, meat and fish.
> - Advise on using salt substitutes (if recommended) to increase potassium intake.
> - Advise the reporting of signs and symptoms of hypokalaemia and regular check-ups with their GP or practice nurse, especially if taking digitalis.

Hyperkalaemia

Hyperkalaemia is defined as plasma potassium in excess of 5 mmol/L. Potassium is the most abundant intracellular cation, with approximately 98% located inside the cell. Hyperkalaemia could occur as a result of:

- Renal impairment
- Increased intake of potassium in diet and medications
- A shift from the intracellular to the extracellular space
- Pseudohyperkalaemia could occur as a result of:
  - Prolonged tourniquet time when taking a sample
  - Difficulty collecting a blood sample
  - The fist may have been clenched
  - Test tube haemolysis, e.g. blood may have been squirted through a needle into the bottle
  - Use of the wrong anticoagulant, especially potassium ethylenediaminetetraacetic acid (EDTA)
  - Sample of blood stored for too long
  - Sample taken from limb receiving intravenous fluids containing potassium.

Pathophysiology

The major causes of hyperkalaemia are kidney disease, diseases of the adrenal gland, potassium leaking out of cells into the circulation, trauma and starvation, and medications such as potassium supplements. Potassium moving out of the cell could occur in acidosis – when hydrogen ions move into the cell, potassium moves out.

Cell membrane function is very susceptible to potassium levels. Even a small difference can affect cardiac muscle function, resulting in cardiac arrest. In diabetes, when patients are treated with insulin for hyperkalaemia, potassium moves into the cell with glucose via the co-transporter system, thus lowering the serum potassium level. Serious consequences may arise for the patient if the treatment is not regulated properly. Bianchi *et al.* (2019) report that moderate hyperkalaemia can also be managed by inducing diarrhoea with regular lactulose, or by using rectal calcium polystyrene sulfonate resin (calcium resonium), thus removing potassium via the gastrointestinal tract.

Investigations and Diagnosis

- *Full blood count*: looking for normocytic, normochromic anaemia (which may suggest acute haemolysis), thrombocytosis and/or leucocytosis.
- Serum urea and electrolytes.
- *ECG*: in hyperkalaemia the ECG may show:
  - Tall T (tented) waves
  - Prolonged PR interval
  - Widening and prolongation of the QRS (Figure 23.9).

Signs and Symptoms

Symptoms are non-specific and include weakness and fatigue. Occasionally, a patient presents with muscular paralysis or shortness of breath. They may also complain of palpitations or chest pain.

Nursing Care and Management

Care of the patient with hyperkalaemia focuses on identifying the problem and taking measures to return potassium within the normal range. Interventions should include preventing fluid imbalance, detecting cardiac problems and monitoring the impact hyperkalaemia has on other body systems.

Fluid and Dietary Management Renal failure and Addison disease are some of the causes of hyperkalaemia (Bianchi *et al.*, 2019). Patients are at risk for fluid retention and other electrolyte imbalances, affecting other systems of the body. If the patient is

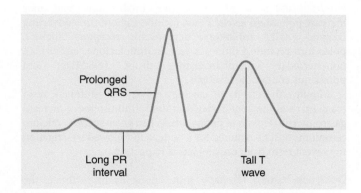

Figure 23.9 ECG pattern of hyperkalaemia, showing prolonged QRS and tall T wave.

in renal failure, then a strict fluid regimen needs to be adhered to as per organisational policy and regulation.

- Daily checks on serum urea and electrolytes should be done to ensure that treatment is effective.
- Weigh the patient daily to ensure that they are not gaining fluid-retaining weight.
- Maintain an accurate fluid input and output chart and advise the patient and their relatives of the importance of monitoring fluid balance.
- Monitor urine output hourly. Oliguria or anuria may indicate renal failure and thus an increased risk for hyperkalaemia and fluid volume excess.
- Ensure that the patient is on a low-potassium diet and avoids consuming fruit juice, fruits, chocolate, fruit gums, biscuits, coffee or potatoes.
- Provide reassurance and support for the patient and their relatives.

What the Experts Say

A man in his 80s was admitted to hospital for management of diabetes complications. His nurse and doctor identified that the man's potassium levels were high (6.9 mmol/L) and he was commenced on treatment for hyperkalaemia. Despite this, his potassium levels remained elevated after several blood tests.

A few days after admission, the man was observed adding three or four sachets of a reduced-sodium salt to his meals. The patient was advised to stop adding these non-prescribed supplements which were, in fact, causing him harm. The patient's blood levels tested at 4.9 mmol/L once the reduced-sodium salt was taken out of his diet.

This type of salt could significantly raise potassium levels in patients with reduced kidney function, or those taking certain drugs.

Protecting the Heart Hyperkalaemia can affect myocardial contraction, resulting in poor cardiac output as high levels of potassium can affect atrial and ventricular depolarisation.

- ECGs should be taken to assess any changes in cardiac function.
- Monitor vital signs hourly, reporting changes in pulse or respiration rates immediately to enable prompt action.

Medications Seek to discontinue medications that may increase potassium levels. These include angiotensin converting enzyme (ACE) inhibitors, angiotensin receptor blockers, potassium-retaining diuretics (e.g. spironolactone, amiloride), non-steroidal anti-inflammatory drugs (NSAIDs) and potassium-containing laxatives.

Monitor the effects of calcium polystyrene sulfonate resin (calcium resonium) enema and lactulose administered to increase gastrointestinal losses of potassium. When given rectally, calcium resonium must be retained for 9 hours and followed by irrigation to prevent resin from causing faecal impaction.

Dextrose/Insulin Therapy Intravenous insulin facilitates the shift of potassium into the cells. This treatment is administered with 50 mL of 50% glucose. It lowers serum potassium within 15 minutes, necessitating regular serum potassium level checks.

Blood glucose should be measured 30 minutes after starting the infusion and then hourly up to 6 hours after completion as delayed hypoglycaemia is possible when less than 30 g of glucose is administered with insulin.

Health Promotion and Discharge

- Advise the patient about foods high in potassium, such as bananas, milk, shellfish, nuts and chocolate.
- Advise the patient to check food labels and over-the-counter prescriptions for their potassium content.
- Discuss the importance of adequate fluid intake to promote renal excretion of potassium.
- Advise the patient to avoid adding salt supplements to their diet.
- Hyperkalaemia is a serious condition. Inform the patient of the signs and symptoms of hyperkalaemia and that they should report to the GP or practice nurse if they recognise these symptoms.

Primary Care

To continue their management at home, advise patients and their relatives on the following.

- Foods rich in potassium, e.g. tea, coffee, wholegrain bread, chocolate.
- Foods low in potassium, e.g. butter, margarine, honey, cranberry juice.
- Avoid potassium supplements.
- Daily weight and reporting gains to practice nurse.
- Carefully read food/dietary supplement labels.
- The importance of maintaining an adequate fluid intake or restriction to maintain renal function.

Hypocalcaemia

Calcium is the fifth most abundant ion in the body. The normal total serum calcium concentration is 2.12–2.62 mmol/L in adults. Ninety-nine percent of calcium is found in the bones, 0.5% in the teeth and another 0.5% in soft tissues.

Pathophysiology

Hypocalcaemia can result from hypoparathyroidism from surgery (parathyroidectomy, thyroidectomy), radiotherapy, acute pancreatitis, systemic disease (e.g. amyloidosis, sarcoidosis), deficiency or abnormal metabolism of vitamin D, hypomagnesaemia and renal failure.

Calcium exists in two forms in the ECF: in plasma, as free ionised calcium, and as a complex bound to protein. It is the free ionised calcium that is important for muscle contraction and conducting nerve impulses. Hypocalcaemia decreases the contractility of cardiac muscle fibres, leading to decreased cardiac output.

Symptoms

The symptoms of hypocalcaemia include:

- Low blood calcium (<2.12 mmol/L)
- Tetany (tonic muscular spasm)
- Painful muscle spasm of hands and feet
- Facial muscle spasms/grimacing
- Lip and mouth paraesthesias (tingling or numbness of the lips or mouth)
- Finger and toe paraesthesias
- Muscle aches/bone pain
- Fracture/deformity.

Nursing Care and Management

Usually, hypocalcaemia is not a major problem in the adult, as there is a large calcium reserve in the bones. However, women are more at risk of calcium loss than men and of developing osteoporosis. Treating the underlying cause is essential.

- Monitor cardiovascular status including heart rhythm/rate, blood pressure and peripheral pulses. Hypocalcaemia can lead to poor cardiac output and hypotension.
- Frequently monitor airway and respiratory status, reporting changes that include respiratory stridor (a high-pitched, harsh inspiratory sound indicative of upper airway obstruction) or increased respiratory rate or effort. These changes may indicate laryngeal spasm due to tetany.
- Advise women of all ages of the importance of maintaining adequate calcium intake through diet or calcium supplements, as needed.
- Discuss hormone replacement therapy and potential benefits during and after menopause.
- Encourage women and men to take regular exercise.

Medications Turner *et al.* (2016) report that in acute hypocalcaemia, the following treatment should be carried out.

- Administer 10–20 mL of calcium gluconate 10% by slow intravenous injection. Repeat as necessary, and follow with an infusion of 100 mL of 10% calcium gluconate in 1 litre of normal saline or 5% dextrose 50–100 mL/h until normocalcaemia is achieved.

Additional guidance in managing hypocalcaemia includes the following points.

- Oral calcium preparations may need to be given to complement intravenous treatment or where IV access is difficult.
- Monitor serum calcium concentrations regularly to assess response.
- Give vitamin D by mouth to assist with calcium absorption in persistent hypocalcaemia.
- Monitor for cardiac arrhythmias during intravenous administrations of calcium.
- If a patient has low magnesium, correcting magnesium levels is necessary before hypocalcaemia will resolve.

A diet high in calcium-rich foods may be recommended for patients with chronic hypocalcaemia. Calcium supplements may be combined with vitamin D, or vitamin D may be given alone to increase gastrointestinal absorption of calcium. If hypocalcaemia is caused by malabsorption, the underlying problem should be treated. Patients with coeliac disease should take oral calcium and vitamin D and adhere to a gluten-free diet.

Health Promotion and Discharge

- Discuss the risk factors and preventive measures related to hypocalcaemia with the patient.
- Advise the patient on calcium supplements and the importance of maintaining good fluid intake.
- Provide information on food sources high in calcium and vitamin D.
- Inform the patient on how to recognise the signs and symptoms of hypocalcaemia and to report to the practice nurse or their GP when symptoms persist.
- Discuss hormone replacement therapy with women during and after menopause.

Primary Care

In preparing the patient with hypocalcaemia for discharge and home care, the nurse should discuss the following with the patient and their relatives.

- Discuss risk factors for hypocalcaemia specific to the patient, and provide information about managing these risk factors to avoid future episodes of hypocalcaemia.
- Advise about prescribed medications, including calcium supplements.
- Provide a list of foods high in calcium, as well as sources of vitamin D if recommended.
- Discuss symptoms to report to the practice nurse/GP and stress the importance of follow-up care.

Hypercalcaemia

Hypercalcaemia is a condition in which the serum calcium is greater than 2.62 mmol/L. Excess ionised calcium in the ECF can have serious widespread effects.

Pathophysiology

Hypercalcaemia occurs when the serum calcium is above 2.62 mmol/L and usually results from increased resorption of calcium from the bones. This may be due to cancer of the bones (bone tissue destruction by a tumour), prolonged immobilisation and milk-alkaline syndrome, usually caused by too much milk and antacid at the same time. Primary hyperparathyroidism results from increased parathyroid hormone production, and malignancy is responsible for more than 90% of cases. Prolonged immobility and lack of weight bearing also cause increased resorption of bone, releasing calcium into extracellular fluids.

Increased absorption of calcium from the gastrointestinal tract can lead to hypercalcaemia because of excess vitamin D, overuse of calcium-containing antacids or excessive milk ingestion. Renal failure and drugs such as thiazide diuretics can interfere with kidney elimination of calcium, causing high serum calcium levels. Endocrine conditions like thyrotoxicosis, phaeochromocytoma and primary adrenal insufficiency can also cause hypercalcaemia.

Investigations and Diagnosis

- Thyroid function test.
- Plain X-rays may show features indicative of bone abnormalities, such as demineralisation, bone cysts, pathological fractures or bony metastases.
- Ultrasound scan, computed tomography (CT) scan or intravenous pyelogram (IVP) may be required to detect abnormalities of the urogenital tract, such as calcification or stones.
- Ultrasound or technetium scan of the parathyroid glands may be indicated if hypertrophy or adenoma is suspected.

Symptoms

- Polyuria
- Polydipsia
- Constipation
- Muscle weakness
- Anorexia
- Nausea and vomiting

Hypercalcaemia can also cause more serious problems, such as depression, dehydration, bone fractures, kidney stones and myocardial infarction.

401

Nursing Care and Management

This can be considered under the headings of the immediate management of acute hypercalcaemia and the longer-term management of the underlying condition.

Fluid and Diet Management Patients with hypercalcaemia are administered 0.9% saline to increase the circulating volume and promote urine excretion of calcium. A loop diuretic such as furosemide is given to enhance the effect by inhibiting the tubular reabsorption of calcium. Hydration is needed because many patients are dehydrated due to vomiting or renal defects in concentrating urine. In addition, loop diuretics tend to depress renal calcium reabsorption, thereby helping to lower blood calcium levels.

Cardiovascular and renal function is carefully assessed prior to fluid therapy; the patient is carefully monitored for evidence of fluid overload during treatment.

Discourage excessive consumption of high-calcium foods such as milk, cheese and leafy vegetables. Ensure that there is adequate roughage in the diet to prevent constipation. If necessary, seek advice from the dietitian regarding low-calcium foods.

Encourage fluids such as blueberry or cranberry juice to help maintain acidic urine. Acidic, dilute urine reduces the risk of calcium salts precipitating out to form kidney stones. Fluids also help to prevent calcium renal stones and urinary tract infection.

Closely monitor and maintain an input and output chart.

Risk for Injury Take necessary precautions when moving or transferring patient; their bones are prone to fracture due to bone resorption.

If the patient is prescribed digoxin, observe them for symptoms of digoxin toxicity: vision changes, anorexia and changes in heart rate and rhythm. Hypercalcaemia increases the risk of digitalis toxicity so monitor serum digitalis levels.

Bed-bound patients should be encouraged to perform passive and active exercises.

Vital signs may indicate if the patient is improving, stable or getting worse. Frequently assess vital signs, respiratory status and heart sounds. Report any changes immediately to the person in charge.

Medications Glucocorticoids (cortisone), which compete with vitamin D, and a low-calcium diet may be prescribed to decrease gastrointestinal absorption of calcium, inhibit bone resorption and increase urinary calcium excretion. Calcitonin may be prescribed to decrease skeletal mobilisation of calcium and phosphorus, and to increase renal output.

Bisphosphonates (sodium clodronate and ibandronic acid) are very effective for helping to reduce calcium levels. They can also help to reduce pain from bone metastases and stop damaged bones breaking.

Health Promotion and Discharge

- Identify risk factors and promote mobility and light exercise. Physical exercise has frequently been shown to induce bone mass gain and prevent osteoporosis. Weight-bearing exercises, such as walking, mainly affect the bones in the legs, hips and lower spine.
- Advise the patient on the effects of smoking. Smoking has been shown to increase bone loss as well as dramatically increasing the risk of a number of serious health problems.
- Advise the patient to drink plenty of fluids, especially water. Drinking fluids can prevent dehydration and formation of kidney stones.

Primary Care

Nurses should offer advice on the following topics when preparing the patient for discharge into the community.

- Avoiding excess intake of calcium-rich foods and antacids.
- Ensuring that the patient understands why they have to continue taking the prescribed medications.
- Encouraging the patient to increase dietary fibre and fluid intake to prevent constipation.
- Maintaining weight-bearing physical activity to prevent hypercalcaemia.
- Encouraging a generous fluid intake of up to 3–4 L per day, if allowed.
- Reporting early symptoms of hypercalcaemia to the practice nurse or GP.
- Promoting mobility in patients as it helps the uptake of calcium.
- Advising the patient on how to recognise the signs and symptoms of hypercalcaemia and how to take preventive measures.

Hypomagnesaemia

Hypomagnesaemia, a low serum level of magnesium, is associated with concomitant electrolyte disturbances like hypokalaemia and hypocalcaemia and is seen in many critically ill patients. If untreated, hypomagnesaemia may also lead to fatal dysrhythmias. Since normal kidneys can excrete large amounts of magnesium, hypermagnesaemia is rarely seen in the absence of renal insufficiency.

Serum magnesium levels should be checked regularly and replaced accordingly, particularly in serious illness (Hansen & Bruserud, 2018).

Shock

Shock is a life-threatening condition that occurs when vital organs are deprived of oxygen due to a problem affecting the circulatory system. Shock develops when oxygen supply to the cells is insufficient to meet metabolic demand.

Pathophysiology

Shock is a state in which there is inadequate tissue perfusion to maintain oxygen supply which is necessary for normal cellular function (Vincent & De Backer, 2013). Shock is divided into:

- *Hypovolaemic*: reduced blood flow resulting from trauma, blood loss through surgery, dehydration
- *Cardiogenic*: due to heart diseases such myocardial infarction and heart failure
- *Obstructive*: obstruction of blood flow, e.g. pulmonary embolism
- *Distributive*: due to impaired utilisation of oxygen and thus production of energy by the cell. Septic, neurogenic and anaphylactic shock all come under this group.

Stages of Shock

Stage I: Early, Reversible and Compensatory Shock

In the early stages, signs and symptoms of shock are non-identifiable. Pulse rate may be slightly elevated. If injury is minor, arterial blood pressure is usually maintained and no further symptoms occur.

However, cellular changes may occur in response to poorer blood flow. At this stage, certain compensatory mechanisms are initiated.

- The release of epinephrine (adrenaline) and norepinephrine (noradrenaline) from the adrenal medulla.
- The renin–angiotensin system causes narrowing of peripheral blood vessels and raises blood pressure. Release of aldosterone from the adrenal cortex stimulates the kidneys to reabsorb sodium and excrete potassium.
- The release of ADH from the posterior pituitary gland increases renal reabsorption of water to increase intravascular volume.
- Glucocorticoids raise blood glucose by a process called gluconeogenesis. In addition, glucocorticoids release amino acids from tissues and decrease protein synthesis.

Stage II: Progressive Shock

If the shock is not successfully treated, it will proceed to the progressive stage. Because of the decreased perfusion of the cells, sodium ions build up within the cell, while potassium ions leak out. This can result in hyperkalaemia, which may in turn cause cardiac arrest. Anaerobic metabolism as a result of inadequate oxygen supply increases the body's metabolic acidosis. The arteriolar smooth muscle and precapillary sphincters relax, such that blood remains in the capillaries. As a result, the hydrostatic pressure will increase and, combined with histamine release, will lead to leakage of fluid and protein into the surrounding tissues. As fluid is lost from the blood vessels, the blood concentration and viscosity increase.

Stage III: Refractory Shock

At this stage, the vital organs have failed and the shock can no longer be reversed. Brain damage and cell death are occurring, and death will occur imminently.

Hypovolaemic Shock

Hypovolaemic shock is the most common type of shock and is caused by insufficient circulating volume. Its primary cause is haemorrhage (internal and/or external) or loss of fluid from the circulation, for example dehydration (Nall, 2021). The aim is to correct the hypovolaemia and hypoperfusion of vital organs such as the heart and the kidneys before irreversible damage occurs. In the early stages of hypovolaemia, the compensatory mechanisms are initiated (see stage I). However, if the fluid loss is great, compensatory mechanisms may not be successful and the patient's condition will deteriorate.

Investigations and Diagnosis

Tests that may be carried out include:

- Blood chemistry, including kidney function tests
- Arterial blood gases/oxygen saturation
- Blood pressure measurements
- *Full blood count*: urea and electrolytes, haemoglobin, cross-match for blood transfusion
- CT scan, ultrasound or X-ray of suspected areas
- Echocardiogram to identify heart problems
- Urinary catheterisation to measure urine output.

Signs and Symptoms

- Tachycardia, as a result of low blood flow. The pulse will be weak and thready.
- Tachypnoea in response to sympathetic nervous stimulation, hypoxia, acidosis.
- Peripheries will be cold from poor perfusion. Capillary refill time will be prolonged. This, however, may be a poor indicator of hypovolaemia.
- Fall in blood pressure or postural hypotension as a result of poor cardiac output.
- Anxiety and restlessness.
- Late features include confusion as a result of decreased brain oxygenation.

Case Study

Maria Baglietto is a widowed 84-year-old women admitted to the acute medical ward following a 3-day history of vomiting and diarrhoea. Maria had gone on an outing with a local club a few days previously and eaten from a buffet. Several other people who went to the same outing have also developed similar symptoms.

Maria's daughter visits her daily and had found her mother very drowsy that lunchtime. Although she responded to questions, it was clear to her daughter that her mother was confused.

A blood test at the hospital reveals a significantly low sodium and potassium count. Maria is severely dehydrated. She is started on a regimen of normal saline with potassium 40 mmol/L, 8 hourly. Oral fluids are to be encouraged when she is more alert.

The nurse prioritises care for the first 12 hours and commences a strict intake and output chart to monitor fluids. She considers inserting a urinary catheter if Maria does not produce urine after 4 hours. She charts observations hourly and performs frequent neurological checks. She follows plans for mouth and pressure area care and documents this. She undertakes a risk assessment for falls, making sure that Maria has her call bell nearby so that she can ask for assistance if she needs to get out of bed.

Practice Assessment Document

The student will need to engage in discussion with their placement supervisor about proficiencies throughout their placement and find proactive ways to demonstrate achievement. For instance, in order to show that you have knowledge and understanding of observations and what to do with abnormal findings, you and your supervisor may decide that you will be undertaking Maria's neurological assessment over a 12-hour shift.

You may need to prepare for this to ensure that you have all the knowledge you require. Before the shift, you may need to review your knowledge of neurological responses and the procedure. At the start of the shift, you will probably need to observe your supervisor undertaking the process once or twice before you attempt it yourself under direction. It is prudent to take notes and to ask questions about anything that needs to be clarified after this has happened. Once your supervisor is sure that you can safely do the procedure on your own, you may discuss when and how you produce information to report on Maria's progress.

Cardiogenic Shock

Cardiogenic shock occurs when there is failure of the heart's pumping action, resulting in reduced cardiac output and consequent hypoperfusion of the tissues and organs despite the presence of adequate intravascular volume. Myocardial infarction is the most common cause of cardiogenic shock (Rathod et al., 2019).

Signs and Symptoms

- Chest pain
- Nausea and vomiting
- Dyspnoea
- Profuse sweating
- Confusion and disorientation
- Palpitations
- Pale, cold skin with slow capillary refill and poor peripheral pulses (paleness may also be noted in the following areas: inner membranes of the lower eyelids, palms of the hands, fingernails, tongue, mucous membranes inside the mouth)
- Hypotension
- Tachycardia or bradycardia
- Peripheral oedema
- Oliguria

Obstructive Shock

Obstructive shock occurs when there is inadequate perfusion of tissues with oxygenated blood resulting from pulmonary embolism, cardiac tamponade or tension pneumothorax.

Signs and Symptoms

- Hypotension
- Weak and rapid pulse
- Cool and clammy skin
- Rapid breathing
- Hypothermia
- Confusion
- Dry mouth
- Fatigue

Distributive (Septic) Shock

Septic shock is a life-threatening condition that happens when blood pressure drops to a dangerously low level due to a serious blood infection (sepsis). If sepsis is not treated, it leads to septic shock. Patients at risk for developing infections leading to septic shock include those who are hospitalised and those who have debilitating chronic illnesses or poor nutritional status.

The condition is often associated with Gram-negative bacteria like *Escherichia coli*, *Klebsiella*, *Proteus* and *Pseudomonas*. Gram-positive bacteria, e.g. streptococci and staphylococci, can also cause sepsis.

Septic shock occurs in two distinct phases: hyperdynamic phase and hypodynamic phase. In the hyperdynamic phase, the patient may present with low cardiac output, low urine output, vasodilation, tachycardia, confusion, agitation and fever with chills. The hypodynamic phase is characterised by hypovolaemia and hypotension, and activity of the compensatory mechanisms results in typical shock manifestations, including cold moist skin, oliguria and changes in mental status. Death may result from respiratory failure, cardiac failure or renal failure.

Neurogenic Shock

Neurogenic shock is the result of an imbalance between parasympathetic and sympathetic stimulation of vascular smooth muscle. It can be caused by an illness, a drug or an injury blocking impulses from the sympathetic nerves and thus increasing parasympathetic activity.

Neurogenic shock causes a dramatic reduction in systemic vascular resistance as the size of the vascular compartment increases. As systemic vascular resistance decreases, pressure in the blood vessels becomes too low to drive nutrients across capillary membranes, and cellular metabolism is impaired.

Signs and Symptoms

- *Blood pressure*: hypotension
- *Pulse*: slow and bounding
- *Respirations*: vary
- *Skin*: warm, dry
- *Mental status*: anxious, restless, lethargic progressing to comatose
- *Urine output*: oliguria to anuria
- *Other*: lowered body temperature

Anaphylactic Shock

Anaphylaxis is a severe, life-threatening, allergic reaction that can affect many systems of the body, including:

- Airways
- Breathing
- Circulation.

There are numerous triggers, including food (peanuts, fish, egg, milk), venom (bee and wasp stings) and drugs (antibiotics, NSAIDs, opioids).

Signs and Symptoms

Signs include itching of the palate or external auditory meatus, dyspnoea, laryngeal oedema (stridor) and wheezing (bronchospasm). General symptoms include palpitations and tachycardia (as opposed to bradycardia in a simple vasovagal episode at immunisation), nausea, vomiting and abdominal pain, feeling faint with a sense of impending doom and, ultimately, collapse, loss of consciousness and cardiac arrest.

What the Experts Say Eleanor's Experience

" When her son, Thomas, was 20 months old, Eleanor discovered that he had a severe food allergy. He was eating a peanut bar at a family party. He took one bite and soon began coughing. His face became swollen and he broke out in hives. Eleanor rushed Thomas to hospital. He was experiencing a life-threatening allergic reaction called 'anaphylaxis' or 'anaphylactic shock'.

By the time medical personnel began treating him, 'he was one huge hive', Eleanor recalls. 'They worked on him for 3 hours before he began to look more like himself again.'

Eleanor's initial reaction was shock. 'I knew nothing about food allergies or anaphylaxis,' she said. 'Now I have to carry an Epipen with me for Thomas should he have another reaction and I have to be really alert over anything he eats that I have not made myself.'

Nursing Care and Management

The nursing care of shock involves identifying patients at risk and taking appropriate measures to detect early signs of shock to safeguard the patient. Currently, hospitals use various early warning tools like NEWS2 (RCP, 2017) to identify patients at risk of developing shock.

- Monitor vital signs (body temperature, pulse and respiration rate, blood pressure, oxygen saturation using a pulse oximeter) half-hourly for patients at risk of developing shock and report and document any changes immediately so that prompt action can be taken. Continuous monitoring will provide information about the patient's respiratory status.
- Ensure that the patient's airway is not obstructed; check their breathing. Administer oxygen as prescribed using a face-mask or nasal cannula and monitor its effect. Nurses should be alert in detecting hyperventilation occurring in respiratory alkalosis leading to fatigue of the respiratory muscle. If this occurs, the patient may need ventilation to assist their breathing.
- The patient may be connected to an ECG monitor to assess cardiac status. Nurses should be familiar with the normal ECG tracing of the heart so that they can detect and report any arrhythmias to the person in charge.
- Communicate verbally with the patient when recording as it is vital to ensure that the patient is conscious and alert. If cerebral perfusion is low, leading to cerebral hypoxia, the patient will gradually become less responsive and eventually unconscious.
- A urinary catheter may be inserted to measure and record hourly urine output. A decrease in circulating blood volume with hypotension and the effect of the compensatory mechanisms associated with shock can cause poor urine production. Urinary output of less than 0.5 mL/kg per hour may indicate reduced renal blood flow and is a sign of early renal failure. Measurement of urine osmolality and specific gravity may point to altered renal function.
- Monitor bowel sounds, abdominal distension and abdominal pain. Check with the patient if they are in any pain and administer any prescribed medication for pain regularly.
- Check with the patient for any chest pain and observe for central (lips) and peripheral (fingernails) cyanosis, anxiety and restlessness.
- Monitor the condition of the skin for colour and temperature, as they may indicate the severity of shock. If the skin is pale and clammy, this indicates overactive sympathetic activity.
- Check for capillary refill. A slow capillary refill suggests that there is vasoconstriction, which would lead to poor delivery of oxygen to the tissues.

Medications

In cardiogenic shock, the aim is to minimise the damage to the myocardium. Apart from oxygen therapy, inotropes (drugs modifying the force or speed of contraction of cardiac muscle) and dopamine, dobutamine, epinephrine (adrenaline) and norepinephrine (noradrenaline) may be administered to improve cardiac contractility and elevate blood pressure. Nurses need to be aware of the side-effects (tachycardia, dysrhythmias, myocardial ischaemia, hyperglycaemia, lactic acidosis and excessive vasoconstriction) which may affect the progress of the patient.

Fluid Replacement

The most effective treatment for the patient in hypovolaemic shock is the administration of intravenous fluids or blood. Normal saline is the fluid of first choice (Guest, 2020). However, regular checks of urea and electrolytes should be carried out, as saline contains a high amount of sodium and if the patient has renal failure then the high levels of sodium could lead to hypernatraemia. Treatment of hypovolaemia depends on its severity. At its most severe, intravenous fluids and blood transfusions are given rapidly to raise blood volume. Medications are used to increase blood pressure, stabilise heart rate and strengthen heart contractions. Any underlying cause of hypovolaemia must also be treated to prevent ongoing fluid loss.

Nurses overseeing an infusion of fluids and monitoring hypovolaemia should be aware of the potential complications and their related symptoms. Complications of infusing large volumes of fluids include hypothermia, acid–base imbalance, hyperkalaemia, hypocalcaemia, clotting problems and allergic reactions. Nurses need to check the patient's blood pressure, temperature, pulse, respiration and mental state hourly.

Blood and Blood Products

If hypovolaemic shock is due to haemorrhage, the transfusion of blood, blood products or plasma volume expanders may be used to treat the hypovolaemia. When using blood and blood products, nurses need to check that they have been cross-matched and that they adhere to organisational guidelines for administering blood. The patient's temperature, heart, respiration rates and blood pressure should be obtained and recorded every 15 minutes for the first blood transfusion.

Blood Transfusion Procedure

Before commencing a blood transfusion, these are some of the action points you should undertake.

- Always have a second nurse with you.
- Positively identify the patient using an open question: 'Can you tell me your full name and date of birth?'.
- Check these details against the patient's ID band for accuracy.
- Check that the transfusion has been prescribed in the treatment chart.
- Check that the blood group and donation number on the compatibility label are identical to the blood group and donation number on the blood component.
- Monitor the patient's vital signs as per trust protocols for blood transfusion.
- Check with the patient if they are comfortable with the transfusion.
- Ask the patient to report any reaction such as body rashes and fever immediately to the nurse.
- Document care interventions and record outcomes.

What to Do If . . .

A patient has a severe blood transfusion reaction (shortness of breath, chest pain, hypotension, nausea/vomiting).

- STOP the transfusion and keep the line open with normal saline.
- Urgent medical review.
- Continuous vital signs until stable.
- Remain by the patient's side and provide comfort and reassurance.
- Always document any intervention and record the outcomes.

Case Study

Morris Casey, 71 years, is admitted to a medical ward with a history of shortness of breath and fatigue. His initial blood results show a low haemoglobin count of 8.4 g/dL and low serum iron count. He is diagnosed with iron deficiency anaemia. His doctor orders 2 units of blood to be transfused over 6 hours and prescribes iron tablets for discharge, expected to be the next day if there are no complications.

The nurse prepares Morris for his transfusion. She makes him comfortable and spends some time explaining the reasons for the transfusion and what he should watch out for as adverse effects. Once Morris has given consent, she collects the first bag of blood and undertakes all the necessary product and identity checks before she starts Morris on the transfusion. The nurse takes a set of observations, and notes a score of 2 on Morris's NEWS2 chart due to a blood pressure of 103/60 mmHg and slightly elevated pulse of 96 beats per minute. These observations may indicate that the heart is compensating for Morris's lack of red blood cells by pumping blood around the body faster. She takes his observations every 15 minutes for the first hour and notes an improvement in blood pressure and pulse after the first unit which has brought his NEWS2 score down to 1.

Morris has the transfusions and experiences no problems. A repeat full blood count 12 hours later delivers a haemoglobin count of 110 g/L. Prior to discharge, the nurse refers Morris to a dietitian so that she can advise him on an iron-rich diet. An appointment is made for him to be reviewed at his family practice in 1 month.

Conclusion

This chapter has provided information regarding fluid and electrolyte imbalance and shock. It is essential for nurses to monitor patients in their care for subtle changes resulting from these imbalances. The elderly and children are at particular risk. Assisting patients with fluid imbalances, whether in the hospital or community setting, presents the nurse with a major challenge. Patients and their relatives will need support and information to help them understand and manage life-threatening situations.

Key Points

- The movement of fluid and electrolytes ensure that the cells have a constant supply of essential electrolytes like sodium, chloride and potassium.
- Fluid and electrolyte imbalance can affect all body systems, especially the cardiovascular, respiratory, renal and central nervous systems.
- The most common electrolyte imbalances relate to sodium, potassium and calcium.
- Both hyperkalaemia and hypokalaemia affect the conducting system of the heart. If not treated promptly, they can be fatal.
- Shock is a life-threatening condition that occurs when vital organs are deprived of oxygen due to a problem affecting the circulatory system. Shock develops when oxygen supply to the cells is insufficient to meet the metabolic demands of the cells.
- Hypovolaemic shock is the most common type of shock and is caused by insufficient circulating volume. Primary causes are haemorrhage or loss of fluid from the circulation. Correcting hypovolaemia and hypoperfusion of vital organs is imperative before irreversible damage occurs.
- Anaphylactic shock results in vasodilation, pooling of blood in the peripheries and hypovolaemia.

References

Bianchi, S., Aucella, F., De Nicola, L., *et al.* (2019) Management of hyperkalemia in patients with kidney disease: a position paper endorsed by the Italian Society of Nephrology. *Journal of Nephrology*, 32(4), 499–516.

Bradford, S. & Rossiter, S. (2020) Working together to improve outcomes for patients with chronic oedema/wet legs. *Wound UK*, 16(1), 52–56.

Care Quality Commission (2012) *Time to Listen in NHS Hospitals: Dignity and Nutrition Inspection Programme 2012.* www.cqc.org.uk/sites/default/files/documents/time_to_listen_-_nhs_hospitals_main_report_tag.pdf (accessed December 2021).

Davis, I., Laybourne, T. & Cronin, C. (2019) Improving the provision of mouth care in an acute hospital trust. *Nursing Times*, 115(5), 33–36.

Guest, M. (2020) Understanding the principles and aims of intravenous fluid therapy. *Nursing Standard*, 35(2), 75–82.

Hamilton, P.K., Morgan, N.A., Connolly, G.M. & Maxwell, A.P. (2017) Understanding acid–base disorders. *Ulster Medical Journal*, 86(3), 161–166.

Hansen, B. & Bruserud, Ø. (2018) Hypomagnesemia in critically ill patients. *Journal of Intensive Care*, 6(21), 1–11.

Health Education England (2016) *Mouth Care Matters.* www.mouthcarematters.hee.nhs.uk/wp-content/uploads/2016/10/MCM-GUIDE-2016_100pp_OCT-16_v121.pdf (accessed December 2021).

King's College London (2011) *The Challacombe Scale of Clinical Oral Dryness*. https://fgdpscotland.org.uk/wp-content/uploads/2018/09/Challacombe-Scale-oral-dryness-ENG.pdf (accessed December 2021).

Ko, S.Y., Esteve Cuevas, L.M., Willeboer, M., *et al.* (2019) The association between intravenous fluid resuscitation and mortality in older emergency department patients with suspected infection. *International Journal of Emergency Medicine*. https://intjem.biomedcentral.com/articles/10.1186/s12245-018-0219-2 (accessed December 2021).

Kozier, B., Erb, G., Berman, A., *et al.* (2012) *Fundamentals of Nursing: Concept, Process and Practice*, 2nd edn. Pearson Education, London.

Messina, Z. & Patrick, H. (2021) *Partial Pressure of Carbon Dioxide*. StatPearls, Treasure Island, FL. www.ncbi.nlm.nih.gov/books/NBK551648/

Nall, R. (2021) *Hypovolemic shock*. www.healthline.com/health/hypovolemic-shock (accessed December 2021).

National Institute for Health and Care Excellence (2015) *Hyponatraemia. Scenario: Management*. https://cks.nice.org.uk/topics/hyponatraemia/management/management/ (accessed December 2021).

Nursing & Midwifery Council (2018a) *Future Nurse: Standards of proficiency for registered nurses*. www.nmc.org.uk/globalassets/sitedocuments/education-standards/future-nurse-proficiencies.pdf (accessed December 2021).

Nursing & Midwifery Council (2018b) *Standards of Proficiency for Nursing Associates*. www.nmc.org.uk/globalassets/sitedocuments/education-standards/nursing-associates-proficiency-standards.pdf (accessed December 2021).

Nursing & Midwifery Council (2018c) *The Code: Professional Standards of Practice and Behaviour for Nurses, Midwives and Nursing Associates*. www.nmc.org.uk/globalassets/sitedocuments/nmc-publications/nmc-code.pdf (accessed December 2021).

Peate, I. & Evans, S. (2020) *Fundamentals of Anatomy and Physiology for Nursing and Healthcare Students*. Wiley-Blackwell, Hoboken, NJ.

Peate, I., Nair, M. & Wild, K. (2012) *Adult Nursing: Acute and Ongoing Care*. Pearson Education, Harlow.

Picetti, D., Foster, S., Pangle, A.K., *et al.* (2017) Hydration health literacy in the elderly. *Nutrition & Healthy Aging*, 4(3), 227–237.

Pierce, J.D., Shen, Q. & Thimmesch, A. (2016) The ongoing controversy: crystalloids versus colloids. *Journal of Infusion Nursing*, 39(1), 40–44.

Rathod, K.S., Sirker, A., Baumbach, A., *et al* (2019) Management of cardiogenic shock in patients with acute coronary syndromes. *British Journal of Hospital Medicine*, 80(4), 204–210.

Royal College of Physicians (2017) *National Early Warning Score (NEWS2)*. www.rcplondon.ac.uk/projects/outputs/national-early-warning-score-news-2 (accessed December 2021).

Turner J., Gittoes, N. & Selby, P. (2016) Emergency management of acute hypocalcaemia in adult patients. *Endocrine Connections*, 5(5), 7–8.

Vincent, J. & De Backer, D. (2013) Circulatory shock. *New England Journal of Medicine*, 369, 1726–1734.

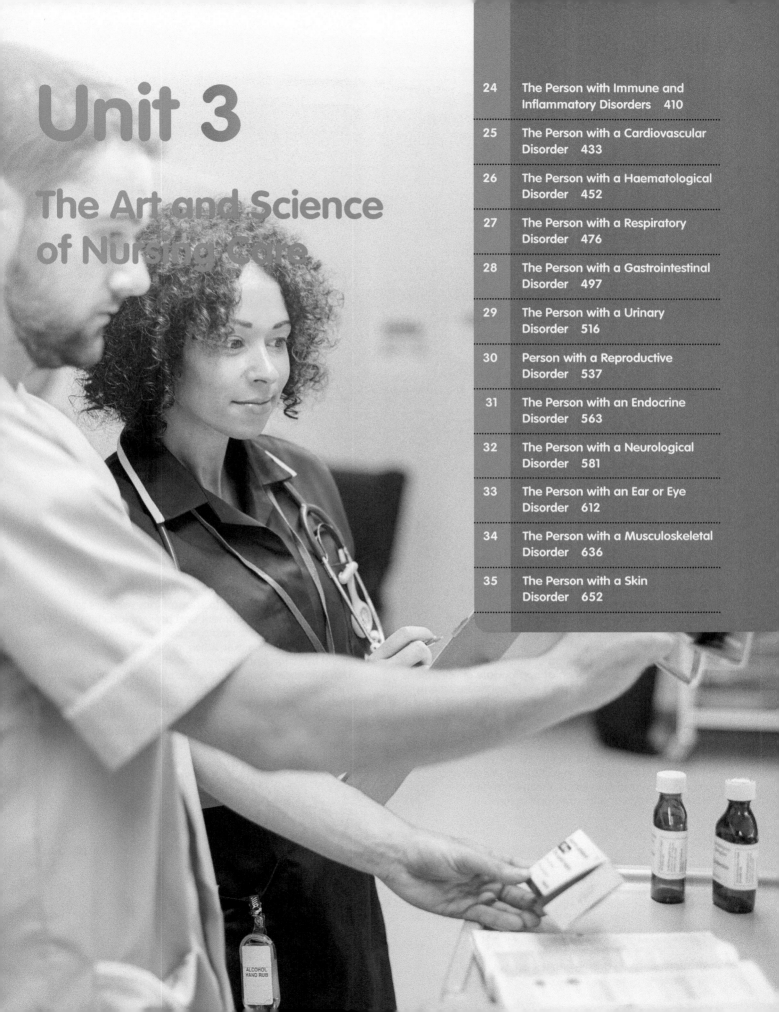

Unit 3

The Art and Science of Nursing Care

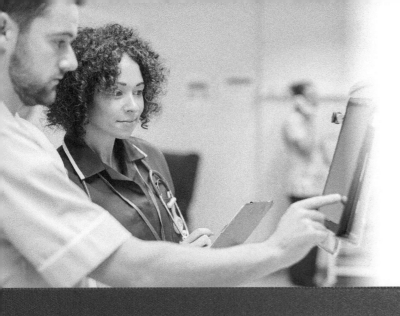

24

The Person with Immune and Inflammatory Disorders

Graeme Measor

Teesside University, UK

Learning Outcomes

On completion of this chapter you will be able to:

- Demonstrate and apply knowledge of the immune system, its form and function
- Describe the functions of the cells and chemical proteins, the tools for protecting the body against foreign invaders
- Understand the classification of micro-organisms to enable the implementation of appropriate interventions to provide a safe environment in a healthcare setting
- Discuss the physiology of innate immunity, explaining how inflammation links to infection and fever and wound healing
- Compare and contrast the processes of cell-mediated and antibody-mediated immunity
- Communicate information regarding the causes, implications and treatment of common health conditions involving the immune system.

Proficiencies

NMC Proficiencies and Standards:

- Protect health through understanding and applying knowledge of microbes to support interventions to provide a safe environment and prevent infection (2.12)
- Observe, assess and respond rapidly to infection risks using best practice guidelines, providing information to avoid infection and promote health (9.1)
- Use evidence-based practice to plan and structure individualised care to protect patients with a compromised immune system (1.20)
- Recognise signs of inflammation and infection (9)
- Evaluate the nursing care of patients with infection and implement effective interventions to promote recovery (3.15).

 Visit the companion website at **www.wiley.com/go/peate/nursingpractice3e** where you can test yourself using flashcards, multiple-choice questions and more.

Nursing Practice: Knowledge and Care, Third Edition. Edited by Ian Peate and Aby Mitchell.
© 2022 John Wiley & Sons Ltd. Published 2022 by John Wiley & Sons Ltd.
Companion website: www.wiley.com/go/peate/nursingpractice3e

Introduction

If microbes are ingested, inhaled or enter tissues through cuts or skin damage, they can cause disease. Despite our constant exposure to microbes, most of us remain relatively healthy, with our immune system taking care of unwanted invaders (*pathogens*). The function of the immune system is to protect the body against attack and build up immunity.

Healthcare professionals must have knowledge of the cells, tissues and organs that make up this system so they can recognise the signs of infection and initiate appropriate and timely care.

This chapter begins with a question, followed by an overview of the classification of microbes and then leads into the structures and functions of the immune system. The mechanisms of innate and acquired immunity are explored and explained. The diseases associated with a malfunctioning immune system are highlighted and discussed throughout the chapter.

Jot This Down

Think back to when you last had a cold or a sore throat. You may have had a runny or blocked nose, felt congested, been sneezing or coughing and had a dry mouth. Your throat may have been sore, your nasal secretions or sputum may have been discoloured. You may have gone to the practice nurse or GP who will have examined you, checked your temperature and felt your neck. They may have listened to your chest with a stethoscope, taken your pulse, asked you about the colour and consistency of any secretions such as sputum, and asked if you had any pain or discomfort anywhere.
- What do you think the practice nurse or GP was looking for?
- What medication did you expect and what medication might you have received?

These clinical signs will be answered and explained once you have explored and understood the anatomy and physiology of innate immunity.

In this exercise, you might have had the following thoughts. The common cold is caused by a viral infection of the upper respiratory tract (nose, sinuses and throat) and the symptoms are related to the inflammatory response of innate immunity, and it is this that the practice nurse or GP would have been looking for. The tissues become inflamed and the mucous membranes secrete excess mucus in order to trap the virus and sneezing then expels it from the body. Coughing is a result of the increased mucus dripping down the back of the throat. Low-grade fevers associated with the symptoms of a cold in young adults are not an indication of infection.

There is no cure for the common cold, and antibiotics will not help. Treatment is given to help relieve the symptoms and support innate immunity by:
- Replacing any fluids lost due to sweating and a runny nose, with plenty of liquids
- Rest
- Eating a healthy well-balanced diet, which is recommended to maintain a healthy immune system, but no specific diet or mineral or vitamin supplementation is necessary (NICE, 2016)
- Steam inhalation
- Gargling with salt water.

Wang *et al.* (2020) suggest that zinc supplements may reduce cold duration by 2.25 days in healthy adults. If the virus manages to overcome these initial defence mechanisms, a secondary infection with a new virus or bacteria can occur, although the risk is low (Ismail & Schellack, 2018). Examples include sinusitis, otitis media, bronchitis and pneumonias, which cause:
- Discoloured secretions (yellow/green)
- Persistent fever with a 'red' inflamed sore throat; white patches on the throat or tonsils
- Painful swelling of neck glands
- Pain in the chest, face, head or ears
- Breathlessness, wheezing.

Inflammation

The symptoms of inflammation are brought about by the organised activity of the immune system. Inflammation has different levels of intensity, varying from mild discomfort and irritability to life-threatening assaults on health. As it is a response to tissue damage, it can be localised or systemic. Signs of inflammation are redness, swelling, heat and pain, which are indicators that the body is initiating the innate immune response. It also indicates the start of the healing process and tissue repair (Figure 24.1).

The Innate Response

The main purpose of this response is to prevent entry of the invader. Skin and mucous membranes are the first line of defence. Immune cells called Langerhans cells in the epidermis and mucosal tissues serve as the first line of immunity. They are referred to as Toll-like receptors as they can recognise potential pathogens and activate the signalling pathways to start the immune response (Fitzgerald & Kagan, 2020).

When the Langerhans cells detect an intruder, they stimulate signalling dendritic cells and natural killer T cells, which are resident in the dermal layer of the skin. These then stimulate inflammatory dendritic cells, which release cytokines which initiate the inflammatory response.

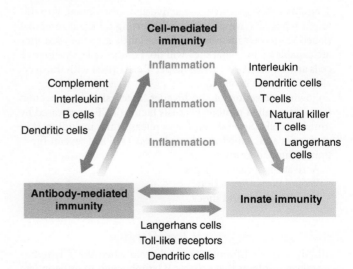

Figure 24.1 **The immune response has three interlinked phases: innate, cell mediated and antibody mediated.**

The inflammatory response can proceed in one of three ways.

1. If the Langerhans cells recognise the antigen, they take a piece of it and present it to the memory B cells archive. The B cells then extract the specific antigen–antibody and send it to the surface. If the antigen is in your nose or gut, the antibody will activate interleukin which will start the relevant mild inflammatory process, such as coughing, sneezing or diarrhoea.

2. If tissue damage occurs and the first-line defence cells do not detect an invader, the inflammatory dendritic cells will orchestrate the inflammatory response and will only use the cells and proteins needed for healing and repair.

3. If the Langerhans cells do not recognise the invader, they send a message to dendritic cells, which start the inflammatory process locally and a number of reactions occur.

   - Neutrophils are the first cells to be called and, by attracting chemical proteins such as histamine and complement, inflammation can isolate the microbe in the tissues. The chemicals in the bloodstream bring about:
     - Vasodilation, which increases the blood flow to the area of damage. This is why inflamed areas look red and swollen
     - Increased blood vessel permeability, allowing the neutrophils and other inflammatory chemicals to pass out of the bloodstream into the tissues to attack the invader.
   - Neutrophils kill the microbe by phagocytosis, ingesting the invader. Several immune system cells can perform phagocytosis such as neutrophils, dendritic cells and macrophages. Cells which perform phagocytosis can also be called phagocytes.
   - Neutrophils expel the remnants of the microbe and waste from the tissue damage, including some dead neutrophils, in the form of pus.
   - The T cells in the tissues also take the invader DNA into the bloodstream and the process of cell-mediated immunity will then proceed to antibody-mediated immunity.

Cell-mediated Immunity

The cell-mediated response begins once the microbe DNA is presented to a T lymphocyte by a macrophage.

- T lymphocytes become more active and differentiate into different types of T lymphocytes by inserting different receptors (labels) into their membranes. These labels indicate what they are capable of and what they will do. For example, cytotoxic T cells are the destroyers while helper T cells assist with the overall continuation of the fight.
- Following detection of the invader, a cell signalling protein (cytokine) called tumour necrosis factor (TNF) is released by immune cells. Several cell types release this, including skin mast cells and activated macrophages. TNF has several functions related to immunity:
  - Activation of macrophages
  - Proinflammatory action
  - Initiating fever and shock.

Antibody-mediated Immunity

Antibody-mediated immunity is achieved when the T lymphocytes release proteins that activate B lymphocytes to differentiate into plasma cells which make antibodies. Once the infection is cleared, the plasma cell will remain dormant as a memory B cell.

If the microbe is a virus, dendritic cells produce an antiviral protein called interferon which interferes with viral replication. A virally infected cell will start to produce interferon as a warning to the immune system, principally shouting 'I've been infected!'. Interferon triggers macrophages and natural killer cells to kill the virally infected cell.

Red Flag

The most effective barrier against microbes is preventing them from becoming pathogens. Health professionals must have sufficient awareness and comprehension of effective infection prevention and control strategies (Figure 24.2).

Jot This Down

What do you think nurses and nursing associates need to know about microbes?

Use tissues when you sneeze	**Harmless bacteria and fungi live naturally on your skin**
A single sneeze propels germs over a distance of 32 feet	If they multiply your skin can become infected – keep skin clean and dry (www.nhs.uk/Conditions/Athletes-foot/Pages/Introduction.aspx)
Wash your hands between patients	
(www.wales.nhs.uk/sites3/Documents/739/rcn%20infection%20control.doc.pdf)	**Wash your hands before any procedures**
Put your hand over your mouth when you cough	e.g. mouth care, eye care, bathing (Collins 2008)
(www.wales.nhs.uk/sites3/Documents/739/rcn%20infection%20control.doc.pdf)	**Drink plenty of fluids** (Eccles 2004)
Cover any cuts or grazes when looking after patients	**Clean surfaces and any spillages**
(Collins 2008)	(Collins 2008)

Safety with microbes – washing your hands with soap and warm water

– the physical action of scrubbing loosens up the microbes, the soap picks them up and binds them together and the water washes them away (Collins 2008)

Figure 24.2 **Simple preventive measures.**

In this exercise, you may have considered the following.

- Many species colonise the human body and are called normal flora.
- Normal flora are found on the skin, mucous membranes and gastrointestinal tract.
- Some benefit the host, as the following examples demonstrate.
  - *Staphylococcus epidermidis* protects against colonisation by pathogenic bacteria on the skin through competitive inhibition. It dominates the location.
  - *Lactobacillus* species, which grow in the vagina and gastrointestinal tract, are 'good germs' as they produce lactic acid as a by-product. This creates an acidic environment that prevents other microbes such as the fungus *Candida* (also known as thrush) from growing on the mucous membranes.
  - *Escherichia coli* in the bowel secretes vitamin K which is required for blood clotting; it also prevents pathogenic bacteria from establishing themselves in the bowel. This organism is the most common cause of urine tract infections (NICE, 2020).

Case Study Urinary Tract Infection

Sophie is a 25 year old who has presented with a stinging pain on urination, frequency of urination and malodorous urine. She has suffered symptoms like this once before, and believes she has a urinary tract infection (UTI).

The nurse should enquire about possible pregnancy and check her vital signs, such as temperature, pulse and respiratory rate. As Sophie is under 65 years and is otherwise healthy, the nurse will use a urine dipstick to aid diagnosis.

If the dipstick is positive for nitrite or leucocyte and red blood cells, then a UTI is likely.

The patient will be prescribed an antibiotic to help clear the infection. She will be advised to increase her fluid intake to flush any microbes in the urethra away (Hooton *et al.*, 2018), and take simple analgesia such as paracetamol (provided there are no contraindications).

She should also be asked to return if symptoms do not improve.

This case study is based on current NICE (2020) guidelines. The case study relates to the NMC Code (2018) 6.1 make sure that any information or advice given is evidence based including information relating to using any health and care products or services.

The Classification of Microbes/Micro-organisms

Eukaryotes

Eukaryotes have a nucleus enclosed within a nuclear envelope. They include all animal cells and fungi.

Jot This Down

Can you think of a common fungal infection?

In this exercise, you might have thought about athlete's foot (tinea pedis). This fungus feeds off dead skin cells and lives in a moist, warm, dark environment. It causes infection when it multiplies. If it is not treated effectively, it can spread to other areas such as toenails, causing fungal nail infections.

What the Experts Say

'As a health professional, you need to be aware of the development, transmission and treatment of athlete's foot. It can be contracted from contaminated towels, clothing and surfaces, such as communal bathrooms and showers.

Preventive measures involve:

- Washing the feet regularly with soap and water and thoroughly drying them, particularly between the toes.
- Advise against mobilising in bare feet
- Change socks regularly and wear cotton socks
- Regular hand washing.

It is usually treated with topical antifungals, but resistant strains may require the addition of oral antifungals.

Nichola, ward nurse

Prokaryotes

Prokaryotes are single-celled organisms that lack an envelope-enclosed nucleus. They include bacteria and Archaea.

Bacteria

Bacteria are cells that are equipped with all the structures and ingredients necessary for reproduction, growth and survival. Bacterial resistance to antibiotics, such as meticillin-resistant *Staphylococcus aureus* (MRSA), is one of the biggest threats to global health (WHO, 2020). It is important to note that it is the bacteria that become resistant to the antibiotic, and not the person.

Archaea

Archaea are within the classification of micro-organisms but no pathogenic archaea have as yet been clearly identified. They tend to be found in extreme environments, such as freezing tundra.

Viruses

Viruses require a living host to multiply and are not considered to be alive. They are a strand of DNA with a protein coat, without a cell or metabolism of their own. Once they are inside a host cell, they use the host DNA to reproduce. Antibiotics do not kill viruses. Prevention is the best strategy against a virus, such as vaccination (see Chapter 16 for a discussion of vaccinations).

The Lymphatic System and Immunity

The lymphatic system (Figure 24.3) is part of the circulatory system and has three basic functions.

- Transporting interstitial fluid, initially formed as a blood filtrate, back into the bloodstream.
- Transporting absorbed fat from the small intestine to the blood.
- Playing a vital role in the immune response.

413

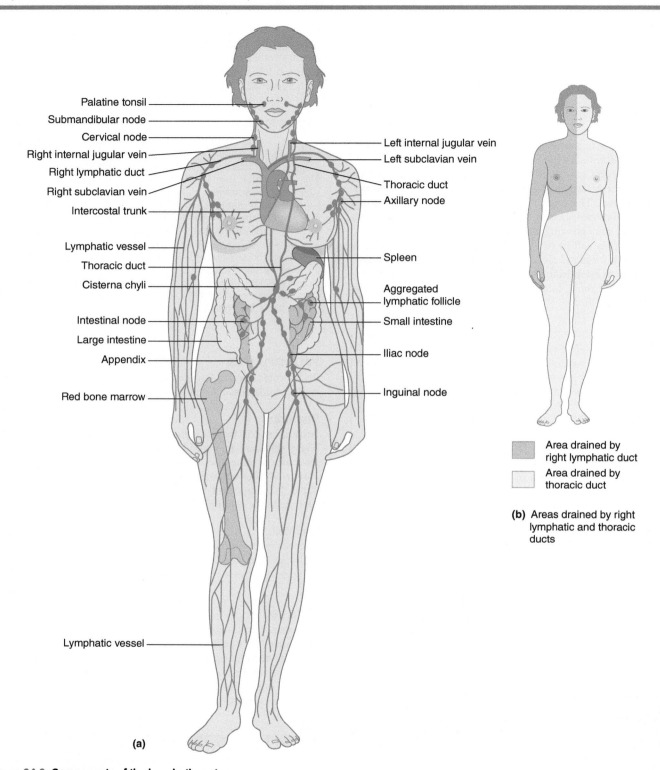

Palatine tonsil
Submandibular node
Cervical node
Right internal jugular vein
Right lymphatic duct
Right subclavian vein
Intercostal trunk

Left internal jugular vein
Left subclavian vein
Thoracic duct
Axillary node

Lymphatic vessel
Thoracic duct
Cisterna chyli

Spleen

Aggregated
lymphatic follicle

Intestinal node
Large intestine
Appendix

Small intestine

Iliac node

Red bone marrow

Inguinal node

Lymphatic vessel

(a)

Area drained by
right lymphatic duct

Area drained by
thoracic duct

(b) Areas drained by right
lymphatic and thoracic
ducts

Figure 24.3 **Components of the lymphatic system.**

The organs and tissues of the lymphatic system serve as storage depots for specialised immune cells and proteins that work to protect the body against invasion by microbes, fight pathogens and build up immunity.

The skin and red bone marrow are associated organs of immunity. The **skin** is composed of a superficial epidermis and a deeper dermis. The epidermis acts as the principal structural barrier to microbes and is the first line of defence. As it is avascular, you do not bleed when you damage the epidermal layer, and microbes on the skin do not have direct access to the blood or lymphatic circulation. Specialised skin immune cells called Langerhans cells work in unison with other cells in the dermis, such as T helper cells, as part of the surveillance network (Guttman-Yassky et al., 2019). The dermis is a deeper, thicker layer of connective tissue containing a network of lymphatic and blood vessels. It contains many resident immune cells including lymphocytes, mast cells, leucocytes, macrophages and proteins such as cytokines.

Repair of the dermis is referred to as 'deep wound healing' and involves a more structured process directed by the inflammatory response.

The *red bone marrow*, a connective tissue located chiefly in cancellous (spongy) bone tissue, contains pluripotent stem cells which have the ability to develop into several different types of cells. The cells that make up the immune system originate in the red bone marrow (Figure 24.4).

Before exploring the organs and tissues of the lymphatic system, we will look at the channels that connect them, which are the lymphatic capillaries and lymphatic vessels.

Lymphatic Capillaries

Lymphatic capillaries are tubes lined with endothelium that run between the cells of connective tissue. Unlike blood capillaries, which are closed tubes with an arterial inflow and a venous outflow, lymphatic capillaries are open-ended. The reason they have an open end is because they are the drains of the interstitial spaces. Most of the components of the blood plasma, apart from red blood cells and proteins, filter from the blood capillary network into the interstitial space at the arterial end of the capillary and are then returned into the bloodstream at the venous end of the capillary. Any excess fluid (about 3 L per day) drains into the lymphatic vessels and is called *lymph*.

Dietary fats and fat-soluble vitamins, absorbed by lymphatic capillaries in the small intestine called 'lacteals', give lymph a milky white colour.

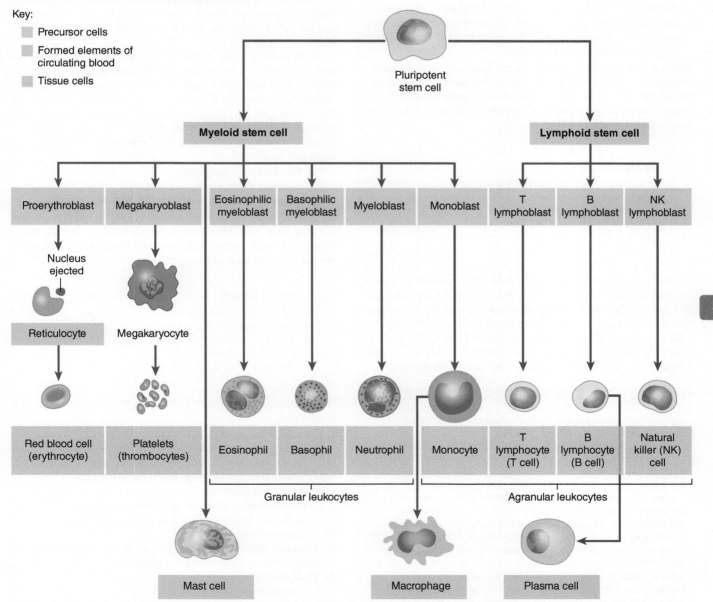

Figure 24.4 **Origin, development and structure of immune cells. Some generations of some cell lines have been omitted.**

Some tissues, including cartilage, the epidermis, central nervous system and red bone marrow, are not drained by lymphatic capillaries.

As well as containing the filtered constituents of plasma, it also provides an exit for any proteins that may have escaped from the bloodstream into the interstitial space. If proteins have leaked out of the bloodstream into the interstitial spaces, they cannot be reabsorbed into the venous capillary because of the concentration gradient across the capillary wall. The proteins become trapped in the interstitial space. They then absorb fluid from the bloodstream by osmosis (see Chapter 23) and the interstitial compartment will swell. The proteins and fluid are returned to the circulatory system via lymphatic ducts.

The flow of lymph is maintained by the:

- 'Milking pump' action of skeletal muscles: as they contract, they compress the vessels and the fluid is pushed forwards
- 'Respiratory pump': when we inhale, the negative pressure in the thoracic cavity pulls the fluid forward; when we exhale, the pressure in the thoracic cavity increases and the valves in the lymphatic vessels prevent backflow.

Valves in the lymphatic capillaries and lymphatic vessels maintain the one-way flow of lymph, which originates in the interstitial spaces and circulates into lymphatic capillaries, lymphatic vessels, lymph nodes and then via lymphatic ducts back into the venous bloodstream.

Jot This Down

Think back to when you may have seen a build-up of proteins in the interstitial compartments and how it may present in a patient.
- What is it called and what care would you implement to help the patient feel more comfortable?

In this exercise, you may have recognised a condition called *oedema*, swelling in the tissues, as the proteins are like sponges and draw the liquid out of the bloodstream into the interstitial space. The fluid has then become trapped in the interstitial space until it can all be drained by the lymphatic vessels. The flow of lymphatic fluid and thus drainage of interstitial fluid is facilitated by increasing venous return, which is achieved with exercise.

Practice Assessment Document

Demonstrate the ability to keep complete, clear, accurate and timely records
Patients with right heart failure have increased pressure in the venous system. This forces fluid out into the interstitial space and this accumulates as oedema at the lowest point, termed dependent pitting oedema. This means, when you gently press the patient's skin, it leaves a pit where you pressed. You will see patients with bilateral swollen ankles. As these patients are being treated for heart failure, it is vital to monitor their daily weight accurately to determine their response to treatment. This relates to the NMC Code (2018) 13.1 accurately identify, observe and assess signs of normal or worsening physical and mental health in the person receiving care. How might you, working with your supervisor, document your findings in an objective manner?

Lymphatic Vessels

Several lymphatic capillary networks empty into lymphatic vessels, which are lined by endothelial cells, and have a thin layer of smooth muscle and an outer adventitia that binds them to the surrounding tissues. In the skin, they lie in the subcutaneous tissue and generally follow the same route as veins. In the deeper tissues, they form plexuses around the arteries.

At intervals along their route, these vessels flow through lymph nodes.

Lymph Nodes

Capsular trabeculae (Figure 24.5) divide the node into compartments, with each compartment containing a superficial cortex and a deeper medulla surrounded by lymphatic sinuses.

Within the cortex, there are aggregates of dividing B lymphocytes called lymphatic nodules. Within the nodules, there is a germinal centre where B lymphocytes proliferate and develop into antibody-producing plasma cells or memory B cells.

Strategically, lymph flows through the node in one direction, entering via a number of afferent lymphatic vessels. Within the node, the lymph flows into a series of channels containing branching fibres called sinuses, which surround the cortex, like an orange in a mesh bag. Lymphocytes and resident macrophages are embedded in the fibres which, in essence, ensures that all lymph fluid will pass through a lymph node and be filtered.

- The fibres trap the pathogens.
- Macrophages destroy some of them.
- Lymphocytes destroy the others with immune responses.

As there are only two efferent vessels via which lymph can flow out of a node, the flow is slow enough to allow the lymph to circulate through several sinuses, which means that it is filtered several times before it can leave the node.

Jot This Down

Think about patients who have had painful and/or swollen lymph glands.
- Why did they have swollen glands?
- What is it called?
- Are all swollen glands painful?

In this exercise, you might have thought about the following possibilities.

1. **Infection:** bacterial, viral, fungal.
   - Localised infection, with either one or two swollen glands; typical examples are common cold, tonsillitis, cellulitis.
   - Systemic infection, with several swollen glands; a typical example is glandular fever. Swollen glands is called 'lymphadenopathy' and is an indication that they are having to work excessively to filter and destroy pathogens and produce antibodies.
2. **Immune disorder:** rheumatoid arthritis with continuous inflammation (autoimmune disease).
3. **Malignancy.**
   - Lymphoma
   - Leukaemia.

Not necessarily painful but 'discomforting'.

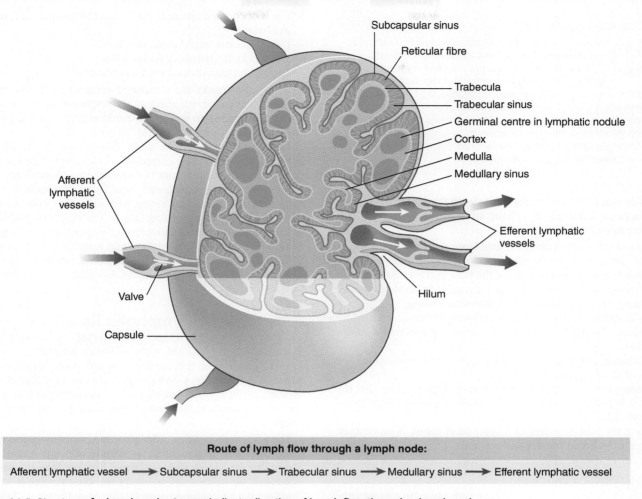

Route of lymph flow through a lymph node:

Afferent lymphatic vessel ⟶ Subcapsular sinus ⟶ Trabecular sinus ⟶ Medullary sinus ⟶ Efferent lymphatic vessel

Figure 24.5 **Structure of a lymph node. Arrows indicate direction of lymph flow through a lymph node.**

417

Lymph nodes are concentrated in several areas around the body, and are simply named after the areas they occupy, e.g. axillary lymph nodes are in the axilla.

Jot This Down

Thinking back to clinical practice and infection, where do you think the locations of lymph glands are in the body?

In this exercise, you may have thought of any of the following.
- Cervical
- Inguinal
- Axillary
- Pelvic
- Abdominal
- Thoracic
- Supratrochlear

All these are in locations where they are needed more readily, which is where pathogens are most likely to enter the body: through the mouth, nose, lungs, gastrointestinal and reproductive tracts.

Jot This Down

The lymphatic system, as with any type of drainage system, can become blocked. Think about any clinical practice situation where you might see a build-up of lymphatic fluid called 'lymphoedema'.

In this exercise, you may have cared for someone with a swollen arm following surgery, which involved the lymph glands in the axilla, such as a 'modified radical' mastectomy. A modified radical mastectomy involves the surgical removal of the breast tissue and most of the axillary lymph nodes. When the lymph nodes are removed, it impairs the drainage of lymph fluid from the interstitial compartments.

The aim of the intervention is to push the excess fluid out of the arm back into the lymphatic and circulatory system. This often takes a few weeks.

- The elastic sleeve covers the arm from the wrist to the top of the arm; care must be taken to make sure it is not too tight under the arm and restricting the flow in the axilla. The arm must be measured and assessed at regular intervals as a badly fitting sleeve can make the lymphoedema worse.
- A 'stretchy' bandage may be more comfortable.
- Manual lymphatic drainage facilitates the movement of the fluid.
- Facilitate and encourage exercises to assist drainage of the fluid from the arm.
- Support the arm on a pillow when resting, ensuring that the arm is not too tight against the chest, as this will impede the drainage.
- Keep the skin clean and dry; apply oil or cream to prevent the skin from becoming dry and cracked.

Lymphatic Follicles

Unlike the lymph nodes, which are encapsulated in a dense connective tissue layer, lymphatic follicles are not surrounded by a capsule and are scattered throughout the mucous membranes. They are referred to as mucosa-associated lymphatic tissue (MALT), which lines the respiratory airways, gastrointestinal, urinary and reproductive tracts, where the follicles intercept microbes that enter the body through external openings. Larger collections of follicles are the tonsils (adenoid and palatine) and the lingual tonsils at the base of the tongue, which are positioned to participate in immune responses against inhaled or ingested microbes. There are also lymphatic follicles called Peyer's patches in the ileum for protecting the intestinal wall and the appendix, which is involved in the production of immunoglobulin A (IgA) antibodies, helping with the maturation of B lymphocytes and the direction of lymphocytes around the body.

Lymphatic Trunks

Lymphatic vessels pass lymph, from node to node, through a sequential chain of lymph nodes. When they exit from this chain, they unite with other vessels from a particular region to form a 'lymphatic trunk'.

- The lumbar trunks drain lymph from the legs, pelvis, kidneys, adrenal glands and abdominal wall.
- The intestinal trunk drains the stomach, intestines, pancreas, spleen and liver.

- The bronchomediastinal trunks drain the thoracic wall, lungs and heart.
- The intercostal trunks drain the chest.
- The subclavian trunks drain the arms.
- The jugular trunks drain the head and neck.

The way the trunks are structured means that if one trunk becomes blocked, it will affect all the respective linked chain of nodes that drain into it. Lymph trunks empty into one of two collecting ducts (see Figure 24.3).

There are two *lymphatic ducts*. The lumbar, intestinal, left bronchomediastinal and intercostal trunks empty into the thoracic duct, which runs from the abdomen up through the diaphragm into the left subclavian vein. This is the main duct for the return of lymph to the blood, with more than two-thirds of the lymphatic system draining into it. The right bronchomediastinal, subclavian and jugular trunks empty the other third of the lymph into the much smaller right lymphatic duct, situated within the right thoracic cavity. This duct returns the lymph into the junction of the right internal jugular and right subclavian veins.

Other Types of Lymphatic Tissue

The *spleen* is the largest single mass of lymphatic tissue, located in the upper left quadrant of the abdomen between the stomach and diaphragm. It is similar to lymph nodes in structure, with the splenic artery and splenic vein entering and exiting through a hilum, but it has blood sinuses instead of lymphatic sinuses. It consists of two distinct tissues called white pulp and red pulp,

- The white pulp consists of lymphocytes, monocytes and macrophages and is structured as islands of white tissue surrounded by blood sinuses. Blood flowing into the spleen through the splenic artery enters the central arteries of the white pulp and pathogens are filtered from the blood. Within the white pulp, the B and T lymphocytes carry out immune responses and the resident macrophages destroy the filtered pathogens by phagocytosis.
- The red pulp is composed of blood-filled venous sinuses and splenic tissue cells arranged into cords (splenic cords), which consist of red blood cells, macrophages, lymphocytes, plasma cells and granulocytes (see Figure 24.4). Within the red pulp, the spleen:
  - Stores platelets
  - Carries out a 'clearing up' role by removing aged, defective, fragile or deformed blood cells and platelets
  - Produces red blood cells during fetal life.

Nursing Fields Child and Family
The spleen is not a vital organ and sometimes has to be removed following damage from trauma. While a splenectomy in adults has much less effect on immunity, why is it more of a problem in children?

In the preceding Nursing Fields box, you might have thought about the building up of immunity. As we age, the body becomes more adept at fighting against invaders and infections that it has seen in the past. This immunity is still being built up in children and it is more difficult for an immature immune system to fight off invaders. A splenectomy will hinder this process.

The *thymus gland* is an encapsulated organ located in the mediastinum, between the aortic arch and the sternum, and extends from below the thyroid in the neck into the thoracic cavity superior to the heart. It is packed with a large number of immature T lymphocytes and provides the environment for these to:

- Mature into immunocompetent T lymphocytes
- Differentiate into their functioning roles such as cytotoxic and helper T lymphocytes.

Apart from the immature and maturing T lymphocytes, the thymus gland consists of the following.

Dendritic cells, which assist in the differentiation process of the T lymphocyte, are derived from monocytes (see Figure 24.4). Because they have a projection similar to that of an axon in the nervous system, they share the name; however, dendritic cells in the lymphatic system have a different function.

Epithelial cells produce hormones called thymosins that stimulate the development of antibodies (immunoglobulins). These cells also possess several long processes that extend outwards in a circle. The dendritic cells use these extending processes like 'pictures' to teach the T lymphocytes how to distinguish between self and foreign tissue.

- Making the markers derived from the 'pictures'.
- Inserting these markers into their membranes, which are now called antigen receptors.
- Being able to recognise these markers as their own label.

This recognition includes detecting whether:

- The markers are made correctly
- The T cell is recognising them as correct, and as 'self'.

If they are incorrectly made or the T cell does not recognise them as self, the T cell is recognised as a malfunctioning T cell and destroyed by the thymic macrophages.

Each epithelial cell has enough 'pictures' for as many as 50 T cells in each session of producing and teaching at any one time.

The thymus gland is large in children and continues to grow until it reaches maturity at puberty. This is because during childhood, the immune system meets and fends off a great number of new infections for the first time. By puberty, it has fought off a large population of infections and has a large archive of antibodies; thereafter, as it expands with experience, so the thymus gland gets smaller. In adulthood, our immunity has matured and become more able to fight off infections and the thymus gland continues to shrink. Before it atrophies and disappears, it has populated the lymphatic tissues with functioning T cells that have the ability to differentiate. Throughout its working life, it is like a T-cell factory, nurturing the developing T cells and then moving them on.

Jot This Down

Write down those autoimmune diseases that you know of and the type of tissue(s) involved.

In this exercise, you might have thought about systemic lupus erythematosus, often referred to as 'lupus', which is an inflammatory connective tissue disorder characterised by the presence of antinuclear antibodies.

Normally, we do not react against our own tissues, which is a concept known as 'self-tolerance'. If the T cell is unable to distinguish self body tissues, it will instigate self-destruction, which is the basis of autoimmune diseases.

While the T cell is growing and maturing, it undergoes several tests and in most cases, when it fails to pass a test, it is destroyed by thymic macrophages. However sometimes a defective T cell slips past and is sent out into the lymphatic tissues and will:

- Be unable to develop an immune response to a specific antigen and will be unable to fight an invader, which means that the individual will have a compromised immunity
- Be intolerant of self, which means that an individual will develop an autoimmune disorder.

Autoimmune disorders or diseases can generally be divided into those that are localised and those that are systemic.

Localised Disorders

Localised disorders occur when the T cells attack specific organs or tissue cells, with examples divided into the following groups.

Dermatological Diseases

- *Psoriasis* is an inflammatory disorder where healthy skin cells are replaced more rapidly than usual and build up on the skin surface, causing red itchy patches that are often flaky and crusty and covered with silvery scales.

Care, Dignity and Compassion

Living with psoriasis can have a profound psychological impact, causing increased anxiety, which can exacerbate the condition. Additionally, patients may develop psoriasis-associated diseases such as psoriatic arthritis, metabolic syndrome and premature cardiovascular disease (Takeshita *et al.*, 2017). Offer the patient the opportunity to discuss how they are feeling about their condition or any other symptoms they have. This relates to the NMC Code (2018) 2.6 recognise when people are anxious or in distress and respond compassionately and politely.

Practice Assessment Document

Platform 'Working in Teams': *demonstrate knowledge of when and how to refer people safely to other professionals or services for clinical intervention or support*

From the above example, if your patient reveals additional health issues, you may need to involve other members of the multidisciplinary team, such as a counsellor, rheumatologist or cardiovascular specialist. This relates to the NMC Code (2018) 3.3 act in partnership with those receiving care, helping them to access relevant health and social care, information and support when they need it.

Whilst working in practice, take an opportunity to become involved in a multidisciplinary meeting. At the meeting, note who the different team members are and what their roles and functions are. Seek feedback on this activity from your practice supervisor, practice assessor or academic assessor.

- *Vitiligo* is characterised by white patches on the skin where the melanocytes that produce melanin are destroyed.
- *Alopecia areata* is the loss of hair in round patches where the hair follicles are the target.

Endocrinological Diseases

- *Primary myxoedema*: thyroid deficiency resulting from destruction of the thyroid gland.
- *Graves disease*: hyperthyroidism resulting from thyroid-stimulating immunoglobulins that stimulate activity of the gland.
- *Addison disease*: characterised by atrophy and hypofunction of the adrenal cortex.
- *Insulin-dependent (type 1) diabetes*: causes impaired insulin secretion as the result of islet cell destruction by antibodies directed at the cell surface or cytoplasm.

Haematological Diseases

- *Idiopathic thrombocytopenic purpura*: a chronic disorder characterised by petechiae, purpura and mucosal bleeding due to antibodies against platelets.
- *Haemolytic anaemia*: caused by destruction of circulating erythrocytes.
- *Antiphospholipid antibody syndrome*: caused by abnormal antibodies that attack proteins on the membranes of cells in the blood and blood vessels, resulting in increased risk of developing clots in the circulation.

Gastrointestinal Diseases

- *Pernicious anaemia*: results from absence of intrinsic factor associated with loss of parietal cells; most individuals have antibodies to parietal cells.
- *Coeliac disease*: intolerance to gluten; the immune system reacts to gluten in the diet and causes inflammation in the intestine.
- *Inflammatory bowel disease*: term used to describe the following conditions.
  - *Ulcerative colitis*: chronic inflammation of the colon and rectal mucosa.
  - *Crohn's disease*: chronic inflammation of the entire gastrointestinal tract.

Systemic Disorders

Systemic disorders affect the whole body and are not restricted to a single organ or body part.

- *Scleroderma*: characterised by the overproduction of collagen.
- *Sjögren syndrome*: a systemic inflammatory disorder in which the glands that secrete fluids are attacked. Characterised by dryness of the mouth, eye and other mucous membranes.
- *Rheumatoid arthritis*: a chronic syndrome with inflammation of joints and generalised manifestations, characterised by infiltration of synovium by lymphocytes and plasma cells.

Case Study Rheumatoid Arthritis

Naga is a 25 year old with rheumatoid arthritis. She has had symmetrical multiple joint pains, with swelling, morning stiffness and restricted movements for the past 5 years.

As the condition progresses, she is likely to develop symmetrical swellings of her finger joints and a characteristic ulnar deviation deformity to her fingers. She may go on to have degenerative rupture of the finger extensor tendons.

This is all caused by the same pathophysiological response of the overproduction of inflammatory synovium which destroys articular cartilage and surrounding tendons.

Naga will receive treatment with disease-modifying antirheumatic drugs (DMARDs) which will slow the progression of the condition but will not cure it. She may go on to need surgeries to replace joints destroyed by the disease. It is therefore of paramount importance that she takes her medications as prescribed and is reviewed regularly by her rheumatology team.

The Nursing Associate

The examples listed above mean that the nursing associate needs to develop appropriate therapeutic relationships with patients with varying and complex needs. Take the time to get to know your patients and how they feel about their condition. The standards of proficiency for the nursing associate (NMC, 2018) state: 1.10 demonstrate the skills and abilities required to develop, manage and maintain appropriate relationships with people, their families, carers and colleagues.

The Cells of Immunity

T lymphocytes and *B lymphocytes* develop from stem cells in the red bone marrow (see Figure 24.4).

T cells are called T cells because they mature in the thymus. Immature T lymphocytes migrate from the red bone marrow to the thymus gland, where they mature into immunocompetent cells. As with B lymphocytes, maturity is signalled when the T cells make and insert proteins into their cell membranes. These cell surface proteins function as receptors and distinguishing protein markers called cluster of differentiation (CD), like a name badge. These define the cell's function and enable it to carry out specific roles in immunity.

Types of T cells include:

- Helper T cell, CD4
- Cytotoxic T cell, CD8
- Suppressor T cell, CD8
- Surveillance T cells, CD3 and CD28
- Memory T cell, which has both CD4 and CD8 proteins on its cell membrane.

CD4 cells are the most numerous of the T lymphocytes, making up 70% of the circulating population.

B cells mature in the bone marrow. Once they have developed and reached the pre-B (precursor B cell) or immunoglobulin stage, they migrate to the thymus gland and lymphoid tissues (spleen, lymph nodes and lymphatic follicles), where they mature and carry out immune responses. Maturity is achieved when they have produced and inserted proteins, called antigen receptors, into their cell surface and they can further differentiate into:

420

- Plasma B cells, which make antibodies (immunoglobulins [Ig])
- Memory B cells.

Immunoglobulins

Immunoglobulins connect themselves to an antigen (a foreign invader, pathogen). They can stick to toxins to neutralise them; they can stick to pathogens and label them for destruction (opsonisation) by other immune cells and they can activate the complement system. The complement system is the 'complementary' immune system which will be discussed later.

There are five types of immunoglobulin which are found in different regions of the body and have different functions:

- IgE
- IgM
- IgG
- IgD
- IgA.

IgE

IgE is secreted by plasma cells in skin, mucous membranes of gastrointestinal and respiratory tracts and tonsils. It is the least common immunoglobulin in serum as it binds tightly to receptors on basophils and mast cells even before interacting with antigens. The binding activity triggers the release of various chemical proteins such as histamine that mediate inflammation.

IgM

IgM is the first immunoglobulin to be made in the foetus and the first to be made by a 'novice' B cell, when it is stimulated by an antigen. This means it is the first immunoglobulin class to be released into the plasma by the plasma B cells during the primary response. It is found in two places:

- Free in the plasma, the third most common in serum
- Attached to the B cell membrane. When it is attached to the B cell, it serves as an antigen receptor. It forms natural antibodies, such as those for ABO blood group antigens, where it presents as a wheel shape with five prongs (Figure 24.6).

It fixes complement and helps in clumping micro-organisms together (agglutination) for elimination.

Jot This Down

In which situation would this property of agglutination be disadvantageous?

In this exercise, you might have thought about blood groups and blood transfusion mismatch. When there is a blood transfusion mismatch, an inflammatory reaction termed 'haemolytic reaction' occurs when the donor red blood cells (erythrocytes) are destroyed by preformed recipient antibodies. The red blood cells stick together (agglutinate) and block the blood flow.

A massive inflammatory reaction can be fatal!

Blood Groups Red blood cells (erythrocytes) are produced in the bone marrow (see Figure 24.4).

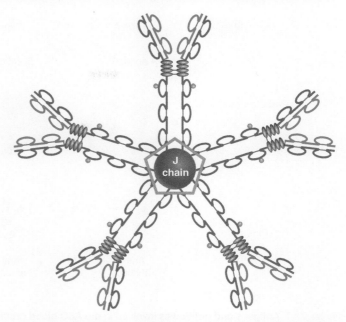

Figure 24.6 The middle J chain of IgM immunoglobulin regulates its five-pronged wheel structure. All immunoglobulins have heavy and light chains (coloured green and blue, respectively) with a hinge or central region.

The surfaces of erythrocytes have genetically determined groups of antigens on their membranes. Based on the combinations of these antigens, there are three main blood groups, A, B and O. Two of the major antigens are designated A and B; those with the A antigen are designated as blood type A, those with blood type B have the B antigen. When neither antigen is found on the erythrocytes, the person is identified as type O. If you are type A, you will have antibodies that react with type B; if you are type B, you will have antibody A in the plasma; if you are type AB, you will have neither antibody; and if you are type O, you will have type A and B antibodies (Figure 24.7).

Sometimes you may get a reaction if a foreign blood group A is introduced to a group A. This is because the antigens are not always assembled in the same way and although two people may be group A, that does not mean that they are exactly the same type of A.

A third major erythrocyte antigen is the Rh antigen. Persons with this antigen are called Rh positive; those without are Rh negative.

IgD

Low levels are found in serum, as it is primarily found on B cell surfaces functioning as a receptor for an antigen, and it is capable of anchoring to the membrane. Significantly, it does not bind complement.

IgG

- Most versatile, as it can carry out all the functions of the immunoglobulins, which makes it the main antibody of both primary and secondary responses.

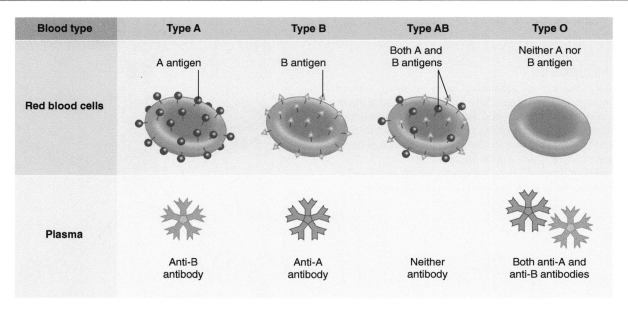

Figure 24.7 Antigens and antibodies involved in the ABO blood groups.

- Most abundant antibody in serum and extravascular spaces; represents 75–85% of circulating antibodies in serum.
- Crosses the placenta mediated by a receptor on placental cells and provides passive immunity to the foetus (the transfer of active antibody-mediated immunity in the form of ready-made antibodies from the mother to the baby).
- Fixes complement.
- Binds to macrophages, monocytes and some lymphocytes.

IgA
- Second most common.
- Major class of immunoglobulin in secretions – tears, saliva, colostrum (first breast milk), intestinal juices and mucus.
- Bathes and protects mucosal surfaces as it prevents pathogens from adhering.

Immunoglobulins vary in structure, but all structures have antigen recognition sites formed by the interaction of light chain and heavy chain variable regions, which provide a conical structure.

It is like a pair of forceps – open them up and pick up a pea! The pea represents the antigen. The open end of the forceps can change its shape to recognise different types and shapes of peas. IgA is the versatile forceps (Figure 24.8) capable of picking up any shape or size of pea. The B cell will then make a more specialised type of forceps, which is now pea shaped.

Natural Killer Cells

Natural killer (NK) cells are lymphocytes that target cells. They reside in the spleen, lymph nodes and red bone marrow and will attack and destroy any body cells that they sense as being imperfect. These imperfect cells are those that display unusual or abnormal plasma membrane proteins. Cells that have become infected or are abnormal, such as tumour cells, become targets. Sometimes the behaviour of NK cells is a little erratic and they target normal uninfected cells, often experienced as a transient irritable throat or runny nose.

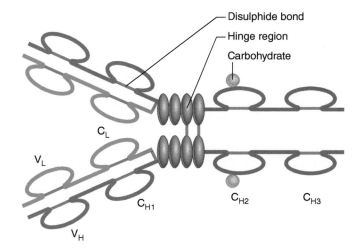

Figure 24.8 Immunoglobulins: blue light chain represents open forceps, green heavy chain represents the forceps fixed end and the hinge region enables the forceps to open and close.

The NK Cell: A Good Cell or a Bad Cell or a Nuisance Cell?

- When a NK cell binds to a target cell, it releases cytotoxic granules such as perforin that perforate the cell membrane of the target cell, which allows excess fluid to flow into the cell and the target cell bursts and dies. This process is called lysis. If it was an infected cell, as it bursts it releases the microbe, which is then destroyed by phagocytosis.
- NK cells release granzymes that digest proteins and induce the target cell to self-destruct by apoptosis. This destroys the cell that is infected but not the microbe inside the cell; however, this can be destroyed by phagocytosis.

Natural Killer T Cells

Natural killer T (NKT) cells are cells that originate from the T lymphocyte and have properties that resemble those of both the T lymphocyte and the NK cell. They are found in the skin and mucous membranes and induce the release and action of interleukin 17 (which amongst other things acts as an inflammatory mediator).

Macrophages (*Macro* – big, *Phage* – eater)

These are modified monocytes, which migrate to tissues such as the skin, liver, lungs, brain, spleen, red bone marrow and lymph nodes. Here they reside as either monocytes or fixed macrophages. They stand guard and are alerted by chemicals telling them of the presence of a pathogen. They can phagocytose pathogens, release chemicals that stimulate inflammatory activity and play a part in wound healing.

Granular white blood cells (see Figure 24.4) are produced in the red bone marrow and are different from the lymphocytes and monocytes, which are agranular.

All granular leucocytes release *chemical proteins*. Chemical proteins act as messengers, which can stimulate body tissues to react by:

- Modifying their structure, such as increasing the spaces between the cells and increasing vascular permeability
- Modifying their behaviour, such as increasing their metabolism, or by
- Releasing further chemical proteins such as histamine and cytokines.

Neutrophils

These circulate in the bloodstream, waiting for an intruder, and their primary function is phagocytosis. They respond swiftly to the alert from the inflammatory dendritic cell when the outer defences are compromised and are the first cells to be attracted to the site of tissue damage.

Jot This Down

When we have an infection or an inflammatory reaction, blood samples are taken. What do you think we are looking for?

A full blood count will tell us which cells have increased in numbers. If the neutrophils are high, it indicates the infection is 'early'. An exception when the neutrophil level may not be raised but a person has an obvious infection is if the red bone marrow is not producing the neutrophils or they were not being developed, as in types of leukaemia or from medication such as chemotherapy.

As soon as the neutrophils arrive, they:

1. Release granules that enhance the inflammatory response by increasing vasodilation and vascular permeability
2. Activate the endothelial cells to express surface proteins, which are 'leg-like' projections that enable the neutrophil to move by diapedesis along the inner lining of the capillary and move into the tissues via gaps in the vascular capillary wall

3. Release extracellular traps (NETs) for the containment of infection and inflammation (Papayannopoulos, 2017)
4. Express complement receptors that aid phagocytosis
5. Begin to destroy any microbes in the tissues by phagocytosis.

Basophils and Mast Cells

Basophils circulate in the bloodstream and their numbers are generally very low unless an active infection is present, when they migrate towards the infected area and release chemical proteins.

Mast cells are not mobile and are found stationed in connective and mucosal tissue. They contain granules rich in histamine.

Eosinophils

Eosinophils counteract the inflammatory response of basophils and mast cells by breaking down the chemicals they release. Their numbers are generally low, unless there is an inflammatory response to a microbe or an allergic antigen.

Their main function is to stop the inflammatory process from going too far. They also have a role in fighting invasion by parasitic worms.

Dendritic Cells

These are modified monocytes and function as weak phagocytes. We have discussed their action in the thymus, where their most important role is as an antigen-presenting cell (APC). They can ingest a foreign cell and display the foreign antigen on their own cell membrane. The dendritic cells then pass through the lymph nodes, displaying the antigen 'like carrying a placard' and searching for the lymphocytes that match that antigen. This APC triggers adaptive immunity as it is like a 'foghorn' shouting for it to 'get active' and is a significant bridge between innate and acquired immunity.

Chemical Proteins Involved in Immunity

C-reactive Protein

C-reactive protein (CRP) is made and released by the liver in response to chemicals discharged by macrophages and adipocytes (fat cells) in the acute phase of inflammation. It binds to a protein on the surface of dead or dying cells and bacterial cells, which activates the complement system. The serum level is raised in the presence of a bacterial infection.

Prostaglandins and Leukotrienes

Prostaglandins are released by the damaged tissue and bring about vasodilation. They also intensify the activity of *histamine* and *kinins*, which further increases vasodilation. There are numerous types of prostaglandins, for example PGE_2, PGD_2 and prostacyclin, all with vascular activities (not discussed in this chapter). They cause pain indirectly by sensitising the C fibres, which makes these pain receptors more sensitive to the effects of the kinins, for example *bradykinin* and *kallikrein*, which are released by the damaged tissues. They induce vasodilation and the contraction of smooth muscle.

The stinging sensation when you prick your finger is caused by the kinins and the prostaglandins.

Leukotrienes produced by white blood cells cause vasodilation and increased vascular permeability.

Lipoxins

Lipoxins are formed by platelets and neutrophils working together and released into the bloodstream. They direct macrophages to clean up dead cells and inhibit chemotaxis, to stop the inflammatory process.

Complement

Complement is a group of 20 proteins that are normally inactive. They are produced by the liver and found in the bloodstream and tissues throughout the body. They are numbered C1–C9, plus factors B, D and P and some other regulatory proteins. When stimulated, they act as a cascade, i.e. C1 activates C2 and so on.

They are activated by tissue damage and the subsequent invasion of a pathogen and act in one of two pathways.

1. *The classical pathway*: depends on antibodies binding to invading microbes to form an antigen–antibody complex, and then one of the C proteins, usually C1, binds to the antigen–antibody complex, which is called complement fixation.
2. *The alternative pathway*: interaction between factors B, D and F with a surface protein on the microbe.

Both these pathways cause an orderly cascade of events. The complement proteins:

- Produce the 'membrane attack complex', which punctures the microbe's cell wall, causing it to burst as it fills with fluid entering through the puncture site
- Stick to the microbe, labelling it for destruction by phagocytes, a process called opsonisation ('ready to eat')
- Encourage further phagocytes and macrophages, which increases inflammation
- Bind to mast cells, which in turn causes them to release histamine.

Cytokines

Cytokines are produced by damaged tissues and leucocytes and help to neutralise the invaders by intensifying the process of inflammation. They do this by attracting phagocytes into the area by chemotaxis (chemical attraction).

Examples of specific cytokines are as follows.

- *Interleukins (IL1–IL30)*: released by leucocytes and act on leucocytes and participate in the regulation of inflammation. They act as messengers and are involved in almost every aspect of immunity.
- *Interferons*: antiviral chemicals produced by cells infected by a virus. They are protective, as they travel to and bind to both neighbour and distant cells that are not infected and stimulate these non-infected cells, 'telling' them to produce chemical proteins. These proteins then either block any potential receptors or cover their cell membrane. They may release chemicals that prevent the virus from approaching the cells, so they become invisible to it. These actions prevent the virus from entering the cell membrane and so protect themselves.

- *Histamine*: released by damaged tissues and increases local vasodilation and vascular permeability and attracts leucocytes by chemotaxis to the site of injury. Plays a core role in the inflammatory response.
- *Tumour necrosis factor (TNF)*: a key regulator in the inflammatory process by attracting neutrophils, monocytes, T and B lymphocytes and macrophages in response to various stimuli. It also stimulates monocytes to secrete interleukins and more TNF, thus playing a role in the continuation of the inflammatory activity.

Fever

Tumour necrosis factor released from stimulated macrophages and T lymphocytes enters the bloodstream, and as an *endocrine hormone* it acts as a *pyrogen* and stimulates further cytokine liberation from mononuclear cells.

These circulating cytokines enter the brain, where they interact with a receptor on the hypothalamus, raising the body's temperature set point – its thermostat.

At first, your body will feel cold and will take action to make you feel warmer, shutting down the peripheries and shivering until the new temperature is achieved. This experience is what is called a 'fever' – feeling cold with an elevated temperature. This is a deliberate tactic by the chemicals that are mediating the fight activity, as the increase in temperature increases the intensity of the inflammatory fight against the pathogen.

> **Jot This Down**
>
> The hypothalamus controls body temperature by resetting the thermostat, which brings about a number of body responses to raise the temperature.
> List these activities and explain what you would do to help the body reach the new set temperature and make the patient comfortable.

In this exercise, you might have listed these suggestions.

- Provide extra clothing if the patient shivers.
- Give extra drinks or sugar if necessary, as the body will need extra fuel. You may need to check blood glucose levels if the patient is beginning to feel tired, the blood pressure is dropping too low and/or the heart rate is too fast. The heart rate will increase with body temperature as it will need to get the fuel round the body so that it can fight.
- Check vital signs.
- Once the body has reached the new set level, the patient will begin to feel more comfortable.

In severe infection, the subsequent systemic overproduction of TNF and cytokines leads to vascular instability and will eventually lead to sepsis.

Inflammation is like a circle of events and will continue to go round and round until it is stopped. Lipoxins stop the inflammatory process and clean up the mess.

Phagocytosis

Phagocytes are specialised cells that perform phagocytosis, which occurs in five steps (Figure 24.9).

1. *Chemotaxis* of phagocyte to the site of damage.
2. *Adhesion*: the attachment of the microbe to the phagocyte.

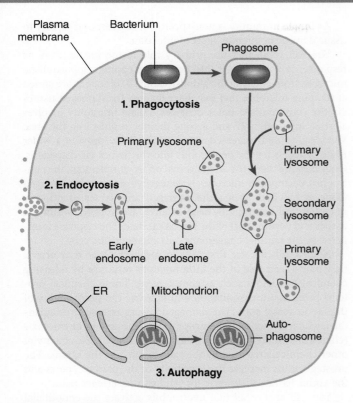

Figure 24.9 Phagocytosis.

3. *Ingestion*: the phagocyte engulfs the microbe and encases it in a phagosome (vesicle) in the cytoplasm.
4. The phagosome then fuses with a lysosome which contains lysosomal digestive enzymes to *digest* the microbe.
5. *Destroyed or stored*: if the phagocyte did not manage to digest all the microbe, it stores the remnants in residual bodies.

If there are many microbes, the red bone marrow is stimulated and will increase the number of neutrophils – 'production increases to meet the demand'.

Immunity in Action

We have looked at the structure of the lymphatic system and all the cells and chemicals it has at its disposal. We will now discuss these structures and cells in action.

Pathogens either feed on our bodies or produce toxic substances. This activity changes the internal environment and upsets the smooth working life of our cells and thus the smooth running of body systems.

Innate Immunity

Recalling the triangle of immunity, we will look at innate immunity first.

Innate immunity consists of two sets of barriers: an outer perimeter and a back-up secondary chemical 'fence'. We are born with all the structures and features of the 'innate' immune system (Figure 24.10), which are our barriers to prevent invasion. They

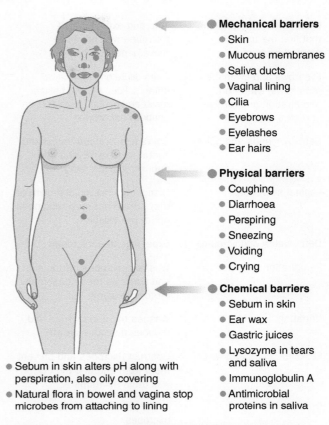

● Sebum in skin alters pH along with perspiration, also oily covering
● Natural flora in bowel and vagina stop microbes from attaching to lining

Figure 24.10 The structures and features of the innate immune system.

are situated in those places that the microbes are likely to target and are divided into three categories of barriers.

- Mechanical
- Physical
- Chemical.

Jot This Down

List the components and functions of the first-line defences that comprise part of the innate immune system.

In this exercise, you might have thought about the following.

EXTERNAL PHYSICAL AND MECHANICAL BARRIERS	CHEMICAL BARRIERS AND INTERNAL DEFENCES
Skin: the outer epidermal tissues and keratinised cells, which strengthen the outer layer of the skin	Sebum provides an oily protective coating that prevents microbes from settling and multiplying
Mucous membranes of upper respiratory tract (nasal passages, pharynx and larynx) and lower respiratory tract (trachea, bronchi and lungs)	Secrete mucus that moistens surfaces and traps microbes, which are then dispelled by coughing and sneezing

Cilia: hair-like projections that line the upper respiratory tract	Trap and expel inhaled microbes with wave-like movements
Eyebrows and eyelashes protect the eyes from perspiration and foreign particles	Tears dilute and wash away irritants, keep the eye tissues moist and contain lysozyme, an antibacterial enzyme
Salivary glands and saliva	Saliva keeps mouth moist and contains lysozyme and IgA, antimicrobial proteins
Vaginal secretions	Discourage microbial growth as they are acidic; move microbes out of the vagina
Defaecation and vomiting	Expel ingested microbes
Perspiration	Washes microbes off the skin and contains the antimicrobial protein lysozyme
Urinating	Washes the urinary tract and reduces microbial growth
Earlobes, hairs and wax	Obstruct microbes and prevent them from entering the ear; wax traps microbes
Stomach	Acidic gastric juices destroy microbes

Jot This Down

List the nursing interventions that may be necessary to support innate immunity and prevent infection.

In the preceding 'Jot This Down' exercise, you may have thought about the following.

1. *Oral hygiene*: keeping the mouth and nasal passages clear and moist. Provide and encourage fluids and assist with drinking if help is required. Give mouth care if the person you are caring for is unable to eat and drink or if the mouth becomes dry for any other reason. For example, you may be caring for someone who is breathless and breathing through their mouth. When oxygen is delivered, it makes the mucous membranes dry. Keep the mouth clean and moist to prevent the salivary ducts becoming clogged and to prevent cracked lips and gums.

2. *Eye care*: prevent the eyes from becoming dry with eye care if required and prevent the tear ducts from becoming clogged.

3. *Maintaining fluid balance* to ensure adequate hydration, which helps to prevent the skin becoming dry with the possible formation of sores. It also aids urination.

4. *Adequate nutrition* to maintain the mucous membranes lining the respiratory and gastrointestinal tracts and outer surface skin tissues.

5. *Personal hygiene*, which promotes general well-being of the skin and prevents microbes from germinating in areas where the skin is creased or hidden (groin, axilla).

As innate immunity is non-specific, it can respond rapidly to tissue damage before the onset of infection.

You will recall that the primary role of the innate immune response is to prevent infection by stopping opportunistic microbes from entering the bloodstream. All its actions are aimed at trapping microbes that may have entered the damaged tissues via the compromised outer defences. Innate immunity involves alerting interleukin 17 and getting the neutrophils into the area. Vasodilation and increased vessel permeability provide a wider route of access for the neutrophils into the tissues via diapedesis. Once they are there, the area is sealed off by complement, the neutrophils destroy the microbes by phagocytosis and the damaged tissue is repaired. When the damaged area is sealed off, any microbes and neutrophils, dead or alive, are trapped within the tissues and become part of the serous exudate. The response is initiated by the sentinel Langerhans cells and dendritic cells.

Neutrophils are the first cells to respond. Once they arrive, they play a lead role in the inflammatory response by releasing chemical mediators such as complement. These chemical proteins bring about vasodilation and increase the permeability of the blood vessel wall. The damaged tissues release prostaglandins, which attract more neutrophils into the area by chemotaxis (chemical attraction). The prostaglandins amplify the activity of other chemicals released by the tissues, such as the kinins. The prostaglandins increase the sensitivity of the pain receptors and the kinins irritate these receptors and you experience pain.

You will also recall that neutrophils activate the endothelial cells to express surface proteins which are 'leg-like' projections that enable the neutrophil to move by diapedesis along the inner lining of the capillary and move into the tissues via gaps in the vascular capillary wall and release extracellular traps (NETs) to trap the microbe.

Red Flag

Vasodilation and increased vascular permeability increase the blood flow to the area of damage, which causes *swelling*, *redness*, *warmth* and *pain*.
The accumulation of prostaglandins and bradykinins increases the sensation of pain. The clinical presentation is classically one of *inflammation*.

Wound Healing

Deep Wound Healing

There are four phases of wound healing: haemostasis, inflammation, proliferation and remodelling.

Following injury (Figure 24.11), there is immediate platelet aggregation, with platelets releasing thromboplastin that facilitates *haemostasis*. After this first phase, when bleeding has been controlled and the tissues are cleaned, optimum wound healing requires a well-structured and orderly progression of tissue repair by: 1. haemostasis, 2. inflammation, 3. proliferation, and finally 4. extracellular matrix deposition and remodelling.

Exudate from the inflammatory process contains neutrophils, some of which will still be active and will continue to kill any microbes by phagocytosis. This means that any exudate is sterile and will promote healing. As part of innate immunity, the damaged tissues release platelet-activating and tissue growth factors,

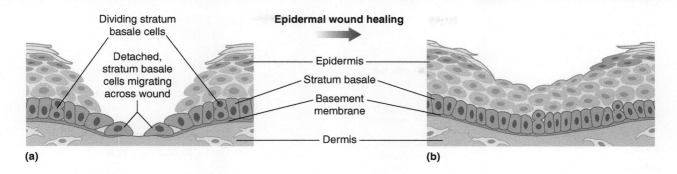

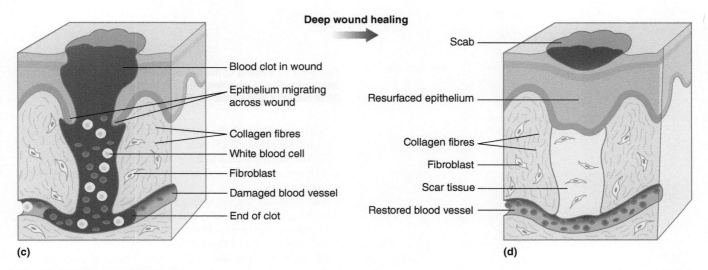

Figure 24.11 Skin wound healing.

and thus wound healing starts immediately following tissue damage with the *inflammatory* phase.

Extracellular matrix deposition (*granulation*) is achieved by the tissues themselves with the use of chemical mediators and growth factors. Granulation starts from 2 days after injury and lasts up to 3 weeks, with fibroblasts laying down beds of collagen and filling the defect with new capillaries. Once granulation has occurred, there is contraction of the skin and the edges of the wound are pulled together. Finally, *epithelialisation* (growth of epithelial cells) crosses moist surfaces; cells travel about 3 cm from the point of origin in all directions, which completes the *proliferative* phase.

At about 3 weeks, the process is completed by the *remodelling* phase, with new collagen forming that increases tensile strength in wounds.

Medicines Management

Medications most likely to impair wound healing and damage skin integrity include some antibiotics, anticonvulsants, angiogenesis inhibitors, steroids and non-steroidal anti-inflammatory drugs. However, drugs such as ferrous sulfate, insulin, thyroid hormones and vitamins may facilitate wound healing (Beitz, 2017). Always check the BNF to investigate any effects medications may have on a patient's wounds.

Cell-mediated Immunity

You will recall that as the need for defence intensifies (Figure 24.12), the neutrophils recruit the help of the monocytes. Monocytes live in the general circulation, but there is a large store of them in the spleen. As the monocytes migrate to the area of invasion, they enlarge and develop into phagocytic cells, termed 'wandering macrophages'. Other stored monocytes are termed 'fixed macrophages', as they stand guard in specific tissues such as the skin, liver, lungs, brain, spleen, lymph nodes and red bone marrow. The macrophages are larger and more aggressive towards microbes in comparison to the size and behaviour of the neutrophils.

Linking Innate Immunity to Cell-mediated Immunity

Following digestion of the microbe, the macrophage retains the microbe's DNA and displays it on its outer membrane surface next to its 'self' marker protein, known as the *human leucocyte antigen (HLA)* or *self-antigen*. When the macrophage presents the DNA to the T lymphocyte, the macrophage is referred to as an antigen-presenting cell (APC). The activity links innate immunity to cell-mediated immunity.

These self-antigens are commonly referred to as the *major histocompatibility complex* (MHC) as they are coded within a large cluster of genes from a region in the genome (DNA) known as the major histocompatibility complex. As chromosomes are

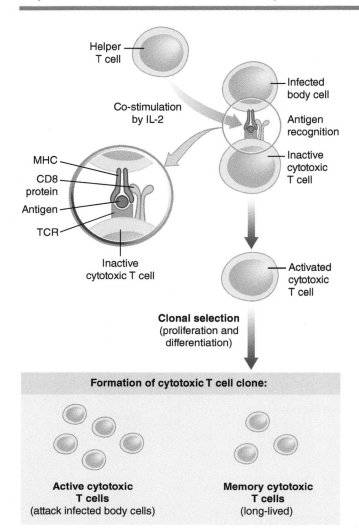

Figure 24.12 **Cell-mediated immunity.**

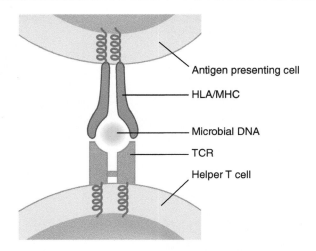

Figure 24.13 **Binding of the helper T-cell receptor (TCR) with major histocompatibility complex (MHC) or human leucocyte antigen (HLA) receptor and microbial DNA.**

– The regulatory T (R) cell to differentiate into memory T (M) and suppressor T (S) cells
– Alerting the B cells to the presence of foreign DNA.
• The memory T cells will now recognise that foreign DNA if it turns up again.
• The cytotoxic T CD8 cells go on the rampage and circulate, looking for infected cells and eliminating them. They do this by releasing granules (granzymes) that puncture the infected cell membrane and the cell dies.
• In addition, cytotoxic cells secrete chemical proteins that attract neutrophils and encourage phagocytosis and prevent them from leaving the area.

The suppressor T cells stop the process when all the infected cells have been destroyed.

After *tissue transplantation*, the donor tissue is sometimes recognised as foreign and macrophages present donor DNA to the interleukin-activated lymphocytes (B and T cells), which brings about both antibody- and cell-mediated effects. Killer T cells bind with cells of the transplanted tissue, resulting in cell cytolysis and death. Helper T cells stimulate the multiplication and differentiation of B cells, and antibodies are produced to graft endothelium. To reduce the chances of this happening, donors and patients must be matched so that their proteins are as similar as possible. The greatest genetic diversity between different individuals occurs in the MHC region and particular care must be taken to match the MHC molecules of patients and donors as accurately as possible.

paired, each person inherits one member of the pair from each parent; because each chromosome pair contains multiple genes, each carrying instructions for the production of one part of the self-antigen, the possibility of two people having the same HLA type is extremely remote (Figure 24.13).

Recall that T-cell maturity is signalled when the T cells make and insert antigen receptors on their cell surface as they develop in the thymus gland. T-cell antigen receptors (TCRs) on the surface of T cells recognise the microbe fragments as foreign only when they are bound to the HLA and form HLA–microbial DNA complexes.

• When the T cell recognises the foreign DNA, it binds to the self-receptor and the microbial DNA on the macrophage and releases interleukin 1, which in turn mobilises the CD4 helper T cells.
• The CD4 cell is activated and releases interleukin 2, a co-stimulator, which enables:
  – The helper T to recognise the microbial DNA as foreign
  – This 'educated' helper T cell to clone, thus creating many more helper T cells that recognise this foreign DNA
  – The helper T cell to differentiate into regulatory T cells and cytotoxic T cells

The Nursing Associate Platform - Promoting health and preventing ill health

Helping a patient make the right choices regarding lifestyle, diet and exercise whilst living in an immunocompromised state is an ongoing challenge. The registered nurse and nursing associate need to be able to advise patients appropriately to empower them to make choices that promote health. This relates to outcome 2.1 which states 'understand and apply the aims and principles of health promotion, protection and improvement and the prevention of ill health when engaging with people',

Antibody-adapted Immunity

The B lymphocytes are the key cells for mediating the antibody-mediated immune response (Figure 24.14). The interleukins, secreted by helper T cells functioning as APCs in the cell-mediated immune response, stimulate the growth and differentiation of B cells into memory cells and plasma cells. They are further activated by contact with an antigen. The plasma B cells produce specific antibodies, which inactivate an invading antigen. The memory B cells 'remember' a specific antigen and, when exposed to it a second time, immediately initiate a large immune response to quickly overwhelm the invading antigen. This is termed the secondary immune response.

Antibodies may bind to viruses or bacteria and inhibit their pathogenic activity. Different B cells generally produce different immunoglobulins, which enables our B-cell repertoire to deal with almost any pathogenic molecule.

Immunological response is the preferred means of studying allergies, even though there may be two types of reaction occurring simultaneously.

Jot This Down

List at least four diseases that you can think of when inflammation is inappropriate.

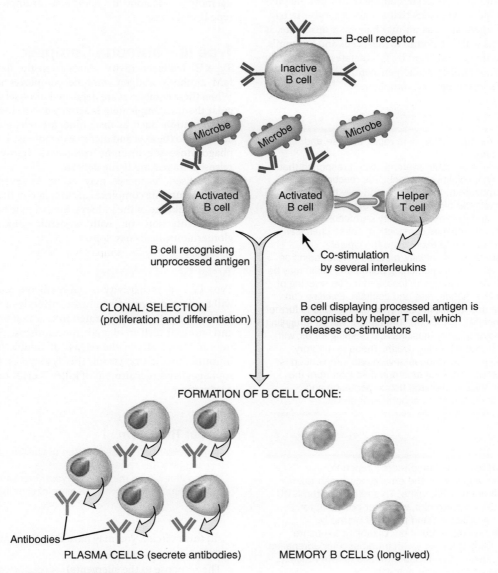

Figure 24.14 Activation and clonal selection of B cells.

B-cell receptor

Inactive B cell

Microbe · Microbe · Microbe

Activated B cell · Activated B cell · Helper T cell

B cell recognising unprocessed antigen

Co-stimulation by several interleukins

CLONAL SELECTION (proliferation and differentiation)

B cell displaying processed antigen is recognised by helper T cell, which releases co-stimulators

FORMATION OF B CELL CLONE:

Antibodies

PLASMA CELLS (secrete antibodies)

MEMORY B CELLS (long-lived)

In this exercise, you might have thought about:

- Arthritis: rheumatoid or joint injury
- Psoriasis
- Crohn's disease
- Asthma: allergy.

Disorders of the Immune System

We have learned how *inflammation* warns, fights, destroys and evicts unwanted residents in our bodies. Recall the classic presentation of inflammation, as redness, swelling, warmth and pain, all of which, in the case of *hypersensitivity*, will be exacerbated in terms of speed of onset, intensity and duration.

There are four types of hypersensitivity reaction.

Type I – Atopic and Anaphylactic

Common hypersensitivity reactions, such as allergic asthma, allergic rhinitis (hay fever), allergic conjunctivitis and anaphylactic shock, are type I hypersensitivity. This response is triggered when an allergen, such as animal hair or a dust mite, is inhaled and interacts with IgE bound to mast cells and basophils. The potency of the threat perceived by IgE dictates the intensity of the response. This antibody–allergen complex prompts the mast cells to release histamine and complement.

Red Flag Anaphylaxis

In anaphylaxis, the response is rapid, intense and life-threatening.

Anaphylaxis is an acute systemic type I response that occurs in highly sensitive persons. The reaction begins within minutes of exposure to the allergen and may be almost instantaneous. The release of histamine and other mediators causes vasodilation and increased capillary permeability, smooth muscle contraction and bronchial constriction. These chemical mediators cause the person to experience the typical manifestations of anaphylaxis. Initially, a sense of foreboding or uneasiness, light-headedness and itching palms and scalp may be noted. Hives may develop, along with localised tissue swelling of the eyelids, lips, tongue, hands, feet and genitals. Swelling can also affect the uvula and larynx, impairing breathing. This is further complicated by bronchial constriction. The patient will be struggling to breathe, using the accessory muscles and gasping for air, with stridor and wheezing, and a barking cough. These respiratory effects can be lethal if the reaction is severe and intervention is not immediately available. Vasodilation and fluid loss from the vascular system can lead to impaired tissue perfusion and hypotension, a condition known as anaphylactic shock.

What to Do If . . .

A patient develops an anaphylactic reaction.
Raise the alarm, alert the emergency/crash team. The patient needs adrenaline. This relates to the NMC Code (2018) 15.2 arrange, wherever possible, for emergency care to be accessed and provided promptly. Use the Airway, Breathing, Circulation, Disability, Exposure (ABCDE) approach. Early treatment with intramuscular adrenaline is the treatment of choice. If your patient has a known reaction, they may be carrying an adrenaline auto-injector.

Type II – Cytotoxic

A haemolytic transfusion reaction to blood of an incompatible type is characteristic of a type II or cytotoxic hypersensitivity reaction. IgG or IgM antibodies are formed to a cell-bound antigen, such as the ABO antigen. When these antibodies bind with the antigen, the complement cascade is activated, resulting in destruction of the target cell. Haemolytic disease of the newborn is caused by this type of reaction.

Type II reactions may be stimulated by an exogenous antigen, such as foreign tissue or cells, or a drug reaction, in which the drug forms an antigenic complex on the surface of a blood cell, stimulating the production of antibodies. The affected cell is then destroyed in the resulting antigen–antibody reaction; for example, haemolytic anaemia is sometimes associated with the administration of drugs such as penicillins.

Endogenous antigens can also stimulate a type II reaction, resulting in an autoimmune disorder such as Goodpasture syndrome, in which antigens are formed to specific tissues in the lungs and kidneys. Hashimoto thyroiditis and autoimmune haemolytic anaemia are additional examples of autoimmune type II reactions.

Type III – Immune Complex

Type III hypersensitivity results from the formation of IgG or IgM antibody–antigen immune complexes in the circulation. When these complexes are deposited in vessel walls and extravascular tissues, complement is activated and chemical mediators of inflammation, such as histamine, are released. Neutrophils are attracted to the area and increase the intensity. When neutrophils phagocytose the immune complexes, lysosomal enzymes are released, increasing tissue damage.

Localised responses may occur at several different sites. Because immune complexes accumulate in the glomerular basement membrane of the kidneys, for example following a streptococcal infection or with systemic lupus erythematosus, glomerulonephritis develops.

Type IV – Delayed

Type IV hypersensitivity is cell mediated and so the response will be slow in comparison to an antibody–antigen interaction. It occurs due to an exaggerated interaction between an antigen and normal cell-mediated mechanisms. This exaggerated interaction results in the release of soluble inflammatory and immune mediators (from the lysozymes within the macrophages) and recruitment of killer T cells, causing local tissue destruction.

Jot This Down

A patient has been admitted to your ward and has told you they have allergies.
What will be the focus of your assessment for this statement? What are the aims of your interventions?

In this exercise, you may have thought about:

- Establishing the allergen
- The response to the allergen(s)
- Minimising exposure to the allergen.

What are the aims of your interventions?

- To prevent a hypersensitivity response.
- Provide prompt, effective interventions if an allergic response occurs.
- Observe for evidence of an allergic response.

With a hypersensitivity response, supportive care is important to relieve discomfort. This may involve the administration of selected antihistamine or anti-inflammatory medications.

NOTE: Reassure the patient that all measures have been implemented to try to stop an allergy reaction. The patient may not trust that all staff will take care to remove the allergen, for example, and may keep asking if all the members of staff know about the allergy and are taking the correct care. To allay the individual's fear, suggest placing the information in a prominent place so that the patient and everyone else can read it.

Red Flag

Identifying allergens for the individual to reduce the likelihood of exposure is a key aspect of management. A complete history of the client's allergies is obtained, including medications, foods, animals, plants and other materials. The type of hypersensitivity response is documented, as are its onset, manifestations and usual treatment.

The nurse in the allergy clinic tells the patient what is going to happen. Allergy clinics do tests to identify allergens and you may have seen patients with red dots in a line on the anterior aspect of the forearm. The potential allergens have been applied on the skin to test for an inflammatory response.

Initially, the blood will be tested before the allergen is put on the skin because if the patient is hypersensitive, it may cause an extreme response even if it is only on the skin.

To identify possible allergens or hypersensitivity reactions, laboratory tests may be ordered such as white blood cell count (WBC), radioallergosorbent test (RAST), blood type and cross-match, indirect and direct Coombs test, immune complex assay or complement assay.

Immunodeficiency

Immunodeficiency is when the inflammatory response is impaired or absent. This may happen if one of the components is missing or damaged.

Genetic and Inherited

Common variable immune deficiency (CVID) is characterised by humoral immunity deficiency. A genetic mutation impairs the development of B cells, resulting in deficient and insufficient numbers of IgG, IgA and IgM.

Jot This Down

A patient has an impaired immunity due to a genetic mutation. What do you think their needs are?

In this exercise, you might have thought about:

- Prevention of infection
- Prenatal diagnosis
- Genetic counselling.

Management involves careful and caring consideration and investigation so the correct information can be provided as it has serious implications for future pregnancies and other relatives. Genetics consultation can help.

Care, Dignity and Compassion

If a patient has impaired immunity due to a genetic condition, the registered nurse as part of the multidisciplinary team will need to help the patient and their family with sensitive communication of information. They will need to:

- Understand the cause of the condition and expected prognosis
- Understand the implications
- Explain the need for genetic testing and how this is done.

Immunodeficiency Acquired Through Infection

Human immunodeficiency virus (HIV) destroys helper T cells, which leads to acquired immune deficiency syndrome (AIDS).

Recall that helper T cells are involved in cell-mediated immunity and that without them, the immune response is 'truncated'. As you know, a virus enters a cell and instructs the cell's nucleus to manufacture more viruses, turning the cell into a virus factory.

Produced by Drug Therapy as an Unwanted Side-effect

Methotrexate (chemotherapy) is an example of a drug which has the potential to impair immunity as it interferes with the production of white blood cells.

Medicines Management

Chemotherapy is the most common cause of a compromised immune system in patients undergoing cancer treatment. There are numerous ways in which this happens which are specific to each drug. In principle, chemotherapy kills cells that divide the fastest but it does not discriminate between normal cells and cancer cells. Consequently, as well as killing the cancer cells, common side-effects of chemotherapy are lowered immunity, hair loss, nausea, mouth ulcers and diarrhoea. Patients will need additional support during this treatment from many members of the multidisciplinary team, including consultants, specialist nurses, counsellors, dietitians and physiotherapy.

Diseases That Reduce the Source of Immunity, Such As Leukaemias

These result in the production of large amounts of abnormal white blood cells that have no immune function, they just occupy space. They essentially crowd out the functioning cells by their sheer numbers, so immunity is impaired. Infection is the most common form of non-cancer death in patients who have cancer (Zarosky *et al.*, 2017).

What the Experts Say

Grace, aged 10 years, has leukaemia. 'Going through cancer treatment is really hard. The worst part is not the hair loss, it's feeling sick and being sick. After that, taking medications every day. I hate taking tablets, some of the tablets make me feel sick, which means I have to take more tablets to stop feeling sick. And I'm scared of getting sepsis because of my low immunity. Two and a half years of treatment, it's a really long time.'

Conclusion

This chapter has provided the reader with an insight into the major organs and tissues of the lymphatic system and their functions. It has explored the basic processes of immunity and discussed all the structures and tools that the body uses to protect itself. There are several examples of when the immune system starts off with a fault, develops a fault or is damaged, and the reader is invited to explore the functions of the cells and chemical proteins that are the tools for protecting the body against foreign invaders.

Eukaryotes, bacteria, archaea and viruses are examined, so that the appropriate interventions can be implemented to provide a safe environment in a healthcare setting, and the reader is provided with examples of applications to nursing interventions. The chapter explores the physiology of innate immunity and explains how inflammation links to infection and fever and wound healing.

Key Points

- The difference between the innate, cell-mediated and antibody-mediated responses.
- The lymphatic system – the structure and its components – how they function and communicate to fight infection.
- The impact of genetics on immunity.
- The chemical proteins involved in immunity.
- Immunoglobulins and antibodies.
- Autoimmune diseases.
- Cancer.

References

Beitz, J.. (2017) Pharmacologic impact (aka 'breaking bad') of medications on wound healing and wound development: a literature-based overview. *Ostomy Wound Management*, 63(3), 18–35.

Collins, A. (2008) Preventing health care-associated infections. In: R. Hughes (ed.) *Patient Safety and Quality. An Evidence-Based Handbook for Nurses.* US Department of Health and Human Services, Rockville, MD.

Eccles, R. (2004) Drink plenty of fluids, a systematic review. *British Medical Journal*, 328, 499.

Fitzgerald, K.A. & Kagan, J.C. (2020) Toll-like receptors and the control of immunity. *Cell*, 180(6), 1044–1066.

Guttman-Yassky, E., Zhou, L. & Krueger J.G. (2019) The skin as an immune organ: tolerance versus effector responses and applications to food allergy and hypersensitivity reactions. *Journal of Allergy and Clinical Immunology*, 144 (2), 363–374.

Hooton, T.M., Vecchio. M., Iroz. A., *et al.* (2018) Effect of increased daily water intake in premenopausal women with recurrent urinary tract infections: a randomized clinical trial. *JAMA Internal Medicine*, 178(11), 1509–1515.

Ismail, H. & Schellack, N. (2018) Colds and flu – an overview of the management. *Professional Nursing Today*, 22(1), 3–12.

National Institute for Health and Care Excellence (2016) *Clinical Knowledge Summaries, The Common Cold.* https://cks.nice.org.uk/topics/common-cold/management/management/ (accessed December 2021).

National Institute for Health and Care Excellence (2020) *Clinical Knowledge Summaries, Urine Tract Infection.* https://cks.nice.org.uk/topics/urinary-tract-infection-lower-women/background-information/causes/ (accessed December 2021).

Nursing & Midwifery Council (2018) *The Code: Professional Standards of Practice and Behaviour for Nurses, Midwives and Nursing Associates.* www.nmc.org.uk/globalassets/sitedocuments/nmc-publications/nmc-code.pdf (accessed December 2021).

Papayannopoulos, V. (2017) Neutrophil extracellular traps in immunity and disease. *Nature Reviews Immunology*, 18, 134–147.

Takeshita, J., Grewal, S., Langan, S., *et al.* (2017) Psoriasis and comorbid diseases: epidemiology. *Journal of the American Academy of Dermatology*, 76(3), 377–390.

Wang, M.X., Win, S.S. & Pang, J. (2020) Zinc supplementation reduces common cold duration among healthy adults: a systematic review of randomized controlled trials with micronutrients supplementation. *American Journal of Tropical Medicine and Hygiene*, 103(1), 86–99.

World Health Organization (2020) *Antibiotic resistance: key facts.* www.who.int/news-room/fact-sheets/detail/antibiotic-resistance (accessed December 2021).

Zarosky, N.G., Churilla, T.M., Egleston, B.L., *et al.* (2017) Causes of death among cancer patients. *Annals of Oncology*, 28, 400–407.

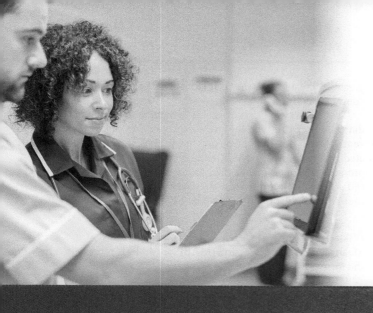

25

The Person with a Cardiovascular Disorder

Carl Clare

University of Hertfordshire, UK

Learning Outcomes

On completion of this chapter you will be able to:

- Discuss the factors affecting blood pressure
- Explore the common components of health promotion in cardiovascular disease
- Describe the common sites of cardiac pain
- Explain the first-line treatment of a myocardial infarction

Proficiencies

NMC Proficiencies and Standards:

- Identify and take the major pulses
- Assess the patient for the common signs and symptoms of heart failure
- Deliver nursing care to patients with a variety of cardiovascular disorders
- Advise patients on lifestyle changes to help manage their pain
- Advise patients on the resumption of daily activities
- Categorise the stage of hypertension a patient is suffering from

Visit the companion website at www.wiley.com/go/peate/nursingpractice3e where you can test yourself using flashcards, multiple-choice questions and more.

Nursing Practice: Knowledge and Care, Third Edition. Edited by Ian Peate and Aby Mitchell.
© 2022 John Wiley & Sons Ltd. Published 2022 by John Wiley & Sons Ltd.
Companion website: www.wiley.com/go/peate/nursingpractice3e

Introduction

Nursing the patient with a cardiovascular disorder can be challenging for the newly qualified nurse or nursing associate. The association of the heart with the centre of the human being and the subsequent fear that any disorder may engender in the patient requires the healthcare professional to be aware of the physical and psychological needs of the patient. Furthermore, health promotion and information giving are crucial to the care of the patient with a cardiovascular disorder and require up-to-date knowledge to enable effective care and partnership working.

The chapter will begin with a brief overview of the factors affecting blood pressure in the clinical setting and how they affect patient presentation. Following on from this will be a review of some of the common conditions that affect the heart or the blood vessels, their epidemiology, risk factors, care and treatment. Where appropriate, health promotion advice will also be provided.

Anatomy and Physiology of the Heart and Circulatory System

For a review of the anatomy and physiology of the heart and circulatory systems, please refer to Peate & Evans (2020).

Blood Pressure

Whilst the anatomy and physiology of the heart and circulatory systems can be reviewed in Peate & Evans (2020), it is useful to the healthcare professional in the practice setting to understand several elements of the physiology of blood pressure as the presentation of various trends in the blood pressure and heart rate can help with diagnosis and/or treatment of the underlying condition, regardless of cause.

Blood pressure is composed of two components.

- *Systolic blood pressure*: the pressure in the arteries when the heart is in systole (contracting).
- *Diastolic blood pressure*: the pressure in the arteries when the heart is in diastole (relaxing).

The difference between the systolic and diastolic pressures is known as the *pulse pressure* (Figure 25.1) and is a reflection of the

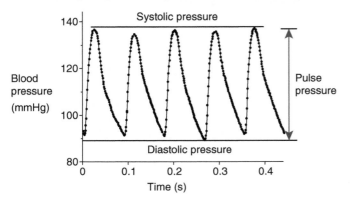

Figure 25.1 The relationship between systolic, diastolic and pulse pressures.

pressure created by the ventricles of the heart when they contract.

The total systolic pressure is dependent on the baseline diastolic pressure plus the pressure created by the contracting ventricles of the heart (pulse pressure). Thus, if the pressure created by the contracting ventricles is 60 mmHg and the diastolic pressure is 80 mmHg, then the systolic pressure will be 140 mmHg (80 + 60 = 140); however, if the diastolic pressure is 60 mmHg, then the systolic pressure would be 120 mmHg (60 + 60 = 120).

Mean Arterial Blood Pressure

Mean arterial blood pressure (MABP or MAP) is represented by the formula:

$$MABP = Cardiac\ output(CO) \times Total\ peripheral\ resistance(TPR)$$

> **Jot This Down**
>
> Total peripheral resistance (TPR) is also known as systemic vascular resistance (SVR).

Therefore, in order to increase blood pressure, there can be an increase in cardiac output or an increase in total peripheral resistance (TPR).

Cardiac Output

The amount of blood the heart pumps out in 1 minute is known as 'cardiac output' and is defined by the following formula.

Cardiac output (CO) = stroke volume (SV) × heart rate (HR)

Thus, the amount of blood the heart pumps out in 1 minute is made up of the amount of blood pumped out of the ventricle in one beat (SV), measured in millilitres, times the heart rate (HR), measured in beats per minute. This gives a total volume. Therefore, if SV was 70 mL and the heart rate was 75, then cardiac output is 70 × 75, which equals 5250 mL (or 5.25 L) per minute.

Stroke volume is affected by several factors (see Peate & Evans, 2020) and a summary is noted below.

- *Preload*: the strength of contraction of the ventricle is partly related to the amount of blood in the ventricle.
- *Force of contraction*: the contractility of the heart muscle can be affected by several factors such as hormones and sympathetic nervous system activity.
- *Afterload*: refers to the pressure in the arteries that the ventricle must overcome in order to pump out blood.

Heart rate is controlled by two main mechanisms.

- *Autonomic nervous system activity*: sympathetic nervous system activity leads to an increase in heart rate and parasympathetic nervous system activity leads to a decrease in heart rate
- *Hormone activity*: the release of epinephrine (adrenaline) or large amounts of thyroxine leads to an increase in heart rate.

Total Peripheral Resistance

Total peripheral resistance (TPR) is most powerfully altered by changing the radius of the lumen of the arteries (particularly the arterioles); other factors that can alter TPR are blood viscosity and total blood vessel length. However, on a minute-by-minute basis, the alteration of TPR is regulated by the relaxation and constriction of the arterial walls, thus affecting the diameter of the tube the blood must flow through.

Assessing the Cardiovascular System

As with the assessment of any of the bodily systems, the healthcare professional must always explain the procedures they are about to carry out and gain consent from the patient.

The first step in assessing the cardiovascular system is to obtain a medical history from the patient. Without this data, the healthcare professional not only risks ignoring the patient's experiences of their disorder and the effect it has on their lives, but also this information can be useful in differentiating between different cardiovascular disorders, some of which can be intermittent.

History taking for the patient with a potential cardiovascular disorder focuses on:

- Chest pain
- Shortness of breath
- Palpitations
- Syncope (fainting)
- Risk factors.

The physical assessment of the cardiovascular system requires the patient to have been resting quietly before examination, so that results such as pulse and blood pressure are not affected by exercise.

Radial Pulse

Pulses can be found at many points on the body (Figure 25.2 shows the major pulse sites). When assessing the cardiovascular system, it is normal to start with the radial pulse, which is found in the wrist on the same side as the thumb (Figure 25.3). To assess the radial pulse, place two fingers on the point of pulsation and, using a watch with a second hand, count the number of beats in 60 seconds.

Once the pulse rate has been taken, then take time to assess the way the pulse feels.

- Is it thready and weak or strong and bounding?
- Is it regular or irregular?
- Is every pulsation the same strength?

The normal resting pulse rate will vary from patient to patient and can be affected by many factors, including the physical fitness of the patient, their age and anxiety levels. The range considered to be normal is 60–100 beats per minute but trained athletes may easily have a heart rate between 40 and 60 beats per minute. A weak and thready pulse may be suggestive of peripheral shutdown in response to shock or a reduced pulse pressure. The regularity of the pulse and changes in pulse strength from beat to beat can be important indicators of the presence of certain disturbances in heart rhythm such as atrial fibrillation.

What To Do If . . . You Cannot Feel a Radial Pulse

If you cannot feel an accurate pulse rate at the radial site, then it is acceptable to move to the brachial site (the same place the stethoscope is put to take a blood pressure) to palpate the pulse. If the pulse remains difficult to feel, then a heart rate can be taken by listening to the heartbeat with a stethoscope placed against the approximate position of the heart on the left side of the chest.

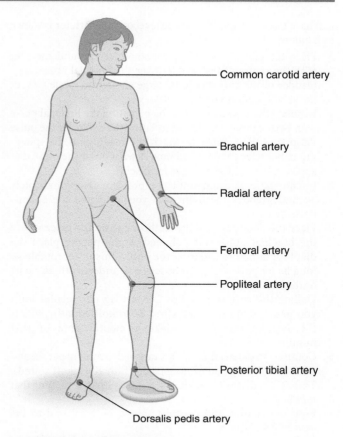

Figure 25.2 Pulse sites on the body.

Common carotid artery
Brachial artery
Radial artery
Femoral artery
Popliteal artery
Posterior tibial artery
Dorsalis pedis artery

Measuring Blood Pressure

In order to take a patient's blood pressure you will need a:

- Manual sphygmomanometer
- Stethoscope.

The patient should be seated and relaxed, having rested for at least 5 minutes. Ensure no tight clothing is restricting the arm

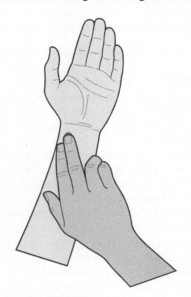

Figure 25.3 Assessing the radial pulse.

and have the arm supported at the level of the heart, for instance by a pillow.

1. Place the cuff of the sphygmomanometer around the arm with the centre of the bladder over the brachial artery. The bladder of the cuff should be large enough to circle 80% of the arm but not more than 100%.
2. Estimate the systolic pressure by palpating the brachial pulse with two or three fingers and inflating the cuff until the pulse disappears. Remember to watch the reading on the sphygmomanometer so that you know at what point the pulse disappears. Release the pressure in the cuff.
3. Inflate the cuff again until the pressure is approximately 30 mmHg above the point that you estimated the systolic pressure to be.
4. Place the diaphragm of the stethoscope on the place where the brachial pulse was palpated. Some people place the diaphragm before inflating the cuff – this is acceptable so long as no part of the stethoscope is underneath any part of the cuff.
5. Deflate the cuff at a rate of 2–3 mmHg per second until you hear a tapping sound (first Korotkoff sound). This is the systolic pressure – make a mental note of that number.
6. Continue to deflate the cuff at a rate of 2–3 mmHg per second until the tapping sound disappears (fifth Korotkoff sound). This is the diastolic pressure – make a mental note of that number.
7. Both the systolic and diastolic should be measured to the nearest 2 mmHg.
8. Deflate the cuff fully and record the systolic and diastolic on the appropriate documentation.

What To Do If . . . The Tapping Sound Never Disappears

This is often due to pressing too hard with the stethoscope. Reassess the blood pressure, trying to be gentler with the stethoscope. If on repeat the tapping noise does not disappear, then use the point where the sounds change as the measurement of diastolic blood pressure and record in the documentation that the fourth Korotkoff sound was used to measure diastolic blood pressure.

If using an electronic blood pressure monitor.

1. The patient should be seated and relaxed, having rested for at least 5 minutes. Ensure no tight clothing is restricting the arm and have the arm supported at the level of the heart, for instance by a pillow.
2. Place the cuff of the sphygmomanometer around the arm with the centre of the bladder over the brachial artery. The bladder of the cuff should be large enough to circle 80% of the arm but not more than 100%.
3. Read the systolic and diastolic blood pressures as displayed and record on the appropriate documentation.

Normal blood pressure readings are considered to be 90–140 mmHg systolic and 60–90 mmHg diastolic. However, patients should be reassured that one reading above these levels does not necessarily mean they have high blood pressure, as blood pressure varies widely throughout the day and unless they have symptoms (such as feeling dizzy), lower blood pressures are not necessarily an indication of a problem.

Assessing the Peripheral Vascular System in the Legs

- Compare the colour and temperature of the two legs, looking for colour changes (such as a blue or purple discoloration).
- Compare the temperature of the two legs using the back of the hand.

Jot This Down

Different parts of the hand are better for different types of assessment.
- The back of the hand is best for assessing temperature.
- The palms are best for assessing vibration.
- The fingertips are best for assessing pulsation.

- Press on the nailbed of the big toe so that it blanches and then note how long it takes for the colour to return. Compare the time taken for both feet.
- Palpate the dorsalis pedis pulse (Figure 25.4) on both feet, assessing strength and comparing the two. The dorsalis pedis pulse can be difficult to palpate and if you cannot find it, this does not mean it is not present.

Jot This Down

Many healthcare professionals who work in areas such as cardiac catheter recovery or on vascular surgery wards mark the dorsalis pedis with a pen once it has been palpated (with the permission of the patient). This makes regular assessment easier.

- Palpate the posterior tibial pulse (Figure 25.5) in both ankles, assessing strength and comparing the two. The posterior tibial pulse can be felt on the inside (big toe side) of the ankle. It is just below and behind the big bony part that sticks out (the medial malleolus).
- Palpate the popliteal pulse in both knees (Figure 25.6), assessing strength and comparing the two. The popliteal pulse is located in the fold behind the knee. The easiest way to find it is to have the patient's leg slightly bent, place your thumbs on the kneecap and then curl your fingers round the knee into the fold behind the knee. This pulse is quite deep and may require some pressure to palpate but be careful not to be too firm.

Pulses should be equal on both sides of the body; any differences should be recorded and reported.

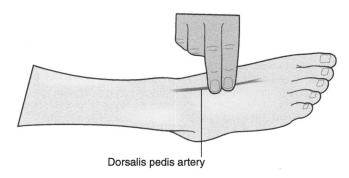

Dorsalis pedis artery

Figure 25.4 **Palpating the dorsalis pedis pulse.**

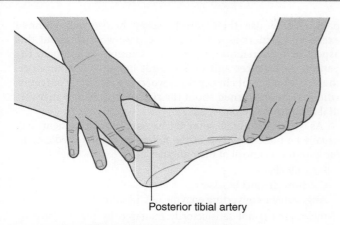

Posterior tibial artery

Figure 25.5 Palpating the posterior tiblal pulse.

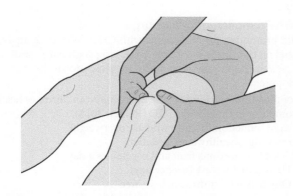

Figure 25.6 Palpating the popliteal pulse.

Disorders of the Cardiovascular System

Coronary Heart Disease

Coronary heart disease (also known as ischaemic heart disease [IHD] or coronary artery disease [CAD]) is the label applied to a group of conditions based on the development of narrowing in the lumen of one or more of the coronary arteries leading to a reduction of blood flow, and therefore oxygen, to the tissues (thus creating ischaemia). The group of conditions are:

- Stable angina
- Unstable angina
- Myocardial infarction.

Risk factors for CHD include:

- Smoking
- High-fat diet
- Lack of exercise
- Family history of CHD
- High serum cholesterol
- High blood pressure
- Diabetes
- Obesity
- Ethnic origin.

Stable Angina

Stable angina is characterised by chest pain/discomfort, jaw pain or pain in the arm (usually the left arm) that usually occurs when the patient is exercising or emotionally distressed.

Pathophysiology

The heart muscle has a high oxygen requirement and the blood flow to the heart muscles is through the coronary arteries. In patients with any form of CHD, the pathophysiology of the early stages is based on the same processes. Cholesterol and other fatty substances are laid down in the artery wall into a structure known as a *plaque*. As the plaques are present between the tunica intima and tunica media, the lumen of the artery becomes narrowed because the thick muscle layer of the tunica media creates a barrier that pushes the plaque into the lumen of the artery (Figure 25.7).

The supply of oxygen to the heart muscle and the demand of the heart muscle for that oxygen are balanced by several factors. When we exercise (or increase our heart rates in other ways), the myocardium requires more oxygen as it is working harder. In people without significant narrowing of the coronary arteries, this demand can be met by increasing blood flow. In the patient with significant atherosclerosis, leading to stable angina, the increased demand for oxygen by the heart muscle cannot be met due to the narrowing of the artery lumen and thus the patient experiences pain due to hypoxia of the myocardium.

Signs and Symptoms

The symptoms of stable angina include the experience of pain or discomfort in the chest, which may radiate into an arm (the left arm is usual), shoulder and jaw. Pain of cardiac origin is commonly described as tightness or heaviness and may be associated with shortness of breath. In stable angina, the pain is brief (usually no longer than 10 minutes), is associated with physical exertion or emotional distress and is normally relieved by rest or a GTN spray (which most patients with angina will have been prescribed). Some patients will experience more episodes of angina

437

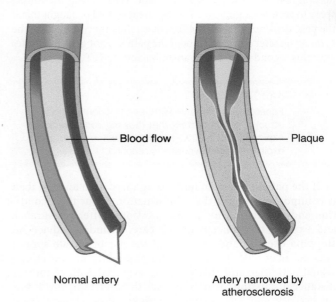

Blood flow   Plaque

Normal artery   Artery narrowed by atherosclerosis

Figure 25.7 Atherosclerosis.

during the cold winter months. Entering the cold air from a warm house appears to be related to a sudden increase in blood pressure, leading to a greater workload for the heart and thus increased myocardial oxygen demand (Ikäheimo, 2018).

Diagnosis and Investigations

The diagnosis of stable angina can usually be made with a good degree of certainty by taking a history from the patient. If they report typical chest pain occurring on exertion, lasting for a short period and relieved by rest, then the diagnosis is almost certainly stable angina. However, certain investigations and physical examination are still required to confirm the diagnosis and to assess the underlying CHD.

- *Full blood count.*
- *12-lead ECG*: this will often be normal but on occasion there may be indicators of previous myocardial damage or other factors related to the structure of the heart.
- *Exercise tolerance test (ETT)*: this involves exercising the patient on a treadmill while they are attached to continuous ECG monitoring. This can give an indication of how much coronary artery disease is present (Gaunt, 2019). A significant result from the ETT may lead to the patient undergoing coronary angiography to assess the degree to which the coronary arteries are narrowed (often referred to as 'stenosis') and how many of the major arteries have narrowing in them.
- *Plasma glucose and cholesterol tests* are also recommended to assess for two of the risk factors of CHD.

Nursing Care and Management

Generally, patients with stable angina are managed by the GP or in the outpatient department and hospitalisation is not required.

Often, episodes of pain can be managed by stopping the activity that has led to the pain and resting.

Patients with stable angina will be prescribed a nitrate spray for use when they have episodes of pain. The spray is administered under the tongue as required by the patient. However, it is best to warn patients who are new to the use of nitrate spray that they need to sit down before using the spray, as it can cause hypotension and then the patient may faint. When using the nitrate spray to treat an angina attack, the patient should be taught that if the pain does not go after the first dose, then they should use the spray again after 5 minutes, and if the pain has not gone 5 minutes after this second dose, to call an ambulance (NICE, 2020).

Medicines Management

Especially for patients with less frequent angina attacks, it is important that they regularly check the expiry date of their GTN spray, as when the spray expires its effectiveness is reduced.

If the patient has been newly diagnosed with angina, then it is important to give them information about their condition and give them time to ask questions. Offer reassurance and explore the concept of self-care, including advice on stopping exercise and resting and the use of nitrate sprays. Patients may wish to explore the possibility of continuing sexual activities and this must be explored with them, for instance discussing the need to pace themselves in any physical activity and recognising the signs of developing chest pain and to use their nitrate spray before any planned exertion. Partners especially can become worried about this aspect of their relationship, as they cannot see the pain the patient experiences and thus cannot judge it. Furthermore, the very concept of chest pain is worrying for many partners, who may be concerned about the risk of triggering a myocardial infarction (Jaarsma, 2017).

As well as the nitrate spray for 'as-required' use, patients will usually be prescribed two of the following regular medications for long-term control of their angina:

- Beta-blocker
- Calcium channel blocker
- Angiotensin-converting enzyme (ACE) inhibitor.

If the angina is not satisfactorily managed by the use of drug therapy, then the patient may be offered some form of revascularisation therapy, such as angioplasty or coronary artery bypass graft (CABG).

Health Promotion and Discharge

Health promotion for all patients with CHD (including angina) is based on risk factor reduction. CHD is a progressive condition and health promotion can help to slow down its further development.

- Stopping smoking is one of the most important forms of health promotion in those with CHD (Reiner, 2018).
- Weight reduction in those who are overweight.
- Promoting a healthy balanced diet.
- At least five portions fruit and vegetables a day.
  - High fibre (at least 18 g per day).
  - Oily fish at least three times a week.
  - Avoid fatty foods.
- Exercising at least 150 minutes per week (moderate intensity).

Red Flag

Patients with coronary heart disease should not start a new exercise regime without consulting their doctor first.

- Patients with high blood cholesterol levels or high blood pressure will need treatment for these conditions.
- Patients with diabetes are especially at risk of heart disease and as well as the health promotion mentioned, stress must be placed on ensuring good control of their diabetes.

Unstable Angina

Unstable angina is a severe form of angina that suggests a greater degree of coronary artery stenosis or instability of the plaques in the coronary arteries.

Pathophysiology

The underlying pathophysiology of unstable angina is based on the same process of atherosclerosis but the plaque has become unstable and clots are developing on the top of the plaque, leading to greater blockage of the artery. These clots will often partially dissolve and then reoccur, with the associated pain waxing and waning as a result.

Signs and Symptoms

The signs and symptoms of unstable angina are:

- Chest pain similar to stable angina but can be more severe
- Often occurs while resting, sleeping or with little physical exertion
- May last longer than stable angina
- Rest or medicine usually do not help relieve it
- May get worse over time.

Diagnosis and Investigations

Diagnosis of unstable angina is based on:

- 12-lead ECG
- Measurement of cardiac enzymes in the blood, such as CK(MB) and troponin I or troponin T
- Coronary angiogram
- Plasma glucose and cholesterol tests are also recommended to assess for two of the risk factors of CHD.

Nursing Care and Management

Nursing care of the patient with unstable angina will be based on the delivery of medical treatment according to prescription, including:

- Intravenous nitrates
- Antiplatelet therapy (such as aspirin or clopidogrel)
- Intravenous infusions of glycoprotein IIb/IIIa inhibitors
- Intravenous infusion of heparin or subcutaneous injections of low molecular weight heparin.

The initial nursing actions should be based around maintaining patient safety. Specific nursing actions include:

- Provision of reassurance and a calm environment to minimise stress
- Implementation of bedrest
- Oxygen delivery as per prescription
- Cardiac monitoring
- Pain relief may be required (such as intravenous morphine).

Further treatment may involve angioplasty or CABG.

Health Promotion and Discharge

Health promotion is the same as that for stable angina in promoting healthy lifestyles and reducing risk factors.

On discharge, the patient should be advised to call an ambulance if they have angina symptoms lasting for more than 10 minutes that are not relieved by rest or their usual medication. Patients should also be referred to the hospital cardiac rehabilitation programme (NICE, 2020). Cardiac rehabilitation is a structured programme of exercise and health promotion, carried out as a group activity under the supervision of a healthcare professional. The programme includes teaching sessions by dietitians and other health professionals.

Patients who have been diagnosed with unstable angina will require information on self-management. For instance, some patients may benefit from attending self-management programmes (previously the NHS expert patient programme), which are provided by a charity (www.selfmanagementuk.org, accessed December 2021). The self-management programme teaches patients skills such as:

- Staging and spacing activities
- Taking appropriate rest
- Taking exercise
- Healthy diet
- Managing pain and fatigue
- Dealing with depression or anger
- Communicating with family, friends and healthcare professionals.

Primary Care

- Denial may involve forgetting to take prescribed medications. Healthcare professionals should advise on the importance of taking the prescribed medications.
- Teach the patient the side-effects of medications prescribed and the importance of not discontinuing medications abruptly.
- Teach the patient how to take and store GTN and advise them to carry some GTN when they go out, in case of emergency.
- Advise the patient not to undertake strenuous exercise and to follow a programme of exercise as planned by their practice healthcare professional.
- Stress the importance of calling 999 (in the UK) when experiencing severe chest pain.

Myocardial Infarction

Myocardial infarction (MI) or acute myocardial infarction is the medical term for an event commonly known as a heart attack. It happens when blood stops flowing properly to part of the heart and the heart muscle is injured due to not getting enough oxygen. Usually, this is because one of the coronary arteries that supplies blood to the heart develops a blockage because of an unstable build-up of white blood cells, cholesterol and fat.

Pathophysiology

The pathophysiology of MI is based on the same underlying development of atherosclerotic plaques as both forms of angina. However, in MI, the plaque in the arterial wall ruptures, exposing the mix of cholesterol, chemicals and fatty substances to the bloodstream, activating platelets and blood cells (Figure 25.8). This leads to the development of a thrombus within the coronary artery that either completely or mostly blocks blood flow through the artery. This cessation of blood flow starves the part of the heart muscle supplied by the artery of oxygen and nutrients and leads to cell death.

Signs and Symptoms

- Central crushing chest pain radiating into the arm, neck and/or jaw; may be epigastric. May be described as crushing, 'band-like', 'like an elephant is sitting on my chest'. See Figure 25.9 for patterns of pain.
- Onset at rest or with exertion.
- Persisting for longer than 15 minutes.
- Sweating.
- Pallor.
- Shortness of breath.
- Nausea and vomiting.

It is important to note that in certain patient groups, pain may be absent as a symptom. This is most likely in women, the elderly

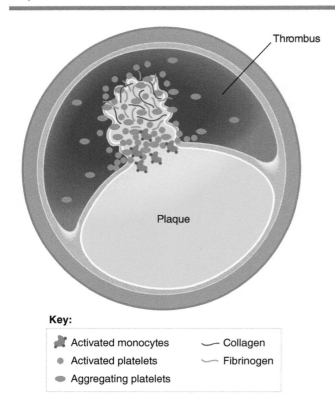

Key:

🔹 Activated monocytes   — Collagen

🔹 Activated platelets   〜 Fibrinogen

🔹 Aggregating platelets

Figure 25.8 **Ruptured atherosclerotic plaque.**

and patients with diabetes or hypertension. In these groups of patients, the most common signs and symptoms (in the absence of chest pain) are excessive sweating, nausea and vomiting, and shortness of breath. In all patients, it is important to note risk factors for, and any history of, CHD as this can aid diagnosis and therefore rapid treatment.

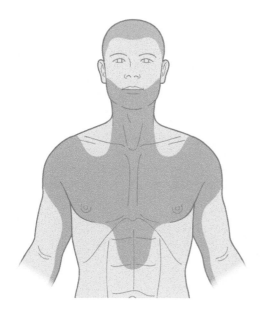

Figure 25.9 **Typical areas where pain associated with myocardial infarction may be reported.**

Diagnosis and Investigations

A common phrase used with regard to acute MI is 'time is myocardium'. The longer it takes to reach diagnosis and subsequent treatment of the MI, the more heart muscle dies and the greater the risk of death or long-term complications, such as heart failure. Therefore, the presentation of a patient with new chest pain is treated as a medical emergency and the patient is assumed to be suffering an MI until proven otherwise.

The diagnosis is based on taking an accurate patient history, including the patient's report of the current condition, past medical history and family history of heart disease. Specific investigations include:

- *Cardiac enzymes*: troponin I or troponin T and CK(MB). Note that negative results from blood tests cannot be considered diagnostic for ruling out MI before 12 hours after the onset of pain
- *Serial 12-lead ECGs*: if the patient has presented very early after the onset of pain injury, patterns may not be obvious on the ECG and thus repeat ECGs are always taken if the first is not conclusive
- *Plasma glucose and cholesterol tests* are also recommended to assess for two of the risk factors of CHD.

Nursing Care and Management

The initial management of acute MI is based on maintaining patient safety, the reduction of myocardial work and the reperfusion of the heart muscle.

Pain relief is paramount; current guidelines recommend the use of morphine (5–10 mg) or diamorphine (2.5–5 mg) titrated to pain. A popular method of titrating pain relief is to make up a 10 mg dose of morphine in 10 mL of water for injection and administer the morphine in 1 mL (1 mg) increments until pain relief is achieved. The benefit of opiate pain relief is that it also acts to relieve anxiety in the patient. However, as opiates are associated with nausea and vomiting, it is advisable to administer an antiemetic at the same time (Ibanez *et al.*, 2018). The patient is also attached to continuous cardiac monitoring as the risk of cardiac arrhythmias and even cardiac arrest are high.

Red Flag

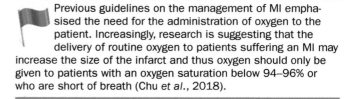

Previous guidelines on the management of MI emphasised the need for the administration of oxygen to the patient. Increasingly, research is suggesting that the delivery of routine oxygen to patients suffering an MI may increase the size of the infarct and thus oxygen should only be given to patients with an oxygen saturation below 94–96% or who are short of breath (Chu *et al.*, 2018).

Some experts still recommend the use of sublingual nitrate spray in the patient suffering from MI. If intravenous morphine is ineffective, then the recommendation is for the use of intravenous nitrates or beta-blocker drugs. Before the use of nitrates or beta-blockers it is necessary to measure the patient's blood pressure as both nitrates and beta-blockers can significantly reduce the blood pressure.

Aspirin is an effective antiplatelet drug. In patients who are not already taking regular aspirin and are not allergic to aspirin, the dose is 300 mg crushed and swallowed or chewed.

Patients suffering from an acute MI will be maintained on bedrest to minimise cardiac work. Reassurance will be necessary for both the patient and relatives, as they will be anxious.

Definitive treatment of MI is based on restoration of blood flow to the myocardium. Previously, this was carried out the use of thrombolytic therapy (otherwise known as fibrinolysis) to break up the blood clot. In the past 18 or more years (since initial UK trials in 2003), there has been growing use of primary angioplasty (also known as primary percutaneous coronary intervention, or primary PCI). The patient has a catheter inserted through a hole made in the femoral or radial artery and the catheter is manoeuvred to the coronary artery, where the blockage is situated. A balloon is then passed through and inflated to push the thrombus into the walls of the artery and, if necessary, a metal cage (a stent) is inserted into the artery to keep the artery open (Figure 25.10). Increasingly, the use of bare metal stents has been phased out in favour of drug-eluting stents (stents coated with a slow-release drug that inhibits the growth of the tunica intima into the lumen of the stent) as long-term outcomes have been shown to be improved with these new stents (Piccolo *et al.*, 2019).

Health Promotion

Health promotion is the same for MI as for angina in that there should be promotion of healthy lifestyles and the reduction of risk factors for CHD. As with other patients suffering from cardiovascular diseases, patients who are to begin exercise regimes should consult with their doctor.

Following MI, patients may need information and education to address misconceptions about cardiac disease and improve medication compliance (Crowley *et al.*, 2015).

Depending on the result of angiography or other testing, if the patient has plaques in one or more arteries, they may be referred for further angioplasty or CABG to help prevent further MI and/or improve quality of life by increasing myocardial oxygen supply and thus reducing symptoms of angina.

Discharge

Patients should be referred to the hospital cardiac rehabilitation programme. Cardiac rehabilitation is a structured programme of exercise and health promotion carried out as a group activity under the supervision of a healthcare professional. The programme includes teaching sessions by dietitians and other health professionals.

Patients who have suffered an MI will often have psychological needs (Kumar & Nayak, 2017) and may suffer from:

- Anxiety
- Depressed mood
- Anger
- Depression
- Exhaustion
- Social withdrawal.

Patients should be made aware of the availability of counselling therapies through their GP or may wish to access local support groups.

Return to work will depend on medical factors and the nature of the work and thus no single specific guideline can be formulated. In the majority of cases, the patient may begin driving 4 weeks after the MI so long as they have made a satisfactory recovery and they must inform their insurance company. Drivers of passenger-carrying vehicles and light or heavy goods vehicles must contact the DVLA for further advice on returning to work. Patients wishing to travel on commercial airplanes as a passenger within 4 weeks of an MI should consult with their doctor and contact the airline and the travel insurance provider.

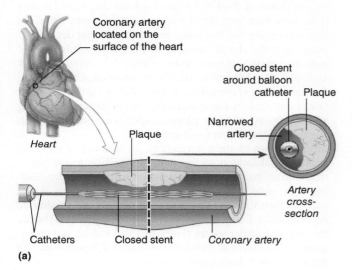

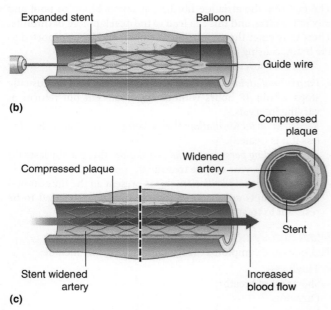

Figure 25.10 Coronary stent insertion.

Primary Care

When a patient has an MI, they report feelings of anxiety and boredom. Healthcare professionals need to take time to talk to the patient and relatives and alleviate the fears and anxieties they may have.
Some of these fears and anxieties may include:
- Lack of self-confidence
- Frustration when unable to do what they previously managed

(Continued)

441

- Inability to return to the normal life to which they are accustomed.

Graduated physical activity should be encouraged in order to return patients to their normal activities of living.

Most patients should be able to resume driving 4–6 weeks after an uncomplicated MI. They should be advised to inform the DVLA of their intentions.

Occupational health and community healthcare professionals should be able to provide support for the patient and family throughout convalescence.

Pericarditis

Pericarditis is inflammation of the pericardium and is a relatively common cause of chest pain.

Pathophysiology

Pericardial tissue damaged by bacteria or other mechanisms releases the chemical mediators of inflammation into the surrounding tissue, thus starting the inflammatory process. As inflammation becomes established, the pericardium will swell and friction occurs as the inflamed pericardial layers rub against each other.

Signs and Symptoms

Chest pain is the primary presenting symptom.

- Progressive.
- Frequently severe.
- Sharp.
- May radiate.
- Worse when supine and relieved by sitting up/forward.
- Fever is possible but not always present.
- Pericardial rub (a creaking or rustling sound that may be heard on auscultation of the heart) may be present but is relatively rarely heard as it is transient.

Diagnosis and Investigations

- A 12-lead ECG: the ECG will often show changes similar to those of an MI with some minor differences and is best reviewed by a cardiologist.
- Troponin I or T may be raised.
- Full blood count often shows an increased white cell count that is indicative of inflammation.
- Raised serum C-reactive protein (CRP) and erythrocyte sedimentation rate (ESR): indicative of inflammation
- Echocardiography may or may not be useful.

Nursing Care and Management

Most cases of pericarditis are self-limiting and respond quickly to non-steroidal anti-inflammatory drugs such as ibuprofen. Anxiety is often a problem and will increase the perception of pain and so the healthcare professional should explain the diagnosis and give reassurance.

Health Promotion and Discharge

Patients who are being discharged following an episode of pericarditis usually require no specialist health promotion or discharge advice unless there is an underlying condition.

Disorders of the Cardiac Rhythm: Atrial Fibrillation

Atrial fibrillation is a common disorder of the cardiac rhythm.

Pathophysiology

Within the normal heart, the heart rhythm is regulated by the sinoatrial (SA) node, leading to a regular heartbeat. The impulse generated in the SA node is rapidly transmitted around the atria and both atria contract in an organised fashion. In atrial fibrillation, there are multiple areas in the atrial wall creating electrical impulses and activating the cardiac muscle in their local area. Thus, the atrial myocardium no longer contracts in a co-ordinated fashion but 'fibrillates' – in essence, viewed from the outside, the atria look like jelly wobbling on a plate – and no co-ordinated contractions occur. This can lead to changes in blood pressure for several reasons.

- The loss of the 'atrial kick' means that the ventricles no longer receive that final third of the blood volume they would receive if the atria were working in a co-ordinated fashion. Thus, the ventricles pump out less blood and cardiac output decreases.
- Sometimes the chaotic number of electrical impulses in the atria may mean that none is strong enough to activate the AV node and thus activate ventricular contraction. Cells lower in the conduction system of the heart will then take over but the rate of ventricular contraction will be lower (potentially falling as low as 20–30 beats per minute) and thus cardiac output falls due to the reduction in heart rate.
- In many cases of atrial fibrillation, the number of electrical impulses transmitted to the ventricles will be much higher than normal but also the transmission will be irregular, leading to a rapid irregular heartbeat. If the heartbeat is fast enough, then the time the heart is in diastole will be shorter. As ventricular filling is reliant on the time in diastole (before the atrioventricular valves close), this will reduce and consequently the volume of blood the ventricles will pump out will decrease, thus reducing cardiac output.

The fact that the atria are fibrillating causes blood to pool and mix in the atria, and this can lead to the development of thrombi. These may enter the circulation as emboli and be transported to the brain, causing a stroke.

There are several classifications of atrial fibrillation.

- *Paroxysmal atrial fibrillation*: this comes and goes and usually stops within 48 hours without any treatment but returns at varying intervals.
- *Persistent atrial fibrillation*: this lasts for longer than 7 days (or less if it is treated).
- *Long-standing persistent atrial fibrillation*: this usually lasts for longer than a year despite treatment.
- *Permanent atrial fibrillation*: this is present all the time and no more attempts are made to convert it as it has proved to be resistant to treatment.

Signs and Symptoms

The signs and symptoms of atrial fibrillation may include:

- Tiredness
- Shortness of breath
- Dizziness
- Fainting
- Palpitations

- Irregular pulse, often with significant differences in pulse strength between beats (commonly this is rapid but may be very slow)
- Low blood pressure.

Diagnosis and Investigations

- *A 12-lead ECG*: atrial fibrillation will show as an irregular ventricular activation (QRS wave) but there will be an absence of atrial waves (P wave). In patients with paroxysmal atrial fibrillation, it may be difficult to 'catch' the atrial fibrillation with a standard ECG recording and therefore the patient may have a 24-hour ECG monitor attached in the outpatient department in an attempt to capture a recording of an episode of atrial fibrillation.
- *Echocardiography*: transthoracic echocardiography (TTE) will be used to assess the function of the heart and the heart valves; this is a non-invasive test involving the use of a transducer placed on the chest wall. Transoesophageal echocardiography (TOE) is a form of echocardiography where the transducer is passed down the patient's throat (in the same manner as endoscopy). The reason for TOE is to assess the atria for the presence of thrombi, which may not be seen by TTE.
- *Chest X-ray*: to assess for potential lung causes of atrial fibrillation.
- *Blood test*: this is especially useful for checking the thyroid hormone levels and the electrolyte levels in the blood.

Nursing Care and Management

Treatment of atrial fibrillation is based on three main components.

Rate Control

This is usually achieved by the use of medicines. The most common drug used in the treatment of atrial fibrillation is amiodarone but beta-blockers are also commonly prescribed. Traditionally, digoxin was prescribed but has increasingly fallen out of use except for patients with associated heart failure (Soar *et al.*, 2021). If patients are administered intravenous amiodarone, then the prescription must be followed closely. The dose is administered in two separate infusions. The first infusion is given over 20–60 minutes and the second over 23 hours. **Under no circumstances should amiodarone be administered as a bolus or rapid infusion except to patients in cardiac arrest, as rapid administration can cause cardiovascular collapse** (Soar *et al.*, 2021). Patients receiving long-term amiodarone therapy (i.e. taking amiodarone tablets) should be warned that the drug can cause changes in skin colour and that they must avoid exposing their skin to the sun.

Digoxin is less commonly used for atrial fibrillation with haemodynamic compromise (unstable blood pressure) as beta-blockers or calcium channel blockers have a faster onset of action, but if it is prescribed, then it should not be administered to patients with a heart rate of less than 60 beats per minute. Patients should be warned to report episodes of vomiting and/or diarrhoea and episodes of dizziness or blurred vision, as these may be symptoms of digoxin toxicity.

Anticoagulation

As noted, atrial fibrillation is a high risk for causing a stroke and thus patients with atrial fibrillation are prescribed warfarin. Patients prescribed warfarin will require education about the purpose of anticoagulation and the importance of regular monitoring of their clotting by blood test. It is also vital that patients are educated to always take their warfarin at the same time every day, not to miss doses or adjust the dose except on medical advice, to avoid alcohol except in moderation and not to drink cranberry juice, as alcohol and cranberry juice can affect the anticoagulant effects of warfarin. Further studies have shown the potential risk of increased risk of bleeding associated with several herbal supplements and foods including Chinese wolfberry, chamomile tea, cannabis, cranberry, chitosan, green tea, *Ginkgo biloba*, ginger, and St John's wort (Tan & Lee, 2021). The exact effect of these supplements and foods is unknown and therefore patients should be advised to consult with a doctor or pharmacist before starting any new herbal or over-the-counter supplement. Patients should be informed to report unusual levels of bruising or bleeding, blackened stools, rashes or hair loss to their doctor.

Cardioversion

This is the restoration of the heart rhythm to normal. It can be attempted by drug therapy (such as amiodarone) or by electrical shock under sedation. In cardioversion for arrhythmias not associated with a cardiac arrest, the electrical shock is delivered by synchronisation of the electrical shock with the 'R' wave of the ECG to prevent the creation of ventricular fibrillation. The majority of electrical cardioversions are undertaken as an elective procedure as a day-case patient and the patient should be treated as a surgical patient, including being nil by mouth, according to protocol (see Chapter 14). Emergency cardioversion may be carried out on patients who are haemodynamically compromised (e.g. a systolic blood pressure below 90 mmHg).

> ### Case Study
>
> ***New-onset atrial fibrillation in an elderly patient***
> Jennifer is an 80-year-old woman who was admitted to the ward with an acute community-acquired chest infection. On admission to the ward, she was assessed and found to have a CURB65 risk of 4 (high risk). Prescribed treatment included supplemental oxygen via facemask titrated to maintain an oxygen saturation of greater than 96% and intravenous antibiotics (for more information on pneumonia please refer to Chapter 27).
>
> Later on the day of admission, Jennifer reports a fluttering feeling in her chest and a feeling of dizziness and light headedness. A 12-lead ECG shows fast atrial fibrillation and medical staff suspect this is related to the pneumonia as it is a known risk factor for the development of atrial fibrillation in the elderly (Nichols, 2017). Previous vital signs on admission to the ward showed a regular heart rate. Her current observations are noted below.
>
> | VITAL SIGN | OBSERVATION | NORMAL |
> | --- | --- | --- |
> | Temperature | 38.0 °C | 36.0–37.9 °C range |
> | Pulse | 130 beats per minute and irregularly irregular | 60–100 beats per minute |
> | Respiration | 22 breaths per minute | 12–20 breaths per minute |
> | Blood pressure | 92/65 mmHg | 100–139 mmHg (systolic) range |
> | O$_2$ saturations | 96% on 40% O$_2$ | 94%–98% |

Jennifer's NEWS2 score is noted below

PHYSIOLOGICAL PARAMETER	3	2	1	0	1	2	3
Respiration rate						22	
Oxygen saturation %				96			
Air or oxygen		O$_2$					
Temperature °C					38		
Systolic BP mmHg		92					
Heart rate							130
Level of consciousness				A			
Score	0	4	0	0	1	2	0
Total		7					

Take time to reflect on this case study and then consider the following.

1. Jennifer's heart rate has increased, and her systolic blood pressure has dropped. What do you think is happening and why? Consider the role of atrial fibrillation and heart rate.
2. What immediate nursing actions could you take? Consider the tension between sitting the patient up for chest expansion and lying them down due to a low blood pressure.
3. What treatment options might be recommended to treat the new-onset atrial fibrillation?
4. Given Jennifer's NEWS2 score of 7, what is the recommended escalation action according your local trust policy?

Practice Assessment Document

In medical settings students often report difficulty getting outcomes associated with the unconscious patient or airway management signed off. The treatment of atrial fibrillation by cardioversion is a perfect opportunity to undertake or be involved with this care as the patient will be anaesthetised for the procedure. Asking to be involved with the cardioversion (usually by accompanying the patient to the theatre recovery department) may allow the student to assist with the care and management of the patient during and after the procedure.

Health Promotion and Discharge

Health promotion and discharge advice will be dictated by the underlying cause of the atrial fibrillation (if known) and advice on medications, as detailed above.

Heart Failure

Heart failure is a syndrome characterised by an inability of the heart to pump blood around the body at a sufficient pressure.

Heart failure can be acute or chronic and right-sided, left-sided or bilateral.

Heart failure is also known as:

- *Congestive cardiac failure (CCF)*: right-sided heart failure
- *Congestive heart failure (CHF)*: right-sided heart failure
- *Left ventricular failure*: left-sided heart failure.

Risk factors for heart failure include:

- Age
- Sex
- Hypertension
- Coronary heart disease
- Diabetes
- Excess alcohol use.

Pathophysiology

The pathophysiology of heart failure is complex and remains the subject of much research.

Heart failure can be roughly categorised into three categories.

- Heart failure due to *left ventricular systolic dysfunction (LVSD)*: the part of the heart that pumps blood around the body (left ventricle) becomes weak, most commonly caused by CHD, especially MI. The incidence of heart failure with reduced ejection fraction (HFrEF) in the UK has reduced as the treatment of myocardial infarction has improved.
- Heart failure with *preserved ejection fraction (HFpEF)*: the incidence of HFpEF is increasing in the UK, probably as a consequence of better treatment of MI but also as an effect of an ageing population (Vasan *et al.*, 2018).
- Heart failure due to *valve disease*.

Primary Care

A study of heart failure in the primary care setting (Marciniak *et al.*, 2017) notes that a significant proportion of patients with suspected heart failure in the community setting have significant associated heart valve disease. Thus, an important aspect of the further care of these patients is a referral for echocardiography to assess valve function. It is important for the healthcare professional to encourage attendance at any appointment for echocardiography as undiagnosed heart valve disease can have a significant impact on prognosis.

As the heart begins to fail and cardiac output is reduced, there is a reduction in blood pressure; in compensation, several mechanisms become active.

- Sympathetic nervous system
- Hormonal outflow (such as adrenaline)
- Renin–angiotensin–aldosterone system

This leads to an increase in total peripheral resistance, which has the short-term effect of increasing tissue perfusion but also of increasing afterload and the work the failing ventricle has to do, thus exacerbating the original problem.

Signs and Symptoms

Some of the signs and symptoms of heart failure can be seen in Figure 25.11 and include the following.

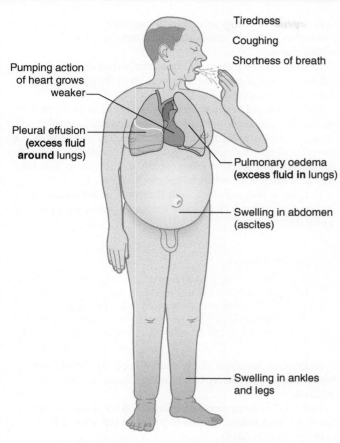

Tiredness

Coughing

Shortness of breath

Pumping action of heart grows weaker

Pleural effusion (excess fluid **around** lungs)

Pulmonary oedema (**excess fluid in** lungs)

Swelling in abdomen (ascites)

Swelling in ankles and legs

Figure 25.11 Signs and symptoms of heart failure.

Shortness of Breath

As the failing left ventricle is unable to empty completely, there is an increase in the left ventricular pressure at the end of diastole (LVEDP). As this pressure increases, the pressure within the pulmonary veins (supplying the left atrium) also increases, leading eventually to pulmonary oedema. The patient will be short of breath on exertion in the beginning but as the heart failure progresses, shortness of breath at rest will also develop. Orthopnoea may also be present (usually first noted at night). As the patient lies down, there is an increase in venous return, leading to an increase in left ventricular pressure and exacerbation of symptoms.

Jot This Down

Orthopnoea is traditionally measured in 'pillows'. That is, the doctor will ask (and record) how many pillows the patient requires to sleep at night. As the shortness of breath increases, the patient will require more and more pillows, as they gradually have to lie more and more at an angle. Eventually, patients may end up sleeping upright in a chair.

As the pulmonary oedema progresses, the patient will develop a cough and produce white frothy sputum.

Oedema

Patients with right-sided heart failure (right ventricular failure) can develop oedema of the tissues supplied by the systemic circulation. These patients may show oedema of:

- Legs: usually starting with foot or ankle oedema but potentially eventually leading to gross oedema of the legs

---

Practice Assessment Document

Ageing often leads to damage of the skin integrity and reduced healing but this is exacerbated by the presence of oedema making the skin more susceptible to damage and tears as the skin is stretched by the swelling tissues (Payne, 2019). Oedematous legs are heavier and thus the temptation for the patient is to drag their legs across the bed or chair, leading to shearing forces that may break the skin. Oedematous skin is more friable and less resistant to damage caused by knocks and minor impacts, leading to an increase in the incidence of broken skin. Associated reduction in healing increases the potential for leg ulcers to develop.

Caring for a patient with leg oedema in any setting is an opportunity to achieve outcomes associated with assessing skin and/or risk assessment. For instance, the patient's bedside environment or home shsould be checked for unnecessary equipment that may lead to bumps and scrapes and the skin should be assessed for rashes or sores when removing compression stockings.

- Sacrum
- Abdomen (ascites)
- Liver: oedema of the liver may lead to jaundice.

Red Flag

Patients with oedema may have impaired drug metabolism and thus caution should be used in both the prescribing and administration of any medication that is metabolised by the liver, as the half-life may be prolonged and blood levels may rise to toxic levels. Monitor patients with liver oedema closely for the known side-effects of any administered medication.

Anorexia

Intestinal oedema may result from severe heart failure, leading to reduced peristalsis and malabsorption of nutrients. Patients with liver failure may feel bloated and nauseous. Appetite and food intake decrease and muscle wastage occurs.

The Nursing Associate

Often the assessment of nutrition is restricted to certain groups of patients but the assessment and planning of nutritional needs and fluid intake of the patient with heart failure is an opportunity for the nursing associate to meet the requirements of outcome 3.9 (specifically nutrition and hydration) (NMC, 2018). Patients with heart failure should be assessed for nutritional intake and plans made for improving intake, for instance by eating small snacks regularly rather than bigger meals as the patient can often feel full quite quickly. Furthermore, patients with heart failure are often asked to restrict fluid intake and promoting the use of dilutable fruit squashes often leads to thirst being quenched more effectively than with plain water. Alternatively, the patient could be encouraged to suck on ice cubes.

Fatigue and Lethargy

A large proportion of patients with heart failure experience fatigue and lethargy. This may result from shortness of breath, poor tissue perfusion, muscle wasting, poor nutrition and a lack of sleep as a result of orthopnoea.

Diagnosis and Investigations

Heart failure is diagnosed when:

1. There are symptoms of heart failure (at rest or on exertion)
2. There is objective evidence of cardiac dysfunction
3. There is a response to treatment for heart failure (Oeing *et al.*, 2016).

For heart failure to be diagnosed, at least points 1 and 2 must be met, as the signs and symptoms of other disease processes (such as pulmonary disease) can be similar to the early stages of heart failure.

The severity of heart failure can be classified using several systems, but the most commonly used is the New York Heart Association (NYHA) Functional Classification (Brennan, 2018).

- *Class I (mild)*: no limitation of physical activity. Ordinary physical activity does not cause undue fatigue, palpitation or dyspnoea (shortness of breath). Essentially well-treated heart failure.
- *Class II (mild)*: slight limitation of physical activity. Comfortable at rest, but ordinary physical activity results in fatigue, palpitation or dyspnoea.
- *Class III (moderate)*: marked limitation of physical activity. Comfortable at rest, but less than ordinary activity causes fatigue, palpitation or dyspnoea.
- *Class IV (severe)*: unable to carry out any physical activity without discomfort. Symptoms of cardiac failure at rest. Patient is essentially housebound.

The tests and investigations undertaken include (NICE, 2014):

- Echocardiography, to assess heart function and the heart valves
- Blood tests for:
  - Electrolytes
  - Albumin
  - Creatinine
  - BNP (B-type natriuretic peptide) or N-terminal pro-B-type natriuretic peptide (NT-proBNP)
- A 12-lead ECG to assess for heart disease
- Cardiac catheterisation to assess for heart disease and assess heart function
- Chest X-ray to assess the heart size and for signs of pulmonary oedema
- Exercise tolerance test to assess for heart disease and exercise ability.

Nursing Care and Management

Treatment of heart failure includes the administration of medications, such as diuretics, ACE inhibitors and beta-blockers.

Patients who are hospitalised with severe heart failure may require treatment with inotropic sympathomimetics, such as dopamine or dobutamine. These drugs create the same response as sympathetic nervous system activation, thus increasing the force of contraction of the ventricles and increasing heart rate. Patients receiving these drugs should be cared for in a

high-dependency unit or coronary care unit and will require continuous cardiac monitoring and hourly blood pressure measurement.

In addition, the patient will be administered diuretic therapy and may be placed on fluid restriction. Strict fluid balance monitoring will be required.

Patients should be cared for in an upright or semi-recumbent position (at the angle the patient finds most comfortable) and oxygen therapy administered, as prescribed. The combination of shortness of breath (including rapid mouth breathing) and oxygen therapy will result in a dry mouth and regular mouth care should be offered, as well as humidified oxygen.

Peripheral oedema along with shortness of breath and lethargy increase the risk of pressure sores and pressure area care is essential.

Jot This Down

When considering pressure areas, it is important to consider the effects of any medical equipment on skin integrity. For instance, always remember to check the ears of patients wearing an oxygen mask and the nose for patients using nasal cannula.

Referral to members of the multidisciplinary team, such as the dietitian, physiotherapist and occupational therapist, will be required.

Heart failure has a worse prognosis than most cancers, and in end-stage heart failure, referral to palliative care should be made a priority (NICE, 2018).

Health Promotion

Patients with heart failure should be given advice on:

- Smoking cessation
- Abstaining from alcohol
- Reducing salt intake
- Having a yearly flu vaccination and pneumonia vaccination
- Exercise and rehabilitation
- Medication compliance.

Discharge and Community Care

Patients with heart failure in the community cannot be asked to monitor their fluid balance. However, daily weights have proven to be an effective method of monitoring fluid retention in heart failure, as weight gain or loss on a daily basis is almost always a reflection of alterations of fluid levels in the body. Patients should be advised to:

- Always use the same scales
- Always wear similar clothing (or be naked)
- Weigh themselves first thing in the morning after going to the toilet but before having anything to eat or drink
- Record the weight in a diary for the doctor to review.

In some circumstances, patients may be monitored remotely using telemonitoring. There is an increasing range of telemonitoring interventions in heart failure. For instance, scales can be connected to the internet and the daily weight is recorded in a centralised database monitored by healthcare staff (Kitsiou *et al.*, 2015).

Increasingly, evidence has shown that the use of specialist heart failure healthcare professionals in the community has improved the community management of heart failure and helped to prevent multiple readmissions (McLaughlin *et al.*, 2015).

Hypertension

Hypertension (commonly known as high blood pressure) is often unnoticed by the patient but is a risk factor for many other cardiovascular conditions and for that reason it is often referred to as the 'silent killer'.

Hypertension is a risk factor for:

- Coronary heart disease
- Stroke
- Renal disease
- Aortic aneurysm
- Heart failure.

Pathophysiology

Hypertension is categorised as either primary or secondary.

- *Primary*: hypertension without a known medical cause, the most common form of hypertension.
- *Secondary*: hypertension with a known medical cause, such as renal disease and certain types of tumour.

Current evidence for the pathophysiology of primary hypertension is complex and involves many physiological systems and processes, including the renin–angiotensin–aldosterone system, endothelial function and the autonomic nervous system.

Signs and Symptoms

Hypertension rarely causes any symptoms, except in rare cases of extremely high blood pressure, which can cause headache, nose bleed and blurred or double vision.

Diagnosis and Investigations

The diagnosis of hypertension is based on a series of blood pressure readings and is never based on a single reading. Current guidance suggests that a repeated blood pressure over 140/90 mmHg should be followed up by ambulatory blood pressure monitoring (a 24-hour automated blood pressure monitor that allows the patient to continue with their everyday activities) to confirm the hypertension and rule out the possibility of 'white coat hypertension' (i.e. transient blood pressure elevation due to the anxiety of being in a healthcare facility). Alternatively, home blood pressure measurement may be used based on an accredited automated blood pressure monitor the patient can use twice a day for 7 days at home (NICE, 2019a).

Hypertension is graded into stages.

- *Stage 1 hypertension*: systolic blood pressure of >140 mmHg and/or diastolic blood pressure of >90 mmHg.
- *Stage 2 hypertension*: systolic blood pressure of >160 mmHg and/or diastolic blood pressure of >100 mmHg.
- *Severe hypertension*: systolic blood pressure of >180 mmHg and/or diastolic blood pressure of >110 mmHg.

Further tests are undertaken to assess cardiovascular risk factors or secondary causes of hypertension.

- Urine dipstick for blood and protein.
- Blood electrolytes and creatinine and eGFR (estimated glomerular filtration rate, a measure of renal function).

- Blood glucose to assess for diabetes (as diabetes carries a greater risk of organ damage in the presence of hypertension).
- Serum cholesterol.
- 12-lead ECG.
- Fundoscopy to assess for potential damage to the retinas.

Nursing Care and Management

Hypertension is managed almost exclusively in primary care and the outpatient department.

Treatment for hypertension is always based on health promotion (see below) and, normally, with medication such as calcium channel blockers, beta-blockers, diuretics or ACE inhibitors. However, treatment choices will be affected by the ethnicity of the patient as it is recommended that patients of African or Afro-Caribbean family origin are prescribed angiotensin receptor blockers rather than ACE inhibitors (NICE, 2019b).

Case Study

Chronic hypertension in a pregnant woman of Afro-Caribbean family background

Benita is a 34-year-old woman of Afro-Caribbean family background. She is known to suffer from chronic hypertension which has improved with lifestyle advice and treatment with angiotensin receptor blockers. The practice nurse is undertaking a health review when Benita admits to being 2 months pregnant. Understandably Benita is concerned about the impact of hypertension on the baby. Chronic hypertension is three times more prevalent in the Afro-Caribbean population and is an independent factor for increased risk of adverse pregnancy outcomes (Panaitescu *et al.*, 2017).

VITAL SIGN	OBSERVATION	NORMAL
Temperature	36.8 °C	36.0–37.9 °C range
Pulse	80 beats per minute	60–100 beats per minute
Respiration	16 breaths per minute	12–20 breaths per minute
Blood pressure	145/90 mmHg	100–139 mmHg (systolic) range
O_2 saturations	98%	94–98%

Take time to reflect on this case study and then consider the following.

1. Reinforcing behavioural changes and health promotion advice is always valuable in any patient interaction. What advice would you give to Benita with regard to her hypertension?
2. Review the NICE guidelines regarding chronic hypertension in pregnancy (NICE, 2019b) which state that angiotensin receptor blockers are contraindicated in pregnancy. What alternatives could be provided?
3. Who could the GP or practice nurse refer Benita to for further care of her hypertension during the pregnancy?

Health Promotion

Health promotion for hypertensive patients includes:

- Losing weight if required
- Exercising regularly
- Eating a healthy diet
- Cutting down on alcohol
- Stopping smoking
- Cutting down on salt and caffeine.

Abdominal Aortic Aneurysm

An aneurysm is a localised dilation of a blood vessel; the most common place for an aneurysm to develop is in the abdominal aorta.

Abdominal aortic aneurysm (AAA) is much more common in men and the incidence increases with age (especially in patients with peripheral vascular disease).

Epidemiology

The risk factors for aortic aneurysm development are:

- Smoking
- Family history of aortic aneurysm
- High blood pressure
- High cholesterol
- Atherosclerosis
- Inherited conditions
- Trauma.

Pathophysiology

The underlying pathophysiology for aortic aneurysm is unclear. While aneurysm formation is commonly associated with atherosclerotic disease, it appears that the underlying disease process is different and atherosclerosis develops after degenerative changes in the wall of the aorta (Kent, 2014).

Regardless of the underlying processes, the result is a dilation of the aorta involving the entire aortic wall (Figure 25.12).

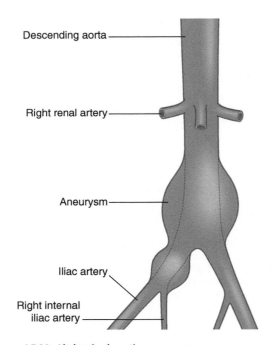

Descending aorta

Right renal artery

Aneurysm

Iliac artery

Right internal
iliac artery

Figure 25.12 Abdominal aortic aneurysm.

In most cases, the patient will not be aware of the aneurysm, but in the event of the aneurysm rupturing, the mortality rate is over 80%.

Signs and Symptoms

Most patients will not be aware of the fact they have an AAA, as there are often no signs or symptoms. If the aneurysm does become large enough to press on nearby structures, the patient may be aware of mild abdominal and/or back pain but there are many causes of mild abdominal or back pain and therefore help is rarely sought. In the event of a rupture, the patient will collapse with intense abdominal and/or back pain and will rapidly go into shock due to blood loss.

Diagnosis and Investigations

Generally, AAAs are diagnosed during assessment of the patient for other reasons, although there is now an NHS screening programme that invites men for screening the year they turn 65 years of age.

Investigations for AAA include:

- Abdominal ultrasound
- CT scan.

The Nursing Associate

The proficiencies for nursing associates (NMC, 2018) include the need to explain the reason for health screening and identify those who are eligible for screening (outcome 2.7). Research into attendance for AAA screening shows that amongst men of Afro-Caribbean descent, attendance for screening is especially poor (Ahmad et al., 2021) and one factor associated with non-attendance is not understanding what the screening is and its importance. By understanding the reason for the screening and its importance for the prevention of serious illness, the nursing associate can discuss the screening with the patient and encourage attendance.

Nursing Care and Management

Treatment of an AAA depends on its size. Small AAAs tend to be managed medically with risk factor control and monitored regularly; however, patients should be encouraged to report new symptoms as a matter of urgency. Larger AAAs (those at much higher risk of rupture) are treated surgically as follows.

- *Open surgical approach*: a traditional large incision is made into the abdomen, and the dilated aorta is removed and replaced with a synthetic graft. In most cases the graft will last the rest of the patient's life. The downside to this form of surgery is that it can be difficult in patients who have multiple risk factors, making surgery under general anaesthesia high risk.
- *Endovascular graft placement*: this is the placement of a tube-shaped graft within the aorta using a similar method to angioplasty. The graft is mounted on a balloon and inserted into the aorta on a catheter via the large arteries. Once in place, the balloon is inflated and the graft is expanded into place. Not every patient is suitable for endovascular placement of their graft and the decision is based on factors such as size and location of the aneurysm.

Following traditional repair of an AAA, the patient should be nursed as per standard postoperative care (see Chapter 14), but most patients will be transferred to an ICU or high-dependency unit immediately after theatre, as a period of support for the heart may be required after surgery (Kohlman-Trigoboff *et al.*, 2020). Patients will require monitoring for shock (in the case of the graft leaking), a sudden reduction in renal output or limb ischaemia (due to the development of emboli) and paralytic ileus. Most patients will return to the general ward within 24–48 hours. Following endovascular repair, the puncture wound must be monitored for bleeding/haematoma formation. The potential risks include damage to the iliac arteries, stent migration within the aorta or bleeding around an undersized stent.

Health Promotion and Discharge

Health promotion and discharge advice for the patient following AAA repair includes:

- Healthy diet
- Exercise
- Lose weight
- Stop smoking
- If the patient has hypertension, diabetes or high cholesterol, then advice should be given specific to those conditions
- May be required to take aspirin, or other antiplatelet therapy, to prevent clot formation.

Peripheral Artery Disease

Peripheral artery disease can affect any of the limbs but is most common in the legs. For that reason, this section only discusses peripheral artery disease in the legs. It is also known as peripheral vascular disease.

Pathophysiology

Peripheral artery disease is caused by the same underlying processes of atherosclerosis as CHD but affects the arteries of the legs. The risk factors for peripheral artery disease are the same as those for coronary artery disease.

Signs and Symptoms

In many cases, peripheral artery disease will not create any symptoms but in others it will lead to intermittent claudication. Intermittent claudication is a cramp-like pain felt in the calf, thigh or buttock during walking or other exercise. It is caused by lack of oxygen to the muscles because of poor blood supply and is relieved by rest.

Diagnosis and Investigations

Examination of the lower limbs may reveal the following.

- The affected leg may be pale and cold, with loss of hair and with skin changes (e.g. the skin may look 'shiny').
- The feet may be cold, pale or mottled and there may be evidence of ulceration.
- There may be poorly healing wounds of the extremities.
- Patients with severe peripheral artery disease or critical lower limb ischaemia may have ulceration or gangrene.
- Palpation of the femoral, popliteal, dorsalis pedis and posterior tibial pulses may reveal weak or absent pulses.

  Investigations include:

- Doppler ultrasound of the arteries
- Angiogram.

Nursing Care and Management

Treatment of peripheral artery disease can include the following.

- *Medical*: for less severe disease, treatment may rely on the reduction of risk factors and use of medication to relieve symptoms (such as peripheral vasodilators).
- *Angioplasty*: the same treatment as used for CHD but in the peripheral arteries.
- *Bypass surgery*: involves the use of veins harvested from the patient's leg to use as conduits to bypass the narrowed section of arteries.

Nursing care will depend on the treatment option undertaken but after angioplasty or bypass surgery, great care must be taken to assess and record limb colour, temperature and pulses, as thrombi and emboli are a risk to the patient's limb. The poor tissue viability of the leg presents a particular risk for the development of pressure sores.

Health Promotion and Discharge

The health promotion and discharge advice for patients who have peripheral vascular disease is the same as for all other conditions based on underlying atherosclerosis, with exercise being especially important.

Venous Insufficiency

Venous insufficiency is a condition in which the flow of blood through the veins is impaired. The most common manifestation of venous insufficiency is varicose veins but as the condition progresses, venous ulcers may develop.

Pathophysiology

The pathophysiology of venous insufficiency is commonly based on venous hypertension due to two factors.

- *Incompetent valves* in the veins leading to increased pressure due to backward flow of blood.
- *Venous obstruction* due to thrombi (often developing on the valves).

Obesity and lack of exercise have also been raised as potential contributing factors (Parker *et al.*, 2015).

Signs and Symptoms

- Dull aching heaviness or cramping in the legs.
- Itching and tingling skin on the legs.
- Aching, burning or throbbing sensations in the legs that get worse when standing.
- Pain that gets better when legs are raised.
- Swelling of the legs.

  People with chronic venous insufficiency may also have:

- Redness of the legs and ankles
- Skin colour changes around the ankles
- Varicose veins on the surface (superficial)
- Thickening and hardening of the skin on the legs and ankles (lipodermatosclerosis)
- Ulcers on the legs and ankles.

If the venous insufficiency becomes chronic, then the patient may develop *venous eczema* (red, scaly, flaky and itchy skin) and finally *venous ulcers*. Venous ulcers are the final stage of skin breakdown due to venous insufficiency. As the pressure in the veins increases, fluid leaks into the tissue and the skin, leading to swelling and eventually skin breakdown.

Diagnosis and Investigations

In most cases, history taking and a physical examination are sufficient to diagnose venous insufficiency. Duplex scanning can be carried out to assess venous hypertension (and has mostly replaced the use of tourniquet tests) and ankle brachial pressure index using Doppler will help to rule out arterial disease.

Chronic venous insufficiency is categorised according to the CEAP classification system (Lurie *et al.*, 2020).

Investigations of a venous ulcer include:

- Measurement of ankle brachial pressure index (ABPI) using Doppler
- *Measurement of the surface area of the ulcer*: this helps in assessing healing
- *Swabs for microbiology culture and sensitivity testing*: only where there are signs of infection
- *Biopsy*: especially if the ulcer has an unusual appearance or fails to heal after 12 weeks.

Nursing Care and Management

The treatment for venous insufficiency will depend on the manifestations of the condition.

The most common form of treatment is compression stockings; patients may also be advised to elevate their legs when resting to aid venous return, to take daily exercise and to lose weight. If there is a background of thrombus development, then the patient may also be commenced on anticoagulants.

Varicose veins can be surgically removed (stripped) from the leg.

Venous eczema is treated with:

- Compression stockings to treat the underlying venous insufficiency
- Moisturising creams to rehydrate the dry itchy skin
- Corticosteroid creams are used to treat severe cases.

Venous Leg Ulcers

Much of the care of venous leg ulcers is carried out in the primary care setting and includes the following.

- *Graduated multilayer compression*: before this treatment is tried, diabetes, neuropathy and peripheral vascular disease should be excluded and any pre-existing swelling controlled by bedrest or elevation. The treatment involves applying bandages to the leg, maximising the pressure at the ankle and reducing the pressure as the bandages go higher up the leg.

Red Flag

At 24–48 hours after the initiation of compression therapy, the patient's skin must be assessed for potential complications (SIGN, 2010).

- *Debridement and cleaning*: adherent slough should be debrided and any trapped pus released.
- *Dressing*: the treatment of choice for most vascular ulcers is a simple non-adherent dressing as there is insufficient evidence for the use of any other dressing (SIGN, 2010).
- *Antibiotics* are only indicated in proven (clinically significant) infection.
- *Pain relief* may be required.

Health Promotion and Discharge

Prior to discharge, healthcare professionals should encourage the patient to discuss any fears and anxieties they may have about coping in the community. Emphasise the importance of taking all medications prescribed and if they experience any unwanted side-effects to see their GP immediately.

- Use compression stockings during waking hours to decrease swelling. The stockings are available on prescription and a new pair will be required every 3–6 months.
- Shower normally and use emollients to moisturise the skin.
- Avoid long periods of sitting or standing. Even moving your legs slightly will help the blood in your veins return to your heart. Preferably begin some form of exercise.
- Elevate the legs when resting to promote venous return.
- Care for wounds if you have any open sores or infections.
- Patients should be made aware of the Lindsay Leg Club Foundation (www.legclub.org) if one is available in their area.
- Stop smoking. Smoking damages the circulation.

Conclusion

This chapter has reviewed the examination of the cardiovascular system and addresses a few of the many conditions that may affect the heart or vascular system.

The cardiovascular system is responsible for the transportation and delivery of oxygen and nutrients to the tissues via the blood and the removal of waste products from the tissues. The system relies on a central pump, the heart, which can be divided into two systems.

- *Right heart pump*, which circulates blood around the pulmonary circulation (the lungs).
- *Left heart pump*, which circulates blood around the systemic circulation (the rest of the body).

A disorder of either of these two pumps may be caused by conditions such as myocardial infarction and lead to the development of oedema in the lungs or the rest of the body.

The blood flow through the body is via tubes called arteries, arterioles, veins and venules.

- Arteries and arterioles channel blood away from the heart to the lungs or the systemic circulation.
- Veins and venules channel blood back to the heart.

Capillaries are the vessels that allow for the passage of oxygen and nutrients into the tissues.

Nursing patients with a cardiovascular disorder requires the healthcare professional to be able to undertake a thorough physical assessment of the patient's circulatory system, to recognise the signs and symptoms of different disorders and to promote health by guided education.

Key Points

- The cardiovascular system is complex and interconnected and particularly disorders of the heart will manifest in signs and symptoms in the circulatory system.
- Examination of the cardiovascular system requires both physical assessment skills and the ability to take a focused history from the patient.
- In myocardial infarction, time is critical but the healthcare professional should remain calm so as not to unduly distress the patient.
- Patients with a disorder of the heart are often anxious and require psychological support and reassurance.
- Health promotion for patients with a cardiovascular disorder is often based on modifiable risk factors, such as diet, exercise and smoking.
- There are many support groups available nationally for patients with a variety of cardiovascular disorders.

References

Ahmad, M., Reading, K. & Gannon, M.X. (2021) Improving abdominal aortic aneurysm (AAA) screening uptake through patient engagement – analysis and outcomes of strategies to improve uptake at a regional program level. *Annals of Vascular Surgery*, 72, 488–497.

Brennan, E.J. (2018) Chronic heart failure nursing: integrated multidisciplinary care. *British Journal of Nursing*, 27(12), 681–688.

Chu, D.K., Kim, L.H., Young, P.J., *et al.* (2018) Mortality and morbidity in acutely ill adults treated with liberal versus conservative oxygen therapy (IOTA): a systematic review and meta-analysis. *Lancet*, 391(10131), 1693–1705.

Crowley, M.J., Zullig, L.L., Shah, B.R., *et al.* (2015) Medication nonadherence after myocardial infarction: an exploration of modifying factors. *Journal of General Internal Medicine*, 30(1), 83–90.

Gaunt, H. (2019) Exercise tolerance testing. *British Journal of Cardiac Nursing*, 14(1), 31–34.

Ibanez, B., James, S., Agewall, S., *et al.* (2018) 2017 ESC Guidelines for the management of acute myocardial infarction in patients presenting with ST-segment elevation: the Task Force for the management of acute myocardial infarction in patients presenting with ST-segment elevation of the European Society of Cardiology (ESC). *European Heart Journal*, 39(2), 119–177.

Ikäheimo, T.M. (2018) Cardiovascular diseases, cold exposure and exercise. *Temperature*, 5(2), 123–146.

Jaarsma, T. (2017) Sexual function of patients with heart failure: facts and numbers. *ESC Heart Failure*, 4, 3–7.

Kent, K.C. (2014) Abdominal aortic aneurysms. *New England Journal of Medicine*, 371(22), 2101–2108.

Kohlman-Trigoboff, D., Rich, K., Foley, A., *et al.* (2020) Society for Vascular Nursing Endovascular Repair of Abdominal Aortic Aneurysm (AAA) Updated Nursing Clinical Practice Guideline. *Journal of Vascular Nursing*, 38(2), 36.

Kitsiou, S., Paré, G. & Jaana, M. (2015) Effects of home telemonitoring interventions on patients with chronic heart failure: an overview of systematic reviews. *Journal of Medical Internet Research*, 17(3), e63.

Kumar, M. & Nayak, P.K. (2017) Psychological sequelae of myocardial infarction. *Biomedicine & Pharmacotherapy*, 95, 487–496.

Lurie, F., Passman, M., Meisner, M., *et al.* (2020) The 2020 update of the CEAP classification system and reporting standards. *Journal of Vascular Surgery: Venous and Lymphatic Disorders*, 8(3), 342–352.

Marciniak, A., Glover, K. & Sharma, R. (2017) Cohort profile: prevalence of valvular heart disease in community patients with suspected heart failure in UK. *BMJ Open*, 7(1), e012240.

McLaughlin, D., Hoy, L. & Glackin, M. (2015) Heart failure nurse specialist crisis interventions and avoided hospital admissions. *British Journal of Cardiac Nursing*, 10(7), 326–333.

National Institute for Health and Care Excellence (2014) *Acute Heart Failure: Diagnosis and Management*. Clinical Guideline No. 187. National Institute for Health and Care Excellence, London.

National Institute for Health and Care Excellence (2018) *Chronic heart failure in adults: diagnosis and management*. NICE Guideline 106. National Institute for Health and Care Excellence, London.

National Institute for Health and Care Excellence (2019a) *Hypertension in adults: diagnosis and management*. NICE Guideline 136. National Institute for Health and Care Excellence, London.

National Institute for Health and Care Excellence (2019b) *Hypertension in pregnancy: diagnosis and management*. NICE Guideline 133. National Institute for Health and Care Excellence, London.

National Institute for Health and Care Excellence (2020) *Acute coronary syndromes*. NICE Guideline 185. National Institute for Health and Care Excellence, London.

Nichols, L. (2017). Pneumonia as a trigger for atrial fibrillation. *Journal of Rural Medicine*, 12(2), 146–148.

Nursing & Midwifery Council (2018) *Standards of proficiency for nursing associates*. NMC, London.

Oeing, C.U., Tschöpe, C. & Pieske, B. (2016) The new ESC Guidelines for acute and chronic heart failure 2016. *Herz*, 41(8), 655–663.

Panaitescu, A.M., Syngelaki, A., Prodan, N., Akolekar, R., & Nicolaides, K.H. (2017) Chronic hypertension and adverse pregnancy outcome: a cohort study. *Ultrasound in Obstetrics & Gynecology*, 50(2), 228–235.

Parker, C.N., Finlayson, K.J., Shuter, P. & Edwards, H.E. (2015) Risk factors for delayed healing in venous leg ulcers: a review of the literature. *International Journal of Clinical Practice*, 69(9), 967–977.

Payne, D. (2019) Leg care: improving assessment and adherence. *Nursing and Residential Care*, 21(7), 370–376.

Peate, I. & Evans, S. (eds) (2020) *Fundamentals of Anatomy and Physiology for Nursing and Healthcare Students*, 3rd edn. Wiley, Oxford.

Piccolo, R., Bonaa, K.H., Efthimiou, O., *et al.* (2019) Drug-eluting or bare-metal stents for percutaneous coronary intervention: a systematic review and individual patient data meta-analysis of randomised clinical trials. *Lancet*, 393(10190), 2503–2510.

Reiner, Ž. (2018) The importance of smoking cessation in patients with coronary heart disease. *International Journal of Cardiology*, 258, 26–27.

SIGN (2010) *Management of Chronic Venous Leg Ulcers*. SIGN Guideline 120. Scottish Intercollegiate Guidelines Network, Edinburgh.

Soar, J., Böttiger, B.W., Carli, P., *et al.* (2021) European Resuscitation Council guidelines 2021: adult advanced life support. *Resuscitation*, 161, 115–151.

Tan, C.S.S. & Lee, S.W.H. (2021) Warfarin and food, herbal or dietary supplement interactions: a systematic review. *British Journal of Clinical Pharmacology*, 87(2), 352–374.

Vasan, R.S., Xanthakis, V., Lyass, A., *et al.* (2018) Epidemiology of left ventricular systolic dysfunction and heart failure in the Framingham study: an echocardiographic study over 3 decades. *JACC: Cardiovascular Imaging*, 11(1), 1–11.

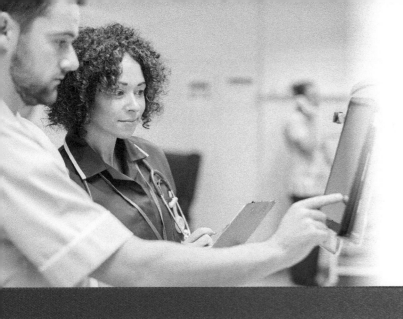

26

The Person with a Haematological Disorder

Marie Jones

Manchester Foundation Trust, UK

Learning Outcomes

On completion of this chapter you will be able to:

- **Describe the function of blood**
- **Explore the pathophysiology of common haematological conditions**
- **Discuss disorders of red and white blood cells, and platelets**
- **Discuss the diagnostic investigations associated with these conditions**
- **Analyse the nursing care associated with haematological conditions**
- **Discuss appropriate treatments**

Proficiencies

NMC Proficiencies and Standards:

- **Assess, monitor, document and deliver care for patients**
- **Using evidence-based practice, identify and prioritise nursing care for patients with haematological disorders**
- **Safely administer treatment prescribed for patients with haematological disorders**
- **Work collaboratively within the multidisciplinary team to provide co-ordinated care**
- **Assess functional health status for patients**
- **Provide health promotion to patients with haematological disorders**

 Visit the companion website at www.wiley.com/go/peate/nursingpractice3e where you can test yourself using flashcards, multiple-choice questions and more.

Nursing Practice: Knowledge and Care, Third Edition. Edited by Ian Peate and Aby Mitchell.
© 2022 John Wiley & Sons Ltd. Published 2022 by John Wiley & Sons Ltd.
Companion website: www.wiley.com/go/peate/nursingpractice3e

Introduction

Blood is a fluid connective tissue and one of the largest organs in the body (Mirza, 2020). Its constant flow provides a transport medium for many essential cells, nutrients, gases, hormones and waste products. Conditions affecting blood can have wide-reaching consequences, and symptoms can range from mild to serious or become life-threatening.

Blood has three main functions.

1. *Protection*: white cells protect the body from invading pathogens; platelets protect the body from bleeding during trauma.
2. *Distribution (transport)*: oxygen, nutrients and hormones are transported in blood. Waste products are transported for disposal.
3. *Regulation*: plasma proteins help to maintain fluid balance. Proteins and solutes dissolved in the blood act as buffers and have a role in maintaining the pH of blood (Peate & Evans, 2020).

Composition of Blood

Blood can be divided into blood plasma and the formed elements.

Plasma contains many dissolved substances, such as gases, hormones, waste products, nutrients, inorganic salts and enzymes. It also contains the plasma proteins that maintain the osmotic pressure of blood. A reduced osmotic pressure will lead to fluid moving out of blood and into tissue, presenting as oedema.

The *formed elements* are red blood cells, white blood cells and platelets. Blood cells originate from haematopoietic stem cells, formed in the bone marrow by a process known as haemopoiesis. Stem cells have the potential to mature into functional blood cells (maturation). The type of cell they become is determined by the body's specific needs at the time and is controlled by hormones and other factors in a supply and demand fashion. Figure 26.1 shows the development of blood cells from stem cell through differentiation into formed elements.

Knowing the normal serum value and the function of each cell types allows health professionals to evaluate conditions that might affect the blood. Table 26.1 provides a summary of this information.

Red Blood Cells

Red blood cells (erythrocytes) contain haemoglobin which is responsible for binding with and transporting respiratory gases. Haemoglobin consists of the protein globin bound to iron-containing haem molecules. The process of producing new red cells is called erythropoiesis and happens continually (Marieb & Hoehn, 2019).

Erythropoiesis requires a supply of iron, vitamin B12, folic acid and the hormone erythropoietin (EPO). Erythropoiesis increases when the body's oxygen demand is not met, for example in tissue hypoxia, when the number of erythrocytes decreases or there is an increased demand for oxygen. During these situations, EPO production is increased by the kidneys, stimulating the erythrocytes to mature more quickly.

During erythropoiesis, the stem cell undergoes several changes. Proerythroblasts become erythroblasts and then reticulocytes. Reticulocytes are full of haemoglobin and within approximately 2 days, will become erythrocytes (Marieb & Hoehn, 2019).

In health, the rate of erythrocyte production remains relatively constant, ensuring cellular oxygenation is maintained. Overproduction of erythrocytes will lead to increased blood viscosity and risk of clot formation.

Destruction of Red Cells

Red blood cells begin to wear out after about 120 days (Tortora & Derrickson, 2020). They are broken down into their constituent parts, some of which are salvaged and reused by the body. Iron is reused in the bone marrow to form new haemoglobin and the remainder is reduced to bilirubin, which becomes a constituent of bile.

Conditions Associated with the Red Cells

Anaemia

The World Health Organization (2021) defines anaemia as: '. . . a condition in which the number of red blood cells or their oxygen carrying capacity is insufficient to meet physiological needs, which may vary by age, sex, altitude, smoking and pregnancy'. It is characterised by abnormally low numbers of circulating red cells or a low haemoglobin level or a combination of both.

Signs and Symptoms

Due to oxygen deficit within the body, patients with anaemia will have associated signs and symptoms.

- Reduced oxygen leading to diminished cell metabolism.
- Peripheral blood vessels constrict to conserve oxygen.
- Lack of oxygen-carrying capacity can cause extreme tiredness and fatigue.
- Increased respiratory rate, tachypnoea, tachycardia or palpitations will occur to compensate for diminished oxygen supply.
- Decreased oxygen delivery to the skin and epithelium can lead to delayed healing and increased risk of ulcer formation.
- Severe acute anaemia can lead to angina, and over a long period of time can lead to congestive cardiac failure.

Anaemia can be due to the following altered pathophysiology.

1. *Nutritional anaemia*: deficiency of nutrients required to produce red blood cells.
2. *Haemolytic anaemia*: excessive destruction or loss of red cells.
3. *Aplastic anaemia*: impaired bone marrow function.

The signs and symptoms of anaemia are the same whatever the pathology.

Investigation and Diagnosis A full blood count (FBC) may be carried out to confirm diagnosis. FBC shows hypochromic microcytic anaemia (there may be a mixed picture with co-existent B12 or folate deficiency).

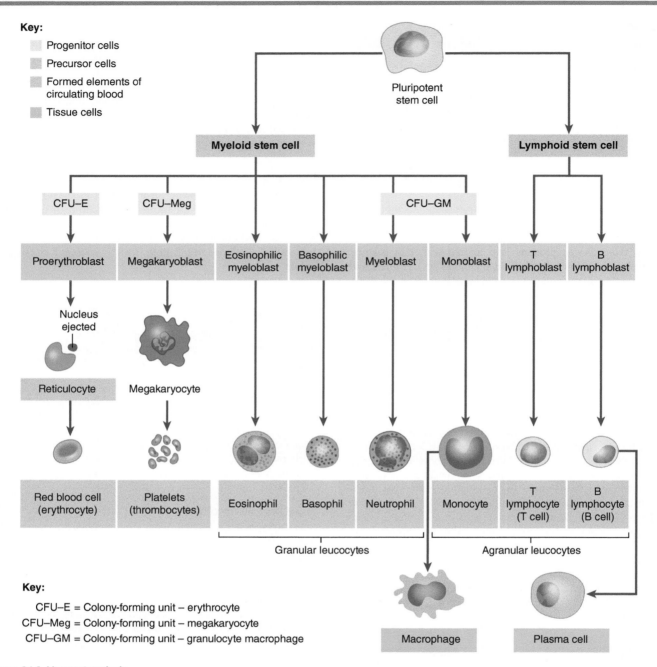

Figure 26.1 **Haematopoiesis.**

- Hypochromia means a low mean corpuscular haemoglobin (MCH).
- Microcytosis means a low mean corpuscular volume (MCV).
- *A haemoglobinopathy will also cause a hypochromic microcytic anaemia.*

Nutritional Anaemia

Iron deficiency anaemia

Iron deficiency anaemia is the most common cause of anaemia diagnosed in primary care (RCN, 2019). Iron is required to produce haemoglobin so if the supply does not match production requirements, then iron deficiency anaemia develops (McCance & Heuther, 2018). This can lead to an insufficient number or malformed cells, i.e. shape, size or colour.

Causes Lack of dietary iron, found in green vegetables, liver, kidney, beef, egg yolks and wholemeal bread. Iron is especially required during pregnancy and in adolescence during growth spurts.

In problems of the digestive tract, iron can be ingested in the correct quantity but malabsorption disorders, such as coeliac disease, prevent it from being absorbed.

Table 26.1 The formed elements of the blood – serum values in health, lifespan and function.

CELL NAME	IDENTIFICATION	NORMAL SERUM VALUE	LENGTH OF TIME TO DEVELOP	NORMAL LIFESPAN	FUNCTION
Erythrocyte (red blood cell, RBC)	Nucleus absent, biconcave disc, pink colour, 7–8 µm in diameter	Man: 4.5–6.5 × 10^{12}/L Woman: 3.8–5 × 10^{12}/L	5–7 days	100–120 days	Transport of respiratory gases
Leucocytes (white blood cells, WBC)	Nucleus present, whole cells	Both: 4–11 × 10^9/L	See type of WBC	See type of WBC	Defence: see type of WBC
Neutrophil	Granulocyte, contains cytoplasmic granules; 10–12 µm in diameter	Both: 2.5–7.5 × 10^9/L	6–9 days	6 hours to a few days	Phagocytose bacteria
Eosinophil	Granulocyte, contains red cytoplasmic granules 10–14 µm in diameter	Both: 0.04–0.44 × 10^9/L	6–9 days	8–12 days	Destroys antigen–antibody complexes; inactivates some of the allergy-associated inflammatory chemicals
Basophil	Granulocyte contains large blue–purple granules, 8–10 µm in diameter	Both: 0–0.1 × 10^9/L	3–7 days	A few hours to a few days	Contains heparin; releases some inflammatory mediators, e.g. histamine
Lymphocytes	Agranulocyte, pale blue cytoplasm, spherical nucleus, 5–17 µm in diameter	Both: 1.3–4 × 10^9/L	Days to weeks	Hours to years	Immune response, can attack cells directly or via antibodies
Monocytes	Agranulocyte, blue–grey cytoplasm, kidney-shaped nucleus, 14–24 µm in diameter	Both: 0.2–0.8 4 × 10^9/L	2–3 days	Months	Phagocytosis; can move into the tissue as a macrophage
Platelets	Cell fragments, deep purple, contain granules, 2–4 µm in diameter	Both: 150–440 × 10^9/L	4–5 days	5–10 days	Required for blood clotting; can seal small tears in blood vessels

455

Iron deficiency anaemia can also be caused by an excessive loss of iron through chronic bleeding. This is commonly seen in women with heavy periods (menorrhagia). It can be caused by cancer or gastrointestinal bleeding from chronic or undiagnosed gastric ulcers. Patients with iron deficiency anaemia often report cravings for unusual substances, known as pica (seen in pregnant women), brittle hair and nails, cracks at the corner of the mouth (angular stomatitis) and a sore tongue.

Patients with iron deficiency anaemia should increase their iron intake in food/diet or by a supplement. Table 26.2 highlights the recommended daily intake. Parenteral iron can be prescribed if the patient cannot tolerate oral iron replacement. Blood transfusion should not be the first line of treatment, unless the anaemia is severe enough to lead to cardiovascular instability (RCN, 2019). If the underlying cause is not obvious, patients should be investigated; the GP may consider gastrointestinal investigations to rule out chronic bleeding or malabsorption disorders.

Signs and Symptoms

Many people with iron deficiency anaemia will only display a few signs or symptoms of the illness. The most common symptoms include:

- Tiredness
- Lethargy
- Shortness of breath.

Vitamin B12 Deficiency Anaemia

Vitamin B12 deficiency anaemia, also known as *pernicious anaemia*, has a slow onset. It is the most common form of megaloblastic anaemia, characterised by very large red blood cells (McCance & Heuther, 2018). It can occur as a result of congenital deficiency of intrinsic factor, gastric mucosa atrophy associated with age or due to gastric surgery, which leads to reduced production of intrinsic factor. Pernicious anaemia can also occur due to lack of vitamin B12 in the diet.

Table 26.2 Foods containing vitamins and minerals associated with anaemia.

VITAMIN/ MINERAL	FOODS	RECOMMENDED DAILY ALLOWANCE (RDA)	TOO MUCH	TOO LITTLE	NOTES
Iron	Liver, meat, nuts, dried fruit, wholegrains, beans, soya flour, fortified breakfast cereals, dark green leafy vegetables	Men: 8.7 mg Women: 14.8 mg	Constipation, nausea and vomiting, stomach pain. Very high doses can be fatal, particularly for children	Anaemia	Tea and coffee reduce iron absorption. Avoid liver in pregnancy; spinach is high in iron but also contains a substance that makes iron absorption harder
Vitamin B$_{12}$	Eggs, cheese, salmon, cod, meat, milk, some fortified breakfast cereals	Adults: 0.0015 mg	Not known	Anaemia, degeneration of nerve fibres of the spinal cord	Vegan diets have low vitamin B$_{12}$
Folic acid	Fortified breakfast cereals, broccoli, Brussels sprouts, spinach, peas, asparagus, chickpeas, liver, brown rice	Adults: 0.2 mg	Can disguise vitamin B$_{12}$ deficiency and this could lead to nervous system damage	Anaemia, increased incidence of spina bifida	Folic acid should be part of the daily diet

Intrinsic factor is essential for absorption of vitamin B12. Ingested vitamin B12 binds with intrinsic factor in the stomach and the resulting complex is absorbed via the ileum and transported to the bone marrow for erythrocyte maturation (Marieb & Hoehn, 2019).

Lack of dietary vitamin B12 occurs in people who have low dietary intake, such as a vegetarian (vegan) diet. Vitamin B12 is found in meat, fish, eggs and dairy produce, although not all vegans will develop evidence of deficiency. Vitamin B12 can be given as a daily supplement. Table 26.2 highlights the recommended daily allowance.

Pernicious anaemia due to lack of intrinsic factor means that a vitamin B12 supplement will not be absorbed by the stomach and have no benefit, so vitamin B12 injections are required every 2–3 months, usually for life.

Folic Acid Deficiency Anaemia

Folic acid (or folate) is essential for erythrocyte maturation and DNA synthesis (Marieb & Hoehn, 2019). Folate is found in dark green vegetables, meat, eggs, fruits and cereals and is metabolised in the liver into folic acid. Alcohol interferes with folate metabolism and folic acid stores become depleted (McCance & Heuther, 2018). Malabsorption disorders and medications can also interfere with the ability to metabolise and store folic acid.

Those with folic acid deficiency anaemia should increase folic acid in their diet or take a supplement. Table 26.2 highlights the recommended daily intake.

Red Flag

Nurses must consider the likely cause of anaemia in elderly patients. Elderly and frail patients may have a poor diet which could be due to social concerns, self-neglect or lack of support in the community. This must be addressed as a package of care may be required before discharge.

Primary Care

Anaemia is a condition usually managed in the community under the care of a GP. People with anaemia should be encouraged to eat a healthy diet rich in vitamins and minerals. Eating smaller amounts more regularly can help.

Admission to hospital may be required if symptoms are severe, poorly managed or exacerbating other medical conditions such as congestive cardiac failure.

Health Promotion and Discharge

People with anaemia can experience tiredness and fatigue; the principles of cancer-related fatigue could be applied, and the following advice given (Fabi *et al.*, 2020).

- Assess your activity; if it is not essential, then do not partake.
- Delegate: let other people help. Be specific, ask them to do the things that you cannot.
- Sleep and rest need to be of good quality. Set a routine, avoid stimulants such as caffeine and television before sleep and rest.
- Manage other symptoms such as pain by taking prescribed pain medication.
- Organise the environment so that items you need are close.
- Tiredness can affect mood, i.e. irritability or depression. Discuss mood changes with your GP.
- Stop activities if there are signs of tachycardia, palpitations, pain or dizziness and get help.

Haemolytic Anaemia

In some instances, anaemia can develop despite normal nutritional intake of vitamins and minerals and the presence of a functioning bone marrow.

Erythrocyte numbers are maintained by a balance between production and destruction. If destruction of erythrocytes occurs before the normal lifespan ends, this is called haemolytic anaemia. This is due to a problem with the erythrocyte (*intrinsic*), such as sickle cell anaemia, or due to disorders not necessarily associated with the erythrocyte (*extrinsic or acquired*) that affects the erythrocyte, such as infection or inflammation.

Intrinsic Haemolytic Anaemia

Sickle cell anaema is a haemaglobinopathy, an inherited condition commonly found in people of African descent but can also be seen in the Caribbean, Mediterranean, India and the Middle East (Bain, 2020). It is a serious, chronic condition, occurring as a result of a mutation on the beta-chain of the haemoglobin molecule. The abnormal form of haemoglobin, HbS, can transport oxygen, but the erythrocyte count and haemaglobin are often low (Bain, 2020).

This small structural change in haemoglobin has a dramatic effect on function. Sickle haemoglobin (HbS) can lead to sickle cell trait or sickle cell disease. In sickle cell trait, 40% of the haemoglobin is HbS; in sickle cell disease, 80–95% of haemoglobin is HbS (Abboud, 2020). A person who inherits the sickle cell gene from both parents (homozygous) will suffer from sickle cell disease. A person who inherits one normal and one sickle cell gene (heterozygous) has sickle cell trait and may remain symptom free.

Those with sickle cell trait are often asymptomatic. During episodes of severe hypoxia, there is a tendency to sickle. When HbS becomes deoxygenated, the erythrocyte is distorted into a characteristic crescent or sickle shape (Figure 26.2). The erythrocyte can return to its normal shape when fully oxygenated again but permanent damage can develop over time (Bain, 2020). The lifespan of the erythrocyte is reduced. The breakdown of haemoglobin leads to hyperbilirubinaemia, presenting as jaundice which can lead to gallstones. The bone marrow struggles to maintain the demand for erythrocytes and aplastic anaemia can develop.

Several conditions can precipitate sickling, including:

- Dehydration
- Infection
- Acidosis
- Hypoxia
- Low body temperature
- Changes in environmental temperature
- Excessive exercise
- Anaesthesia
- Stress: physical and emotional.

Symptoms The symptoms of severe anaemia are often seen, such as pallor, fatigue, weakness, irritability, tachycardia and dyspnoea. In Black, Asian and minority ethnic groups (BAME), pallor can be identified by pale palms, oral mucosa or conjunctivae.

In severe sickling, blood viscosity increases, blood flow is reduced and blood vessels can become occluded. This is called sickle cell crisis. Sickle cell crisis typically lasts 4–6 days. Vessel occlusion means that the tissue supplied by these vessels does not receive oxygen and ischaemia, infarction and potentially necrosis can occur.

Because the sickled cells stick to the blood vessel endothelium, activator substances are released that lead to hypercoagulation, platelet and thrombin activation and the formation of clot, and vasoconstriction also occurs – all of which further occlude the vessel. Vessel occlusion may occur anywhere in the body and is accompanied by very severe pain (Abboud, 2020). The most common sites are joints, bones, chest and abdomen. Repeated vessel occlusions (infarcts) can lead to damage of major organs, including the heart, kidneys, liver and spleen. Cerebral vessel occlusion can lead to stroke and transient ischaemic attack (TIA).

Sickle cell disease is incurable but supportive treatment has improved the life expectancy of those who have it. This includes oxygen therapy, analgesia, bedrest, hydration, warmth, good diet rich in iron and supplements that promote erythrocyte production.

Patients with sickle cell disease experience pain, which can be chronic or acute. Hospital admission could be required during crisis episodes due to hypoxia or severe pain (Abboud, 2020).

Investigation and Diagnosis The following tests diagnose sickle cell anaemia.

- Haemoglobin electrophoresis.
- FBC to determine haemoglobin and serum iron levels.

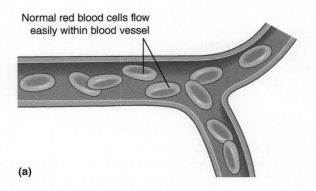

Normal red blood cells flow easily within blood vessel

(a)

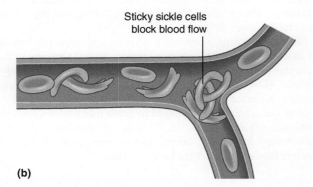

Sticky sickle cells block blood flow

(b)

Figure 26.2 **The differences between normal red blood cells and sickled red blood cells, and the effects at the smaller blood vessels.**

Jot This Down

Haemoglobinopathy is the generic term used to describe genetic faults of haemoglobin. Sickle cell disease and thalassaemia are recessively inherited genetic conditions which affect the haemoglobin molecule.

457

What the Experts Say

Patients with haemaglobinopathies should be managed in a specialist centre. NHS England has commissioned specific centres in the UK to provide specialist care to patients and expert advice to other healthcare providers (NHS England, 2021).

The Nursing Associate Standards 1.11, 2.4, 3.5, 4.1, 6.1, 6.2, 6.5

Shiraz is 19 years old and recently moved to the UK for university; he lives in student accommodation. He is admitted with a sickle cell crisis, severe pain and dehydration. He has no family in the UK and has had anxiety due to exams. He has not been hospitalised in the UK before and is frightened. He is not known to the haemaglobinopathy team and has little support here. You recognise that he has a chronic health condition and may be unfamiliar with the services available. You refer him to the haemaglobinopathy specialist nurse and haematology social worker; they undertake an assessment of his physical and psychological care needs and put a care plan in place. This could prevent future sickle cell crisis and hospital admission.

What role does the nursing associate play in ensuring that Shiraz has safe and patient-centred care?

Thalassaemia is an inherited disorder affecting haemoglobin synthesis; the alpha (α) or beta (β) chains of adult haemoglobin can be affected, leading to anaemia.

The α-thalassaemias are caused by the deletion of a gene leading to production of defective α-chain synthesis. The severity of this condition and the intervention required are dependent on the number of defective genes.

The β-thalassaemias occur due to a mutation in the β-globin gene, which leads to a defect in β-chain synthesis. β-thalassaemia is sometimes called 'Mediterranean' or 'Cooley's anaemia'. It is prevalent in the Mediterranean regions of southern Italy and Greece. The α- and β-thalassaemias are common in the African and African-American community (Bain, 2020). The severity of this condition is dependent on the number of defective genes. Thalassaemia minor can be asymptomatic while those with thalassaemia major can have severe anaemia. It is evident from a young age (6–9 months old) and the patient becomes dependent on blood transfusions.

Mild thalassaemia can lead to the following symptoms

- Mild/moderate anaemia.
- Bone marrow hyperplasia.
- Mild splenomegaly.

Major thalassaemia is more serious and can lead to the following symptoms.

- Severe anaemia, requiring repeated blood transfusions.
- Liver and spleen enlargement due to increased red cell destruction.
- Long bone fractures associated with bone marrow thinning.
- Repeated blood transfusions can lead to an accumulation of iron (iron overload) in the heart, liver and pancreas leading to organ failure.

Acquired Haemolytic Anaemia

Factors extrinsic to red blood cell production can also lead to haemolysis. Autoimmune disorders, infection (e.g. malaria), blood transfusion reactions and some drugs are examples of acquired haemolytic anaemia. Mechanical destruction of red cells can occur secondary to trauma, prosthetic heart valves, vasculitis, chemotherapy/radiation, haemodialysis or severe burns. Haemolytic anaemia can be associated with severe blood loss due to trauma; the bleeding must be stopped and lost blood replaced with transfusion.

Practice Assessment Document

Monitor and manage blood component transfusions For some it may be challenging to achieve this competency as a student nurse. The registered nurse is responsible for safe administration of blood products, which includes following policy and procedures for checking and administering blood products. Appropriate training and competency assessments are necessary to ensure patient safety.

With your supervisor, you could discuss the following points.

- Why administer blood products. *What are the alternatives?*
- Checking patients' details correctly. *What are the consequences of administering the wrong blood product?*
- Monitoring observations before, during and after transfusion. *What abnormalities might be detected? What observations should be monitored?*
- Monitoring for transfusion reactions? *What symptoms might the patient experience?*
- Actions taken if a transfusion reaction occurs. *Why must the transfusion be stopped immediately?*
- What would your next steps be? *Who needs to be informed?*

You could review the transfusion policy and write a reflective account of your learning or write a case study for a patient you have cared for.

Aplastic Anaemia: Impaired Bone Marrow Function

Impaired bone marrow function leads to aplastic anaemia, which is a rare condition. Bone marrow failure can lead to reduced production of all blood cells. Full blood count demonstrates pancytopenia – reduced red blood cells, white blood cells and platelets. Normal bone marrow is replaced by fat. The condition may be permanent but is often temporary, depending on the cause (Furlong & Carter, 2020).

Idiopathic aplastic anaemia accounts for approximately half of the cases where the cause is not known. Aplastic anaemia can occur due to viral illnesses such as hepatitis A, B and C, cytomegalovirus (CMV) and mononucleosis (Epstein–Barr virus) (Furlong & Carter, 2020).

Stem cells can also be damaged by some medications, such as antibiotics (chloramphenicol), NSAIDs or chemotherapy and radiotherapy for cancer. Some autoimmune diseases, such as systemic lupus, can affect the bone marrow.

Signs and Symptoms The signs and symptoms of aplastic anaemia are the same as for other anaemias. If white blood cells are also low, infection can occur and reduced platelets can lead to bleeding. Treatment involves immunosuppression or allogeneic stem cell or bone marrow transplant. This will depend on the severity of the condition, age of the patient and availability of a suitable donor (Carreras *et al.*, 2019).

Investigation and Diagnosis of Anaemia

The diagnosis of anaemia is often made following a FBC taken by the GP. Table 26.3 highlights the normal values for red blood cells obtained from an FBC. Further tests, including a blood film, can identify abnormal or immature red blood cells. Irregularities may include variable sizes of red blood cells (anisocytosis) – small cells are referred to as microcytosis and large cells macrocytosis.

The shape of the red blood cell is also important and if cells are of different shapes, this is called poikilocytosis; sickle cells can also be identified in this way.

If iron deficiency anaemia is suspected, the following investigations should be undertaken.

- Serum iron: normal values, 60–170 µg/dL
- Total iron-binding capacity (TIBC): normal values, 240–450 µg/dL
- Ferritin: normal value, 20–50%

Table 26.3 Normal red blood cell values in full blood count.

TEST	NORMAL RANGE[a]	WHAT IS MEASURED
Red cell count (RCC)	Men: 4.5–6.5 × 10^{12}/L Women: 3.8–5 × 10^{12}/L	Number of red cells per microlitre of blood
Reticulocytes	25–100 × 10^9/L	Number of reticulocytes per microlitre of blood
Haemoglobin (Hb)	Men: 130–180 g/L Women: 110.5–160.5 g/L	Haemoglobin per 100 mL of blood
Haematocrit (Hct)	Men: 40.7–50.3% Women: 36.1–44.3%	Percentage of the volume of blood that is red cells
Mean cell volume (MCV)	76–96 femtolitres	Average volume of the individual red blood cell
Mean cell haemoglobin (MCH)	27–32 picograms	Average weight of haemoglobin per red cell
Mean cell haemoglobin concentration (MCHC)	30–36 picograms	Average concentration of haemoglobin per red cell

[a] Normal range may vary between laboratories.

A low serum iron level and a raised TIBC can be indicative of iron deficiency anaemia.

Ferritin is an iron storage protein produced by the liver and its role is to mobilise iron stores when the body's demand for iron is not being met by dietary intake. When the iron reserves are depleted, the ferritin level will be low.

Vitamin B12 deficiency anaemia can be caused by a poor dietary intake of vitamin B12 or lack of intrinsic factor. The Schilling test is used to identify which type of vitamin B12 deficiency is present.

The sickle cell test examines the haemoglobin in erythrocytes to identify HbS present in sickle cell trait or sickle cell disease. Haemoglobin electrophoresis will differentiate sickle cell trait and sickle cell disease. It is also used to identify other haemoglobin abnormalities such as thalassaemia or haemolytic anaemia.

A bone marrow biopsy can also be examined to identify abnormalities within the bone marrow.

Treatment of Anaemia

Vitamin and mineral deficiency anaemias are resolved by increasing the intake of these by either diet or supplements. Pernicious anaemia does not respond to oral supplements of vitamin B12 as the lack of intrinsic factor will prevent the oral vitamin from being absorbed; monthly injections of vitamin B12 are usually required for life.

> **Medicines Management**
>
>
> Iron tablets can be better tolerated if taken with food. Reducing side-effects may prevent the patient from discontinuing treatment and improve concordance with treatment prescribed.
>
> Advise people (especially mothers of young children) about the safe storage of iron supplements, as they have potentially toxic effects and are a common cause of accidental overdose in children.

Nursing Care and Management of Anaemia

The nursing care of the patient with anaemia will depend on the severity of symptoms. Many patients with anaemia are managed at home under the care of the GP and community nurses. Nursing assessment should consider the patient's ability to manage at home and be alert for more serious symptoms. Table 26.4 summarises the nursing interventions and goals required for managing anaemia.

Although the type of anaemia can vary, similar symptoms are experienced by most patients. The most serious of these is an inability to provide oxygenated blood to the tissues. Mild anaemia can lead to fatigue and shortness of breath on exertion as the body tries to increase the oxygen intake. In its most severe form, where blood loss occurs, this can lead to circulatory collapse.

Fatigue is also experienced, and patients often feel too tired or weak to undertake activities of living. Support might be necessary until the anaemia has responded to treatment.

Polycythaemia

An increase in red cell concentration in blood is known as polycythaemia or *erythrocytosis*. There are different mechanisms for

Table 26.4 **Nursing care: Anaemia.**

ASSESSMENT	RATIONALE	INTERVENTION/HEALTH PROMOTION	EVALUATION
Respiratory system	Dyspnoea (shortness of breath) due to reduction in the oxygen-carrying capacity of red cells	Severe dyspnoea: hospital admission may be required for oxygen therapy. Oxygen will help symptoms but not stop the underlying cause. A blood transfusion may be considered until the anaemia improves with diet or supplements	Oxygen therapy is no longer required
Nutritional intake	Ensure diet contains B12, folate and iron	Health promotion: educate patients on appropriate dietary intake. Monitor for concordance with oral supplements	Normal haemaglobin level in full blood count
Activity tolerance	Inadequate tissue oxygenation precipitates fatigue	Advise on fatigue management: · Reduce activity and rest frequently · Increase activity as symptoms improve · Assistance with activities of living may be required	Usual level of activity is achieved
Skin	Inactivity and reduced oxygen supply to the tissues can lead to increased risk of skin breakdown	Activity as tolerated. If bed bound, use pressure-relieving mattress and reposition regularly. Promote good skin hygiene practices	Absence of pressure sores
Oral care	Oral mucosa: tongue and lips become dry and cracked	Oral assessment, hygiene and care	Intact oral mucosa

developing polycythaemia. An increase in red cells with a normal plasma volume is called 'absolute' polycythaemia. If plasma volume is reduced with a normal number of red cells, this is 'relative' polycythaemia, often due to dehydration or secondary to fluid loss.

Absolute polycythaemia can be divided into two categories:

- Primary polycythaemia (polycythaemia vera)
- Secondary polycythaemia.

Primary Polycythaemia (Polycythaemia Vera)

There is an increase in the production of red cells; white blood cells and platelets are also increased but to a lesser extent. This is usually caused by a mutation of a protein called JAK2. This signalling protein increases the production of red cells and has been found in 95% of patients with this type of polycythaemia (Randolph, 2020). Polycythaemia vera (PV) affects more men than woman and progresses over 10–20 years; it can develop into leukaemia or myelofibrosis. The increased red cells increase blood volume and viscosity, leading to sluggish blood flow and congestion. Sluggish blood flow leads to clot formation within the blood vessels and the deprivation of nutrients and oxygen to the underlying tissue can cause necrosis. Increased viscosity can cause hypertension (Moench, 2020). This condition is often diagnosed following routine blood tests.

Signs and Symptoms Signs and symptoms include hypertension, full and bounding pulse, dyspnoea, headaches and fatigue. Vision and hearing disturbances can also occur. Sluggish blood flow can lead to cyanosis but reddening of hands and face can develop (plethoric). Pruritus is common and accompanied by painful joints in the fingers and toes. Weight loss and drowsiness occur, and delirium can develop.

Sluggish blood flow causes congestion in the spleen and liver, leading to hepatomegaly and splenomegaly; congestive heart failure can also develop.

Thrombosis associated with PV can affect the extremities as well as organs, such as the brain, heart and liver; venous thromboembolism (VTE), TIAs, angina and portal hypertension can also develop (Hubert & VanMeter, 2018).

Diagnosis Serum EPO levels are measured and are usually low, while the red cell count is high. Bone marrow aspiration shows an increase in proliferation of all the blood cells. Haematocrit is raised.

Nursing and Management Polycythaemia is incurable and therefore treatment is aimed at symptom control, minimising clot and bleeding risks and reducing plasma volume (Moench, 2020). Treatment will depend on risk stratification, but could include:

- Venesection to remove 250–500 mL of blood, lowering the haematocrit
- Cytoreductive therapies such as hydroxycarbamide to slow production of blood cells and lower blood counts
- Aspirin, prescribed to reduce the risk of thrombosis, unless anticoagulation is already prescribed.

The nursing care is aimed at prevention, recognition, early intervention and management of symptoms. Baseline observations of blood pressure, pulse, respiratory rate and oxygen saturation should be taken and monitored regularly. Dyspnoea should be managed by encouraging sitting up, physiotherapy and oxygen therapy if required. Cardiovascular assessment should include prevention of VTE such as physiotherapy, leg elevation and antithrombosis stockings (if prescribed); smoking cessation and weight loss are also important to reduce the risk of thrombosis. Pain should be assessed, and regular analgesia prescribed if necessary. Hepatomegaly and splenomegaly can lead to the patient feeling full with reduced appetite, so small frequent meals may be preferable (Randolph, 2020).

What the Experts Say

'Encourage the patient undergoing venesection to increase their fluid intake before and after. Patients should be advised to rise slowly from a sitting position to avoid fainting from orthostatic hypotension.'
Dr Rachel Brown, haematology consultant

Secondary Polycythaemia

Secondary polycythaemia is the most common form and occurs when red cell production is increased in response to increased EPO production by the kidneys. This occurs during hypoxia, due to renal tumours or renal disease, due to smoking, in chronic lung conditions such as chronic obstructive pulmonary disease (COPD) or in heart disease.

Treatment will depend on the cause; therefore, treatment of renal and cardiac diseases should alleviate the symptoms. Venesection can improve secondary polycythaemia, and patients should be advised to stop smoking.

Red Flag COVID-19 and Blood

People with COVID-19 have a higher risk of developing VTE and pulmonary embolism.
People who have had or are having treatment for blood cancer:
- have a higher risk of hospitalisation and mortality if they contract COVID-19
- are less likely to develop appropriate antibodies/immune response to the COVID-19 vaccine
- will probably have cancer treatment postponed if they become COVID-19 positive. This can increase the risk of disease progression or relapse.

White Blood Cells and Lymphoid Tissue Disorders

White blood cells are also called *leucocytes* and account for less than 1% of whole blood. The function of leucocytes is to defend the body from invading pathogens, toxins and tumour cells (Marieb & Hoehn, 2019).

White blood cells develop from haematopoietic stem cells in the bone marrow; their production is controlled by hormones. White blood cells can migrate from the blood into tissue, where they contribute to the immune or inflammatory response

(Marieb & Hoehn, 2019). When white blood cells react to an attack or tissue damage, the body responds by increasing their production. Within hours, the number of white blood cells in the blood will increase. White blood cells can be divided into two types: *granulocytes* and *agranulocytes*.

The granulocytes include neutrophils, basophils and eosinophils, while agranulocytes include lymphocytes and monocytes. Granulocytes mature fully in the bone marrow. Agranulocytes leave the bone marrow not fully mature and enter the bloodstream.

Neutrophils account for 50–70% of the total number of white blood cells. They are mobile, attracted to sites of inflammation and particularly effective against bacteria and some fungi. Neutrophil granules contain hydrolytic enzymes, and some contain antibiotic-like proteins (defensins) (Marieb & Hoehn, 2019). Neutrophils are efficient phagocytes. During bacterial infections, the number of neutrophils in the blood will increase.

Eosinophils can attack pathogens that are too large to be phagocytosed, such as parasites. Eosinophils phagocytose antigen–antibody complexes involved in allergy responses, reducing the severity of reactions often seen in asthma and allergy. They neutralise histamine production and have a significant role in the control of inflammatory responses.

Basophils contain histamine, heparin and platelet activating factor. During inflammatory responses, and in the presence of an allergen, basophils release the contents of their granules. Basophils are involved in anaphylaxis and hypersensitivity reactions. Mast cells are similar to basophils and located in the tissues. Histamine is a vasodilator and its release produces a drop in blood pressure and heart rate.

Monocytes leave the bloodstream and enter the tissues where they mature into *macrophages*. They form part of the reticuloendothelial system (RES) in the spleen, liver, lymph nodes and bone marrow (Mirza, 2020). Macrophages destroy bacteria, foreign material, dead cells and protozoa. They also participate in the immune response.

Lymphocytes are found in lymphoid tissue with only a small proportion found in the bloodstream (Figure 26.3). Lymphocytes mature in the lymph tissue and become one of two specialist cells:

- *T lymphocytes (T cells)*: defend the body against cells infected by viruses or tumour cells
- *B lymphocytes (B cells)*: are involved in the immune response and the production of antibodies.

The Lymphatic System

The lymphatic system consists of lymphatic vessels, tissue and organs, located throughout the body (see Figure 26.3). The *lymphatic vessels* return fluid that has escaped from the vascular system back to the blood. When this fluid is located inside the lymphatic vessels, it is known as lymph (lymphatic) fluid. Lymphatic capillaries can allow pathogens, cancer cells and cell debris into the lymphatic system where they can travel throughout the body, threatening unaffected areas. The lymphatic fluid is filtered through the lymph nodes, where the immune system can take action and some of the pathogens can be acted upon (Waugh & Grant, 2018).

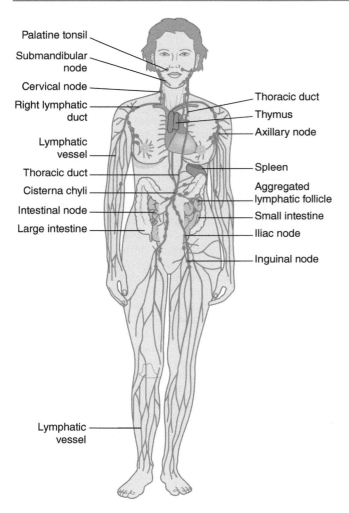

Palatine tonsil

Submandibular node

Cervical node

Right lymphatic duct

Lymphatic vessel

Thoracic duct

Cisterna chyli

Intestinal node

Large intestine

Thoracic duct

Thymus

Axillary node

Spleen

Aggregated lymphatic follicle

Small intestine

Iliac node

Inguinal node

Lymphatic vessel

Figure 26.3 The location of lymphoid tissue.

Lymphoid tissue is usually loose connective tissue, except for the thymus. Lymphoid tissue is the site for proliferation of lymphocytes and is found in many organ systems throughout the body.

Lymphoid organs include the spleen, thymus and tonsils. The spleen is a site for lymphocyte proliferation; the macrophages located here remove pathogens, foreign matter and debris from the blood passing through the spleen. It also has a role in the breakdown of red cells. The thymus is most active in early life. It secretes hormones responsible for ensuring that T lymphocytes become immunocompetent. The tonsils deal with pathogens that are trapped there.

Conditions Associated with the White Blood Cells

Leucopenia and Neutropenia

In *leukopenia*, the total number of white blood cells is less than 4×10^9/L. As neutrophils make up the largest group of white blood cells, reduced neutrophils are often seen when the count is low.

Neutropenia is a decrease in the number of neutrophils to less than 2×10^9/L. Neutropenia can be moderate ($<1 \times 10^9$/L) or severe (0.5×10^9/L).

Neutropenia can be caused by some medications or haematological conditions such as aplastic anaemia or leukaemia. Autoimmune disorders such as systemic lupus or rheumatoid arthritis can result in low neutrophils (Table 26.1 highlights cells' normal life expectancy). Anorexia nervosa and starvation can lead to a pseudo-neutropenia where the neutrophils are not adequately distributed. In conditions such as severe sepsis, the production of new neutrophils does not meet the body's demand for neutrophils, so they are consumed more quickly.

A drastic reduction in the neutrophil count can be caused by chemotherapy, which interferes with haematopoiesis in the bone marrow, or drugs that suppress the bone marrow. Neutropenia is also associated with haemodialysis, an immune response or infection (McCance & Heuther, 2018).

Neutropenia increases the risk of infections, often in the respiratory, digestive or urinary tract, as the body's defence is reduced. Severe neutropenia can lead to life-threatening infections that require hospital admission.

Nurses should be vigilant for signs and symptoms of infection such as pyrexia, tachycardia, malaise and sepsis.

Morbidity and mortality are increased by neutropenia-related infections particularly if the neutropenia is secondary to cancer therapy (NICE, 2016).

> **The Nursing Associate** Standards 1.13, 2.9, 3.7, 3.11, 5.3, 6.2
>
> Patients with neutropenia are at increased risk of developing neutropenic sepsis. If not treated quickly, this can become life-threatening and lead to multiorgan failure or death. Patients with neutropenia may not develop a temperature, so it is important to recognise other signs that indicate sepsis, including hypotension, tachycardia or increased respiration rate. Concerns must be highlighted to a senior colleague or doctor immediately so treatment can be commenced.
>
> What is the role of the nursing associate in the detection of sepsis in the neutropenic patient?

Investigation and Diagnosis

Diagnosis will be based on the result of the white cell count. Suspected sources of infection should be investigated through microbial analysis, for example blood culture, sputum, swabs and urine or faeces specimens.

The National Institute for Health and Care Excellence (NICE, 2016) recommends educating patients and their relatives on signs and symptoms of sepsis so help can be sought urgently. NICE also recommends that secondary and tertiary care have appropriate pathways in place to assess high-risk patients promptly and manage suspected and confirmed sepsis. Educating staff and the use of an appropriate scoring system are advocated to improve recognition and management of patients with sepsis (NICE, 2016). Patients presenting with a pyrexia of 38 °C or above and/or clinical signs should have antibiotic therapy commenced within 1 hour. Prompt initiation of treatment can prevent severe sepsis and death (Hird, 2020).

If patients are neutropenic, chemotherapy treatment might be postponed or treatment dose reduced until counts improve; this can lead to psychological concerns for cancer patients and their families.

Nursing Care and Management

Nursing care of neutropenic patients has three main goals.

1. Protect the patient from potential infections.
2. Observe for any signs of infection.
3. Treat infection promptly.

Primary Care

Neutropenic patients in the community should be educated on the importance of reducing the risk of infection and recognising signs and symptoms. Patients and their families should know when and where to get help.

Advice should include the following.

- The importance of hand washing
- Ensure eggs and meats are well cooked
- Wash fruit and vegetables before eating (peel if possible)
- Avoid unpasteurised products
- Avoid crowded places, i.e. cinema or supermarket
- Limit visitors, particularly children
- Pay attention to personal and oral hygiene
- Be careful with pets and avoid cleaning up after them
- Use gloves when cleaning or gardening
- Monitor for signs of infection and check body temperature daily
- Contact the hospital, specialist nurse or GP immediately if there are concerns about infection

The nurse caring for a neutropenic patient in any healthcare setting should take the following into consideration.

- Educate patients, visitors and staff on the importance of good hand hygiene to avoid cross-infection.
- Friends or family should be asked not to visit if they know or suspect that they have an infection, including cough, runny nose or diarrhoea.
- Monitor pressure areas to reduce the risk of infection through pressure ulcers.
- Appropriate precautions should be used when undertaking invasive procedures, i.e. aseptic non-touch technique (ANTT).
- Oral hygiene should be carried out regularly using a soft tufted toothbrush and a saline rinse/mouthwash.
- Avoid unpasteurised foods (low-immunity diet may be suggested; consider referral to a dietitian).
- Avoid damage to the rectal mucosa by preventing constipation. Offer stool softeners and aperients. Rectal digital examinations should not be performed.
- Avoid using urinary catheters to reduce the risk of urinary tract infection.
- Neutropenic patients should be nursed in protective isolation (side room) to reduce the risk of cross-infection.
- Observations including temperature, heart rate, blood pressure, respiration rate and oxygen saturations should be checked; if abnormal, antibiotic therapy should be prescribed and commenced within 1 hour.

Leukaemia

Leukaemia is a malignant disorder or cancer of white blood cells (Waugh & Grant, 2018). The stem cells are reduced and fail to mature, and the bone marrow is replaced with proliferating immature cells. This reduces opportunity or space for normal blood cells such as red cells and platelets to grow (McCance & Heuther, 2018). Immature malignant white cells do not function normally and can infiltrate other organs such as the spleen, liver and lymph nodes. They cannot protect the body from infections, which can lead to sepsis that can be fatal. There are several types of leukaemia but many of the signs, symptoms, treatments and nursing care are similar.

Signs and Symptoms

These are common for all types of leukaemia.

- *Infections*: can be prolonged and difficult to treat. Infection can present in the oral mucosa, gastrointestinal tract, upper respiratory tract or urinary tract. Pyrexia and night sweats can also be present.
- *Anaemia*: due to the inability to produce enough red blood cells.
- *Thrombocytopenia*: a reduced number of platelets leads to increased bruising and bleeding. Bleeding gums and petechial rash may develop.
- *Infiltration of the liver, spleen and lymph nodes*: causes pain, swelling and organomegaly that can be palpable on physical examination.
- *Infiltration of the meninges of the brain*: leads to headache, raised intracranial pressure, altered levels of consciousness and nausea.
- *Increased metabolism and weight loss.*
- *Fatigue.*

In the UK around 10 000 new cases of leukaemia are reported each year (Cancer Research UK, 2021a).

The four main types of leukaemia are:

- Acute myeloid leukaemia
- Acute lymphoblastic leukaemia
- Chronic myeloid leukaemia
- Chronic lymphocytic leukaemia.

Acute Myeloid Leukaemia

Acute myeloid leukaemia (AML) is the most common type of leukaemia in adults, particularly those over 65 years old. It develops quickly over days and weeks as there is an increased production of cancer cells called myeloblasts. The 5-year survival varies from 40% to 60% in the under 50s and as low as 5% in those over 65 where outcome is poorer (Cancer Research UK, 2021b). Many patients with AML will achieve remission with chemotherapy alone but there is a high risk of disease relapse. Treatment such as stem cell transplant is used with curative intent and can significantly improve overall outcome (Heuser *et al.*, 2020).

Acute myeloid leukaemia is classified into various subtypes based on cytogenetic and molecular analysis, and this can help determine prognosis and treatment strategy. Acute promyelocytic leukaemia (APML) is a rare subtype of AML that requires a different treatment approach. Patients with APML are initially at increased risk of disseminated intravascular coagulation (DIC) which can be life-threatening. Patients with APML who respond to treatment have a high chance of being cured.

The cause of AML is largely unknown but there is an association with exposure to high levels of radiation, benzene and smoking. Undergoing chemotherapy or radiotherapy treatment for other cancers has been seen to increase the risk of developing AML, although this risk is small. Myelodysplasia or other haematalogical disorders can transform into AML. There is also a genetic link, as children with Down syndrome are more likely to develop AML.

Acute Lymphoblastic Leukaemia

Acute lymphoblastic leukaemia (ALL) is the most common type of acute leukaemia in children and young adults although some adults will also develop ALL. The risk factors are similar to those for AML but it is thought passive smoking and some viruses can also increase the risk of developing ALL (Cancer Research UK, 2019a). It occurs due to a proliferation of lymphoblasts in the bone marrow that inhibit the growth of normal cells, leading to side-effects seen in AML.

Complete remission is possible following combination chemotherapy treatment, although some cases have a poorer prognosis, such as Philadelphia chromosome-positive (Ph-positive) ALL where more intensive treatment and stem cell transplant would be necessary.

Nursing Fields Children

When caring for a child with leukaemia, the whole family must be considered. Implications of diagnosis and treatment are extensive and include growth, nutrition, isolation, fear and pain, psychological/psychosocial, educational, sexuality, hospitalisation and procedures.

Case Study

Four-year-old James is taken to the emergency department by his mother. He has a 1-week history of fever, fatigue, bone pain and poor appetite. He was seen in primary care and his mother was told that he probably had a viral infection. Worsening symptoms for 2 days with bruising and nosebleed.

Past medical history
Normally fit, well and active. Chicken pox age 2 years, no other previous medical history. Not on regular medications.

On examination
Pallor, purpura rash on body and limbs, fatigued, short of breath. Abdominal tenderness and palpable spleen.

Investigations
Full blood count: WBC >100 × 10^9/L, haemoglobin 80 g/L, platelets 13 × 10^9/L

Bone marrow biopsy: confirms diagnosis of acute lymphoblastic leukaemia with excessive immature lymphoblasts. Additional tests on the bone marrow including immunophenotyping, cytogenetic and molecular analysis help to classify the ALL and stratify treatment.

Treatment
Combination chemotherapy treatment is commenced urgently. This is divided into five phases, some of which will be inpatient and some outpatient and will usually take 2–3 years to complete. High-risk ALL might require treatment with a stem cell transplant (Blood Cancer UK, 2021).

- What are the implications for James and his family?
- What support might be required throughout his diagnosis and treatment?

Chronic Myeloid Leukaemia

Chronic myeloid leukaemia (CML) is a rare condition. In the UK, approximately 800 people are diagnosed with CML annually, and the risk increases with age (Cancer Research UK, 2019b). CML is associated with the Philadelphia chromosome, an abnormality involving a translocation of chromosomes 22 and 9. The onset of CML is slower and more insidious. Some signs and symptoms can be present but often the disease is detected during routine screening.

The disease staging is described in three phases.

- *Chronic phase*: mild symptoms, such as tiredness and weight loss. FBC usually shows raised white cell and platelet counts.
- *Accelerated phase*: fatigue, abdominal distension with enlarged spleen leads to heavy uncomfortable abdomen. An increasing number of blood cells in the bone marrow are immature.
- *Blast phase* (*blast crisis*): presents like acute leukaemia, with large numbers of immature white cells. Leukaemia cells spread and affect other organs. Deterioration in condition occurs rapidly and even with treatment the prognosis is poor in this stage.

Treatment of CML with medicines called tyrosine kinase inhibitors (TKI) such as imatinib or nilotinib can lead to remission. Stem cell transplant is also an option for those who do not respond to TKIs (BSH, 2020).

Chronic Lymphocytic Leukaemia

Chronic lymphocytic leukaemia (CLL) is the most common leukaemia and involves mature B lymphocytes. Over 3000 people in the UK are diagnosed annually with CLL. Large numbers of B lymphocytes are seen but do not function effectively, leaving patients prone to recurrent infections (Cancer Research UK, 2020a).

Chronic lymphocytic leukaemia is staged using the Binet system. Patients can be asymptomatic in 70–80% of cases, although those presenting with stage C disease can have nosebleeds and bruising due to a low platelet count. Symptoms such as tiredness and fatigue are associated with anaemia, while weight loss and night sweats are commonly associated with enlarged lymph nodes and splenomegaly. Infection is common.

Investigations and Diagnosis of Leukaemia

A thorough assessment of the patient's history, medications, presenting symptoms, clinical examination, blood tests and bone marrow biopsy is required.

An FBC looks at the number, size and shape of cells in the peripheral blood and the maturity of white blood cells. Leukaemia is confirmed following a bone marrow biopsy (BMB). The BMB demonstrates abnormalities in the numbers and development of red and white blood cells and platelets. In all leukaemias, the haemoglobin and platelet count are usually low, while the white blood cell count can be very high or very low.

Primary Care

People with blood cancer should have a thermometer at home so temperatures can be monitored. An 'alert card' should be carried to highlight the increased risk of infection and sepsis to other healthcare professionals.

Nursing Care and Management of Leukaemia

Leukaemia is a life-threatening condition. Nurses must be skilled in managing the complications and side-effects of treatment required for leukaemia.

Most leukaemias are treated using chemotherapy, which usually involves an intensive regimen. The aim of chemotherapy is to kill the leukaemia cells in the bone marrow. Radiotherapy is used in some cases: it damages the cells' DNA and stops cell division and multiplication, but the cells can still function. Normal cells can also be damaged by chemotherapy and radiation treatment but, unlike the cancer cells, they can recover.

Key areas of nursing include managing the risk of infection, haemorrhage, side-effects of chemotherapy and radiotherapy treatments and psychological support.

- Patients should be nursed in a side room. Hospital infection prevention and control policies and guidelines must be followed.
- Checking observations is critical for detecting early signs of infection. A low white cell count increases the risk of infection. Complaints of chills, fever or coughs should be reported promptly for immediate action.
- The patient's room and mattress must be cleaned, and bedding changed daily in keeping with local policy and guidelines.

Table 26.5 summarises the types of leukaemia.

Red Flag

 A body temperature of 38 °C for more than 1 hour requires immediate treatment.

Table 26.5 **Summary of the types of leukaemia.**

LEUKAEMIA	WHO DOES IT AFFECT?	RISK FACTORS	SIGNS AND SYMPTOMS	TREATMENT (WILL DEPEND ON STAGE OF CANCER AND AGE OF PATIENT)
Acute myeloid leukaemia (AML)	Adults of any age more common in >65 years	Largely unknown. Association with exposure to radiation and benzene, previous chemotherapy, smoking	Weakness/fatigue Fever Weight loss Infections Bleeding and bruising Bone pain Breathlessness Gum infiltration/ swelling	Chemotherapy Stem cell transplant Supportive care only in elderly patients who may not tolerate intensive chemotherapy
Acute lymphoblastic leukaemia (ALL)	Most common type of leukaemia in children and young adults. Can also affect adults	Same risk factors as AML. Associated with previous chemotherapy and some genetic conditions	Weakness/fatigue Fever Weight loss/night sweats Infections Bleeding/bruising/purpura Bone pain Breathlessness Swollen lymph nodes and abdominal discomfort Organomegaly Central nervous system involvement	Chemotherapy Radiotherapy in some cases Stem cell transplant CART-T therapy
Chronic myeloid leukaemia (CML)	A rare leukaemia more common in men	Philadelphia chromosome Previous radiotherapy	Infections Poor appetite Weight loss Swollen lymph nodes Pale and tired appearance Easily bruises or bleeds Night sweats Headache Bone pain Large spleen	Tyrosine kinase inhibitor (TKI) Chemotherapy Stem cell transplant in some cases
Chronic lymphocytic leukaemia (CLL)	Adults over 60 years old. More common in men	Family history	May be asymptomatic Swollen lymph nodes Abdominal discomfort Weight loss Infection Anaemia Fatigue Fever	Chemotherapy Monoclonal antibody therapy Supportive care

Lymphomas

Lymphoma is a malignant condition involving lymphatic tissue and cells of the immune system. Damaged cells proliferate, leading to development of cancer in the lymphatic system and some organs such as the spleen or bone marrow. Lymphoma is the fifth most common cancer diagnosed in the UK (Lymphoma Action, 2021). Although there are many types of lymphoma, Hodgkin lymphoma (Hodgkin disease) and non-Hodgkin lymphoma are the most common. The symptoms, investigations and diagnosis are similar for both.

Hodgkin Lymphoma

An abnormal cell called a Reed–Sternberg cell is seen in Hodgkin lymphoma. This cell is a cancerous type of B lymphocyte. The first symptoms are enlargement of lymph nodes but this is not usually associated with any pain. It is usually progressive and can easily spread if left untreated. It commonly begins in the lymph nodes above the diaphragm. It can also be seen in the spleen and liver, although bone marrow involvement is rare (Lymphoma Action, 2021). Hodgkin lymphoma is a rare condition, with 1800 cases diagnosed per year; it occurs in those aged 20–34 years and in those over 70 (Cancer Research UK, 2021c). Survival is good, with 80% of those diagnosed in England and Wales expected to live for 10 years or more.

Previous treatment for non-Hodgkin lymphoma or a lowered immune system due to antirejection drugs, immunosuppression or other autoimmune illness increase the risk of developing Hodgkin lymphoma. There are also links with Epstein–Barr virus and some genetic factors are recognised.

The disease is staged according to the Ann Arbor classification, which is critical in determining an appropriate treatment pathway.

As the disease progresses, organs such as the liver can become affected, leading to jaundice. If the lungs are affected, breathlessness and a cough may be present. Pressure from enlarged lymph nodes can affect the nervous system.

Non-Hodgkin Lymphoma

Malignant transformation of B or T cells in lymphoid tissue leads to the development of non-Hodgkin lymphoma (NHL), of which there are more than 60 different types. B-cell lymphoma accounts for most cases of NHL, while T-cell lymphoma affects young adults and teenagers. Annually, over 13 000 people are diagnosed with NHL in the UK; 60% of those diagnosed will be over 65 years old (Cancer Research UK, 2021d).

Around 75% of adults will present with lymphadenopathy of the neck, axilla or femoral region, which is usually painless and superficial (Cancer Research UK, 2021d). NHL can spread quickly to other lymphoid tissues and organs. Additional symptoms include frequent fevers, night sweats and significant weight loss. For some patients, pruritus will also be present. Not everyone with a diagnosis of NHL will have these symptoms.

If lymphoma has spread to bone marrow, there will be evidence of suppression of the other blood cells, leading to anaemia, bruising or bleeding and infections. Other symptoms can be present if there is extranodal spread, such as enlarged tonsils, liver and spleen; breathlessness if the chest lymph nodes are involved; and weight loss, nausea, vomiting and abdominal pain if gastrointestinal lymph nodes are involved. Extranodal involvement is more common in NHL than Hodgkin lymphoma.

Lymphoma Diagnosis

An FBC is often normal until later stages of the disease. Chest X-ray will demonstrate any lung involvement or enlarged lymph nodes such as a mediastinal mass. CT or positron emission tomography (PET) scan are usually undertaken to explore the extent of the disease and for staging. A lymph node biopsy is undertaken to differentiate between NHL and Hodgkin lymphoma.

Lymphoma Treatment

Cycles of combination chemotherapy are used to kill cancer cells and can be used in conjunction with radiotherapy and other treatments. Radiotherapy can be targeted at specific lymph nodes. Monoclonal antibodies can also be used as they target specific cell types. Stem cell transplant is only considered when other lines of treatment have been unsuccessful.

Multiple Myeloma

Myeloma is a type of cancer that develops from cells in the bone marrow called plasma cells, found wherever bone marrow is located, including the spine, pelvis and ribcage. The condition is often called multiple myeloma as it can develop at several sites in the body. It is an incurable clonal B-cell malignancy where proliferations of plasma cells accumulate and secrete monoclonal paraproteins. Plasma cells form part of the immune system and produce proteins called antibodies (also called immunoglobulins). Antibodies are made by the plasma cells when there is an infection and are important in attacking bacteria and viruses. Myeloma accounts for 10% of all haematological malignancies and is often seen in older patients, with the median age at diagnosis being 66 (Cancer Research UK, 2020b).

Signs and Symptoms

In the early stages of myeloma, it can be detected on routine blood tests in asymptomatic patients. Symptoms develop when the bone marrow fills with abnormal plasma cells; these cells damage bones and prevent the production of other blood cells, resulting in:

- *Low blood counts*: increased risk of infections, bruising, bleeding and anaemia
- *Bone pain and irreversible damage*, including pathological fractures.
- *Hypercalcaemia*: calcium is released into the bloodstream when bones are damaged
- *Renal impairment or failure*: large amounts of protein pass through the kidneys, causing damage.

Investigation and Diagnosis

Investigations include blood tests, urine analysis, bone marrow biopsy and X-ray or MRI scan. The results are used to stage the disease using the International Staging System (ISS), which gives an indication of expected survival and prognosis (NICE, 2018).

Treatment

The aim of treatment is to bring the myeloma under control; if no active signs of myeloma are detected, it is said to be in remission. Chemotherapy, steroids and biological therapies are the recommended treatments. Stem cell transplant is not curative but is recommended in patients who respond to treatment and are fit enough as survival can be improved (NICE, 2018). Radiotherapy is used to eradicate pain. Bisphosphonates are given regularly to prevent further bone damage and to relieve pain.

Nursing Care and Management During Chemotherapy

Haematological malignancies are normally treated with chemotherapy-based protocols; steroids, monoclonal antibodies, targeted therapies and radiotherapy can also be used. Patients may be offered treatment as part of a clinical trial. This can give patients access to new or experimental treatments.

Medicines Management

Nausea is a common side-effect of chemotherapy. Advising patients to have antiemetics before food or other medications can prevent worsening nausea or vomiting.

Chemotherapy

Cytotoxic chemotherapy acts on cells that divide and multiply rapidly, either stopping the division of cells or destroying the cells and preventing replication. Chemotherapy drugs are designed to interfere with the natural cell cycle and are often given in combination as different drugs work at various stages within the cell cycle. Chemotherapy also interferes with the cell division of healthy cells, leading to unwanted side-effects experienced by patients. Chemotherapy is given in cycles, with a specific gap between each cycle to allow normal cell and bone marrow recovery. Treatment can be given orally or intravenously, and therefore a central line may be required for some treatments. The aim of chemotherapy is to eradicate the cancer, induce remission and treat cancer-related symptoms (Carreras *et al.*, 2019).

Care, Dignity and Compassion

Consider the psychological implications for patients undergoing cancer treatment: infection risk, being nursed in protective isolation, hair loss, fertility and insertion of central line.

Psychosocial Care

A cancer diagnosis and the prospect of chemotherapy can be terrifying for patients and their relatives, so it is important that they are supported throughout the process. Patients can be anxious about treatment, prognosis and the future. Giving an opportunity to discuss concerns can help patients regain control of the situation and gather strength to cope.

The nurse has a vital role in supporting patients, and careful explanation of treatment and side-effects is necessary to reduce anxiety and fear (Kerr *et al.*, 2021). Table 26.6 highlights chemotherapy side-effects. Written information should be offered to ensure the patient is well informed and reassured.

Some treatment regimens are administered in an inpatient setting, so patients have access to support from the multidisciplinary team. Many treatment regimens are now managed in the outpatient setting, so it is important that access to the same level of support is available for all patients. Patients should be

Table 26.6 Advice for chemotherapy patients.

SIDE-EFFECTS ASSOCIATED WITH CHEMOTHERAPY	ADVICE/TREATMENT
Neutropenia and increased risk of infection	Patients should monitor for signs of infection, i.e. temperature. Most chemotherapy units have a 24-hour helpline to advise patients who are unwell. Antibiotics should be commenced within 1 hour of presentation
Anaemia	Blood transfusion may be necessary if haemoglobin <80 g/L. Symptoms include dizziness, fatigue, pallor, breathlessness or dyspnea. Rest and sleep are encouraged
Thrombocytopenia	Low platelets can lead to bruising and bleeding. Platelet transfusion may be required
Hair loss	Hair loss can be distressing for men and women. Psychological support including advice on head coverings and wig referral is essential
Nausea and vomiting	A common side-effect of chemotherapy. Antiemetics should be prescribed throughout treatment
Loss of appetite/ anorexia	This includes taste changes, dry mouth and poor appetite. High-calorie supplements can be prescribed. Encourage small frequent meals. Referral to dietitian might be necessary
Diarrhoea and constipation	Both should be treated promptly to prevent additional discomfort. Stool samples must be obtained to rule out infective causes
Fatigue	Fatigue is often experienced. Advise patients to conserve energy, include sleep and rest in their routine and limit visitors
Psychological support	Patients can feel isolated throughout treatment. It is important they feel supported by family and friends. Refer patients to clinical nurse specialist who can signpost to additional support

allocated a cancer specialist nurse who will act as a key worker (Kerr *et al.*, 2021).

Before each cycle of treatment, patients are assessed for side-effects, toxicity of treatment and baseline blood tests. Occasionally, treatment is postponed if blood levels are too low and more time is needed for recovery. It is important that this is communicated to patients and reassurance given to minimise anxiety and fear. Following treatment, patients discharged into the community should have a point of contact to discuss any concerns. Most chemotherapy units have a 24-hour emergency helpline where advice can be given over the telephone if patients become unwell. The specialist nurse is also a point of contact.

Radiotherapy

Radiotherapy is sometimes used in haematological cancers. The purpose of radiotherapy is to use X-rays to damage the DNA within the cancer cells. Radiotherapy can also temporarily damage healthy cells, causing unwanted side-effects. The radiotherapy can be applied externally or it can be implanted internally, depending on the place and nature of the cancer being treated. Radiotherapy can be given as part of the treatment or for symptom management, sometimes referred to as 'palliative radiotherapy'.

Patients can be anxious about radiotherapy, so support and information about treatment and side-effects are essential. Side-effects of radiotherapy should be discussed, so patients know what to expect; nurses have a vital role in this. Side-effects include:

- Tiredness
- Skin soreness
- Hair loss at the radiotherapy site.

> **Jot This Down**
>
> Patients having radiotherapy should be advised not to use lotions, perfumes and some deodorants prior to radiotherapy to minimise skin reactions, sensitivity or burning.

Haemopoietic Stem Cell Transplants from Bone Marrow or Cord Blood

Haemopoietic stem cell transplant (HSCT) is the replacement of abnormal or damaged bone marrow with healthy bone marrow to restore normal blood cell production. HSCT is a treatment used for some malignant and non-malignant conditions. The decision to transplant and the type of transplant will depend on diagnosis, prognosis, age and co-morbidities of the patient. (Carreras *et al.*, 2019). The cells required to undertake HSCT can be collected in one of three ways: bone marrow harvest, peripheral blood stem cells or cord blood cells. There are three potential sources of haemopoietic stem cells.

- *Autologous*: stem cells taken from the patient at a time when the disease has been treated and is in remission. Cells are frozen and used later when HSCT is planned. Cells can be collected from bone marrow or peripheral blood.
- *Allogeneic*: stem cells taken from a volunteer donor. Tissue typing is the process of matching recipient and donor tissue. Siblings have a 25% chance of being a suitable match. If there are no matched siblings, a matched unrelated donor can normally be identified through the donor registries. Cells can be collected from bone marrow or peripheral blood.
- *Cord blood cells*: stem cells collected from umbilical cord which are stored in blood banks worldwide. The cord blood registry is searched to ensure the tissue typing is adequately matched.

Preparing the Patient

Before HSCT, patients are given a preparative regimen called 'conditioning', which comprises chemotherapy, immunosuppressive drugs, antirejection drugs and, in some cases, total body irradiation (TBI radiotherapy). The aim of conditioning is to empty the damaged bone marrow and kill any cancerous cells. Immunosuppressive drugs are given to suppress the immune system to prevent rejection of the stem cells. The stem cells are infused through a central line like a blood transfusion. It takes 2–3 weeks for the transplanted cells to grow in the bone marrow and produce healthy blood cells, including white blood cells important in fighting infection (Babic & Murray, 2019). While the patient has low blood counts, they are at risk of infection, bleeding and the side-effects of chemotherapy and radiotherapy. Patients are nursed in isolation and will usually remain in hospital for 4–6 weeks.

Allogeneic HSCT carries an additional risk of graft-versus-host disease (GVHD), where the transplanted cells see the recipient as foreign and attack the recipient tissue. Immunosuppressants and steroids are used to prevent and treat GVHD (Michonneau & Socié, 2019). Table 26.7 lists the side-effects and treatment associated with HSCT.

> **Care, Dignity and Compassion**
>
> It can take considerable time to recover from cancer treatment. Patients can have long-term physical, medical and psychological side-effects (Babic & Murray, 2019). Patient-centred care and rehabilitation following treatment are essential, including exercise and psychological support to help regain normality and quality of life.

Chimeric Antigen Receptor Therapy

Chimeric antigen receptor therapy (CAR-T) is a highly complex and innovative new treatment, which is a targeted therapy aimed at specific cancer cells. CAR-T is a type of immunotherapy which involves using the patient's own immune system to fight their cancer, including lymphoma, leukaemia and myeloma (Freyer & Porter, 2020). CAR-T cells are also known as advanced therapy medicinal products (ATMPs).

The patient's T cells are collected using an apheresis machine, and are then manufactured in a laboratory. Manufacturing CAR-T cells is a complex process; the T cells are 'infected' with a virus that contains a genetic code to produce a CAR, designed to target specific cancer cells. They are engineered and expanded in a laboratory and then transported to a specialist centre where they will be infused back to the patient (Freyer & Porter, 2020) (Figure 26.4).

Once the CAR-T cells are manufactured, the patient is admitted to a specialist centre and given a preparative regimen using lymphodepleting chemotherapy; the CAR-T cells are then infused into the patient. The cells can recognise and bind to specific cancer cells and kill them. Side-effects of this treatment include cytokine release syndrome (CRS), neurotoxicity, tumour lysis syndrome, low blood counts or coagulation disorders and infections. Patients are monitored closely for these side-effects for 30 days following cell infusion (Miao *et al.*, 2021).

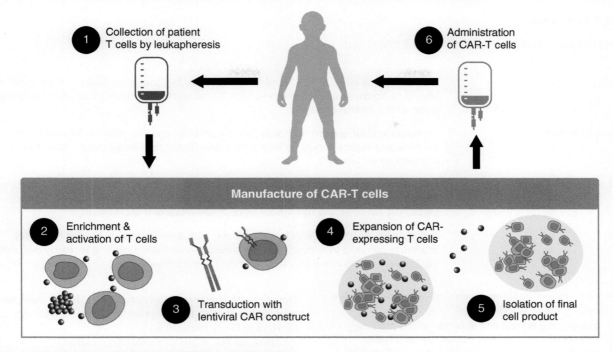

Figure 26.4 Collection, manufacturing and infusion of CAR-T cells.

Table 26.7 Advice to patients undergoing haemopoietic stem cell transplant (HSCT).

SIDE-EFFECTS ASSOCIATED WITH HSCT	ADVICE/TREATMENT
Graft-versus-host disease (GVHD) (allogeneic transplant only)	Can affect the liver, bowel or skin. Ciclosporin throughout transplant to prevent GVHD. Immunosuppressants and steroids are used to treat GVHD. Patient should monitor for rash, diarrhoea or sickness
Infection	Antibiotics, protective isolation, daily cleaning of the room and changing linen, strict hand washing and limiting of visitors, daily shower and attention to mouth care, low-immunity diet, monitoring of vital signs, particularly temperature and monitoring of blood results. Potential infection sites should be swabbed for microscopy. Central lines should be treated as a potential source and strict ANTT must be used
Anaemia	Blood transfusion will be required when haemoglobin <70g/L. The nurse must assess the patient for signs and symptoms of anaemia
Bleeding	Bleeding and bruising may be evident. Platelets will be transfused if platelet count ≤10 × 10^9/L in afebrile patients and ≤20 × 10^9/L in febrile patients
Mucositis and oesophagitis	Oral mucous membranes are damaged by treatment and can be painful. Oral care is essential: soft tufted toothbrush and regular mouthwashes. Analgesia, intravenous fluids or parenteral nutrition may be necessary. Mouth swab should be taken to investigate secondary infection
Nausea and vomiting	Both are common. Antiemetics should be prescribed prior to commencing treatment and are usually required throughout treatment.
Loss of appetite/weight loss	Loss of appetite is common. Small frequent meals should be encouraged. A nutritional assessment and plan should be made by the dietitian, including supplement recommendation. Parenteral nutrition may be necessary as calories are essential for healing. Patient must be weighed daily and maintain a strict fluid balance chart. Food charts can be helpful

(Continued)

469

Table 26.7 (*Continued*)

SIDE-EFFECTS ASSOCIATED WITH HSCT	ADVICE/TREATMENT
Diarrhoea	A common side-effect of HSCT and GVHD. Personal hygiene is important. A stool chart should be commenced, and samples sent for microscopy and virology. Loperamide can be given once infection ruled out
Lethargy and fatigue	Tiredness and fatigue are normal following transplant and can continue for several months. Exercise and activity should be increased gradually and rest encouraged. Physiotherapy referral may be helpful
Protective isolation	Patients are nursed in isolation and visitors limited to prevent cross-infection. Contact with friends and relatives should be encouraged by telephone or social networking/internet/skype. The nurse should monitor for signs of low mood and depression
Infertility	Fertility must be discussed before transplant. High-dose chemotherapy and total body irradiation can lead to infertility and early menopause. Sperm banking is readily available. Egg/embryo preservation may be available in some centers

Practice Assessment Document

Interpreting normal and abnormal blood profiles
It is unlikely that student nurses will undertake venipuncture or cannulation on a haematology ward, but there will be opportunities to discuss blood results, interpretation and actions required. Take time to consider the questions below or your supervisor could write other scenarios.

- Make a list of the most common blood test requested on haematology patients. *What are the normal values? What are the possible causes for the abnormal blood results?*
- When interpreting an abnormal full blood count, *what are the consequences of abnormally low white blood cells, red blood cells and platelets? What could be done to improve/correct these blood results?*
- A patient with low platelets is at increased risk of bleeding. *What interventions might be put in place to reduce the harm risk associated with trips, slips and falls? What advice could be given to reduce the risk of bleeding?*
- Your patient on the ward is anaemic. *What advice should be given for managing activities of living? When would a blood transfusion be given? Are there alternatives?*
- The white blood cell count is low. *What interventions should be put in place to reduce infection risk? What assessments should be undertaken?*
- A patient has a nosebleed that won't stop. *What blood tests could be checked? What else could you do?*
- Consider the consequences of abnormal blood results in relation to the patients you are caring for. *What action was taken? What was the outcome and how was the response measured?*

As a student nurse, what is your role in improving the patient's experience and ensuring delivery of safe and harm-free care when a patient has abnormal blood results?

Disorders of Haemostasis and Platelets

Platelets are essential for blood clotting; they originate from stem cells and require thrombopoietin for their development. *Haemostasis* is the sequence of responses that stops bleeding.

Disorders of haemostasis occur because blood does not clot sufficiently or clots inappropriately within the vascular system (Tortora & Derrickson, 2020).

There are five stages to normal haemostasis.

1. *Vessel spasm*: endothelial injury results in vessel constriction, reducing blood flow to the damaged area.
2. *Platelet plug formation*: platelets aggregate in the area and form a plug to seal off the damaged vessel wall.
3. *Blood coagulation*: blood is transformed from a liquid to a gel. The soluble plasma protein fibrinogen is converted to the insoluble fibrin, which forms a mesh and eventually becomes a blood clot. Blood coagulation relies on activation of the blood coagulation pathway. Figure 26.5 illustrates the complexity of the blood clotting process and the clotting factors involved.
4. *Clot retraction*: the clot usually stabilises within 30 minutes. It then retracts as the trapped platelets contract. The platelets release growth factors which stimulate tissue repair at the site of the damaged vessel.
5. *Clot dissolution*: a permanent repair occurs and blood flow is re-established. This is called fibrinolysis. Plasminogen, an enzyme that promotes fibrinolysis, is converted to plasmin. Plasmin dissolves the fibrin strands that make up the clot.

There are many clotting factors involved in haemostasis and the clotting pathway (Table 26.8). Any interruption to this pathway or reduction in clotting factors can interfere with the normal coagulation pathway. An absence of vitamin K can also disrupt the blood coagulation pathway. A smooth and intact endothelium and naturally occurring anticoagulants such as heparin (secreted by the endothelial tissue) and antithrombin prevent platelets aggregating and clotting when not required (McCance & Heuther, 2018). Anticoagulants are products that inhibit blood clotting.

When patients present with bleeding of unknown aetiology, blood is tested for its ability to clot and the presence of indicators of clotting (Table 26.9). Table 26.10 highlights clinical features often seen in clotting disorders.

What To Do If . . .

A patient tells you he has been having frequent nosebleeds (epistaxis) lately. Given this patient is on warfarin, what would your next steps be?

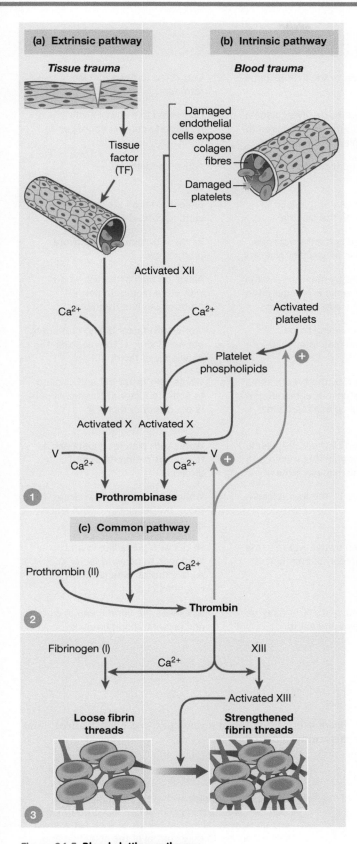

Figure 26.5 Blood clotting pathways.

Inherited Bleeding Disorders

This is a disorder where there is a lack of or deficiency in clotting factors, including von Willebrand disease and haemophilia A and B. Haemophilia A and B are inherited, sex-linked recessive disorders that are passed from mother to son. The defect is a mutation in a gene on the X chromosome. Figure 26.6 demonstrates how this disorder occurs.

Haemophilia A is the most common haemophilia and occurs due to deficiency in factor VIII. Bleeding pattern, severity and treatment required are dependent on the classification of the condition from mild to severe.

- *Mild*: 5–50% of normal concentration of factor VIII. These patients will probably only need treatment due to surgery or trauma. No risk of spontaneous bleeding.
- *Moderate*: 1–5% of normal concentration of factor VIII. These patients will require treatment due to surgery or trauma. Some risk of spontaneous bleeding.
- *Severe*: <1% of normal concentration of factor VIII. These patients would be prescribed a prophylactic treatment regime of factor VIII concentrate. They will spontaneously bleed without prophylaxis.

Haemophilia B is less common and occurs as a result of deficiency in factor IX; it is also known as 'Christmas disease'. Severity grading and treatment are the same as for haemophilia A.

Von Willebrand disease is an inherited bleeding disorder. People with this condition have a deficiency of a protein produced by the endothelial cells called *von Willebrand factor*. The role of this protein is to promote platelet adhesion and to carry factor VIII. Von Willebrand disease is the most common of the inherited bleeding disorders (Fritsma, 2020). Treatment is based on the severity of the condition and includes desmopressin (DDAVP), tranexamic acid or clotting factor concentrate.

What the Experts Say

> 'The aim of treatment is to help patients self-manage their bleeding disorder, reduce bleeding risk and achieve a good quality of life. Newer targeted therapies are used as prophylaxis to prevent bleeding, improve patient quality of life, improve adherence to treatment and psychological well-being.'
> Paula Grey, haemophilia specialist nurse

Immune thrombocytopenic purpura is an immune disorder referred to as ITP. The immune system produces antibodies against platelets leading to destruction and removal in the spleen. This lowers the platelet count, leading to excessive bruising and bleeding. The immune system also appears to interfere with cells responsible for normal platelet production, which can further lower the platelet count (DeChristopher & Jeske, 2020).

In children, ITP often develops acutely following a virus and in adults, it usually develops over time. ITP can be classified as primary, occurring on its own, or secondary, occurring alongside another condition. Autoimmune diseases, chronic infections, medications, pregnancy and certain cancers are common

Table 26.8 Blood clotting factors and their functions.

FACTOR NUMBER	FACTOR NAME	SITE OF FORMATION	ACTIONS
I	Fibrinogen	Synthesised by the liver (plasma protein)	Converted to fibrin for clot formation
II	Prothrombin	Synthesised by the liver (plasma protein); vitamin K is required to produce this plasma protein	Converted to thrombin, which is required to convert fibrinogen to fibrin
III	Tissue factor (TF) (thromboplastin)	Released from damaged tissue (lipoprotein)	Activates factor VII
IV	Calcium ions	Present in diet or released by the bone into the plasma	Essential for all stages of the clotting cascade
V	Platelet accelerator (proaccelerin/labile factor)	Synthesised by the liver (plasma protein); also released by platelets	Works with factor X to activate prothrombin
VII	Serum prothrombin conversion accelerator	Synthesised by the liver (plasma protein); vitamin K is required to produce this plasma protein	Activates factor X, which works with other factors to convert prothrombin into thrombin
VIII	Antihaemophilic factor A (AHF)	Endothelium lining blood vessels and platelets (plug)	Works with factor IX and calcium to activate factor X. Haemophilia A is deficiency of factor VIII
IX	Plasma thromboplastin component (PTC) or Christmas factor or antihaemophilic factor B	Synthesised by the liver (plasma protein); vitamin K is required to produce this plasma protein	Works with factor VIII and calcium to activate factor X. Haemophilia B is deficiency of factor IX
X	Stuart–Prower factor	Synthesised by the liver (plasma protein); vitamin K is required to produce this plasma protein	Works with platelet phospholipids to convert prothrombin into thrombin
XI	Plasma thromboplastin antecedent (PTA) or antihaemophilic factor C	Synthesised by the liver (plasma protein)	Works with calcium to activate factor IX. Deficiency of PTA leads to haemophilia C
XII	Hageman factor	Synthesised by the liver (plasma protein; proteolytic enzyme)	Works with prekallikrein and kininogen to activate factor XI. Also activates plasmin which degrades clot
XIII	Fibrin stabilising factor (FSF)	Synthesised by the liver (plasma protein). Also present in platelets	Stabilises the fibrin mesh of clots and prevents fibrin breakdown

secondary triggers. Treatment can include immunosuppression, immunoglobulin replacement or antibody treatments. Thrombopoietin receptor agonists, which encourage the bone marrow to produce more platelets, may also be used.

Patients diagnosed with these conditions bleed or bruise easily. Bleeding can be prolonged or extensive and can happen spontaneously or in relation to an injury (Fritsma, 2020). Bleeding can occur from the gums, gastrointestinal system, nose (epistaxis), and bleeding into the central nervous system, joints and muscles. Bleeding into the joints is called *haemarthrosis* and can eventually cause permanent joint deformity and disability.

Care, Dignity and Compassion

Encouraging patients with a bleeding disorder to learn about their condition, self-manage treatment and understand the implications of their actions will give autonomy to take control of the condition and make informed choices.

Case Study

Lisa is 28 years old and in the second trimester of her first pregnancy. She attends clinic for routine antenatal assessment.

Past medical history
Nil

Medications
Oral multivitamin

Assessment
Blood pressure and weight – normal
FBC – demonstrates low platelets 60 × 10⁹/L, other counts normal

Diagnosis
Suspected gestational ITP, asymptomatic, no bleeding

Management plan
Joint management in specialist centre by obstetrician and haematology
Regular platelet monitoring throughout remainder of pregnancy
Safe for vaginal delivery if platelets remain >50 × 10⁹/L
Planned/urgent caesarean section or epidural platelets should be >80 × 10⁹/L
Platelet transfusion may be required during labour

Treatment
Steroids or intravenous immunoglobulin will only be given if platelets drop <20 × 10⁹/L or bleeding is evident

Outcome
Platelet count usually recovers spontaneously post partum
Follow-up as an outpatient by the haematology team

Patient education
What advice might be required if Lisa is considering subsequent pregnancies?

Table 26.9 The blood test, normal range and what is being measured.

TEST	NORMAL RANGE	USE
Platelets	150–400 × 10⁹/L	Number per 1 L of blood
Prothrombin time (PT)	12–14 seconds	Measures the time it takes for blood to clot
Activated partial thromboplastin time (APTT)	26–33.5 seconds	Measures the time it takes for a clot to form
Thrombin time	10–17 seconds	Time taken for fibrinogen to form fibrin
Fibrinogen	2.0–4.0 g/L	Amount of fibrinogen in the plasma
D-dimer	<500 ng/mL	Predictor of recent clot formation

Health Promotion and Education

Due to the risk of bleeding, patients will be given health promotion and lifestyle advice as it is easier to reduce the risk of bleeding than to manage active bleeding. Patients should be advised as follows.

Table 26.10 Visual signs associated with bleeding disorders.

TERM	MEANING
Haematoma	Bleeding into soft tissue: the blood becomes trapped and forms a haematoma
Petechiae	Tiny pinpoint haemorrhages seen on the skin
Purpura	Red/purple spots caused by bleeding under the skin

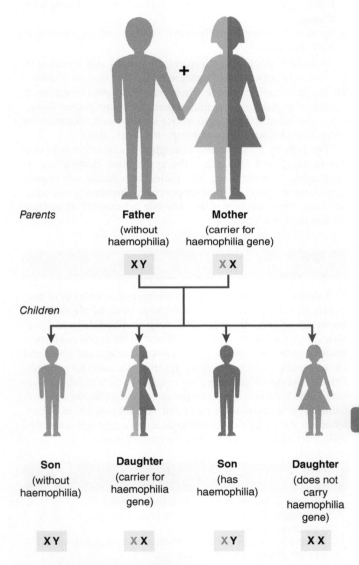

Figure 26.6 **Haemophilia inheritance.**

- Be aware of the signs of bleeding, how to manage bleeding and when to seek urgent medical help.
- Inform medical practitioners, e.g. dentist, prior to any treatment.
- Take care with personal hygiene, e.g. cutting nails and wet shaving.

473

- Ensure good oral hygiene and attend regular dental checks to reduce the need for invasive dental procedures.
- Recognise the signs of haemarthrosis and seek medical advice.
- Exercise caution when using medications that can affect blood clotting such as aspirin, antiplatelet drugs and intramuscular injections.
- Sporting activities: non-contact sports are preferable. Extreme sports should be avoided.
- Non-invasive procedures such as tattooing should be avoided.
- Carry a 'health alert card', bracelet or neck pendant.
- Learn about your medications; good compliance with prophylactic regimes will prevent spontaneous bleeds and long-term damage.
- Speak to your specialist haemophilia centre when planning to have children.

Patients with clotting disorders are usually self-managed in the community but should be registered with a specialist haemophilia centre; serious bleeding may require hospital treatment. It is important that the nurse undertakes a thorough patient assessment and identifies the significance of any bleed. Examine the patient for obvious signs and symptoms of bleeding.

The priority for any nurse managing this situation is to stop the bleeding and administer the appropriate clotting factors required to treat the bleed. The patient and family will require emotional and psychological support from the nursing and medical team. Physiotherapy plays a key role in preservation of muscle and joint function.

Conclusion

This chapter has provided information regarding a variety of haematological disorders. A good knowledge of blood physiology is important in order to understand the pathophysiology and provide appropriate nursing care. It is essential for registered nurses, student nurses and nursing associates to understand abnormal blood results and the implications this can have for patients. Patients should be monitored for changes in their condition that could indicate a serious or life-threatening complication of their hematological diagnosis or treatment. It is not possible in a chapter of this size to fully cover this topic and the reader is advised to seek other texts that can support the content here.

Key Points

- Anaemia is the most common disorder of red blood cells. Signs and symptoms of anaemia are the same regardless of cause.
- An increase in red cell concentration in the blood is known as polycythaemia or erythrocytosis.
- Leukaemia and lymphoma are malignancy or cancer of the white blood cells.
- Care of the patient with leukaemia, lymphoma and myeloma focuses on the risk of bleeding, infection and managing side-effects of treatment.
- Care, education and health promotion are undertaken by nursing associates, student nurses and qualified staff nurses.
- Bleeding and clotting disorders can result from low platelet production or a deficiency in clotting factors.

References

Abboud, M.R. (2020) Standard management of sickle cell disease complications. *Hematology/Oncology and Stem Cell Therapy*, 13(2), 85–90.

Babic, A. & Murray, J. (2019) Role of nursing in HSCT. In: E. Carreras, C. Dufour, M. Mohty, & N. Kroger (eds) *The EBMT Handbook; Hematopoietic Stem cell Transplantation and Cellular Therapies*. Springer Open. www.ebmt.org/education/ebmt-handbook (accessed December 2021).

Bain, B. (2020) *Haemoglobinopathy Diagnosis*, 3rd edn. Wiley, Chichester.

Blood Cancer UK (2021) *Childhood acute lymphoblastic leukaemia (ALL) treatment*. https://bloodcancer.org.uk/understanding-blood-cancer/leukaemia/childhood-leukaemia/childhood-acute-lymphoblastic-leukaemia-all/childhood-all-treatment/ (accessed December 2021).

British Society of Haematology (BSH) (2020) A British Society of Haematology guideline on the diagnosis and management of CML. *British Journal of Haematology*, 191(2), 171–193.

Cancer Research UK (2019a) *Risk and causes for acute lymphoblastic leukaemia (ALL)*. www.cancerresearchuk.org/about-cancer/acute-lymphoblastic-leukaemia-all/risks-causes (accessed December 2021).

Cancer Research UK (2019b) *Chronic myeloid leukaemia (CML) statistics*. www.cancerresearchuk.org/health-professional/cancer-statistics/statistics-by-cancer-type/leukaemia-cml (accessed December 2021).

Cancer Research UK (2020a) *Chronic lymphoblastic leukaemia (CLL)*. www.cancerresearchuk.org/about-cancer/chronic-lymphocytic-leukaemia-cll (accessed December 2021).

Cancer Research UK (2020b) *What is myeloma?* www.cancerresearchuk.org/about-cancer/myeloma/about (accessed December 2021).

Cancer Research UK (2021a) *Leukaemia (all subtypes combined) statistics*. www.cancerresearchuk.org/health-professional/cancer-statistics/statistics-by-cancer-type/leukaemia (accessed December 2021).

Cancer Research UK (2021b) *Acute myeloid leukaemia (AML) statistics*. www.cancerresearchuk.org/health-professional/cancer-statistics/statistics-by-cancer-type/leukaemia-aml (accessed December 2021).

Cancer Research UK (2021c) *Hodgkin lymphoma: risks and causes*. www.cancerresearchuk.org/about-cancer/hodgkin-lymphoma/risks-causes (accessed December 2021).

Cancer Research UK (2021d) *Non-Hodgkin lymphoma*. www.cancerresearchuk.org/about-cancer/non-hodgkin-lymphoma (accessed December 2021).

Carreras, E., Dufour, C., Mohty, M. & Kroger, N. (2019) *The EBMT Handbook; Hematopoietic Stem cell Transplantation and Cellular Therapies*. Springer Open. www.ebmt.org/education/ebmt-handbook (accessed December 2021).

DeChristopher, P.J & Jeske, W.P. (2020) Thrombocytopenia and thrombocytosis. In: E.M. Keohane, C.N. Otto & J.M. Walenga (eds) *Rodak's Hematology Clinical Principles and Applications*, 6th edn. Elsevier, St Louis, MO.

Fabi, A., Bhargava, R., Fatigoni, S., *et al.* (2020) Cancer-related fatigue: ESMO Clinical Practice Guidelines for diagnosis and treatment. *Annals of Oncology*, 31, 713–723.

Freyer, C. & Porter, D. (2020) Advances in CAR T therapy for hematologic malignancies. *Pharmacotherapy*, 40(8), 741–755.

Fritsma, G.A. (2020) Hemorrhagic disorders and laboratory assessment. In: E.M. Keohane, C.N. Otto & J.M. Walenga (eds) *Rodak's Hematology Clinical Principles and Applications*, 6th edn. Elsevier, St Louis, MO.

Furlong, E. & Carter, T. (2020) Aplastic anaemia: current concepts in diagnosis and management. *Journal of Paediatrics and Child Health*, 56, 1023–1028.

Hird, S. (2020) Early diagnosis and effective management of sepsis. *Nursing Standard*, 35, 59–66.

Hubert, R. & VanMeter, K. (2018) *Gould's Pathophysiology for the Health Professions*, 6th edn. Saunders Elsevier, St Louis, MO.

Hucks, G. & Rheingold, S.R. (2019) The journey to CAR T cell therapy: the pediatric and young adult experience with relapsed or refractory B-ALL. *Blood Cancer Journal*, 9, 10.

Kerr, H., Donovan, M. & McSorley, O. (2021) Evaluation of the role of clinical nurse specialist in cancer care: an integrative literature review. *European Journal of Cancer Care*, 30, e13415.

Lymphoma Action (2021) *What is lymphoma?* www.lymphomas.org.uk/about-lymphoma/what-lymphoma (accessed December 2021).

Marieb, E.N. & Hoehn, K. (2019) *Human Anatomy & Physiology, Global Edition*, 11th edn. Pearson, Harlow.

McCance, K.L. & Heuther, S.E. (2018) *Pathophysiology. The Biologic Basis for Disease in Adults and Children*, 8th edn. Mosby Elsevier, St Louis, MO.

Miao, L., Zhang, Z., Ren, Z. & Li, Y. (2021) Reactions related to CAR-T cell therapy. *Frontiers in Immunology*, 12, 663201.

Michonneau, D. & Socié, G. (2019) GVHD prophylaxis (immunosuppression). In: E. Carreras, E., C. Dufour, M. Mohty & N. Kroger (eds) *The EBMT Handbook; Hematopoietic Stem cell Transplantation and Cellular Therapies*. Springer Open. www.ebmt.org/education/ebmt-handbook (accessed December 2021).

Mirza, K.M. (2020) Hematopoiesis. In: E.M. Keohane, C.N. Otto & J.M. Walenga (eds) *Rodak's Hematology Clinical Principles and Applications*, 6th edn. Elsevier, St Louis, MO.

Moench, S. (2020) Assessment and management of patients with polycythemia vera. *Oncology Nurse Advisor*. www.oncologynurseadvisor.com/home/cancer-types/myeloproliferative-neoplasms/assessment-and-management-of-pts-with-pv/ (accessed December 2021).

National Institute for Health and Care Excellence (2016) *Sepsis: recognition, diagnosis and early management*. NG51. NICE, London. www.nice.org.uk/guidance/ng51 (accessed December 2021).

National Institute for Health and Care Excellence (2018) *Myeloma: diagnosis and management*. NG35, NICE, London. www.nice.org.uk/guidance/ng35 (accessed December 2021).

NHS England (2021) *Specialised haemoglobinopathy services*. www.england.nhs.uk/commissioning/spec-services/npc-crg/blood-and-infection-group-f/f05/specialised-haemoglobinopathy-services/ (accessed December 2021).

Peate, I. & Evans, S. (2020) *Fundamentals of Anatomy and Physiology for Nursing and Healthcare Students*. Wiley, Oxford.

Randolph, T.R. (2020) Myeloproliferative neoplasms. In: E.M. Keohane, C.N. Otto & J.M. Walenga (eds) *Rodak's Hematology Clinical Principles and Applications*, 6th edn. Elsevier, St Louis, MO.

Royal College of Nursing (2019) *Iron Deficiency and Anaemia in Adults: RCN guidance for nursing practice*. RCN, London.

Tortora, G.J. & Derrickson, B. (2020) *Principles of Anatomy and Physiology*, 16th edn. Wiley, Hoboken, NJ.

Waugh, A. & Grant, A. (2018) *Ross and Wilson Anatomy and Physiology in Health and Illness*, 13th edn. Elsevier Churchill Livingstone, Edinburgh.

World Health Organization (2021) *Anaemia*. www.who.int/topics/anaemia/en/ (accessed December 2021).

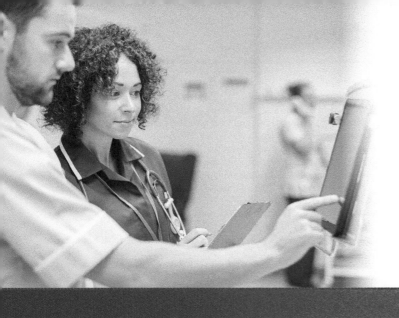

27

The Person with a Respiratory Disorder

Anthony Wheeldon

University of Hertfordshire, UK

Learning Outcomes

On completion of this chapter you will be able to:

- Recognise the importance of respiratory rate and oxygen saturation as part of a comprehensive patient assessment
- Demonstrate the ability to perform a comprehensive assessment of an individual's respiratory status
- Recognise the cardinal signs and symptoms of acute deterioration in patients with severe and life-threatening respiratory diseases
- Plan effective care strategies for individuals with respiratory disorders
- Work with other members of the multidisciplinary team to ensure that patients receive care interventions that are based on the best available evidence
- Promote self-management strategies with individuals living with chronic respiratory disease

Proficiencies

NMC Proficiencies and Standards:

- Use evidence-based, best practice approaches for meeting needs for respiratory care and support, accurately assessing the person's capacity for independence and self-care and initiating appropriate interventions
- Share information and check understanding about the causes, implications and treatment of a range of common health conditions, including respiratory disease
- Undertake a whole body systems assessment including respiratory status
- Manage airway and respiratory processes and equipment

Visit the companion website at **www.wiley.com/go/peate/nursingpractice3e** where you can test yourself using flashcards, multiple-choice questions and more.

Nursing Practice: Knowledge and Care, Third Edition. Edited by Ian Peate and Aby Mitchell.
© 2022 John Wiley & Sons Ltd. Published 2022 by John Wiley & Sons Ltd.
Companion website: www.wiley.com/go/peate/nursingpractice3e

Introduction

The earth's atmosphere contains many pollutants, meaning that respiratory diseases are highly prevalent throughout the world. Respiratory disease accounts for a significant number of deaths and places a heavy burden on health services economically as well as the burden it brings to individuals, families and communities. A major influencing factor on the development of respiratory disease is socioeconomic status. People with lower socioeconomic status are far more likely to develop and live with respiratory disease. This chapter looks at respiratory disease and its associated nursing care.

Respiratory Anatomy

The respiratory system is divided into the upper and lower respiratory tract (Figure 27.1). The structures found deep within the lower respiratory tract are microscopic, very fragile and easily damaged by infection. For this reason, both the upper and lower respiratory tracts are designed to protect these fragile structures from invading airborne pathogens. The nasal cavity, for instance, is lined with a mucous membrane made from pseudostratified ciliated columnar epithelium, which contains a network of capillaries and a plentiful supply of mucus-secreting goblet cells. Mucus traps and covers any passing dust particles, which are then propelled by the cilia towards the pharynx where they can be swallowed or expectorated. For further protection, the upper respiratory tract is lined with irritant receptors, which when stimulated by invading particles (dust or pollen, for example) force a sneeze, ensuring the expulsion of the offending material through the nose or mouth. The pharynx also contains five tonsils (Figure 27.2). Tonsils are lymph nodules and part of the immune system. The epithelial lining of their surface has deep folds, called crypts, which trap inhaled pathogens.

The lower respiratory tract includes the larynx, the trachea, the right and left primary bronchi and all the constituents of both lungs (Figure 27.3). The lungs are two cone-shaped organs that almost fill the thorax. They consist of a massive network of airways of ever decreasing size. For this reason, the structure of the lungs is often referred to as the bronchial tree.

The first branch of the bronchial tree is the trachea (or windpipe), which carries air from the larynx down towards the lungs. The trachea and the bronchi contain irritant receptors, which stimulate a cough, forcing large invading particles upwards towards the oesophagus and pharynx. The trachea is also lined with pseudostratified ciliated columnar epithelium which traps smaller inhaled debris and propels them upwards into the upper respiratory tract where they are swallowed or expectorated. The outermost layer of the trachea contains connective tissue that is reinforced by a series of 16–20 C-shaped cartilage rings, which prevent the trachea from collapsing due to the pressure changes that occur during an active breathing cycle. Before entering the lungs, the trachea divides into two primary bronchi at a point known as the carina.

Within the lungs, the primary bronchi divide into the secondary bronchi, each serving a lobe (there are three lobes in the right lung and two in the left). The secondary bronchi split into tertiary bronchi, which eventually lead to a terminal bronchiole. The section of the lung supplied by a terminal bronchiole is referred to as a lobule, which contains sphere-like structures called alveoli (Figure 27.4). The lobule is the site of gaseous exchange, where oxygen is transferred from the lungs into circulation.

For a more detailed overview of respiratory anatomy, please see Wheeldon (2020).

Respiratory Physiology

The functions of human cells are dependent upon the transfer of energy between molecules. The substance that provides the energy source is adenosine triphosphate (ATP). At any one time a human cell will contain around 1 billion molecules of ATP, but each molecule will only survive around 1 minute before being used. Oxygen (O_2) is fundamental in the production of ATP and therefore cells only survive if they receive a continuous supply of oxygen. The manufacture of ATP also produces carbon dioxide (CO_2). If allowed to build up, carbon dioxide can affect cellular activity and disrupt homeostasis. The principal function of the respiratory system therefore is to ensure that the body extracts enough oxygen from the atmosphere whilst simultaneously eliminating excess carbon dioxide. In addition to the exchange of oxygen and carbon dioxide, the respiratory system also filters inspired air, excretes small amounts of water and heat, articulates vocal sounds, provides the sense of smell and plays a major role in the regulation of arterial blood pH.

Key Concepts of Respiratory Physiology

It is important for nurses to have in-depth understanding of the key concepts of respiration in order to assess and plan care for people living with respiratory disease. This chapter will explore

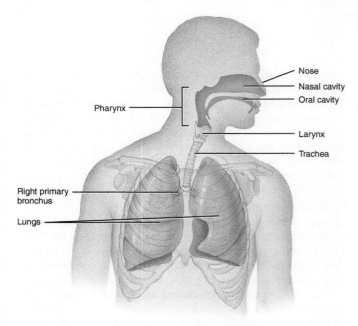

Pharynx

Nose
Nasal cavity
Oral cavity

Larynx

Trachea

Right primary bronchus

Lungs

Anterior view showing organs of respiration

Figure 27.1 Upper and lower respiratory tracts.

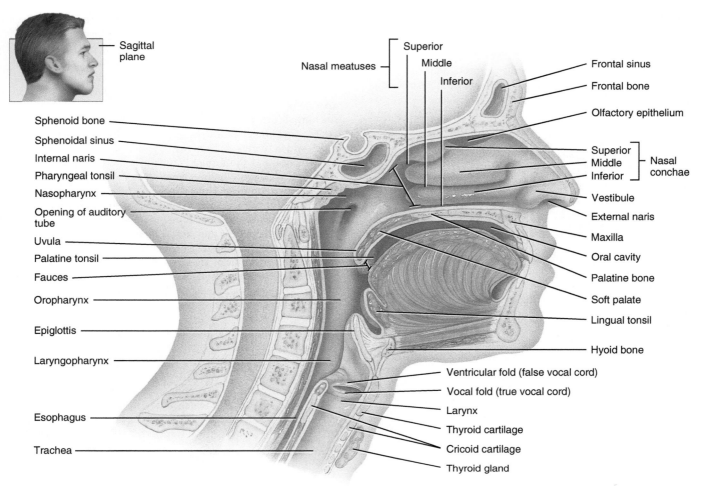

Sagittal plane

Nasal meatuses
- Superior
- Middle
- Inferior

Frontal sinus
Frontal bone
Olfactory epithelium

Nasal conchae
- Superior
- Middle
- Inferior

Sphenoid bone
Sphenoidal sinus
Internal naris
Pharyngeal tonsil
Nasopharynx
Opening of auditory tube
Uvula
Palatine tonsil
Fauces
Oropharynx
Epiglottis
Laryngopharynx
Esophagus
Trachea

Vestibule
External naris
Maxilla
Oral cavity
Palatine bone
Soft palate
Lingual tonsil
Hyoid bone
Ventricular fold (false vocal cord)
Vocal fold (true vocal cord)
Larynx
Thyroid cartilage
Cricoid cartilage
Thyroid gland

Sagittal section of the left side of the head and neck
showing the location of respiratory structures

Figure 27.2 **Structure of the upper airways.**

the concepts listed below. Readers may also find it useful to refer to Wheeldon (2020), which contains a more detailed exploration of respiratory anatomy and physiology.

- *Work of breathing*: the amount of energy required to breathe.
- *Control of breathing*: how the brain controls the rate and depth of breathing.
- *External respiration*: how oxygen moves from the lungs into circulation.
- *Transport of gases*: how oxygen is transported from the lungs to the tissues.

Work of Breathing

During inspiration, respiratory muscles, such as the diaphragm and intercostal muscles, must overcome the elastic recoil of lung tissue and natural resistance to airflow through very small airways. The energy required by the respiratory muscles to overcome these hindering forces is referred to as the *work of breathing*. The actual amount of energy expended is kept to a minimum by the ease with which lungs can expand. This ease of expansion is referred to as lung compliance. Lung compliance is aided by a detergent-like substance called surfactant, which is produced by type 2 alveolar cells found within the alveoli. Surfactant reduces the surface tension that occurs where alveoli meet pulmonary capillary blood flow in the lobule, thereby reducing the amount of energy required to inflate the alveoli. Despite these opposing forces, the work of breathing accounts for less than 5% of total body energy expenditure. However, many lung diseases can affect lung compliance and airway resistance and therefore increase work of breathing (Lumb & Thomas, 2020).

Control of Breathing

The rate and depth of breathing are controlled by respiratory centres within the medulla oblongata and pons in the brainstem. The respiratory centres contain specialised chemoreceptors that continually analyse carbon dioxide levels within cerebrospinal fluid (CSF). As levels of CO_2 rise, the phrenic and intercostal nerves are innervated and messages are sent to the diaphragm and intercostal muscles instructing them to contract. Rising levels of carbon dioxide detected by central chemoreceptors are the main stimulus for inspiration. As it relies solely on fluctuations in carbon dioxide, this stimulus for inhalation is often referred to as the *hypercapnic drive*. Another set of chemoreceptors referred

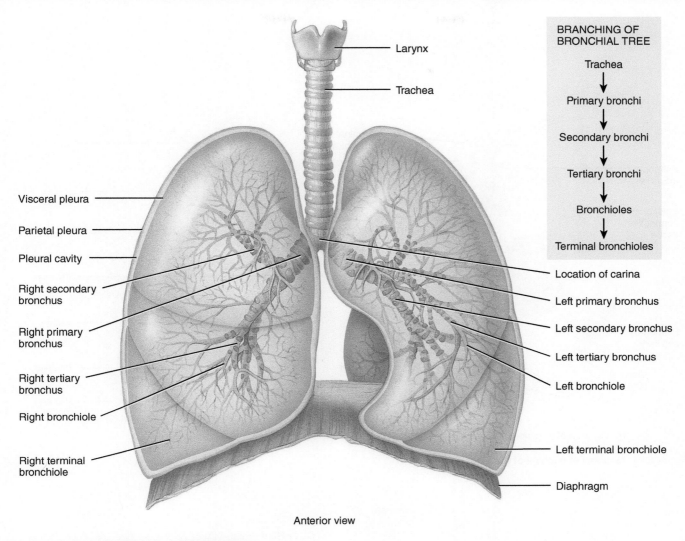

BRANCHING OF BRONCHIAL TREE

Trachea
↓
Primary bronchi
↓
Secondary bronchi
↓
Tertiary bronchi
↓
Bronchioles
↓
Terminal bronchioles

Larynx

Trachea

Visceral pleura

Parietal pleura

Pleural cavity

Right secondary bronchus

Right primary bronchus

Right tertiary bronchus

Right bronchiole

Right terminal bronchiole

Location of carina

Left primary bronchus

Left secondary bronchus

Left tertiary bronchus

Left bronchiole

Left terminal bronchiole

Diaphragm

Anterior view

Figure 27.3 Anatomy of the lower respiratory tract.

to as the peripheral chemoreceptors are found in the aorta and carotid arteries. The peripheral chemoreceptors analyse levels of O_2 as well as CO_2. If arterial levels of oxygen fall or arterial levels of carbon dioxide rise, the glossopharyngeal and vagus nerves are innervated, stimulating further contraction. As this stimulus for inhalation relies mostly on fluctuations of oxygen, it is referred to as the *hypoxic drive*.

Although breathing is essentially a subconscious activity, the rate and depth of breathing can be controlled voluntarily or even stopped all together, when swimming under water for example. Breathing can also be influenced by state of mind. The inspiratory area of the respiratory centres can be stimulated by both the limbic system and hypothalamus, two areas of the brain responsible for processing emotion. Fear, anxiety or even the anticipation of stressful activities can cause an involuntary increase in the rate and depth of breathing. Other factors that can affect breathing include pyrexia and pain. Because breathing is largely beyond an individual's control, any changes in respiration rate are clinically significant (Rolfe, 2019).

Jot This Down

Take some time to think about how anxiety may influence a patient's respiratory rate and consider what nursing interventions you could utilise in order to help reduce anxiety and breathlessness.

479

External Respiration

External respiration is the diffusion of oxygen from the alveoli into pulmonary circulation and the diffusion of carbon dioxide from pulmonary circulation to the alveoli. This diffusion of oxygen and carbon dioxide occurs because gas molecules always move from areas of high concentration to low concentration.

Each lobule of the lung has its own arterial blood supply, which originates from the pulmonary artery. The pulmonary artery originates from the right ventricle of the heart and the blood within it has been collected from systemic circulation. It is therefore low in O_2 and relatively high in CO_2. The amount (and therefore pressure)

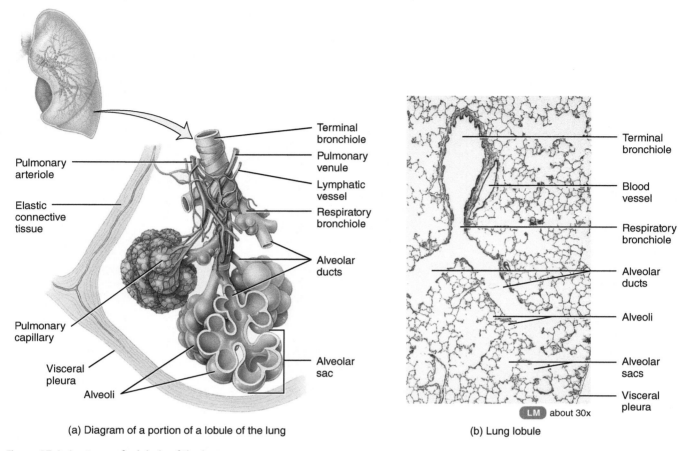

(a) Diagram of a portion of a lobule of the lung

(b) Lung lobule

Figure 27.4 Anatomy of a lobule of the lungs.

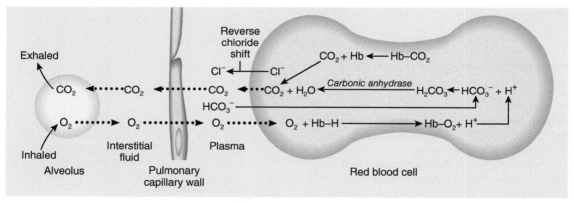

Exchange of O$_2$ and CO$_2$ in pulmonary capillaries (external respiration)

Figure 27.5 External respiration – exchange of oxygen and carbon dioxide within the lungs.

of oxygen in the alveoli is far greater than in the passing arterial blood supply. Oxygen therefore moves passively through the wall of the alveoli, through interstitial fluid, through the capillary wall and into pulmonary circulation, a process which takes approximately 0.25 seconds. This swift process ensures that the blood flowing away from the lungs, through the pulmonary veins and towards the left atrium of the heart has been reoxygenated.

While oxygen is being transferred from the alveoli into blood, carbon dioxide makes the reverse journey. Because there is less carbon dioxide in the alveoli than in pulmonary circulation, carbon dioxide diffuses through the capillary wall, across interstitial space and through the wall of the alveoli ready to be exhaled (Figure 27.5).

Transport of Gases

Both oxygen and carbon dioxide are transported in blood plasma and attached to haemoglobin within erythrocytes (red blood cells). The vast majority of oxygen, around 98.5%, is transported attached to haemoglobin in the erythrocyte. Each erythrocyte contains around 280 million haemoglobin molecules, each of which has the potential to carry four oxygen molecules. Pulse oximetry is used to measure how much oxygen is attached to haemoglobin. This measurement, commonly referred to as oxygen saturation, is the percentage of haemoglobin in arterial blood that is carrying oxygen. In health, this measurement should be around 97–99% and should be expressed as SpO_2. The remaining 1.5% of oxygen is dissolved in blood plasma; this volume of oxygen is measured in terms of the pressure it exerts (kilopascals – kPa). This measurement of oxygen is expressed as PaO_2 and in health should be around 11–13.5 kPa.

Just like oxygen, a small amount of carbon dioxide, around 10%, is transported in plasma. The normal pressure levels of carbon dioxide in arterial plasma ($PaCO_2$) are between 4.5 and 6 kPa. Carbon dioxide is also transported attached to haemoglobin (Hb), although only around 20% is transported that way. Nevertheless, haemoglobin has a greater affinity for carbon dioxide than oxygen. Within the tissues, this facilitates the release of oxygen as carbon dioxide is being created. The remaining 70% of carbon dioxide combines with water to form carbonic acid.

Jot This Down

Take some time to think about how anaemia (a blood condition) may affect distribution of oxygen throughout the body. How might a low haemoglobin (Hb) level change a nurse's view of their patient's oxygen saturation reading.

Respiratory Disease

Respiratory disease has many causes. Some diseases, such as tuberculosis, pneumonia, influenza and COVID-19, are contracted via the inhalation of a pathogen. Others are associated with lifestyle or occupation. Chronic obstructive pulmonary disease and lung cancer, for example, are caused by smoking and pneumoconioses develop due to consistent exposure to harmful occupational agents. Other respiratory diseases, such as asthma, are associated with allergy or hyper-responsive airways. Some respiratory diseases are described as being obstructive because airflow in and out of the respiratory system is obstructed. Other respiratory conditions are referred to as being restrictive, in that airflow through the lungs is restricted. This section will explain the pathophysiology of respiratory infection, obstructive and restrictive lung disorders, lung cancer and respiratory conditions associated with the pleura.

Nursing Fields High Prevalence of Respiratory Illness: Learning Disabilities

Respiratory illness is a leading cause of mortality for people with a learning disability, with pneumonia accounting for 41% of premature deaths (NHS, 2021a). This may be explained by swallowing, eating and gastrointestinal problems among some people with multiple needs. Often, people living with learning disabilities experiencing difficulties in communicating their symptoms and nurses need to be vigilant for evidence of irritability, lack of engagement or communication, lethargy and loss of appetite when conducting a respiratory assessment.

Respiratory Failure

Respiratory failure occurs when the individual's respiratory disease has altered lung function to the extent that they are no longer able to maintain adequate oxygen saturation levels and are at risk of developing hypoxaemia (Paramothayan, 2019). In some instances, the individual's condition deteriorates to the extent that they are also no longer able to expel excess carbon dioxide. Respiratory failure therefore is categorised into two types, labelled type 1 and type 2. Individuals unable to maintain adequate oxygen levels are said to be in respiratory failure type 1, whereas those patients who deteriorate further and are unable to expel excess carbon dioxide are described as being in respiratory failure type 2.

Respiratory Failure Type 1

Hypoxaemic patients, with oxygen saturation readings lower than 90% or a partial pressure oxygen reading of less than 8 kPa, will be in respiratory failure type 1. Ultimately the management of patients in respiratory failure type 1 will focus on treating the underlying causative respiratory disease/disorder and the provision of oxygen to maintain oxygen saturations above 92% or 88% in patients with chronic carbon dioxide retention (British Thoracic Society, 2017).

Respiratory Failure Type 2

Respiratory disease often leads to increased respiratory effort (work of breathing) and therefore acute exacerbation of any underlying respiratory disease can lead to respiratory muscle fatigue. Respiratory muscle fatigue may lead to shallow and weak rate and depths of breathing. A reduction in ventilation leads to an increased accumulation of carbon dioxide (hypercapnia). Elevated arterial blood carbon dioxide levels above 6 kPa will lead to a reduction in arterial blood pH. For this reason, respiratory failure type 2 is also referred to as respiratory acidosis. Ventilation is the only way to reduce carbon dioxide. Patients with respiratory failure type 2 may be placed on a mechanical ventilator, which will increase their depth of breathing. One common example of mechanical ventilation used in both hospital and community settings is non-invasive positive pressure ventilation (NIPPV). NIPPV is delivered by a special portable machine that delivers breaths via a flexible hose and special facial mask (British Thoracic Society and Intensive Care Group, 2016).

Red Flag

Individuals with chronic obstructive pulmonary disease (COPD) may have chronic carbon dioxide retention, which may desensitise their hypercapnic drive. As a result, such patients may rely more on their hypoxic drive. Excess oxygen may reduce respiratory effort and care should therefore be taken when administering oxygen to individuals with COPD.

Respiratory Assessment

A comprehensive respiratory assessment must include an initial assessment, to establish severity of condition and to detect early signs of acute deterioration, and a patient history. It must include assessment of respiratory rate, an inspection of presentation, peak flow and oxygen saturation, cough and expectoration and a patient history.

Respiratory Rate

On initial assessment, the nurse must establish the severity of the patient's condition. Respiratory rate plays a pivotal role in this assessment. An adult's respiratory rate should remain between 12 and 20 respirations per minute at rest (Hill & Annesley, 2020). Any changes in respiratory rates are clinically significant. Respiration rates less than 12 respirations per minute at rest can be associated with opiate overdose, respiratory fatigue, central nervous system depression and hypothermia. Raised respiratory rates greater than 24 respirations per minute (tachypnoea) at rest are a key indicator of acute deterioration and are associated with high mortality rate. When assessing respiratory rate, the nurse must also observe for signs of respiratory distress or dyspnoea (difficulty in breathing). Dyspnoea may be positional and patients may find relief if positioned appropriately. Table 27.1 details some common positional dyspnoeas.

Assessing respiratory rate alone will not provide all the necessary information for a comprehensive respiratory assessment. In order to fully establish a patient's respiratory status, the nurse must check the following.

- Respiratory rate in respirations per minute.
- Inspiration/expiration ratio.
- Shape of chest expansion.
- Added sounds.
- Use of accessory muscles.

Many conditions can alter a patient's breathing pattern and if the nurse identifies such a change, they are better placed to plan appropriate and effective care. Table 27.2 details some of the more common abnormal respiratory patterns and their causes.

Care, Dignity and Compassion

Patients often describe dyspnoea (difficulty in breathing) as breathlessness. Breathlessness can be very distressing and frightening. Breathless patients will therefore require comfort, reassurance and explanations of oxygen and prescribed respiratory medication.

Jot This Down

One of the signs of severe life-threatening asthma is an inability to speak in sentences. In terms of a comprehensive respiratory assessment, why is it so important for the nurse to establish whether their patient can speak in complete sentences?

What to Do If . . . The patient coughs when I'm counting respirations

It is important that your record of respiratory rate is accurate and if your patient does cough while you are counting respirations, once the patient has recovered, you should restart your respiration count from the beginning – remember to count for a full minute.

Inspection

On initial assessment, the nurse must observe for signs of cyanosis, a bluish or darkish hue, which could indicate hypoxaemia. Peripheral cyanosis, visible in the fingers and toes and mucous membranes, is caused by deficient delivery of oxygenated blood to the peripheries. Because peripheral cyanosis is caused by deficient blood flow, its presence does not necessarily indicate hypoxaemia. Heart failure, vascular occlusion or vasoconstriction (as occurs in extreme cold conditions, for example) could be the root cause of peripheral cyanosis. Central cyanosis, which is visible in the lips and mouth, occurs when haemoglobin is carrying reduced amounts of oxygen, often as a result of respiratory failure. Oxygen saturations usually have to fall below 90% (or plasma levels of <8 kPa) before central cyanosis is visible. However, patients with anaemia may not display signs of cyanosis as their depleted levels of haemoglobin may still be fully saturated with oxygen. Central cyanosis may also be present in patients with polycythaemia, a condition which stimulates the overproduction of erythrocytes (red blood cells).

Other useful assessments include the presence of finger clubbing, an indicator of respiratory disease, and halitosis, which could be a sign of respiratory tract infection. Cyanosis can be difficult to detect on people with darker skin tones and healthcare professionals should inspect the nails, eyes, lips and gums where changes are more easily observed.

Peak Flow and Spirometry

Other essential assessments include peak expiratory flow rate (PEFR) or 'peak flow' and spirometry. PEFR is the force of expiration in litres per minute and it measures the extent of airway resistance. An inability to meet a predicted value based on age, sex and height could indicate increased airway resistance as occurs during an asthma attack (Hill, 2019). Spirometry is a measurement of expiration, which is used by the multidisciplinary team to measure the extent of airway obstruction. Spirometry measures the force and volume of a maximum expiration after a full inspiration, a volume referred to as forced vital capacity (FVC). The volume expired by the patient after 1 second

Table 27.1 Common types of positional dyspnoea, their characteristics and causes.

POSITIONAL DYSPNOEA	CHARACTERISTICS	CAUSES
Orthopnoea	Difficulty in breathing when lying down	Severe asthma Congestive heart failure Chronic obstructive pulmonary disease Mitral valve disease
Trepopnoea	Patient is more comfortable lying on their side	Congestive heart failure
Platypnoea	Difficulty in breathing sitting up	Arterial hypoxaemia

Table 27.2 Abnormal respiratory patterns, their characteristics and causes.

RESPIRATORY PATTERN	CHARACTERISTICS	CAUSES
Cheyne–Stokes respiration	Cyclic respiratory pattern which fluctuates between fast and slow respiratory rates interspersed with periods of apnoea	Increased intercranial pressure Severe heart failure Renal failure Drugs overdose Meningitis End of life
Tachypnoea	Rapid, shallow, respiratory rate greater than 24 respirations per minute	Exercise Fear and anxiety Respiratory failure Acidosis and alkalosis Brainstem lesions
Bradypnoea	Slow respiratory rate, less than 10 respirations per minute	Drug overdose Brainstem lesions Coma
Hypoventilation	Slow, shallow respiration rate	Drug overdose Anaesthesia Chest, pleuritic pain
Hyperventilation Kussmaul breathing (air hunger)	Increase in respiration rate and depth	Exercise Fear and anxiety Respiratory failure Acidosis and alkalosis Brainstem lesions
Biot respiration	Irregular rate and depth interspersed with periods of apnoea	Head trauma Brain abscesses Heat stroke Spinal meningitis Encephalitis

is called forced expiratory volume in the first second (FEV_1). By comparing FEV_1 with FVC, the FEV_1:FVC ratio, the severity of airway obstruction can be ascertained. An FEV_1:FVC ratio of less than 75% is indicative of an obstructive airways disease (Heuer & Scanlon, 2018).

Oxygen Saturations

Pulse oximeters are used to gauge the percentage of arterial haemoglobin that carries oxygen. This reading is called 'oxygen saturation' (SpO_2), which in health should be between 97% and 99%. The pressure of oxygen dissolved in arterial plasma (PaO_2) provides practitioners with a more accurate reflection of oxygenation. Arterial blood gas readings are attained by placing a sample of the patient's arterial blood into a blood gas analyser. A printed or visual result is produced, which provides information on arterial blood pH, carbon dioxide, bicarbonate and oxygen. An oxygen saturation produced via blood gas analysis is referred to as SaO_2.

Red Flag

Certain factors affect the accuracy of pulse oximeter readings. Tremors, anaemia, polycythaemia, cold extremities, acrylic nails and nail varnish can all jeopardise an accurate reading. For this reason, SpO_2 should only be used in conjunction with other nursing observations.

Table 27.3 Characteristics of sputum and possible diagnoses.

SPUTUM CHARACTERISTICS	POSSIBLE DIAGNOSIS
Mucoid: clear, grey or white	Asthma Chronic bronchitis
Serous: watery or frothy	Pulmonary oedema
Mucopurulent: yellowish Purulent: dark green/yellow Foul smelling	Respiratory tract infection
Bloodstained	Carcinoma Pulmonary embolism Trauma

Cough and Sputum

Ascertaining the nature of a patient's cough can aid diagnosis. A cough which is worse during the night, for example, is an indicator of asthma whereas a cough with a sudden onset suggests inhalation of a foreign object. If the patient has a productive cough, samples should be collected for microscopy and culture in order to determine the presence of infection. However, the colour and consistency of a patient's sputum could provide a clue to the nature of the patient's respiratory problem (Table 27.3). The presence of blood is also significant as haemoptysis may indicate the presence of tuberculosis.

Patient History

A patient history could help the multidisciplinary team to establish the nature and severity of the patient's respiratory complaint. Childhood respiratory disease could be a precursor to adult lung problems and a family history could determine potential congenital respiratory disease. Use of vaccines could rule out influenza and recent foreign travel may suggest tropical disease. The patient's age could also help determine diagnosis. Respiratory distress in individuals under 30 years would suggest asthma, pneumothorax or cystic fibrosis whereas dyspnoea in those over 50 years is more likely to suggest cancer, pneumoconiosis or COPD. Information on appetite and weight changes can also be of significance. Reduced appetite and weight loss are indicative of lung cancer and tuberculosis, for example.

It is also vital that the nurse establishes some of the patient's living conditions and lifestyle choices. Many respiratory infections are exacerbated by damp and overcrowded living conditions; the patient may also work in a profession that exposes them to irritant substances such as paint fumes, dust and animal dander. The latter is also true of patients with pets; a common example is pneumoconiosis caused by the dander of birds, a condition called bird fancier's lung. Smoking is the major cause of COPD and lung cancer and an accurate smoking history could aid diagnosis, as could the volume of alcohol the patient drinks. Alcoholism is a risk factor for the development of pneumonia.

If the patient already uses respiratory medication, it is vital that the nurse establishes the patient's compliance and in some instances their inhaler technique. Medication misuse or omissions may exacerbate their respiratory problems.

Medicines Management

It is very important that patients with asthma use their steroid inhaler regularly and that their inhaler technique is correct. The regular correct use of steroid inhalers is recognised as a major way of preventing/reducing the incidence of asthma attacks.

The Nursing Associate Provide and monitor care

Nursing associates must provide compassionate, safe and effective support to people experiencing respiratory distress.

This is of particular relevance to Platform 3 – Provide and monitor care.

Specifically:

3.2   demonstrate and apply knowledge of body systems and homeostasis, human anatomy and physiology, biology, genomics, pharmacology, social and behavioural sciences when delivering care

3.8   demonstrate and apply an understanding of how people's needs for safety, dignity, privacy, comfort and sleep can be met

3.12 demonstrate the knowledge and skills required to support people with commonly encountered symptoms including anxiety, confusion, discomfort and pain

3.16 demonstrate the ability to recognise the effects of medicines, allergies, drug sensitivity, side effects, contraindications and adverse reactions.

Source: NMC (2018a)

Professional and Legal Issues

Comprehensive respiratory assessment is closely aligned to many of the key aspects of the NMC's Code (NMC, 2018b).

Prioritise people

Breathlessness is beyond an individual's control and can be a frightening experience.

Respiratory illness is, therefore, a psychological as well as a physiological experience.

Prioritise alleviation of symptoms of breathlessness and promote comfort and well-being.

Practise effectively

Nurses should only recommend or implement interventions to alleviate breathlessness and promote comfort that are based on the best available evidence.

It is vital that all members of the multidisciplinary team are aware of patient preferences and the nature of the patient's respiratory dysfunction.

Preserve safety

You must continue to assess and re-evaluate individuals experiencing respiratory difficulties.

Ensure you are adequately knowledgeable to undertake a respiratory assessment. If you are not, seek guidance from a more experienced member of staff.

Nurses must act if they feel a patient's breathlessness is not being adequately assessed or dealt with.

Bronchodilator therapies, including inhaled, oral, subcutaneous or intravenous, must be administered safely and nurses must keep an accurate record of all drugs administered.

Promote professionalism and trust

Ensure that the well-being of patients is promoted and protected.

Nurses must work at all times to ensure that patients requiring assistance with alleviating breathlessness have a positive experience.

Practice Assessment Document

Able to make a holistic, person-centred and systematic assessment of physical, emotional, psychological, social, cultural and spiritual needs

By demonstrating the ability to carry out a thorough and holistic respiratory assessment, you can reassure practice assessors that you are looking at the impact of respiratory illness on an individual's physical and psychological well-being. When discussing respiratory assessment with your practice assessor, highlight the need to explore your patient's psychosocial history and its impact on their health and well-being.

Platform 3 – Assessing needs and planning care

Registered nurses prioritise the needs of people when carrying out a respiratory assessment.

Specifically:

3.2   demonstrate and apply knowledge of body systems and homeostasis, human anatomy and physiology, biology, genomics, pharmacology and social and behavioural sciences when undertaking full and accurate person-centred nursing assessments and developing appropriate care plans

(Continued)

3.4   understand and apply a person-centred approach to nursing care, demonstrating shared assessment, planning, decision making and goal setting when working with people, their families, communities and populations of all ages

3.15   demonstrate the ability to work in partnership with people, families and carers to continuously monitor, evaluate and reassess the effectiveness of all agreed nursing care plans and care, sharing decision making and readjusting agreed goals, documenting progress and decisions made

3.16   demonstrate knowledge of when and how to refer people safely to other professionals or services for clinical intervention or support.

Respiratory Tract Infection

Influenza

Influenza is a highly infectious viral respiratory infection. Although it can be contracted at any time of year, in the northern hemisphere influenza is most predominantly active during the winter months. New strains of the influenza virus could lead to global outbreaks or pandemics.

Pathophysiology

The influenza virus is found within aerosol particles and droplets produced by via coughs and sneezes. The viruses that cause influenza are called orthomyxoviruses. Typically there are three types of orthomyxovirus: type A, type B and type C. Type A influenza viruses are found in both animals and humans. The outer lipoprotein layer of the type A influenza virus normally displays three proteins: haemagglutinin, neurominidase and M2. There are 16 identified subtypes of haemagglutinin and nine subtypes of neurominidase and type A influenza viruses are classified according to which subtypes are present. For example, the most common variation of type A influenza is H1N1, which displays haemagglutinin subtype 1 and neurominidase subtype 1 on its outer lipoprotein layer.

As type A influenza viruses are found in both animals and humans, infections can occasionally transfer between species. Examples of this are 'swine flu', which is a variation of the H1N1 virus, and 'avian' or 'bird flu', which is caused by a H5N5 influenza strain. Type B influenza viruses are considered less severe than type A and almost exclusively affect humans only. Type C infections are thought to cause only mild or even asymptomatic infections (Hubert & VanMeter, 2018).

Individuals Most at Risk

- Children under 5 years old.
- The older person.
- Immunocompromised individuals.
- Women in the later stages of pregnancy.
- People with chronic health conditions, such as diabetes, respiratory, heart and renal disease, cancer.
- Young adults (in flu pandemics).

Signs and Symptoms

- Fever (sudden onset).
- Headache.
- Sore throat.
- Muscle aches.
- Dry cough.
- Weakness and malaise.
- Fatigue.
- Loss of appetite.

Nursing Care and Management

Mild and uncomplicated cases of influenza can be treated with rest, antipyretic drugs (e.g. paracetamol and ibuprofen) and plenty of fluids. For those living with or caring for individuals with influenza, effective hand washing and appropriate use of tissues should be promoted. Antiviral drugs such as oseltamivir or zanamivir are usually only prescribed to vulnerable or 'at-risk' individuals. Such drugs are also mainly reserved for prophylactic cover for people with 'risk factors' who have been exposed to contagious individuals. The most effective management strategy for the minimisation of the impact of influenza is vaccination.

Complications/Prognosis

Infection with influenza viruses can lead to the development of lower respiratory tract infections such as bronchitis and pneumonia. Mortality rates for influenza arise almost exclusively as a result of secondary lower respiratory tract infection. The development of lower respiratory tract infections is greater in individuals with suppressed immune systems or those living with chronic illnesses such as diabetes, respiratory disease, heart disease or renal disease.

Coronavirus (COVID-19)

Coronaviruses cause mild to severe respiratory infections in humans. Around 15% of common colds are caused by coronaviruses and are considered mild infections. However, the following novel (or new) strains of coronavirus can cause severe respiratory disease associated with a high mortality rate.

- Severe acute respiratory syndrome (SARS–CoV). First identified 2002.
- Middle East respiratory syndrome (MERS-CoV). First identified 2012.
- Severe acute respiratory syndrome (SARS-CoV-2). First identified 2019.

SARS-CoV-2 is commonly referred to COVID-19 and this section will address its impact and related nursing care.

Pathophysiology

The COVID-19 virus is spread from person to person via airborne respiratory droplets. Once inside the respiratory tract, the virus binds to nasal epithelial cells. For a short while, individuals are asymptomatic but highly infectious. After a few days, the virus spreads through the upper respiratory tract, causing a dry cough, pyrexia and lethargy. In around 20% of infected individuals, the infection migrates into the lower respiratory tract, triggering an immune response. The subsequent inflammation results in respiratory distress syndrome (Parasher, 2020).

Individuals Most Vulnerable to Severe Ill Health

Everyone is at risk of contracting COVID-19 because it is a novel (new) virus and as such there is very little immunity within communities. Risk of severe illness increases with age and obesity, and pregnancy and ethnicity are also significant risk factors However, people who fit the following criteria are at the greatest risk of developing severe symptoms or death.

- Individuals living with long-term illness.
- People living with dementia.
- People with type 1 or type 2 diabetes.
- People who have had an organ transplant.
- People living with cancer or undergoing chemotherapy.
- Individuals who are immunosuppressed.
- People on dialysis.
- People with liver disease.
- An adult with Down syndrome (NHS, 2021b).

Signs and Symptoms

There are many reported symptoms of COVID-19 but the following are the most common.

- Fever.
- Cough.
- Shortness of breath and difficulty in breathing.
- Loss of taste or smell.
- Muscle aches.
- Headache.
- Sore throat.
- Fatigue.
- Nausea and vomiting.
- Diarrhoea.

Nursing Care and Management

The location of care of people with COVID-19 is dependent on the severity of infection. Only 20% of individuals will experience severe symptoms and the majority of people will have mild-to-moderate symptoms and will be able to self-care at home. Indicators of severe and critical COVID-19 include development of pneumonia, respiratory distress, respiratory rates greater than 30 respirations per minute and oxygen saturations of less than 90%. People with symptoms of severe to critical COVID-19 should be cared for in hospital environments.

Key care considerations include the following.

- Isolation and staff to wear full personal protective equipment (PPE) (see Chapter 16).
- Oxygen therapy.
- Non-invasive ventilation.
- Steroid therapies.
- Antibiotics (British Medical Journal Best Practice, 2021).

Complications/Prognosis

While for many people, COVID-19 is a mild illness (around 17–20% of people infected with COVID-19 experience no symptoms at all), around 1 in 5 will become seriously unwell and require hospital admission. COVID-19 is associated with a high mortality rate and in 2020, 72 178 people died after testing positive for the virus in England, a death rate of 128.2 per 100 000 people (Public Health England, 2021). While the majority of people who recover from COVID-19 make a full recovery, a small proportion continue to suffer symptoms weeks and months after testing negative. This phenomenon, known as long COVID, is not well understood but it is estimated that around 660 000 people in the UK had experienced symptoms that lasted longer than 12 weeks after becoming

---

> **Box 27.1 Common reported symptoms associated with long COVID**
>
> | | |
> |---|---|
> | Fatigue | Dizziness |
> | Shortness of breath | Pins and needles |
> | Chest pain or chest tightness | Joint pain |
> | Loss of memory or difficulty in concentrating | Depression and anxiety |
> | | Tinnitus/earache |
> | Insomnia | Nausea, loss of appetite |
> | Palpitation | Abdominal pain, diarrhoea |
> | Loss of smell and taste | Rashes |
> | Pyrexia, sore throat, headaches | |
>
> *Source:* NHS (2021b).

---

unwell with COVID-19. Box 27.1 lists symptoms that are currently associated with long COVID.

Pulmonary Tuberculosis

Pulmonary tuberculosis (TB) is a lower respiratory tract infection, which is predominantly caused by *Mycobacterium tuberculosis*, an air-borne slow-growing bacillus. The disease typically has two phases: primary and secondary infection.

Pathophysiology

During the primary infection, lymphocytes and neutrophils congregate at the infection site, usually in the upper lobes. The bacilli are then trapped and walled off by fibrous tissue. During the primary infection phase of TB, the infected individual is often asymptomatic and unaware they have TB. Until secondary infection, the bacilli remain latent and the individual is not infective. Secondary infection occurs at some point after primary infection and is caused by re-exposure to TB or another form of bacteria. The bacilli are then reactivated and quickly multiply and as a result the patient soon becomes symptomatic and infectious. Bacilli are very hardy and can survive trapped in fibrous tissue for long periods. Individuals can remain unaware that they have TB for many years.

Over recent years, many strains of TB have become resistant to the first-line pharmacological treatments (see Nursing Care and Management). TB that is resistant to one or more first-line drug is referred to as multidrug-resistant TB (MDR-TB). Some strains of TB have become resistant to almost all the second-line pharmacological treatments, a condition called extensively drug-resistant TB (XDR-TB).

Risk Factors

According to the National Institute for Health and Care Excellence (2016), there are *under-served* and *high-risk* groups of people that are vulnerable to exposure to tuberculosis. People at high risk could be any age and from any ethnic background and include:

- Close contact with infected individuals
- New migrants from countries with high prevalence of TB
- People with suppressed immune system (i.e. human immunodeficiency virus [HIV])
- People from 'under-served' groups (see below).

Certain individuals are 'under-served' by healthcare providers and therefore are at greater risk of infection. People considered under-served include:

- People who are homeless and their children
- People who misuse substances and their children
- People in prison and their children
- Vulnerable migrants and their children
- Children from Gypsy or Travelling communities.
- Looked-after children.

Signs and Symptoms
- Chronic cough.
- Haemoptysis.
- Weight loss.
- Pyrexia.
- Fatigue.
- Night sweats.

Investigations
Tuberculosis is diagnosed by chest X-ray and a sputum acid-fast staining test, which determines the presence of the bacteria that cause TB. Further culture tests will determine whether the species of TB infection is *Mycobacterium tuberculosis*, *Myobacterium bovis* or *Myobacterium africanum*. The possible outcomes of both tests are:

- Acid-fast bacillus positive/culture positive – these individuals are infective and will need to isolate
- Acid-fast bacillus negative/culture positive – in the majority of cases these individuals may not be infective
- Acid-fast bacillus negative/culture negative – although the test is negative, patients displaying symptoms may still receive a positive diagnosis of TB from their X-ray.

Nursing Care and Management
Tuberculosis is treated with a 6-month medication regimen that consists of 2 months of rifampicin, isoniazid, pyrazinamide and ethambutol followed by a further 4 months of rifampicin and isoniazid. Infective patients will remain infective for the first 2 weeks of treatment.

In the main, individuals with TB are cared for in the community, with the main nursing focus being infection control, prevention and compliance with drug therapy. Only if there is a medical or socioeconomic reason should be the patient being cared for in hospital. Individuals with suspected pulmonary tuberculosis who need to remain in hospital must be cared for in a side room and away from wards where immunosuppressed patients are cared for. Individuals with confirmed tuberculosis must be risk assessed for the presence of MDR-TB and if found to be MDR-TB positive or at high risk of having MDR-TB, they should be nursed in a negative pressure isolation room (NICE, 2016).

Health Promotion and Discharge
Pulmonary TB remains very treatable if the individual complies with the 6-month drug regimen. Non-compliance could lead to the further development of MDR-TB or even XDR-TB. As XDR-TB is resistant to almost all pharmacological treatment options, it has a high mortality rate. It is for this reason that support with drug compliance is the key to the control and prevention of TB (Paramothayan, 2019).

Primary Care Tuberculosis

As most patients with TB are cared for in the community, the main focus of the primary care nurse will be:

- Advice and support with treatment compliance
- Advice on the reduction of transmission
- Restriction on visitors, especially young children, in the first 2 weeks of treatment
- Remaining away from work or study for the first 2 weeks of treatment
- Avoiding public transport
- Cough etiquette – covering mouth when coughing or sneezing and disposing of tissues safely. Maintaining good hand hygiene
- Maintaining good ventilation at home by opening windows.

Jot This Down
Individuals with infective TB will be nursed in isolation. Take time to consider how this might impact on their psychological well-being.

Case Study Shirley

Shirley is a 42-year-old homeless woman, who currently lives in a city centre hostel. She has been suffering with a productive cough for many months. One morning she coughed up a small amount of blood, which she found frightening. She decided to go to a local accident and emergency department, where she explained to one of the nurses that in addition to the haemoptysis, she had also been experiencing night sweats. Shirley is admitted to hospital with suspected pulmonary tuberculosis. She is commenced on oral rifampicin, isoniazid, pyrazinamide and ethambutol and placed in isolation. After 10 days, Shirley begins to feel much better and is prepared for discharge back into the community.

What advice and guidance should the nurse provide for Shirley?

Pneumonia
Pneumonia is a lower respiratory tract infection caused by a variety of inhaled pathogens. Infected individuals mainly contract pneumonia by inhaling a bacterium, virus or fungus. Pneumonia can also be caused by the aspiration of secretions such as vomitus or by transmission of blood-borne pathogens from an infection elsewhere in the body.

Pneumonia is classified by its cause and location. Some pneumonia infections are localised in one or more lobes and are described as lobular while other pneumonia infections are spread or diffuse throughout the lungs. Pneumonia can also be categorised as community or hospital acquired (nosocomial). Community-acquired pneumonia can be caused by both viral and bacterial infections. Although individuals with chronic cardiorespiratory disorders are at risk, healthy individuals can also be affected, especially following an influenza infection. Hospital-acquired (nosocomial) infection affects patients with low immune resistance, the older person or an immunosuppressed individual, for example. Such cases are normally caused by bacterial infections, such as *Klebsiella pneumoniae* or *Pseudomonas aeruginosa* (Hubert & VanMeter, 2018).

Pathophysiology

Lobular Pneumonia Pneumonia infections which are localised to one or more lobes are referred to as lobular infections. Lobular pneumonia is normally caused by bacterial infections such as *Streptococcus pneumoniae* or *Pneumococcus* and it is associated with a sudden and acute onset of symptoms. Once the invading bacteria reach the lower respiratory tract beyond the trachea, they multiply quickly in the warm and moist confines of deep lung tissue. The resultant inflammatory response causes vasodilation of capillaries, which causes the alveoli to fill with debris and exudate. The exudate quickly fills with neutrophils, erythrocytes and fibrin and a solid mass called consolidation soon forms. Consolidation in the alveoli disturbs external respiration and less oxygen diffuses from the alveoli into pulmonary circulation.

Bronchopneumonia Bronchopneumonia infections are characterised by diffuse affected areas, which are spread throughout both lungs. It has an insidious onset with symptoms developing over time. Many pathogens can cause bronchopneumonia but the infection normally starts in the bronchi before spreading to the alveoli. The resultant alveoli inflammation causes a build-up of exudate within the alveoli walls and gaseous exchange is reduced as a result.

Legionnaire's Disease Community- and hospital-acquired pneumonias caused by *Legionella pneumophila*, a Gram-negative bacterium found in natural water sources, are called Legionnaire's disease. Contraction of Legionnaire's disease usually occurs when people come into contact with infected in-built water sources, i.e. cooling systems. Legionnaire's disease causes severe lung consolidation with lung necrosis and has a high risk of mortality.

Primary Atypical Pneumonia (PAP) PAP is caused by bacterial or viral infection. Bacterial infections include *Chlamidiya pneumoniae* and *Mycoplasma pneumoniae*, miniscule bacteria found within the upper respiratory tract. Viral pneumonia usually occurs as a result of influenza, when upper respiratory tract inflammation descends into the lower respiratory tract causing diffuse inflammation of interstitial tissue rather than the alveoli themselves.

Pneumocystis carinii Pneumonia (PCP) PAP is considered to be a fungal infection, which when inhaled causes alveolar necrosis and diffuse interstitial tissue inflammation. The alveoli fill with exudate as a result. PCP is an opportunistic and often deadly infection, which preys on individuals with weakened immune systems (Hubert & VanMeter, 2018).

Risk Factors

- Age – the very young and the older person are at greater risk.
- Individuals living with chronic cardiorespiratory disease.
- Immunocompromised individuals.
- Smoking.
- Alcoholism and drug abuse.

- Intubation – unconscious patients have increased risk of developing pneumonia.
- Patients at risk of aspiration – i.e. patients with dysphagia, stroke, gastric reflux.

Signs and Symptoms

- Hypoxaemia.
- Tachypnoea and dyspnoea.
- Tachycardia.
- Pyrexia – in response to bacterial infection.
- Dehydration – pyrexia causes fluid loss; also the body loses humidified air on expiration.
- Reduced lung expansion – consolidation makes it hard to expand the lungs and breathing becomes difficult.
- Pain – inflammation could spread to the pleura, causing pleuritic pain.
- Productive cough – the exudate present in the alveoli often produces rusty-coloured sputum.
- Lethargy.

Investigations

A diagnosis of pneumonia can be confirmed by sputum cultures that identify the causative agent. An X-ray can also establish the extent of lung tissue damage. In order to determine the severity of pneumonia, healthcare professionals use an assessment called CURB-65 (or CRB-65), which is a six-point range that determines how unwell an individual is. A point is scored for the presence of new **c**onfusion, blood **u**rea greater than 7 mmol, a **r**espiratory rate greater than 30 respirations per minute, low **b**lood pressure (i.e. systolic blood pressure less than 90 mmHg or diastolic blood pressure less than 60 mmHg) and an individual greater than **65** years of age. A score of 3 or more indicates a severe pneumonia infection (NICE, 2019a).

Nursing Care and Management

Pneumonia is treated by the administration of antibiotics and most cases will be nursed in the community. Nurses caring for individuals with pneumonia in hospital settings play a vital role in the early detection of deterioration. The main care goals include the following.

- Safe administration of prescribed antibiotics.
- Safe administration of prescribed oxygen – to correct hypoxaemia and maintain oxygen saturations above 90%.
- Patient positioning – placing the patient in an upright position will promote diaphragm and intercostal muscle activity and enhance ventilation.
- Establishing and minimising pain levels – to make the patient more comfortable and enhance respiratory effort.
- Temperature management – safe administration of antipyretic agents, such as aspirin, paracetamol or ibuprofen, electric fans, reducing bed clothing.
- Close monitoring of vital signs – respiration rate greater than 30 respirations per minute, new hypotension (systolic less than 90 mmHg or diastolic less than 60 mmHg) and new mental confusion could indicate life-threatening pneumonia in those aged 65 years or more. Vital signs should therefore be recorded hourly until the patient's condition stabilises.
- Fluid balance – as the patient may be dehydrated. A minimum of 2.5 L every 24 hours is required. Fluids may be administered intravenously if required.
- Communication – to reduce anxiety and promote comfort.

Jot This Down

Patients with pneumonia may experience pleuritic pain. Take time to consider how pain may affect pulmonary ventilation and gaseous exchange.

Primary Care Pneumonia

A sizeable proportion of patients with pneumonia will be cared for in the community and the main focus of primary care is ensuring a safe recovery. The nurse should ensure that the following occur.

- Regular assessment – nurses should be alert for the signs of acute deterioration.
- Review patient's well-being regularly.
- Refer any patient with signs of severe or life-threatening pneumonia to a hospital setting.
- Advise the patient to use over-the-counter cough suppressants.
- Advise the patient to increase fluid intake and ensure they maintain a good diet.
- Monitor for side-effects of antibiotic therapy, such as diarrhoea.
- Advise patients to refrain from smoking.
- Treat pleuritic pain with over-the-counter paracetamol or non-steroidal anti-inflammatory drugs.
- Ensure family or significant others know who to contact should there be deterioration (Moreton, 2019).

Obstructive Lung Disorders

Obstructive lung disorders obstruct airflow in and out of the lungs. In conditions such as asthma and COPD, the obstruction to airflow occurs as a result of airway narrowing and an increased resistance to airflow, especially during expiration. For many, airway resistance can be overcome by increasing respiratory muscle work. However, normal passive expiration may not be enough to promote adequate alveoli emptying and resultant forced expiration may generate high intrathoracic pressures that force smaller airways to close, trapping air in the chest.

Asthma

Asthma is a chronic inflammatory airways disease. Individuals with asthma are said to have hypersensitive or hyper-responsive airways resulting in periods of reversible inflammation and constriction in the bronchi and bronchioles. Increased airway inflammation and constriction obstructs airways, resulting in a characteristic wheeze.

Pathophysiology

The pathophysiology of asthma is complicated and intricate. The walls of the bronchi and bronchioles contain smooth muscle and are lined with mucus-secreting glands and ciliated cells. Large quantities of mast cells are found adjacent to the airways' blood supply. Once stimulated, the mast cells release several cytokines (chemical messengers), which cause physiological changes to the linings of the bronchi and bronchioles. The three main cytokines are histamine, kinin and prostaglandin, which cause smooth muscle contraction, increased mucus production and increased capillary permeability. As a result, the airways soon narrow and become flooded with mucus and fluid leaking from blood vessels (see Figure 27.2). As the airways become obstructed, it becomes increasingly difficult to breathe and to expectorate the mucus. If left unresolved, fatigue can occur, resulting in a weak and inadequate respiratory effort which may cause hypoxaemia and in severe cases hypercapnia.

Risk Factors

Individuals with asthma periodically react to triggers, substances or situations that would not normally cause airway inflammation and constriction. Traditionally, individuals are divided into those who suffer with extrinsic asthma and those with intrinsic asthma. In individuals with extrinsic asthma, airway inflammation is thought to occur because of hypersensitive reactions associated with allergy, i.e. pollen, dust mites or foodstuffs. Intrinsic asthma is linked to hyper-responsive reactions to other forms of stimuli, infection, sudden exposure to cold, exercise, stress or cigarette smoke, for example. In reality, many people have a combination of both intrinsic and extrinsic asthma and irrespective of the causative agents, the pathophysiological changes, symptoms and treatments are the same.

Signs and Symptoms

The main symptoms of asthma are:

- Cough, which may become productive with thick sticky mucus
- Dyspnoea and chest tightness
- Wheeze
- Peak flow less than predicted or best.

Acute-severe asthma is suspected when one or more of the following is present.

- Peak flow 33–50% of predicted or best.
- Dyspnoea accompanied by an inability to complete sentences in one breath.
- Tachypnoea – respiratory rate 25 breaths per minute or higher.
- Tachycardia – heart rate greater than 110 beats per minute.

Life-threatening asthma is suspected when any of the following is present in an individual with acute-severe asthma.

- Peak flow less than 33% of predicted or best.
- Oxygen saturation (SpO_2) less than 92%.
- Silent chest.
- Poor respiratory effort.
- Cyanosis.
- Hypotension.
- Exhaustion.
- Arrhythmia.
- Altered conscious level.
- Arterial oxygen level (PaO_2) less than 8 kPa.

Near-fatal asthma is deemed to be present when arterial carbon dioxide ($PaCO_2$) is high (hypercapnia) or mechanical ventilation with raised pressures is required (British Thoracic Society and Scottish Intercollegiate Guidelines Network, 2019).

Diagnosis/Investigations

A diagnosis of asthma is complicated by the fact that many of its main symptoms are also indicators of other respiratory diseases. The British Thoracic Society and Scottish Intercollegiate

Guidelines Network (2019) state that clinicians should consider a diagnosis of asthma based on the following.

- Episodic problems with asymptomatic periods and variable peak flow readings.
- Symptoms of wheeze, cough, chest tightness and breathlessness that fluctuate.
- Family history of atopic conditions, such as eczema, dermatitis and rhinitis.

Nursing Care and Management

Nurses must be aware of the signs of severe and life-threatening asthma (see above). Asthma is reversible and care should focus on close monitoring and health promotion. The main care goals are as follows.

- Continuous monitoring of vital signs until the patient has stabilised.
- Safe administration of prescribed oxygen to maintain oxygen saturation above 92%.

- Safe administration of prescribed bronchodilators and steroids – to alleviate dyspnoea (see Tables 27.4 and 27.5).
- Communication – as speaking requires a constant flow of air, patients experiencing acute breathlessness are only able to talk for very short periods before the need to breathe interrupts them. The patient's inability to complete a sentence therefore provides a sensitive measure of the extent of their respiratory distress.
- Regular peak flow (PEFR) measurement.
- Comfort and reassurance – dyspnoea can be a traumatic experience and fear and anxiety also promote hyperventilation. Listen to the patient's anxieties and provide continuous explanations for the multidisciplinary team's actions.
- Sputum collection – yellow or green sputum can indicate infection.
- Health promotion – avoidance of triggers, compliance with prescribed pharmacological therapies, smoking cessation and weight reduction in obese patients may reduce the frequency of asthma attacks.

Table 27.4 Summary of corticosteroids used in the treatment of respiratory disease. *Source*: Adapted from Joint Formulary Committee (2021).

INDICATION	CORTICOSTEROIDS[a]	ROUTE	CARE CONSIDERATIONS
Prophylaxis and reduction of frequency of exacerbations	Beclametasone Budesonide Fluticasone Mometasone Furoate	Inhaler	Inhaled corticosteroids can cause hoarseness, loss of voice and candidiasis. Advise patients to rinse out their mouths after taking these inhalers
Exacerbation	Prednisolone Hydrocortisone	Oral Intravenous	Steroids can irritate the lining of the stomach and gastrointestinal tract. Many preparations of prednisolone have an enteric coat, but patients must be advised not to take them on an empty stomach

[a] Corticosteroids are potent anti-inflammatory agents. They are used to reduce bronchial hyperactivity in patients with asthma, chronic obstructive pulmonary disease and other respiratory diseases where reversibility is present. The table shows the main corticosteroids currently utilised.

Table 27.5 Summary of bronchodilator therapies given in asthma and chronic obstructive pulmonary disease. *Source*: Adapted from Joint Formulary Committee (2021).

TYPE	ACTIONS	EXAMPLES	ROUTES	CARE CONSIDERATIONS
Beta-2 agonists	Mimic the actions of adrenaline. Beta-2 agonists stimulate beta-2 receptor sites in the airways, promoting rapid bronchodilation within 15 minutes, with a duration of 4–8 hours, depending on dose	Salbutamol Terbutaline Fenoterol Salmeterol	Inhaler Nebuliser Oral Subcutaneous	Patient must be advised of the potential for tachycardia and hand tremor
Anticholergenics	Block the action of acetylcholine, a neurotransmitter released by the parasympathetic nervous system. Acetylcholine promotes bronchoconstriction and bronchial secretion. Peak bronchodilator effects occur within 1 hour, with a duration similar to beta-2 agonists	Ipratropium bromide	Inhaler Nebuliser	Patient may need frequent mouthwashes May cause dry mouth and a bitter taste
Methylxanthines	Increase concentration of intracellular cyclic adenosine monophosphate (cAMP). Increased cAMP causes bronchodilation	Theophylline	Oral Intravenous (as aminophylline)	Optimal effects occur when plasma theophylline levels are between 10 and 20 mg/L. Regular blood tests are required

Red Flag

Singular or infrequent peak flow measurements will not accurately reflect the patient's status; PEFR should be measured every 15–30 minutes after commencement of treatment until conditions stabilise. PEFR can also be used to measure the effectiveness of bronchodilator therapy; therefore, PEFR should be measured before and after inhaled or nebulised beta-2 agonists at least 4 times a day throughout their stay in hospital.

Primary Care Asthma

The major role of the primary care nurse will be to promote self-management in patients with asthma. This should entail:

· A written personalised action plan
· Regular reviews by trained asthma clinicians
· Regular reviews of medication usage to optimise treatments
· Promotion of appropriate use of steroid inhalers
· Advice on smoking cessation.

Medicines Management Side-effects of steroids

Patients taking oral or intravenous steroids will need careful monitoring as they can cause a range of significant side-effects. Nurses should advise patients of the potential for the following to occur and monitor for their presence.

· Osteoporosis.
· Diabetes.
· Weight gain.
· Increased body hair.
· Altered mood and irritability.

Practice Assessment Document

Applies knowledge of basic pharmacology and how medicines interact with body systems
Knowing how bronchodilator therapies work and their major side-effects is vital if patient safety is to be maintained. Demonstrating an understanding of the differences between inhaled and nebulised bronchodilators and their major side-effects may enable your practice assessor to establish your safety in the administration of medicines. When looking to achieve skills associated with pharmacology, explaining the impact bronchodilators have on people is a good way of demonstrating knowledge.

Chronic Obstructive Pulmonary Disease

Chronic obstructive pulmonary disease (COPD) is often defined as airflow obstruction that is progressive, not fully reversible and does not change markedly over several months. Patients diagnosed with chronic bronchitis and emphysema are collectively regarded as having COPD. People with chronic asthma sufferers are also at risk of developing fixed airway obstruction as their airways become remodelled over time.

Pathophysiology

Emphysema Emphysema is the permanent enlargement of the airspaces beyond the terminal bronchiole and the destruction of the elastic recoil of the alveolar wall. This degeneration of lung tissue is thought to be related to the action of destructive enzymes called proteases. Proteases are released from neutrophils and macrophages during respiratory infections. To minimise the effects of proteases, lung tissue produces a substance called alpha-1-antitrypsin, which counteracts the destructive action of protease. Individuals with emphysema produce less effective alpha-1-antitrypsin and alveolar destruction is allowed to continue unabated. This reduction in the efficacy of alpha-1-antitrypsin is predominantly caused by smoking. The resultant damaged alveoli lack the elastic recoil that is required for exhalation, often resulting in overinflation and air trapping. Increased intrathoracic pressure pushes the diaphragm downwards, disturbing its natural concave shape and making breathing difficult. Respiratory infections can easily develop as individuals find it increasingly difficult to expectorate secretions. Also further destruction of the alveolar walls and nearby capillaries will result in reduced surface area for external respiration, rendering the patient at risk of hypoxaemia and hypoxia (Hubert & VanMeter, 2018).

Chronic Bronchitis Chronic bronchitis is defined as the presence of a productive cough lasting for 3 months in each of 2 consecutive years when other pulmonary and cardiac causes of cough have been ruled out (Devereux, 2017). Chronic bronchitis is characterised by increased mucus production and damaged bronchial cilia in the bronchi. The increase in mucus stimulates airway irritant receptors, resulting in a chronic cough. Constant airway irritation produces inflammation and a thickening of the bronchial wall and the destruction of cilia makes mucus clearance difficult and mucus collects and blocks the smaller airways as a result. The individual is then susceptible to further infections which cause yet more irritation and inflammation. Over time, increasing numbers of airways become blocked, reducing external respiration. The increased mucus production and cilia dysfunction found in chronic bronchitis occur in response to a constant bombardment of inhaled pollutants such as cigarette smoke (MacNee & Rabinovich, 2017).

Risk Factors

· Smoking.
· Occupational pollutants.
· Alpha-1-antitrypsin syndrome.

Signs and Symptoms

· FEV_1 less than predicted.
· Dyspnoea, due to airway obstruction and air trapping.
· Productive cough.
· Reduced exercise tolerance.
· Cor pulmonale – chronic hypoxia causes hypertension within the pulmonary circulation. Eventually, the right ventricle becomes enlarged and fails, ultimately leading to peripheral oedema.

Diagnosis/Investigations

The symptoms of chronic asthma may be indistinguishable from COPD and many COPD patients may also have asthma. Accurate diagnosis therefore is often problematic (Devereux, 2017).

However, the following investigations can help MDT members when a diagnosis of COPD is being considered.

- Spirometry – an FEV_1 of less than 80% of FVC indicates airway obstruction.
- Chest X-ray (to exclude other respiratory disease, e.g. lung cancer).
- CT scan – can determine the presence of emphysema.
- Arterial blood gas readings – to determine precise levels of arterial oxygen and carbon dioxide.
- Sputum examination.
- Lung function tests.
- Exercise testing.

Nursing Care and Management

The main management goals for COPD are:

- Smoking cessation advice.
- Education on prescribed oxygen and bronchodilator therapies – to maximise relief of breathlessness.
- Immunisation – to minimise frequency of exacerbations.
- Dietary advice – severe weight loss is a feature of both emphysema and chronic bronchitis.
- Pulmonary rehabilitation.
- Promotion of self-management techniques – COPD is associated with high levels of anxiety and depression.

Care, Dignity and Compassion

COPD is a diverse and varied condition and its management requires a holistic approach centred upon self-management and symptom control. Wherever possible, the patient should be cared for in their own home.

Health Promotion and Discharge

Chronic obstructive pulmonary disorder is a chronic irreversible respiratory disorder. Management should focus on holistic interventions for self-management and symptom control. Patients with COPD can experience exacerbations of their condition and the following are factors that may lead to hospitalisation (NICE, 2018).

- Inability to cope at home.
- Severe breathlessness.
- Deteriorating condition.
- Confined to bed or limited activity.
- Cyanosis.
- Worsening peripheral oedema.
- Impaired levels of consciousness.
- Already receiving long-term oxygen therapy.
- Poor social circumstances.
- Acute confusion or disorientation.
- Rapid onset of exacerbation.
- Acute co-morbidities (e.g. heart disease or diabetes).
- SpO_2 less than 90%.
- Raised arterial carbon dioxide levels ($PaCO_2$) greater than 7 kPa or adverse changes in arterial blood pH.
- Chest X-ray changes.

What the Experts Say Smoking Cessation

'Smoking tobacco poses serious health risks to not only the individual who smokes but those around them, through second-hand smoke. Smoking is the most preventable cause of death and consequently smoking cessation, in which nurses help people to achieve abstinence from smoking, is a key public health goal.'
Adelle, community nurse

Primary Care Chronic Obstructive Pulmonary Disease

One of the major care concepts for patients living with COPD is the maintenance of well-being through the active utilisation of coping strategies. This should entail:

- Regular reviews by trained respiratory clinicians
- Regular reviews of medication usage to optimise treatments
- Promotion of self-management and coping strategies
- Referral to pulmonary rehabilitation services
- Advice on smoking cessation.

Bronchiectasis

Bronchiectasis is chronic airway dilation caused by chronic inflammation. The inflammation is often caused by inadequate clearance of micro-organisms or chronic/frequent lung infections. Patients with bronchiectasis have thickened bronchial walls and suffer frequent sputum production and chronic coughs.

Pathophysiology

In bronchiectasis, lung function deteriorates over many years. Patients become locked in a vicious cycle of infection, inflammation and damage. Once infected, the patient's inability to clear the pathogen leads to an inflammatory response. While inflammation protects against pathogens, in patients unable to clear micro-organisms the inflammatory response may become chronic and counterproductive, leading to bronchial wall damage and irreversible dilation of the airways.

Risk Factors/Causes

The most common causes of bronchiectasis are cystic fibrosis and childhood respiratory disease. Other risk factors include viral, bacterial and fungal infections, aspiration, airway obstruction, inhalation of toxic substances and immunosuppression. Many lung conditions such as COPD, allergic bronchopulmonary aspergillosis (ABPA) and bronchiolitis can lead to the development of bronchiectasis, as can autoimmune or inflammatory disorders such as coeliac disease, rheumatoid arthritis, systemic lupus erythematosus, ankylosing spondylitis, Sjogren syndrome and inflammatory bowel disease. Patients with congenital conditions may also be at risk, especially cardiorespiratory disease such as Marfan syndrome, tracheobronchomegaly, pulmonary ciliary dyskinesia or chest wall deformities such as scoliosis and pectus excavatum.

Signs and Symptoms

- Chronic cough.
- Increased sputum production.
- Lethargy and malaise.
- Haemoptysis.
- Weight loss.
- Dyspnoea.
- Chest pain.
- Bronchospasms.
- Reduced exercise tolerance.
- Reduced respiratory function.

Diagnosis/Investigations

- Lung function test.
- Spirometry.
- Sputum cultures.
- Chest X-ray.
- CT scan.

Nursing Care and Management

Bronchiectasis is a chronic respiratory condition and as with other chronic respiratory diseases such as COPD, its management requires a holistic approach centred upon clearance of secretions, self-management and symptom control. The main management goals are:

- Physiotherapy to assist the clearance of mucus and other respiratory secretions
- Pulmonary rehabilitation
- Antibiotic therapy
- Education on prescribed oxygen and bronchodilator therapies – to maximise relief of breathlessness
- Promotion of self-management techniques.

What the Experts Say Pulmonary Rehabilitation

'Pulmonary rehabilitation (PR) programmes involve physical exercises and advice and guidance from a range of healthcare professionals. They are an excellent way of enabling people living with respiratory disease to manage their condition and well-being.

People who undertake pulmonary rehab find that they have more stamina and feel fitter. They feel able to cope with breathlessness and tell us that they feel better psychologically as well. I recommend pulmonary rehabilitation to all my patients who are struggling to cope with their long-term respiratory condition.'

Halima, respiratory nurse specialist

The Nursing Associate Being an accountable professional

Nursing associates act in the best interests of people living with a long-term respiratory condition, putting them first and providing nursing care that is person centred, safe and compassionate.

This is of particular relevance to Platform 1 – Being an accountable professional. Specifically:

1.4   demonstrate an understanding of, and the ability to, challenge or report discriminatory behaviour

---

1.11   provide, promote, and where appropriate advocate for, non-discriminatory, person-centred and sensitive care at all times. Reflect on people's values and beliefs, diverse backgrounds, cultural characteristics, language requirements, needs and preferences, taking account of any need for adjustments

1.12   recognise and report any factors that may adversely impact safe and effective care provision.

Source: NMC (2018a)

Restrictive Lung Disorders

Restrictive lung disorders impede lung expansion and therefore reduce ventilation. The causes of reduced lung expansion can be either anatomical or pathological. Anatomical causes include conditions such as kyphosis or scoliosis, in which malformations of the spine affect the individual's ability to fully expand their thorax. Pathological reasons for reduced lung expansion include diseases which affect lung compliance, cause muscle paralysis or restrict lung function. Poliomyelitis, amyotrophic lateral sclerosis and botulism, for example, can cause respiratory muscle paralysis, whereas muscular dystrophy causes muscle weakness.

Respiratory diseases that restrict lung function are in the main chronic conditions caused by the inhalation of industrial or commercial pollutants. This group of respiratory diseases is called the pneumoconioses. The different types of pneumoconiosis are often named after the job or pastime that generated them, for example coal worker's lung or bird fancier's lung (Hubert & VanMeter, 2018).

Practice Assessment Document

Able to promote health and well-being, self-care and independence by teaching and empowering people to make choices in coping

There is a correlation between well-being and the ability to cope with a long-term respiratory problem. Demonstrating to your practice assessor that you are able to listen to your patients and devise care plans that recognise coping strategies and promote well-being will reassure them that you are able to work with your patients to promote self-care.

Lung Cancer

Lung cancer is the development of tumours within the lung tissue. The vast majority of lung cancers (95%) develop in bronchial tissue. There are two major types of bronchial carcinoma: *non-small cell* and *small cell*. Non-small cell carcinomas account for 70% of all lung cancers. Non-small cell carcinomas can be subdivided again into *squamous cell carcinomas*, and *adencarcinmoas or large cell carcinomas*. Squamous cell carcinomas tend to develop within the larger bronchi whereas other non-small cell carcinomas are found in the smaller airways, making them much harder to detect. Small cell carcinomas tend to grow near the large bronchi and are the most aggressive bronchial carcinomas.

Pathophysiology

Smoking or other irritants (e.g. asbestos) damage the pseudostratified epithelium of lung tissue, rendering the lungs more susceptible to inflammation. Certain chemicals present within cigarette smoke are carcinogenic and promote the development of tumours within the lung tissue.

Risk Factors

- Smoking.
- Passive smoking.
- Exposure to occupational pollutants.

Signs and Symptoms

The following signs and symptoms are considered indicative of lung cancer in patients who smoke tobacco.

- Cough.
- Haemoptysis.
- Dyspnoea.
- Chest pain.
- Wheeze.
- Finger clubbing.

Diagnosis/Investigations

- Biopsy.
- CT scan.
- Chest X-ray.

Nursing Care and Management

- Safe administration of chemotherapy.
- Minimisation of impact of the side-effects of chemotherapy.
- Working with the patient and family to adjust to the diagnosis of cancer through good communication and teaching skills.
- Providing practical information and support for patients and families.

Care, Dignity and Compassion

The diagnosis of cancer is likely to be a traumatic event not only for the person concerned but also for their family and friends. It is vital the nurse does not make assumptions about their patient and ensures that the planning and implementation of care are based on the individual.

Primary Care Lung Cancer

For patients with a new diagnosis of lung cancer, primary care nurses must ensure that the following aspects of care are provided.

- Represent the patient's perspective – ensure that the patient's opinions and wishes are accounted for in all care decisions.
- Ascertain whether or not the patient has any advance decisions relating to their care and treatment.
- Refer all patients with a cancer diagnosis to a relevant clinical nurse specialist.
- Promote self-care and coping strategies, e.g. coping with breathlessness.

- Monitor the patient for the following signs of deterioration or co-morbidities.
  - Weight loss.
  - Loss of appetite.
  - Dysphagia.
  - Depression.
  - Increased breathlessness.
- Ensure patient receives adequate pain relief.
- Monitor and treat cough with opiate analgesia.

Source: NICE (2019b)

Case Study

Isaac is a 63-year-old solicitor who lives with his wife Mercy, who is a primary school teacher. They have four grown-up children who no longer live with them and they now share a detached house in the suburbs. They share passions for ballroom dancing and gardening. They also both play an active role in their local church. Isaac has smoked tobacco since he was 18 years old and while he has cut down considerably in recent years, he still smokes 10–15 cigarettes a day.

For many weeks, Isaac has had an annoying, irritating cough that would not go away. His GP has also prescribed two courses of antibiotics for chest infections in the past 6 months. He has also noticed that he often experiences chest pain, particularly when he walks, coughs or laughs. Mercy has noticed that he appears to have lost weight and gets breathless easily when they are dancing. She is also worried that he seems more tired and lethargic than normal normally and lacks his usual energy and enthusiasm for church activities.

What may Isaac's symptoms and smoking history be indicative of?

Pleural Disorders

Any condition that causes air or fluid to collect in the pleural space can cause the lung to partially or fully collapse. Air within the pleural space is referred to as a pneumothorax. Fluid within the pleural space is called a pleural effusion, unless the fluid in question is blood in which case the patient has a haemothorax.

Pathophysiology

The pleural space between parietal and visceral pleura only contains a thin film of fluid. Any air or extra fluid entering the pleural space will cause the lung to collapse, resulting in areas of underventilated lung, a phenomenon known as atelectasis. The surface area for external respiration is dramatically reduced and the patient may develop hypoxaemia (West & Luks, 2021). Trauma is the major cause of a haemothorax but cancer can also cause bleeding within lung tissue.

Pleural effusions can originate from within lung tissue or from pulmonary circulation. Exudate pleural effusions occur from within lung tissue as a result of respiratory disease. Diseases such as lung cancer, pneumonia or tuberculosis cause inflammation which can result in the generation of fluid that is rich in protein and white blood cells. Inflammation also increases pulmonary capillary permeability, allowing fluid to leak out of blood vessels and into the pleural space. Transudate pleural effusions occur as a result of a problem within the circulation. Conditions such as left ventricular heart failure cause increases in capillary hydrostatic pressure, forcing fluid out of circulation and into the pleural space. A decrease in blood osmotic pressure will also force fluid from blood vessels into the pleural space. Causes of reduced blood osmotic pressure include hypoproteinaemia.

The presence of air in the pleural cavity is called a pneumothorax. Pneumothoraces are mainly caused by trauma or chronic respiratory disease. However, some individuals have a congenital defect or bleb within the alveolar wall which can rupture spontaneously.

Risk Factors
- Trauma.
- Chronic respiratory disease.
- Heart failure.
- Tall young men are at particular risk of spontaneous pneumothorax.

Signs and Symptoms
Small pneumothoraces may not produce noticeable symptoms but the larger the pneumothorax, the more severe the symptoms. Patients with a pneumothorax may present with the following.
- Sudden-onset dyspnoea.
- Sharp pleuritic pain, which is worse on inspiration.
- Chest auscultation may reveal diminished or absent breath sounds.

Diagnosis/Investigations
The main investigation for pleural disorders is a chest X-ray; the critically ill patient, however, may require a CT scan. Oxygen saturations and arterial blood gas readings can also determine deterioration.

Nursing Care and Management
Chest drains are often used to assist the reinflation of the affected lung. The main care responsibilities therefore centre on the monitoring of both the patient and the drain and attention should be paid to the following.
- Patient positioning – placing the patient in an upright position will encourage drainage and aid expansion of the thorax.
- Position of the chest drain – the drainage bottle must be kept below the patient's chest level to prevent fluid re-entering the pleural space. Coiled and looped tubing should also be avoided as it can impede drainage flow and lead to a tension pneumothorax or surgical emphysema.
- Continuous monitoring of vital signs until the patient's condition stabilises.
- Close monitoring of the chest drain.
  - Swinging – the level of the fluid in the underwater seal of the drain should fluctuate between 5 and 10cm when the patient breathes. Absence of swinging could indicate a kink or blockage in the tubing.
  - Bubbling – bubbles often occur in the water seal bottle without suction when the patient exhales or coughs. Continuous bubbling indicates a problem with the drain or insertion site.
- Administration of prescribed analgesics for pleuritic pain.

- Accurate recording of drainage – the health professional should note the quantity, colour and consistency of the fluid being drained.

Infection control – the insertion site should be checked daily for signs of infection, i.e. redness, swelling, heat, pain and discharge (adapted from Davison et al., 2021).

Complications/Prognosis
Patients with pleural disorders are at risk of developing an empyema, which is the formation of pus in the pleural effusion.

Health Promotion and Discharge
Prior to discharge, patients should be taught how to clean and re-dress their chest insertion wound site if they are deemed able to do so. Patients should also be advised to continually assess the chest drain insertion site for signs of infection. If a suture is in place, arrangements must be made for removal by a community nurse.

Platform 4 – Providing and evaluating care

Registered nurses take the lead in providing evidence-based, compassionate and safe nursing interventions when caring for an individual living with respiratory disease.

Specifically:

4.1 demonstrate and apply an understanding of what is important to people and how to use this knowledge to ensure their needs for safety, dignity, privacy, comfort and sleep can be met, acting as a role model for others in providing evidence based person-centred care

4.5 demonstrate the knowledge and skills required to support people with commonly encountered physical health conditions, their medication usage and treatments, and act as a role model for others in providing high-quality nursing interventions when meeting people's needs

4.8 demonstrate the knowledge and skills required to identify and initiate appropriate interventions to support people with commonly encountered symptoms including anxiety, confusion, discomfort and pain

4.14 understand the principles of safe and effective administration and optimisation of medicines in accordance with local and national policies and demonstrate proficiency and accuracy when calculating dosages of prescribed medicines.

Conclusion

Respiratory disease places a heavy burden on the health services and it also impacts negatively on individuals, families and communities. Its impact on services, however, can be reduced by good-quality, holistic nursing care. Whatever the cause, be it life-style choice, occupation or opportunistic infection, the main areas of care include clearance of secretions, enhancement of ventilation and oxygenation as well as more psychosocial factors such as self-management and coping mechanisms for those living with chronic respiratory illness and breathlessness. Patients living with or experiencing respiratory disorders are at risk of acute exacerbation and deterioration. The nurse must therefore be skilled in accurate comprehensive respiratory assessment.

Key Points

- The absorption of oxygen and disposal of carbon dioxide follow four distinct processes.
- The rate and depth of breathing are dependent upon:
  - Optimum oxygen and carbon dioxide levels
  - Hydrogen ions
  - Body temperature
  - Cognitive well-being.
- Changes in respiratory rate at rest are always clinically significant.
- An inability to maintain adequate oxygen levels constitutes respiratory failure, of which there are two types.
  - Respiratory failure type 1 – inadequate oxygenation.
  - Respiratory failure type 2 – inadequate oxygenation and hypercapnia.
- Nurses must be able to perform a comprehensive respiratory assessment, which must include the following.
  - Respiratory rate.
  - Assessment of symmetry and depth of breathing.
  - Listening for added sounds.
  - Oxygen saturation.
- Nurses must be able to recognise the cardinal signs of acute deterioration in patients with acute respiratory disorders.
  - Tachypnoea.
  - Tachycardia.
  - Hypoxia and hypoxaemia.
  - Cool clammy peripheries.
  - Confusion, disorientation, agitation.
  - Loss of consciousness.
- Patients living with long-term respiratory disorders will require psychosocial care strategies that promote self-care and coping interventions.

References

British Medical Journal Best Practice (2021) *Coronavirus 2019 (COVID-19) and differentials.* https://bestpractice.bmj.com/info/coronavirus_covid-19/ (accessed December 2021).

British Thoracic Society (2017) Guideline for emergency oxygen use in adult patients. *Thorax,* 72, supplement 1.

British Thoracic Society and Intensive Care Group (2016) BTS/ICS guidelines for the ventilatory management of acute hypercapnic respiratory failure in Adults. *Thorax,* 71, supplement 2.

British Thoracic Society and Scottish Intercollegiate Guidelines Network (2019) *SIGN 158 British Guideline on the Management of Asthma: A National Clinical Guideline.* BTS, London.

Davison, L., McSporran, W., Brady, G., Forsythe, C. & Ratcliffe, O. (2021) Respiratory care, CPR and blood transfusion. In: S. Lister, J. Hofland, H. Grafton & C. Wilson (eds) *The Royal Marsden Manual of Clinical Nursing Procedures,* 10th edn. Wiley, Chichester.

Devereux, G.S. (2017) Definition, epidemiology and risk factors. In Currie, G.P. (ed.) *ABC of COPD,* 3rd edn. Wiley-Blackwell, Chichester.

Heuer, A.J. & Scanlan, C.L. (2018) *Wilkins' Clinical Assessment in Respiratory Care,* 8th edn. Elsevier, St Louis, MO.

Hill, B. (2019) Measuring peak flow in adults with asthma. *British Journal of Nursing,* 28(14), 924–926.

Hill, B. & Annesley, S.H. (2020) Monitoring respiration rates in adults. *British Journal of Nursing,* 29(1), 12–16.

Hubert, R.J. & VanMeter, K.C. (2018) *Gould's Pathophysiology for the Health Professions,* 6th edn. Elsevier, St Louis, MO.

Joint Formulary Committee (2021) *British National Formulary,* 81st edn. Pharmaceutical Press, London.

Lumb, A. & Thomas, C. (2020) *Nunn and Lumb's Applied Respiratory Physiology,* 9th edn. Elsevier, Edinburgh.

MacNee, W. & Rabinovich, R.A. (2017) *Pathology and Pathogenesis.* In: G.P. Currie (ed.) *ABC of COPD,* 3rd edn. Wiley-Blackwell, Chichester.

Moreton, T. (2019) Challenges of diagnosing and managing pneumonia in primary care. *Nursing Times,* 115(9), 34–38.

National Institute for Health and Care Excellence (2016) *Tuberculosis.* NG33. NICE, London.

National Institute for Health and Care Excellence (2018) *Chronic obstructive pulmonary disease in over 16s: diagnosis and management.* NICE, London.

National Institute for Health and Care Excellence (2019a) *Pneumonia (community acquired): antimicrobial prescribing.* NICE, London.

National Institute for Health and Care Excellence (2019b) *Lung cancer: diagnosis and management.* NICE, London.

NHS (2021a) *Learning Disability Mortality (death) Review Programme.* www.england.nhs.uk/learning-disabilities/improving-health/mortality-review/ (accessed December 2021).

NHS (2021b) *Coronavirus (COVID-19).* www.nhs.uk/conditions/coronavirus-covid-19/ (accessed December 2021).

Nursing & Midwifery Council (2018a) *Standards of proficiency for nursing associates.* www.nmc.org.uk/globalassets/sitedocuments/education-standards/nursing-associates-proficiency-standards.pdf (accessed December 2021).

Nursing & Midwifery Council (2018b) *The Code: professional standards of practice and behaviour for nurses, midwives and nursing associates.* www.nmc.org.uk/standards/code/ (accessed December 2021).

Paramothayan, S. (2019) *Essential Respiratory Medicine.* Wiley-Blackwell, Chichester.

Parasher, A. (2020) Covid-19: current understanding of its pathophysiology, clinical presentation and treatment. *British Medical Journal,* 97. 312–320.

Public Health England (2021) *COVID-19 confirmed deaths in England (to December 2020): Report.* www.gov.uk/government/publications/covid-19-reported-sars-cov-2-deaths-in-england/covid-19-confirmed-deaths-in-england-to-31-december-2020-report (accessed December 2021).

Rolfe, S. (2019) The importance of respiratory rate monitoring. *British Journal of Nursing,* 28(8), 504–508.

West, J.B. & Luks, A.M. (2021) *Pulmonary Pathophysiology: The Essentials,* 10th edn. Wolters-Kluwer, Philadelphia.

Wheeldon, A. (2020) The respiratory system. In: I. Peate & S. Evans (eds) *Fundamentals of Anatomy and Physiology for Nursing and Healthcare Students,* 3rd edn. Wiley-Blackwell, Chichester.

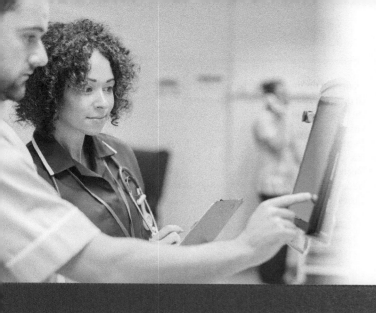

28

The Person with a Gastrointestinal Disorder

Louise McErlean

Ulster University, UK

Learning Outcomes

On completion of this chapter you will be able to:

- Describe the pathophysiology of commonly occurring disorders of the gastrointestinal system, and the accessory organs
- Understand the assessment of the gastrointestinal system
- Identify the nursing care and treatment required for commonly occurring gastrointestinal disorders
- Describe the complications associated with commonly occurring gastrointestinal disorders
- Consider the medications given for commonly occurring digestive system conditions

Proficiencies

NMC Proficiencies and Standards:

- Assess and document a health history for persons who present with or are at risk of gastrointestinal dysfunctions
- Involve the patient to formulate a person-centred care plan
- Assess physical and psychological care needs of those in their care
- Evaluate the nursing care delivered to those living with elimination disorders
- Work in partnership with the interprofessional team for the safe delivery of care in all settings

 Visit the companion website at www.wiley.com/go/peate/nursingpractice3e where you can test yourself using flashcards, multiple-choice questions and more.

Nursing Practice: Knowledge and Care, Third Edition. Edited by Ian Peate and Aby Mitchell.
© 2022 John Wiley & Sons Ltd. Published 2022 by John Wiley & Sons Ltd.
Companion website: www.wiley.com/go/peate/nursingpractice3e

Introduction

The gastrointestinal (GI) system is also known as the digestive system or alimentary canal or tract. The main function of the GI system is to break down nutrients from the diet into the essential materials required by the cells of the body so that they can carry out their specific functions. The GI system does this by digesting the dietary intake, absorbing the required nutrients obtained from the process of digestion and eliminating any unwanted material. The digestive system is a long tube that begins in the mouth and ends at the anus. It is supported by the accessory organs – the salivary glands, pancreas, gallbladder and liver (Figure 28.1). As a large system, there is opportunity for disorder along its vast length. This chapter will focus on commonly occurring conditions of the gastrointestinal tract.

Peate & Evans (2020) provide much detail regarding the anatomy and physiology of the gastrointestinal tract, so the reader is advised to consult this text.

Peptic Ulcer

A peptic ulcer is an area of damage to the inner lining (mucosa) of the stomach and/or the duodenum (Figure 28.2). In some cases, the ulceration can penetrate to the muscle layer. A bacterium,

Helicobacter pylori, and the use of non-steroidal anti-inflammatory drugs (NSAIDs) are the main causes of peptic ulcers. There is an increased risk of developing a peptic ulcer associated with smoking, excessive alcohol intake and obesity (McErlean, 2021). Peptic ulcer can affect people of any age, including children, but the condition is most common in people over 60 years of age. Both sexes are equally affected by peptic ulcer. Peptic ulcers can occur secondary to the psychological stress associated with critical illness and major trauma.

Medicines Management

Make a list of medicines that are non-steroidal anti-inflammatories (NSAIDs) and note if they are a prescription-only medication or available over the counter at the pharmacist.

Pathophysiology

'Peptic ulcer' is a term used to define the formation of an ulcer in the stomach and/or the duodenum. Ulcers in the stomach (gastric ulcers) are found in any part of the stomach but are most commonly seen on the 'lesser curve' (see Figure 28.2) and duodenal ulcers are found after the pyloric sphincter. The ulcers may be superficial or deep, affecting all layers of the mucosa extending into the muscle layer. Ulcers can be single or multiple.

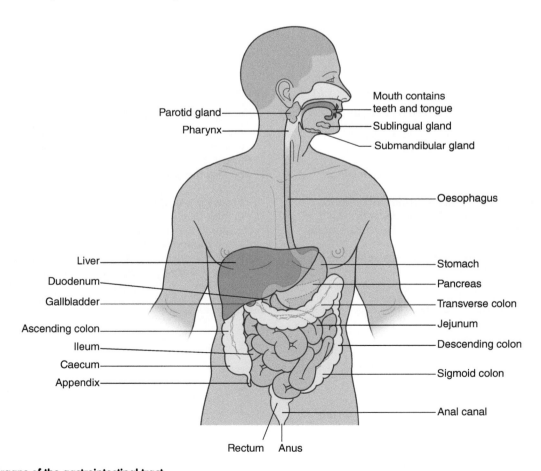

Figure 28.1 Organs of the gastrointestinal tract.

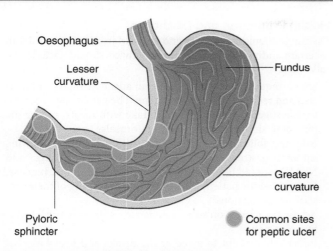

Oesophagus

Lesser
curvature

Fundus

Greater
curvature

Pyloric
sphincter

Common sites
for peptic ulcer

Figure 28.2 Common sites for peptic ulcer.

The pathophysiology of the condition is different depending on the cause. *Helicobacter pylori* produces urease which changes the acidity within the stomach. It produces toxins which affect the integrity of the mucosal cells and exposes them to more acidity and damage.

Non-steroidal anti-inflammatory medications inhibit cyclo-oxygenase. Cyclo-oxygenase produces prostaglandins that have a role in protecting the mucosa from the harsh acidic environment, hence the reduction in prostaglandins leaves the mucosa vulnerable to effects of hydrochloric acid.

Red Flag

 An adverse effect associated with NSAID medications is hypersensitivity reactions, for example bronchospasm or angio-oedema.

Investigation and Diagnosis

- Tests for *H. pylori*, including ^{13}C urea breath test and blood test to detect immunoglobulin G (IgG) antibodies.
- Stool *Helicobacter* antigen test (SAT).
- Barium swallow may be used to identify any ulcer formation.
- Endoscopy and biopsy of gastric lining to detect changes resulting from *H. pylori* infection.
- Stool test for occult blood.

If symptoms persist, endoscopy may be required to examine the digestive tract. An endoscope (a thin flexible tube with a camera and light) is inserted into the oral cavity and down into the digestive tract via the oesophagus. The endoscopist can visualise and photograph the upper digestive tract, looking for any abnormalities. Tissue samples can be taken for laboratory analysis. The procedure can be uncomfortable and sedation can be given.

Signs and Symptoms

Signs and symptoms of peptic ulcer include the following.

- Epigastric pain usually 1–3 hours after eating a meal.
- Heartburn as a result of gastro-oesophageal reflux.

- Occult or obvious blood in the stool.
- Haematemesis is present if the ulcer is bleeding (vomit is described as resembling coffee grounds when altered blood is present).
- Fatigue, weakness, dizziness associated with blood loss.
- Dyspepsia (indigestion).

Nursing Care and Management

A full history should be obtained in order to formulate a care plan to meet the specific needs of the person. Nursing assessment should consider the symptoms, the trigger for symptoms, body mass index (BMI), medication history and lifestyle factors. Testing for *H. pylori* is required. A proton pump inhibitor may be prescribed. The healthcare provider should help the patient identify any lifestyle factors that may be associated with the ulcer, such as stress, heavy alcohol consumption, smoking or consuming a lot of caffeine. Care should include dietary advice, altering lifestyle, avoiding stressful situations and adherence to the medications prescribed.

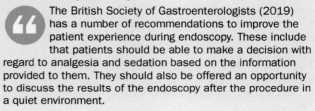

What the Experts Say

The British Society of Gastroenterologists (2019) has a number of recommendations to improve the patient experience during endoscopy. These include that patients should be able to make a decision with regard to analgesia and sedation based on the information provided to them. They should also be offered an opportunity to discuss the results of the endoscopy after the procedure in a quiet environment.

Nutrition Dietary advice should be offered to the patient. Small regular meals are encouraged (approximately five small meals per day) to prevent hunger pain. It is important to advise the patient that bland or restrictive diets are no longer necessary. Alcohol intake in moderation is not harmful but binge drinking could lead to peptic ulcer. Smoking should be discouraged because the ulcer may not heal or may take longer to heal.

Medications The medications used to treat peptic ulcer include drugs to eradicate *H. pylori*, to decrease gastric acid content and to protect the GI mucosa. Medications prescribed may include the following.

- Proton pump inhibitors (PPIs) such as omeprazole and lansoprazole to inhibit the release of hydrochloric acid from the parietal cells in the stomach. If endoscopy is indicated, PPIs should be stopped at least 2 weeks before the procedure as these drugs may mask any underlying serious pathology.
- Antacid for the relief of dyspepsia and alginates to protect the lining of the stomach.
- Antibiotics such as amoxicillin, clarithromycin and metronidazole to treat *H. pylori* infection.

Complications The complications associated with peptic ulcer disease includes gastrointestinal bleeding. This is an emergency and the person may have to have a surgical or endoscopic intervention to treat the haemorrhage.

Red Flag

 Many people take anti-inflammatory drugs for their anti-inflammatory, antipyretic and analgesic effects. It is important to consider the other medications the person may be prescribed. People who are prescribed warfarin, for example, are at an increased risk of bleeding. NSAIDs can also reduce the effects of some antihypertensive medications.

Surgery For the majority of patients presenting with peptic ulcer, the treatments are conservative; the medications used are generally very effective. For a minority of patients where the ulcer fails to respond or there is evidence of bleeding, a surgical procedure is indicated. The procedure of choice is vagotomy and pyloroplasty or distal subtotal gastrectomy. For general preoperative and postoperative care, refer to Chapter 14. NICE (2020a) has produced perioperative care guidance for adults based on best practice.

The following postoperative care is required.

- The patient's vital signs and early warning scores are monitored and acted upon as per the NEWS2 chart.
- If a nasogastric tube is inserted, ensure that it is draining freely and aspirate every 2–4 hours. Note the colour and amount aspirated. Regular nasal care is required and ensure that the nasogastric tube is comfortably positioned and secured. The position of the NG tube should be noted and documented according to local policy and procedure.
- The patient will be nil by mouth for the first 24 hours. Sips of water are introduced slowly and cautiously and this is gradually increased to free fluids once bowel sounds are normal.
- Provide oral hygiene as required by offering frequent mouthwashes.
- Assess the patient for pain and administer analgesia as prescribed.
- Ensure that all documentation is completed (NMC, 2018a).

What To Do If . . .

What would you do if the patient you were looking after suddenly developed secondary haemorrhage postoperatively? The nursing actions should include the following.

- Seek help.
- Assess using the ABCDE and record on the NEWS2 chart.
- Check the wound and any drains.
- Reinforce the dressings.
- Report to the person in charge, and if necessary escalate your findings according to local policy.
- Prepare the patient in case a return to theatre is required.
- Ensure there is intravenous (IV) access for the administration of prescribed fluids or blood products.

Health Promotion and Discharge

Discharge should be planned and initiated in advance in order to ascertain individual patient needs. Advice should include the following.

- Small frequent meals may enable an adequate intake of nutrients and reduce dumping syndrome. The patient should avoid simple sugars and reduce fluid intake with meals. Advise the patient to sit upright, especially after meals.
- Iron and folic acid supplements may be required following subtotal gastrectomy, and aspirin-containing drugs and NSAIDs should be avoided as they irritate the gastric mucosa. Ensure that the patient has a good understanding of their prescribed medications.
- Advise the patient on stress avoidance, as stress is a risk factor for some patients.
- Inform the patient to avoid acidic drinks and heavy alcohol consumption.
- Ensure that the patient has a relative or friend with them and if necessary transport to go home, particularly if the patient is elderly. Referral to a social worker or home care may be required.
- Provide letters for the appropriate community healthcare providers, for example GP and community nurse, to explain the care given in the hospital and the follow-up care. Nurses should adhere to local policy with regard to discharging patients into the community; hospital and community teams should work together to ensure the best possible outcome for the patient.

Jot This Down

It is not certain how people contract *H. pylori*, but researchers think it may be through food or water. The organism is also found in the saliva of some infected people, so mouth-to-mouth contact can spread the bacterium.

Care, Dignity and Compassion

A cancer diagnosis can have a devastating effect on the person affected and their loved ones. A person-centred approach to the services available both in hospital and in primary care is essential to reduce the stress and anxiety for all. Macmillan Cancer Care recommends a holistic needs assessment as well as personalised care and support plans to ensure that care, dignity and compassion are maintained (Macmillan Cancer Care, no date).

Carcinoma of the Stomach

There were 6595 new cases of stomach cancer in the UK between 2015 and 2017. Stomach cancer accounts for 2% of UK cancers (Cancer Research UK, 2021). Stomach cancer is the 17th most common cause of cancer-related death in the world. It is a difficult disease to cure in Western countries, mainly because most patients present with advanced disease. Stomach cancer affects the pylorus (50% of cases), the lesser curvature (25% of cases) and the cardia (10% of cases).

Areas Affected and Proliferation

Most stomach cancers (around 95%) are adenocarcinomas. The remaining 5% are lymphomas, sarcomas or carcinoids. Adenocarcinomas can spread along the stomach wall (Figure 28.3a) to the duodenum and to other organs in the abdominal cavity. If the tumour infiltrates the lymphatic system (Figure 28.3b) and blood vessels, then other organs, such as the liver (Figure 28.3c), lungs and ovaries, the bones and the peritoneum become affected. Lymphomas arise from the lymphatic tissue within the wall of the stomach, sarcomas arise from the muscle or connective tissue within the wall of the stomach and carcinoids arise from cells in the stomach lining that synthesise hormones.

Risk Factors

Non-environmental and environmental risk factors are associated with the development of stomach cancer (McCance et al., 2018). Non-environmental risk factors include those who have a diagnosis of pernicious anaemia or a family history of gastric cancer. Environmental risk factors include:

- Lifestyle: alcohol, smoking.
- Diet: food additives (nitrates), salted foods, high red meat intake.
- Infection: *H. pylori*.
- Age and gender: over 55 years, more men than women.

It is generally assumed that food preservation by refrigeration and not by salting is an important factor in the declining incidence of gastric adenocarcinoma. Increasing the amount of fresh fruit and vegetables and reducing red meat and salted foods in the diet can decrease the risk.

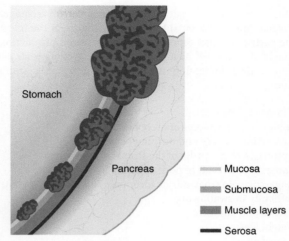

Mucosa
Submucosa
Muscle layers
Serosa

(a) Tumour growth in stomach wall

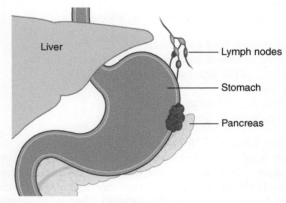

Lymph nodes
Stomach
Pancreas

(b) Stomach cancer spreads to lymph nodes

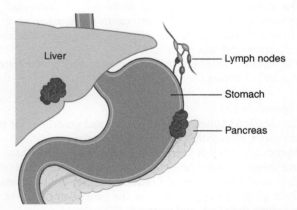

Lymph nodes
Stomach
Pancreas

(c) Stomach cancer spreads to other organs (e.g. liver metastasis)

Figure 28.3 (a) Tumour affecting the layers of the stomach. (b) Tumour has spread into neighbouring lymph nodes. (c) Tumour has spread to the liver.

Pathophysiology

Continuous and severe gastritis and *H. pylori* infection lead to changes in the gastric mucosa which increases the risk of developing both gastric and duodenal carcinomas. The use of dietary salt can lead to chronic gastritis. Nitrates are converted to nitrosamines in the presence of salt. Nitrosamines are carcinogenic. Prostaglandins are essential for the maintenance of the integrity of the gastric mucosa. Smokers have a decreased production of prostaglandins as well as a higher risk of developing *H. pylori* infection, thus increasing their risk of developing stomach cancer.

Signs and Symptoms
- Initially few symptoms are reported.
- Indigestion, acidity and burping (eructation).
- Dysphagia if the cardia of the stomach is involved.
- Anorexia as a result of poor appetite.
- Epigastric pain (may mimic ulcer pain) and loss of appetite.
- Difficulty in swallowing.
- Nausea and vomiting.
- Weight loss.
- Loss of appetite.
- Change in bowel habit.
- Anaemia.
- Haemorrhage (if blood vessels are affected).

Investigation and Diagnosis
- Medical history of eating and bowel elimination habits.
- Physical and clinical examination.
- CT scan.
- Fibreoptic gastroscopy and biopsy.
- Barium meal.

Nursing Care and Management
Surgery is indicated when the stomach cancer is diagnosed at an early stage. The removal of the stomach is called *gastrectomy*. This could be either a partial gastrectomy (half of the stomach) or a total gastrectomy (all of the stomach). The type of operation needed depends on the size of the tumour and where it is located in the stomach. Traditionally, gastrectomy was performed as open surgery but increasingly, gastrectomy for stomach cancer is performed laparoscopically by surgeons who have undertaken specific training in this procedure.

For detailed principles of preoperative and postoperative care, refer to Chapter 14.

Preoperative Care
- Nurses should adhere to local policies and guidelines for the safe preparation of the person for gastric surgery.
- Psychological care is paramount in the preoperative phase to give the patient confidence in the aftercare in the community. Visits from Marie Curie or Macmillan nurses can be invaluable in giving the opportunity for the patient and relatives to talk about their fears and worries.

Postoperative Care Post gastrectomy, routine postoperative care is required. In some instances, the patient may be nursed in intensive care for a short period of time. The nurse should observe the patient for any signs of deterioration using a National Early Warning Scoring 2 (NEWS2) system. Any signs of deterioration should be reported as per the guidance (Royal College of Physicians, 2017). A full top-to-toe assessment should be undertaken using the ABCDE approach. Postoperatively, there is likely to be a nasogastric tube *in situ* as well as wound drains and a urinary catheter. A jejunostomy tube may also be placed to allow

for postoperative feeding that bypasses the anastomosed area to allow healing to occur.

Initially patients are nil by mouth. In some instances, a contrast swallow test may be conducted prior to the introduction of diet to check the anastomosis. Bowel function slowly returns over a period of days. The presence of bowel sounds and the passing of flatus are good indicators that bowel function is returning.

The Nursing Associate

Nursing associates can help patients with eating and drinking. They should also undertake malnutrition universal screening tool (MUST) reviews and complete food and fluid charts. If the patient does require jejunal feeding, the nursing associate can support the delivery of this, reporting any concerns to the nurse in charge.

Practice Assessment Document Bowel sounds

There has been controversy over the value of auscultation of bowel sounds as an indicator of intestinal functioning returning to normal. There is little supporting evidence for this activity and a lack of consensus about correct technique (Felder *et al.*, 2014). Adhere to local policy procedure at all times.

Have a discussion regarding the pros and cons of auscultation of bowel sounds with your practice supervisor and identify any alternatives to listening for bowel sounds.

Red Flag

Nasogastric tubes are easily dislodged and usually easily replaced. Post gastric surgery, if the tube does dislodge, do not attempt to reposition it, as this could lead to potential complications at the site of the anastomosis. Seek help from the medical team.

Clear liquids are offered slowly and cautiously; there may be borborygmi (sounds as if the stomach is rumbling). If fluids are tolerated, the nasogastric tube can be removed and diet is gradually introduced. Initially diet will be liquid and will progress to soft and then normal diet as tolerated by the person.

Jot This Down

Please revise the functions of the stomach.

The stomach has many important functions that are now missing. Food now enters the oral cavity and moves directly into the duodenum. The duodenum does not have the same storage capacity as the stomach so there could be some discomfort after eating. This can be relieved by eating smaller, more frequent meals. There may be a requirement to adjust diet as previously enjoyed foods may now be difficult to digest. Diet may present a challenge after a total gastrectomy. The dietary changes may be temporary, until the digestive system adjusts, or they may be permanent.

Fluid balance is assessed in the immediate postoperative period and when the risk of dehydration is lessened then this can be stopped and the urinary catheter removed. The surgeon will decide when it is appropriate to remove any wound drains and the nasogastric tube.

Pain assessment is crucial in the immediate postoperative period and beyond. Analgesia should be prescribed and administered to ensure the patient is comfortable and can participate in their own care. Acute pain is a common complication postoperatively with patients reporting pain even after discharge (Rockett et al., 2017).

Complications Dumping syndrome is a complication following gastric surgery that may occur 10–30 minutes after eating. The symptoms associated with dumping syndrome include epigastric fullness, discomfort, excessive sweating and feeling unwell. Following ingestion of a meal, resting for 30 minutes in a semi-recumbent or recumbent position may alleviate symptoms.

Vitamin B12 is absorbed in the presence of intrinsic factor which is usually produced by the stomach. An absence of intrinsic factor means that vitamin B12 injections will continue for life. Vitamin B12 is a water-soluble vitamin responsible for the development of myelination in the central nervous system, red blood cell formation and DNA synthesis.

Iron levels may also reduce post gastrectomy due to rapid gastric emptying, preventing the absorption of iron.

Both iron and vitamin B12 are required for the production of erythrocytes. Therefore anaemia can be a complication. Pernicious aneamia is the term used for anaemia caused by a lack of vitamin B12.

Health Promotion and Discharge

Prior to discharge, nurses need to discuss some of the risk factors associated with stomach cancer. Advise the patient on the following.

- The relationship between gastric cancer and consumption of foods preserved with nitrates (such as bacon and other processed meats); encourage limited consumption of these products.
- Smoking is also a risk factor for stomach cancer. Smoking cessation preoperatively enhances postoperative recovery. Smoking cessation services should be offered pre- and postoperatively.
- Wash fruits and vegetables thoroughly before eating.
- Advise the patient to take regular small meals and to rest in a reclining position after each meal for approximately 30 minutes.

- Reinforce the information from the physiotherapist regarding gentle exercises and deep breathing.
- Ensure that the patient has all the necessary outpatient appointments before being discharged home.
- The patient will be referred to the oncology team who will assess the requirement for any future adjuvant treatment such as chemotherapy.

Hepatitis

Hepatitis is inflammation of the liver. Hepatitis can occur due to viral illness or the effects of alcohol, drugs and toxins. It can be acute or chronic. Inflammation of the liver leads to the destruction of hepatocytes and a reduction in liver function. (Bauldoff et al., 2019). Please review the functions of the liver.

Viral Hepatitis

There are a variety of different strains of the virus that affect the liver in different ways. The strains are hepatitis A virus (HAV), hepatitis B virus (HBV), hepatitis C virus (HCV), hepatitis D virus (HDV) and hepatitis E virus (HEV).

Hepatitis A Infection with HAV, or infectious hepatitis, often occurs by the faecal–oral route via contaminated food, water, shellfish and direct contact with an infected person. It can be associated with living in unsanitary conditions. It can also be transmitted sexually. Lifetime immunity probably results after the infection has run its course. Serum IgG may remain elevated for life.

Hepatitis B Hepatitis B, sometimes referred to as serum hepatitis, is transmitted by contaminated blood and blood products (prior to 1991), tattoos or a virus-contaminated needle, and also from mother to foetus via the placenta (Lister *et al.*, 2020). HBV is a DNA virus. A person can be a carrier without suffering any symptoms and is capable of spreading it to others. Hepatitis B is a risk factor for primary liver cancer and decompensated liver disease. HBV has been implicated in 60–90% of cases of liver carcinoma when the disease has reached its chronic phase.

Hepatitis C Hepatitis C, formerly known as non-A, non-B hepatitis, is the primary worldwide cause of chronic hepatitis, cirrhosis and liver cancer (Bauldoff *et al.*, 2019). It is an RNA virus that may be transmitted through parenteral, faecal–oral or sexual routes. Acute hepatitis C is usually asymptomatic; if symptoms do develop, they are often mild and non-specific. Hepatitis C is unique in that it does not produce lasting immunity to reinfection. Only about 15% of acute infections completely resolve; most progress to chronic active hepatitis (Bauldoff *et al.*, 2019).

Hepatitis D This is caused by a defective RNA virus distinct from all the others. The onset is sudden and the symptoms similar to those for HBV. Co-infection with HBV is necessary for the efficient replication of HDV. It is transmitted parenterally and often overlooked, as the person is infected with HBV.

Hepatitis E Hepatitis E is an RNA virus transmitted via the faecal–oral route. It can be severe in pregnant women.

Pathophysiology and Signs and Symptoms

Exposure to a virus leads to an inflammatory process that causes destruction of hepatocytes and associated scarring as well as affecting the liver macrophages – the Kupffer cells. The inflammatory process can obstruct the bile canaliculi, the narrow channels that allow the transportation of bile from the hepatocyte. This leads to obstructive jaundice (McCance & Huether, 2018).

There are four phases associated with viral hepatitis.

Incubation Phase This phase can last from 15 to 180 days depending on which virus is present.

Prodromal Phase Usually commences about 14 days after exposure to the virus and symptoms can be seen. Symptoms are:

- Nausea and vomiting
- Fatigue
- Headache
- Malaise
- Low-grade fever
- Anorexia.

Each virus presents differently and HCV may not display any symptoms in this stage.

Icteric Phase This phase is seen after the prodromal phase and can last between 2 and 6 weeks. Dark urine and clay-coloured stools (lack of bile pigment) can precede the onset of jaundice.

Jaundice occurs as the occluded passage of bile leads to bilirubin being absorbed into the bloodstream. The serum bilirubin levels rise, causing yellowing of the skin and the sclera.

Jaundice can cause pruritus as a result of bile salts in the skin. The liver is enlarged (hepatomegaly) and there may be abdominal pain and fatigue. An abnormal liver function test may be evident as well as changes to blood clotting. HBV may not present with jaundice.

Recovery Phase Usually occurs between 6 and 10 weeks after exposure. Jaundice resolves and liver function tests normalise.

At this stage, acute hepatitis can develop into chronic hepatitis.

Chronic Hepatitis The exact cause of the disease is unknown but a number of different possibilities are thought to be responsible, including infectious hepatitis, HBV, HCV and HDV, drug reactions, alcohol poisoning, autoimmune hepatitis and haemochromatosis (a disorder of the body's iron metabolism). Many patients have no symptoms, while some may experience malaise, fatigue and aching muscles and joints. Jaundice is a very late symptom of the disease and is a sign that the liver is damaged. Liver enzymes, such as serum aminotransferase levels, are elevated. Chronic active hepatitis usually leads to cirrhosis of the liver and end-stage liver failure.

Investigations and Diagnosis

Investigations that may be carried out to confirm the diagnosis include:

- Full blood count and electrolyte levels
- Polymerase chain reaction (PCR) test
- Urinalysis for the presence of bilirubin and urobilinogen
- Renal function test
- Alpha-1-antitrypsin
- Liver biopsy
- Ultrasound, CT or MRI scan of the liver (NICE, 2020b).

The Nursing Associate

Nursing associates who have been deemed proficient in venepuncture can draw blood and therefore send the required bloods to the lab.

Nursing Care and Management

The nursing care and management of hepatitis are dependent on the type of infection. Vaccination programmes are available for hepatitis A and B.

Nursing care should consider reducing demand on the liver, while promoting physical care, preventing complications and providing information about the disease, prognosis and treatment. Most hepatitis patients do not need isolation unless they present a health risk to other patients.

Infection Prevention An important goal when caring for persons with acute viral hepatitis is preventing spread of the infection. Use the local trust and Health Protection Agency guidelines in the care of patients. Use the recommended personal protective equipment (PPE) when managing bodily fluids and adhere to hand hygiene protocols.

What To Do If . . .

Needlestick injuries can occur in clinical practice and are a source of anxiety in relation to infection prevention. When administering an intramuscular injection to a patient, you sustain a needlestick injury. What should you do?

- Encourage the wound to bleed while holding it under running water.
- Wash the wound using soap and water.
- Do not scrub the wound.
- Cover the wound with a plaster.
- Seek help from the occupational health department or your GP.
- Report the incident using the usual reporting mechanisms.
- Revise the correct procedure for giving an intramuscular injection to prevent this from happening again.

Fatigue Fatigue is common in acute hepatitis. Ensure the patient is aware of this and advise them to work within their capability with regard to fatigue. Extra assistance may be required to carry out the activities of living. Promote rest times and if the patient is at risk of falls due to fatigue, ensure a falls risk assessment is completed. As recovery progresses, increasing activity levels are tolerated with less fatigue.

Medications The medications used to treat hepatitis depend on the viral infection.

Health Promotion and Discharge

Nurses play an important role in preventing the transmission of hepatitis. Emphasis on personal hygiene measures, such as hand washing after toileting and before all food handling, is important.

Advise the patient to avoid alcohol to prevent further damage to the liver and encourage high-calorie soft drinks as a high intake of calories is essential to promote healing. Small, regular meals are preferable; a low-fat diet is required if there is a bile flow obstruction.

Discuss recommendations for hepatitis A and hepatitis B vaccination with people in high- or moderate-risk groups for these infections.

Primary Care

Before the patient is discharged, nurses should ensure that they and their relatives are given the necessary information for home care.

- Advise the patient and their relatives on maintaining personal hygiene, strict hand washing when preparing food and not sharing eating utensils.
- Advise the patient to rest when fatigue sets in.
- Encourage good nutritious fluid intake.
- Avoid alcohol consumption as alcohol is a risk factor for liver damage.
- Offer advice on the medications they are discharged with, and the importance of continuing with the drugs until further notice.
- Inform the patient about any outpatient appointments and the importance of adhering to these.
- Always seek advice from the pharmacist or the GP when buying over-the-counter medications.
- Offer counselling and information on support groups in the community.

Alcohol-related Liver Disease

Alcohol-related liver disease (ARLD) refers to liver damage caused by excess alcohol intake. Regular heavy drinking of alcohol can interfere with many of the vital functions of the liver, ultimately leading to damage to liver cells. There are several stages of severity.

Initially, large amounts of fat accumulate between the hepatocytes, causing fatty liver disease (steatosis). This condition rarely causes symptoms and is reversible if the person stops drinking. However, many heavy drinkers will progress from fatty liver disease to alcohol-related hepatitis. This is unrelated to infectious hepatitis although both conditions can co-exist. Alcohol-induced hepatitis is reversible during the early stages, but for many people the condition progresses to become life-threatening.

Cirrhosis and liver failure is the end-stage of ARLD, where patients start to demonstrate life-threatening complications such as:

- Internal (variceal) bleeding
- Build-up of toxins in the brain (encephalopathy)
- Fluid accumulation in the abdomen (ascites)
- Liver cancer
- Liver failure.

Health Education and Promotion

- Advise men and women not to regularly drink more than 14 units of alcohol per week.
- If consuming 14 units every week, drink these over 3–4 days rather than binge drinking.
- Have several drink-free days per week.
- Provide information about local self-help groups.
- Opportunistic screening at well persons clinics.

Mental Health While the physical health and management of those living with alcohol dependence is important, the affects on their mental health and well-being must be given parity of esteem. O'Connor (2020) notes that there are 589 000 people in the UK living with alcohol dependence and one-quarter of these will be using mental health medications for anxiety, depression, sleep disorders and metal health issues such as psychosis or bipolar disorder. There is also an increased risk of suicide for those who depend on alcohol. A large section of the population is thought to be managing alcohol dependence without seeking help. It is therefore important to ask people who come into your care about their alcohol intake and recommend the appropriate mental health services to recognise and treat the associated mental health risks.

Case Study

Adele Johnstone is 48 years old and has been homeless for several months. She has been sofa surfing and due to her alcohol dependence, she finds it difficult to stay in the one place. After a recent night at the hostel, one of the volunteers persuaded Adele to seek medical help as she appeared slightly jaundiced. After 3 days in hospital, Adele appears confused and seems to be suffering from acute alcohol withdrawal symptoms. She is seen by a specialist team for acute alcohol withdrawal and prescribed a benzodiazepine in the short term

Source: Based on NICE (2021).

Gallbladder Disorders

The most common disorders of the gallbladder are cholecystitis (inflammation of the gallbladder), cholelithiasis (stones in the gallbladder) and cancer of the gallbladder.

Pathophysiology

Cholecystitis Cholecystitis is defined as inflammation of the gallbladder, which causes severe abdominal pain. It may result from bacterial infection or irritation from the stones in the gallbladder. Dietary factors, including high fat intake, have been associated with cholecystitis. However, gallstones in the cystic duct have been identified as the main cause of acute cholecystitis resulting in biliary colic, which affects the shoulder, back and right scapula (Bauldoff *et al.*, 2019). If it is untreated and there are repeated attacks of acute cholecystitis, the person can develop chronic cholecystitis. The obstruction of the cystic duct by the gallstones leads to distension of the gallbladder. The pressure within the gallbladder can result in some severe complications, for example ischaemia caused by decreased blood flow, necrosis and perforation of the gallbladder.

Signs and symptoms that present include:

- Fever
- Pain
- Abdominal guarding
- Rebound tenderness
- Raised serum alkaline phosphatase and bilirubin levels.

Pain management is required as well as correction of any fluid and electrolyte imbalance. Antibiotics are prescribed. Cholecystectomy may be required if the condition becomes chronic or the gallbladder perforates.

Cholelithiasis Cholelithiasis, also known as gallstones, occurs when stones develop in the gallbladder and biliary tract (cystic and common bile ducts). Gallstones differ in size, shape and composition. Approximately 80% of gallstones are composed of cholesterol with some calcium, 2–3% are pigmented stones and 10% consist of only cholesterol.

Gallstones form in the bile through a process of crystal formation. As they become increasingly crystallised, they form macrostones (McCance & Huether, 2018). The gallstones can cause no issues unless they move and they can lodge in either the common bile duct or the cystic duct. The signs and symptoms associated with gallstones are:

- Pain (biliary colic) on the right side of the abdomen
- Pain often associated with ingestion of fatty foods
- An intolerance to fatty foods
- Heartburn and flatulence
- Cholecystitis.

Gallstones are often detected by abdominal ultrasound. NICE (2014) recommends the use of magnetic resonance cholangio-pancreatography (MRCP) if gallstones are suspected but not visible on ultrasound and if the bile duct is dilated and liver function tests are abnormal. If a diagnosis is not made after MRCP then endoscopic ultrasound can be used.

Gallstones located in the gallbladder often do not require treatment until they are symptomatic and then the treatment of choice is laparoscopic cholecystectomy. However, common bile duct stones should be treated by laparoscopic cholecystectomy whether symptomatic or not.

Until the gallbladder or gallstones have been removed, the patient should avoid the foods that cause the symptoms to appear.

Untreated gallstones can lead to potential complications, for example pancreatitis.

Cancer of the Gallbladder The most common form of cancer of the gallbladder is adenocarcinoma. Although this cancer is rare, it is aggressive and if not treated can infiltrate neighbouring tissues such as the hepatic ducts, the liver (Figure 28.4) and the surrounding lymph nodes and pancreas. This cancer is more common in females than males and the survival rates are poor as a result of the metastases.

Investigations and diagnosis

- Full blood count: the white cell count is likely to be raised if there is an infection.
- Liver enzymes for any abnormality.
- Ultrasound of the gallbladder wall and for pericholecystic fluid and stones.
- Endoscopic retrograde cholangiopancreatography (ERCP) is currently the only reliable and widely available investigation for common bile duct stones.
- CT may be useful when filling the bile duct is unsuccessful in ERCP, or when the procedure cannot be used for other reasons.
- Cholecystograms if necessary but ultrasound is now more commonly carried out.
- Urinalysis, chest X-ray and ECG to exclude other diseases.
- Hydroxyiminodiacetic acid (HIDA) scan is an effective method of diagnosing acute cholecystitis.

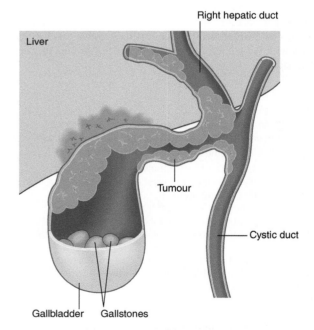

Figure 28.4 **Carcinoma of the gallbladder. The tumour has spread into the hepatic ducts and is partially blocking the right hepatic duct and the liver. Note some gallstones in the gallbladder.**

Signs and Symptoms

Some of the signs and symptoms of gallbladder disorders include the following.

- Biliary colic.
- Scleral jaundice (yellow coloration of the eye) and systemic jaundice (skin).
- Intolerance to fatty food, leading to nausea and vomiting, belching, pain after eating.
- Abdominal distension after eating.
- Strong yellow-coloured urine when the stones block the common bile duct.
- Pyrexia (a high temperature), which is usually mild and no higher than 38 °C.

Jot This Down

Explain why the urine is dark yellow in the patient with obstructive jaundice.

Nursing Care and Management

The patient with a gallbladder disorder can be very ill and may be in shock as a result of severe pain, nausea and vomiting. The priority is to admit the patient and administer appropriate analgesic, antiemetic and antispasmodic drugs; nil by mouth is recommended due to nausea and vomiting. The patient should be monitored until the condition stabilises; give fluids by intravenous infusion to prevent dehydration and monitor serum amylase, urea and electrolyte levels and liver function. The patient is then prepared for surgery. For detailed principles of preoperative and postoperative care, refer to Chapter 14.

Surgery Cholecystectomy is carried out either laparoscopically or through open cholecystectomy. Unless the patient requires an open cholecystectomy, the preferred surgical procedure is laparoscopic cholecystectomy for gallbladder disorders, as only small cuts are needed in the abdomen with small scars remaining afterwards. The operation is done with the aid of a special telescope that is pushed into the abdomen through one small cut. This allows the surgeon to see the gallbladder. Instruments pushed through another small cut are used to cut out and remove the gallbladder. The recovery of the patient following this procedure is much quicker than when open surgery is performed.

An open cholecystectomy is an effective method of treating acute cholecystitis but has a longer recovery time than laparoscopic cholecystectomy. Most people take approximately 6 weeks to recover from an open cholecystectomy. Open cholecystectomy is carried out for patients who:

- Are in the last 3 months of pregnancy
- Are obese (very overweight, with a body mass index of 30 or more)
- Have cirrhosis (scarring of the liver)
- Have a condition that affects the blood's ability to clot, such as haemophilia.

Preoperative Care For the principles of preoperative and postoperative care, refer to Chapter 14.

- Patients are informed that following keyhole surgery, they are allowed to drink and have a light meal on the same day if they

do not have any complications from the anaesthetic. In the case of open surgery, fluid and diet may be introduced slowly and cautiously.

- The nurse should discuss pain management and the type of analgesia that may be prescribed following surgery.
- Allow the patient and their relatives time to discuss any fears or worries they might have about the surgery.
- The length of stay in hospital varies. For laparoscopic cholecystectomy, the length of stay may be between 1 and 3 days, while for an open cholecystectomy it may be a couple of days longer.

Postoperative Care Postoperative care for the patient who has had an open cholecystectomy involves monitoring of blood pressure, pulse, respiration and temperature. Breathing tends to be shallow as a result of the effect of anaesthesia and the patient's reluctance to breathe deeply due to the pain caused by the proximity of the incision to the muscles used for respiration. Advise the patient to support the operative site when breathing deeply and coughing, and give pain medication as necessary.

A small drain may be inserted for 24 hours and then removed as a precautionary measure to monitor excess fluid loss. Nurses must document all fluid loss on a fluid balance chart and should report any excess loss immediately for prompt action.

Fluid intake and urine output are measured and recorded and the operative site is observed for colour and amount of wound drainage. Fluids are given intravenously until the patient is allowed to take oral fluids, and when bowel sound returns, diet is introduced.

Pain management should commence with an assessment of the patient's pain at regular intervals. Nurses can use any of the pain assessment tools such as the visual analogue scale. The patient should be asked to indicate their personal level of pain and appropriate prescribed analgesia administered. The effect of the analgesia should be recorded in the patient's care plan.

To prevent postoperative complications, early mobility is encouraged. The patient should be encouraged to take active exercises to prevent venothrombus embolism and to improve circulation.

Measures to manage the patient's anxiety should be implemented preoperatively and continued throughout the postoperative recovery period, until discharge. This should include the provision of adequate levels of information for patients and their relatives.

Depending on the surgeon's preferences, some types of sutures/clips will need to be removed by either the community nurse or the practice nurse; others will dissolve on their own over the course of several weeks. Patients should be informed exactly what type of wound closure has been used and if it needs to be removed and by whom.

Alternative Treatments *Extracorporeal shockwave lithotripsy (ECSL):* shock waves are used to break up or dissolve the stone, so that it can be passed via the GI tract.

- *Oral dissolution therapy:* gallstones composed of cholesterol can sometimes be treated using a medication called ursodeoxycholic acid, which slowly dissolves gallstones. Ursodeoxycholic acid is also sometimes prescribed as a precaution against gallstones if it is thought that the patient has a high risk of developing them. Ursodeoxycholic acid is taken orally (in tablet form), and a course of treatment can last up to 2 years.

- *Contact dissolution therapy*: drugs to dissolve the stones are introduced into the gallbladder via a tube through the skin.

Diet After a cholecystectomy there is no need to follow a low-fat diet. A low-fat diet may result in weight loss. However, due to the role that cholesterol appears to play in the formation of gall-stones, it is recommended that patients avoid eating fatty foods that have a high cholesterol content. These foods include:

- Meat pies
- Sausages and fatty cuts of meat
- Butter and lard
- Cakes and biscuits.

A low-fat, high-fibre diet is recommended. This includes eating wholegrains and at least five portions of fresh fruit and vegetables a day. A low-fat diet is advisable for everyone to follow as a healthy option.

Health Promotion and Discharge

Prior to discharge, nurses need to advise the patient on the following points.

- *Pain relief*: the patient can take over-the-counter analgesics, such as paracetamol or ibuprofen. Advise the patient to read the information leaflet that comes with the medicine and if they have any questions to ask the pharmacist for advice.
- *Regular exercise and lifting* must be introduced slowly, to avoid any discomfort and to avoid complications such as secondary bleeding.
- *Driving*: due to discomfort from the seatbelt, patients should be advised not to resume driving until approximately 2 weeks after the surgery. Some insurance companies may not insure drivers for a number of weeks after surgery, so it is best to check with the insurance company before starting to drive.
- *Outpatient appointments*: advise the patient on the importance of attending the outpatient appointments as arranged.
- If the patient has a *dressing*, this can be removed after 2 days and no further dressing over the wound is necessary. They can have a bath or shower daily to keep the wound clean. If there are sutures or clips to be removed, an appointment with the practice nurse is made to remove them.

Primary Care

Most patients can continue to eat a healthy well-balanced diet after they have their gallbladder removed. However, if they develop side-effects, such as mild diarrhoea, it may be advisable to eat more high-fibre foods and avoid foods that make the diarrhoea worse.

If the patient is unduly worried about going back to work or doing physical activities such as lifting, the nurse should advise them to seek advice from the GP or the practice nurse.

If the patient is assessed as requiring additional support in the community, a referral should be made to the social worker and the community nurse to arrange a package of care to meet the needs of the patient.

Practice Assessment Document

Nurses and nursing associates must document and maintain all records in accordance with *Future Nurse: Standards of proficiency for registered nurses* (NMC, 2018b) or *Standards of proficiency for nursing associates* (NMC, 2018c).

The Nursing Associate

The NMC (2018c) requires that nursing associates write accurate, clear, legible records and documentation. Think about how you would document the care of a patient awaiting a cholecystectomy.

Inflammatory Bowel Disease

Inflammatory bowel disease (IBD) is a term that includes Crohn's disease (CD) and ulcerative colitis (UC). These are common diseases, predominantly occurring in the Western world and affecting mainly young adults. They are chronic conditions characterised by periods of relapse or remission.

Inflammatory bowel disease should not be confused with irritable bowel syndrome (IBS), although some people with inflammatory bowel disease also have irritable bowel syndrome. Inflammatory bowel disease is an idiopathic disease caused by an immune system response to the host's microflora. It is thought to result from a complex interplay between environmental factors and a genetic predisposition (NICE, 2015a).

Pathophysiology

Crohn's Disease The ulceration of the mucosa that occurs in CD can affect the entire length of the digestive tract from the mouth to the anus. The areas most commonly affected are the distal part of the small intestine (ileum) and the proximal part of the large intestine (ascending colon). It can affect both men and women and occurs between the ages of 10 and 30 years old. Family history is a risk factor associated with CD. Inflammation begins in the submucosa of the intestine and spreads across the intestinal wall. The entire intestinal wall can be affected. Abscesses can form and the granulomas formed are described as having a cobblestone appearance. The affected lumen will narrow due to inflammation and oedema and fibrotic strictures can occur, which can lead to a possible bowel obstruction. In CD fistulae can form in the perianal area, between loops of bowel and even into the bladder.

Abdominal pain is common. Diarrhoea, which may contain blood and mucus, is also common, with patients passing five or more stools per day. This is due to decreased colonic absorption of water but could also be associated with medications. Depending on the area of the digestive tract affected, vitamin and mineral deficiencies can occur. This can lead to other problems, for example bone disease due to lack of calcium or aneamia due to lack of vitamin B12. Chronic blood loss can also lead to anaemia. Poor absorption of the products of digestion plus a loss of appetite can lead to weight loss. Bowel obstruction can occur.

Ulcerative Colitis Ulcerative colitis affects the mucosa of the colon and rectum (Larsen, 2015). It can affect both men and women and occurs between the ages of 10 and 40 years old. Family history is a risk factor and there are some suggestions that factors such as infection, immunity and diet may contribute to its development (McCance & Huether, 2018). Continuous lesions develop in the affected mucosa. They tend not to affect the bowel wall. The mucosal barrier is damaged by the lesions and the mucosa becomes oedematous. The appearance is red and velvety. In severe disease, the lesions can merge together to form larger lesions and the mucosa can become haemorrhagic. Pseudopolyps can develop in the epithelium. The muscularis mucosa can become thickened and along with the presence of oedema, this can lead to the possibility of bowel obstruction.

The signs and symptoms will depend on the severity of the disease but include diarrhoea – large volumes of watery diarrhoea can be produced. This is due to loss of function of the large intestine mucosa as well as the reduced amount of time available for the absorption of water. The diarrhoea may contain blood and pus due to the inflammatory processes occurring within the bowel. The patient complains of crampy pain. Pyrexia as a result of infection and tachycardia associated with dehydration also occur. Weight loss and anaemia are common. Complications of ulcerative colitis include anal fissures, toxic megacolon, strictures, obstruction and an increased risk of colon cancer (McCance & Huether, 2018).

Investigations and Diagnosis

- Sigmoidoscopy of the lower intestine and taking biopsy samples from the bowel wall. Since the lower bowel is involved in all those with UC and about half of those with CD, this is a helpful investigation for inflammatory bowel disease.
- Colonoscopy of the large intestine and terminal ileum using a flexible tube inserted via the anus. Colonoscopy has reduced the need for barium enema examinations. It can also be used to determine how much of the large intestine is involved and the extent and severity of disease. It also has the advantage of allowing biopsies to be taken from the bowel wall during the procedure.
- Histopathology is the detailed microscopic examination by a pathologist of tissue samples, biopsies, taken during sigmoidoscopy and colonoscopy. Histopathology can be very helpful in confirming the diagnosis and indicating whether inflammatory bowel disease is active or not.
- CT or MRI scan of the abdomen.
- Blood tests to eliminate the presence of anaemia.

Signs and Symptoms

- Pain and discomfort: the duration of the pain can vary a great deal. Many patients with IBS describe the pain as a spasm, colic or crampy.
- Bloating and swelling of the abdomen.
- Diarrhoea or constipation: sometimes the stools become small and pellet-like, or watery or ribbony. At times, mucus and blood may be mixed with the stools.
- Other symptoms include poor appetite, nausea, belching, headache, quick fullness after eating, heartburn.
- Pyrexia.
- Tachycardia.
- Dehydration.

Complications

The two most common complications are:

- *Bowel obstruction*: severe inflammation that causes sections of the bowel to narrow and harden, leading to intestinal obstruction
- *Fistula (Crohn's disease)*: a channel that develops between the anus and the skin near the anus.

For both these complications, surgery may be needed to prevent further complications, such as perforations and rupture of the colon.

Nursing Care and Management

Relieving pain is one of the primary goals. Some patients may complain of severe colicky pain, while others may have intermittent pain. The analgesia prescribed will need to treat the type of pain described by the patient. Before and after the administration of medication, a pain assessment tool should be used to check the effectiveness of the analgesia.

Due to the increased risk of malnutrition, a nutritional risk assessment should be carried out using the Malnutrition Universal Screening Tool (MUST) (BAPEN, 2016). Regular weights and the use of a food chart may be required. The dietitian should be involved to ensure that any oral nutritional supplements are prescribed appropriately.

Complications such as anaemia should be treated. Blood transfusion may be required.

The patient may be prescribed supplementary intravenous fluid in acute stages of the disease. Ensure that the patient does not become dehydrated as a result of the diarrhoea and vomiting. Record intake and output accurately on a fluid balance chart. Where necessary, maintain a stool chart and monitor the frequency and whether there is any blood in the stool.

Medications Both CD and UC are treated with medications such as corticosteroids, which help reduce inflammation, and immunosuppressants, which block the harmful activities of the immune system. Budesonide and prednisolone are steroids that are often used to treat CD. Anti-inflammatory drugs such as sulfasalazine are used to treat inflammation in the early stages of CD. Immunosuppressants such as azathioprine and mercaptopurine may be prescribed to reduce inflammation and suppress the immune system.

Medicines Management

Steroids come in different forms: injections, enteric-coated tablets, inhalers and ointments. Many people take glucocorticoids (steroids) and may not be aware that one of the side-effects is type 2 diabetes. Can you list the other side-effects of steroids?

Infliximab and adalimumab are treatment options for adults with severe active CD whose disease has not responded to conventional therapy (including immunosuppressive and/or corticosteroid treatments) or who are intolerant of, or have contraindications to, conventional therapy (NICE, 2015b).

Nutrition During an acute episode, most patients find a diet lower in fibre and residue helps to relieve symptoms such as cramping and wind. It can also reduce the number of times the patient defaecates. A low-residue diet aims to rest the bowel and allow it to heal.

A low-residue diet involves avoiding roughage (insoluble fibre) that the body cannot break down. Roughage is found in skins, pips, seeds, wholegrain cereals, nuts and raw fruit and vegetables. Other food or drinks that can increase bowel motions are spices, greasy food, alcohol, caffeine and fizzy drinks. Often, these dietary changes are temporary and once the disease has resolved, efforts should be made to reintroduce fibre gradually.

Surgery Surgery may be required for CD when the symptoms cannot be controlled using medication alone. An estimated 80% of people living with CD will require surgery at some point in their life. Surgery may be required for management of the complications of CD, for example fistula, strictures or obstruction. Surgery can be performed to remove diseased areas of bowel where there is multiple stricture formation.

Surgery for UC may be required if there is a poor response to conventional treatment, to reduce the risk associated with the complications of ulcerative colitis, for example severe bleeding or toxic megacolon. Subtotal colectomy with formation of an ileostomy is the most common type of surgery for UC. For some patients, this can proceed to a restorative proctocolectomy with ileo-anal pouch procedure, removing the need for a stoma.

Health Promotion and Discharge

Prior to discharge, nurses should advise the patient on the following points.

- Minimise consumption of sugars and refined foods, as they tend to exacerbate inflammation of the bowel, and avoid alcohol and caffeine.
- Encourage the patient to drink approximately 2–3 L of fluid per day to prevent dehydration.
- Eat a health-promoting diet. After identifying and removing any allergenic foods from the diet, choose a balanced diet composed of whole, unprocessed, preferably organic foods, especially plant foods (fruits, vegetables, whole grains, beans, nuts, especially walnuts, and seeds) and coldwater fish, such as salmon and mackerel. Fish are rich in omega-3 fatty acids, which are a good source of anti-inflammatory substances.
- Advise on vitamin and mineral supplements as they are essential for tissue healing; the absorption of these substances, especially vitamin B12, may be affected by inflammatory bowel disease.
- Only use antibiotics when absolutely necessary.
- Take regular exercise, as it helps tone muscles and improve bowel function.
- Advise the patient to see their GP if the symptoms of inflammatory bowel disease are affecting their physical and mental status.
- Advise the patient to keep all outpatient appointments as organised, even if they feel better.

What the Experts Say

Young women may have concerns about inflammatory bowel disease and pregnancy. This is what a consultant gastroenterologist advises.

'Generally, fertility is not affected by having inflammatory bowel disease. However, it is important to keep the disease under control before and during pregnancy as it maximises the chance of conceiving and avoiding complications during pregnancy. If unduly worried, always discuss your plans with the gastroenterologist.'

Primary Care

Inflammatory bowel disease is a chronic condition and the patient and their relatives will need advice on support services and daily self-management. Advise the patient and their family about the following.

- The disease process and the signs and symptoms associated with the illness.
- A significant number of patients who have inflammatory bowel disease suffer from malnutrition. Therefore, advice on nutritional intake and diet is important when patients are discharged into the community.
- Some patients will have had surgery and may have a colostomy/ileostomy and will therefore need advice on the care of ostomies and the resources available in the community for stoma care. See the following sections on ileostomy and colostomy for detailed nursing care.
- The adherence to prescribed medications, such as steroids, to control inflammation.
- If necessary, encourage the intake of nutritional supplements such as Ensure® to maintain weight and nutritional status.
- The importance of maintaining a fluid intake of at least 2–3 L/day, increasing fluid intake during warm weather, exercise or strenuous work.

Stomas

A stoma is a surgically created opening between the intestine and the abdominal wall that allows faecal material to flow out into a stoma bag (Bauldoff *et al.*, 2019). There are two types of stoma: ileostomy and colostomy. Stomas may be required in patients with inflammatory bowel disease or cancer of the colon.

Pathophysiology

Ileostomies An ileostomy is formed when a portion of the ileum is brought out of the abdominal wall. In an ileostomy, the colon, rectum and anus are usually completely removed (Lister *et al.*, 2020). The surgery may be carried out in patients with IBD or carcinoma of the colon and rectum. The anal canal is closed, and the end of the terminal ileum is brought to the body surface through the right abdominal wall to form the stoma (Figure 28.5). Ileostomies can either be temporary (loop ileostomies) or permanent. Permanent ileostomies are formed following total colectomy (total removal of the colon) and loop ileostomies are formed to allow time for healing to take place after an anastomosis (surgical joining) of the bowel.

Colostomies A colostomy can be formed along any section of the colon. Colostomies take the name of the portion of the colon from which they are formed: ascending, transverse, descending and sigmoid colostomies (Figure 28.6). The most common site for a colostomy is in the sigmoid colon. Colostomies can either be temporary or permanent. Permanent colostomies are formed following removal of colorectal cancers. The surgery is often termed abdominoperineal resection. Temporary colostomies are formed to allow time for healing to take place after an anastomosis (surgical joining) of the bowel.

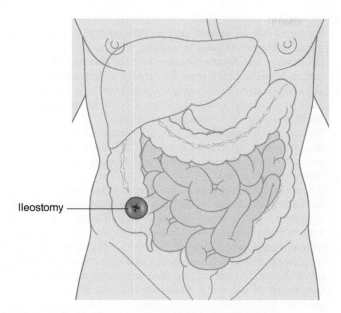

Ileostomy

Figure 28.5 Ileostomy on the right side of the abdomen.

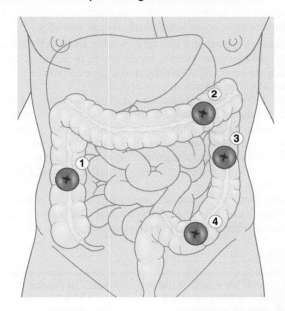

1. Ascending colostomy   3. Transverse colostomy
2. Descending colostomy   4. Sigmoid colostomy

Figure 28.6 Types of colostomy.

Bowel Cancer

Bowel cancer is the fourth most common cancer in the UK (Cancer Research UK, 2021). Most tumours develop in the rectum and sigmoid colon, although any portion of the colon may be affected.

Pathophysiology
Nearly all colorectal cancers are adenocarcinomas that begin as adenomatous polyps that develop from the epithelial tissue.

Polyps are often benign but some will undergo a change due to genetic mutations which allow it to become malignant. If the adenoma crosses into the muscularis mucosa, it becomes invasive and malignant. The tumours develop slowly over 10–15 years (McCance & Huether, 2018), hence the importance of colorectal cancer screening. As the tumours grow, they cause severe intestinal obstruction and, in advanced cases, can infiltrate other organs such as the liver, lungs, brain, bones and kidneys via the portal or lymphatic circulation. Spread to other areas of the peritoneal cavity can occur when the tumour extends through the serosa or during surgery.

The surgery is performed either by open surgery or through a laparoscope. Both techniques are thought equally effective in removing cancer and have similar risks of complications. Laparoscopic colectomies have the advantages of a faster recovery time and less postoperative pain.

Bowel cancer screening is offered in all four nations of the UK. Bowel screening programmes continue to evolve based on the best evidence available.

Investigations and Diagnosis
- Physical examination.
- Digital rectal examination.
- Sigmoidoscopy and biopsies.
- Colonoscopy and biopsies.
- CT scan to detect metastases.

Signs and Symptoms
- Rectal bleeding without other haemorrhoid symptoms.
- Change in bowel habit.
- Diarrhoea or constipation.
- Pain.
- Anorexia.
- Weight loss.
- Anaemia from occult bleeding, which can result in tiredness, feeling weak and breathless.

Staging of the Cancer
During the surgery, tissue will be taken and sent to the laboratory for staging.

Patients face an anxious wait for the results of this test.

Staging of bowel cancer is based on the TNM (tumour, node, metastasis) system.

Tumour Size (T)
- T1: tumour is only present in the inner layer of the bowel.
- T2: tumour has grown into the muscle layer of the bowel wall.
- T3: tumour has grown into the outer lining of the bowel wall.
- T4: tumour has grown through the outer lining of the bowel wall. It may have grown into another part of the bowel or other nearby organs or structures. Or it may have broken through the membrane covering the outside of the bowel (the peritoneum).

Node (N) There are three possible stages describing whether cancer cells are present in the lymph nodes.
- N0: no lymph nodes contain cancer cells.
- N1: one to three lymph nodes close to the bowel contain cancer cells.
- N2: cancer cells in four or more nearby lymph nodes.

Metastasis (M) This refers to whether the cancer has spread to different sites in the body.

- M0: cancer has not spread to other organs.
- M1: cancer has spread to other parts of the body.

The TNM results indicate the stage of the cancer. For example, a cancer described as T2N0M0 would indicate that:

- The tumour has grown into the muscle layer of the bowel wall
- There is no evidence of cancer cells in the lymph nodes
- There is no evidence of any spread to other parts of the body.

The Dukes' staging system is another method of describing the cancer and is based on the examination of biopsies. For colorectal cancer:

- A: tumour is in the mucosa and submucosa
- B: tumour has advanced to the serosa but not the lymph nodes
- C: tumour has now infiltrated the lymph nodes
- D: tumour has now spread to other organs and tissues, resulting in metastasis.

The stage of the tumour will dictate future treatment options for the patient and this should be discussed with both the surgeon and the oncologist.

Nursing Care and Management

Enhanced Recovery Programme An enhanced recovery surgical programme should be used for most bowel cancer patients (NICE, 2020a). In enhanced recovery, patients are involved in their own care. They choose what is best for them throughout their treatment with help and advice from their GP and healthcare team. This programme differs from traditional care by:

- Ensuring patients are in the best possible physical condition before surgery
- Minimising the trauma patients go through during surgery, for example better pain control following surgery
- Ensuring patients experience the best possible rehabilitation after surgery.

For detailed principles of preoperative and postoperative care, refer to Chapter 14. In planning and implementing care, consider both physical and psychosocial care needs of the patient. In the preoperative phase, there are some major considerations that should be taken into account. The potential for formation of a stoma is stressful for the patient. They are worried about altered body image as well as the success of the surgery in relation to removal of the tumour. Psychological care needs should be considered with both the patient and their significant others in the preoperative phase.

Give the patient and their relatives time to express their concerns and worries. Nurses should give all the necessary information and build a trusting relationship with the patient. Some of their anxieties may include loss of control of normal bodily function and restrictions on current lifestyle and daily activities (Vujnovich, 2008; Nadesalingam, 2020). Other concerns that should be considered include sexual activities, socialising and travelling. All these worries should be addressed in the preoperative phase to ensure an uneventful recovery. Not all colorectal surgery will result in stoma formation but some resections will. The possibility of adjuvant therapy such as radiotherapy or chemotherapy should be discussed with the patient before treatment begins.

Preoperative Care in Relation to Stoma Formation

- If a stoma is to be formed, preoperative referral to a specialist stoma nurse practitioner is advised. The nurse can provide information and discuss concerns with the patient. It is important to begin teaching prior to surgery to facilitate learning and acceptance of the stoma postoperatively. This provides an ideal opportunity to discuss altered body image, grieving, family relationship, depression and anger.
- Discuss the availability of support groups or associations, and provide a referral as necessary or desired. A support group can help with information and support with regard to living with a stoma.
- If necessary, refer the patient and their relatives to the dietitian for dietary advice and to answer any questions they may have regarding food the patient can eat or should avoid.
- Any verbal preoperative information should be supported with written information for the patient to take away and read; supplement this where appropriate with other media, e.g. reliable websites. The patient and their relatives should have contact details of voluntary colostomy societies for advice and guidance and also know how to contact the stoma nurse.

Postoperative Care in Relation to Stoma Formation The specific care for a stoma patient includes the following.

- Checking the stoma for bleeding, viability and function. In the early postoperative period, small amounts of blood in the pouch are expected. A healthy stoma appears pink or red and moist as a result of mucus production.
- After 4–5 days, the stoma may start to function. Teach the patient how to empty and change the stoma bag. Encourage the patient to participate in the cleaning of the stoma and changing of their stoma bag. If the patient agrees, involve their relatives when caring for the stoma. Preparation for discharge and the resources in the community should also be discussed.
- Ensure that the patient has sufficient dressings, stoma bags and deodorisers to effectively manage the stoma, thereby reducing some of the patient's anxiety.

What To Do If . . .

 What will you do if the patient refuses to change the stoma bag and refers to their stoma as a foreign object? Some nursing considerations include:

- Talking to the patient about their anxieties
- Giving time for the patient to come to terms with the altered body image
- With the patient's consent, involving their relatives in stoma care.
- Seeking advice and support from the specialist stoma nurse practitioner.

- There may be changes in the amount and consistency of faeces. With ileostomies, faeces are produced approximately 4 hours after a main meal and are loose, whereas with a colostomy faeces are produced the following morning and are formed. Ileostomies are associated with increased output (Larsen, 2015). Often, patients have to change their diet to control wind and malodour, for example that caused by fizzy drinks and fish, respectively.

- Ileostomies usually have a very high output and thus there is a risk of dehydration. Patients need to have a good intake of fluid and take an extra 1 L above the usual intake of fluid. However, advise the patient to avoid fizzy drinks and beer as these may cause flatulence.
- During the first few weeks following the formation of a colostomy or ileostomy, patients may experience sudden urges to defaecate. This is known as the 'phantom rectum' and can be very distressing for them. Nurses need to reassure and inform patients that it is normal to have such a feeling and that over time it will subside.

Jot This Down

List some of the complications that may be associated with living with a stoma.

Red Flag

 In abdominoperineal resection, the anus is closed and sutured. Nurses should be aware that patients who have undergone abdominoperineal resection cannot have rectal suppositories or any other medications, such as analgesia, rectally.

Acute Pain   In the early postoperative period, a patient-controlled analgesia infusion (PCA) is often used to manage pain. The infusion contains morphine sulfate which is administered intravenously. The patient can control the administration of the analgesia but the pump is set up to prevent any chance of accidental overdose. As well as monitoring the pump and the pain assessment for the patient, the nurse/nursing associate should monitor for the side-effects associated with the administration of opioid analgesia.

As well as using a numeric rating as a pain assessment, the nurse should also observe for other indicators of pai,n for example non-verbal signs such as grimacing, muscle tension, apparent dozing, changes in pulse or blood pressure and rapid shallow respirations.

Practice Assessment Document

 The NMC (2018b,c) expects that both nurses and nursing associates can recognise side-effects of the medicines being administered to those in their care:
Nurse: 'demonstrate knowledge of pharmacology and the ability to recognise the effects of medicines, allergies, drug sensitivities, side effects, contraindications, incompatibilities, adverse reactions, prescribing errors and the impact of polypharmacy and over the counter medication usage'
Nursing associate: 'demonstrate the ability to recognise the effects of medicines, allergies, drug sensitivity, side effects, contraindications and adverse reactions'

The side-effects associated with the administration of opioid analgesia are respiratory depression, confusion, drowsiness, constipation, dry mouth, hallucination, nausea, vomiting, palpitations and arrhythmias.

Diet   Diet is an important consideration for those recovering from cancer surgery. It can be further complicated when also managing a stoma. A range of foods should be available to prevent weight loss and malnutrition. For those patients with a stoma, the dietitian can discuss the foods that increase odour and gas, such as fish, cabbage, egg, cauliflower and beans. For those worried about loose stools, advise the patient on foods that help to thicken stool, for example bananas and rice, and that some food may be undigested, such as corn, tomato skin and pips (Lister *et al.*, 2020). Patients should be encouraged to drink 2–3 L of water per day to avoid becoming constipated.

Altered Body Image   Altered body image through stoma formation creates a lot of issues for the patient and their relatives. Nurses need to be sensitive when dealing with the patient's questions and worries. Nichols & Riemer (2011) state that the patient's angst about altered body image is often overlooked and that they struggle to come to terms with their condition (Gallacher, 2017). Thus, nurses need to be sensitive when answering questions about the stoma and body image.

Jot This Down

Think about a patient you have nursed following stoma surgery for bowel cancer. How did they react to their altered body image? Was there anything further you could have done to help the patient to come to terms with their condition?

Cultural and Religious Considerations   These issues should be discussed with patients. In Black's (2004) seminal work, she states that, in some cultures, the left hand is considered dirty and is used for cleaning and hygiene and the right hand for eating and touching clean items. The stoma nurse needs to consider this when discussing stoma care with the patient, choosing stoma equipment and the siting of the stoma. In certain cultures, having a stoma may be regarded as 'unclean', adding to the patient's difficulties in adjusting.

Sexuality   There are several issues that need to be addressed when offering advice to patients after stoma surgery. The impairment for both men and women depends on the complications during the procedure. Women who have their rectum removed may find having sex in the traditional 'missionary position' painful because the rectum is no longer available to support the vagina during sex. A different position may be one way to overcome this problem. After surgery, some women may find that their vagina is much dryer and therefore having sex may be uncomfortable. Advice on the use of lubricants should be offered to the patient.

Some men may find erectile dysfunction an issue postoperatively, as a result of nerve and blood vessel damage to the penis during surgery. They should be referred to a urology specialist to discuss medication options that may help with this.

Work   Once the bowel has returned to normal function, there is no reason why the patient should not return to work. The stoma nurse will advise on appliances that are suitable for the work they do; for some patients it may be necessary for the employer to make reasonable adjustments to enable the patient to continue working. Stoma patients do not need to inform their work colleagues of their surgery unless they want to; some patients like to share their experience with others and this is perfectly normal.

Chemotherapy and Radiotherapy

Patients may need chemotherapy and/or radiotherapy treatment following stoma surgery. The tumour may have invaded other tissues and organs and this treatment is used to destroy any cancerous cells in these areas. Soreness of the skin and general tiredness are common side-effects of these treatments. Nurses should inform the patient that the skin around the genitals and anus can be very sore following radiotherapy. Patients should be advised to refrain from any sexual activities until the skin around that region heals.

Chemotherapy drugs affect patients in different ways. No two patients experience the same side-effects with the same chemotherapy drugs. Common side-effects include the following.

- Nausea and vomiting.
- Diarrhoea.
- Hair loss and thinning.
- Fatigue.
- Reduction in blood cells (red and white blood cells and platelets).
- Some drugs can affect the lining of the mouth and make it sore and temporarily alter the sense of taste. Some may even cause mouth ulcers.

Unfortunately, as well as causing short-term side-effects, radiotherapy to the rectum can cause some long-term side-effects. These include:

- Frequent bowel movements and sometimes diarrhoea
- Frequency as a result of shrinking of the bladder from radiotherapy
- Loss of fertility in both men and women
- Early menopause in women
- Erectile dysfunction in men.

Case Study

Carlos received his bowel screening test in the post 1 month after his 60th birthday. The first test was found to be incorrectly completed and a second test was sent to Carlos. Carlos did not wish to engage with the second test but was persuaded by his family to complete it. His test was positive and Carlos underwent a colonoscopy procedure. After the procedure, Carlos was informed that there was a suspicious polyp that had been sent to the laboratory for confirmation of a colorectal cancer diagnosis. One month later, Carlos was in hospital having a resection of his bowel. Following recovery and at the outpatient appointment, Carlos was informed that his cancer was caught in time, it had not spread and the surgeon was confident that it had been removed. Carlos was referred to oncology but no further cancer treatment was required. The importance of screening in early identification and treatment of cancer cannot be overestimated.

Health Education and Discharge

Early detection of colorectal cancer is an important part of the nursing care, as the prognosis is much better if the cancer is detected early. Nurses, in collaboration with dietitians, are well placed to advise patients on diets that may be considered risk factors in colorectal cancer. These include red meat and sugar and the fat content of food, and patients should be advised to increase fibre intake in their diet. Preventive measures should also include health screening and providing advice on all dietary intake.

Advise the patient to seek medical advice if they see blood in their stool and experience alterations in their bowel habit.

Discharge planning should be carried out on the day the patient is admitted for surgery. Implementing the advanced recovery pathway, nurses should set a provisional discharge date and put into action the care needs of the patient in the community. As Gluyas (2015) discusses, with the fragmentation of healthcare, the patient will have contact with a number of healthcare professionals. Therefore effective communication between healthcare professionals, in both the acute and primary care sectors, is key to psychological adaptation and successful rehabilitation of the patient. Care needs include the following.

- Visits by the stoma nurse and their contact details.
- Contact details of colostomy societies.
- Stoma supplies and advice on further prescriptions.
- Compliance on prescribed medications.
- Advice on diet, fluid intake, exercise and work.
- Contact details of counsellors in stoma care if necessary.
- Referral to cancer support groups and social services as necessary.
- Listen and give time for the patient and their relatives to express worries and concerns about living with a stoma.

What the Experts Say

Stoma care nurses run stoma care clinics at which they see people at various points post surgery. It is important to provide this service to help patients recover physically and mentally from the surgery and to provide a point of contact and source of information. Stoma care nurses receive specific stoma care training, making them an excellent source of information and advice in the postsurgical period and beyond.

Conclusion

This chapter has provided an insight into some of the common conditions associated with gastrointestinal disorders. Nurses play an important role in supporting patients with physical, emotional and psychosocial issues surrounding gastrointestinal disorders. Nurses need to work with the patient, their relatives and other healthcare professionals to provide high-quality care. Continuity of care following discharge is crucial for patients who have altered body image as a result of surgery. Effective communication and collaboration between healthcare professionals, both in the acute and primary sectors, is important to successful rehabilitation for the patient following discharge.

Key Points

- A bacterium, *Helicobacter pylori* (*H. pylori*), is the main cause of peptic ulcers. Peptic ulcer can affect people of any age, including children, but the condition is most common in people who are 60 years of age or over.
- The most common cause of peptic ulcer is *H. pylori* infection. It is a Gram-negative, spiral-shaped bacterium. The next most common cause is excessive use of NSAIDs.
- Around 95% of stomach cancers are adenocarcinomas and 5% are lymphomas, sarcomas and carcinoids. Adenocarcinomas can spread along the stomach wall to the duodenum and can also spread to other organs in the abdominal cavity.
- There is a correlation between diet and stomach cancer. High intakes of red meat, salt, pickled and smoked foods have been associated with stomach cancer, while eating a lot of fruit and green vegetables can reduce the risk.
- Hepatitis, regardless of the cause, can have devastating effects. Preventing the spread of hepatitis is an important nursing responsibility.
- The formation of a stoma results in altered body image and can affect both the patient and their relatives. Nurses should give the patient and their relatives time to express their concerns and worries, and should give all the necessary information and build a trusting relationship with them. Some of their anxieties may include loss of control of normal bodily functions, restrictions on current lifestyle and daily activities.
- During the first few weeks following the formation of a stoma, the patient may experience sudden urges to defaecate. This is known as 'phantom rectum' and can be very distressing for the patient. Nurses need to reassure and inform the patient that it is normal to have such a feeling and that over time it will lessen.

References

BAPEN (2016) *Introducing MUST*. www.bapen.org.uk/screening-and-must/must/introducing-must (accessed December 2021).

Bauldoff, G., Gubrud, P. & Carno, M. (2019) *LeMone & Burkes Medical-Surgical Nursing. Critical Reasoning in Patient Care*, 7th edn. Pearson, London.

Black, P.K. (2004) Psychological, sexual and cultural issues for patients with a stoma. *British Journal of Nursing*, 13(12), 692–697.

British Society of Gastroenterology (2019) *British Society of Gastroenterology position statement on patient experience of GI endoscopy*. www.bsg.org.uk/wp-content/uploads/2019/12/Patient-Experience-GI-endoscopy_2019.pdf (accessed December 2021).

Cancer Research UK (2021) *Stomach cancer incidence and statistics*. www.cancerresearchuk.org/health-professional/cancer-statistics/statistics-by-cancer-type/stomach-cancer/incidence#heading-Eight (accessed December 2021).

Felder, S., Margel, D., Murrell, Z. & Fleshner, P. (2014) Usefulness of bowel sound auscultation: a prospective evaluation. *Journal of Surgical Education*, 71(5), 768–773.

Gallacher, R. (2017) Altered body image. *Nursing Standard*, 31(50), 64–65.

Gluyas, H. (2015) Improving healthcare outcomes. *Nursing Standard*, 30(4), 50–57.

Larsen, P.D. (2015) *Lubkin's Chronic Illness: Impact and Intervention*, 9th edn. Jones and Bartlett Publishers, Burlington, MA.

Lister, S., Hofland, J. & Grafton, H. (2020) *The Royal Marsden Manual of Clinical Nursing Procedures*, 10th edn. Wiley Blackwell, Chichester.

Macmillan Cancer Care (no date) *Personalised Care for People Living with Cancer*. www.macmillan.org.uk/healthcare-professionals/innovation-in-cancer-care/personalised-care (accessed December 2021).

McCance, K.L. & Huether, S.E. (2018) *Pathophysiology. The Biologic Basis for Disease in Adults and Children*, 8th edn. Elsevier, St Louis, MO.

McErlean, L. (2021) The gastrointestinal system and associated disorders. In: Peate, I. (ed.) *Fundamentals of Applied Pathophysiology. An Essential Guide for Nursing and Health Care Students*, 4th edn. Wiley Blackwell, Chichester.

Nadesalingam, M. (2020) Pharmaceutical considerations for patients with stomas. www.pharmaceutical-journal.com/article/ld/pharmaceutical-considerations-for-patients-with-stomas (accessed December 2021)

National Institute for Health and Care Excellence (2014) *Gallstone disease: diagnosis and management*. CG188. NICE, London.

National Institute for Health and Care Excellence (2015a) *Inflammatory bowel disease*. QS81. NICE, London.

National Institute for Health and Care Excellence (2015b) *Review of NICE Technology Appraisal Guidance No. 187: Infliximab and Adalimumab for the Treatment of Crohn's Disease*. NICE, London.

National Institute for Health and Care Excellence (2020a) *Perioperative care in adults*. NG180. NICE, London.

National Institute for Health and Care Excellence (2020b) *Virtual Touch Quantification to Diagnose and Monitor Liver Fibrosis in Chronic Hepatitis B and C*. MTG27. NICE, London.

National Institute for Health and Care Excellence (2021) *Acute Alcohol Withdrawal Pathway*. https://pathways.nice.org.uk/pathways/alcohol-use-disorders/acute-alcohol-withdrawal (accessed December 2021).

Nichols, T.R. & Riemer, M. (2011) Body image perception: the stoma peristomal skin condition. *Gastrointestinal Nursing*, 9(1), 22–26.

Nursing & Midwifery Council (2018a) *The Code. Professional standards of practice and behaviour for nurses, midwives and nursing associates*. www.nmc.org.uk/globalassets/sitedocuments/nmc-publications/nmc-code.pdf. (accessed December 2021).

Nursing & Midwifery Council (2018b) *Future nurse: Standards of proficiency for registered nurses*. www.nmc.org.uk/globalassets/sitedocuments/education-standards/future-nurse-proficiencies.pdf (accessed December 2021).

Nursing & Midwifery Council (2018c) *Standards of proficiency for nursing associates*. www.nmc.org.uk/globalassets/sitedocuments/education-standards/nursing-associates-proficiency-standards.pdf (accessed December 2021).

O'Connor, R. (2020) Alcohol dependence and mental health. https://publichealthmatters.blog.gov.uk/2020/11/17/alcohol-dependence-and-mental-health/ (accessed December 2021).

Peate, I. & Evans, S. (eds) (2020) *Fundamentals of Anatomy and Physiology for Nursing and Healthcare Students*, 3rd edn. Wiley, Oxford.

Rockett, M., Vanstone, R., Chand, J. & Waeland, D. (2017) A survey of acute pain services in the UK. *Anaesthesia*, 72, 1237–1242.

Royal College of Physicians (2017) *National Early Warning Score (NEWS) 2*. www.rcplondon.ac.uk/projects/outputs/national-early-warning-score-news-2 (accessed December 2021).

Vujnovich, A. (2008) Pre- and post-operative assessment of patients with a stoma. *Nursing Standard*, 22(19), 50–56.

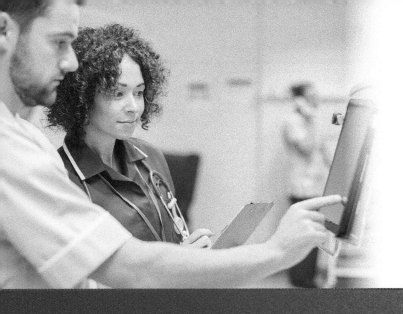

29

The Person with a Urinary Disorder

Jamie Swales

East Lancashire Hospital NHS Trust, UK

Learning Outcomes

On completion of this chapter you will be able to:

- Describe the structure and functions of the urinary system
- Describe the microscopic structures of the urinary system
- Explain how the urinary system maintains homeostasis
- Explain urine production and its composition
- Discuss the pathophysiology of common urinary tract disorders encountered in practice
- Outline the nursing care, management and interventions of the disorders described

Proficiencies

NMC Proficiencies and Standards:

- Take responsibility for collaborative assessment, planning and delivery of care for patients with urinary disorders, with the patient and, where applicable, their relatives and carers
- Assess the holistic health status of the patient with urinary tract disorders, using data collected to determine nursing diagnoses and interventions
- Apply research-based evidence in implementing nursing care for patients with urinary tract disorders
- Provide safe and effective nursing care for patients undergoing surgery of the urinary tract
- Recognise and provide appropriate health promotion for prevention and self-care of urinary disorders and associated interventions
- Evaluate nursing care outcome, revising the care as needed to promote, maintain or restore the health of patients with urinary disorders

 Visit the companion website at www.wiley.com/go/peate/nursingpractice3e where you can test yourself using flashcards, multiple-choice questions and more.

Nursing Practice: Knowledge and Care, Third Edition. Edited by Ian Peate and Aby Mitchell.
© 2022 John Wiley & Sons Ltd. Published 2022 by John Wiley & Sons Ltd.
Companion website: www.wiley.com/go/peate/nursingpractice3e

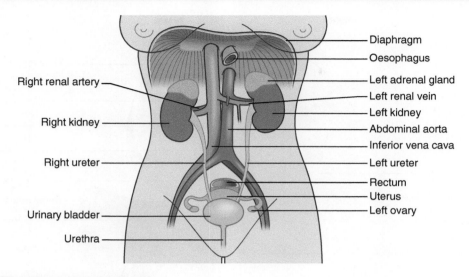

Figure 29.1 Organs of the urinary system in a female.

Introduction

The urinary system (also called the *renal system*) plays an important role in maintaining homeostasis by regulating body fluids, filtering metabolic wastes from the bloodstream, selectively reabsorbing substances and water into the bloodstream, and eliminating metabolic wastes and water as urine. Therefore, any disease relating to the urinary system affects the whole body. The kidneys (part of the urinary system) also have an endocrine function: production and release of hormones such as renin and erythropoietin. This chapter discusses the structure and functions of the urinary system, and nursing care management and interventions of some common disorders that nurses/nursing associates might come across in practice.

Anatomy and Physiology

The urinary system (renal system) typically consists of paired kidneys, the paired ureters, the urinary bladder and the urethra (Figure 29.1). The kidneys perform the major work of the urinary system, with the other structures being mainly passageways and storage areas.

In order to have sufficient knowledge, skills and competency in the care of urological disorders, it is imperative nurses/nursing associates have a good understanding of anatomy and physiology which in turn will promote safety and wellbeing (NMC, 2018a,b).

The Kidneys

The two kidneys are located in the abdominal cavity and lie at a slightly oblique angle on either side of the vertebral column (just above the waist) at the levels of T12 to L3 (Figure 29.2). They are approximately 10–12 cm long, 5–7 cm wide and 3–4 cm thick (Jenkins & Tortora, 2013). They are bean-shaped organs, where the outer surface is convex and the inner surface is concave in shape. Near the centre of the concave border is an indentation

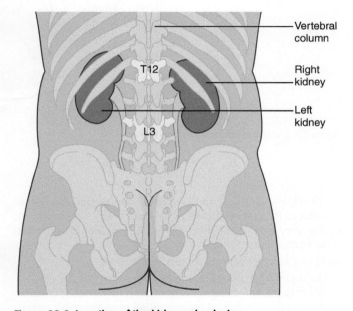

Figure 29.2 Location of the kidneys: back view.

called the *renal hilum* through which the ureter, renal artery, renal vein, lymphatic vessels and nerves enter and exit the kidney.

Jot This Down

Name the gland that sits on top of each kidney like a crown. What are some of its functions?

The kidneys are surrounded by three layers of tissue.

- The *renal fascia*: a thin outer layer of fibrous connective tissue that surrounds each kidney (and the attached adrenal gland) and attaches it to surrounding structures.

517

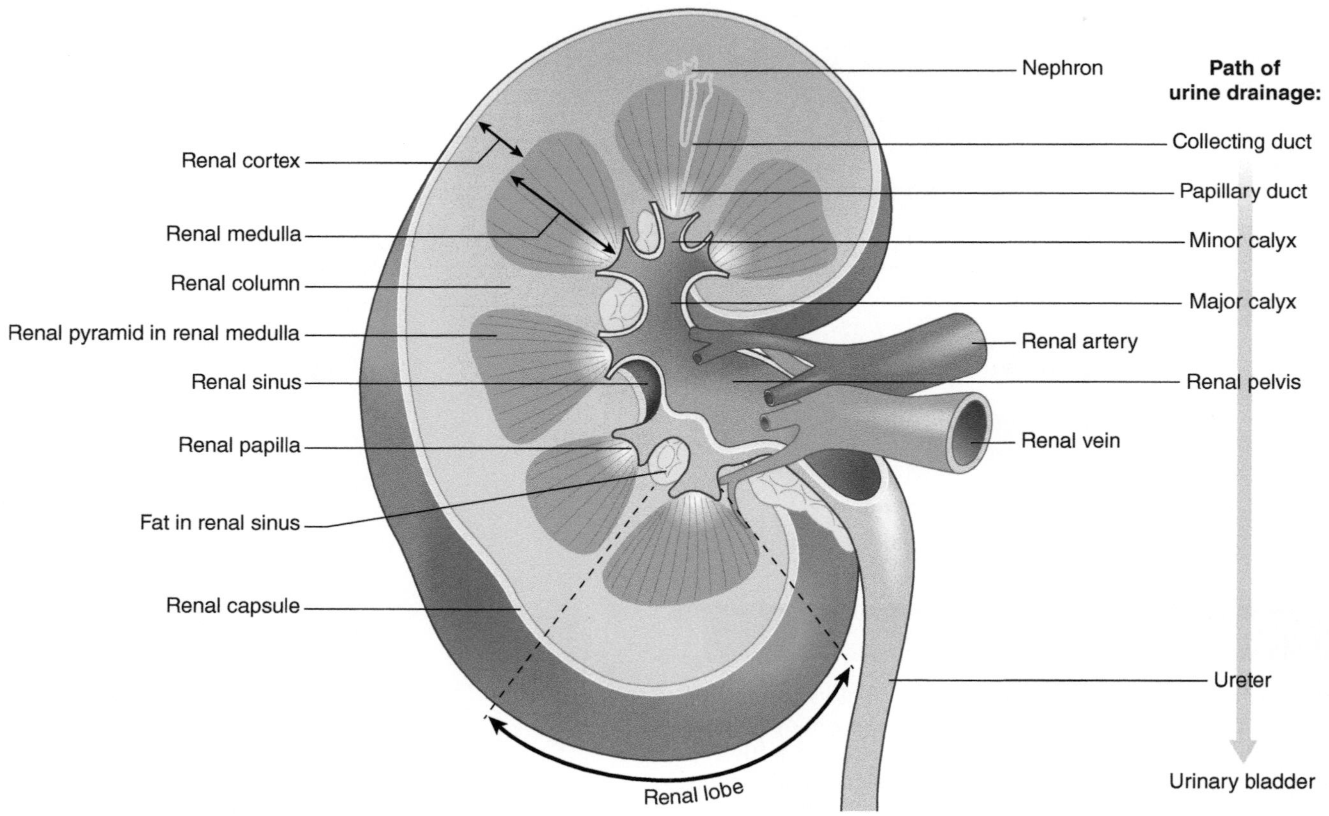

Figure 29.3 Internal structures of the kidney.

- The *adipose capsule*: a middle layer of adipose (fat) tissue that cushions the kidneys and helps to retain heat.
- The *renal capsule*: the inner fibrous membrane that prevents the entrance of infections.

Inside the kidney, there are three major sections.

- The *renal cortex* along the convex side.
- The *renal medulla* lying adjacent to the renal cortex. It consists of striated, cone-shaped regions called renal pyramids (medullary pyramids). The peaks, called *renal papillae*, face inward (Figure 29.3). The unstriated regions between the renal pyramids are called *renal columns*.
- The *renal sinus*: a cavity that lies adjacent to the renal medulla. The other side of the renal sinus, bordering the concave surface of the kidney, opens to the outside through the renal hilus. The renal pelvis is situated in the renal sinus, a funnel-shaped structure that merges with the ureter. Branches of the renal pelvis, known as the major and minor calyces, extend toward the medulla. They collect and convey urine to the pelvis of the kidney.

The renal pelvis is continuous with the ureter as it leaves the hilum. From the pelvis, urine is propelled, by peristalsis, through the ureter and into the bladder for storage (see Figure 29.3).

Renal Blood Supply

The kidneys receive their blood supply directly from the aorta via the renal arteries and blood is returned to the inferior vena cava via the renal veins. The kidneys receive approximately 20%

of the cardiac output. The blood supply to the kidneys arises from the paired renal arteries at the level of L2. The hilum, located where the kidney curves inwards in a concave shape, is the opening where the renal artery enters. The renal veins return the blood from the kidneys and lie anterior to the renal artery at the hilum (see Figure 29.3). The left renal vein is longer than the right, as it crosses the midline to reach the inferior vena cava. For more detail on blood flow to the kidney see Figure 29.4.

Nephron

There are approximately 0.8–1 million nephrons in each kidney and it is these structures that filter the blood to produce urine (Jenkins & Tortora, 2013). The nephron consists of a cup-shaped glomerular capsule (Bowman capsule) and, immediately below the capsule, a twisted region called the proximal convoluted tubule. This is followed by a long hairpin-like section called the loop of Henle, which runs deep into the medulla and then back into the cortex. This is followed by another twisted region, called the distal convoluted tubule (Figure 29.5). The distal convoluted tubules of several nephrons empty into a single collecting duct in the medulla of the kidney that then converges to a renal papilla, which represents the apex of the renal pyramid. Urine then collects into 9–12 minor calyces, which then converge into approximately 3–4 major calyces (Jenkins & Tortora, 2013). The major calyces then empty into the renal pelvis, which passes urine through the ureteropelvic junction and into the ureter, which

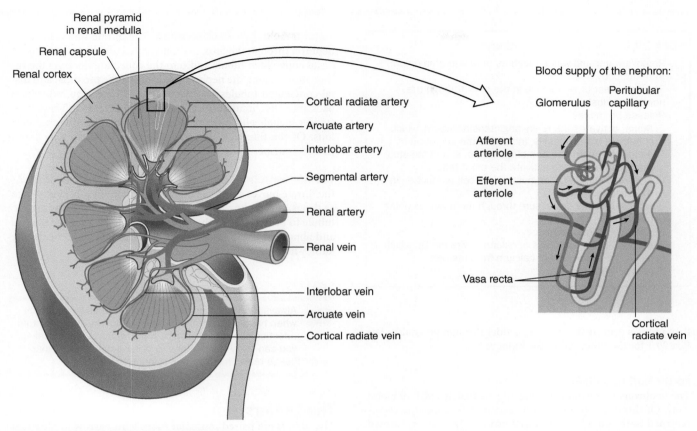

Figure 29.4 Blood flow through the kidney.

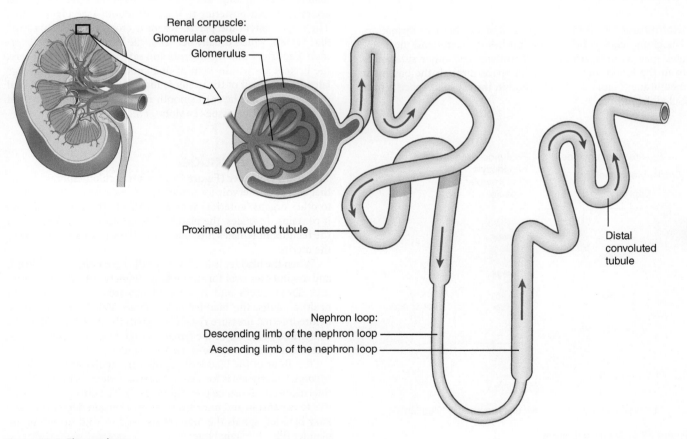

519

Figure 29.5 The nephron.

Box 29.1 Functions of the kidneys

- Remove water and waste (such as urea and ammonium) from the body.
- Regulate electrolyte balance in the body through the hormone aldosterone.
- Release hormones.
  - *Renin*: activates the renin–angiotensin system, which constricts blood vessels, increases the secretion of antidiuretic hormone and aldosterone, and stimulates the hypothalamus to activate the thirst reflex.
  - *Erythropoietin (EPO)*: stimulates red cell production in the bone marrow.
- Help maintain blood pressure through the renin–angiotensin system.
- Regulate acid–base balance.
- Play a role in the synthesis of calcitriol (vitamin D), which helps in the absorption of calcium from the diet.
- Synthesise glucose.

then propels urine distally to the bladder through peristalsis. See Box 29.1 for the functions of the kidneys.

Formation of Urine

The nephrons of the kidneys filter approximately 190 L of blood daily. Of this amount, only 1% is excreted as urine; the rest is returned to the circulation (Silverthorn, 2015). Urine is formed from the filtered blood by glomerular filtration, tubular reabsorption and tubular secretion.

Glomerular Filtration This is the first step in urine formation. The glomerular blood pressure pushes the water and most solutes such as urea, uric acid, electrolytes and other substances from the blood into the capsular space through the basement membrane (Figure 29.6). The fluid in the capsular space is now called the *filtrate*.

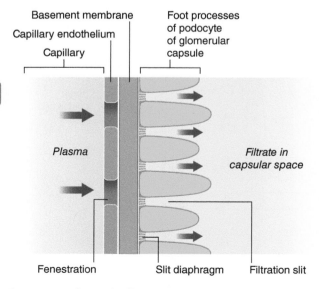

Figure 29.6 **Glomerular filtration.**

Tubular Selective Reabsorption The filtrate flows along the nephron through the proximal convoluted tubule, loop of Henle, distal convoluted tubule and into the collecting duct. As the filtrate moves along the nephron, cells lining the proximal and distal convoluted tubules selectively reabsorb the required solutes back into the circulation to maintain homeostasis. These substances include glucose, amino acids, lactate, vitamins and most ions. Of the filtered water, 99% is reabsorbed and only 1% is passed as urine.

Tubular Secretion The final stage in the formation of urine. As the filtrate moves along the nephron, unwanted substances such as drugs, metabolic waste and excess ions are secreted into the tubule to be expelled in the urine. See Table 29.1 for the normal and abnormal composition of urine. Through this process, the kidney helps to maintain homeostasis.

Red Flag

Always wear appropriate personal protective equipment when handling body fluids; this is imperative to maintain infection control standards. If precautions are not taken, you can carry the bacteria to other patients or to your family. Please read Chapter 16 in relation to this.

The Ureters

The ureters are paired muscular tubes with narrow lumina that carry urine from the kidneys to the bladder. They are approximately 26–30 cm long. The ureter begins at the level of the renal artery and vein posterior to these structures (see Figure 29.1). The ureter enters the pelvis, where it crosses anteriorly to the iliac vessels, which usually occurs at the bifurcation of the common iliac artery into the internal and external iliac arteries. Here, the ureters are within 5 cm of one another before they diverge laterally. The wall of the ureter is made up of an inner epithelial mucosa, a middle layer of smooth muscle and an outer layer of fibrous connective tissue (LeMone *et al.*, 2011).

The Urinary Bladder

The urinary bladder (Figure 29.7) is a musculomembranous sac that acts as a reservoir for urine. Its size, position and proximity to other organs (anterior) vary according to the amount of fluid it contains. In males, the bladder lies immediately anteriorly to the rectum; in females it is anterior to the vagina and inferior to the uterus.

When the bladder is moderately full, it contains about 500 mL and assumes an oval form; the long diameter of the oval measures about 12 cm and is directed upwards and forwards. In healthy adults, the bladder holds about 300–500 mL of urine before internal pressure rises and signals the need to void urine. The urinary bladder in the female is slightly smaller because the uterus occupies the space above the bladder.

The floor of the bladder is a small triangular area called the *trigone*. The trigone is formed by the two ureteral orifices and the internal urethral orifice (see Figure 29.7). The area is very sensitive to expansion and once stretched to a certain degree, the urinary bladder signals the brain of its need to void urine. As the bladder fills, this signal intensifies.

Table 29.1 **Normal and abnormal findings in the urine.**

URINALYSIS	NORMAL FINDINGS	ABNORMAL FINDINGS
Colour	Yellow to amber	This can vary depending on diet, hydration, medications and any diseases
Odour	Aromatic smell	Early morning urine may smell a bit strong because it is concentrated
Leucocytes (white blood cells)	Negative	If present, may indicate bladder or kidney infection, fever or kidney diseases
Urobilinogen	Normally found in urine	If elevated, may indicate liver diseases or excessive destruction of red blood cells
Bilirubin	Negative	This may be positive in hepatic diseases
Glycosuria (glucose in urine)	Negative	May be positive in diabetes mellitus, long-term steroid therapy and acute pancreatitis
Ketones	Negative	Found in patients with diabetes, high protein diet and in starvation
Haematuria (blood in urine)	Negative	Positive in patients with urinary tract infection (UTI), kidney diseases, cancer of the bladder; possible contamination from menstruation in females and kidney or pelvic trauma
Protein	A trace may be present	If present in larger amounts, may be due to UTI, kidney diseases such as nephrotic syndrome, toxaemia of pregnancy, septicaemia and side-effects of some drugs, such as neomycin, barbiturates and sulfonamides, and in patients receiving total parenteral nutrition
Nitrites	Negative	Positive when dietary nitrate is converted to nitrites by Gram-negative bacteria
pH	Normal range 4.5–8	A pH of less than 4 may indicate dehydration, uncontrolled diabetes or starvation. A pH >8 may indicate UTI or be due to intake of drugs such as kanamycin, sodium bicarbonate and potassium citrate. The pH range is also dependent on the dietary intake of the patient. A person eating a lot of red meat may present with strong acid urine, while a vegan or vegetarian may present with alkaline urine
Specific gravity (SG)	Normal range 1005–1030	High SG may indicate dehydration, fever, diabetes mellitus, vomiting or diarrhoea. A low SG may result from overingestion of fluid, diabetes insipidus or renal disease

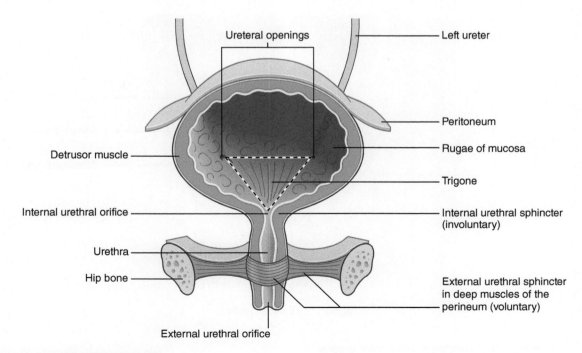

Figure 29.7 **Urinary bladder in the female.**

The Urethra

The urethra is a thin-walled muscular tube that channels urine to the outside of the body. It extends from the base of the bladder to the external urinary meatus. In males, the urethra travels through the penis and carries semen as well as urine (Figure 29.8), and is approximately 20 cm long. The prostate gland encircles the urethra at the base of the bladder in males. The male urinary meatus is located at the end of the glans penis. In females, the urethra is shorter and emerges above the vaginal opening (Figure 29.9). The female urethra is approximately 3–5 cm long, and the urinary meatus is anterior to the vaginal orifice.

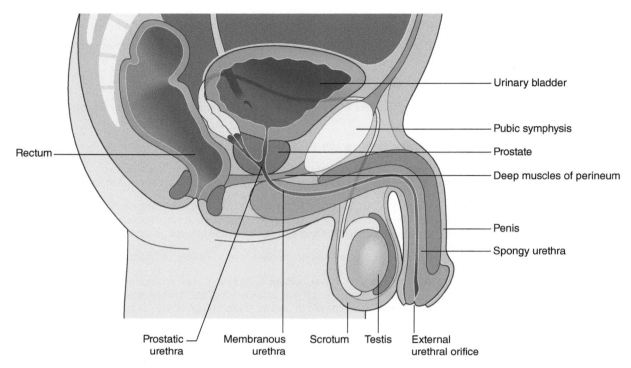

Figure 29.8 The male urethra in relation to other pelvic organs.

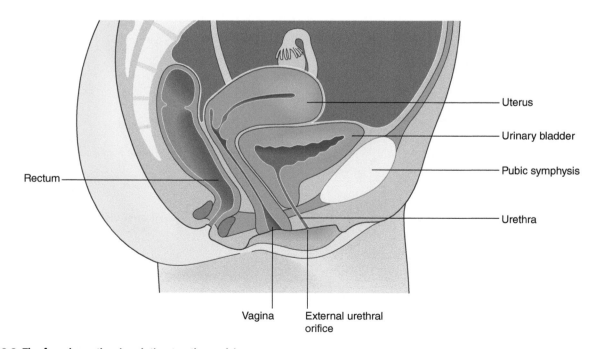

Figure 29.9 The female urethra in relation to other pelvic organs.

Urinary Tract Infection

Urinary tract infection (UTI) is the presence and multiplication of micro-organisms in one or more structures of the urinary tract with organisms invading the surrounding tissue (Health Protection Agency, 2012). The organisms that cause UTIs include *Escherichia coli*, common Gram-negative enteral bacteria, *Proteus*, *Klebsiella*, *Serratia* and *Pseudomonas*. A UTI is normally described as either upper or lower infection. An upper UTI or *pyelonephritis* is an infection in the kidneys. A lower UTI or *cystitis* is an infection in the bladder.

Pathophysiology

The two main common UTIs are cystitis and pyelonephritis. Cystitis is more common in women, as they have a short urethra compared with men (see Figures 29.8 and 29.9). The urethra's opening is also located very close to the anus, which makes it easy for bacteria from the anal region to reach the bladder and cause an infection. Although men are less prone to cystitis, it could be more serious because cystitis may be the result of prostatitis or other problems associated with an enlarged prostate or an obstruction such as kidney stones. Cystitis can be either acute or chronic. In acute cystitis, the patient may experience painful or burning frequency, urgency and suprapubic pain/low back pain. In chronic cystitis, the patient may not have symptoms, except pyuria.

Pyelonephritis relates to inflammation of the parenchyma and the pelvis of the kidney and it is usually associated with bacterial infection. Pyelonephritis can be either acute or chronic. Acute pyelonephritis is a bacterial infection of the kidney, which may start from the lower urinary tract and ascend to one or both kidneys. Chronic pyelonephritis is associated with non-bacterial infections and inflammatory processes that may be metabolic, chemical or immunological in origin (Porth, 2015).

Chronic pyelonephritis involves chronic inflammation and scarring of the tubules and interstitial tissues of the kidney and can lead to chronic kidney disease (CKD). It can result from renal diseases, UTI, recurrent episodes of acute pyelonephritis or obstruction of the ureter. The kidney becomes scarred and irregular and the calyces and renal pelvis are deformed. There are some people who are at increased risk of UTIs, for example those with pre-existing kidney disease, diabetes or a compromised immune system, in pregnancy and the frail elderly.

Signs and Symptoms

- Dysuria.
- Urgency.
- Nocturia.
- Urine that smells unpleasant.
- Haematuria.
- Pyrexia (especially in pyelonephritis).
- Rigors (especially in pyelonephritis).
- Pyuria (pus in the urine).
- Low back pain (especially in pyelonephritis).
- Malaise (especially in pyelonephritis).
- Older adults may present with confusion.

Investigations

Investigations for UTI may include the following.

- *Urinalysis*: see Table 29.1 for some of the positive findings.
- *Urine culture*: for high-risk patients, e.g. pregnant or immuno-suppressed patients, or those who have failed to respond to earlier antibiotic treatment. Urine culture should always be done in men with a history suggestive of UTI, regardless of the results of the urinalysis.
- An *ultrasound* of the upper urinary tract should be carried out to rule out urinary obstruction or renal stone disease in acute uncomplicated pyelonephritis in premenopausal non-pregnant women.

Nursing Care and Management

The main objective in UTI is to identify the cause and offer appropriate treatment. The patient will need reassurance and psychological support and health education. In the patient with acute pyelonephritis, bedrest should be encouraged until symptoms of pyrexia and severe groin pain subside. It is important for nurses/nursing associates to report signs of groin pain such as restlessness, sweating and tachycardia for prompt action.

Medications Trimethoprim and nitrofurantoin (NICE, 2018a,b) are currently the first choice for lower UTI in the UK, because they are cost-effective, well tolerated and work in 80% of infections. Second-line antibiotics should be prescribed in line with urine culture sensitivities.

For the treatment of pyelonephritis, those who can be managed within primary care should be treated initially with cefalaxin 500 mg BD-TDS and further treatment should be tailored utilising available urine culture sensitivities (NICE, 2021a).

Pain Pain is a common symptom of both lower and upper UTIs. In cystitis, inflammation causes a sensation of a full bladder, dull constant suprapubic pain and possibly low back pain. The inflamed bladder wall and urethra cause dysuria (difficult or painful micturition), and pain and burning when voiding urine. Bladder spasms may develop, causing periodic severe stabbing discomfort. Pain associated with pyelonephritis is often steady and dull, localised to the outer abdomen or flank region. Urological disorders rarely cause central abdominal pain (LeMone *et al.*, 2011). Nurses/nursing associates (NMC, 2018a) should:

- Assess the timing, quality, intensity, location and duration using an appropriate pain assessment tool. A change in the nature, location or intensity of the pain could indicate an extension of the infection or a related but separate problem
- Administer the prescribed analgesia or antispasmodic medication and note its effect. Paracetamol and/or non-steroidal anti-inflammatory drugs (NSAIDs) are used for symptomatic relief (NICE, 2021a)
- Advise the patient to see their GP if pain and discomfort persist after 24 hours of treatment. Continued discomfort may indicate a complicated UTI or other urinary tract disorder.

Urinary Tract Infections and Dementia People with dementia who develop a UTI may exhibit a noticeable change in behaviour known as delirium. The person may become agitated or restless, have difficulty concentrating, have delusions or hallucinations or become withdrawn and very sleepy. These people may not be able to express their symptoms, so it is important for the nurse/nursing associate to be aware of the possibility of a UTI.

Fluid and Diet Intake Encourage daily fluid intake of 2.5–3 L unless contraindicated. Increased fluid dilutes urine, reduces irritation of the inflamed bladder and urethral mucosa, and helps to flush out bacteria from the bladder.

- Monitor hourly urine output and record the amount, colour, clarity and odour of urine. Urine should return to normal colour (light yellow or amber) after 48 hours of treatment. If changes do not occur, report any findings immediately for prompt action.
- Probiotic bacteria in foods such as yoghurt and sauerkraut can help prevent UTIs by promoting the growth of beneficial bacteria and inhibiting overgrowth or infection by pathogens.

Health Promotion and Discharge

Prior to discharge, nurses/nurse associates should advise on measures to prevent UTI. Encourage the patient to drink approximately 2.5–3 L daily and advise them on the type of fluid to drink and which to avoid. Encourage the patient to empty their bladder every 3–4 hours and not to retain urine over a longer period. Nurses/nurse associates should teach women to clean the perineal region from front to back after voiding and defaecating. Voiding urine before and after sexual intercourse, to flush out bacteria, should be encouraged; it may be appropriate to recommend a change in the method of contraception if UTIs are recurrent.

Health promotion is a fundamental role of nursing staff (NMC, 2018a), and ensuring a clear understanding of this is relation to urinary disorders is fundamental in your care of this group of patients.

Primary Care

Both upper and lower UTIs are usually managed in the community and therefore it is important that nurses/nursing associates ensure that patients are well informed on the care and management of UTI in the community. Nurses/nursing associates should discuss:
- Risk factors for UTI and how to eliminate these factors through patient education
- Signs and symptoms of UTI and the need to seek advice when preventive measures are not effective
- Appropriate fluid and diet intake and importance of monitoring urine output
- Importance of compliance with any prescribed medications and completing antibiotics as prescribed
- The importance of maintaining personal hygiene and the need to wash hands before and after attending to toilet needs.

Case Study

A 34-year-old female presents to the GP practice with dysuria, offensive smelling urine and lower suprapubic abdominal pain. She has noted an increased frequency of urine with intermittent urgency to empty her bladder. She is systemically well with no fever.

An initial assessment of this patient including full vital signs, physical examination and urinalysis would be undertaken.

If the urinalysis was positive for signs of infection, a prescription for appropriate antibiotics and analgesics would be given. Prior to discharge, safety netting information and self-care advice would be given.

Renal Calculi

Renal calculi are formed when waste products accumulate in the renal tract as crystals; over a period of time, the crystals form hard stones called calculi. Stones can form from any of the following substances.

- Calcium – make up about 80% of urinary stones (NICE, 2020).
- Uric acid (a waste product of food metabolism).
- Cystine (an amino acid that helps build protein).
- Formation of struvite stones as a result of UTI.

Risk Factors

- Family history of renal calculi.
- Chronic dehydration.
- Sex (3:1 ratio of men to women).
- Excess dietary intake of calcium, oxalate, proteins.
- Gout (results in a chronically increased amount of uric acid in the blood and urine and can lead to the formation of uric acid stones).
- Hyperthyroidism.
- Obesity.
- Recurrent UTIs.
- Carcinoma of the bone.
- Some medications also increase the risk of kidney stones.

Pathophysiology

The formation of stones within the urinary tract is called urolithiasis (NICE, 2020). The kidneys filter and excrete salts, including calcium oxalate, uric acid, cystine and xanthine. These salts can become extremely concentrated if there is insufficient urine production (e.g. due to dehydration) or if unusually high amounts of crystal-forming salts are present. When salt concentration levels reach the point at which they no longer dissolve, these salts form crystals. These crystals eventually form kidney stones.

Often, the cause of calcium stones is not known. The condition is then called idiopathic nephrolithiasis. Research suggests that nearly all stones result from problems in the breakdown and absorption of calcium and oxalate. Genetic factors may play a part in the formation of these stones. Several medical conditions (dehydration) and drugs (calcium supplement tablets) can also affect digestion and intestinal absorption. Some drugs, for example loop diuretics and acetazolamide, increase the risk of calcium stones. Diet has also been identified in the formation of calcium stones, for example dairy products, particularly cheeses that contain high levels of calcium.

Human body tissues, and certain foods, contain substances called purines. Purine-containing foods include dried beans, peas and liver. When the body breaks down purines, it produces uric acid. The presence of a certain level of uric acid in the body is normal, but excess uric acid can lead to stones. Some drugs, such as allopurinol and salicylates, promote uric acid stone formation.

Struvite stones are almost always caused by UTIs due to bacteria that produce certain enzymes. These enzymes raise the concentration of ammonia in the urine. Ammonia makes up the crystals that form struvite stones. The stone-promoting bacteria are usually *Proteus* but may also be *Pseudomonas, Klebsiella, Providencia, Serratia* and staphylococci. Women are twice as likely to have struvite stones as men.

Cystine stones develop from genetic defects that cause abnormal transport of amino acids in the kidney and the gastrointestinal system, leading to a build-up of cystine, one of these amino acids.

Investigations and Diagnosis
- Abdominal X-ray to identify urinary obstruction.
- Ultrasound.
- Non-contrast CT urogram.
- Serum creatinine.
- Serum urate.
- Serum calcium and phosphate.
- Full blood count.
- Urinalysis to detect UTI.
- Urea and electrolytes to detect imbalance.

Signs and Symptoms
- Sometimes asymptomatic.
- Dull, aching flank pain.
- Microscopic haematuria.
- Renal colic.
- Acute, severe flank pain on affected side, radiating to the suprapubic region, groin and external genitals.
- Nausea, vomiting, pallor and cool clammy skin.

Nursing Care and Management
Nursing care should include identification of the cause of renal stones in conjunction with the wider MDT and the provision of appropriate treatment and care. Initial management can either be done as an inpatient or on an urgent outpatient basis, usually depending on how severe the pain is and if the patient is presenting with complications such as retention of urine or excessive bleeding.

Medications
- NSAIDs (e.g. diclofenac) are the first-line treatment, administered intramuscularly, intravenously or orally if the patient is tolerating food. If the pain is severe, then a suitable opioid analgesic should be prescribed (e.g. morphine) and administered with a suitable antiemetic for nausea. Caution should be exercised in patients with existing renal impairment as NSAIDs can cause a build-up of nephrotoxic metabolites (BNF, 2021).

- Nurses/nursing associates should document the outcome of the analgesia in the patient's notes. Reassess the patient's pain level every 1–2 hours using a suitable pain assessment tool such as the pain scale. Encourage the patient to lie in a comfortable position that brings relief.

Diet and Fluid Management
- Dietary modifications may be necessary to prevent further episodes of renal calculi formation. This may include reduced intake of dietary calcium and vitamin D for calcium stones and limiting intake of foods high in purines such as sardines, kidneys and red meat.
- Protein increases uric acid, calcium and oxalate levels in the urine, and reduces citrate levels. Diets high in protein, particularly meat protein, have been consistently connected with kidney stones. (Meat protein has higher sulfur content and produces more acid than vegetable protein.) Where stones contain calcium oxalate, advice should be given to reduce the amount of salt in the diet and avoid food that is rich in oxalate such as tea, chocolate, spinach and peanuts.
- Encourage the patient to drink 2.5–3 L of fluid daily to promote urine production and to avoid the formation of kidney stones, thereby preventing acute kidney injury. Increasing urine volume decreases the concentration of minerals in the urine, which makes it less likely that a stone will form. However, during the time that stones are being passed, care is needed with fluid intake. Excessive fluid intake will increase urine output, which leads to an elevated pressure within the renal system causing increased pain; this in turn will cause hydronephrosis (distension of the ureter and kidney).

Invasive Procedures Small calculi, 5 mm or less in diameter, will pass through the urinary tract without any intervention. Some stones become stuck in a kidney or the ureter and cause persistent symptoms or problems such as pain, haematuria and UTI. In these cases, the pain usually becomes severe, and the patient may need to be admitted to hospital. There are various treatment options.

- *Extracorporeal shock wave lithotripsy (ESWL)*: this is the least invasive of procedures, where high-energy shock waves are focused onto the stones, causing them to disintergrate. The technique is used when stones are considered inaccessible via retrograde or percutaneous routes. The stone fragments are then passed in the urine. Adverse effects can include pain and heamaturia.
- *Percutaneous nephrolithotomy (PCNL)* is generally performed when the stones are larger than 20 mm or when there are staghorn calculi (these stones generally fill the pelvis of the kidney). A nephroscope (a thin telescope-like instrument) is passed through the skin and into the kidney. The stone is broken up and the fragments of stone are removed via the nephroscope; adverse effects include sepsis and a risk of haemorrhage. The procedure is usually performed under general anaesthesia.
- In *uretero-pyeloscopic laser lithotripsy*, a telescope is passed up into the ureter via the urethra and bladder and a laser is used to break up the stone. This technique is used for most types of kidney stones and has a high stone clearance rate; however, there is a greater risk of infection, haematuria, more postoperative pain and, more rarely, ureteric injury.

525

Red Flag

A stone that completely obstructs the ureter can lead to hydronephrosis and damage to the affected kidney. As the other kidney continues to function normally, urine output may not fall significantly with the obstruction of one ureter.

Health Promotion and Discharge

Prior to discharge, the nurse/nurse associate should discuss the following points.

- The importance of maintaining good fluid intake, for example 2.5–3 L of fluid daily. This is to ensure that there is good urine production and to prevent UTI. The patient should void urine into a container to catch any stones that may be passed. Advise the patient to drink cranberry juice as it increases citrate excretion and reduces oxalate and phosphate excretion.
- Offer dietary advice on the importance of low salt intake. Reduce intake of oxalate-rich (e.g. chocolate, rhubarb and nuts) and urate-rich (e.g. offal and certain fish) foods.
- The patient may be discharged home with medications to prevent further stone formation and these may include thiazide diuretics (for calcium stones), allopurinol (for uric acid stones) and calcium citrate (for oxalate stones). Stress the importance of taking the medication regularly.

Primary Care

Prior to discharge, nurses/nursing associates should discuss the following topics to prepare for self-care at home.

- The importance of maintaining adequate fluid intake of 2.5–3 L per day.
- If the patient is discharged home with medications, the importance of taking the medications as prescribed.
- Reduce salt intake to no more than 3 g (about half a teaspoonful) daily, as higher amounts may raise the level of calcium in the urine.
- The signs and symptoms of UTI and the preventive measures to avoid recurrence.
- The importance of keeping well hydrated during exercise.
- Advise the patient to keep any outpatient appointments as booked and to see their GP if they are concerned or if they experience any severe pain as a result of stones blocking the urinary tract.

Bladder Cancer

Bladder cancer is more common in men than women and usually takes a long time to develop and is therefore rarely seen in people under 40 years, generally occurring in those over 60. Most bladder cancers are formed from the lining (known as the transitional cell lining) and this cancer is often referred to as transitional cell carcinoma. It is currently called urothelial carcinoma (about 90% of bladder cancers).

Other rarer types of bladder cancer include squamous cell carcinomas (5% of cases) and adenocarcinomas (1–2% of bladder cancers) (Cancer Research UK, 2021).

Risk Factors

Possible risk factors include the following.

- Smokers are up to four times more likely to develop bladder cancer and passive smoking may also increase the risk. Cancer Research UK (2021) found that approximately half of all bladder cancers could be related to smoking.
- Exposure to certain industrial chemicals (e.g. in the rubber, paint, dye, printing and textile industries, gas and tar manufacturing, iron and aluminium processing) and radiation.
- Repeated episodes of bladder infection may also slightly increase the risk.

Pathophysiology

Bladder cancer develops in the lining or the wall of the bladder. It is caused by the uncontrolled growth of cells. Most cases of bladder cancer appear to be caused when the tissue of the bladder is exposed to harmful substances, which, over the course of many years, leads to abnormal biological changes in the bladder's cells. The most common harmful substance is tobacco smoke. It is estimated that half of all cases of bladder cancer are caused by smoking.

Carcinogenic breakdown products of certain chemicals and from cigarette smoke are excreted in the urine and stored in the bladder, possibly causing a local influence on abnormal cell development. Squamous cell carcinoma of the urinary tract occurs less frequently than transitional epithelial cell tumours.

Transitional cell carcinoma is the most common bladder cancer and develops in the top layer of cells that line the bladder wall. These cells come into contact with waste products in the urine that may cause cancer. Squamous cell carcinoma develops in the flat cells that line the bladder wall. Adenocarcinoma is a rare type of bladder cancer that develops in the mucus-producing cells that line the bladder wall.

Bladder tumours are rated by cell type and grade. Grade I tumours are highly differentiated and rarely progress to become invasive, whereas grade III tumours are poorly differentiated and usually progress. The staging of bladder tumours is outlined in Table 29.2; for tissue involvement see Figure 29.10.

Investigations and Diagnosis

- *Cystoscopy*: an invasive procedure using a cystoscope to look into the bladder.
- *Intravenous urogram (IVU)*: a special type of X-ray procedure used to look inside the bladder and urinary system.
- *Ultrasound, MRI or CT scan*: these can help doctors to check the urinary system to see if the cancer has spread.

Table 29.2 Staging of bladder tumour.

STAGES	ORGANS AFFECTED
Ta	Affects the bladder mucosa
T1	Bladder mucosa and submucosal layers
T2	Superficial muscle of bladder wall
T3a	Deep muscle affected
T3b	Involvement of perivesicular fat
T3–4N1	Lymph node and adjacent organs affected

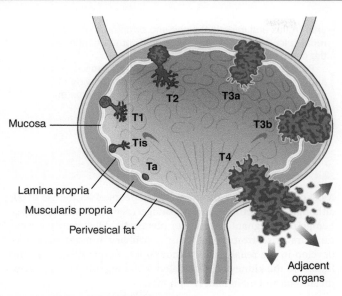

Figure 29.10 Stages of bladder cancer.

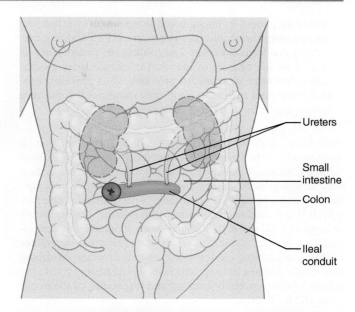

Figure 29.11 Formation of an ileal conduit. A section of the terminal ileum is used to form a stoma, where both ureters are implanted and for the urine to flow into. The stoma protrudes from the skin to minimise skin irritation from the urine.

Signs and Symptoms

- Haematuria is the presenting sign in 80% of urinary tract tumours.
- Frequency.
- Urgency.
- Dysuria.

Nursing Care and Management

The most widely used type of surgery in bladder cancer is transurethral resection of bladder tumour (TURBT) which is considered to be the first treatment that many patients require following diagnosis of a non-muscle invasive bladder cancer. The aim is to remove the cancerous cells and seal the surrounding tissue to prevent recurrence. In the event of the cancer returning, the procedure can be repeated. Prior to discharge, most patients require a single chemotherapy treatment, which is instilled directly into the bladder via a urethral catheter to prevent recurrence. When the cancer has invaded into the muscle (see Figure 29.10), it is necessary to remove the whole bladder (cystectomy), the surrounding lymph nodes and the prostate gland in men and perform a urinary diversion (Figure 29.11).

Preoperative Care

- *Psychological preparation*: nurses/nursing associates should provide both verbal and written information about the surgery, pain management and contact numbers for the patient and their families to get in touch when in difficulties.
- *Information about altered body image*: nurses/nursing associates should encourage the patient to discuss any concerns they may have about returning to their usual activities, perceived relationship changes and resumption of sexual relations. Offer information about support groups or contact with someone who has successfully adjusted to a urinary diversion.
- *Arrange visits by the stoma nurse* to discuss appliances that are available and to advise the patient on the care of the stoma and answer any questions they may have regarding caring for the stoma at home.

- *Physical preparation of the patient*: the nurse/nursing associate should adhere to local and professional guidelines in the safe preparation for urinary diversion.

Postoperative Care

- Postoperative care should include monitoring vital signs, pain management, fluid management, risk assessment for deep vein thrombosis, pressure sores, personal hygiene, nutrition, and other routine postoperative care.
- Maintain a closed drainage system if a catheter is attached to the urostomy bag and ensure that the bag is not blocked. Impaired urine flow can lead to urinary retention and distension of the bladder, a newly created reservoir or the renal pelvis (hydronephrosis). Although urine is sterile, bacteria can multiply rapidly if the closed system is compromised, resulting in UTI.
- When the patient is allowed to eat and drink normally, encourage them to increase fluid intake to approximately 2.5–3 L per day. Increased fluid intake results in good urine production and prevents UTI. Monitor urine output hourly for the first 24 hours postoperatively, then every 4–8 hours.
- Empty the catheter bag or the urostomy bag every 2 hours as overfilling may damage the seal, allowing leakage and contact of urine with the skin.
- Assess colour and consistency of urine. Urine may be cloudy due to mucus production by bowel mucosa. Bright red blood in the urine from a urinary diversion may indicate haemorrhage as a complication, and excessive cloudiness or malodorous urine may indicate UTI.
- Check the stoma site and surrounding skin every 2 hours for the first 24 hours or as often as deemed necessary. Assess the skin for redness, excoriation or signs of breakdown, as impaired skin integrity may lead to local or systemic infection and impaired healing.

Advise the patient on the signs and symptoms of infection and the measures they could take to prevent UTI. Following cystectomy and formation of an ileal conduit, the patient is at risk of UTI for life because of impaired urinary defence mechanisms. Following strict aseptic protocols when providing urostomy care and increasing fluid may minimise the risk to a certain degree but does not eliminate it.

Radiation and Chemotherapy Treatment Radiation is another adjunctive therapy used in the treatment of urinary tumours. Although radiation alone is not curative, it can reduce tumour size prior to surgery and is used as palliative treatment for inoperable tumours and for those who cannot tolerate surgery. It is also used in combination with systemic chemotherapy to improve local and distant relapse rates. If radiation or chemotherapy is used as adjunctive therapy, the patient may experience hair loss, stomatitis, nausea and vomiting or other disturbing side-effects. Nurses/nursing associates should be sensitive to the patient's feelings, actively listening and responding to their concerns (NMC, 2018b).

Health Promotion and Discharge

Prior to discharge, nurses/nursing associates need to discuss the following with the patient and their family.

- Offer dietary advice and if necessary, refer to a dietitian.
- Encourage 2.5–3 L of fluid intake per day. Increased fluid intake promotes urine production and helps to prevent UTI.
- Encourage the patient not to smoke. Provide referral to smoking cessation programmes or clinics for people who wish to stop smoking.
- Advise the patient of the importance of keeping follow-up appointments as organised and compliance with medications prescribed.
- Advise the patient to engage, when necessary, with the stoma nurse in order to anticipate and deal with any problems which may occur; this can prevent or minimise complications and avoid a great deal of patient anxiety.

Red Flag

Nurses/nursing associates must measure urine output hourly following any invasive procedure. This ensures close observations of the kidneys during postoperative care of a patient.

Primary Care

Individual and family teaching for the patient who has had surgery to create a urinary diversion is important. They need to come to terms with altered body image and therefore nurses/nursing associates need to be sensitive when providing stoma care and answering any questions the patient or their family may have. The patient should be informed of the importance of being well hydrated during exercise and in hot weather, as dehydration results in poor urine output and increases the chance of developing UTI.

The patient who has had a urinary diversion needs teaching about care of the stoma and surrounding skin, prevention of urine reflux and infection, signs and symptoms of UTI and renal calculi, and, in some cases, self-catheterisation using the clean technique.

Provide information about the Urostomy Association and support groups. Joining a support group will provide the patient with the opportunity to form new friendships and explore what it is like to live with a stoma.

Renal Tumour

Most cases of kidney cancer develop in people over the age of 60, although it sometimes affects younger people. It can be either benign or malignant, primary or metastatic. Most primary renal tumours arise from renal cells; a primary tumour also may develop in the renal pelvis, although less frequently. Metastatic lesions to the kidney are associated with lung and breast cancer, melanoma and malignant lymphoma.

Pathophysiology

Most renal tumours are renal cell carcinomas. These tumours arise from tubular epithelium and can occur anywhere in the kidney. The affected kidney tends to become larger. In time, the tumour may grow through the wall of the kidney and invade nearby tissues and organs, such as the muscles around the spine, the liver and the renal blood vessels. The tumour, which can range in size up to several centimetres, has clearly defined margins and contains areas of ischaemia, necrosis and haemorrhage. Some cells may break off into the lymph circulation or the bloodstream. The cancer may then spread to nearby lymph nodes or to other areas of the body (metastasise). Some rare types of cancer arise from other types of cell within the kidney. For example, transitional cell (urothelial) cancers arise from transitional cells which line the renal pelvis, ureters and bladder. Transitional cell cancer is common in the bladder but, in some cases, it develops in the renal pelvis.

Risk Factors

- Most cases develop in people over the age of 55 and kidney cancer is more common in men.
- People who smoke have an increased risk of developing kidney cancer. Some of the chemicals from tobacco get into the body and are passed out in the urine. These chemicals in the urine can be carcinogenic to kidney tubule cells.
- Industrial chemicals, such as asbestos, cadmium and some organic solvents, have been linked to an increased risk of kidney cancer.
- Obesity is a risk factor for kidney cancer. About one-quarter of kidney cancer cases are due to being overweight.
- Genetic factors may play a role in some cases. People with some rare genetic disorders, such as von Hippel–Lindau syndrome and Birt–Hogg–Dube syndrome, have a higher risk of developing kidney cancer.

Investigations and Diagnosis

- Physical examination and detailed history-taking, e.g. lifestyle, previous illnesses and occupation.
- An ultrasound scan of the kidney can usually detect a kidney cancer. This is often one of the first tests carried out to diagnose kidney cancer.

- Blood chemistry studies, including estimated glomerular filtration rate (eGFR), liver function tests, etc.
- A CT scan may be used if there is doubt about the diagnosis.
- Urinalysis to check the colour of urine and its contents, such as sugar, protein, red blood cells and white blood cells.
- Intravenous pyelogram (IVP): this is an X-ray of the kidneys using a contrast dye to identify if there are any blockages within the renal tubules.
- Biopsy to check for signs of cancer. To perform a biopsy for renal cell cancer, a thin needle is inserted into the tumour and a sample of tissue is withdrawn.

Signs and Symptoms
- Heavy haematuria.
- Flank pain that is not relieved with over-the-counter analgesics.
- Palpable abdominal mass.
- Fever without signs of infection.
- Fatigue.
- Unexplained weight loss.
- Anaemia.
- Loss of appetite.

Staging of the Cancer
Factors that can affect the chance of recovery and treatment options include age at the time of diagnosis, general health and also the stage of the disease.

Tumour size (T)
T0   No evidence of a primary tumour in the kidney.
T1   The tumour is under 7 cm and is contained within the kidney.
T2   The tumour is greater than 7 cm and remains contained within the kidney.
T3   The tumour has penetrated the other covering of the kidney to invade major blood vessels and adrenal glands.
T4   The tumour has spread further than the tissues and blood vessels around the kidney.

Node (N)
N0   Lymph nodes are clear of the cancer.
N1   Cancer has spread to one nearby lymph node only.
N2   Cancer has infiltrated more than one lymph node.

Metastasis (M)
M0   There is no metastatic spread of the cancer.
M1   There is metastatic spread to other organs.

Nursing Care and Management
Nephrectomy (removal of the kidney) or partial nephrectomy (may be done to prevent the loss of kidney function) is carried out for kidney tumours. In cases where the tumour is advanced, a radical nephrectomy is performed; this includes the removal of the adrenal gland, upper ureter, fat and fascia surrounding the kidney, as well as the entire kidney,

External and/or internal radiation therapy is sometimes used as an adjunct to surgery or in place of it. Chemotherapy may also be prescribed to stop the growth of cancer cells.

Preoperative Care For the principles of preoperative and postoperative care, refer to Chapter 14.
- Nurses/nursing associates need to adhere to local policies and trust guidance in the safe preoperative preparation of the patient for theatre, including giving information and identifying any special needs.
- Discuss postoperative care, including pain management, with the patient. Preoperative teaching about postoperative expectations reduces anxiety for the person and family during the early postoperative period,
- Although deep breathing and coughing may be painful due to the proximity of the incision to the diaphragm, breathing exercises are encouraged to prevent pneumonia,
- Discuss operative and postoperative expectations as indicated, including the location of the incision and anticipated tubes, stents and drains.

Postoperative Care
- Monitor vital signs using the National Early Warning Score, which includes temperature, blood pressure, heart rate, oxygen saturation and respiration rate hourly, until the condition of the patient is stable.
- The location of the incision, combined with the respiratory depressant effects of narcotic analgesics, increases the risk for respiratory complications in the person who has had a nephrectomy. Change position frequently and mobilise as soon as possible with the help of a physiotherapist. Encourage frequent (every 1–2 hours) deep breathing, spirometer use and coughing. Support the incision with a pillow when coughing, as it helps to reduce pain.
- Monitor urine output and note the colour and amount and any haematuria, pyuria or sediment. Promptly report oliguria (reduced urine output) or anuria (absence of urine), as well as changes in urine colour or clarity. It is important to monitor the function of the remaining kidney. The urine output should be greater than 30 mL/hour
- Postoperative pain can be a problem due to the location and size of the surgical incision. Using a pain assessment tool, check with the patient every 2 hours for the severity, quality and duration of the pain. Observe other signs of pain, such as restlessness, facial expressions, guarding and changes in vital signs. It is helpful to complete this assessment before and after the administration of analgesics, as well as non-pharmacological interventions.
- Ensure all tubes and wound drains are clearly labelled and record all output on a fluid balance chart. Attend to and report any excess bleeding to the person in charge for prompt action and escalate according to trust policy. Maintaining drainage tube patency is vital to prevent potential hydronephrosis. Bright bleeding or unexpected drainage may indicate a surgical complication.
- Fluid management is also crucial to postoperative management. The patient may be at risk for fluid deficit or excess. Close monitoring to ensure adequate renal and cardiac function can identify changes early and prevent or minimise complications. Accurate recording of all intake and output, daily weights, blood pressure and pulse assessments, and monitoring of serum creatinine and blood urea levels provide important information on renal status. Once the patient can tolerate oral fluid, slowly increase fluid intake to 2–3 L per day. This helps prevent dehydration and maintains good urine flow.

529

- Report signs and symptoms of UTI such as dysuria, frequency, urgency, nocturia or cloudy malodorous urine to the person in charge. Prompt treatment of postoperative infection is vital to allow continued healing and prevent compromise of the remaining kidney.

Red Flag

Nurses/nursing associates should be aware that pneumothorax is a possible complication of nephrectomy. Hourly monitoring of vital signs is needed during the early stages to detect any respiratory complications.

- Nurses/nursing associates should demonstrate respect for cultural, spiritual and religious values and beliefs. Values and belief systems can provide a structure and form for dealing with the grieving process as a result of altered body image.
- Assist family members to share concerns with one another. Sharing of fears and concerns among family members promotes involvement and support of the entire family unit so that the individual is not left to cope alone.
- Refer to cancer support groups, social services or counselling as appropriate. Support groups and counselling services provide additional resources for coping.

Health Promotion and Discharge

Prior to discharge, nurses/nursing associates should:

- Discuss any worries patients may have regarding the surgery and aftercare. Allow the patient time to ask questions and respond in a sympathetic and empathetic manner
- Ensure that outpatient appointments are booked and advise the patient of the importance of keeping the appointment
- If necessary, arrange transport to and from the hospital after the outpatient appointment
- Advise the patient of the importance of taking medications that may be prescribed as part of the treatment
- Encourage the patient to drink approximately 2.5–3 L of fluid daily and to monitor their urine output. Advise the patient on the signs and symptoms of UTI, such as frequency or burning sensation when voiding urine, and to see the GP if any of these symptoms occur.

Primary Care

If renal cancer was detected at an early stage and cure is anticipated, teaching for home care focuses on protecting the remaining kidney. Include the following measures to prevent infection, renal calculi, hydronephrosis and trauma.

- Maintain a fluid intake of 2.5–3 L per day, increasing the amount during hot weather or strenuous exercise.
- Encourage the patient to urinate when the urge is perceived, and before and after sexual intercourse.
- Properly clean the perineal area to prevent infection.
- Observe for symptoms of UTI, and understand the importance of early and appropriate evaluation and intervention.
- If the patient is an elderly male, he should observe for symptoms of prostatic hypertrophy, a major cause of urinary tract obstruction. Stress the importance of routine screening examinations.

Renal Failure

Acute kidney injury (AKI) has now replaced the term 'acute renal failure' (NICE, 2018c). The incidence of AKI is increasing, with stage 1 AKI occurring in 15% of acute hospital admissions, with an estimated cost of over £1 billion.

Clinically, AKI is a condition in which the kidneys are unable to remove accumulated metabolites from the blood, leading to altered fluid, electrolyte and acid–base balance with a build-up of urea and nitrogenous waste products in the blood. The cause may be a primary kidney disorder, or renal failure may be secondary to a systemic disease or other urological defects. AKI may be either acute or chronic. AKI has an abrupt onset and, with prompt intervention, is often reversible.

Chronic kidney disease (CKD) has now replaced the term 'chronic renal failure'. It has a slow onset, with few symptoms until the kidneys are severely damaged and unable to meet the excretory needs of the body.

Acute Kidney Injury

Acute kidney injury is a rapid decline in renal function with azotaemia (excess of urea and other nitrogenous waste in the blood) and fluid and electrolyte imbalances. The most common causes of AKI are ischaemia and toxins in the blood. The kidney is particularly vulnerable to both because of the amount of blood that passes through it. A fall in blood pressure or volume can cause ischaemia of kidney tissues.

NICE (2018) recommends that AKI can be diagnosed using the following criteria:

- A rise in serum creatinine of 26 mmol/L or greater in 48 hours
- A 50% or greater rise in serum creatinine in the previous 7 days
- A decline in urine output to 0.5 mL/h for 6 hours (adults).

The stage of AKI affects both the management and the prognosis, hence the importance of defining consistent stages.

Risk Factors

- Age 65 and above.
- Previous history of AKI.
- Chronic kidney disease (eGFR less than 60 mL/min/1.73m²).
- Chronic conditions such as heart failure, liver disease and diabetes.
- Neurological or cognitive impairment or disability (which may limit fluid intake because of reliance on a carer).
- Sepsis.
- Symptoms or history of urological obstruction or conditions which may lead to obstruction.
- Hypovolaemia.
- Oliguria (urine output less than 0.5 mL/kg/h).
- Nephrotoxic drug use within the last week (especially if hypovolaemic), for example NSAIDs, angiotensin-converting enzyme (ACE) inhibitors, angiotensin II receptor antagonists (ARBs) and diuretics.
- Exposure to iodinated contrast agents within the past week.
- Cancer and cancer therapy (risk will depend on the type of cancer, proposed treatment and premorbid risk factors).
- Immunocompromise (for example, HIV infection).
- Toxins (for example, some herbal remedies, poisonous plants and animals).

Pathophysiology

The causes and pathophysiology of AKI are commonly categorised as pre-renal, intrinsic and postrenal. Pre-renal AKI is the most common. In pre-renal AKI, hypoperfusion leads to AKI without directly affecting the integrity of kidney tissues. Intrinsic (or intrarenal) AKI is caused by direct damage to functional kidney tissue. Urinary tract obstruction with resulting kidney damage is the precipitating factor for postrenal AKI, the least common form.

Pre-renal Pre-renal AKI results from conditions that affect renal blood flow and perfusion. Any disorder that significantly decreases vascular volume, cardiac output or systemic vascular resistance can affect renal blood flow. Pre-renal AKI is rapidly reversed when blood flow is restored, and the renal parenchyma remains undamaged. Causes include:

- Volume depletion as a result of haemorrhage, severe vomiting or diarrhoea, burns, inappropriate diuresis
- Oedematous states resulting from cardiac failure, cirrhosis, nephrotic syndrome
- Hypotension
- Renal hypoperfusion from the use of NSAIDs or selective cyclo-oxygenase (COX)-2 inhibitors, renal artery stenosis or occlusion, hepatorenal syndrome
- Septic shock.

Intrarenal Intrinsic or intrarenal failure is characterised by acute damage to the renal parenchyma and nephrons. Intrarenal causes include diseases of the kidney itself and acute tubular necrosis (ATN), the most common intrarenal cause of AKI.

- Glomerular disease, such as glomerulonephritis, thrombosis, haemolytic uraemic syndrome.
- Vascular disease, such as renal artery stenosis, renal vein thrombosis, malignant hypertension.

Postrenal Any condition that prevents urine excretion can lead to postrenal AKI. This results in retention of urine, which could result in AKI. These conditions include:

- Calculus
- Blood clot
- Papillary necrosis
- Urethral stricture
- Prostatic hypertrophy or malignancy
- Bladder tumour
- Radiation fibrosis
- Pelvic malignancy
- Retroperitoneal fibrosis.

Investigations and Diagnosis

- *Urinalysis*: blood and/or protein suggest a renal inflammatory process. Microscopy for cells, casts, crystals: red cell casts are diagnostic in glomerulonephritis; tubular cells or casts suggest ATN.
- Osmolality of urine is over 500 mmol/kg if the cause is pre-renal and 300 mmol/kg or less if it is renal; patients with ATN lose the ability to concentrate and dilute the urine and will pass a constant volume with inappropriate osmolality.
- Serum urea, creatinine and electrolytes.
- Full blood count.

- Renal ultrasonography to determine renal size, symmetry, evidence of obstruction.
- Chest X-ray (pulmonary oedema); abdominal X-ray if renal calculi are suspected.
- Contrast studies, such as IVU and renal angiography, should be avoided because of the risk of contrast nephropathy.
- Doppler ultrasound of the renal artery and veins: assessment of possible occlusion of the renal artery and veins.
- Magnetic resonance angiography: for more accurate assessment of renal vascular occlusion.
- ECG: recent myocardial infarction, tented T waves in hyperkalaemia.
- Renal biopsy.

Signs and Symptoms

- *Urine output*: AKI is usually accompanied by oliguria or anuria, but polyuria may occur. Abrupt anuria suggests an acute obstruction, acute and severe glomerulonephritis or acute renal artery occlusion. Gradual diminution of urine output may indicate a urethral stricture or bladder outlet obstruction, e.g. benign prostatic hyperplasia.
- Nausea, vomiting.
- Dehydration.
- Confusion.
- Hypertension.
- *Abdomen*: may reveal a large painless bladder typical of chronic urinary retention.
- Dehydration with postural hypotension and no oedema.
- Fluid overload with raised jugular venous pressure (JVP), pulmonary oedema and peripheral oedema.
- *Pallor, rash, bruising*: petechiae, purpura and nosebleeds may suggest inflammatory or vascular disease, emboli or disseminated intravascular coagulation.
- Pericardial rub.
- Possible back pain/abdominal pain.

Phases

The course of AKI due to ATN typically includes three phases: initiation, maintenance and recovery.

Initiation The initiation phase may last hours to days. During this period, kidney function is suppressed. The patient may present with oliguria or anuria. Bleeding from the kidneys may be a problem if there is tubular damage. If AKI is recognised and the initiating event is effectively treated during this phase, the prognosis is good. The initiation phase of AKI has few symptoms; in fact, it is often identified only when symptoms of the maintenance phase develop.

Maintenance The maintenance phase of AKI is characterised by a significant fall in eGFR and tubular necrosis. This phase may last 1–2 weeks (Peate *et al.*, 2012). Oliguria may develop, although many persons continue to produce normal or near-normal amounts of urine (non-oliguric AKI). Even though urine may be produced, the kidney cannot efficiently eliminate metabolic wastes, water, electrolytes and acids from the body during the maintenance phase of AKI. Fluid and electrolyte imbalances occur during this phase and the specific gravity of urine is the same as plasma. Serum creatinine and blood urea nitrogen (BUN) levels are elevated. The patient may present with oedema and hypertension, confusion, disorientation, agitation or lethargy, hyper-reflexia and possible seizures or coma, due to azotaemia and electrolyte and acid–base imbalances.

Recovery The final phase is the recovery phase. Diuresis may occur as the nephrons and eGFR recover, and retained salt, water and solutes are excreted. Serum creatinine, BUN, potassium and phosphate levels remain high and may continue to rise despite increasing urine output. Renal function improves rapidly during the first 5–25 days of the recovery phase and continues to improve for up to 1 year. During this phase, the patient may pass approximately 4–6 L of urine per day depending on fluid retention. Dehydration is a problem, as a result of increased fluid loss and the inability of the kidneys to perform selective reabsorption.

Red Flag

> If AKI is not treated promptly, it could lead to ischaemic ATN and intrarenal or intrinsic AKI.
> Restoration of blood pressure and blood flow to the kidneys reverses pre-renal AKI.

Nursing Care and Management

A full nursing assessment of vital signs, weight, fluid intake and output, nursing history and assessment of the patient's knowledge of the disease process should all be carried out in order to provide high-quality care. It is important to alleviate the patient's and relatives' worries and anxieties. Healthcare professionals should give the patient time to ask questions and respond appropriately. Psychological care is important in the management of the patient with AKI.

Medications The primary focus in drug management for AKI is to restore and maintain renal perfusion and to eliminate drugs that are nephrotoxic from the treatment regimen. The patient may be prescribed the following medications.

- Furosemide to induce diuresis.
- Antihypertensives such as ACE inhibitors to control hypertension.
- Antacids to prevent gastric ulcers. The person with AKI has an increased risk of gastrointestinal bleeding, probably related to the stress response and impaired platelet function. Regular doses of antacids, histamine H_2-receptor antagonists (e.g. ranitidine) or a proton pump inhibitor such as omeprazole are often prescribed to prevent gastrointestinal haemorrhage.
- A potassium-binding exchange resin may be given orally or by enema to treat hyperkalaemia. Dextrose (50%) and insulin may be given intravenously to reduce serum potassium levels by moving potassium into the cells.

Fluid Management Adequate hydration is of paramount importance to the patient's management (NICE, 2018). Once vascular volume and renal perfusion are restored, fluid intake is usually restricted. Nurses/nursing associates need to follow local policy in the fluid management of a patient with AKI. Fluid balance is carefully monitored, using accurate weight measurements and the serum sodium as the primary indicators.

In AKI, the kidneys often cannot excrete adequate urine to maintain a normal extracellular fluid balance. Rapid weight gain and oedema indicate fluid retention and, in addition, heart failure and pulmonary oedema may develop, which can present a significant management problem.

Nutrition Strict nutritional status should be maintained. Protein intake should be limited to minimise the increase of nitrogenous wastes. Carbohydrates are increased to maintain adequate calorie intake and provide a protein-sparing effect. Where necessary, the dietitian may be involved in the care of the patient with AKI. In some cases, parenteral nutrition is prescribed to provide essential amino acids, carbohydrates and fats when the patient cannot take an adequate diet as a result of nausea and vomiting. The disadvantages of parenteral nutrition in the patient with AKI include the risk of developing fluid overload and infection through the venous line.

Dialysis for AKI In oliguric or anuric patients, the fluid intake required for maintaining hydration generally means that dialysis will be necessary. This may be offered as peritoneal dialysis or as haemofiltration. Because excess fluid and solutes are removed more gradually in peritoneal dialysis, it poses less risk; however, this slower rate of metabolite removal can be a disadvantage in AKI. In peritoneal dialysis there is also an increased risk for developing peritonitis.

Health Promotion and Discharge

Prior to discharge, nurses/nursing associates should advise the patient and relatives of the importance of maintaining adequate fluid intake. During exercise and hot weather, encourage the patient to keep well hydrated. Inform the patient to adhere to the dietary advice offered by the dietitian. Monitor urine output and advise the patient to see the GP if symptoms of UTI, such as haematuria, frequency and a burning sensation when voiding urine, occur. If medications are prescribed to take home, inform the patient and their relatives of the importance of taking the medications as prescribed and to avoid overdosing on any medications that are nephrotoxic.

Primary Care

Acute kidney injury is a serious condition. The patient is often critically ill, which puts a lot of stress on their family. Nurses/nursing associates need to show empathy when dealing with the patient and family (NMC, 2018a,b). Include family members in teaching during the initial stages to promote understanding of what is happening and the reasons for specific treatment measures. Inclusion of the family reduces their anxiety and provides a valuable resource for reinforcing teaching about care after discharge.

Patient teaching needs for home care include the following.

- Advise the patient and their relatives to avoid medications purchased over the counter that could lead to kidney damage.
- Monitor their urine output to ensure that the patient does not develop a UTI. Encourage oral fluid, approximately 2.5–3 L per day.
- Monitor weight, blood pressure and pulse.
- Continue dietary restrictions as per advice by the dietitian.
- Advise the patient to contact their GP when necessary.

Case Study

A 78-year-old male presents to the emergency department following a 4-day history of increasing loose stool, some noted intermittent vomiting and general lethargy. He has had a reduced oral fluid intake over the last 48 hours due to nausea.

A full assessment of this patient would need to be undertaken, including vital signs, physical examination, a detailed history and blood tests, including specific ones to look at kidney function.

Treatment would include, but is not limited to, intravenous fluids, antiemetics and close observation of urine output.

Chronic Kidney Disease

Although the kidneys usually recover from AKI, many chronic conditions can lead to progressive renal damage, resulting in CKD. The functional units of the kidneys (nephrons) are lost and renal mass decreases, with progressive deterioration of glomerular filtration, selective reabsorption and tubular secretion. CKD can develop slowly for many years without any symptoms as the body can tolerate/compensate for a relatively large reduction in kidney function. It is often detected when the kidneys are in the final stage of CKD or by chance when blood tests and urinalysis are checked as part of health screening. The kidneys are unable to excrete metabolic wastes and regulate fluid and electrolyte balance adequately.

Jot This Down

Diabetes is one of the leading possible causes of CKD. Can you name any other conditions that cause CKD?

Pathophysiology

Any condition that destroys renal function can lead to CKD (NICE, 2021b). The pathophysiology of CKD involves a gradual loss of entire nephron units. CKD is divided into five stages of increasing severity. In the early stages, as nephrons are slowly destroyed, remaining healthy nephrons take over their functions but become hypertrophied. The blood pressure and filtration in the remaining healthy nephrons increase to compensate for the loss of nephrons, resulting in damage to the remaining healthy nephrons. This process of continued loss of nephron function may continue even after the initial disease process has resolved. See Table 29.3 for some of the common diseases leading to nephron destruction and end-stage renal disease.

As the number of sclerosed glomeruli increases, the symptoms of CKD can be observed. They include:

- Progressive fall in renal excretory function (assessed by eGFR). eGFR is a measure of how many millilitres of waste fluid the kidneys can filter from the blood in a minute. A healthy pair of kidneys should be able to filter more than 90 mL/minute
- Proteinuria: detected by urine protein/creatinine ratio (PCR) or albumin/creatinine ratio (ACR)
- A tendency to hypertension
- Renal shrinkage: detected with renal ultrasound.

The course of CKD is variable, progressing over a period of months to many years. There are three phases of CKD (early,

Table 29.3 Pathophysiology of chronic kidney disease.
Source: Peate *et al.* (2012).

CAUSE	EXAMPLES
Diabetic nephropathy	Changes in the glomerular basement membrane, chronic pyelonephritis and ischaemia lead to sclerosis of the glomerulus and gradual destruction of the nephron
Hypertensive nephrosclerosis	Long-standing hypertension leads to renal arteriosclerosis and ischaemia, resulting in glomerular destruction and tubular atrophy
Chronic glomerulonephritis	Bilateral inflammatory process of the glomeruli leads to ischaemia, nephron loss and shrinkage of the kidney
Chronic pyelonephritis	Chronic infection commonly associated with an obstructive or neurological process and vesicoureteral reflux leads to reflux nephropathy (renal scarring, atrophy and dilated calyces)
Polycystic kidney disease	Multiple bilateral cysts gradually destroy normal renal tissue by compression
Systemic lupus erythematosus	Basement membrane damage by circulating immune complexes leads to focal, local or diffuse glomerulonephritis

second and third phases). In the early phase, BUN levels are elevated (2–5 mg/mL) and the eGFR is greatly reduced. During this phase, the unaffected nephrons compensate and the patient may be asymptomatic. In the second phase, BUN levels are above 10 mg/mL and creatinine is above 0.4 mg/mL. In the third phase, BUN levels are above 20 mg/mL and creatinine is above 0.5 mg/mL.

As CKD progresses, the patient presents with the symptoms of CKD (see later section). Further damage to the kidneys at this stage, as a result of infection, dehydration or urinary tract obstruction, can precipitate the onset of renal failure.

Risk Factors

- Hypertension.
- Diabetes (type 1 or type 2).
- A history of cardiovascular disease.
- A family history of renal disease.
- Structural abnormality of the renal tract.
- A history of renal stone disease.
- Prostatic hyperplasia.
- Autoimmune disease (systemic lupus erythematosus, SLE).
- Polycystic kidney disease.
- Long-term use of regular medicines such as NSAIDs.
- Chronic glomerulonephritis/pyelonephritis.

Investigations and Diagnosis

- Urinalysis to detect abnormalities and specific gravity.
  - Haematuria may indicate glomerulonephritis.
  - Glycosuria with normal blood glucose is common in CKD.
- Blood urea and electrolyte levels to determine renal function: 24-hour urine creatinine is useful in assessing the severity of renal failure.
- Ultrasound of the kidneys to determine the size of the kidneys.
- Renal biopsy.
- Urine cultures to detect UTI.

Signs and Symptoms

In the early stages of CKD, the person may be asymptomatic. As the disease progresses, the patient may present with the following.

- Symptoms of anaemia.
  - Pallor.
  - Lethargy.
  - Breathlessness.
- Platelet abnormality.
  - Epistaxis.
  - Bruising.
- Haematuria, polyuria.
- Oliguria, anuria.
- Polyneuropathy.
- Confusion, coma.
- Hypertension, heart failure.
- Diarrhoea and vomiting.
- Oedema due to salt and water retention and heart failure.
- Muscle cramps.
- Insomnia.
- Itchy skin.
- Weight loss/poor appetite.
- Increased need to urinate.
- Erectile dysfunction in men.

Complications

Anaemia Several causal factors for anaemia have been identified.

- Bone marrow fibrosis.
- The kidneys produce erythropoietin (hormone). A deficiency in this hormone affects the production of red blood cells.
- Increased red blood cell destruction.
- Bleeding from the gastrointestinal tract or even blood loss during haemodialysis.
- Nutritional deficiencies (iron and folate) and increased risk of blood loss from the gastrointestinal tract also contribute to anaemia.
- Anaemia contributes to symptoms such as fatigue, weakness, depression and impaired cognition.
- Renal failure impairs platelet function, increasing the risk of bleeding disorders, such as epistaxis and gastrointestinal bleeding. The mechanism of impaired platelet function associated with renal failure is poorly understood.

Fluid and Electrolyte Imbalance Loss of functional kidney tissue impairs the kidney's ability to regulate fluid, electrolyte and acid–base balance. In the early stages of CKD, impaired filtration and reabsorption lead to proteinuria, haematuria and decreased urine-concentrating ability. Salt and water are poorly conserved, and risk for dehydration increases. Polyuria, nocturia and a fixed specific gravity of 1.008–1.012 are common. As the GFR decreases and renal function deteriorates further, sodium and water retention are common, necessitating salt and water restrictions (Peate et al., 2012).

Cardiovascular Disease Cardiovascular disease, such as myocardial infarction and heart failure, is a common cause of death in CKD. Coronary artery calcification is common in patients with end-stage renal failure. Hypertension, hyperlipidaemia and glucose intolerance all contribute to the process. Hypertension results from excess fluid volume, increased renin-angiotensin activity, increased peripheral vascular resistance and decreased prostaglandins. Increased extracellular fluid volume can also lead to oedema and heart failure. Pulmonary oedema may result from heart failure, resulting in blood pooling in the lung capillaries, which leads to fluid accumulation in the alveolar sac.

Immune System The immune system is affected as a result of high levels of urea and a build-up of metabolic wastes. This increases the risk of developing infection. The white cell count is low, humoral and cell-mediated immunity are impaired, and phagocyte function is defective. Both the acute inflammatory response and delayed hypersensitivity responses are affected.

Gastrointestinal Tract Anorexia, nausea and vomiting are the most common early symptoms of uraemia. Hiccups are also commonly experienced. Gastroenteritis is frequent. Ulcerations may affect any level of the gastrointestinal tract and contribute to an increased risk of gastrointestinal bleeding. Peptic ulcer disease is particularly common in uraemic persons. Uraemic fetor (urine-like breath odour), often associated with a metallic taste in the mouth, may develop. Uraemic fetor can further contribute to anorexia.

Nervous System Severe uraemia causes depressed CNS function. CNS symptoms include difficulty in concentrating, fatigue, convulsions, seizures and insomnia. Asterixis, tremor and myoclonus are also features of severe uraemia. Peripheral neuropathy is also common in advanced uraemia. As uraemia progresses, motor function is impaired, causing muscle weakness, decreased deep tendon reflexes and gait disturbances.

Bone Disease Hyperparathyroid bone disease, osteomalacia, osteoporosis and osteosclerosis are some of the diseases associated with CKD. Parathyroid hormone causes increased calcium resorption from bone. In addition, osteoblast (bone-forming) and osteoclast (bone-destroying) cell activity is affected. This bone resorption and remodelling, combined with decreased vitamin D synthesis and decreased calcium absorption from the gastrointestinal tract, are all associated with bone diseases.

Endocrine Abnormalities These include:

- Hyperprolactinaemia: may occur in both men and women
- Increased levels of luteinising hormone in men and women
- Decreased testosterone levels with decreased spermatogenesis
- Abnormal thyroid hormone levels
- Absence of the normal menstrual cycle.

Skin Disease Anaemia and retained pigmented metabolites cause pallor and a yellowish hue to the skin in uraemia. Dry skin with poor turgor, a result of dehydration and sweat gland atrophy, is common. Bruising and excoriations are frequently seen. Metabolic wastes not eliminated by the kidneys may be deposited in the skin, contributing to itching or pruritus. In advanced uraemia, high levels of urea in the sweat may result in crystallised deposits of urea on the skin, called uraemic frost.

Nursing Care and Management

Nursing care requires careful planning to help the patient and relatives come to terms with the condition. The aim is to ensure that the patient has a good quality of life by developing ways to cope with the illness, the treatment and the complications that may occur as a result of CKD and its treatment.

Pain Management

- Nurses/nursing associates should assess each pain fully before administering analgesics. The use of a pain assessment tool is recommended.
- Record a pain score and review the patient every 2 hours for the effect of analgesics.
- Nurses/nursing associates should be aware that patients with pain may also have significant emotional, social or spiritual problems. These need to be considered when providing care. Agree goals for pain management with patient and family.
- Administer prescribed analgesia for continuous pain on time and note its effect.
- Most people taking regular opioids need a laxative, as one of the side-effects of opioids analgesia is constipation. Renal and hepatic impairment affect opioid metabolism and excretion.
- Paracetamol is recommended as first-line treatment for mild-to-moderate pain. The maximum 24-hour dose for adults is 4 g but this should be reduced in patients with a low body mass index or severe liver impairment due to chronic alcohol dependence. Regular paracetamol may not improve analgesia in patients also receiving regular strong opioids.

Other Medications Diuretics such as furosemide or other loop diuretics may be prescribed to reduce extracellular fluid volume and oedema. This also helps to lower blood pressure and potassium levels. Hypertension is present in 80–85% of people diagnosed with CKD. Maintaining blood pressure control is the most important goal in trying to slow the progression of CKD; antihypertensive drugs such as ACE inhibitors are used to regulate blood pressure, slow the progress of renal failure and prevent complications of coronary heart disease and cerebral vascular disease. Most patients may require two or three drugs to control their hypertension. The choice of other antihypertensives used will depend on existing co-morbidities. Following an ACE and ARB, a diuretic may be used (often a thiazide but in CKD stages 4 and 5, a loop diuretic may be needed, such as furosemide, possibly at high doses if there is fluid overload). Next choice would be a calcium channel blocker (e.g. amlodipine), then a beta-blocker and then an alpha-blocker. Folic acid and iron supplements are given to combat anaemia associated with chronic renal failure.

Nutrition and Fluid Management Where dietary intervention is agreed, this should occur within the context of education, detailed dietary assessment and supervision, to ensure malnutrition is prevented. In CKD, the body is unable to store excess proteins, unlike carbohydrates and fats. Any unused protein is broken down as urea and nitrogenous waste, which are normally excreted by the kidneys. In CKD, these waste products are retained by the body, resulting in a toxic build-up, in turn causing uraemic symptoms. However, prolonged dietary protein restriction should be avoided. Once dialysis has commenced, a high-protein diet is recommended. Water and sodium intake are regulated to maintain the extracellular fluid volume at normal levels. Strict water and sodium restrictions may be necessary as CKD progresses.

Dialysis Patients with CKD usually require dialysis. This may be peritoneal dialysis, continuous ambulatory peritoneal dialysis (CAPD) or haemodialysis. Long-term dialysis has a higher risk for complications, for example fluid overload, electrolyte imbalance and the risk of death resulting from complications such as infection (peritonitis, *Staphylococcus aureus* infection) and cardiovascular disease (endocarditis, stroke and peripheral vascular disease). Kidney transplantation has become the treatment of choice for many persons with end-stage renal disease. It allows freedom from dietary and fluid restriction and complications of anaemia.

> ### Nursing Fields Paediatric
> Many children worry about what dialysis will feel like, whether it will hurt and how they might look or feel after dialysis. It is normal to be scared of needles at first. They might be nervous about how they will get along with the other patients and the staff. The physicians, the nurses, the social worker and the child life specialists will be there for help and support while they are being treated. Nurses/nursing associates should be able to answer most questions.

Health Promotion and Discharge

Prior to discharge of the patient with CKD into the community, nurses/nursing associates need to focus on measures to reduce complications from CKD treatment and to provide information to help the patient and family to lead a healthy lifestyle.

- Discuss measures to reduce the risk of UTIs and stress the importance of prompt treatment to eradicate the infecting organism. Inform the patient that keeping well hydrated is important to ensure that they do not develop a UTI.
- If dietary restrictions have been prescribed, ensure that the patient and family understand the need for these restrictions.
- If the patient has been prescribed medications, ensure that they understand the need to take the medications as prescribed. Discuss any side-effects and what to do if these symptoms occur.
- Encourage the patient to take regular exercise.

The patient with CKD will require dialysis. It may be haemodialysis with an arteriovenous fistula or shunt or peritoneal dialysis with a permanent peritoneal catheter. Nurses/nursing associates should:

- Include the patient in decision making and encourage self-care. Increased autonomy enhances the patient's sense of control, independence and confidence
- Help the patient develop and achieve realistic goals. Realistic goals allow the person to see progress

535

- Facilitate contact with a support group or other community members affected by renal failure. The person benefits by providing and receiving support in a group of people going through similar circumstances
- Refer for counselling as indicated or desired. Counselling can help the person develop effective coping and adaptation strategies
- Stress the importance of keeping the fistula sites clean, observing for any signs of infection, such as inflammation, swelling and pain, and reporting these signs and symptoms to the stoma nurse/GP/practice nurse immediately for prompt action.

Conclusion

Caring for patients with a urinary disorder is challenging and demanding. The disorders associated with the urinary system can be either acute or chronic. Treatment varies depending on the type of kidney or urinary disease present. In general, the earlier kidney or urinary disease is recognised, the more likely it is to be treatable and potentially reversible which improves patient outcomes.

With information on leading a healthy lifestyle and following the doctor's advice on treatment for high blood pressure and other conditions, it is possible to live without symptoms or further deterioration of kidney function. At all stages of kidney disease, one can help reduce the chances of the kidneys getting worse and the risk of cardiovascular disease by adopting a healthier lifestyle.

Self-care is an integral part of daily life. It means the individual takes responsibility for their own health and well-being, with support from the people involved in their care, such as the GP, practice nurse and other support workers. Self-care includes daily activities to stay fit, maintain good physical and mental health, prevent illness or accidents and deal effectively with minor ailments and long-term conditions.

Patients and their relatives should be informed that, in most cases, CKD cannot be completely prevented, although preventive measures can be taken to reduce the chances of the condition developing.

Practice Assessment Document

In your role as a student nursing associate, you should endeavour to observe and assess patients who present with a wide range of urological disorders, ensuring you undertake appropriate skills under supervision, to support your newly acquired knowledge around this group of patients. You could ask to undertake spoke placements with urology nurse specialists and other related areas within clinical practice.

Key Points

- The two main UTIs are cystitis and pyelonephritis. Cystitis is more common in women, as women have a short urethra compared with men. For an uncomplicated UTI, a short course of antibiotic therapy should treat the problem.

- Nurses/nursing associates should advise the patient on measures to prevent UTI. Encourage the patient to drink approximately 2.5–3 L per day and advise on the type of fluid to drink and avoid.
- Kidney stones can obstruct any section of the urinary tract. Some obstructions may cause severe pain, such as renal colic, while others may be without any symptoms in the early stages, such the formation of stones in the kidney.
- AKI is a frequent complication of critical illnesses, typically occurring in individuals with no prior history of kidney disorder. There may be no symptoms or signs, but oliguria (urine volume less than 400 mL in 24 hours) is common. There is an accumulation of fluid and nitrogenous waste products demonstrated by a rise in blood urea and creatinine.
- People with any stage of CKD have an increased risk of developing heart disease or a stroke. This is why it is important to detect even mild CKD, as treatment may not only slow down progression of the disease but also reduce the risk of developing heart disease or stroke.

References

BNF (2021). *Morphine*. https://bnf.nice.org.uk/drug/morphine.html#renalImpairment (accessed December 2021).

Cancer Research UK (2021) *Types*. www.cancerresearchuk.org/about-cancer/bladder-cancer/types-stages-grades/types (accessed December 2021).

Health Protection Agency (2012) *Primary care guidance: diagnosing and managing infections*. www.hpa.org.uk/Topics/Infectious Diseases/InfectionsAZ/PrimaryCareGuidance/ (accessed December 2021).

Jenkins, G.W. & Tortora, G.J. (2013) *Anatomy and Physiology: From Science to Life*, 3rd edn. John Wiley & Sons, Hoboken, NJ.

LeMone, P., Burke, K. & Bauldoff, G. (2011) *Medical–Surgical Nursing: Critical Thinking in Client Care*, 4th edn. Prentice Hall, Upper Saddle River, NJ.

National Institute for Health and Care Excellence (2018a) *Urinary Tract Infection (Lower) Women*. NICE, London.

National Institute for Health and Care Excellence (2018b) *Urinary Tract Infection (Lower) Men*. NICE, London.

National Institute for Health and Care Excellence (2018c) *Acute Kidney Injury*. NICE, London.

National Institute for Health and Care Excellence (2020) *Renal or Ureteric Coli: Acute*. NICE, London.

National Institute for Health and Care Excellence (2021a) *Pyelonephritis*. NICE, London.

National Institute for Health and Care Excellence (2021b) *Chronic Kidney Disease*. NICE, London.

Nursing & Midwifery Council (2018a) *The Code: Professional standards of practice and behaviour for nurses, midwives and nursing associates*. NMC, London.

Nursing and Midwifery Council (2018b) *Standards of proficiency for nursing associates*. NMC, London.

Peate, I., Nair, M., Hemming, L. & Wild, K. (2012) *LeMone and Burke's Adult Nursing: Acute and Ongoing Care*. Pearson Education, Harlow.

Porth, C. (2015) *Pathophysiology: Concepts of Altered Health States*, 4th international edn. Lippincott, Philadelphia, PA.

Silverthorn, D.U. (2015) *Human Physiology: An Integrated Approach* (ebook). Prentice Hall, Englewood Cliffs, NJ. content, perms

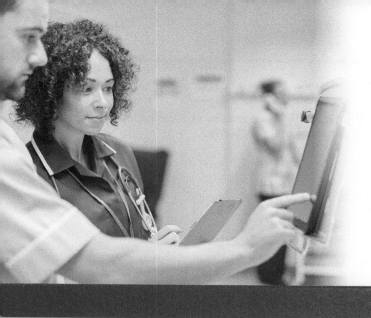

30

The Person with a Reproductive Disorder

Hazel Ridgers

University of Brighton, UK

Learning Outcomes

On completion of this chapter you will be able to:

- Explain some of the most common normal and abnormal changes that can occur in the female and male reproductive systems
- Use the nursing process as a framework for providing care for several reproductive health conditions, including cervical and testicular cancers
- Identify risk factors and key screening and diagnostic tests for these conditions
- Describe the main presentations of the three common sexually acquired infections (SAIs)

Proficiencies

NMC Proficiencies and Standards:
Platform 2 Promoting Health and Preventing Ill Health:

- Understand and apply the aims and principles of health promotion, protection and improvement and the prevention of ill health when engaging with people.
- Promote and improve mental, physical, behavioural and other health related outcomes by understanding and explaining the principles, practice and evidence base for health screening programmes.

Annexe A: Communication and Relationship Management Skills

- Be aware of own unconscious bias in communication encounters

Platform 2 Promoting Health and Preventing Ill Health:

- Understand and apply the aims and principles of health promotion, protection and improvement and the prevention of ill health when engaging with people.
- Understand the factors that may lead to inequalities in health outcomes.
- Explain why health screening is important and identify those who are eligible for screening.

(Continued)

Nursing Practice: Knowledge and Care, Third Edition. Edited by Ian Peate and Aby Mitchell.
© 2022 John Wiley & Sons Ltd. Published 2022 by John Wiley & Sons Ltd.
Companion website: www.wiley.com/go/peate/nursingpractice3e

Proficiencies (Continued)

Annexe A: Communication and Relationship Management Skills

- Be aware of the possibility of own unconscious bias in communication encounters.

 Visit the companion website at www.wiley.com/go/peate/nursingpractice3e where you can test yourself using flashcards, multiple-choice questions and more.

Introduction

One unifying characteristic of all living things is the potential ability to reproduce. The reproductive system is composed of organs involved in the propagation of the species and, for many, the joy of sexual arousal and excitement.

Reproductive health is often closely linked to the way that people express themselves, their sexual identity, sexual behaviours and sexual orientation. A wide range of factors including genetics, social and cultural norms, personal attitudes and health beliefs can affect a person's reproductive health. Nurses must be aware of these factors and consider how they may influence both an individual patient's reproductive health knowledge and their preferences and goals for their care. Nurses must also be aware that perceived social and cultural norms affect the organisation and provision of reproductive healthcare services and mean that services are often tailored to the needs of heterosexuals. As such, reproductive health services can marginalise the health needs of gay, lesbian, bisexual, transgender people and others. An awareness of this and endeavouring to provide care that is high quality, inclusive, non-judgemental and patient centred will allow you to demonstrate to the Nursing & Midwifery Council (NMC, 2018a) that you fulfil its expectation that registrants will provide care that is accessible to all, across a range of settings, at all times.

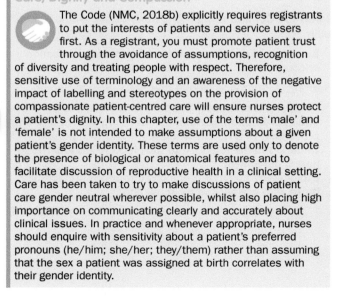

Care, Dignity and Compassion

The Code (NMC, 2018b) explicitly requires registrants to put the interests of patients and service users first. As a registrant, you must promote patient trust through the avoidance of assumptions, recognition of diversity and treating people with respect. Therefore, sensitive use of terminology and an awareness of the negative impact of labelling and stereotypes on the provision of compassionate patient-centred care will ensure nurses protect a patient's dignity. In this chapter, use of the terms 'male' and 'female' is not intended to make assumptions about a given patient's gender identity. These terms are used only to denote the presence of biological or anatomical features and to facilitate discussion of reproductive health in a clinical setting. Care has been taken to try to make discussions of patient care gender neutral wherever possible, whilst also placing high importance on communicating clearly and accurately about clinical issues. In practice and whenever appropriate, nurses should enquire with sensitivity about a patient's preferred pronouns (he/him; she/her; they/them) rather than assuming that the sex a patient was assigned at birth correlates with their gender identity.

The physiological and anatomical aspects of the reproductive tract are mainly linked to procreation. However, nurses must consider the psychological and social aspects of reproduction, demonstrating an understanding of the impact these aspects may have on a patient's desire to conceive or not conceive as well as the sexual pleasure often provided by the reproductive organs.

Untreated sexually acquired infections (SAIs) can lead to serious long-term health consequences for individuals, communities and nations. Nurses are at the forefront of promoting safer sex messages among the general population and those at particularly increased risk of SAIs. It is a requirement of registration with the NMC (NMC, 2018b) to pay special attention to promoting well-being, preventing ill health and meeting the changing health and care needs of people during all life stages. Those who are interested in developing their understanding and skill acquisition further should seek out health professionals who are practising in the sexual health field as well as accessing relevant texts on the subject.

Understanding the anatomy and physiology of a person's reproductive system is required to enable the nurse to undertake a detailed patient history and competently recognise and assess normal and abnormal internal and external genitalia. Applying this knowledge enables nurses to educate patients about their reproductive systems, provide care that is safe and effective, promote optimum health and function and reduce the transmission of SAIs. For a detailed presentation of anatomy and physiology of the reproductive system, see Peate & Evans (2020).

This chapter provides general information on undertaking a reproductive health assessment. It also offers instruction on undertaking reproductive health assessments of both sexes. Several female and male reproductive health-related conditions and their associated nursing care are discussed. For ease of reference, the chapter focuses on female and male reproductive health separately. Finally, the chapter provides a very brief overview of some common SAIs. HIV is often considered alongside SAIs but due to space constraints, this disorder of the immune system will not be discussed here.

Overview of the Assessment of a Person's Reproductive System

The ability of the nurse to assess a patient's reproductive system without judgement and with compassion and sensitivity is important to the patient from both physical and psychological perspectives.

Practice Assessment Document

Demonstrating caring and compassion and protecting dignity

Intimate examinations can cause excessive stress and anxiety for patients. Being exposed with people observing can be distressing. You can demonstrate that you care, you are compassionate, and you are respecting the person's dignity by exposing only the part of the person's body that needs to be uncovered to facilitate examination. Usually no more than one part of a patient's body should be exposed at one time during a reproductive health assessment.

Take care to ensure the person is warm and comfortable and that they are given every opportunity to request that the examination stops if they are unsure about any aspect of it. Protect their privacy – ensure doors are closed, screens and curtains are effective in providing dignity and that only those people necessary for the examination should attend. Provide chaperones; read the local chaperoning policy and demonstrate your knowledge of it to your practice assessor.

Skills of assessment are perfected over years of practice; the nurse must demonstrate competence and confidence and provide care in line with The Code (NMC, 2018b). This requires the nurse to employ a person-centred approach and endeavour to create an environment that enhances patient comfort and encourages and empowers them to share in decisions about their care and treatment.

The nurse must also provide reassurance that the patient is owed a duty of confidentiality (NMC, 2018b) and therefore their information and the results of examination will be treated as confidential. This is vital to engender patient trust in reproductive and sexual healthcare staff and services, ensuring that patients return for any follow-up treatment or future care.

Jot This Down Confidentiality

The NMC (2018a) requires nurses to respect people's right to privacy and confidentiality and all NHS employees are bound by a legal duty of confidence to protect personal information. Take some time to think why the duty of confidentiality might be important to a patient accessing reproductive or sexual health services.

For patient comfort and ease of examination, the nurse should offer the patient the opportunity to empty their bladder before the examination. Always check to see if a urine specimen is required prior to this. It is usual for a gown to be worn after the patient has removed their clothing, a drape cover for genitalia can also be used; the patient may prefer to keep their underwear on until the examination is imminent. Care should be taken to reveal only those body parts that are being examined to demonstrate respect and preserve dignity.

The nurse should adapt the method of assessment to suit the circumstances. Assessment may be undertaken as part of a holistic appraisal or can be specifically focused where the problem is known or suspected. If the examination is part of a total physical assessment, then it is usual for the reproductive system to be the last system to be assessed. Both reproductive and urinary systems are assessed.

The assessment phase of the nursing process also reviews information from diagnostic tests and a patient's general medical history alongside the objective findings of any physical assessments. Chapter 4 of this book describes the nursing process in more detail.

Assessment of the Female Reproductive System

A comprehensive health assessment of the female reproductive system will include gathering subjective and objective data (see Chapter 4). Physical assessment of the female reproductive system begins with inspection and palpation of the external genitalia (Figures 30.1 and 30.2). A speculum is used to visualise the inner vagina and cervix and when collection of specimens is needed. The uterus, fallopian tubes and ovaries are palpated during physical assessment.

Collection of the woman's past medical history and experiences specific to her reproductive health will aid assessment (Box 30.1).

Examining the Female Genitalia

You can show the patient the speculum or any other equipment that is to be used for the physical assessment. Some patients may wish to self-insert the speculum; this may alleviate anxiety. Where this is appropriate and preferred by the patient, support them to do so.

Ask that they empty their bladder. This promotes comfort and makes the examination easier, as a full bladder may make palpation of the internal organs uncomfortable for the woman and difficult for the nurse; note that you may be required to obtain a urine specimen as part of the total assessment. Ask them to wear a gown (facilitating privacy and protection of dignity) and remove all clothing except for socks, which can be left on for comfort.

What to Do If . . .

During the examination, the patient says they do not want their partner present, but the partner insists they will stay. How would you deal with that?

Equipment

The equipment required depends on the purpose of the examination. This should be readily available so the examination proceeds smoothly, without unnecessary pauses or interruptions, recognising the impact such interruptions may have on the patient's anxiety, distress, privacy and dignity. The equipment listed in Box 30.2 should be available to examine female genitalia.

Position

The patient is usually asked to assume, or is helped into, the supine lithotomy position. It must be noted that other positions can be used if this is what they prefer or what their circumstances dictate.

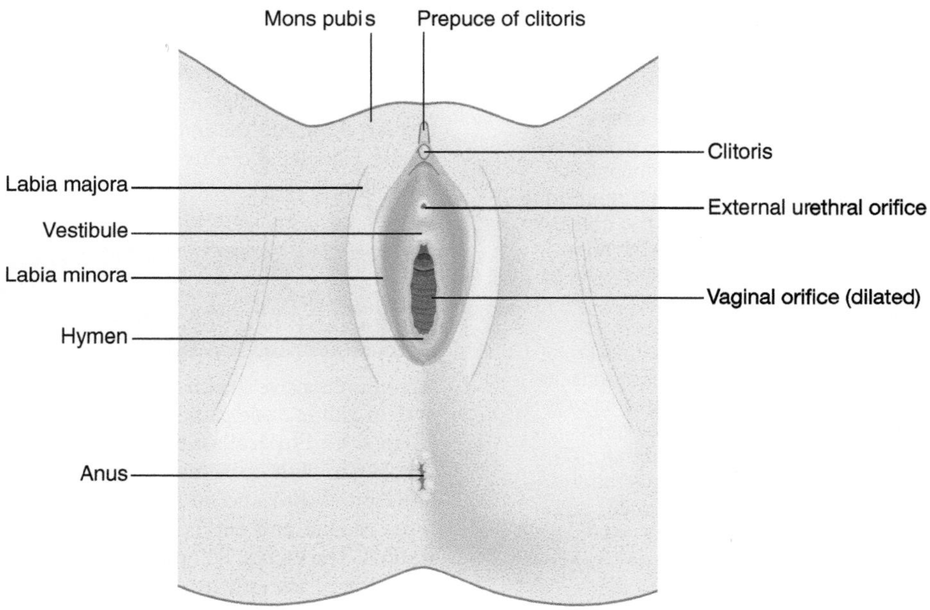

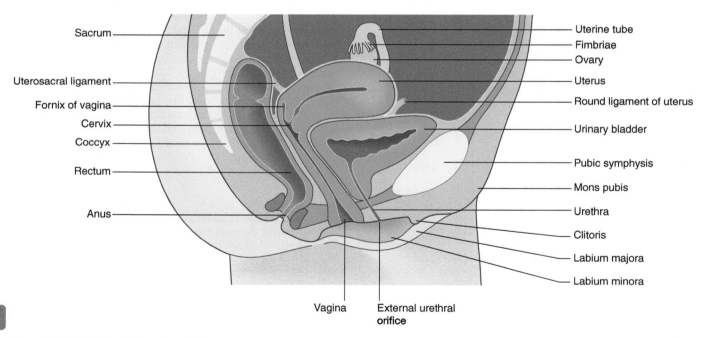

Mons pubis   Prepuce of clitoris

Clitoris

Labia majora

Vestibule

Labia minora

Hymen

Anus

External urethral orifice

Vaginal orifice (dilated)

Figure 30.1 **The external female genitalia.**

Sacrum

Uterosacral ligament

Fornix of vagina

Cervix

Coccyx

Rectum

Anus

Uterine tube

Fimbriae

Ovary

Uterus

Round ligament of uterus

Urinary bladder

Pubic symphysis

Mons pubis

Urethra

Clitoris

Labium majora

Labium minora

Vagina   External urethral orifice

Figure 30.2 **The internal female genitalia.**

Age-related Changes

As a part of the normal ageing process, several age-related changes occur throughout the female body, specifically in response to a decrease in size of the reproductive organs. Reduced oestrogen affects the reproductive system, and neuroendocrinological, biochemical and metabolic changes occur throughout the body (Table 30.1).

Digital Bimanual Palpation

A bimanual examination completes the pelvic examination. External genitalia are observed, noting lumps or ulcers, discoloration or discharge and signs of obvious prolapse. Standing, the nurse uses gloved fingers and a water-soluble lubricant, gently inserting the first two fingers of the dominant hand into the vagina; inside the introitus, the fingers are advanced along the

Box 30.1 Past History and Experiences Specific to the Woman's Health

· Menstrual history
· Pregnancies
· Medications
· Pain with menses
· Symptoms of vaginitis
· Problems with urinary function
· Bowel problems
· Sexual history
· Current or previous sexual abuse or physical abuse
· Contraceptive history
· Past surgical history (including female genital mutilation)
· Long-term conditions
· Genetic disorders

Box 30.2 Equipment Required for Genital Examination

· Personal protective equipment
· Light source
· Vaginal speculae
· Alcoholic hand rub
· Disposable examination gloves
· Lubricant
· Various types of sampling devices (i.e. swabs, loops, cytobrush, cervix brush)
· Glass slides, slide container
· Pencil for labelling slides
· Fixative solution
· Specimen forms and bag
· Tissue paper
· Clinical waste container

vaginal canal vertically and the vaginal wall is palpated. Place the other hand above the symphysis pubis, gently pushing down towards the pelvis. Examine the cervix, uterus and adnexa, noting irregularities such as masses or abnormal tenderness.

Document all examinations and outcomes according to local policy and procedure. Give the patient clear explanations of any findings and the proposed next stages of care and treatment.

It is unwise to base treatment decisions on one diagnostic approach (i.e. digital bimanual examination). Abnormal findings should always be followed up using further assessment and/or screening techniques.

Nursing Fields Learning Disabilities

Patients with learning disabilities should have equality of access to cervical screening. However, a report from NHS Digital (2016) shows lower screening coverage in eligible people with learning disabilities. Screening programmes must ensure that all patients have access to information about screening, presented in a way they can understand, and that staff in the screening programmes adopt good practice, enabling all patients who choose to attend for screening to be screened successfully. Public Health England produces a guide to cervical screening for people with learning disabilities to support them to make an informed decision about screening (NHS, 2019).

Heavy Menstrual Bleeding

Heavy menstrual bleeding (HMB), or menorrhagia, is defined as excessive menstrual blood loss that occurs over several consecutive cycles. It can significantly affect physical and psychosocial well-being as well as material quality of life (NICE, 2020). Quantifying levels of menstrual blood loss is challenging.

Table 30.1 Some changes associated with ageing and the female reproductive system.

CHANGES TO STRUCTURE	CHANGES IN FUNCTION	PHYSICAL IMPACT
Ovarian function ceases	Decreased ovulation	Infertility increases
Decreased oestrogen production	Menopause begins	Ability to conceive decreases or is absent
Urinary and genital tracts become thinner	Hormonal fluctuation and vasomotor instability	Menses become erratic with eventual cessation
Pubic hair thins out	Bone formation decreases and disturbed homeostasis	Night sweats, hot flushes and flashes, sleep disturbance, fatigue, mood swings
Labia shrink	Vaginal secretion/lubrication decreases	Risk of osteoporosis as a result of bone loss, osteopathic fractures and height loss
Pelvic musculature relaxes	Vaginal pH alters (decreases)	Dyspareunia can result in loss of libido and lack of interest in sex
	Uterine prolapse	Increased risk for urinary tract infection
	Cystocoele	Vaginitis, itching, discharge, vulval burning
	Rectocoele	Dyspareunia
		Incontinence
		Feeling of pressure in perineal region

Changes in blood chemistry occur at two levels of menstrual blood loss: 60 mL and 120 mL.

Pathophysiology

The pathophysiology of HMB is not always identifiable, but possible causes include:

- *Uterine pathology and lesions*: polyps, fibroids, carcinoma, infection, including pelvic inflammatory disease (PID), endometriosis
- *Systemic disease*: hypothyroidism, liver disease, obesity, polycystic ovarian syndrome (PCOS), haematological disorders
- *Iatrogenic causes*: intrauterine device, anticoagulant treatment, oral injectable steroids for contraception or hormone replacement, tranquillisers or other psychotropic drugs.

Signs and Symptoms

An in-depth history is taken to ascertain the signs and symptoms, and the following should be considered.

- *Menstrual history*: cycle length, number of bleeding days, intermenstrual or postcoital bleeding, amount of blood loss, passage of clots; pain associated with bleeding.
- *Contraception*: current method; patient's need.

Symptoms suggesting an underlying pathology include the following.

- *Metabolic disorders*: symptoms suggesting PCOS and hypothyroidism.
- *Haematological disorders*: excessive bleeding postpartum or tooth extraction, easy bruising.
- *Pelvic inflammatory disease (PID)/infection*: pelvic pain, dyspareunia, vaginal discharge.
- *Endometriosis*: pelvic pain, dysmenorrhoea.
- *Postcoital and intermenstrual bleeding* can suggest pelvic pathology.

Age is an important factor in the assessment; the nurse should aim to rule out any pregnancy-related complications.

Examination

When carrying out an examination, look for signs of underlying pathology.

- Bruising.
- Typical hypothyroid features.
- Features of PCOS (hirsutism, acne, overweight).
- Pallor.
- Koilonychia (spoon-shaped fingernails with longitudinal ridging).
- *Abdominal examination*: there may be tenderness, palpable masses (uterine, ovarian).
- *Pelvic examination*: vulval inspection, speculum examination, bimanual palpation for masses.
- *Cervical smear*: if appropriate.
- *Infection screening*: high vaginal and endocervical swabs as appropriate.

What To Do If . . .

During the examination, you notice that a patient has signs of an infestation with pubic lice.
Tips for practice: sensitively raise your concern with the patient and ensure immediate treatment to ensure eradication of the infestation and reduce the risk of further transmission. Although not always the case, pubic lice are usually acquired from close physical contact with an affected person. A sexual history may be necessary to ascertain the need for a sexual health screen to test for other SAIs. Ensure adequate decontamination of any non-disposable equipment, gowns or drapes once patient care is completed.

Investigations and Diagnosis

The in-depth history facilitates definitive diagnosis. The nurse should enquire about the use of medications, ruling out their interference with normal menstruation. The physical examination may reveal an underlying systemic disorder. Genitourinary or gastrointestinal bleeding, for example from urinary tract infection or haemorrhoids, can be mistakenly interpreted by the woman as vaginal bleeding.

Manual pelvic examination can reveal an obviously abnormal structural irregularity, for example a cervical polyp.

Guidance from NICE (2020) suggests that every woman presenting with HMB should have a full blood count taken. Serum ferritin, coagulation and hormone testing, however, are not routinely recommended and should only be carried out if there is clinical suspicion of underlying pathology.

Endometrial biopsy (in non-pregnant women) or hysteroscopy may offer further information that helps make a detailed assessment of the uterus. If the cause of bleeding cannot be confirmed, a pelvic ultrasound may be required as this may help to diagnose structural abnormalities and endometrial thickness.

Nursing Care and Management

There are complications of HMB that the nurse needs to be aware of, including:

- The presence of iron deficiency anaemia
- Psychological sequelae, e.g. depression, embarrassment
- Social implications, e.g. increased social isolation, impact on intimate relationships
- Financial implications, e.g. cost of sanitary products, time off work.

Most women with HMB can be successfully treated using a medical approach, especially when there is no structural lesion. NICE (2020) advises that treatments should be considered in the following order.

1. *First-line*: levonorgestrel-releasing intrauterine system provides long-term use (at least 12 months is expected).
2. *Second-line*: tranexamic acid or non-steroidal anti-inflammatory drugs (NSAIDs) or combined oral contraceptive pills (COCPs).
3. *Third-line*: cyclical oral progestogens.

If hormonal treatments are unacceptable, either tranexamic acid or NSAIDs may be used.

Medicines Management Ibuprofen

You are about to administer the prescribed dose of ibuprofen to the patient when they inform you that they vomited yesterday, and it looked like there was blood in it. What should you do?

Surgical Management of HMB

Structural abnormalities may require surgical intervention to alleviate symptoms; this should only be considered in the following situations.

- Pharmacological management fails
- There is a severe impact on quality of life
- The patient has no desire to conceive
- The uterus is normal (or there are small fibroids less than 3 cm).

Endometrial ablation can dramatically reduce the amount of cyclic blood loss. Potential complications include:

- Vaginal discharge
- Increased period pain even if no further bleeding
- Need for additional surgery
- Infection
- Rarely perforation.

Contraception after endometrial ablation should still be advised even though fertility is usually not retained.

Hysterectomy should not be used as first-line surgical management for HMB; this is usually reserved for patients with structural lesions not responding to medical treatment and should usually only be considered when:

- Other treatments have failed, are contraindicated or the patient has declined them
- There is a wish for amenorrhoea
- The patient requests it
- No desire to retain the uterus and fertility.

First-line treatment is vaginal hysterectomy, second-line is abdominal hysterectomy. Healthy ovaries should not be removed.

There are potential adverse outcomes, including:

- Infection
- Intraoperative haemorrhage
- Damage to other organs (urinary tract and bowel)
- Urinary dysfunction
- Venous thromboembolism (VTE)
- Menopausal-like symptoms if ovaries are removed.

Menopause

The menopause is defined as the cessation of menstruation for 12 months and marks the end of a female's reproductive capacity. With menopause, the ovaries are no longer active and reproductive organs become smaller. Ovarian follicular development ceases, a finite number of ovarian follicles is depleted and gonadotropin (FSH, LH) levels increase (Peacock & Ketvertis, 2021).

Menopause is not usually a pathological occurrence but rather part of the normal ageing process. It is discussed in detail here in an endeavour to give this fundamental reproductive health issue, with which many patients struggle, the attention it deserves and does not always get.

What The Experts Say. . .

" 'A lot of patients come to see me because their menopausal symptoms are debilitating and having a serious impact on their quality of life. They have often suffered in silence for a while before seeking help or have sought help from other healthcare staff who they feel haven't taken their concerns seriously. I listen carefully to the patient during my assessment. I don't think I can overemphasise how important that is. We then make a diagnostic, treatment and management plan together, focusing on their priorities for their menopausal health.'
Specialist gynaecologist

Climacteric (Perimenopause)

The climacteric, the menopausal transition stage or perimenopause, is the period of change leading up to the last period. It is a retrospective diagnosis from the time when menstruation stops permanently and can only be defined with confidence 12 months after spontaneous amenorrhoea.

Premature menopause (i.e. before 40 years of age) can occur in primary ovarian failure, surgically induced menopause (hysterectomy with or without bilateral oophorectomy), radiation-induced menopause and chemotherapy-induced menopause.

The signs and symptoms of menopause with obvious bodily effects can range from a few years to 10 years or longer. The final menstrual period usually occurs between the ages of 45 and 58 years. In the UK, the most recent research available suggests that the mean age of the natural menopause is 51 years, although this can vary between different ethnic groups (National Collaborating Centre for Women's and Children's Health, 2015). Smoking and socioeconomic factors are linked with premature menopause. Other factors that affect the age at which the final menses occurs may include:

- Age at menarche
- Parity
- Previous oral contraceptive history
- Body mass index (BMI)
- Ethnicity
- Family history.

Signs and Symptoms

The National Institute for Health and Care Excellence (2019a) notes the following symptoms commonly associated with menopause. However, it is important to note that current health status and socioeconomic status have been shown to worsen the experience and range of symptoms experienced (Monteleone et al., 2018).

- Vasomotor symptoms, e.g. hot flushes and sweats.
- Musculoskeletal symptoms, e.g. joint and muscle pain.
- Mood changes, e.g. low mood and anxiety.
- Urogenital symptoms, e.g. vaginal dryness, urogenital atrophy.
- Sexual difficulties.

As oestrogen levels fall, the following additional changes can occur.

- Nails become brittle.
- Thinning of skin.
- Hair loss.
- Widespread aches and pains.

Investigations and Diagnosis

When oestrogen levels start dropping, the pituitary gland releases more follicle-stimulating hormone (FSH), encouraging more oestrogen production in the ovaries. Thus, an elevated FSH may indicate menopause. However, FSH levels vary during the perimenopause, so testing can be an unreliable measure. Instead, a detailed history is required to make a diagnosis. NICE (2019a) advises the diagnosis of perimenopause without laboratory tests in otherwise healthy women aged over 45 years based on their report of vasomotor symptoms and irregular periods. Menopause can be diagnosed in women who have not had a period for at least 12 months and are not using hormonal contraception.

In those aged 40–45 years with menopausal symptoms, including a change in their menstrual cycle, and in women aged under 40 years in whom menopause is suspected, NICE (2019a) recommends testing of FSH levels because of the implications of premature ovarian failure.

Follicle-stimulating hormone levels should be tested when the woman is not taking oestrogen-based contraception or hormone replacement therapy (HRT). Consistently elevated FSH levels >30 IU/L are considered to be in the postmenopausal range; estimates should be repeated in 4–8 weeks to confirm this.

Nursing Care and Management

The nurse should approach issues around the menopause as part of a normal period of physiological adaptation, expressing this as a usual aspect of the ageing process.

Peate & Evans (2020) suggest that regular sustained aerobic exercise improves menopausal symptoms, although the evidence is limited. Engaging in exercise can improve quality of life and symptoms such as mood and insomnia as well as providing cardiovascular and other benefits.

By identifying the patient's most challenging symptoms, the nurse can negotiate individualised care and management options.

Red Flag

Some cases of VTE are asymptomatic but possible symptoms of deep vein thrombosis include:
- Pain, swelling, tenderness in one of the legs (usually the calf)
- Heavy ache in the affected area
- Warm skin around the clot
- Redness of skin, particularly on the back of the leg, below the knee.

Treatment for vasomotor symptoms with hormone replacement therapy (HRT) is usually considered in both the shorter term (5 years) and longer term (>5 years). There are no set time limits on the use of HRT and each patient should be assessed individually regarding their personal risk profile. HRT can be stopped suddenly or gradually but either way, the nurse should inform the patient that for a short time after stopping HRT, symptoms might recur. The nurse should also ensure that the patient is aware that HRT does not provide contraception. Sexually active patients should be advised to continue using contraception for 1 year after their final menses if this occurs after the age of 50 years. For those whose last menses occurs before 50 years of age, the nurse should advise that they continue using contraception for 2 years (Royal College of Obstetricians and Gynaecologists, 2018).

Oral and topical HRT work well for menopausal atrophic vaginitis causing urinary and vaginal symptoms and the nurse can suggest the use of lubricants for comfort (particularly during intercourse). Vaginal moisturisers (which have a longer duration of action) are available without prescription.

Hormone replacement therapy can be used if sleep or mood disturbance symptoms are caused by hot flushes and night sweats. Cognitive behavioural therapy should be considered for low mood or anxiety associated with the menopause. There is no clear evidence that selective seratonin reuptake inhibitors (SSRIs) alleviate these symptoms in menopausal people who have not been diagnosed with depression (NICE, 2019a).

The British Menopause Society (2019) suggests that where libido is reduced or lost, testosterone (patches and implants) may help to improve sexual desire.

Disorders of the Female Reproductive System

The following section provides an overview of some disorders of the female reproductive system. In association with this chapter, gynaecological texts should be consulted for further detailed information.

Pelvic Organ Prolapse

Pelvic organ prolapse (genitourinary prolapse) occurs when one or more pelvic organs descends through the pelvic floor into the vaginal canal, for example:
- Uterus
- Rectum
- Bowel (small or large)
- Vaginal vault.

When pelvic organ prolapse occurs, it is often accompanied by urinary, bowel, sexual or local pelvic symptoms. The nurse needs to understand the pathophysiological and psychological issues involved.

Pathophysiology The levator ani muscles and the endopelvic fascia (connective tissue network connecting organs to pelvic muscles and bones) provide most support to the pelvic organs (Figure 30.3 shows the muscles of the female pelvic floor).

Prolapse occurs when the support structure is weakened; this may be due to direct muscle trauma, neuropathic injury, disruption or stretching. There are many potential causes.

The location and shape of the bones of the pelvis have also been connected to the pathogenesis of pelvic organ prolapse.

Known risk factors include:
- Age: risk doubles with each decade of life
- Vaginal delivery
- Increasing parity
- Overweight and obesity
- Spina bifida.

Potential risk factors include:
- Intrapartum variables:
  - Foetal macrosomia (newborn with larger birthweight)
  - Prolonged second stage of labour
  - Episiotomy
  - Anal sphincter injury
  - Epidural anaesthesia
  - Forceps delivery
  - Use of oxytocin
  - Younger than 25 years at first delivery
- Ethnicity

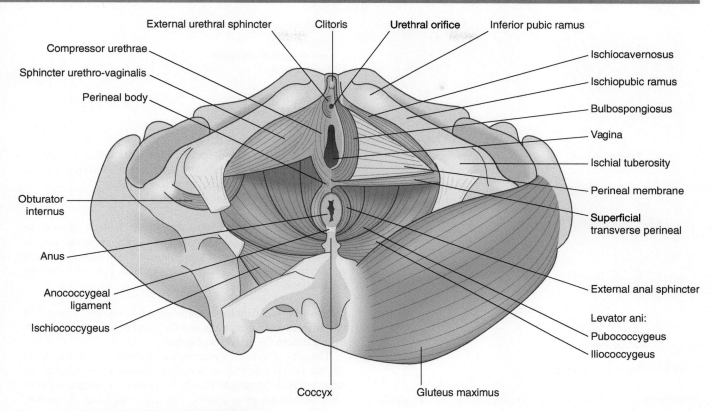

Figure 30.3 The muscles of the female pelvic floor.

- Family history of prolapse
- Constipation
- Connective tissue disorders such as Marfan syndrome
- Previous hysterectomy
- Menopause
- Occupations involving heavy lifting.

It is difficult to determine the incidence of genital prolapse, as not all those affected seek medical advice. It is acknowledged that there is some loss of uterovaginal support in most females, but there is no consensus concerning the level of loss, or what is normal or abnormal.

Types of Pelvic Organ Prolapse Prolapse can occur in the anterior, middle or posterior compartment of the pelvis (Table 30.2). Figure 30.4 provides a diagrammatic representation of the types of prolapse.

Cystourethrocoele is the most common type of prolapse, followed by uterine prolapse and rectocele. Urethrocoeles are rare.

Table 30.2 Types of prolapse. *Source:* Adapted from Norwitz & Schorge (2014).

ANTERIOR COMPARTMENT	MIDDLE COMPARTMENT	POSTERIOR COMPARTMENT
Urethrocoele: prolapse of urethra into the vagina Often associated with urinary stress incontinence	Uterine prolapse: descent of uterus into the vagina	Rectocoele: prolapse of rectum into the vagina
Cystocoele: prolapse of bladder into the vagina. An isolated cystocoele seldom causes incontinence and leads to few or no symptoms. A large cystocoele may cause increased urinary frequency, frequent urinary infections and a pressure sensation or mass at the introitus	Vaginal vault prolapse: descent of vaginal vault post hysterectomy. Usually associated with cystocoele, rectocoele and enterocoele. With complete inversion, the urethra, bladder and distal ureters may be included	
Cystourethrocoele: prolapse of urethra and bladder	Enterocoele: herniation of the pouch of Douglas (including small intestine/omentum) into the vagina. Can occur following pelvic surgery	

545

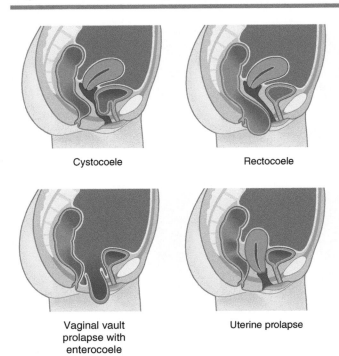

Cystocoele

Rectocoele

Vaginal vault prolapse with enterocoele

Uterine prolapse

Figure 30.4 **Types of prolapse.**

Classification of Pelvic Organ Prolapse Degree of uterine descent can be graded as follows.

1. *First degree*: cervix observable when the perineum is depressed, prolapse contained within the vagina.
2. *Second degree*: cervix prolapsed through the introitus with the fundus remaining in the pelvis.
3. *Third degree*: procidentia (complete prolapse); entire uterus is outside the introitus.

Signs and Symptoms Genital prolapse may be an incidental finding when prolapse is asymptomatic or symptoms are mild. However, symptoms can have a severe impact on quality of life. The most distressing symptom is usually bulging at the vaginal introitus. As a result of gravity, minimal symptoms may be experienced in the morning but symptoms may increase as the day goes on.

Symptoms are related to the site and type of prolapse. Vaginal/general symptoms can be common to all kinds of prolapse.

Vaginal/General Symptoms
- Sensation of pressure, fullness or heaviness.
- Sensation of a bulge/protrusion or 'something coming down'.
- Noticing or feeling a bulge/protrusion.
- Difficulty retaining tampons.
- Spotting (when there is ulceration of the prolapse).

Urinary Symptoms
- Incontinence.
- Frequency.
- Urgency.
- Feeling of incomplete bladder emptying.
- Weak or prolonged urinary stream.
- Need to reduce the prolapse manually before voiding.
- Need to change position to start or complete voiding.

Sex Difficulties
- Dyspareunia.
- Loss of vaginal sensation.
- Vaginal flatus.

Bowel Symptoms
- Constipation/straining.
- Urgency of stool.
- Incontinence of stool, flatus.
- Incomplete or feeling of incomplete evacuation.
- Need to apply pressure to the perineum or posterior vaginal wall to enable defaecation (known as splinting).
- Digital evacuation required to pass a stool.

Investigations and Diagnosis Every patient should be treated as an individual and assessed to determine the nature, severity and progression of symptoms and any current medical conditions, previous obstetric history and past and current medications.

Examination A detailed holistic history is needed to ascertain the patient's main symptoms and the effect of these on their ability to perform the activities of living.

The patient should be examined in a standing position and in the left lateral position. A speculum examination will also be required, and the patient should be given clear explanations of what the examination entails. The nurse supports the patient throughout the procedure.

A rectal examination may be required if there are bowel symptoms.

Investigations A diagnosis is made based on the clinical examination and history. If the patient is experiencing urinary symptoms, NICE (2019b) recommends the following.

- Assessing pelvic floor muscles.
- Urinalysis and, if appropriate, a midstream specimen of urine.
- Postvoid residual urine volume testing using catheter or bladder scan.
- Bladder diaries.
- Symptom and quality of life scoring.

If bowel symptoms are present, consider the following.

- Anal manometry.
- Defaecography.
- Endoanal ultrasound scan (identifies anal sphincter defect if faecal incontinence).

Nursing Care and Management The current management options for women with symptomatic genitourinary prolapse include the following.

- Watchful waiting may be the most appropriate approach if the patient reports few symptoms. They should be observed for the development of new symptoms and provided with information as to what to do should new symptoms develop.
- Non-surgical treatment may be needed if there is evidence of obstructed defaecation or urination, the presence of hydronephrosis or if vaginal erosions develop. All decisions will be made in conjunction with the patient's wishes and individual needs. NICE (2019b) recommends the following

non-surgical interventions for urinary incontinence or overactive bladder.

- *Lifestyle modifications*: caffeine intake reduction; fluid intake management and weight reduction where the patient's BMI is >30.
- *Pelvic floor muscle training*: a supervised trial of at least 3 months and continuation where the effects are positive.
- *Bladder training*: a minimum of 6 weeks should be offered.
- Vaginal pessaries can be used as an alternative to surgery (NICE, 2019b). Inserted into the vagina, a pessary reduces the prolapse, provides support and relieves bladder and bowel pressure. Pessaries need to be carefully managed and regularly removed to avoid complications. Women who opt for a pessary should be referred to a urogynaecology service if pessary care is not available locally.

Surgery Surgery is indicated when a pessary is not effective, the patient requests definitive treatment or if the prolapse is combined with urinary or faecal incontinence.

The risks of surgery for some patients, even for advanced prolapse, may not be warranted. Urinary incontinence can be caused by surgery and some procedures may result in a prolapse in another compartment. Choice of procedure depends on whether the patient is sexually active, the fitness of the patient and the surgeon's assessment. If the prolapse remains corrected and the patient conceives, an elective caesarean section should be advised.

The nurse should advise that patients should avoid heavy lifting after surgery and avoid sexual intercourse for 6–8 weeks. Rigorous internal masturbation may also need to be avoided.

There are several surgical options for urinary stress incontinence as a result of genitourinary prolapse, including colposuspension, rectus fascial sling and in some cases retropubic mid-rethral mesh/tape sling. The use of mesh repair in anterior or posterior vaginal wall prolapse has recently resulted in concerns regarding the extent of complications experienced by those who have had this procedure, the extent of which is not yet fully understood (NICE, 2019b). There are a range of patient decision-making aids published by NICE (2021a) to support informed decision making regarding surgical options. In the light of these concerns and uncertainties, these aids must be included in an open discussion of the harms and benefits of surgical intervention.

Data should be collected on interventions using mesh/tape. The data should include the type of surgery, and its long- and short-term effects must be followed up and documented. The type of mesh/tape used should also be documented and the name of the manufacturer and the inserting surgeon's details should be given to the patient.

Complications and Prognosis

- Ulceration and infection of organs prolapsed outside the vaginal introitus.
- Stress incontinence.
- Chronic retention and overflow incontinence.
- Recurrent urinary tract infections.
- Bowel dysfunction (with rectocoele).

Left untreated, uterine prolapse will gradually worsen. Younger patients in good health and a BMI within normal limits have a better prognosis. Poorer prognosis is associated with older age,

poor physical heath, those with respiratory problems (e.g. asthma or chronic obstructive pulmonary disease) and obesity.

Preventive Measures There is limited evidence to support possible preventive measures.

- Good intrapartum care includes avoiding unnecessary instrumental trauma and prolonged labour.
- Pelvic floor exercises may prevent prolapse occurring secondary to pelvic floor laxity; they are strongly advised after childbirth.
- Smoking cessation reduces chronic cough.
- Weight loss.
- Avoidance of heavy lifting occupations.
- Treatment of constipation throughout life.

Ovarian Cyst

The ovary is a common site for cysts. Most patients who still have a monthly period and one in five of those who have been through the menopause will have one or more ovarian cysts. It is unusual for cysts to affect a person's ability to conceive. Even if the cyst is large and requires removal through laparoscopy, fertility is preserved.

Benign ovarian tumours are divided into three groups.

1. Functional
2. Benign
3. Malignant

Ovarian cysts (fluid-filled sacs) do not usually cause any symptoms, resolving spontaneously.

Ovarian cysts occur in people with regular and irregular menses. Benign ovarian tumours are unusual in premenarchal and postmenopausal people. Benign neoplastic cystic tumours of germ cell origin are most common in young people, accounting for 15–20% of all ovarian neoplasms.

There are two types of functional ovarian cyst: follicular and luteal.

- *Follicular cysts*: these are the most common. The follicle enlarges and fills with fluid, becoming a follicular ovarian cyst, which usually disappears without treatment after a few weeks.
- *Luteal cysts*: less common than follicular cysts, luteal cysts develop when the tissue left behind after an egg has been released (corpus luteum) fills with blood. These usually disappear on their own but can rupture, causing internal bleeding and sudden pain.

Pathological Cysts The most common type of pathological cyst in patients under 40 years old is a dermoid cyst. Over 40 years, the most common type is a cystadenoma.

Signs and Symptoms There may be a dull ache or pain in the lower abdomen and lower back. If there is torsion or rupture, this results in severe abdominal pain and pyrexia. The patient may experience:

- Dyspareunia
- Distended abdomen with palpable mass arising out of the pelvis
- Pressure effects on the bladder, causing urinary frequency
- Pressure effects on venous return, causing varicose veins and/ or leg oedema.

Torsion, infarction or haemorrhage can lead to:

- Severe pain
- Intermittent episodes of severe pain (as a result of intermittent torsion).

Rupture can lead to:

- Peritonitis and shock
- Rupture of mucinous cystadenomas, which may disseminate cells that continue to secrete mucin, causing death by binding the viscera (pseudomyxoma peritonei)
- Ascites
- Endocrine sequelae, for example hormone-secreting tumours may cause virilisation (abnormal development of male sexual characteristics), menstrual irregularities and postmenopausal bleeding.

Conditions That Cause Ovarian Cysts The presence of endometriosis can increase the risk of developing ovarian cysts. Endometriosis occurs when fragments of the endometrium are found outside the uterus, for example in the:

- Fallopian tubes
- Ovaries
- Bladder
- Bowel
- Vagina
- Rectum.

Blood-filled cysts can sometimes form in these tissues.

Polycystic ovarian syndrome (PCOS) can also cause numerous small, harmless cysts to develop on the ovaries, as a result of ovarian hormonal imbalance.

Nursing Care and Management Simple ovarian cysts (<50 mm) based on ultrasound findings do not usually require treatment or follow-up appointments, as most will resolve within a few menstrual cycles.

Larger simple ovarian cysts may require yearly ultrasound follow-up. Those with larger simple cysts should be considered for either further imaging (MRI) or surgical intervention. Monitoring with serial ultrasonography examinations may be required for a postmenopausal patient.

Surgical intervention for benign ovarian tumours is generally very effective, providing a cure with minimal effect on reproductive capacity for those who have been unsuccessful with conservative management.

Laparoscopic surgery for benign ovarian tumours is associated with reduced risk of any unfavourable effect of surgery, reduced pain and fewer days in hospital compared with laparotomy. The outcome is variable, depending on the type and size of the tumour, associated complications and age. Prognosis following surgically removed cysts will depend on the histological results.

Medicines Management Combined Oral Contraceptive Pill (COCP)

Over 15 methods of contraception are available in the UK. The risk of VTE caused by the combined contraceptive pill is very low, despite news reports that using the pill is unsafe. These reports need to be put into context. It must be acknowledged that thrombosis can be a serious side-effect of taking COCPs, but it is extremely rare.

For those who have concerns about taking the oral contraceptive pill, the nurse needs to offer them advice: they should not stop using it, and they can make an appointment to discuss risks with their practice nurse or family planning clinic. There is a low incidence rate of thrombosis associated with the pill. The risk of thrombosis in women using the pill is much less than the risk of blood clots related to pregnancy.

Nurses need to be aware that there has been some misinformation circulating on social media platforms about the risks of concurrent use of combined hormonal contraception (CHC) and vaccination against COVID-19, following the reporting of cases of cerebral venous sinus thrombosis (CVST). The Faculty of Sexual and Reproductive Health (2021) recommends that those using CHC attend for vaccination when it is offered and emphasise that there is no evidence currently to suggest there is an increased risk of thrombosis in those using CHC. Patient should be reminded of the potential risks of COVID-19 infection and missing doses/removing their hormonal contraception to prevent pregnancy.

It must be remembered that COCPs are not suitable for every female; risks differ depending on each person's medical history. Consider alternative options to best suit the person's conception goals and preferences where there are concerns about COCPs.

Cervical Cancer

Globally, gynaecological cancer diagnoses are increasing yearly. The reasons are multifactorial, driven in part by the ageing population and factors including diet, obesity, genetics, economics and the availability of and access to national screening programmes. For reasons of space, the focus in this section is on cervical cancer. For further information see Chapter 15.

In 2018, cervical cancer was the 14th most common cancer in the UK (Cancer Research UK, 2020) and the fourth most common female cancer globally (WHO, 2020).

Risk factors for cervical cancer include:

- Human papillomavirus (HPV)
- Smoking
- Socioeconomic status.

Cervical cancers are theoretically completely preventable, by eradicating infection with HPV, which is present in all cervical cancers. Smoking plays a part in causing some cervical cancers, increasing the likelihood of infection with HPV, or causing HPV infection to be more persistent.

Nursing Fields Children

All children in England aged 12–13 years are offered HPV vaccination as part of the NHS childhood vaccination programme. This vaccine offers protection against cervical, anal and genital cancers. It is usually given in year 8 at school. The HPV vaccine is delivered predominantly through secondary schools and consists of two injections into the upper arm spaced at least 6 and not more than 24 months apart. If a child in year 8 misses their vaccine, the NHS will make vaccination available any time up until their 25th birthday.

People with HIV have an increased risk of cervical cancer and those who have undergone organ transplant have more than double the risk, strongly suggesting that immunosuppression plays a role. Bowden *et al.* (2021) implicate the role of genetics in susceptibility to cervical cancer.

The persistence and degree of severity of dyskaryosis determine whether the woman will need to undergo a further procedure (colposcopy) to provide a histological diagnosis.

Pathophysiology There are two main types of cervical cancer; both are treated in the same way. The most common type of cervical cancer (75–90%) is squamous cell carcinoma. Adenocarcinomas (which develop from the glandular cells lining the endocervix) account for 20–25%; these are more difficult to detect and are becoming more prevalent (Cancer Research UK, 2020).

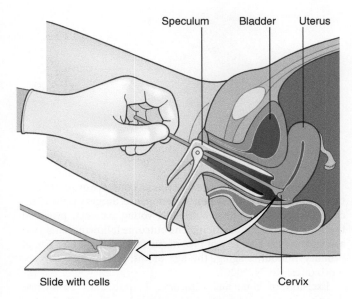

Figure 30.5 Taking a sample of cells.

Labels: Speculum, Bladder, Uterus, Slide with cells, Cervix

Systems of grading are used to determine the extent of changes in the cervix. Knowing the stage of the cancer helps to plan treatment. The stage of a cancer describes its size and whether it has spread beyond its original site. See Chapter 15 for more information on this topic.

Squamous cell cancers spread by direct invasion of accessory structures, including the vaginal wall, pelvic wall, bladder and rectum. Metastatic spread is usually limited to the pelvic area although distant metastasis may occur through the lymphatic system.

Case Study

Elif Sahin is a 26-year-old customer services assistant. Elif presents for an annual learning disability health check with the GP who notes that Elif is overdue for a first cervical smear test. Elif has autistic spectrum disorder (ASD) and a learning disability. Elif thinks she received letters about 'checking for cancer inside' but wasn't sure what they meant. Elif is accompanied by her male partner with whom she is sexually active and who she has asked to accompany her for support during her health check. Elif has had annual health checks before in her early 20s and is familiar with, and consents to, a general health assessment. However, she is unsure about having a cervical smear. The GP sensitively reviews a leaflet with Elif on the cervical cancer screening programme, written specifically for people with learning disabilities. The GP also shows Elif the equipment involved and describes what happens during sampling using the pictures in the leaflet. Elif is still unsure. In line with Elif's wishes, the screen is delayed until the following week when an appointment is made with the practice nurse, allowing Elif to discuss the test with her mother who she would also like to accompany her if she decides to go ahead with screening.

Signs and Symptoms Many cases of cervical cancer are detected by screening. Early symptoms of established cervical carcinoma include:

- Vaginal discharge: may be intermittent or continuous
- Bleeding: can be spontaneous, postcoital, on micturition or defaecation. Occasionally, vaginal bleeding is severe
- Vaginal discomfort/urinary symptoms
- Examination can be relatively normal; there may be white or red patches on the cervix.

Later symptoms can include:

- Painless haematuria
- Chronic urinary frequency
- Painless fresh rectal bleeding
- Changed bowel habit
- Leg oedema, pain and hydronephrosis
- Pelvic discomfort or pain, poorly localised, described as dull or boring into the suprapubic or sacral regions, similar to menstrual discomfort; may be persistent or intermittent
- Rectal examination may reveal a mass or bleeding due to erosion
- Bimanual palpation may uncover pelvic bulkiness/masses due to pelvic spread
- Leg oedema may progress due to lymphatic or vascular obstruction
- Hepatomegaly may develop indicating liver metastases

- Pulmonary metastases are normally only detected if they cause pleural effusion or bronchial obstruction
- Abnormal appearance of the cervix and vagina, related to erosion, ulcer or tumour.

Investigations and Diagnosis Investigations should be tailored to the unique needs of the patient. The nurse assists the patient whilst either undertaking or working alongside other healthcare staff undertaking the relevant investigative and diagnostic procedures.

Those premenopausal patients presenting with abnormal vaginal bleeding should be tested for *Chlamydia trachomatis* according to good practice; many of the signs and symptoms suggestive of cervical cancer are common to genital *Chlamydia trachomatis* infection (RCN, 2020). Postmenopausal patients should be referred urgently to gynaecology services for assessment.

Colposcopy (Figure 30.6) allows for visualisation of the cervix, including the transformation zone (Figure 30.7). The cervix is cleaned with acetic acid, then inspected, biopsied and treated if necessary.

A cone biopsy may be performed (Figure 30.8). A full blood count (FBC) is undertaken to assess for anaemia; renal and liver function tests are also carried out.

A chest X-ray determines metastatic spread and an intravenous urogram is performed. CT scan is used to stage disease, with appropriate biopsies. Barium enema or proctoscopy is performed to assess rectal compression/invasion. Cystoscopy can assess bladder invasion. MRI provides images of a primary tumour, local invasion and nodal enlargement.

Nursing Care and Management The patient must be consulted at each stage of their care programme. The nurse should provide information in a way that allows the patient to make informed decisions and they should be given time to think about the decisions they are making.

If the patient is pregnant, treatment may be delayed until a viable foetus can be delivered (depending on the length of delay required) or a therapeutic abortion may require discussion.

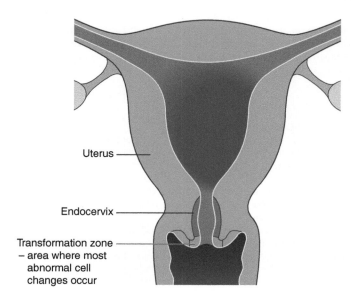

Figure 30.7 **The transformation zone.**

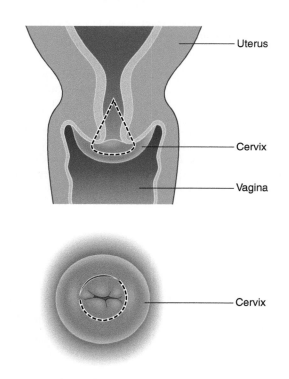

Figure 30.8 **Cone biopsy.**

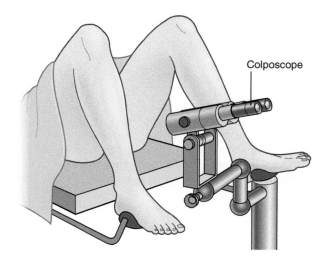

Figure 30.6 **Colposcope.**

Surgery during early-stage disease can conserve ovarian function, avoiding the effects of early menopause. Surgery is the clinically preferred treatment option in young patients, provided there are no contraindications. The outcome following surgery is associated with a variety of prognostic factors, including size of primary tumour, staging, the age of the patient and any co-morbidities (RCN, 2020).

Excision of abnormal ectocervical epithelium performed during colposcopy is used for intraepithelial neoplasia confined to the visible ectocervix; loop diathermy (Figure 30.9) is considered

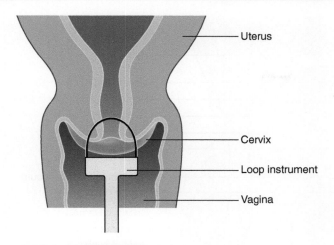

Uterus

Cervix

Loop instrument

Vagina

Figure 30.9 **Loop diathermy.**

the best approach (and provides a specimen for histology) (RCN, 2020).

Pelvic lymph nodes may need to be removed, depending on the staging of the disease. This is performed laparoscopically.

If histology shows the presence of more extensive disease than expected, the patient will be offered postoperative radiotherapy. There is a low risk of postoperative complications.

Chapter 15 of this book discusses the care of people with cancer. The nurse has a central role to play in helping people navigate and make sense of the different treatment options available, as well as providing impartial advice, which people can use to help them make decisions.

Female Genital Mutilation

Female genital mutilation (FGM) is also known as female circumcision. The World Health Organization (2018) defines FGM as any procedure involving partial or total removal of the external female genitalia, or other injury to the female genital organs for non-medical reasons.

FGM is carried out for a wide range of reasons, across a wide geographical area using a range of techniques and in a range of settings from informal to clinical. There is no single religious or cultural basis for this activity and FGM presents in a wide variety of ways. These have been classified into four types by the WHO (2018).

For some patients who have experienced FGM, this has been a traumatic experience that has resulted in significant dermatological, gynaecological, obstetric and infectious disease complications. However, the nurse must also be aware of the status of FGM as a rite of passage imbued with cultural meaning.

Nurses providing care for patients who have had FGM must avoid assumption and judgement about an individual patient's experience, using sensitive communication to support the patient to raise any health or well-being concerns resulting from FGM. This will allow the nurse to provide appropriate clinical care while discharging their professional responsibilities regarding safeguarding. In the UK, FGM is classed as child abuse and the practice is illegal and all healthcare professionals have a mandatory reporting duty (HM Government, 2020). Nurses must also be mindful of the impact that the status of FGM in the UK may have on patients

---

who have experienced it and their resulting apprehension about accessing the healthcare services in light of this. The healthcare professional should offer referral to community groups for support, clinical intervention or other services as appropriate, for example through an NHS FGM clinic. The woman's wishes must always be respected. If the woman is pregnant, the welfare of the unborn child or others in the extended family must also be considered at this point as they are potentially at risk and action must be taken accordingly (HM Government, 2020).

Assessment of the Male Reproductive System

Because of the dual role of some male reproductive organs (with the urinary system), assessment will result in data collection about reproductive and elimination functions. Many of the same diagnostic procedures will be used to evaluate both. The nurse will be required to carry out an assessment of the male reproductive system and an assessment of the patient's needs in several clinical situations, with the intention of making a diagnosis, to plan care and evaluate interventions. See Figure 30.10 for an overview of the male genitalia.

Gender Dysphoria

Gender dysphoria is the distress associated with the experience of gender identity being inconsistent with the phenotype or the gender role typically associated with that phenotype. It is where an individual experiences discomfort or distress because there is a mismatch between their biological sex and gender identity.

At birth, biological sex is assigned depending on genital appearance. Gender identity is the gender that a person 'identifies' with or feels themselves to be. For most people, biological sex and gender identity are the same, but this is not everyone's experience. For example, some people may have the anatomy of a male but identify themselves as a woman, while others may not feel they are definitively either man or woman. Gender dysphoria is a recognised medical condition, for which treatment is sometimes appropriate. Medicalisation of gender dysphoria is the subject of debate and it is important to understand that gender dysphoria is not usually a mental illness. It is important that nurses are aware that only some gender non-conforming people experience gender dysphoria. Identifying as gender non-conforming is a matter of diversity, and not an indication of a disease and does not mean the person is experiencing gender dysphoria.

The condition is also sometimes known as gender incongruence or transgenderism. Some people with gender dysphoria have a strong and determined longing to live according to their gender identity as opposed to their biological sex and sometimes identify as transsexual or trans people. Some trans people have treatment to make their physical appearance more consistent with their gender identity. Transvestism or 'cross-dressing' is not the same as gender dysphoria and is not related to sexual orientation. People who experience gender dysphoria may identify as

(continued)

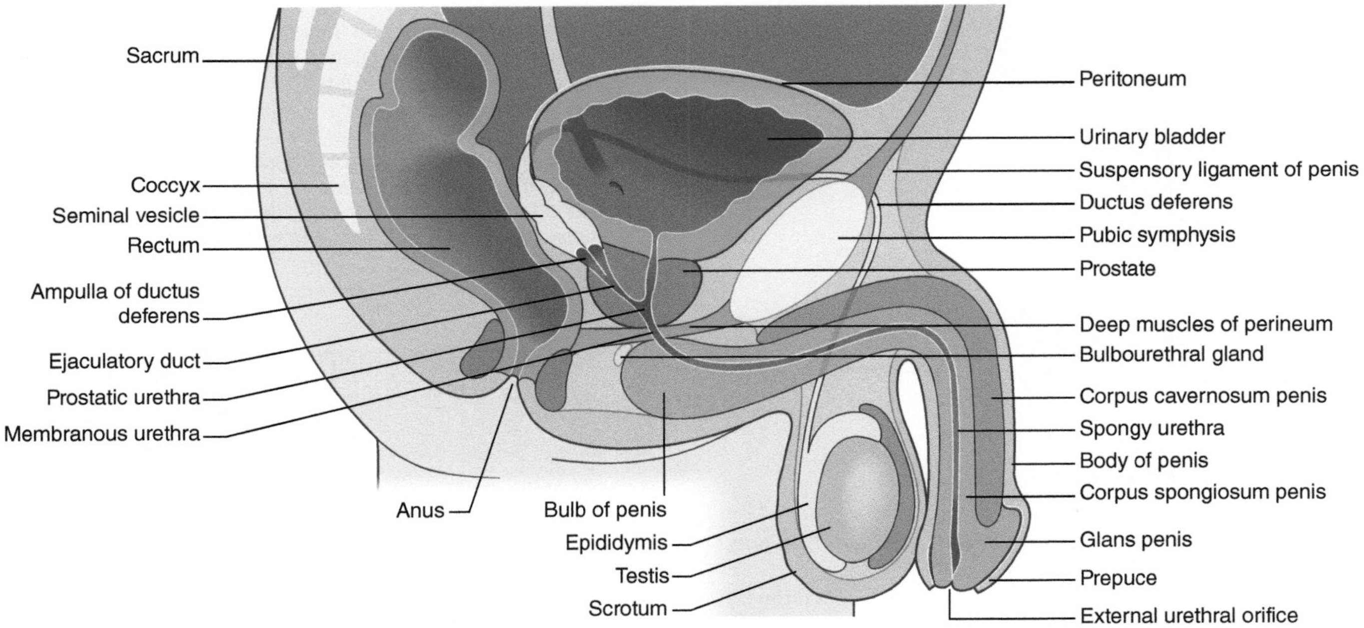

Figure 30.10 **The male genitalia**

straight, gay, lesbian, bisexual or asexual and this may change with treatment.

Key definitions are evolving and may vary between patients and at times the range of terms may cause the nurse confusion. Ask the patient you are caring for what term they would prefer you use.

It can help to distinguish between the meanings of different gender-related terms.

- *Gender dysphoria*: discomfort or distress caused by a mismatch between an individual's gender identity and their biological sex assigned at birth.
- *Transsexualism*: the desire to live and be accepted as a member of the opposite sex, often accompanied by the wish to have treatment to make the physical appearance more consistent with the gender identity.
- *Genderqueer*: an umbrella term that describes gender identities other than man and woman, for example those who are both man and woman, or neither man nor woman, or moving between genders.

Taking a Patient's Health History

The health interview provides an additional method for assessing and determining problems. Several situations arise whereby an interview may be undertaken, for example during a health screening, or it may focus on a chief complaint (i.e. pain in the groin) or occur as part of an in-depth holistic health assessment. Using a holistic approach, you should consider issues from a psychological, social and cultural perspective that can impact negatively and positively on sexuality and sexual activity. The choice of words used when carrying out the health interview should be given careful consideration; choose words that the patient can understand and be aware of the impact that demonstrating offence or embarrassment may have on building patient rapport.

Begin the interview with general questions about the patient's overall health status and then move on to specific questions, using verbal and non-verbal cues that encourage them to explain behaviours, signs and symptoms.

The examination should be carried out in a systematic manner. The penis, scrotum, pubis and groin should be inspected in turn. The nurse should:

1. Communicate
2. Inspect
3. Palpate
4. Examine.

After taking a history, each symptom identified is assessed. It is advisable to offer permission in the approach taken to questioning, for example 'Some patients with diabetes find it difficult to achieve an erection. Have you experienced this?'. Time should be taken to ascertain if there have been any problems with the urinary stream.

Put on gloves before beginning and wear them throughout the examination. Provide the patient with an explanation for everything you do. Bear in mind that the patient may be anxious and the examination itself may cause discomfort. An overview of the male examination is detailed in Table 30.3.

Along with taking a detailed history and a physical examination, other investigations may be required.

- Dipstick urine should be undertaken as appropriate and microscopy for blood, protein, white blood cells and casts undertaken where indicated.
- Microbiology swabs should be taken if there is suspected infection, e.g. *Candida* or any sexually acquired infection.
- Laboratory tests may include:
  - Alpha-fetoprotein
  - Prostate-specific antigen
  - Semen analysis
  - Plasma and serum testosterone levels.

Table 30.3 **Overview of the examination process.**

	INSPECTION	PALPATION AND EXAMINATION
Penis	The skin of the penis should be slightly wrinkled, pink to light brown in white men and light brown to dark brown in black men. Inspect the penile shaft and glans for lesions, nodules, inflammation and oedema. When inspecting the urethral meatus, gently compress the tip of the glans to open. The urethral meatus should be located in the centre of the glans, pink and smooth with no discharge; if discharge is present, a specimen should be taken	Gently use your thumb and forefinger to palpate the shaft of the penis. It should be firm and skin should move unrestricted and be smooth. Palpate to determine if there are any nodules or indurations
Scrotum	With the patient standing, hold the penis away from the scrotum so that you are able to clearly observe the size of the scrotum and its appearance. It is normal for one testis to hang lower (usually the left). The skin on the scrotum is often darker than the skin on the rest of the body. Gently spread the skin of the scrotum and inspect for swelling, nodules, redness, ulcerations and distended veins	
Testes		When palpating the testes, they should be equal in size, move freely, and feel firm, smooth and rubbery. If there are any hard or irregular areas or lumps, then use a torch and transilluminate the scrotal sac by darkening the room and pressing the head of the torch against the scrotum, behind the lump. If there are any lumps, masses, warts or blood-filled sacs, they will appear as opaque shadows. The same test should be carried out on the other testis to make a comparison
Epididymis		The epididymis is usually located in the posterolateral area of the testis. It should be gently palpated and appear smooth, easily identified, non-tender and free from swelling and induration
Spermatic cords		Palpate both spermatic cords, located on top of the testes. Palpate them from the base of the epididymis to the inguinal canal. You can use transillumination if you feel any irregularity or the presence of nodules. If there is any serous fluid present, there will be no glow from transillumination
Inguinal femoral areas	Ask the patient (still in the standing position) to perform the Valsalva manoeuvre (hold his breath and bear down) as you inspect the inguinal and femoral areas	Palpate for a direct inguinal hernia during the Valsalva manoeuvre and you will feel a bulge if a hernia is present
Prostate gland		Explain how you are going to examine the prostate gland. Help the patient to lie on their left side with their right knee and hip flexed. Inspect the skin in the perineal, anal and posterior scrotal regions. The skin should be smooth and unbroken with no protrusions. Explain that you are lubricating your index finger and you will insert this gently into the rectum. Ask the patient to relax, taking deep breaths, so as to ease the insertion of the finger. With the pad of the index finger, palpate the prostate gland on the anterior rectal wall past the anorectal ring. The gland should feel a smooth, rubbery and about the size of a walnut

- Imaging studies can include:
  - Magnetic resonance imaging
  - Ultrasonography.
- Other tests can include:
  - Prostate gland biopsy
  - Urinary flow test
  - Urodynamic studies.

A number of these tests may be used to help make a definitive diagnosis.

Care, Dignity and Compassion

The patient must be offered a chaperone during the assessment, regardless of the sex of the examiner, and nurses must adhere to local protocol, policy and procedure.

To reduce or lessen the patient's anxiety, provide them with explanations for the procedures; taking a matter-of-fact approach may help reduce embarrassment. You can use diagrammatic representations or models of the genitalia that demonstrate those parts that will be examined, if appropriate.

Testicular Disorders

Disorders of the testis include:

- Ectopic testis
- Cryptorchidism
- Testicular torsion
- Testicular cancer.

As the testes are the sites of spermatogenesis and androgen production, these disorders may have a potentially negative effect on fertility and secondary sex characteristics.

Cryptorchidism and Ectopic Testis

These are similar congenital conditions in which descent of the testis is incomplete (in cryptorchidism) or has taken an abnormal route (ectopic). In cryptorchidism, the descending testis stops in the pelvic cavity, inguinal canal or upper end of the scrotum. An ectopic testis ends up in the perineal or suprapubic region or just beneath the skin of the thigh.

Testicular Torsion

Testicular torsion occurs with twisting of the testis on the spermatic cord. This can occur spontaneously or as a result of trauma or vigorous exercise. It occurs most often during puberty but may happen at any time of life. Twisting the testicular blood vessels causes testicular ischaemia and necrosis of the testis. Unless it is corrected within 4–6 hours, damage to the testis can permanently impair fertility. It is therefore treated as a medical emergency (Royal College of Surgeons, 2016).

Testicular torsion may result in scrotal swelling that is not eased by rest or support of the testis. The patient may complain of severe pain and nausea and may vomit. Pyrexia is common.

Testicular Cancer

Testicular cancer accounts for less than 1% of male cancers. Germ cell tumours (GCTs) are the most widespread type of testicular cancer; their incidence has risen over the past two decades, as has the most prevalent risk factor for GCT, an undescended testis (cryptorchidism) (Box 30.3).

Box 30.3 Some Risk Factors Associated with Testicular Cancer

- Cryptorchidism
- Hypospadias
- Family history
- Previous testicular cancer
- Some men with fertility problems
- Men with HIV/AIDS
- Ethnicity (white men are more prone to testicular cancer than black men or men from other ethnic groups in the UK)
- Microlithiasis (the presence of calcium specks in the testes)
- Height (taller than average men have an increased risk compared with shorter men)
- Testicular injury (this can mask the presence of a pre-existing testicular swelling)
- Maternal hormones and pregnancy factors

Source: Adapted from Cancer Research UK (2018).

The following are signs of testicular cancer:

- Painless swelling on one testicle
- Dull ache in pelvis or scrotum that may come and go
- A feeling of heaviness in the scrotum
- Painless nodule on one testicle
- Acute pain in scrotum
- Infertility
- Gynaecomastia
- Malaise and fatigue.

Signs and symptoms associated with metastatic spread include:

- Neck mass
- Respiratory symptoms (including cough, dyspnoea, haemoptysis)
- Gastrointestinal disturbance
- Back pain
- Lower extremity oedema
- Back pain
- Dizziness.

Investigations and Diagnosis

The patient's history and a physical examination will be undertaken. The nurse may be required to act as chaperone to provide physical and emotional support before, during and after the procedures.

Several laboratory investigations will be undertaken to make a definitive diagnosis. Analysis of blood will be undertaken to determine if there are any tumour markers present. Raised biochemical markers provide a strong indication of testicular cancer. Tumour markers are also assessed after surgery, helping establish the presence of residual disease. If these levels are persistently raised, this may indicate the need for further therapy. Serum lactate dehydrogenase (LDH) levels are increased in testicular cancer and if there is metastatic spread, the level will be significantly elevated.

An ultrasound of both testes will be performed. This can demonstrate if there is a solid lump or a fluid-filled cyst; the latter is less likely to be a cancer. A man with suspected urological cancer (when in the primary care setting) should be urgently referred to urology oncology services (NICE, 2021b).

Nursing Care and Management

The treatment offered reflects the man's individual needs and desires, and the stage of the cancer. Care of the person with cancer and undergoing radiotherapy or chemotherapy is discussed in Chapter 15.

There are several treatment modalities including surgical intervention, radiation therapy and chemotherapy. The first line of treatment is surgical removal of the testis (orchidectomy) and following this surgery, the patient may be referred to a psychosexual counsellor for support if they wish.

Red Flag

Alopecia (hair loss) is a common side-effect of some chemotherapy. It usually begins 1–3 weeks after the first chemotherapy dose. Most people have significant hair loss after 1–2 months. Hair loss can occur on other parts of the body, including the arms, legs and face. Hair loss can be very distressing. The nurse should prepare the patient for this event.

Care of a person postoperatively will include managing pain and observing and responding to the man's physiological and emotional needs (see Chapter 15 on the principles of cancer care and Chapter 22 on the principles of pain management).

The diagnosis will be communicated to the patient postoperatively following histological confirmation. A diagnosis of testicular cancer, regardless of how much preoperative preparation has been undertaken, will usually have a huge impact. The extent of the disease and the presence of any metastatic spread will be detected by increased levels of tumour markers and these will be used to aid diagnosis as well as the management of further treatment.

Many patients worry that losing one testicle will affect their ability to have sexual intercourse or make them infertile; however, a person with one healthy testicle can still have a normal erection and produce sperm.

The patient should be offered the option of a prosthetic device once treatment is complete as it may support self-esteem and body image.

Surgery to remove the lymph nodes will not change a patient's ability to have an erection or an orgasm; however, the procedure can cause temporary or permanent infertility as it may interfere with the nerves involved in ejaculation.

Health Promotion

Nurses play a central role in educating men about testicular cancer and self-examination. Nurses also have a duty to raise awareness about factors that put men at risk, as well as providing psychological support to the patient and his family. The nurse must be sufficiently informed about testicular cancer risk, symptoms, testicular self-examination technique (Box 30.4), assessment procedures, treatment regimens and support services.

Discharge Advice

See Box 30.5 for discharge advice that the nurse should give the patient following surgery.

Referral to the community nursing services may be required to care for the patient's wound. Explain that the patient should not remove any dressings until the community nurse has made their assessment. The patient may be advised to wear a scrotal support to provide comfort.

Box 30.4 Advice to Men Concerning Testicular Self-examination

To notice changes in your testicles, you need to know what is normal for you.

- Hold your scrotum in the palms of your hands, so that you can use the fingers and thumbs on both hands to examine your testicles.
- Note the size and weight of the testicles. It is common to have one testicle slightly larger, or which hangs lower than the other, but any noticeable increase in size or weight may mean something is wrong.
- Gently feel each testicle individually.
- You should feel a soft tube at the top and back of the testicle. This is the epididymis. It may feel slightly tender. Do not confuse it with an abnormal lump.
- You should be able to feel the firm, smooth tube of the spermatic cord, which runs up from the epididymis.
- Feel the testicle itself.
- It should be smooth with no lumps or swellings. It is unusual to develop cancer in both testicles at the same time, so if you are wondering whether a testicle is feeling normal or not, you can compare it with the other.
- Remember: if you do find a swelling in your testicle, make an appointment and have it checked by your practice nurse as soon as possible.

Box 30.5 Discharge Advice

You should contact your general practice if:

- You are nauseous or vomiting
- You have a cough, feel weak and you are aching
- You have a fever or chills
- Your skin becomes itchy or swollen or you develop a rash after taking your medicines
- You have questions or concerns about your surgery, condition or care.

You should seek immediate advice (go to an accident and emergency department or call 999) if:

- You have chest pain, feel lightheaded or are having trouble breathing
- You have more pain when you take deep breaths or cough; you cough up blood
- You have severe pain in your legs or your legs become very swollen
- You have lower stomach or back pain that does not go away even after taking your medicines
- You have trouble passing urine or having a bowel movement
- Your incision is swollen, red, bleeding or pus is coming from it
- Your stitches come apart
- Your leg feels warm, tender and painful: it may look swollen and red.

Prostate Disease

The term 'prostate disease' covers several prostate-related conditions. There are three main conditions that can affect the prostate gland.

- Prostatic hypertrophy
- Prostatitis
- Cancer of the prostate

Prostatic hypertrophy is discussed here. A detailed discussion of prostate cancer can be found in Peate & Evans (2020).

Enlargement of the prostate gland, also called benign prostatic hypertrophy (BPH), is a very common condition associated with ageing and is not usually a threat to the man's health.

The prostate gland becomes enlarged for a number of reasons – the exact cause is unknown but may be due to changing levels of testosterone and oestrogen. Younger males produce high levels of testosterone and much lower levels of oestrogen. However, as they age, testosterone levels decrease, resulting in a higher proportion of oestrogen; the increase in oestrogen may be responsible for stimulating prostate growth. As the prostate gland enlarges, it can cause pressure on the urethram which can affect the passing of urine. It may cause:

- Hesitancy
- Frequency
- Difficulty emptying the bladder fully.

These symptoms range from mild to severe. Those with prostate enlargement do not have a higher risk of prostate cancer compared with those without an enlarged prostate. Treatment options include:

- Making lifestyle changes, such as reducing the amount of liquid the man drinks before going to bed; avoiding caffeinated drinks
- The use of alpha-blockers (medications to help relax the muscles within the prostate gland); these include tamsulosin or alfuzosin
- Medications to reduce the size of the prostate, making it easier to urinate (finasteride or dutasteride block the effects of dihydrotestosterone) (NICE, 2019c).

When lifestyle changes and the use of medicines fail, surgery can be used to remove the inner part of the gland. Transurethral resection of the prostate (TURP) and prostatectomy are surgical interventions used for moderate-to-severe symptoms that have not responded to medical treatment.

Following surgery, a urinary catheter usually remains in place for 24–48 hours. The nurse must monitor urinary output every 2–4 hours. The patient is encouraged to drink 2000–3000 mL of fluids daily (if there are no contraindications) to relieve initial dysuria and resolve haematuria.

Jot This Down

You are encouraging a patient to drink 2000–3000 mL of fluid a day.
- How will you know if he has drunk this?
- How would you encourage this?
- How would you involve the patient and his family?

Discomfort after TURP is usually associated with bladder distension, irritation from the catheter or irrigation solution or bladder spasm. Smooth muscle relaxants may be prescribed if bladder spasms persist. Prescribed analgesia should be given, and its efficacy noted.

TURP syndrome is an associated complication; nursing interventions focus on management and prevention of complications. TURP syndrome usually occurs within the first 24 hours. Abnormal vascular absorption of irrigating fluid during surgery causes severe dilutional hyponatraemia and hypervolaemia. The nurse carefully assesses the patient for symptoms of TURP syndrome, which can include:

- Dramatic increase in blood pressure
- Full, bounding pulse
- Bradycardia
- Tachypnoea
- Confusion
- Agitation
- Temporary blindness.

The nurse must seek help immediately if the patient experiences any of the above. Stay with the patient and provide reassurance.

Haemorrhage is the most common complication after TURP. Bladder spasms or movement may initiate bleeding. Nursing interventions include the monitoring of:

- Vital signs as the patient's condition dictates
- Urinary output for colour and consistency of bladder returns every hour.

Increase the rate of bladder irrigation flow as needed to ensure urine flows and prevent obstruction. Instruct the patient to remain flat or at a slight incline immediately postoperatively; sitting may increase venous and bladder pressure, causing bleeding.

You must immediately escalate as required if there is any increase in bleeding or change in vital signs that may indicate haemorrhage. Surgical intervention may be needed if the bleeding continues. Hypovolaemia may develop due to extensive bleeding; the patient may require intravenous fluids or blood transfusion.

Surgical intervention and the presence of an indwelling urinary catheter can lead to urinary tract infection. Careful monitoring is required, and the nurse must perform meticulous catheter care and maintain a closed urinary drainage system.

Clots or tissue debris can obstruct the urinary catheter. By assessing the colour and consistency of bladder returns, patency of inflow and outflow tubing and rate of irrigation, the nurse can prevent urinary retention postoperatively. Bladder irrigation may be required initially to flush out debris and clots. Further saline flushing or milking of the catheter may be used to troubleshoot a blocked or slow-flowing catheter but the nurse must ensure that local policy, procedure and protocol are adhered to.

The surgical team must be notified immediately if an obstruction cannot be resolved or if frank haematuria or new, unexpected clotting is observed.

Health Promotion

Nothing can prevent the development of BPH. Patient education and awareness of the signs and symptoms of BPH should be provided to all males and targeting of at-risk groups should be considered. Nurses working in primary and secondary care settings are ideally placed to offer opportunistic or planned information-giving sessions.

It is important that health promotion emphasises that men should not wait to seek treatment if they experience any of the signs and symptoms associated with BPH. Delay could result in severe obstruction of the urinary system and subsequent kidney damage.

Discharge Advice

Advise the patient to drink twice as much fluid as they usually would for the first 24–48 hours and to avoid the use of alcohol, caffeinated beverages and spicy foods that can irritate the bladder.

Bleeding can occur in 20% of patients 10–14 days post surgery due to scabs detaching from the prostate cavity. If this occurs, patients should be encouraged to increase fluid intake and contact their GP if it does not resolve. Severe bleeding or sudden difficulty in passing urine should immediately be reported to the GP and may require emergency readmission.

The person can return to work when they feel able to do so and the GP is happy with their progress. The British Association of Urological Surgeons (BAUS, 2017) advises that most people need 3–4 weeks restful recuperation at home before returning to work.

Explain what the signs and symptoms of urinary tract infection might be and advise the patient to inform his GP if they occur as antibiotic therapy may be required.

If the person is sexually active prior to surgery, sexual activity (and this includes masturbation) can usually be resumed 2–4 weeks after surgery, as long as there is no bleeding in the urine (which indicates that the prostate still has some healing to do). After TURP, some patients have less or no semen after sexual intercourse. There may be retrograde ejaculation (dry climax). This should not impact desire for, or the ability to have, sex. Some find their erection is poorer following TURP. If this is a problem, then encourage the patient to speak to the community nurse or GP.

Initiation of pelvic floor exercises is recommended to reduce the likelihood or manage the potential loss of bladder control post TURP (BAUS, 2017). Information for patients on how to undertake pelvic floor exercises can be found on the BAUS website or a referral to a urological specialist nurse can be made to support this important part of the person's recovery.

Erectile Dysfunction

For most people, sex is an important aspect of everyday life. The ability to attain and maintain an erection for many demonstrates male potency and is bound closely to constructs of gender and masculinity.

Erectile dysfunction (ED) is only one of a range of male sexual dysfunctions, but it is perhaps the most spoken about. The taboo that was once associated with this condition has been dramatically reduced, because of the advent of easily available and well-tolerated oral treatments. Despite the increased understanding, coupled with advances in the field, the disorder can still be very distressing for both the patient and their partner. The nurse can help to alleviate the distress caused; however, to do this effectively, they must understand the condition and the possible options available to help the patient manage their health and sexual well-being.

Erectile dysfunction can affect males at any age. It is a psychophysiological disorder impacting on sexual arousal. Being aware of the psychological and physical consequences of ED for the patient and their partner may help provide a service that meets the needs of those affected by the condition.

Sociocultural norms and behaviours traditionally associated with masculinity can affect men's willingness to seek healthcare. Discussion of issues of a sexual nature with healthcare providers may be particularly challenging for some people. Many of those affected do not find it easy to discuss ED with their sexual partners, let alone with a nurse. Nurses should be proactive and provide ways which encourage the sharing of anxiety, fears and concerns.

Practitioners must provide accurate information and continue to demystify and challenge stereotypes associated with ED and those who experience it. ED that is not diagnosed and treated can be a cause of physical as well as psychological morbidities, including low self-esteem, anxiety, depression and a diminished quality of life.

Definitions

Erectile dysfunction is defined as an inability to obtain or maintain an erection sufficient for penetration and for the satisfaction of both sexual partners (BAUS, 2021).

Pathophysiology

The British Association of Urological Surgeons (2021) notes that ED is a very common disorder, with incidence increasing with age and affecting up to 55% of males aged 40–70 years. However, whilst increasing ED incidence is age related, it is not an age-dependent disorder.

A patient may present with physical symptoms; they may also have feelings that affect their psychological well-being concerning inadequacy, as well as experiencing feelings of emasculation.

The nurse should be aware of the pathophysiology of erection and how erections occur and are maintained sufficiently to permit satisfactory sexual performance.

Penile erection is a multifaceted physiological process that is the result of co-ordinated neurological, vascular and hormonal events. Erection and detumescence are associated with complex interactions involving several haemodynamic events that cause muscle relaxation and vasoconstriction, resulting in the accumulation of blood under pressure and, usually, end-organ rigidity (see Figure 30.11).

Erection occurs as a result of an assortment of changes associated with:

- The vascular system
- The endocrine system
- Psychological factors.

If alteration in one of the above occurs, there is a potential for erectile failure.

The vascular process can be divided into six phases.

1. Flaccidity
2. Filling phase

557

Figure 30.11 **The male sexual response.** *Source*: Heffner & Schust (2014). Reproduced with permission of John Wiley & Sons Ltd.

3. Tumescence
4. Full erection
5. Rigidity
6. Detumescence.

The male sexual response is shown in Figure 30.11.

Risk Factors Associated with ED

Erectile dysfunction is often multifactorial; the causes can be related to organic or inorganic disorders or a combination of both factors. Organic causes are related to physiological disorders; inorganic causes are psychological in nature. Psychogenic factors are involved in the majority of cases, in spite of the fact that in the majority of men with ED, the dominant pathophysiology is organic. See Table 30.4 for a list of organic factors.

Investigations and Diagnosis

Patients are becoming more aware that simple effective treatments are available and as result are requesting them from health professionals or accessing them independently from online pharmacies.

Primary Care

Most cases of ED are treated in the primary care setting without the need to refer the patient to specialist secondary care.

A diagnosis will need to be made prior to offering treatment and providing the man with a choice concerning treatment options. Treatment options are based on the underlying cause. Table 30.5 outlines the differences between the psychogenic and organic origins of ED.

History taking, physical examination and clinical investigation help to make a diagnosis. ED is now regarded as an independent risk factor for cardiovascular disease and can be the presenting feature of diabetes so the British Society for Sexual Medicine (BSSM, 2017) advises that serum lipids, fasting plasma glucose and/or glycated haemoglobin should be measured in all patients presenting with ED. Further investigations will vary, depending on the patient's history and findings from the physical examination. Individual patients' willingness regarding investigations should always take precedence.

Table 30.4 **Some potential organic causes of ED.**
Source: Adapted from Dick *et al.* (2017).

FACTOR	POTENTIAL COMPONENTS
Vasculogenic	Hypertension Atherosclerosis Venogenic Ischaemia
Neurogenic	Spinal injury Multiple sclerosis Dementia Spinal tumour Parkinson disease Cerebrovascular disease Cauda equina compression Prolapsed intravertebral disc
Endocrinological	Hormone deficiency Hypogonadism Thyroid disease Hyperprolactinaemia
Drug related	Certain antihypertensives Some psychotropics Some hormonal agents
Systemic	Diabetes mellitus Malignancy Chronic renal failure
Surgery	Transurethral and radical prostatectomy Cystectomy Pelvic surgery (abdominoperineal resection) Radiotherapy
Lifestyle	Smoking Alcohol Recreational drugs Trauma to the perineum Bicycling Horse riding
Other	Arthritis Aetiology unknown

Other investigations may include:
- Testosterone
- Prolactin
- Glucose
- LH/FSH
- T4 and TSH
- Liver and renal function
- Neurological tests
- Intracavernous injection test to assess for penile deformities
- Colour Doppler ultrasound to assess vascular integrity
- Phalloarteriography to confirm the presence of vascular abnormality
- Cavernosometry/cavernosography to assess the mechanism of venous occlusion
- Nocturnal penile tumescence and rigidity (NPTR) monitoring to differentiate between psychogenic and organic causes (BSSM, 2017).

Nursing Fields   Mental Health

There is a pressing need to improve the physical health are of people with serious mental illness (SMI) (Department of Health, 2016), indicating that current services are not responsive to the needs of people living with SMI. To provide patient-centred high-quality care, nurses are required to ensure that people with mental health problems have all their health needs met. This should include both baseline and regular assessment of their reproductive and sexual health needs, to promote good physical health and prevent the avoidable increased burden of disease falling on patients living with SMI.

Table 30.5 **Psychogenic versus organic causes of ED.**

PSYCHOGENIC ORIGIN	ORGANIC ORIGIN
Sudden onset	Gradual onset
Good-quality or better spontaneous/self-stimulated/nocturnal erections/waking erections	Lack of tumescence
Premature ejaculation or inability to ejaculate	Normal libido (except in hypogonadal men) and ejaculation
Relationship problems or changes	Risk factor in current or past history in particular with reference to cardiovascular, endocrine and neurological systems
Major life events	Operations, radiotherapy or trauma to the pelvis or scrotum
Psychological problems	Use of medications recognised as being associated with ED
Specific situations	All circumstances
	Lifestyle factors, such as smoking, high use of alcohol, use of recreational drugs or body-building drugs

Nursing Care and Management

Treatments are provided on individual assessment; they vary and can include the increasingly popular oral pharmacological therapies. The primary goal in the management of ED is to enable the patient and their partner to enjoy a satisfactory sexual life. This involves:

- Identifying and treating any curable causes of ED
- Initiating lifestyle change for modifiable risk factors, including psychological factors
- Providing education and psychological therapies to patients and their partners.

Other treatments are also offered dependent on identification of underlying causes:

- Hormonal treatment
- Mechanical/physical devices, e.g. vacuum devices
- Surgical treatment.

All treatment options have the potential to harm, and all have advantages and disadvantages, discussion of which is vital to ensure the patient provides informed consent for their individual treatment pathway.

A non-judgemental approach is essential to caring for a patient with ED, as is supporting understanding of possible underlying causes. A lack of understanding on the part of the patient may result in blame being placed on unrelated factors, such as age, medications, illness or sexual partner.

Erectile dysfunction can be triggered or sustained by performance anxiety. This involves a complex interplay of cognitive, affective, behavioural and physiological responses throughout a sexual situation. It can be triggered by any sexual stimulus that the person associates with their sexual inadequacy. The excessive stimulation that results counteracts both initiation and maintenance of an erection and can also reduce a patient's response to therapies. This in turn can lead to chronic erectile failure, sexual avoidance and decreased sexual arousal (BSSM, 2017).

Jot This Down

What do you think are the dangers of buying drugs such as Viagra (sildenafil) on the internet?

It is not expected that the nurse be an expert in the various psychosexual approaches for patients with ED of psychogenic origin; however, understanding is expected with respect to the pharmacological and other potential interventions. The worldwide availability of drug treatment for ED in the form of phosphodiesterase type 5 (PDE5i) inhibitors (e.g. sildenafil) has transformed the way men with ED are treated. Other forms of non-invasive, non-biological treatments are also available. The nurse must ensure that the patient is provided with information about all treatment options prior to making a final decision for their preferred treatment.

Case Study

Jorge Lopes is a 43-year-old bar manager. He attends a sexual health clinic for an appointment with a nurse practitioner (NP). Jorge tells the NP that he has been in a relationship with his male partner for 15 years, and they have previously enjoyed a fulfilling sexual relationship, but over the last year he has had difficulty maintaining an erection. Jorge's partner was initially supportive, but he and Jorge are now arguing a lot; Jorge's partner thinks Jorge no longer wants to have sex with him and he feels hurt and angry. Jorge feels guilty, depressed and confused as to why this has happened. The NP takes a detailed health history, noting that Jorge has no significant medical history or indicators of organic causes of ED and has spontaneous morning erections. The NP does note that Jorge is experiencing very serious work-related stressors; Jorge was furloughed during each COVID-19 lockdown, had to make a large number of his team redundant (many of whom were friends) and has struggled financially for over a year. His alcohol intake increased significantly during this time. Although Jorge is back at work now and is drinking less, there is uncertainty whether the bar he manages will stay in business. The NP explains how stress, depression and excessive alcohol use can be precipitating factors in erectile dysfunction. The NP offers Jorge a referral for psychosexual counselling (for which there is likely to be an extensive wait) alongside the more immediate option of self-referring to the local cognitive behavioural therapy service.

Treatment Availability

For patients diagnosed with ED within the NHS, sildenafil is available via NHS prescription. Sildenafil is also available over the counter in pharmacies following discussion with a pharmacist or via online pharmacies. Patients should be counselled about the potential risks of purchasing sildenafil, or indeed any medication, online.

Sexually Acquired Infections

Untreated sexually acquired infections (SAIs) can lead to serious long-term health consequences for individuals, communities and nations. Nurses are at the forefront of promoting safer sex messages among the general population as well as being able to focus health promotion on those most at risk of SAIs.

In England, the sexual health of the nation has deteriorated over the last decade. Numbers of new diagnoses of SAIs rose by 5% in 2019, with chlamydia, gonorrhoea and genital warts being most diagnosed (Table 30.6). The impact of poor sexual health remains greatest in young heterosexual adults, black ethnic minorities and in gay, bisexual and other men who have sex with men and this is where the greatest burden falls (PHE, 2020).

Geographically, there is considerable variation in the distribution of SAIs; the highest rates are seen in urban areas, reflecting concentrations of the population who are at greatest risk.

Prevention efforts, for example greater SAI screening coverage and providing easier access to sexual health services, should be sustained and continue to focus on groups who are at the highest risk. Health promotion and education remain the foundations of SAI and HIV prevention, providing improved public awareness of SAIs and HIV and encouraging safer sexual behaviours, including consistent condom use.

Red Flag

Human sexual behaviour is diverse. The nurse should avoid moral or religious judgement of the person's behaviour. Efforts should be concentrated instead on managing their health-related needs, which will include their psychological and emotional needs. The nurse should also take time to address any concerns the individual may have. Any requests for clinician gender that are based on cultural or religious grounds, or which are due to personal preference, should where possible be accommodated.

Care, Dignity and Compassion

The choice of language used when communicating with patients about reproductive and sexual health should be given much thought. The aim should be to encourage the person to speak openly about issues that concern them. The nurse's body language may give away the fact they are feeling uncomfortable when the patient is sharing details about their reproductive or sexual history, and this is unacceptable.

Table 30.6 Key information on the commonly diagnosed SAIs in England.

SEXUALLY ACQUIRED INFECTION	CHLAMYDIA	GONORRHOEA	GENITAL WARTS
Prevalence (PHE, 2020)	Most commonly diagnosed SAI in England. Accounted for 49% of all new SAI diagnoses in 2019	Second most commonly diagnosed SAI in England. Accounted for 15% of all new SAI diagnoses in 2019	Third most commonly diagnosed SAI in England. Accounted for 15% of all new SAI diagnosis in 2019
Pathophysiology	Caused by infection with the bacterium *Chlamydia trachomatis*	Gonorrhoea is the clinical disease resulting from infection with the Gram-negative diplococcus *Neisseria gonorrhoeae*	Around 90% of all cases of genital warts (condylomata acuminata) are caused by two strains of HPV: type 6 and type 11
Signs and symptoms	Urethritis and cervicitis in females are often concurrent. Symptoms include abdominal pain, bleeding between menses, dysuria, urgency, frequency and/ or burning. Symptoms of urethritis in men may include penile discharge and dysuria. Depending on the site of infection, a patient may present with fever, lower abdominal pain or tenderness, rectal discharge and/ or pruritus. If untreated, can cause infertility due to tubal adhesions, ectopic pregnancy and pelvic inflammatory disease (PID)	Urethral infection usually causes urethral discharge in males and may be accompanied by dysuria 2–5 days after exposure. In some cases, urethral infection may be asymptomatic. Rectal infection is often asymptomatic but may cause anal discharge or perianal/anal pain or discomfort. Pharyngeal infection is usually asymptomatic. In females endocervical infection may result in altered vaginal discharge or lower abdominal pain and dysuria may be the result of urethral infection	Lesions around the genital area or noted during examination of the patient's vagina or cervix and may have a smooth-domed, cauliflower or keratotic-like appearance. Lesions are usually asymptomatic, although they may be associated with itching or irritation and may bleed. Lesions can be single or multiple

Prevention of SAIs

Abstinence from any sexual activity greatly reduces the risk of chlamydia, gonorrhea and genital HPV infection but is not an option for most sexually active people. Condoms for penetrative sex and/or oral sex and/or for covering shared sex toys and/or the use of dental dams reduce the risk of SAI, but are not 100% effective. Regular screening for SAIs, reflecting an individual's SAI risk profile, should be recommended. Symptoms indicative of an SAI should be assessed and treated by specialist sexual health services.

What The Experts Say

'The one thing I would say to a student working with people who have sexual health needs is to treat them as you would like to be treated yourself. We are all human and we all have needs and lots of these are diverse and sometimes complex.'
Consultant nurse

Conclusion

This chapter has provided information and discussion of the care that patients who experience normal and abnormal reproductive health changes may need. Reproductive health conditions can be complex and require skilled, sensitive, and compassionate patient-centred nursing care. There are numerous screening and diagnostic tests available to help offer patients care that is responsive and appropriate.

The nurse must use a framework, a systematic approach to guide assessment, diagnosis, planning, implementation and the evaluation of care provision. When applying a systematic approach, the physical, psychological and cultural needs of the patient should be taken into consideration.

The role of the nurse in reproductive health is multifaceted and will include acting as patient advocate. The nurse has a duty to provide care in a non-judgemental manner that recognises and respects diversity and avoids assumptions about patient's reproductive and sexual health needs and preferences.

Key Points

- This chapter has provided information and discussion of the care that patients who experience normal and abnormal reproductive health changes may need. Reproductive health conditions can be complex and require skilled, sensitive and compassionate patient-centred nursing care.
- There are numerous screening and diagnostic tests available to help offer patients care that is responsive and appropriate.
- The nurse must use a framework, a systematic approach to guide assessment, diagnosis, planning, implementation and the evaluation of care provision. When applying a systematic approach, the physical, psychological and cultural needs of the patient should be taken into consideration.
- The role of the nurse in reproductive health is multifaceted and will include acting as patient advocate. The nurse has a duty to provide care in a non-judgemental manner that recognises and respects diversity and avoids assumptions about patients' reproductive and sexual health needs and preferences.

References

Bowden, S., Bodinier, B., Kalliala, I., *et al.* (2021) Genetic variation in cervical preinvasive and invasive disease: a genome-wide association study. *Lancet*, 22, 548–557.

British Menopause Society (2019) *Testosterone replacement in menopause. A guide for GPs and health professionals.* https://thebms.org.uk/wp-content/uploads/2020/04/08-BMS-ToolforClinician-Testosterone-replacement-in-menopause-APR2020.pdf (accessed December 2021).

British Association of Urological Surgeons (2017) *Prostate cancer. What does the treatment involve?* www.baus.org.uk/_userfiles/pages/files/Patients/Leaflets/TURP%20for%20cancer.pdf (accessed December 2021).

British Association of Urological Surgeons (2021) *Erectile dysfunction.* www.baus.org.uk/patients/conditions/3/erectile_dysfunction_impotence/ (accessed December 2021).

British Society for Sexual Medicine (2017) *Guidelines on the management of erectile dysfunction in men.* www.bssm.org.uk/wp-content/uploads/2018/09/BSSM-ED-guidelines-2018-1.pdf. (accessed December 2021).

Cancer Research UK (2018) *Risk factors for testicular cancer.* www.cancerresearchuk.org/about-cancer/testicular-cancer/risks-causes (accessed December 2021).

Cancer Research UK (2020) *Cervical cancer statistics.* www.cancerresearchuk.org/health-professional/cancer-statistics/statistics-by-cancer-type/cervical-cancer#heading-Zero (accessed December 2021).

Department of Health (2016) *Improving the physical health of people with mental health problems: actions for mental health nurses.* https://assets.publishing.service.gov.uk/government/uploads/system/uploads/attachment_data/file/532253/JRA_Physical_Health_revised.pdf (accessed January 2022).

Dick, B., Reddy, A., Gabrielson, A. & Hellstrom, W. (2017) Organic and psychogenic causes of sexual dysfunction in young men. *International Journal of Medical Reviews*, 4(4), 102–111.

Faculty of Sexual and Reproductive Health (2021) *FSRH and CEU statement: Thrombosis with thrombocytopenia, AstraZeneca COVID-19 vaccination and combined hormonal contraception May 2021.* www.fsrh.org/documents/fsrh-recommendation-astrazeneca-vaccine-combined-contraception/ (accessed December 2021).

Heffner, L.J. & Schust, D.J. (2014) *The Reproductive System at a Glance*, 3rd edn. Wiley Blackwell, Oxford.

HM Government (2020) *Multi-agency statutory guidance on Female Genital Mutilation.* https://assets.publishing.service.gov.uk/government/uploads/system/uploads/attachment_data/file/912996/6-1914-HO-Multi_Agency_Statutory_Guidance_on_FGM__-_MASTER_V7_-_FINAL__July_2020.pdf. (accessed December 2021).

Monteleone, P., Mascagni, G., Giannini A., *et al.* (2018) Symptoms of menopause – global prevalence, physiology and implications. *Nature Reviews Endocrinology*, 14, 199–215.

National Collaborating Centre for Women's and Children's Health (2015) *Menopause full guideline: methods, evidence and recommendations.* www.nice.org.uk/guidance/ng23/evidence/full-guideline-pdf-559549261 (accessed January 2022).

National Institute for Health and Care Excellence (2019a) *Menopause: diagnosis and management.* NG 23. www.nice.org.uk/guidance/ng23/chapter/Recommendations#diagnosis-of-perimenopause-and-menopause. (accessed December 2021).

National Institute for Health and Care Excellence (2019b) *Transvaginal mesh repair of anterior or posterior vaginal wall prolapse.* IPG599. www.nice.org.uk/guidance/IPG599/chapter/1-Recommendations (accessed December 2021).

National Institute for Health and Care Excellence (2019c) *Prostate cancer: diagnosis and management.* NG 131. www.nice.org.uk/guidance/ng131 (accessed December 2021).

National Institute for Health and Care Excellence (2020) *Heavy menstrual bleeding: assessment and management*. NG88. www.nice.org.uk/guidance/ng88/chapter/Recommendations#investigations-for-the-cause-of-hmb (accessed December 2021).

National Institute for Health and Care Excellence (2021a) *Surgery for uterine prolapse – patient decision aid*. www.nice.org.uk/guidance/ng123/resources/patient-decision-aids-and-user-guides-6725286109 (accessed December 2021).

National Institute for Health and Care Excellence (2021b) *Scenario: Testicular Cancer*. https://cks.nice.org.uk/topics/scrotal-pain-swelling/management/testicular-cancer/#management (accessed December 2021).

NHS (2019) *Having a smear test: an easy guide about a health test for women aged 25–64*. https://assets.publishing.service.gov.uk/government/uploads/system/uploads/attachment_data/file/790791/CSP05_an_easy_guide_to_cervical_screening.pdf (accessed December 2021).

NHS Digital (2016) Health and care of people with learning disabilities; experimental statistics 2015–16. https://digital.nhs.uk/data-and-information/publications/statistical/health-and-care-of-people-with-learning-disabilities/health-and-care-of-people-with-learning-disabilities-experimental-statistics-2016-to-2017 (accessed December 2021).

NHS England (2019) *Confidentiality Policy*. www.england.nhs.uk/publication/confidentiality-policy/ (accessed December 2021).

Norwitz, E. & Schorge, J. (2014) *Obstetrics and Gynecology at a Glance*, 4th edn. Wiley Blackwell, Chichester.

Nursing & Midwifery Council (2018a) *Future nurse: Standards of proficiency for registered nurses*. www.nmc.org.uk/globalassets/sitedocuments/standards-of-proficiency/nurses/future-nurse-proficiencies.pdf (accessed December 2021).

Nursing & Midwifery Council (2018b) *The Code. Professional standards of practice and behaviour for nurses, midwives and nurse associates*. www.nmc.org.uk/globalassets/sitedocuments/nmc-publications/nmc-code.pdf (accessed December 2021).

Peacock, K. & Ketvertis, K. (2021) *NCBI StatPearls: Menopause*. www.ncbi.nlm.nih.gov/books/NBK507826/ (accessed December 2021).

Peate, I. & Evans, S. (eds) (2020) *Fundamentals of Anatomy and Physiology for Nursing and Healthcare Students*, 3rd edn. Wiley, Oxford.

Public Health England (2020) *Sexually transmitted infections including screening for chlamydia in England in 2019*. https://assets.publishing.service.gov.uk/government/uploads/system/uploads/attachment_data/file/914184/STI_NCSP_report_2019.pdf (accessed December 2021).

Royal College of Obstetricians and Gynaecologists (2018) *Treatments for the symptoms of menopause*. www.rcog.org.uk/globalassets/documents/patients/patient-information-leaflets/gynaecology/pi-treatment-symptoms-menopause.pdf (accessed January 2022).

Royal College of Nursing (2020) *Human Papillomavirus (HPV), Cervical Screening and Cervical Cancer*. www.rcn.org.uk/professional-development/publications/rcn-hpv-cervical-screening-cervical-cancer-pub007960 (accessed December 2021).

Royal College of Surgeons (2016) *Management of Paediatric Testicular Torsion*. RCS, London.

World Health Organization (2018) *Care of women and girls living with female genital mutilation*. www.who.int/reproductivehealth/publications/health-care-girls-women-living-with-FGM/en/ (accessed December 2021).

World Health Organization (2020) *Human papillomavirus (HPV) and cervical cancer*. www.who.int/news-room/fact-sheets/detail/human-papillomavirus-(hpv)-and-cervical-cancer (accessed December 2021).

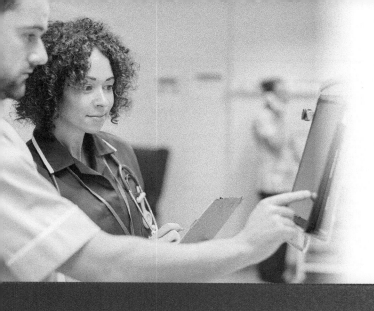

31

The Person with an Endocrine Disorder

Carl Clare

University of Hertfordshire, UK

Learning Outcomes

On completion of this chapter you will be able to:

- List the potential disorders of the endocrine system
- Discuss the role of self-care in the management of endocrine disorders
- Discuss the treatment of each of the endocrine disorders
- Explain the need for regular health checks for patients with diabetes

Proficiencies

NMC Proficiencies and Standards:

- Carry out a basic physical survey for signs of an endocrine disorder
- Ask focused questions to aid in the diagnosis of a particular endocrine disorder
- Provide advice to a patient about their endocrine disorder
- Make referrals to the appropriate members of the multidisciplinary team
- Promote health for patients with diabetes
- Recognise and treat a hypoglycaemic episode

 Visit the companion website at www.wiley.com/go/peate/nursingpractice3e where you can test yourself using flashcards, multiple-choice questions and more.

Nursing Practice: Knowledge and Care, Third Edition. Edited by Ian Peate and Aby Mitchell.
© 2022 John Wiley & Sons Ltd. Published 2022 by John Wiley & Sons Ltd.
Companion website: www.wiley.com/go/peate/nursingpractice3e

Introduction

The endocrine system is a diffusely distributed system of glands and organs. It is a relatively slow-acting and yet very powerful system that acts in concert with the nervous system to maintain homeostasis. In human physiology, *homeostasis* refers to the regulation of the internal environment to maintain normal physiological balance and functioning within the body. In attempting to maintain homeostasis, the endocrine and nervous systems act together to regulate several different aspects of the internal environment, such as fluid balance and blood pressure.

The nervous system reacts rapidly to stimuli and effects its changes over a period of seconds or minutes, and thus is involved in the immediate and short-term maintenance of homeostasis. Because of its rapid onset of action, the nervous system is responsible for the control of rapid bodily processes, such as breathing and movement. The endocrine system is mostly involved in the longer-term regulation of homeostasis; some of the hormones released can exert an effect within seconds but mostly the effects are slower in onset but have a longer-term effect. As the endocrine system is generally slower in the onset of its action and often has a long-term effect, these factors can affect the manner in which endocrine disorders present and the onset of symptoms.

For further details of the anatomy and physiology of the endocrine system refer to Peate & Evans (2020).

Assessing the Endocrine System

Assessing the endocrine system is often based on a general interview of the patient's perceptions of their own health and symptoms, followed by a targeted, problem-focused assessment based on an interpretation of the findings of the initial interview. Therefore, in assessing the endocrine system the initial history taking is essential.

The initial history is structured and includes the following steps.

1. Establish a rapport with the patient and their family, including preparation of oneself and the environment.
    - Ensure that you are presenting a professional, caring and attentive attitude. Show interest in the patient and what they have to say. There is little more off-putting for a patient than an obviously uninterested healthcare worker. The patient is less likely to fully disclose to you either because they feel you do not care or because they feel inhibited by your attitude.
    - The environment should be comfortable and private with no interruptions. Patients are less likely to disclose personal information if they feel they may be overheard, and constant interruptions disrupt the flow of the interview.
2. Gather information on:
    - *The patient's overall health status*: ask open and general questions at this point. Try not to focus too much on one symptom or concern, as this may narrow the discussion; at the same time allow the patient to talk about whatever they feel is important.

The Nursing Associate

Interviewing the patient to gather information is an opportunity to show a range of appropriate communication behaviours, such as open and closed questioning, active listening and non-verbal communication (NMC, 2018b). Whilst often considered routine, the admission of a patient to a ward or unit must never be underestimated as an opportunity to gather information that may be important for the patient's diagnosis and care.

- *The current concern*: most patients will access healthcare with a particular concern/set of concerns. Let the patient use their own words to explore their concerns. This will often be the point where the focus of the interview will be identified.
- *The symptoms experienced and how they affect the patient*: following on from the identification of the main concern (and often at the same time), the patient should be questioned on any symptoms they experience, what makes the symptoms worse, what makes them better and when they occur. Often this will be the point at which the history taker will begin to suspect the potential cause(s) of the symptoms and will wish to ask the patient about potential symptoms related to the suspected condition. For instance, a patient who is reporting constantly feeling tired and lethargic may be suffering from hypothyroidism. The nurse may then explore this by prompting the patient about their appetite and weight loss/gain, as these are also common symptoms of hypothyroidism. For a list of common clinical features that may aid diagnosis, see Table 31.1.
- *Medical history, emotional health and medication*: relevant medical history and current medication should be ascertained and recorded to aid the maintenance of previous care. Emotional history is valuable as changes in emotional state can be a symptom of an endocrine disorder and/or can give an indication of how the disorder is affecting the patient's psychological state.

Table 31.1 Common clinical features and the potential endocrine causes.

CLINICAL FEATURE	ASSOCIATED ENDOCRINE DISORDER(S)
Weight gain	Hypothyroidism Cushing's disease
Weight loss	Hyperthyroidism Diabetes mellitus Adrenal insufficiency
Menstrual disturbance	Thyroid disorders
Excessive thirst	Diabetes insipidus Diabetes mellitus
Sweating	Hyperthyroidism
Erectile dysfunction	Diabetes mellitus
Muscle weakness	Cushing's disease Hyperthyroidism

- *Family history*: many endocrine disorders have a genetic component and thus family history is a valuable aid in assessing the endocrine system.
3. Systematic enquiry using systems of the body and activities of daily living.
   - Systematically asking the patient about the various bodily systems and activities of daily living may discover information that the patient did not regard as important or may attribute to other aspects of health (such as ageing).
4. The patient's perception of their well-being.
   - It is always important to discover the patient's perspective on both their concern/condition and what they hope the healthcare system can do for them. Only the patient can assess how much a symptom affects their life or which symptoms they feel are more important.

Following the history taking, a physical examination can be undertaken. Aspects of physical assessment that may give particular indicators of an endocrine disorder include the following.

General Observations

- *Demeanour and mental state*: agitation may be a sign of hyperthyroidism; depression and apathy may be a sign of hypothyroidism.
- *Appearance*: for instance, central obesity with thin arms and legs may be a sign of Cushing's disease.
- *Pallor*: especially with a yellowish tinge, suggests hypopituitarism.
- *Hair distribution*: for instance, absent axillary and pubic hair may be a sign of hypopituitarism.
- *Vitiligo*: not normally a sign of an endocrine disorder but vitiligo is an autoimmune-based condition and it is more likely that the patient will develop an autoimmune-based endocrine disorder.
- *Hirsutism*: a potential sign of Cushing's syndrome.

Hands

- Skin crease pigmentation is a potential sign of Addison's disease.
- Tremor may be a sign of hyperthyroidism.
- Large fleshy hands are a potential sign of acromegaly.

Pulse and Blood Pressure

- Tachycardia and/or atrial fibrillation may be a sign of hyperthyroidism.
- Hypertension may be a sign of Cushing's disease.
- Hypotension may be a sign of Addison's disease.

Eyes

- Exophthalmos may be a sign of hyperthyroidism.

Face

- A 'moon face' may be a sign of Cushing's disease.
- A large elongated face is associated with acromegaly.

Neck

- A goitre (swollen neck) may be a sign of hyperthyroidism.

Hypopituitarism (Pituitary Insufficiency)

Hypopituitarism is a condition in which the pituitary gland does not produce enough hormones for normal functioning (Higham *et al.*, 2016).

Pathophysiology

Hypopituitarism can be caused by disorders of the pituitary gland itself or by a reduction in hypothalamic-releasing hormones due to a disorder of the hypothalamus, thus reducing the stimuli for pituitary gland activity. The most common cause of hypopituitarism is a tumour of the hypothalamus or pituitary gland or a tumour in the region of the hypothalamus or pituitary gland that is large enough to cause pressure and prevent normal functioning. In the majority of cases, these tumours are benign (non-cancerous) and pose no risk of spread to other parts of the body. However, the role of direct damage to the pituitary is increasingly being recognised.

Causes of direct damage to the hypothalamus or the pituitary gland include stroke, surgery and radiation therapy. In pregnancy, the pituitary can double, and even triple, in size and as a result a drop in blood pressure (for instance, due to a large postpartum haemorrhage) can result in infarction of the pituitary gland, known as Sheehan syndrome, though there is an increasing school of thought that suggests there may be an autoimmune component (González-González *et al.*, 2018) or that there may actually be a chronic syndrome present before the acute presentation (Jose *et al.*, 2019). Whilst the incidence of pituitary insufficiency increases with age, it can be present in children.

Signs and Symptoms

The signs and symptoms of hypopituitarism are related to the reduction of pituitary hormone production and will vary depending on the hormones affected and the speed of onset of the condition. A summary of potential signs and symptoms is given in Table 31.2.

Approximately 50% of patients with pituitary insufficiency will have deficits in 3–5 pituitary hormones (Alexandraki & Grossman, 2019) and thus patients presenting with possible hypopituitarism should be tested for deficits of all the pituitary hormones.

Investigations and Diagnosis

The diagnosis of hypopituitarism is based on clinical examination, detailed history taking, biochemical tests and investigations of the potential cause. Potential biochemical tests are summarised in Table 31.3.

Red Flag

 Insulin tolerance tests are potentially very dangerous and should only be carried out in strictly controlled circumstances. Patients with heart disease, stroke or epilepsy and elderly patients should not undergo an insulin tolerance test.

Investigation of the potential cause of hypopituitarism is mostly based around the radiographic imaging of the hypothalamus and pituitary regions by magnetic resonance imaging (MRI) in order to detect and assess any potential tumour.

Nursing Care and Management

The treatment of hypopituitarism is based on treating the cause (where possible) and hormone replacement therapy for decreased hormone levels. Surgical removal of tumours may result in remission if the tumour is pressing on the hypothalamus or

Table 31.2 Signs and symptoms of hypopituitarism categorised by hormone deficiency.

HORMONE DEFICIENCY	POTENTIAL SIGNS AND SYMPTOMS
Growth hormone	Reduced energy Reduced muscle mass and strength Increased central fat deposition Decreased sweating Reduced bone density In children, a reduction in growth hormone production leads to lack of growth (height), increased body fat and poor bone density
Adrenocorticotropic hormone	Fatigue Weakness Poor appetite Weight loss Nausea and vomiting Abdominal pain Acute circulatory collapse if sudden in onset Loss of pubic and axillary hair in women
Gonadotropins	**Men** Erectile dysfunction Reduced muscle mass Reduced energy **Women** Menstrual changes Breast atrophy **Both** Loss of libido Flushes Infertility
Thyroid-stimulating hormone	Fatigue Apathy Cold intolerance Constipation Weight gain Slow reflexes and cognition
Antidiuretic hormone (diabetes insipidus)	Polyuria Polydipsia Nocturia
Prolactin	Inability to breast-feed

Table 31.3 Potential biochemical tests and investigations for pituitary hormone insufficiency.

POTENTIAL HORMONE DEFICIENCY	BIOCHEMICAL TESTS
Growth hormone	Insulin tolerance test (growth hormone is secreted in response to the intentionally created hypoglycaemia)
Adrenocorticotropic hormone	Insulin tolerance test or Synacthen® test
Gonadotropins	*Men:* testosterone levels and gonadotropin levels *Women:* oestradiol levels and gonadotropin levels
Thyroid-stimulating hormone	TSH levels and thyroid hormone levels
Antidiuretic hormone	Normally based on 24-hour urine collection, blood sodium levels and urine osmolality. Occasionally, a water deprivation test may be carried out in hospital

- Enable the patient to monitor their own condition and report deviations that may be attributed to a worsening state or poor control
- Encourage concordance with treatment regimens.

Nurses must be aware of the signs and symptoms of pituitary hormone insufficiencies in order to educate patients as to what signs and symptoms they should be monitoring for and reporting. It is possible for endocrine disorders to be poorly controlled but no report is made to healthcare professionals because the patient did not know what aspects of bodily functioning may be related to their condition. Information giving and encouraging patients to be involved with their healthcare increases patients' sense of control over their lives, creates a greater sense of well-being and reduces feelings of depression/anxiety and hopelessness.

Nurses must also be aware of the psychological impact of certain signs and symptoms on the patient. Body image may be altered by loss of hair, changes in body fat and the need to take lifelong medication. Depression may be related to loss of the previously healthy person (prior to the onset of the condition), loss of erections or the possibility of infertility. Couples may also require direction to relationship counselling due to changes in sexual relationships due to altered body image, loss of libido or depression.

Patients must be made aware of the need to take lifelong medication and undergo regular blood tests. The importance of attending clinic appointments and ensuring compliance with medication must be reinforced.

The need for multiple replacement medications with many potential routes of administration creates a complex regime of management for the patient, leading to the potential for poor medication compliance. Medication compliance is not always fully in the control of the patient as polypharmacy, poor understanding, cognitive decline and a lack of information giving reduce the potential for self-management, leading to under- or overtreatment. The role of the endocrine specialist nurse with

pituitary gland but not invading them. Medical or radiation therapy will also be considered to reduce tumour size.

Common to all the endocrine conditions, patients with hypopituitarism share a need for psychological support and information, as will their relatives and significant others. Patients will require information on the particular disorders that they experience and the signs and symptoms that they can expect the condition to manifest. Providing the patient with a clear understanding will:

- Reduce anxiety as to what the future may hold
- Allow the patient to attribute signs and symptoms to their condition rather than enduring them
- Give the patient control of their health and illness

advanced understanding of the treatment of hypopituitarism and the complexities of self-management is a valuable addition to the multidisciplinary team around the patient (Llahana, 2021).

Red Flag

 All patients with an endocrine disorder should be encouraged to register with the MedicAlert foundation and wear a MedicAlert talisman: www.medicalert.org.uk/

Health Promotion and Discharge

 Primary Care

Pituitary disorders are relatively rare and it is possible that a GP may only ever see one or two patients with such a disorder in their entire career. However, it is essential that both GPs and practice nurses are aware of the need for a multidisciplinary approach to pituitary disorder care.

Primary care professionals should also be aware of the signs and symptoms of inadequate hormone replacement and the potential side-effects of excess replacement.

Primary care practitioners have a significant role to play in reinforcing the need for treatment compliance and in the ordering and interpretation of blood tests.

Disorders of the Thyroid Gland

Disorders of the thyroid gland are categorised as either hypersecretion of thyroid hormones (excessive thyroid gland activity, known as *hyperthyroidism*) or hyposecretion of thyroid hormones (reduced thyroid gland activity, known as *hypothyroidism*). Thyroid disorders can be further categorised by the underlying mechanism leading to the change in thyroid hormone secretion.

- *Primary*: due to a disorder of the thyroid gland itself.
- *Secondary*: alterations in thyroid function due to an increase or decrease in the production of either thyrotropin-releasing hormone (TRH) from the hypothalamus or thyroid-stimulating hormone (TSH) from the pituitary gland.

This section will review the primary disorders of the thyroid gland.

Hyperthyroidism

Excessive production and release of thyroid hormone.

Pathophysiology

Hyperthyroidism is commonly caused by an autoimmune disorder known as Graves' disease (Wemeau *et al.*, 2018). This is a condition where antibodies mimic the effect of TSH (normally released from the pituitary gland) leading to excessive production of thyroid hormone. Graves' disease is often diagnosed alongside other autoimmune disorders, such as diabetes. The exact reasons for the development of the antibodies are unknown but the peak incidence appears to be between 20 and 40 years of age and there is strong evidence for the interaction of genetic and environmental

causes, including smoking (Antonelli *et al.*, 2020). Other causes of hyperthyroidism include thyroid cancer, thyroid nodules (usually non-cancerous), viral thyroiditis (inflammation of the thyroid gland), postpartum thyroiditis and patients taking iodine-containing drugs (such as amiodarone) (Antonelli *et al.*, 2015).

Signs and Symptoms

The signs and symptoms of hyperthyroidism are related to the activity of thyroid hormone and include:

- Nervousness, restlessness
- Tremors
- Fatigue
- Insomnia
- Tachycardia, palpitations (atrial fibrillation is common in the elderly)
- Shortness of breath
- Weight loss despite an increased appetite
- Frequency of passing stools
- Nausea and vomiting
- Muscle weakness, tremors
- Warm, moist flushed skin
- Fine hair
- Staring gaze, exophthalmos (bulging or protrusion of the eyes): only related to Graves' disease
- Goitre: swelling of the neck, usually due to a swollen thyroid gland
- Heat intolerance.

Jot This Down

Exophthalmos is often slow and insidious in onset, so it may not be noted by the patient or their relatives. Photographing the patient on each clinic visit may be a useful method of assessing its development and progression.

Diagnosis and Investigations

Diagnosis relies on detailed history taking, physical examination and diagnostic tests.

Blood will be taken to assess TSH and free T_4 levels. As the thyroid gland is overproducing thyroid hormone, the negative feedback to the hypothalamus and pituitary gland will lead to a reduction in TSH production. A reduced TSH level in the blood is the most important biochemical result in diagnosing hyperthyroidism. Free T_4 levels may be normal or may be raised.

Isotope thyroid scans are commonly undertaken. The patient is asked to swallow small amounts of a radioactive substance as a capsule or liquid and then a scan is performed to assess how much of the isotope is absorbed by the thyroid gland. A high rate of absorption indicates Graves' disease or thyroid nodules, whereas low uptake may be related to inflammation, excess iodine in the diet or thyroid cancer. Potential cancer of the thyroid may require fine-needle aspiration cytology (taking cells from the swollen lump) to assess for the presence of cancerous cells.

Nursing Care and Management

Treatment of hyperthyroidism is focused on decreasing the excessive production of thyroid hormone. There are three main methods of treating hyperthyroidism.

Antithyroid Drugs Carbimazole is the most commonly used drug in the UK (Weetman, 2013). Antithyroid drugs usually have a slow onset of action due to the storage of thyroid hormone in the thyroid gland, which is released despite the reduction in thyroid hormone production. All antithyroid drugs have significant side-effect profiles and patients must be made aware of these.

- Pruritus
- Rash
- Joint pains
- Diarrhoea
- Altered taste

Remission after stopping antithyroid drugs is very common, with about 50–60% of patients relapsing within 3–6 months (Piantanida, 2015).

Red Flag

Patients taking antithyroid drugs should be advised that if they develop fever, chills and a sore throat, they should seek immediate medical assistance as they require a full blood count to assess for the potential development of agranulocytosis (suppression of white blood cell production).

Radioactive Iodine This treatment relies on the fact that the most active cells in the thyroid gland will take up the most iodine and thus be destroyed. In the first few weeks after treatment, there is often a need to take antithyroid drugs as there may be a sudden release of thyroid hormones and patients must be monitored for thyrotoxic crisis (thyroid storm). Following radioactive iodine treatment, the patient may become hypothyroid as there is little control over the amount of thyroid gland that is destroyed. Radioactive iodine is contraindicated in pregnancy (Lee & Pearce, 2021).

Surgical Removal of Part, or All, of the Thyroid Gland
Thyroidectomy or partial thyroidectomy is the least used of the treatment options as it carries risks of damage to the parathyroid glands and vocal cords, and as the thyroid gland is very vascular there is also a risk of major haemorrhage.

Symptom relief may be required to treat certain symptoms or consequences of hyperthyroidism.

- Atrial fibrillation, tachycardia and heart failure should all be treated with appropriate medication.
- Nutritional deficits may be present due to the excessive metabolism in hyperthyroidism. Frequent snacks should be encouraged to prevent weight loss. High-calorie, high-protein diet should be encouraged until thyroid function is normalised and vitamin supplements (particularly A, thiamine, B_6 and C) should be advocated (Week,s 2005).
- Anxiety can be managed with the use of beta-blocking drugs, which may also be of use in the treatment of tremors. Provision of a quiet, calm environment will also be of value.

Exophthalmos will require monitoring by an ophthalmologist and may require treatment with steroids, radiotherapy or surgery. Patients may also benefit from:

- Raising the head of their bed (e.g. by using extra pillows), which could help reduce some of the puffiness around the eyes

- Stopping smoking because smoking can significantly increase the risk of the thyroid condition affecting the eyes
- Wearing sunglasses if they have photophobia (sensitivity to light)
- Using eye drops to help relieve soreness and to moisten their eyes if they have dry eyes
- Wearing a patch over one eye if they have double vision
- Taking selenium supplements, which may help people with mild thyroid eye disease that has recently started (selenium is a mineral found in Brazil nuts, meat and fish).

Further nursing care includes:

- Encouraging fluid intake in patients who are perspiring excessively
- Provision of fan therapy for comfort
- Light daytime clothes and bed clothes
- Providing a quiet comfortable environment to encourage rest and sleep
- Regular assessment of vital signs
- Regular assessment of mental state.

Nurses should also be aware of, and monitor for, the potential for thyrotoxic crisis (thyroid storm), as this is a medical emergency. Thyroid storm is due to the effect of high blood levels of thyroid hormone in association with increased sympathetic nervous system activity. There are several known causes of thyroid storm, including infection, surgery, myocardial infarction, cerebrovascular events and other serious illness (Chiha *et al.*, 2015). Patients with thyroid storm may present with the following signs/symptoms.

- Very high temperature (over 40 °C).
- Very high heart rate (atrial fibrillation is common).
- Will be very agitated and confused.
- Vomiting and diarrhoea.

Management of this condition will require:

- Nursing in a critical care environment
- Beta-blockade for tachycardia
- Continuous heart monitoring
- Intravenous fluids for dehydration with strict fluid balance monitoring
- Active cooling therapies
- Control of thyroid hormone levels.

Health Promotion and Discharge

Hypothyroidism

Insufficient production and release of thyroid hormone for bodily functioning.

Pathophysiology

There are many causes of hypothyroidism including:

- Treatment for hyperthyroidism
- Radiation therapy of the neck
- Lack of iodine in the diet
- Viral infection of the thyroid gland
- Autoimmune disease.

The most common cause of hypothyroidism in the UK is auto-immune destruction of the thyroid gland, known as Hashimoto's thyroiditis (Caturegli *et al.*, 2014).

Jot This Down

An underactive thyroid can be caused by a problem with the immune system, the body's natural defence system, which can attack the body's own cells, including the thyroid.

Signs and Symptoms

The signs and symptoms of hypothyroidism include:

- Confusion, memory loss, depression
- Lethargy
- Bradycardia, enlarged heart (cardiomegaly), pericardial effusions
- Constipation
- Weight gain
- Muscle cramps, myalgia (generalised muscle aches), stiffness
- Dry cool skin
- Brittle nails
- Coarse hair, hair loss
- Oedema of hands and eyelids
- Cold intolerance
- Vacant expression
- Hoarse voice.

Jot this down

Symptoms can develop slowly over several years and are often non-specific. The following symptoms have the greatest diagnostic value.

- Current or increased constipation
- Current or increasingly hoarse voice
- Current deep voice
- Feeling colder
- Puffy eyes
- Weaker muscles.

Investigations and Diagnosis

Diagnosis relies on detailed history taking, physical examination and diagnostic tests.

Blood will be taken to assess TSH and free T_4 levels. As the thyroid gland is no longer producing thyroid hormone, the negative feedback to the hypothalamus and pituitary gland will be absent and TSH levels will be increased. Free T_4 levels will be normal or reduced.

Red Flag

TSH levels are elevated in patients with untreated primary adrenal insufficiency. Prescribing thyroxine in this situation may precipitate an adrenal crisis.

Nursing Care and Management

The treatment for hypothyroidism is replacement of thyroid hormone with levothyroxine. Levothyroxine should be taken at the same time each day and about an hour before breakfast if possible (Weetman, 2013) as concomitant food intake can affect the bioavailability of levothyroxine (Wiesner *et al.*, 2021). Patients should be warned that symptoms will not disappear immediately, and weight loss will only occur when treatment is combined with a healthy dietary intake and exercise.

Patients must be advised that it may take months to find the correct dose of levothyroxine and frequent blood tests will be required in the first year. Over-replacement of thyroid hormones is a common cause of hyperthyroidism and patients should be made aware of the possible symptoms of hyperthyroidism but warned not to titrate their own levothyroxine dose.

Red Flag

Elderly patients and those with heart disease will require a lower starting dose of levothyroxine (Duntas & Yen, 2019).

Once the correct dose for the patient has been found, they will require yearly blood tests to ensure that their needs have not changed.

Monitoring of concordance with replacement therapy and the use of strategies to encourage and maintain concordance are essential as many patients are reluctant to take long-term thyroxine therapy (Biondi & Wartofsky, 2014). Patients should be informed of the possible side-effects of thyroid replacement therapy, including temporary hair loss (Roberts & Ladenson, 2004), as this will affect concordance with treatment. Patients should be given information regarding the need for adherence to the replacement therapy and what to do in the event of prolonged gastrointestinal disturbance that prevents the taking of the daily levothyroxine dose. Acute illness or trauma may precipitate myxoedemic coma and patients must be made aware of the need to seek medical help.

Red Flag

Levothyroxine is known to interact with multivitamin preparations and they should be taken 4 hours apart.

Antacids and proton pump inhibitors are known to reduce the absorption of levothyroxine and should be taken several hours apart.

Levothyroxine enhances the anticoagulant effect of warfarin.

Myxoedemic coma or crisis is an acute life-threatening emergency that can be brought on by acute events such as stroke, myocardial infarction, infection or trauma or by a lack of concordance with replacement therapy (Kapoor *et al.*, 2017). Signs and symptoms include:

- Hypothermia (temperature less than 35.5 °C)
- Bradycardia (slow heart rate)
- Bradypnoea (slow respiratory rate) and hypoventilation (shallow breathing) leading to hypoxia
- Potentially hypotension
- Deterioration in mental state
- Psychosis
- Swollen puffy face with oedema around the eyes
- Low sodium levels in the blood.

Treatment requires admission to a critical care area and:

- Intravenous thyroid hormone replacement
- Sodium replacement and fluid restriction
- Ambient warming and warm blankets (aggressive rewarming should be avoided)
- Vital signs monitoring and heart monitor
- Potentially respiratory support by intubation and ventilation.

Medicines Management Drug Interactions

Drugs that prevent absorption of levothyroxine include:
- Calcium salts: calcium-containing products
- Ferrous sulfate: iron-containing product
- Aluminium hydroxide: antacid
- Cholestyramine: bile acid sequestrant.

Health Promotion and Discharge

Primary Care

Hypothyroidism is the most common endocrine disorder in primary care but is often underdiagnosed as the symptoms are vague and diverse, and in the elderly many signs and symptoms may be attributed to age. Primary care practitioners should be alert for the possibility of hypothyroidism in patients with more than one potential symptom.

Most patients with hypothyroidism are managed in primary care and education and information giving are vital for ensuring concordance with treatment. Elderly patients may require regular community nursing follow-up to assess pill counts or to review dosset boxes and monitor concordance.

Patients should be referred to specialist care if they:
- Are younger than 16
- Are pregnant or trying to get pregnant (hypothyroidism in the mother can have significant effects on the foetus)
- Have just given birth
- Have another health condition, such as heart disease
- Are taking amiodarone or lithium medication (both drugs interfere with blood tests for TSH).

Disorders of the Parathyroid Glands

Disorders of the parathyroid glands are rare and include *hyperparathyroidism* and *hypoparathyroidism*.

Hyperparathyroidism
Excessive production of parathyroid hormone.

Pathophysiology
Hyperparathyroidism is usually caused by a benign tumour of the parathyroid gland.

Signs and Symptoms
Hyperparathyroidism is often present without any symptoms; if symptoms do occur, they are normally very mild and include:

- Depression
- Fatigue
- Increased thirst
- Polyuria
- Nausea
- Muscle weakness
- Constipation
- Abdominal pain
- Loss of concentration
- Mild confusion.

Investigations and Diagnosis
Hyperparathyroidism is diagnosed by blood tests showing:
- High levels of parathyroid hormone
- High levels of blood calcium
- Low levels of blood phosphorus.

Treatment and Management
Often, hyperparathyroidism does not need treatment but if required, the current treatment is surgical removal of the overactive parathyroid gland(s) (Udelsman *et al.*, 2014).

Patients should be advised to avoid a high-calcium diet (but not avoid calcium altogether) and to drink plenty of fluids to prevent dehydration.

Hypoparathyroidism
Reduced production of parathyroid hormone.

Pathophysiology
Causes of hypoparathyroidism include:
- Damage to the parathyroid glands during neck surgery
- Radiotherapy to the neck
- Autoimmune destruction of the parathyroid glands.

Signs and Symptoms

The symptoms of hypoparathyroidism are partially dependent on the speed at which the disorder develops (Shoback *et al.*, 2016).

- Sudden onset (for instance, due to damage during surgery)
  - Tingling sensation around the mouth or in the hands or feet
  - Jerking, twitching or muscle spasms
  - Muscle cramps
  - Lethargy
  - Irritability
- Slow onset (for instance, due to autoimmune destruction of the glands)
  - Eye problems (especially cataracts)
  - Dry thick skin
  - Coarse hair that may fall out
  - Brittle fingernails with horizontal ridges

Diagnosis and Investigations

Hypoparathyroidism is diagnosed by blood tests showing:

- Low blood calcium levels
- High blood phosphorus levels
- Low blood parathyroid hormone levels.

A urine sample is also tested for high levels of calcium.

Nursing Care and Management

Treatment is with oral calcium and vitamin D supplements. Patients should also be advised to eat a healthy diet including:

- High-calcium foods such as:
  - Milk, cheese and other dairy foods
  - Green leafy vegetables, such as broccoli, cabbage and okra, but not spinach
  - Soya beans
  - Tofu
  - Soya drinks with added calcium
  - Nuts
  - Bread and anything made with fortified flour
  - Fish where you eat the bones, such as sardines and pilchards
- Low-phosphorus foods such as:
  - Red meat
  - Dairy foods
  - Fish
  - Poultry
  - Bread
  - Rice
  - Oats.

Patients should be advised that if they develop muscle spasms, they should seek medical advice immediately as they may require intravenous calcium.

Disorders of the Adrenal Glands

Disorders of the adrenal glands are classified as either *hypersecretion* or *hyposecretion* disorders. Disorders of the adrenal glands can be further categorised by the underlying mechanism leading to the change in hormone secretion.

- *Primary*: due to a disorder of the adrenal glands themselves.
- *Secondary*: alterations in adrenal gland function due to an increase or decrease in the production of either corticotropin-releasing hormone (CRH) from the hypothalamus or adrenocorticotropic hormone (ACTH) from the pituitary gland.

The effects on the body of primary or secondary disorders of the adrenal glands are different and these differences will be noted within this section.

Hypersecretion Disorders of the Adrenal Glands

Hypersecretion disorders of the adrenal glands include:

- Phaeochromocytoma
- Conn syndrome
- Cushing's syndrome
- Cushing's disease.

Both phaeochromocytoma and Conn syndrome are rare in the general setting and will not be discussed in this section. Both can be related to drug-resistant hypertension and are potential diagnoses in the hypertension clinic.

Cushing's disease is a subset of the disorder known as Cushing's syndrome and the symptoms are almost the same; they are otherwise known as *hypercortisolism*. This section will review Cushing's syndrome, noting where Cushing's disease differs in pathophysiology.

Pathophysiology

The pathophysiology of Cushing's syndrome is generally classified as endogenous (caused by factors within the body) or exogenous (caused by factors outside the body).

Endogenous causes of hypercortisolism are either primary or secondary (Prague *et al.*, 2013).

- *Primary hypercortisolism* is caused by a tumour of the adrenal gland, which leads to hypersecretion of cortisol.
- *Secondary hypercortisolism* is caused by a tumour of the pituitary gland leading to hypersecretion of ACTH and the subsequent production of high levels of cortisol from the adrenal glands. It is known as Cushing's disease. Cushing's disease is the leading cause of secondary hypercortisolism.

Exogenous hypercortisolism is the most common cause of Cushing's syndrome and is the result of administration of high doses of corticosteroids for conditions such as arthritis, asthma and other inflammatory conditions.

Signs and Symptoms

The signs and symptoms of all the causes of hypercortisolism (Cushing's syndrome) are the same. Common symptoms are:

- Weight gain
- High blood pressure
- Poor short-term memory
- Irritability
- Excess hair growth (women)
- Red ruddy face
- Extra fat deposition at the neck and shoulders ('buffalo hump')
- Round face (otherwise referred to as a 'moon face')
- Fatigue
- Poor concentration
- Menstrual irregularity

- Slow wound healing
- Depression and rapid mood swings.

Less common symptoms include:

- Insomnia
- Recurrent infections (especially fungal infections such as thrush)
- Thin skin and stretch marks (often showing as purple striations)
- Easily bruising skin
- Weak bones
- Acne
- Hair loss (women)
- Hip and shoulder weakness
- Swelling of feet/legs due to oedema
- Diabetes mellitus.

Diagnosis and Investigations

The diagnosis of hypercortisolism is based on detailed history taking, a physical examination and a number of diagnostic investigations.

History taking will focus on the development of symptoms and must include a full drug history to review the patient for the use of exogenous steroids. Signs and symptoms of hypercortisolism without a history of steroid use will lead on to the use of a number of potential investigations.

- *Late-night salivary cortisol*: a sample of saliva is taken late at night (often around midnight) and tested for cortisol levels. As cortisol production is diurnal, cortisol levels at midnight should be very low. If they are high, then this suggests Cushing's syndrome.
- *24-hour urine collection* that is then tested for cortisol levels.
- *Dexamethasone suppression test*: the patient is administered a synthetic version of cortisol and the cortisol levels in the blood are measured after a suitable time period. The administration of dexamethasone should suppress the production of cortisol by the body. If cortisol levels do not fall, then it is likely the patient is suffering from Cushing's syndrome.

If any one of these tests is negative, then Cushing's syndrome is unlikely. A positive test result often leads to the repeat of that test and the administration of at least one more of the other tests. Repeated positive results usually confirm a diagnosis of Cushing's syndrome and the patient will require a blood test for ACTH levels to assess for a pituitary cause (Cushing's disease). Further investigations will include scanning the pituitary and adrenal glands for tumours.

Treatment and Management

Treatment of hypercortisolism is dependent on the initial cause (Pivonello *et al.*, 2015).

Reducing Steroid Use For those patients who are taking high doses of steroids, the treatment is to gradually reduce the steroid dose to the lowest possible while still maintaining control of the disease the steroids were prescribed for. This must be done in conjunction with medical staff as the dose reduction must be tailored to the individual.

Red Flag

Patients who have been taking steroids for more than a few days must never stop taking their steroids suddenly, as this may precipitate a hypoadrenal crisis. Patients who take steroids for more than 3 weeks must be issued with, and carry, a steroid treatment card.

www.england.nhs.uk/publication/national-patient-safety-alert-steroid-emergency-card-to-support-early-recognition-and-treatment-of-adrenal-crisis-in-adults/

Cortisol-inhibiting Medications Often used for a short period before a more definitive treatment, cortisol-inhibiting medications block the effects of cortisol in the body.

Radiotherapy and/or Surgery Definitive treatment of endogenous hypercortisolism is based on removal of the affected gland or radiotherapy of the pituitary gland if surgery is not possible. Surgery to remove the pituitary gland will leave the patient with hypopituitarism, which will require hormone replacement therapy. If the tumour is affecting the adrenal gland, then often only one of the adrenal glands will need to be removed but removal of both may be necessary.

Nursing Care and Management

- Decrease the risk of injury by removing slip and trip hazards and helping unstable patients to mobilise.
- Refer to the dietitian for advice on diet to promote muscle mass and bone density.
- Minimise the risk of infection. Advise the patient to avoid contact with people suffering from infectious diseases. Have a high suspicion for infection as the symptoms are often masked.
- Promote moderate activity to prevent excessive muscle wasting.
- Provide a quiet comfortable environment to promote sleep.
- Maintain good skin care: avoid adhesive tapes, which may tear skin, and monitor vulnerable areas of skin, such as the shins, for damage.
- Explain to the patient and their family the reasons for their mood swings.
- Provide information and support for issues such as changes in body image.
- Ensure patients who are reducing steroid doses understand the need to follow the reduction plan and not stop the steroids suddenly.
- Ensure patients taking steroids have been given, and carry, the steroid treatment card.

Medicines Management

Steroids that are targeted to a particular part of the body (such as inhaled steroids and steroid creams) are generally safe and have a much lower risk of side-effects.

Patients taking steroids should monitor for the potential signs of Cushing's syndrome but should always seek medical advice and not stop the medication if they suspect they have symptoms.

Patients taking steroids who have never had chickenpox should avoid anyone suffering from chickenpox or shingles.

The Medicines and Healthcare products Regulatory Agency (MHRA) has developed a number of eLearning modules, including one on corticosteroids for healthcare staff. These can be found here (login required): www.gov.uk/government/publications/e-learning-modules-medicines-and-medical-devices/e-learning-modules-medicines-and-medical-devices#corticosteroids

Primary Care

Primary care practitioners have a vital role to play in the prevention of, and monitoring for, Cushing's syndrome.

Cushing's syndrome is often missed as a diagnosis, as it is slow in onset with a non-specific set of symptoms that are easily confused with other conditions such as obesity and hypertension. The average time from the first symptom to diagnosis is 6 years (Prague et al., 2013). As the most common cause of Cushing's syndrome is exogenous steroids, primary care staff should be alert for the syndrome in any patient taking steroids.

Courses of steroid treatment may be prescribed in the hospital setting but are often continued in the community and primary care health professionals should be aware of the need to titrate steroid doses to the lowest effective dose.

Prolonged use of steroids can predispose patients to diabetes mellitus and thus patients should have a blood sugar taken once a year as urine dipsticks are not sufficiently accurate in non-diabetic patients.

https://bestbets.org/bets/bet.php?id=311

Hyposecretion Disorders of the Adrenal Glands

Otherwise known as adrenal insufficiency.

Pathophysiology

Adrenal insufficiency, the reduced production and release of corticosteroids from the adrenal glands, is divided into two types (Bancos et al., 2015).

- *Primary adrenal insufficiency (Addison's disease)* is due to a disorder of the adrenal glands. The leading cause of Addison's disease in the Western world is autoimmune adrenalitis (Saverino & Falorni, 2020), leading to destruction of the glands. Other causes include tuberculosis, and fungal infection in immunosuppressed patients (such as HIV/AIDS or therapeutic suppression of the immune system).
- *Secondary adrenal insufficiency* is most commonly due to the sudden cessation of steroid therapy; however, disorders affecting the hypothalamus or the pituitary gland can also be a cause of secondary adrenal insufficiency.

In primary adrenal insufficiency, the adrenal glands no longer function and thus the production of adrenaline, glucocorticoids and mineralocorticoids is absent.

In secondary adrenal insufficiency, either secretion of CRH from the hypothalamus or secretion of ACTH from the pituitary gland ceases. Either of these situations leads to a lack of ACTH production and thus stimulation for the production and secretion of glucocorticoids by the adrenal glands is removed. However, as mineralocorticoid and adrenaline production is stimulated by factors other than ACTH, their production is preserved.

Patients who have been taking high-dose steroid therapy are at risk of developing temporary adrenal gland atrophy. The steroid treatment leads to negative feedback to the hypothalamus and pituitary gland, thus reducing stimulation for adrenal gland glucocorticoid production. The adrenal gland atrophies and sudden cessation of the steroid therapy leads to insufficient glucocorticoid levels in the blood as the adrenal glands require a gradual period of recovery. The patient can present with the signs and symptoms of adrenal insufficiency and even an acute adrenal crisis.

Signs and Symptoms

The signs and symptoms of all forms of adrenal insufficiency are:

- Fatigue, lack of stamina, loss of energy
- Reduced muscle strength
- Increased irritability
- Nausea
- Weight loss
- Muscle and joint pain
- Abdominal pain
- Low blood pressure
- Women may report a reduction in, or loss of, libido due to lack of adrenal sex hormones.

Because of loss of aldosterone production and high levels of ACTH in primary adrenal insufficiency, these patients may also present with:

- Dehydration
- Hypovolaemia
- Postural hypotension
- Low levels of blood sodium
- High levels of blood potassium
- Hyperpigmentation of the skin, often a darkening in the skin creases (such as the palms, knuckles, inner elbow) or the waist (where clothes rub) but may be an all-over suntan
- Vitiligo (pale patches of skin).

The loss of adrenaline and noradrenaline production from the adrenal medulla in primary adrenal insufficiency does not create any symptoms as endocrine production of adrenaline and noradrenaline is complementary to the nervous system production of these chemicals.

Investigations and Diagnosis

The signs and symptoms of Addison's disease are vague and may be slow and insidious in onset, so that patients may be showing signs and symptoms for up to a year before diagnosis. Occasionally, an acute adrenal crisis may be precipitated by trauma or infection and the patient will present with acute symptoms of severe hypotension, dehydration, hypovolaemic shock, acute abdominal pain and vomiting.

The definitive test for Addison's disease is a Synacthen (artificial ACTH) test. Serum cortisol is measured before and after the administration of intramuscular Synacthen. If the adrenal glands are working, there will be a rise in blood cortisol levels in response to Synacthen.

If secondary adrenal insufficiency is suspected, then blood ACTH and renin levels will be assessed. Both of these will be high in Addison's disease but in secondary insufficiency, ACTH will be low and renin levels will be normal.

If tuberculosis or other infection is suspected as the cause of Addison's disease, then CT or MRI scans will be used to image the adrenal glands.

Nursing Care and Management

Treatment of adrenal insufficiency is normally begun by an endocrinologist but is continued in primary care with routine follow-up in the outpatient clinic.

Treatment for Addison's disease is based on the replacement of glucocorticoid and mineralocorticoid hormones; androgen replacement is not usually prescribed in the UK; although there is some evidence to suggest that the use of dehydroepiandrosterone (DHEA) in premenopausal women may be of benefit, the evidence remains uncertain (Saverino & Falorni, 2020). Replacement therapy in secondary adrenal insufficiency is only required for glucocorticoid hormones.

Medicines Management

Replacement doses of glucocorticoid hormones are based on the patient's body weight and vary between 15 and 25 mg of hydrocortisone taken orally in divided doses (Mukherjee et al., 2017). Doses are split to try to mimic normal cycles of glucocorticoid release but there is still debate as to which regimen is best.

Patients working shifts (especially nights) should have a regimen tailored to their daily routine, not based on the clock. For instance, the first dose is normally taken in the morning but patients on night shift should take their first dose when they get up after sleep.

Glucocorticoid replacement in children is difficult and requires frequent adjustment as they grow.

Mineralocorticoid replacement doses vary between 50 and 200 µg of fludrocortisone once a day (Esposito et al, 2018). Children's doses of fludrocortisone are much higher than the equivalent adult dose and children may need an additional salt supplement.

In hot weather (or episodes of long-lasting exercise), some endocrinologists recommend that the mineralocorticoid dose is increased to compensate for the increase in sweating (Bornstein et al., 2016).

It is important for healthcare staff, or patients, to check the storage requirements of the particular fludrocortisone formulation supplied as some formulations may require refrigeration.

Replacement therapy is titrated by patient symptoms as there is no definitive test to assess correct replacement levels. Therefore, patients will need to be reviewed for the signs and symptoms of Cushing's disease (in the case of over-replacement) and for the signs and symptoms of Addison's disease (in the case of under-replacement).

Alteration of the standard replacement regimen must only be carried out by an endocrinologist, but patients must be made aware of the need for glucocorticoid dose adjustment in certain circumstances, known as 'sick day rules' (Brooke & Monson, 2017).

- If the patient has a fever of 37.5 °C or higher, then the normal replacement dose should be doubled.

- If the patient is taking antibiotics for an infection, hydrocortisone doses should be doubled until the course of antibiotics is finished.
- After vomiting, the patient should take 20 mg hydrocortisone and an oral rehydration solution.
- If the patient is injured, they should take 20 mg hydrocortisone.
- If vomiting persists, the patient should be administered an emergency hydrocortisone injection and medical advice sought.
- Advice regarding alterations of hydrocortisone doses in preparation for physical exercise varies and should be discussed with the endocrinologist.

Red Flag

Patients should be educated about the signs and symptoms of adrenal crisis and both they and family members must be taught how to administer emergency hydrocortisone injections.

The Addison's Disease Self-Help Group has clear instructions for patients on how to administer emergency injections on its website: www.addisonsdisease.org.uk/the-emergency-injection-for-the-treatment-of-adrenal-crisis

Patients undergoing surgical or dental treatment may need to take extra hydrocortisone to cover the treatment period. Insufficient steroid replacement in the event of illness, injury or other physiological stress will lead to shock and potentially death if untreated. Reports have made it clear that hospital doctors and nurses do not always understand the need for hydrocortisone in Addison's disease, leading to avoidable deaths (Simpson et al., 2020) and it is important that healthcare staff heed the requests of patients for hydrocortisone (Wass & Arlt, 2012) as the patient will often know their own requirements.

Patients with any form of adrenal insufficiency will require education and counselling on the need to take regular medication and to monitor for the signs of poor control.

Practice Assessment Document

All types of endocrine disorders require replacement therapies but patients with adrenal insufficiency require special consideration regarding the understanding of sick day rules and the adjustment of glucocorticoid doses in the event of significant exercise or invasive medical procedures. Confirming the understanding of these rules by a patient under your care meets the requirements for ensuring the patient is able to self-manage their own medication regimes (NMC, 2018a).

Health Promotion and Discharge (If Relevant)

Primary Care

The role of the primary care practitioner in the diagnosis and management of adrenal insufficiency is of great importance. Undiagnosed Addison's disease is universally fatal, and deterioration can be rapid. Primary care practitioners should have a suspicion of Addison's disease if the patient presents with being constantly fatigued, losing weight without dieting, has postural hypotension, unusual skin pigmentation and low blood sodium levels.

Patient reports have frequently highlighted the reluctance of primary care practitioners to prescribe more than the absolute minimum amount of oral hydrocortisone or an emergency injection kit, leaving the patient with no ability to self-manage their dose when required or to deal with intermittent supply problems. Patients must be prescribed an extra month's supply of hydrocortisone as a 'back-up' and an emergency injection kit for the first-line treatment of potential crisis.

Patients with adrenal insufficiency should be strongly advised to wear a MedicAlert talisman and carry a steroid card, as emergency treatment in the event of a traumatic event must include intravenous steroids or the situation may become rapidly fatal (Rahman *et al.*, 2017).

Case Study Potential Adrenal Crisis

Andrew was a 52-year-old man admitted to the ward for a routine hip replacement due to degenerative arthritis. The operation proceeded without difficulty and the patient was returned to the ward with no problems. Steroid cover had been given in theatres in the form of 100 mg hydrocortisone IV. The following day, Andrew's hydrocortisone dose was returned to his standard daily dose (10 mg bd) rather than be increased for the postoperative period. Later in the day, the patient began to feel dizzy and reported a pain in his abdomen; he made a request for his hydrocortisone dose to be increased immediately. His observations are noted below.

Following his request, the registered nurse asked the medical staff to attend the ward and Andrew's hydrocortisone was increased to 20 mg twice daily for the remainder of his stay, with a reducing dose back to 10 mg twice a day after a week. The medical staff also prescribed a stat dose of 20 mg of hydrocortisone PO and this resolved Andrew's abdominal pain and dizziness. His heart rate reduced and his systolic blood pressure increased.

VITAL SIGN	OBSERVATION	NORMAL
Temperature	36.9 °C	36.0–37.9 °C range
Pulse	110 beats per minute and irregularly irregular	60–100 beats per minute
Respiration	20 breaths per minute	12–20 breaths per minute
Blood pressure	91/55 mmHg	100–139 mmHg (systolic) range
O$_2$ saturations	96%	94–98%

Andrew's NEWS2 score is noted below.

PHYSIOLOGICAL PARAMETER	3	2	1	0	1	2	3
Respiration rate				20			
Oxygen saturation %				96			
Air or oxygen				Air			

Temperature °C				36.9			
Systolic BP mmHg		92					
Heart rate						110	
Level of consciousness				A			
Score	0	2	0	0	1	0	0
Total	3						

Jot This Down

Take time to reflect on this case study and then consider the following.

1. What is happening to Andrew (consider the hydrocortisone dosing)?
2. If untreated, what will happen to Andrew's blood pressure and heart rate?
3. Consider the role of the expert patient in the management of rare diseases and how working in partnership with the patient can improve outcomes and satisfaction.
4. Given Andrew's NEWS2 score of 3, what is the recommended escalation action according your local trust policy?

Diabetes Mellitus

Diabetes mellitus is a disorder of the endocrine system characterised by high blood glucose levels.

Pathophysiology

There are two types of diabetes.

Type 1 Diabetes Type 1 diabetes develops most commonly in childhood or early adulthood and comprises about 15% of the total incidence of diabetes in the UK; however, the rate of type 1 diabetes is increasing, particularly in children less than 5 years of age (Dabelea *et al.*, 2014). Type 1 diabetes is normally caused by autoimmune destruction of the beta cells of the pancreas and is therefore associated with a severe reduction in, or complete loss of, insulin production (Atkinson *et al.*, 2014).

Type 2 Diabetes Type 2 diabetes is the most common form of diabetes and is generally considered to develop in patients over the age of 40; however, the rates of juvenile-onset type 2 diabetes appear to be rising (Dabelea *et al.*, 2014). Type 2 diabetes is normally characterised by the development of resistance to the effects of insulin in the tissues (especially body fat and skeletal muscles) and the continued production and release of glucose by the liver. These tissues are unable to respond effectively to insulin and absorb glucose from the blood. Recent developments suggest that beta-cell dysfunction is already present in patients at risk of type 2 diabetes, especially those with a family history of diabetes, and this may be the underlying factor in many cases. Furthermore, the impact of environmental factors (such as dietary intake and type of diet) is almost certainly a factor in the increase of type 2 diabetes (Kahn *et al.*, 2014).

Regardless of the primary cause, an increasing blood glucose level results, which leads to toxic damage of the beta cells, further reducing the production of insulin in an ongoing vicious circle. Insulin production is rarely completely stopped in type 2 diabetes. Risk factors for type 2 diabetes include being overweight, lack of exercise, genetic inheritance and increasing age. Genetic predisposition to type 2 diabetes appears to be especially strong in patients from South Asian or Afro-Caribbean backgrounds (Goff, 2019).

Signs and Symptoms

The signs and symptoms of diabetes are common to both forms of diabetes and are mostly related to the high blood glucose levels and include:

- Passing urine more often than usual, especially at night
- Increased thirst
- Extreme tiredness
- Unexplained weight loss (usually only in type 1 diabetes)
- Genital itching or regular episodes of thrush
- Slow healing of cuts and wounds
- Blurred vision
- Abdominal pain
- Increased blood glucose
- Glucose in the urine
- Ketones in the urine.

In both forms of diabetes, the increased blood glucose leads to excretion of glucose in the urine. The glucose has an osmotic effect, drawing water into the renal tubules and increasing urine production. The increased excretion of glucose in the urine leads to water depletion and increased thirst.

In type 1 diabetes, and occasionally in advanced type 2 diabetes, the inability of the cells to utilise glucose leads to the use of fats and amino acids as the primary fuel source in the cells, leading to weight loss and the production of ketones as a by-product. Ketones are strong acids which are passed into the urine. As the ketones are negatively charged, there is usually a simultaneous excretion of positively charged sodium and potassium ions, leading to electrolyte imbalance and abdominal pain.

Diagnosis and Investigations

The rapid onset of type 1 diabetes means that patients rarely remain undiagnosed for long. Many patients will present to their GP due to their symptoms; however, in some cases, the onset is so rapid or is precipitated by an acute illness that the patient develops diabetic ketoacidosis (DKA) and is admitted to hospital as an emergency.

Type 2 diabetes is more insidious in onset and many patients will remain unaware of the fact they have diabetes for years before they are diagnosed, by which point they may have developed complications.

The diagnosis of type 1 diabetes is based on the presence of the classic symptoms of high blood glucose on fingerprick test, weight loss, thirst and increased urine output. Formal diagnosis can then be confirmed by one laboratory blood glucose measurement.

Type 2 diabetes is often diagnosed after opportunistic screening or as a chance finding while being treated for another condition. Current guidance is focused on identifying people at risk of developing type 2 diabetes and encouraging them to have a risk assessment

and risk identification (NICE, 2017). NICE recommends the following strategy.

1. Identify those at risk and either administer a validated risk assessment tool or encourage those potentially at risk to self-administer a risk assessment tool such as the one found on the Diabetes UK website: **https://riskscore.diabetes.org.uk/start**.
2. Those found to have high-risk scores should be offered formal blood tests, such as HbA_{1c}, fasting blood glucose or glucose tolerance test.
3. Those found to be at risk but who have not developed diabetes should be offered guidance on managing risk, such as healthy eating, losing weight and exercise. Guidance on recommendations can be found on the NICE website at **www.nice.org.uk/guidance/ph38/chapter/1-Recommendations**

Nursing Care and Management

The treatment of type 1 diabetes is based on the replacement of insulin by the subcutaneous injection of insulin. There are several forms of insulin, but they are all classified by:

- How soon they start working (onset)
- When they work the hardest (peak time)
- How long it lasts in the body (duration).

Medicines Management

Insulin
On the ward, insulin is often stored in the fridge. However, note that cold insulin increases the pain of the injection and decreases insulin absorption, so for patient comfort and insulin efficacy it is advisable to take the insulin out of the refrigerator a minimum of 1 h prior to injection.

Insulin pens
Patients should be advised not to store opened insulin pens in the fridge.

Unopened pen cartridges are stored in a fridge but once inserted into an insulin pen, the pen should be kept out of the fridge. The insulin can be stored at room temperature for 28 days (International Diabetes Federation, nd) but should be kept in a closed container to minimise temperature changes.

Premixed insulins
When a patient (or nurse) is going to administer a cloudy, or premixed, insulin, it is important that the pen or vial is rotated end over end 20 times (not shaken), otherwise the insulin may not be mixed correctly (Frid *et al.*, 2016). Research has shown that patients are often confused about this technique, and the actual mixing of insulin by patients has a large variation that may affect glycaemic control (Frid *et al.*, 2016).

Injection sites
The most common injection sites are the thighs, abdomen (above and below the umbilicus), upper arms or buttocks. However, it has been observed that patients will repeatedly inject into the abdomen below the umbilicus as this is an easy area to access when clothed. Repeated use of the same injection sites can lead to the development of lipohypertrophy (fatty lumps) that are not only unsightly but can affect insulin absorption at the injection site. It has been clearly shown that the rotation of injection site at every injection reduces the risk of lipohypertrophy so it is recommended that at every clinic appointment, time is taken to remind patients to rotate the site of injection and that healthcare staff carry out a skin assessment to assess for the development of lipohypertrophy (Deeb *et al.*, 2019).

The decision about which insulin to choose is based on the individual's lifestyle and blood sugar levels, and the physician's preference and experience. Newly diagnosed patients will require education regarding self-injection and insulin doses. This should be reviewed, and skills reassessed with the patient regularly. Patients should be advised regarding the storage of insulin and the rotation of injection sites.

People with newly diagnosed type 1 diabetes should be offered a structured programme of education delivered by a qualified health professional and the opportunity for education and information should be offered on a regular basis (NICE, 2020a).

Temperature °C	36.9						
Systolic BP mmHg	100						
Heart rate	80						
Level of consciousness							P
Score	0	0	0	0		0	0	3
Total	3						

Case Study Hypoglycaemia

Jacinta is a 34-year-old woman admitted to the ward for fibroid removal. She has been starved from midnight and has a 5% dextrose infusion running over 12 hours as she is a type 1 diabetic. Unfortunately, Jacinta's morning operation has been pushed back to the afternoon due to an acute emergency being admitted via accident and emergency and she has remained nil by mouth. During the afternoon, it is noted that Jacinta has become increasingly drowsy, but on checking the drug chart there is no record of the administration of any pre-meds. Jacinta's vital signs are noted below. Her conscious level is P on the AVPU score, and her capillary blood sugar is 2.6 mmol/L.

Once the increasing drowsiness is noted, the registered nurse administers glucose gel to Jacinta (as per trust policy) and asks a colleague to get the ward 'hypo box' (hypoglycaemia kit) and to call for urgent medical help. A glucagon injection is considered but as intravenous access is available, Jacinta is commenced on an infusion of 10% glucose (200 mL over 15 minutes) (Joint British Diabetes Societies for Inpatient Care, 2018). Nursing staff continue to monitor Jacinta's airway due to her reduced conscious level and repeat the blood sugar measurement until Jacinta's glucose level increases and her conscious level improves.

VITAL SIGNS	OBSERVATION	NORMAL
Temperature	36.9 °C	36.0–37.9 °C range
Pulse	80 beats per minute	60–100 beats per minute
Respiration	12 breaths per minute	12–20 breaths per minute
Blood pressure	100/55 mmHg	100–139 mmHg (systolic) range
O₂ saturations	96%	94–98%

Jacinta's NEWS2 score is noted below.

PHYSIOLOGICAL PARAMETER	3	2	1	0	1	2	3
Respiration rate				12			
Oxygen saturation %				96			
Air or oxygen				Air			

Jot This Down

Take time to reflect on this case study and then consider the following.
1. What is happening to Jacinta and why?
2. What is the potential first aid that could be delivered as an immediate response?
3. What follow-up treatment should be instituted (remember Jacinta needs to remain nil by mouth)?
4. Given Jacinta's NEWS2 score of 3, what is the recommended escalation action according your local trust policy?
5. With the potential danger to Jacinta but a NEWS2 score of only 3, consider the need of the nurse to use their own knowledge as a basis for escalating care.

Self-monitoring of blood glucose levels is essential using capillary blood glucose testing in the home environment. Education about testing should be offered at diagnosis and skills reassessed regularly.

Dietary advice for all type 1 diabetic patients should include:
- Discussion of the hyperglycaemic effects of different foods and ensuring adequate insulin to cover them
- Types, timing and number of snacks taken between meals and at bedtime
- Healthy eating to reduce arterial risk
- If the person wants it, information on:
  - Effects of alcohol-containing drinks on blood glucose and calorie intake
  - Use of high-calorie and high-sugar 'treats'
  - Use of foods with a high glycaemic index.

Patients with type 1 diabetes will also require education on the recognition and management of *hypoglycaemia* (often called 'hypos').

Red Flag

Hypoglycaemia is a potentially life-threatening condition characterised by a low blood sugar. The patient will present with:
- Hunger
- Nervousness and shakiness
- Perspiration
- Dizziness or light-headedness
- Sleepiness
- Confusion
- Difficulty speaking
- Feelings of anxiety or weakness.

If possible, the patient should be encouraged to eat glucose (in the form of jam, chocolate, etc.) or glucose paste (such as Glucogel®) rubbed into the gums. The glucose will be short-acting and must be followed with a longer-acting carbohydrate (such as brown bread) if the patient is able to eat safely. Semiconscious and unconscious patients will require the administration of glucagon or intravenous glucose.

Treatment of type 2 diabetes will depend on the severity of the condition. Treatment will always include dietary adjustments (healthy diet with reduced fat and sugar) and lifestyle changes (such as exercise and losing weight if required), and in some patients with type 2 diabetes this will be enough to maintain normal blood glucose levels. Dietary advice for patients with type 2 diabetes includes:

- Include high-fibre, low-glycaemic index sources of carbohydrate
- Include low-fat dairy products and oily fish
- Control the intake of foods containing saturated fats and trans-fatty acids
- Avoid the use of foods marketed specifically for people with diabetes as they often contain fructose as a substitute for sucrose. Fructose still affects blood glucose levels.

However, type 2 diabetes may require oral medication. Drugs for type 2 diabetes generally have one of three potential actions:

- Reducing the amount of glucose released by the liver
- Increasing the cells' ability to utilise insulin (decreasing insulin resistance)
- Promoting the production of insulin by the pancreas.

Self-monitoring of type 2 diabetes is occasionally advised, and the patient will need to be educated in the use of capillary blood measurement of glucose. More commonly, the primary care provider will monitor the HbA_{1c} (long-term blood glucose measurement) every 2–6 months.

Patients with both types of diabetes will require advice on:

- *Regular physical activity*: however, strenuous exercise can reduce blood glucose levels and people with type 1 diabetes will need to monitor blood glucose levels and adjust insulin doses accordingly. Exercise regimes should be agreed with appropriate healthcare staff
- *Stopping smoking*: smoking is a risk for anybody, but diabetic patients have an increased risk of cardiovascular disease, which is compounded by smoking
- *Monitoring cholesterol levels* and managing cholesterol intake
- *Reducing salt* in the diet
- *Weight loss*, if required: weight loss improves diabetic control in both types of diabetes.

Furthermore, patients will require regular (usually annual) checks and Diabetes UK has created a list of 15 healthcare essentials that patients should be receiving every year.

1. Blood glucose levels: HbA_{1c} should be measured at least once every year.
2. Blood pressure recorded at least once a year.
3. Cholesterol levels tested every year.

The Nursing Associate

Patients with diabete that patients with diabetes are educated regarding the use of appropriate, well-fitting, footwear at all times (including in the home).

This is an appropriate role for the nursing associate to ensure that the patient in hospital or the community setting is encouraged to wear footwear (such as slippers) and to have regular foot checks by a qualified podiatrist (Chapman, 2017), thus allowing the nursing associate to meet the outcome for appropriate risk assessments and promote preventive health behaviours (NMC, 2018b).

4. Eye test for signs of retinopathy (damage to the retina of the eye).
5. Foot and leg check: people with diabetes have a higher risk of problems with the feet and therefore they should be checked by a professional at least once a year
6. Kidney function test: a urine test for protein and a blood test to measure kidney function.
7. Ongoing, individual, dietary advice from a healthcare professional with relevant expertise in nutrition. Weight should also be monitored.
8. Ongoing emotional and psychological support. Living with diabetes can have an effect on emotional and psychological health, so people with diabetes should be able to talk to specialist healthcare professionals about their concerns. Patients with both types of diabetes have an increased risk of depression and healthcare professionals can use two simple questions to screen for potential depression, e.g. 'During the last month, have you often been bothered by:
   - Feeling down, depressed or hopeless?
   - Having little interest or pleasure in doing things?'
   If the answer to either of these questions is 'yes', then more detailed depression screening may be required
9. Health courses: people with diabetes should be offered the opportunity to attend a course that could help them understand and manage their condition. For instance, Diabetes UK runs two courses for patients with type 2 diabetes.
10. Access to specialists: all people with diabetes need to see specialist diabetes healthcare professionals to help them manage their condition, including access to ophthalmologists, podiatrists and dietitians.
11. Annual flu vaccination.

Practice Assessment Document

One of the outcomes considered more difficult to achieve from the NMC Future Nurse standards (NMC, 2018a) is Outcome 2.11: understand and explain the principles of pathogenesis and immunology as applied to vaccinations. Whilst it is often possible to achieve this outcome in the GP practice where vaccination is a common event, it is much more difficult in other settings. Any interaction with any patient with an endocrine disorder (including diabetes) is a good time to discuss annual flu vaccination as all patients with an endocrine disorder benefit from the protection it provides (Shang *et al.*, 2018).

12. High-quality hospital care: people with diabetes who need to stay in hospital should receive care from specialist diabetes healthcare professionals, whether or not they have been admitted because of their diabetes.

13. Have the opportunity to discuss and receive support for any ongoing sexual problems. Diabetes increases the incidence of sexual dysfunction in men and women.

14. Smokers should receive support and advice on how to quit. Smoking increases the risk of heart disease and cerebrovascular events, which is already raised in people with diabetes.

15. Specialist pregnancy care: diabetes has to be more highly controlled and monitored during pregnancy, so people with diabetes who are planning to have a baby should have the care they need from specialist healthcare professionals.

Red Flag

Women of childbearing age who are pregnant (or wish to become pregnant) will require close management of their diabetic control, as there is an increased risk of miscarriage and stillbirth (NICE, 2020b).

Primary Care

As noted, primary care providers are at the forefront of risk assessment and screening for type 2 diabetes. The vast majority of people with type 2 diabetes are managed in primary care and NICE has set a number of Quality Statements for diabetes care, including blood pressure measurement and control, foot examination, referral to a structured education programme and HbA$_{1c}$ levels (NICE, 2016).

Conclusion

This chapter has reviewed the physiology of the endocrine system and its related conditions. The major functions of the endocrine system are based around four main areas:

- The maintenance of homeostasis
- Metabolism and energy management
- Growth and development
- Reproduction.

The secretion of hormones can be stimulated by nervous impulses, hormones or changes in the body levels of ions and nutrients and further regulation of hormone release is then often controlled by negative feedback loops. Hormones can only have an effect on a cell if that cell has a receptor for the hormone; however, there appears to be virtually no cell within the body that is not affected by the endocrine system. Any part of the endocrine system can become disordered, but the effects of the disorder may be subtle and difficult to diagnose. Management of endocrine disorders requires the multidisciplinary team to work around the patient and with the patient to provide the best outcomes for health.

Key Points

- Endocrine disorders can be slow and insidious in onset with vague symptoms.
- Management of patients with an endocrine disorder requires skills in education and counselling.

- Most patients with an endocrine disorder will be required to carry out self-care activities in managing their disorder and many patients become experts in their own disorder.
- All patients with an endocrine disorder should be strongly advised to wear a MedicAlert talisman.
- Most endocrine disorders have an associated support group and patients should be made aware of any specific to their condition.
- Endocrine disorders are always managed in a shared care agreement between primary care and the hospital consultant.
- The care of patients with diabetes involves the management of risk for long-term complications as much as short-term hormone replacement.

References

Alexandraki, K.I. & Grossman, A.B. (2019) Management of hypopituitarism. *Journal of Clinical Medicine*, 8(12), 2153.

Antonelli, A., Ferrari, S.M., Corrado, A., Di Domenicantonio, A. & Fallahi, P. (2015) Autoimmune thyroid disorders. *Autoimmunity Reviews*, 14(2), 174–180.

Antonelli, A., Ferrari, S. M., Ragusa, F., *et al.* (2020) Graves' disease: epidemiology, genetic and environmental risk factors and viruses. *Best Practice & Research Clinical Endocrinology & Metabolism*, 34(1), 101387.

Atkinson, M.A., Eisenbarth, G.S. & Michels, A.W. (2014) Type 1 diabetes. *Lancet*, 383(9911), 69–82.

Bancos, I., Hahner, S., Tomlinson, J. & Arlt, W. (2015) Diagnosis and management of adrenal insufficiency. *Lancet Diabetes and Endocrinology*, 3(3), 216–226.

Biondi, B. & Wartofsky, L. (2014) Treatment with thyroid hormone. *Endocrine Reviews*, 35(3), 433–512.

Bornstein, S. R., Allolio, B., Arlt, W., *et al.* (2016) Diagnosis and treatment of primary adrenal insufficiency: an endocrine society clinical practice guideline. *Journal of Clinical Endocrinology & Metabolism*, 101(2), 364–389.

Brooke, A.M. & Monson, J.P. (2017) Addison's disease. *Medicine*, 45(8), 492–496.

Caturegli, P., De Remigis, A. & Rose, N.R. (2014) Hashimoto's thyroiditis: clinical and diagnostic criteria. *Autoimmunity Reviews*, 13(4), 391–397.

Chapman, S. (2017) Foot care for people with diabetes: prevention of complications and treatment. *British Journal of Community Nursing*, 22(5), 226–229.

Chiha, M., Samarasinghe, S. & Kabaker, A.S. (2015) Thyroid storm: an updated review. *Journal of Intensive Care Medicine*, 30(3), 131–140.

Dabelea, D., Mayer-Davis, E.J., Saydah, S. *et al.* (2014) Prevalence of type 1 and type 2 diabetes among children and adolescents from 2001 to 2009. *Journal of the American Medical Association*, 311(17), 1778–1786.

Deeb, A., Abdelrahman, L., Tomy, M., *et al.* (2019) Impact of insulin injection and infusion routines on lipohypertrophy and glycemic control in children and adults with diabetes. *Diabetes Therapy*, 10(1), 259–267.

Duntas, L.H. & Yen, P.M. (2019) Diagnosis and treatment of hypothyroidism in the elderly. *Endocrine*, 66(1), 63–69.

Esposito, D., Pasquali, D. & Johannsson, G. (2018) Primary adrenal insufficiency: managing mineralocorticoid replacement therapy. *Journal of Clinical Endocrinology & Metabolism*, 103(2), 376–387.

Frid, A.H., Kreugel, G., Grassi, G., *et al.* (2016) New insulin delivery recommendations. *Mayo Clinic Proceedings*, 91(9), 1231–1255.

Goff, L.M. (2019) Ethnicity and type 2 diabetes in the UK. *Diabetic Medicine*, 36(8), 927–938.

González-González, J.G., Borjas-Almaguer, O.D., Salcido-Montenegro, A., *et al.* (2018) Sheehan's syndrome revisited: underlying autoimmunity or hypoperfusion? *International Journal of Endocrinology*, 2018, 8415860.

Higham, C.E., Johannsson, G. & Shalet, S.M. (2016) Hypopituitarism. *Lancet*, 388(10058), 2403–2415.

International Diabetes Federation (n.d.) *Storage of Insulin*. https://idf.org/images/IDF_Europe/Storage_of_Insulin_-_IDF_Europe_Awareness_Paper_-_FINAL.pdf (accessed December 2021).

Joint British Diabetes Societies for Inpatient Care (2018) *The Hospital Management of Hypoglycaemia in Adults with Diabetes Mellitus*. http://diabetestimes.co.uk/wp-content/uploads/2018/03/JBDS_HypoGuideline.pdf-FINAL-08.03.181.pdf (accessed December 2021).

Jose, M., Amir, S. & Desai, R. (2019) Chronic Sheehan's syndrome – a differential to be considered in clinical practice in women with a history of postpartum hemorrhage. *Cureus*, 11(12), e6290.

Kahn, S.E., Cooper, M.E. & Del Prato, S. (2014) Pathophysiology and treatment of type 2 diabetes: perspectives on the past, present, and future. *Lancet*, 383(9922), 1068–1083.

Kapoor, D., Kapoor, R. & Dhingra, M. (2017) Thyroid emergencies. *Principles and Practices of Thyroid Gland Disorders*, 297.

Lee, S.Y. & Pearce, E.N. (2021) Testing, monitoring, and treatment of thyroid dysfunction in pregnancy. *Journal of Clinical Endocrinology & Metabolism*, 106(3), 883–892.

Llahana, S. (2021) The role of nurses in supporting self-management for patients with hypopituitarism. In: J. Honegger, M. Reincke & S. Petersenn (eds) *Pituitary Tumors* (pp. 157–171). Academic Press, New York.

Mukherjee, A., Sandeep, L., Choudhury, S., Chakraborty, D.S. & Rajasree, S. (2017) Steroid therapy in adrenal insufficiency. *Journal of Analytical and Pharmaceutical Research*, 6(2), 00171.

National Institute for Health and Care Excellence (2016) *Diabetes in Adults*. QS6. NICE, London.

National Institute for Health and Care Excellence (2017) *Type 2 Diabetes: Prevention in People at High Risk*. PH38. NICE, London.

National Institute for Health and Care Excellence (2020a) *Type 1 Diabetes in Adults: Diagnosis and Management*. NG17. NICE, London.

National Institute for Health and Care Excellence (2020b) *Diabetes in Pregnancy: Management from Preconception to the Postnatal Period*. NG3. NICE, London.

Nursing & Midwifery Council (2018a) *Future nurse: Standards of proficiency for registered nurses*. NMC, London.

Nursing & Midwifery Council (2018b) *Standards of proficiency for nursing associates*. NMC, London.

Peate, I. & Evans, S. (eds) (2020) *Fundamentals of Anatomy and Physiology for Nursing and Healthcare Students*, 3rd edn. Wiley, Oxford.

Piantanida, E., Lai, A., Sassi, L., *et al.* (2015) Outcome prediction of treatment of Graves' hyperthyroidism with antithyroid drugs. *Hormone and Metabolic Research*, 47(10), 767–772.

Pivonello, R., De Leo, M., Cozzolino, A. & Colao, A. (2015) The treatment of Cushing's disease. *Endocrine Reviews*, 36(4), 385–486.

Prague, J.K., May, S. & Whitelaw, B.C. (2013) Cushing's syndrome. *British Medical Journal*, 316, 945.

Rahman, S., Walker, D. & Sultan, P. (2017) Medical identification or alert jewellery: an opportunity to save lives or an unreliable hindrance? *Anaesthesia*, 72(9), 1139–1145.

Roberts, C.G.P. & Ladenson, P.W. (2004) Hypothyroidism. *Lancet*, 363(9411), 793–803.

Saverino, S. & Falorni, A. (2020) Autoimmune Addison's disease. *Best Practice & Research Clinical Endocrinology & Metabolism*, 34(1), 101379.

Shang, M., Chung, J. R., Jackson, M. L., *et al.* (2018) Influenza vaccine effectiveness among patients with high-risk medical conditions in the United States, 2012–2016. *Vaccine*, 36(52), 8047–8053.

Shoback, D.M., Bilezikian, J.P., Costa, A.G., *et al.* (2016) Presentation of hypoparathyroidism: etiologies and clinical features. *Journal of Clinical Endocrinology and Metabolism*, 101(6), 2300–2312.

Simpson, H., Tomlinson, J., Wass, J., Dean, J. & Arlt, W. (2020) Guidance for the prevention and emergency management of adult patients with adrenal insufficiency. *Clinical Medicine*, 20(4), 371.

Udelsman, R., Åkerström, G., Biagini, C., *et al.* (2014) The surgical management of asymptomatic primary hyperparathyroidism: proceedings of the Fourth International Workshop. *Journal of Clinical Endocrinology and Metabolism*, 99(10), 3595–3606.

Wass, J.A. & Arlt, W. (2012) How to avoid precipitating an acute adrenal crisis. *British Medical Journal*, 345, e6333.

Weeks, B.H. (2005) Graves' disease: the importance of early diagnosis. *Nurse Practitioner*, 30(11), 31–45.

Weetman, A. (2013) Current choice of treatment for hypo- and hyperthyroidism. *Prescriber*, 24(13–16), 23–33.

Wemeau, J.L., Klein, M., Sadoul, J.L., Briet, C. & Vélayoudom-Céphise, F.L. (2018) Graves' disease: introduction, epidemiology, endogenous and environmental pathogenic factors. *Annales d'Endocrinologie*, 79(6), 599–607.

Wiesner, A., Gajewska, D. & Paśko, P. (2021) Levothyroxine interactions with food and dietary supplements – a systematic review. *Pharmaceuticals*, 14(3), 206.

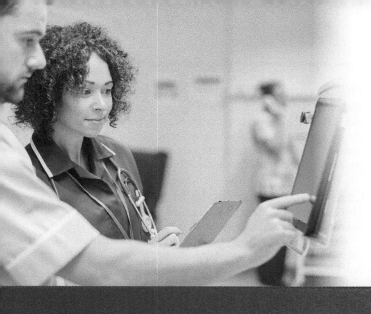

32

The Person with a Neurological Disorder

Mary E. Braine

University of Salford, UK

Learning Outcomes

On completion of this chapter, you will be able to:

- **Understand and apply a person-centred approach to nursing care, demonstrating shared assessment, planning, decision making for patients with neurological problems**
- **Demonstrate the ability to accurately process all information gathered during the assessment process to identify needs for individualised nursing care and develop person-centred, evidence-based plans for nursing interventions with agreed goals**
- **Demonstrate and apply knowledge of common neurological health conditions, medication usage and treatments**
- **Demonstrate knowledge of epidemiology, demography, genomics and the wider determinants of common neurological conditions**

Proficiencies

NMC Proficiencies and Standards:

- **Evidence-based, best practice approaches to communication for supporting people of all ages, their families and carers in preventing ill health and in managing their care:**
  - **Share information and check understanding about the causes, implications and treatment of a range of common health conditions including neurological disease.**
  - **Undertake a whole body systems assessment including neurological status**
  - **Undertake, respond to and interpret neurological observations and assessments**

 Visit the companion website at www.wiley.com/go/peate/nursingpractice3e where you can test yourself using flashcards, multiple-choice questions and more.

Nursing Practice: Knowledge and Care, Third Edition. Edited by Ian Peate and Aby Mitchell.
© 2022 John Wiley & Sons Ltd. Published 2022 by John Wiley & Sons Ltd.
Companion website: www.wiley.com/go/peate/nursingpractice3e

Introduction

The nervous system is one of the most complex body systems, regulating, controlling and integrating all other body systems and maintaining homeostasis. Because of the nervous system's complexity, it is often difficult to understand and can be very challenging; however, nurses will meet patients with neurological disorders in a wide variety of situations. Thus, an understanding of this complex system is crucial in providing safe and effective care for this varied large group of patients, with over 1000 neurological disorders affecting millions of people worldwide.

This chapter provides a brief overview of the functions of the central and peripheral nervous systems, the assessment processes to facilitate diagnosis and management planning, and key nursing care considerations for a few commonly encountered neurological disorders.

Anatomy and Physiology

The nervous system receives, processes and initiates actions through an intricate network of billions of specialised cells called neurones (nerves). It is anatomically divided into two main subdivisions (Figures 32.1 and 32.2).

The Brain and Central Nervous System

The brain is the control centre of the nervous system and is protected from the external environment by three barriers: the skull, the meninges and the cerebrospinal fluid (CSF). The main divisions of the brain include the cerebral cortex, diencephalon, brainstem and cerebellum (Table 32.1).

Coverings of the Brain and Spinal Cord

Three connective tissues (the meninges) cover the brain and spinal cord: the dura, arachnoid and pia mater (Figure 32.3).

Cerebrospinal fluid is a clear colourless liquid that moves in the subarachnoid space in a unidirectional flow. Its protective functions are:

- *Mechanical*: lubricating the meninges and providing a cushioning effect
- *Chemical*: providing the optimum chemical environment for accurate neuronal signalling
- *Circulation*: carrying nutrients and removing waste and potentially noxious substances.

Blood–Brain Barrier

The blood–brain barrier (BBB) is a highly selective membrane located at the interface between the capillary walls and the brain tissue and acts to isolate the brain from the rest of the body.

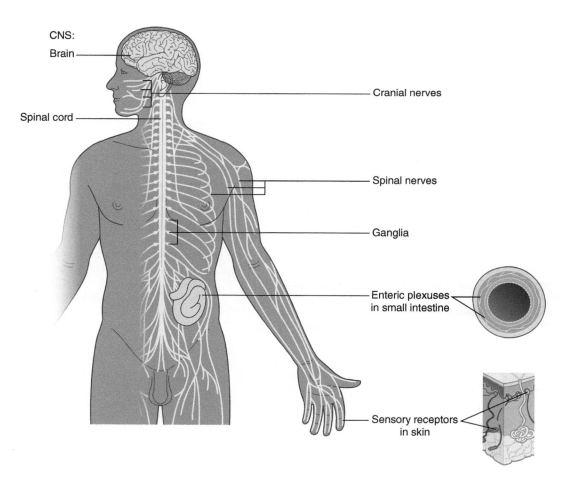

CNS:
Brain
Spinal cord
Cranial nerves
Spinal nerves
Ganglia
Enteric plexuses in small intestine
Sensory receptors in skin

Figure 32.1 The main parts of the nervous system.

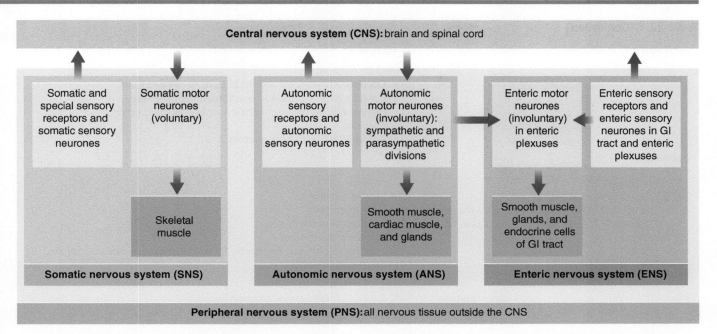

Figure 32.2 Organisation of the nervous system. Grey boxes represent sensory components of the peripheral nervous system (PNS). Yellow boxes represent motor components of the PNS. Red boxes represent effectors (muscles and glands).

Table 32.1 General functions of the four main parts of the brain.

MAIN PART	FUNCTIONS
Cerebral cortex	
• Largest part • Divided into right and left hemispheres connected by the corpus callosum • Each hemisphere is divided into four lobes • Hemispheres are composed of outer cerebral cortex, grey matter, internal white matter	• Receives sensory (afferent) impulses • Initiates motor (efferent) impulses • Controls skeletal muscle activity • Contains the seat of consciousness • Processes sensory information • Responsible for language and information processing • Governs intelligence, reasoning, learning, memory and other complex behaviours
Diencephalon	
• Provides a structural connection between the cerebrum and brainstem, in particular the midbrain. Important structures: • thalamus • hypothalamus	*Thalamus* • Main synaptic relay centre, processes motor information • Receives and relays sensory information to and from the cerebral cortex *Hypothalamus* • Overall homeostasis • Regulates and produces hormones • Regulates autonomic nervous system, water balance and thirst, appetite, circadian rhythm, body temperature • Part of the arousal/alerting mechanism
Brainstem	
Consists of the: • midbrain, • pons • medulla oblongata	*Midbrain* • Conducts impulses from the motor areas in the cerebral cortex to the brainstem • Reflex centre for pupils and eye movement *Pons* • Co-ordinates voluntary movements • Helps control breathing • Nuclei for several cranial nerves

(Continued)

583

Table 32.1 (*Continued*)

MAIN PART	FUNCTIONS
	Medulla oblongata · Controls voluntary movement of lower limbs and trunk · Controls heart rate, blood pressure, respiration rate · Reflexes for vomiting, coughing, swallowing, hiccupping, yawning and sneezing · Nuclei for several cranial nerves
Cerebellum	
· Second largest area · Consists of two hemispheres · Receives information from the cortex via the pons and outgoing information goes to the cortex via the thalamus	· Balance · Muscle tension · Eye movement · Equilibrium of the trunk · Spinal nerve reflexes · Provides information necessary for balance, posture and co-ordinated muscle movement

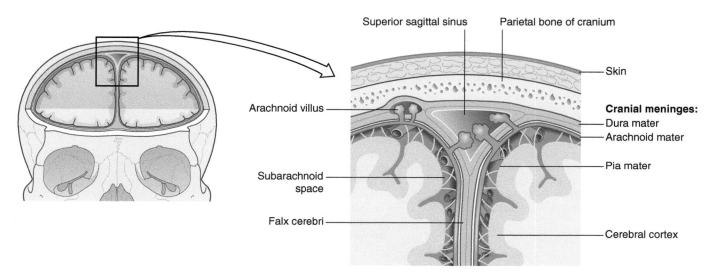

Figure 32.3 The protective coverings of the brain.

It regulates the exchange of substances entering the brain for normal brain activities. In addition, the BBB acts to protect the brain from potentially harmful substances.

Blood Supply to the CNS

The central nervous system (CNS) is one of the most metabolically active systems in the body and thus requires a constant blood supply. Blood flow to the brain is maintained at a constant rate via cerebral autoregulation. Even a brief interruption of blood flow (seconds) can cause serious neurological disturbances and cell death in minutes.

Blood supply to the brain comes from two main sources: two internal carotid arteries and two vertebral arteries which give rise to the unique arrangement of arteries supplying the brain called the circle of Willis (Figure 32.4).

Venous Drainage of the Brain Cerebral drainage is dependent on a system of valveless superficial and deep veins entering the three main dural sinuses (superior sagittal, cavernous and transverse sinuses), which then empty into the right and left internal jugular veins (Figure 32.5).

Spinal Cord

The spinal cord is a long cylindrical segmented structure that extends from the medulla oblongata and terminates, in adults, at the first lumbar vertebra. It receives sensory information from the limbs, trunk and internal organs and contains somatic motor tracts that supply the skeletal muscles, visceral smooth muscles and glands. The spinal cord does not reach the end of the vertebral column; as a result, the lumbar and sacral nerve roots travel inferiorly through the vertebral canal for some distance before

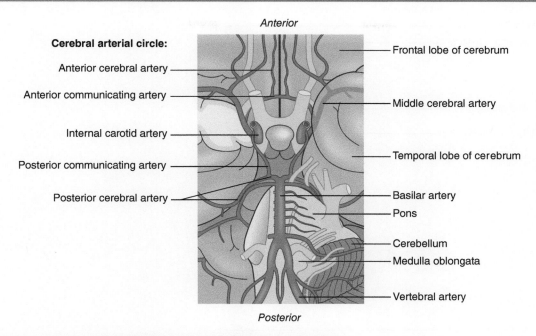

Figure 32.4 Inferior view of the base of the brain showing the cerebral arterial circle.

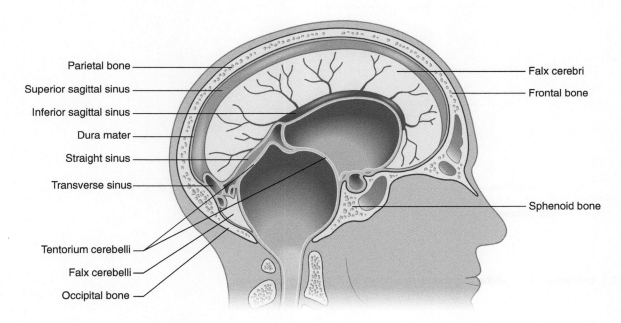

Figure 32.5 Sagittal view of the extension of the dura mater.

exiting the vertebral column through their associated interverte-bral foramina. This collection of descending nerve roots is called the *cauda equina* (Figure 32.6).

The Peripheral Nervous System

The peripheral nervous system (PNS) links the CNS with the rest of the body. The PNS includes the neuromuscular structures out-side the skull and vertebral column, spinal nerves and cranial nerves, neuromuscular junction and receptors. The 31 pairs of spinal nerves (their names relate to where they enter/exit the ver-tebra column) emerge from the cord each containing motor and sensory fibres which can be myelinated or unmyelinated. Each spinal nerve innervates a specific skin area called a dermatome. Some of these branches form complex clusters of nerves called plexuses (Figure 32.7). The 12 pairs of cranial nerves (I–XII) all emerge from the brain, except cranial nerve IX, which emerges from the spinal cord (Figure 32.8).

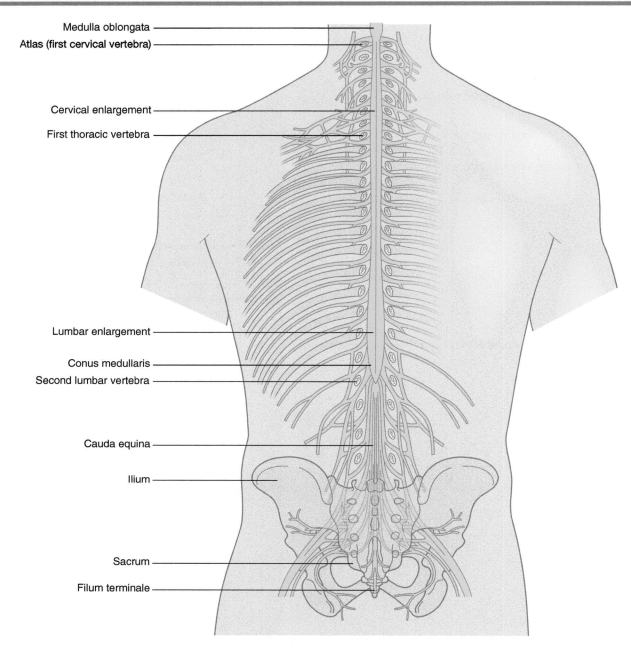

Figure 32.6 External anatomy of the spinal cord. See Figure 32.7 for the spinal nerves.

The PNS provides input form about the external environment via the sensory neurones (afferent) and output information via motor neurones (efferent) to the CNS which can be further subdivided into the somatic nervous system (nerves that transmit information from the skeletal muscles), autonomic nervous system and enteric nervous system (see Figure 32.2).

Autonomic Nervous System

The autonomic nervous system is subdivided into sympathetic and parasympathetic nervous systems and controls many body processes and acts without conscious effort. Along with the endocrine system, the autonomic nervous system regulates homeostasis. The enteric nervous system, found in the wall of the gut, is involved in co-ordinating the contractions of the gut musculature, resulting in gastrointestinal motility (peristalsis).

The major sensory system consists of somatic, visual, auditory, vestibular, taste and olfactory systems. The somatic sensory system includes sensations for pain, tactile sensation (touch, pressure and vibration), temperature, perception of joint position and movement. The human body gathers information from the environment via peripheral sensory nerve receptors and specialised sensory cells and relays this to the primary somatosensory area in the cerebral cortex.

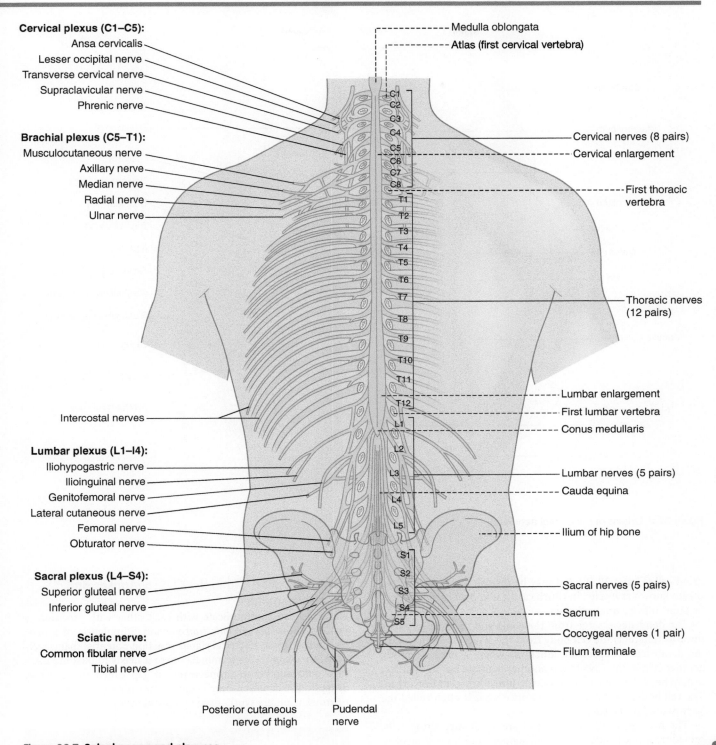

Cervical plexus (C1–C5):
Ansa cervicalis
Lesser occipital nerve
Transverse cervical nerve
Supraclavicular nerve
Phrenic nerve

Brachial plexus (C5–T1):
Musculocutaneous nerve
Axillary nerve
Median nerve
Radial nerve
Ulnar nerve

Intercostal nerves

Lumbar plexus (L1–I4):
Iliohypogastric nerve
Ilioinguinal nerve
Genitofemoral nerve
Lateral cutaneous nerve
Femoral nerve
Obturator nerve

Sacral plexus (L4–S4):
Superior gluteal nerve
Inferior gluteal nerve

Sciatic nerve:
Common fibular nerve
Tibial nerve

Posterior cutaneous nerve of thigh
Pudendal nerve

Medulla oblongata
Atlas (first cervical vertebra)

Cervical nerves (8 pairs)
Cervical enlargement

First thoracic vertebra

Thoracic nerves (12 pairs)

Lumbar enlargement
First lumbar vertebra
Conus medullaris

Lumbar nerves (5 pairs)
Cauda equina

Ilium of hip bone

Sacral nerves (5 pairs)
Sacrum
Coccygeal nerves (1 pair)
Filum terminale

Figure 32.7 Spinal nerves and plexuses.

Cells of the Nervous System

Nervous tissue consists of two major classes of cells: neurones and neuroglia. The neurone is the basic anatomical and functional unit of the nervous system, forming a complex processing network communicating with other neurones and cells within the brain and spinal cord. Most neurones consist of a soma (cell body) and two types of neuronal processes: dendrites and an axon (only one per neurone) (Figure 32.9). Cell bodies are found in clusters in the PNS, known as *ganglia;* in the CNS these clusters are called a *nucleus.*

The axon is a long process that conducts impulses away (efferent) from the cell body towards another neurone, muscle fibre or

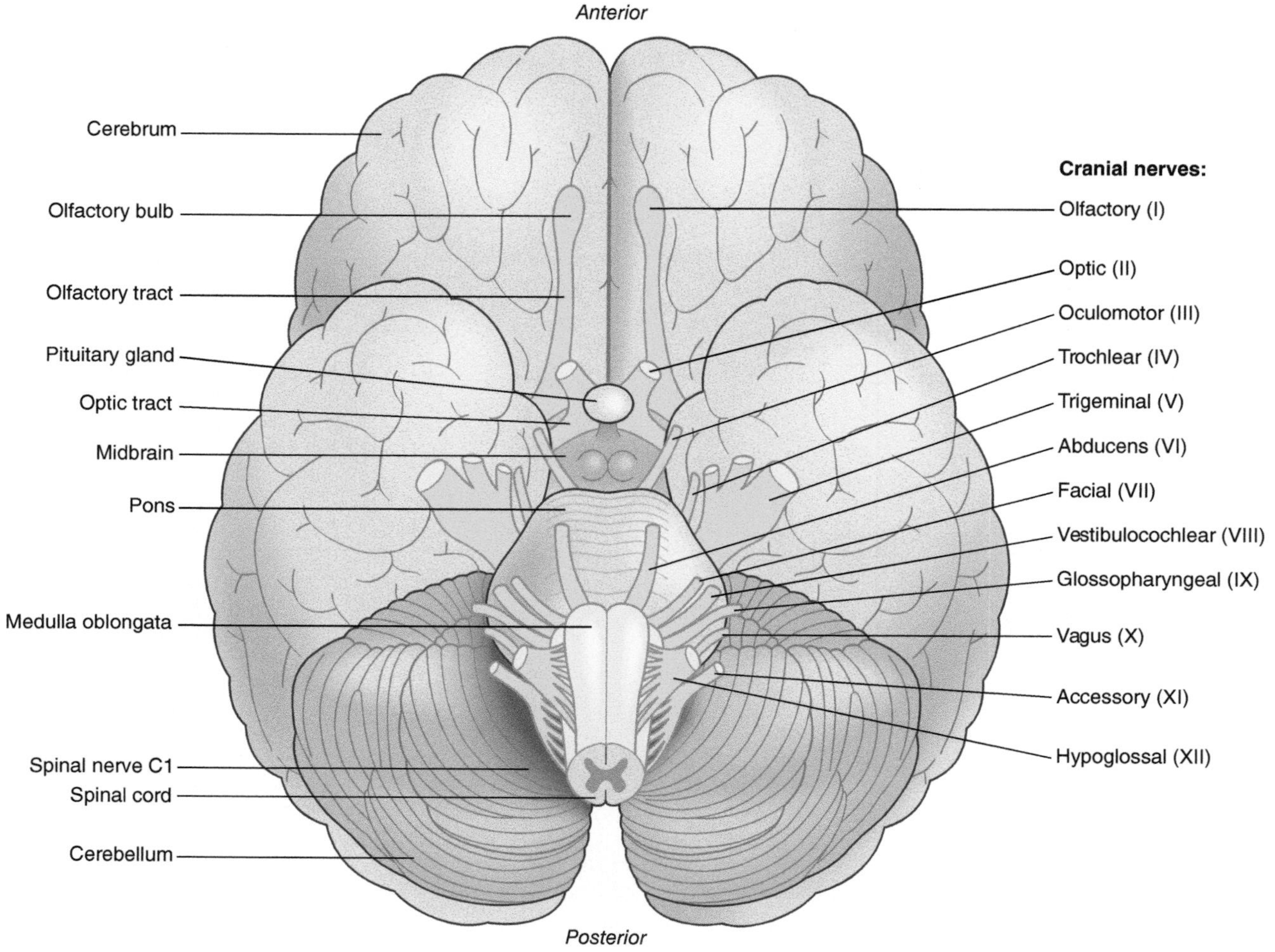

Anterior

Cerebrum

Olfactory bulb

Olfactory tract

Pituitary gland

Optic tract

Midbrain

Pons

Medulla oblongata

Spinal nerve C1

Spinal cord

Cerebellum

Cranial nerves:

Olfactory (I)

Optic (II)

Oculomotor (III)

Trochlear (IV)

Trigeminal (V)

Abducens (VI)

Facial (VII)

Vestibulocochlear (VIII)

Glossopharyngeal (IX)

Vagus (X)

Accessory (XI)

Hypoglossal (XII)

Posterior

Figure 32.8 **Origins of the cranial nerves.**

gland cell (Figure 32.10) and may be insulated by a white lipid sheath known as _myelin_, in which case it is known as myelinated, or axons may be unmyelinated.

The dendrites emerge from the soma and conduct impulses towards (afferent) the cell body from the synapses at the end of the dendrites. Synapses are junctions where a neurone meets another cell; in the CNS this is another neurone but in the PNS, it may be a muscle (neuromuscular junction), gland or organ. The cell bodies and dendrites comprise what is often called the 'grey matter' of the CNS.

The neuroglia (also called 'glia') are small supporting cells, providing homeostatic protection, support and nourishment to the neurones and maintaining homeostasis in the interstitial fluid that bathes them. They also play important roles in CNS functions but are different from nerve cells in that they cannot conduct impulses (Figure 32.11) but are involved in the signalling process. Neuroglia make up about half of the brain mass and outnumber the neurones 10-fold. There are several different types of glial cells (Table 32.2).

Communication within the CNS: Synapses and Neurotransmitters

Neurones can communicate with each other with precision, a process known as _synaptic transmission_. Stimulation of a neurone results in an electrical signal or action potential that travels down the axon to the terminal, where it needs to pass the message onto another neurone across a gap called the synapse. Synaptic transmission may occur electrically or chemically via neurotransmitters synthesised by the neurones.

Nursing Assessment of the Neurological System

Neurological assessment requires a nurse who is a competent and skilled practitioner to recognise changes. This assessment begins at the first encounter with the patient and includes gathering information about the past and current state of health and

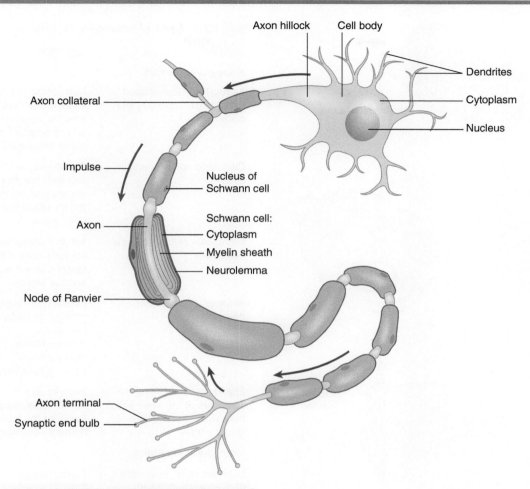

Figure 32.9 **Structure of a typical motor neurone and Schwann cell.**

a comprehensive physical assessment. Accurate assessment helps determine the extent of the cerebral dysfunction and improvement or deterioration of cerebral function. Assessment of the neurological system involves assessing the following five areas.

- Level of consciousness
- Vital signs: respiration and pulse rate, temperature and blood pressure
- Pupil reactivity
- Motor function
- Sensory function

Assessing Consciousness

The precise neurobiology of consciousness is unknown. However, it can be viewed as having two main components: arousal and awareness. Consciousness is a function of the reticular formation (RF), a network of neurones that connect with the spinal cord, cerebellum, thalamus and hypothalamus. Awareness is the result of the combined activity of the RF and cortical function; both are dependent on a complex network of activating pathways. Consciousness can be defined as a state of general awareness of oneself and the environment and is the most sensitive indicator of neurological change.

Altered states of consciousness exist due to damage to neural pathways, while coma is caused by disordered arousal rather than impairment of the content of consciousness. Regular neurological assessments identify trends and changes in loss of consciousness (LOC), and specific signs and neurological function are critical for early detection; even subtle changes may be clinically significant.

The Glasgow Coma Scale (GCS) (Teasdale & Jennett, 1974) is a universal gold standard instrument for assessing consciousness. It indicates the initial severity of trauma to the brain and its subsequent changes over time. The GCS does not diagnose the cause of the altered state of consciousness but is a rating score to grade the best possible central (brain) response.

Individual components of the assessment should be adequately described and communicated, both verbally and orally. The GCS comprises three scales all scored separately, with a numerical value for each, with a total (sum) score ranging from 3 (deep coma and unresponsive) to 15 (fully conscious, alert and orientated) (Table 32.3).

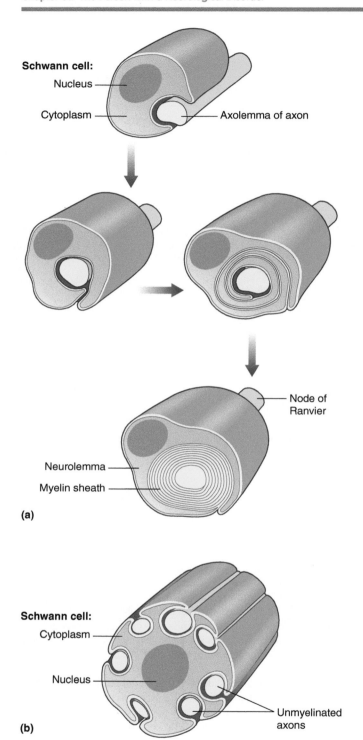

Schwann cell:
- Nucleus
- Cytoplasm — Axolemma of axon

- Neurolemma
- Myelin sheath
- Node of Ranvier

(a)

Schwann cell:
- Cytoplasm
- Nucleus
- Unmyelinated axons

(b)

Figure 32.10 Schwann cells and myelinated and unmyelinated axons in the PNS.

Table 32.2 **Types of neuroglia, location and function.**

TYPE OF NEUROGLIA	FUNCTION
Neuroglia in the CNS	
Astrocytes – star-shaped cells; most numerous glia cells	Maintaining the right extracellular chemicals and ions for nerve signalling and helping to form the blood–brain barrier
Oligodendrocytes – small cells	Provide support to axons and form the myelin sheath and are involved in the growth of damaged CNS axons
Microglia – cells with spiny processes	Act as macrophages or immune cells in the nervous system, phagocytosing debris and pathogens
Aldynoglia – specialist neuroglial cells	Pituitary glia assist in the storage and release of hormones Retinal (Müller) glia support the neurones in the retina and act as a light filter
Ependymal cells lining the ventricles of the brain and the central canal of the spinal cord	Involved with the directional flow of cerebrospinal fluid and facilitate the transport of nutrients and waste
Neuroglia in the PNS	
Schwann cells – equivalent of oligodendrocytes in the PNS	Provide support to axons and form the myelin sheath and are involved in the growth of damaged axons
Satellite cells	Regulate the environment and provide protection and structural support for the neurones

CNS, central nervous system; PNS, peripheral nervous system.

supraorbital pressure or trapezium pinch (Braine & Cook, 2016). It is critical when assessing LOC to do this accurately and take appropriate action promptly, otherwise this may lead to irreversible and serious clinical implications with harmful consequences, especially in the acutely or critically ill. In addition, the nurse should consider the moral and ethical implications when applying a painful (noxious) stimulus. The stimulus should be applied appropriately and should not cause the person harm.

The AVPU scale can give information easily and quickly about the patient's LOC (Box 32.1). Although AVPU is incorporated into the systems of early-warning scores and is ideal in the initial rapid ABCDE assessment, it is not an evidence-based tool and is inadequate in assessing patients with neurological conditions and is not a replacement for the GCS.

The nurse must first observe any spontaneous responses to these three scales and use an auditory stimulus if the patient is to be roused, for example, speech. If this does not elicit a response, then a noxious stimulus is applied. It is generally recommended that central pain is used as a stimulus and the source is either

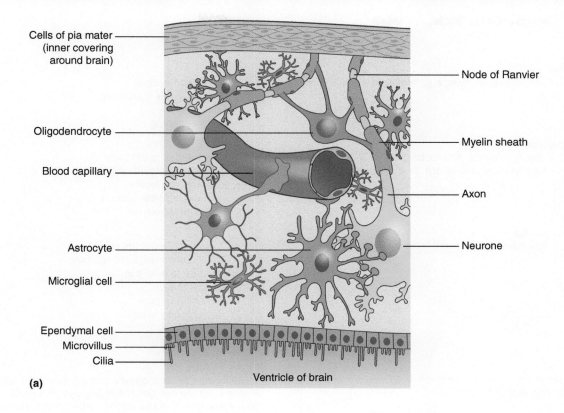

Cells of pia mater
(inner covering
around brain)

Oligodendrocyte

Blood capillary

Astrocyte

Microglial cell

Ependymal cell
Microvillus
Cilia

Node of Ranvier

Myelin sheath

Axon

Neurone

Ventricle of brain

(a)

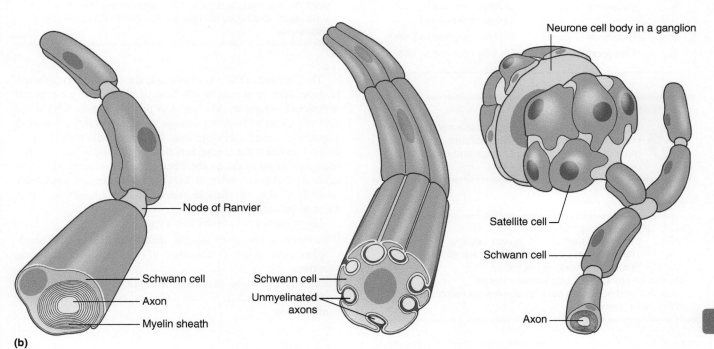

Node of Ranvier

Schwann cell

Axon

Myelin sheath

Schwann cell

Unmyelinated
axons

Neurone cell body in a ganglion

Satellite cell

Schwann cell

Axon

(b)

Figure 32.11 **Neuroglia of the (a) central nervous system and (b) peripheral nervous system.**

591

Table 32.3 **Glasgow Coma Scale.**

FEATURE	RESPONSE	SCORE
Best eye response (Record 'C' if unable to open eyes, e.g. from orbital swelling or facial fractures)	Open spontaneous	4
	Open to verbal commands	3
	Open to pain	2
	No eye opening	1
Best verbal response (Record 'ET' if the person has an endotracheal or 'T' for a tracheostomy tube in place and record 'D' if the person is dysphasic)	Orientated to questions	5
	Disorientated/confused	4
	Inappropriate words	3
	Incomprehensible sounds	2
	No verbal response	1
Best motor response (Record best upper arm response)	To verbal commands obeys	6
	To painful stimuli localises pain	5
	Withdrawal from pain	4
	Flexion to pain	3
	Extension to pain	2
	No response to pain	1

Box 32.1 The AVPU Scale

A	Alert	Are they alert?
V	Responds to voice	Do they respond to verbal stimulation?
P	Responds to pain	Do they respond to pain?
U	Unresponsive	Do they respond at all?

The Nursing Associate

Demonstrate an ability to recognise when a person's condition has improved or deteriorated . . . Interpret (promptly respond, share findings and escalate as needed). (NMC, 2018b)

Red Flag

GCS may be affected if:
· Eyes are closed due to severe swelling
· The verbal and motor responses are absent or reduced because of intubation
· Muscle relaxants have been administered
· Sedation or other drugs such as alcohol and recreational drugs have been taken.

Practice Assessment Document

Undertakes, responds to and interprets neurological observations and assessments. Performs neurological observations using the Glasgow Coma Scale, pupil responses, vital signs and motor function and discusses the recognition of abnormal neurological observations.

Being able to demonstrate that you have met this outcome in a care setting can be challenging due to a range of factors. Take some time to focus on the various types of neurological observation and assessments. Prepare an overview of two types of neurological observations and present these to your supervisor, offering a rationale for the observations being discussed.

The function of the brain, especially the cerebral hemispheres, is dependent on a continuous flow of blood with unimpeded supplies of oxygen and glucose. Any process that disrupts blood flow can cause widespread damage to the cerebral hemispheres, impairing arousal and cognition. LOC may be altered by processes that affect the arousal functions of the brainstem, the cognitive functions of the cerebral hemispheres, or both. There are acute and chronic states of LOC: acute states are potentially reversible, whereas chronic states indicate underlying brain damage and thus are irreversible.

Major causes include the following.

- Intracranial lesions or injuries that affect the cerebral hemispheres or cause dysfunction of the reticular activating system.
- Extracranial causes that cause acute LOC include metabolic disturbances such as alcohol and drug misuse, blood glucose alterations.

Vital Signs

In the neurological patient, changes in vital signs are not consistent with early-warning signals. Vital signs are more useful in detecting progression to late symptoms. As both respiratory and cardiac centres are in the brainstem, compression of the brainstem due to raised intracranial pressure will cause changes in vital signs; see the section on raised intracranial pressure (ICP).

Temperature elevation in the neurological patient can be caused by direct damage to the hypothalamus or traction on the hypothalamus, the primary regulating centre. Cerebral tissue generates a large amount of heat due to high metabolic activity and due to the relatively high blood flow and volume, compared with other organs. Temperature is important, as a 1 °C increase in temperature increases the cerebral metabolic rate by 10%, which could affect neurological recovery.

Assessing Pupillary Reaction

Pupillary assessment is a vital component of neurological assessment. Changes in the size, equality and reactivity of the pupils can provide vital diagnostic information in the critically ill patient. Assessment is performed by shining a light (pen torch) from the direction of the temple into each eye in turn and observing and recording the pupillary reaction or via a pupillometer which uses infrared technology to assess objective pupillary variables including size and constriction velocity.

Under normal conditions, the pupils of both eyes respond identically to a light stimulus, regardless of which eye is being stimulated. Light entering one eye produces brisk constriction of the pupil of that eye, the direct light reflex, as well as constriction of the pupil of the unstimulated eye, the consensual light reflex (pupils are equal and reactive to light, or PEARL); this is recorded as '+', while unreactive pupils are recorded as '−'. Withdrawal of the light should produce an immediate and brisk dilation of both pupils.

The size of the pupil is recorded according to the millimetre scale (as indicated on the neurological observation chart or pen torch). It is also important to note the shape of the pupil: a normal pupil should be round; abnormal pupil shapes may be described as ovoid, keyhole or irregular. Any change in reaction, shape or size of the pupil should be reported and documented immediately.

Motor and Sensory Assessments

Motor function assessment starts with the upper limbs and then progresses to the legs. Assess each limb separately, including assessment of the three 'Ss'.

S Symmetry: observing that both sides of the body move the same.
S Size of the muscle (bulk): observing for wasting, atrophy and hypertrophy.
S Strength of the muscles (power).

In addition, muscle tone is assessed; a soft flabby muscle that fatigues easily is referred to as *flaccidity*, whereas increased tone, evident by increased resistance to passive movement, is referred to as *spasticity*. Assessing for symmetry is the most important consideration when identifying focal findings, i.e. comparing one side of the body with the other. Asymmetrical spontaneous movement and lateralisation (e.g. hemiparesis and hemiplegia) suggest a focal mass lesion on the side of the brain opposite to the side of motor weakness.

Sensory function is an important component of the neurological assessment in people with conditions or diseases that affect the spinal cord or spinal nerves. Assessment involves the ability to perceive various sensations, including touch and sense of position.

Assessing the System: Diagnostic Tests

To enable effective neurological nursing and medical care, an accurate diagnosis is essential. Following physical and neurological examination, several diagnostic tests may be ordered to investigate any abnormal findings, commencing with the least invasive procedures and proceeding to more invasive investigations. Nurses need to be able to provide both emotional support and relevant nursing care before, during and after the procedure.

The Unconscious Patient

Nursing care for an unconscious person is both general and specific. More specific nursing care considerations include the following.

Maintaining a Patent Airway

Support of the airway and respiration is vital in the person with an altered LOC and presents difficulties of ineffective airway clearance and risk of aspiration. A patient who has an altered LOC, who is semi-conscious and unable to maintain their airway, may require an oral pharyngeal airway such as an oropharyngeal or nasopharyngeal airway. However, more severe alterations in consciousness may require endotracheal intubation or a tracheostomy to maintain airway patency. Patients may have a depressed or absent gag and swallowing reflex due to depression of the medullary centres; this presents a high risk for aspiration and increases the risk of pneumonia. Mechanical ventilation is indicated when hypoventilation or apnoea is present. Specific nursing care includes:

- Monitoring breath sounds and rate and depth of respirations and reporting signs and symptoms of aspiration: crackles and wheezes, dyspnoea, tachypnoea and cyanosis
- Suctioning to clear the oropharyngeal airway/tracheostomy of secretion that might otherwise be aspirated
- Positioning the person to allow secretions to drain from the mouth rather than into the pharynx, e.g. lateral position
- Maintaining oxygen saturation levels via prescribed oxygen therapy, monitoring oxygen levels via pulse oximetry and arterial blood gas analysis.

Maintaining Hydration and Nutrition

The patient with reduced consciousness may not be able to maintain normal nutritional status due to reduced intake of nutrients, swallowing problems or cognitive inability to initiate eating. In nutritional assessments, early dietetic advice is crucial and enteral nutrition is important to minimise the effect of protein catabolism and the ensuing loss of lean body mass, by providing sufficient energy and protein. Patients may commence nasogastric feeding, but longer-term enteral feeding regimens are supported with percutaneous endoscopic gastrostomy (PEG) feeding.

Maintaining Mobility and Skin Integrity

Unconscious patients are unable to maintain normal musculoskeletal movement and thus are at high risk for contractures related to decreased movement and inability to maintain skin integrity. Because the flexor and adductor muscles are stronger than the extensors and abductors, flexor and adductor contractures develop quickly without preventive measures. Passive range-of-motion motion exercises (unless contraindicated) must be performed routinely to maintain muscle tone and function, to prevent additional disability and to help restore impaired motor function. Removable orthoses to hold limbs in position may be employed under the direction of the physiotherapist or occupational therapist.

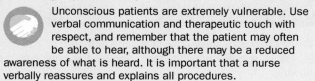

Care, Dignity and Compassion

Unconscious patients are extremely vulnerable. Use verbal communication and therapeutic touch with respect, and remember that the patient may often be able to hear, although there may be a reduced awareness of what is heard. It is important that a nurse verbally reassures and explains all procedures.

The Patient with Raised Intracranial Pressure

In the adult, the rigid, enclosed, inelastic cranial cavity created by the skull is normally filled with three non-compressible interchangeable components (the Monro–Kellie hypothesis): brain parenchyma (85%), blood (7%) and CSF (8%). The pressure exerted by these three non-compressible constituents is referred to as intracranial pressure (ICP). Normal pressure is 0–10 mmHg; sustained elevated pressure of 10 mmHg or higher within the cranial cavity is referred to as increased intracranial pressure (IICP). Transient increases in ICP occur with normal activities, such as coughing, sneezing, straining or bending forward; these are not normally harmful. However, sustained IICP alters cerebral perfusion and oxygenation of brain cells and can result in significant tissue ischaemia and damage to delicate neural tissue. A significant number of neurological patients are at risk of developing increased ICP.

Pathophysiology

The *Monro–Kellie hypothesis* states that the sum of the intracranial volumes of blood, brain and CSF is constant. An increase in volume in any one of the intracranial components must be offset by a decrease in one or more of the others or be associated with a rise in ICP. The body has a limited ability to reduce the volume of these components. The early compensatory mechanisms include moving CSF out of the cranial vault to the spinal subarachnoid space and increased CSF absorption; the venous system is also compressed and cerebral arteries constrict to reduce blood flow. Once these compensatory mechanisms are exhausted, then ICP rises, there is a decrease in cerebral blood flow (CBF) and a subsequent reduction in cerebral perfusion pressure (CPP). Cerebral tissues become ischaemic, and signs and symptoms of cellular hypoxia appear.

The acute physiological response to acute elevations of ICP is known as Cushing's triad. The body's response to the IICP and decrease in CBF triggers a response that increases the arterial pressure to try to overcome the IICP and reduced CBF. Signs of Cushing's triad (response) include:

- Hypertension and widening pulse pressure
- Bradycardia
- Bradypnoea.

If treatment does not stabilise the IICP, then herniation of the brainstem occurs, referred to as tentorium herniation or 'coning', and occlusion of CBF will occur with serious consequences, i.e. severe, permanent neurological deficits or death.

Increased ICP results from three main causes.

- A rise in CSF pressure resulting in dilation of the ventricular system, referred to as *hydrocephalus* ('water on the brain') due to overproduction, decreased absorption or obstruction of flow.
- Increased pressure within the brain caused by a mass (space-occupying lesion), often referred to as the *mass effect*, e.g. tumour, haemorrhage, abscess.
- Swelling within the brain matter itself, due to abnormal accumulation of fluid, which subsequently impedes CBF due to compression of the blood vessels, referred to as *cerebral oedema*.

Signs and Symptoms

These may differ according to the speed and cause of the increased ICP and include:

- Headache, classically worse on rising in the morning, and may worsen with changes of position, coughing and straining
- Vomiting caused by pressure on the vomiting centre
- Oculomotor dysfunction: inability to move the eye(s) upward; ptosis (drooping) of the eyelid due to compression of the cranial nerve III (oculomotor)
- Papilloedema (swelling of the optic discs)
- Double vision (diplopia)
- Progressive deterioration in loc due to displacement of the brainstem
- Late signs: decreased LOC, seizures and pupillary dysfunction, i.e. sluggish response to light progressing to fixed pupils (pupillary dysfunction is first noted on the ipsilateral side)
- Other late signs include *Cushing response*.

Red Flag

Acutely increased intrathoracic pressure causes a significant increase in ICP and a decrease in cerebral perfusion pressure (CPP).

An increase in intrathoracic pressure can occur during the following.

- Valsalva manoeuvre that accompanies straining on defaecation
- Coughing (intra-abdominal pressure), sneezing, vomiting
- Bladder distension
- Extreme hip flexion

Diagnosis and Investigations

A patient presenting with signs of raised ICP requires an urgent CT scan to identify its presence and its underlying cause and to evaluate therapeutic options.

Nursing Care and Management

Primary management is directed at removing the underlying cause of the ICP, if possible. This may involve intracranial surgical techniques to remove a mass, medical treatment of cerebral oedema associated with tumours with dexamethasone (corticosteroid) and strategies to manage hydrocephalus, such as insertion of shunts to redirect the CSF. In addition, treatment is aimed at maintaining adequate CPP, maximising venous return, and reducing blood and CSF volumes. Other treatment options include the following.

- The use of medication to induce an osmotic diuresis (hypertonic saline, mannitol and diuretics).
- Controlled ventilation.
- In some circumstances, when all other measures to reduce ICP prove ineffective, decompressive craniotomy is performed; this involves removal of part of the skull.

Specific Nursing Strategies

Meticulous assessment and monitoring are vital to ensure early detection of signs of IICP and to thus improve patient outcomes. Any changes must be promptly reported for early interventions to be implemented. Multimodal monitoring to detect changes in intracranial dynamics includes measurement of mean arterial pressure (MAP), central venous pressure, pulse, ICP and temperature.

- Elevation of the head of the bed to 30° to promote venous return via the jugular veins.
- Avoiding positions that may obstruct venous return, for example, tracheotomy tapes and cervical collars secured too tightly, and neck rotation and neck and head flexion.
- Maintain normovolaemia through accurate fluid balance, as hypovolaemia causes hypotension and a fall in CPP. Avoid dextrose solutions as these increase cerebral metabolism and oedema, thus increasing ICP.
- Avoid the patient becoming constipated by monitoring and recording bowel movement.
- Monitor for signs of a seizure and administer antiepileptic drugs (AEDs); seizures will result in increased CBF, which could further increase ICP.
- Keep the patient comfortable and pain free to prevent rises in blood pressure and subsequent ICP.
- Treat pyrexia: an increase in body temperature of 1 °C increases cerebral metabolism by up to 10% and therefore increases ICP.
- Maintain nutritional support: this may require enteral feeding (nasogastric tube or PEG).

Traumatic Brain Injury (Head Injury)

Traumatic brain injury (TBI) is defined as an alteration in brain function because of injury from external causes. External causes include the head striking, or being struck by, an object, which may penetrate the brain, and the brain undergoing acceleration or deceleration. Severity can range from a mild concussion to coma or death. TBI is a leading cause of mortality and morbidity in young people and is a worldwide public health problem that can cause long-term disability even in mild TBI, with impairments including physical, cognitive and psychological disabilities. It disrupts not only the patient's life but also the lives of their families/caregivers and socioeconomic costs are high. Although many patients are transferred to specialist neuroscience centres, many TBI patients are managed in general critical care units.

Epidemiology

Epidemiological data are inconsistent and difficult to collate, partly because the majority of TBIs are classified as mild (80%), are not admitted to hospital and many do not seek medical assistance. However, data indicate that over 1 000 000 people will attend emergency departments with a TBI in the UK, with a predominance of adolescent and young adult men and the elderly population. The main causes of a TBI include road traffic accidents, assaults, fall (from any height) and accidents at work or home.

Pathophysiology

Each TBI has a unique set of circumstances and consequences for the patient. The most common method of classifying a TBI uses the labels 'mild', 'moderate' and 'severe'; this classification is dependent on certain characteristics including GCS, period of loss of consciousness, and length of time (post injury) patients remain in a post-traumatic amnesic state, which is a period of confusion and disorientation after emergence from a coma (Table 32.4). It is important to make the distinction between minor, moderate and severe TBI because of the morbidity associated with severe trauma to the head.

In addition to classifying the injury according to severity, a TBI can be classified according to the mechanism of injury, the location of the injury (either focal or diffuse), and whether the injury is open or closed.

Mechanisms of Injury The mechanism of injury is often referred to as the 'primary injury' induced by a mechanical force such as being struck by an object, which may penetrate the brain, and the brain undergoing an acceleration/deceleration movement.

Location of the Injury This refers to the area of the brain which may be localised or focal such as bruising or contusions and haemorrhages. Diffuse or global ischaemic injury occurs due to hypotension, or secondary to raised ICP or shearing and stretching of the neurones called diffuse axonal injury (DAI).

Table 32.4 Classification of TBI by severity.

TBI GRADE	GCS SCORE	SYMPTOMS
Mild, often referred to as concussion	GCS 13–15	LOC <30 minutes, PTA <1 hour Transient symptoms, e.g. dizziness, confusion, headache and vomiting
Moderate	GCS 9–13	LOC 1–24 hours PTA 30 minutes to 24 hours Lethargic or stuporous
Severe	GCS 3–8	LOC severe 1–7 days PTA Very severe 1–4 weeks, extremely severe >4 weeks

LOC, loss of consciousness; PTA, post-traumatic amnesia.

Open Versus Closed *Closed* refers to when the integrity of the skull is not compromised, whereas *open* (penetrating) is when the outer layer of the meninges is breached.

Secondary Injuries These occur after the initial injury has occurred; the brain progressive response is both complex and multifaceted and may include cerebral oedema, vascular injury, seizures and infection.

Diagnosis and Investigations

Radiological examinations include skull X-rays (to identify skull fractures and assess penetrating objects) and CT or MRI (to detect contusions). Other investigations include oxygen saturations and arterial blood gases, with particular attention paid to oxygen and carbon dioxide levels. TBI patients are at high risk of an associated cervical spine injury and should have their neck immobilised until further investigations can be carried out (e.g. cervical spine X-ray).

Signs and Symptoms

Signs and symptoms are varied according to the area of the brain that has been injured. Compression of the brain tissue may result in seizures.

Red Flag

The following red flag signs and symptoms are markers of a more severe TBI.
- Loss of consciousness at any time
- GCS <15 on initial assessment
- Focal neurological deficit
- Retrograde or anterograde amnesia
- Persistent headache
- Vomiting or seizures post injury

When the brain is injured, the response is also complex and multifaceted. The entire spectrum of TBI, from mild to severe, can change a person's function in three major areas: physical (including language), cognitive and emotional/behavioural. However, it is the unseen cognitive, behavioural and emotional sequelae that cause the most serious long-term morbidity and are most important in determining independence, social functioning and family adjustment. These difficulties can negatively impact patients' ability to establish productive and satisfying lifestyles, and affect family members and caregivers, causing caregiver burden, distress and a sense of loss.

Nursing Care and Management

The management of TBI patients is aimed at re-establishing the equilibrium of the intracranial contents and preventing secondary injury (from ischaemia, hypoxia and cerebral compression). Neurological observations (see GCS earlier) are essential, providing a baseline for comparison with future observations and immediate evidence of any deterioration or responses to treatment strategies. The person with a TBI is at high risk for raised ICP (see earlier).

Box 32.2 The ABCDE

A *Airway*: intubation is required for severe TBI patients (GCS <8)
B *Breathing*: maintain oxygenation and normocapnia
C *Circulation*:
- Measure heart rate and blood pressure
- Treat hypotension, aiming for a target MAP of >80 mmHg (Brain Trauma Foundation, 2014)

D *Disability*: assess consciousness using the GCS for baseline and to detect changes in conscious level, and assess the severity of the injury
E *Exposure and environment*: look for signs of injury, e.g. scalp wounds, bleeding from ears and nose

---

Early assessment and management involve:
- Assessment and stabilisation of the airway, breathing and circulation (Box 32.2)
- Assessment of neurological status
- Ascertaining the degree of injury to initiate appropriate levels of care.

Surgery may include the following:
- Surgical evacuation of a clot via either burr holes made into the skull or a craniotomy
- Decompressive craniectomy: removal of part of the cranium (skull) to relieve pressure on the underlying brain and allow the brain to swell upward rather than downward, where it will compress the brainstem, leading to brain death.

Traumatic brain injury provokes hypercatabolism and if left unmanaged, the ensuing malnutrition accentuates immune compromise, so increasing the risk of infection. To ensure nutritional requirements are met, early nutritional assessment and referral to a dietitian for feeding regimens such as enteral feeding are critical.

Red Flag

Never suction a person nasally if they have a basilar skull fracture or have CSF draining from the ears or nose, as catheters could be inadvertently advanced into the cranial cavity.

Case Study

Saeed is a 17 year old who has been admitted to emergency department (ED) after being hit with a cricket ball at school. Upon arrival to the ED, Saeed is conscious with a GCS of 14 (E4 V4 M6) and it is noted he is having trouble recalling the events immediately before or after the accident (post-traumatic amnesia [PTA]).

As Saeed has sustained a significant mild TBI, he is admitted for close neurological observations using the GCS. The following day his GCS is reported to be 15 and he is discharged home.

Adjustment following TBI is a dynamic process and changes over time and Saeed may have residual deficits for

(Continued)

several months. Following mild TBI, if symptoms persist beyond the typical recovery period of 3 months, the term *postconcussion syndrome* is used. It is important to note here that in Saeed's recovery, two processes are occurring at the same time: recovery from brain injury and normal developmental changes in cognitive, behavioural, emotional and social functioning, so the full effects of his injury may not manifest until schoolwork demands a higher level of performance. Providing support and information is important for both Saeed and his family and should include:

- that he should make a full recovery without permanent deficits with time
- take plenty of rest
- not to train or play sport for at least 3 weeks without seeking medical advice as it is dangerous to risk a secondary injury whilst still recovering as a second injury may result in *secondary impact syndrome* – a phenomenon that occurs when a secondary TBI occurs before the initial TBI has not healed, which may be fatal
- inform the school nurse/community nurse for review and further advice
- signpost to support organisations such as Headway (**www.headway.org**).

Stroke

A stroke is a preventable and treatable disease, characterised by a gradual or rapid onset of neurological deficits due to a sudden decrease in CBF to an area of the brain. It is a major medical emergency, requiring rapid treatment to prevent avoidable death and long-term disability.

Epidemiology
Stroke is a major healthcare problem in the UK, is the second most common cause of death in Europe and the leading cause of disability (Wilkins *et al.*, 2017). Few stroke victims will make a full recovery, and most are left with some form of disability. An estimated 20–30% of people who have had a stroke will die within 1 month. The risk of recurrent stroke is 10.4% within 1 year of a first stroke and 12.9% at 10 years (Lin *et al.*, 2021).

Pathophysiology There are two main types of strokes, ischaemic and haemorrhagic.

- *Ischaemic*: up to 80–85% of all strokes are caused by blockage of one of the arteries in the brain, with reduced oxygen supply to brain cells, which can lead to irreversible brain damage and death of brain cells; also known as *infarction*.
- *Haemorrhagic*: a bleed in the brain (burst blood vessel) known as *cerebral haemorrhage* (about 15–20% of all strokes); also referred to as intracranial haemorrhage (ICH).

Potential Risk Factors There are several risk factors for stroke, summarised in Box 32.3. Transient ischaemic attack (TIA), often referred to as a *ministroke*, is a clinical syndrome presenting as acute loss of focal cerebral or monocular function due to inadequate cerebral or ocular blood supply and lasting less than 24 hours; there is rarely loss of consciousness and patients make a complete recovery. TIAs may be an indication that a stroke may occur.

Red Flag

Ischaemic stroke and TIAs are commonly more likely to occur:
- When blood pressure is at its lowest, i.e. waking from sleep
- When there is a sudden change in blood pressure, which may dislodge an embolism in the arterial circulation, e.g. getting out of bed.

Box 32.3 Risk Factors for Stroke

Controllable factors
- Lifestyle habits, e.g., smoking, sedentary lifestyle, drug abuse
- Dietary factors, hyperlipidaemia, excessive alcohol
- Exceeding the recommended daily alcohol limit
- Certain diseases, e.g. diabetes mellitus, carotid artery disease, heart disease

Uncontrollable factors
- Age: incidence of stroke increases dramatically over the age of 55 years
- Gender: more common in men than women
- Race: higher incidences found in South Asia, Africa and the Caribbean
- Family history of stroke or TIA
- Fibromuscular dysplasia

Signs and Symptoms
The constellations of signs and symptoms of the neurological deficits reflect the vessel affected, along with the size and areas of the brain affected and the length of time blood flow is decreased or stopped. Signs and symptoms include:

- Loss of consciousness, nausea and vomiting
- Localised (focal) sensory and motor deficits, usually one-sided
- Dysphagia: can be the sole and over-riding symptom
- Seizure activity
- Communication difficulties
- Visual field deficits 20–57% (Pollock *et al.*, 2019)
- Behavioural and emotional changes.

As the motor pathways cross at the junction of the medulla and spinal cord (decussation), loss or impairment of sensory motor functions occurs on the side of the body opposite to the side of the brain that is damaged. Hemiplegia that develops because of loss of descending motor control may occur in two stages: initially, reduced tone with a flaccid limb (hypotonia); if muscle tone recovers, this may result in a spastic limb (hypertonia), known as spastic paralysis.

Diagnosis and Investigations
Early assessment and diagnosis are crucial for effective management decisions. This may begin outside the hospital when a person suddenly develops neurological symptoms, with screening using the FAST tool to confirm likely stroke or TIA (Box 32.4). Nearly half of the stroke risk following a TIA occurs within the first 48 hours, so people who have had a TIA require urgent referral to the stroke service so that early interventions can be implemented if necessary to reduce the risk of stroke. If confirmed

FAST-positive within 4 hours of onset of symptoms, then the patient should be transferred to a hyperacute stroke unit (HASU) where they will undergo rapid assessment and investigations, treatment and monitoring 24 hours a day.

Box 32.4 FAST Assessment

F   Face:
  · Has their face fallen on one side?
  · Can they smile?
A   Arms:
  · Can they raise both arms and keep them up?
S   Speech:
  · Is their speech slurred?
T   Time to call 999:
  · If you see any single one of these signs

Source: NHS (2021)

Nursing Care and Management

Urgent assessment is particularly crucial for those who have suffered an acute ischaemic stroke and require intravenous thrombolysis with alteplase to dissolves the thrombus, administered up to 4.5 hours from onset of stroke. Alternatively, mechanical clot retrieval (thrombectomy) within 6 hours of the onset of symptoms may be used for large clots and for those patients in whom thrombolysis is contraindicated. Both procedures aim to remove the clot and restore blood flow to cells starved of oxygen and thus minimise brain tissue damage.

Close monitoring in the initial period following a stroke is critical and monitoring for complications post thrombolysis treatment, such as haemorrhage, is also important. Nurses need to be able to appropriately assess the patient and recognise early signs of raised ICP (see earlier).

Management of haemorrhagic strokes (ICH) in acute stroke units is just as crucial as for ischaemic strokes. This may include acute lowering of blood pressure following ICH in people with hypertension, although the optimal approach to the management of elevated blood pressure in patients with acute stroke remains controversial; this is partly because lowering the blood pressure compromises cerebral perfusion in the context of acute stroke.

Swallow screening is an important consideration because dysphagia (difficulty in swallowing) is a common and potentially serious complication of stroke and is associated with an increased risk of aspiration, due to the prolonged transit time, and of associated bronchopulmonary infections, dehydration and malnutrition. The *National Clinical Guideline for Stroke* (Rudd *et al.*, 2017) recommend that this is carried out by a specialist with appropriate skills and training. Nurses are in key positions to undertake early screening.

Following a swallowing assessment, those people with dysphagia may require consistency modifications of diet and fluid (i.e. in a form they can swallow). This may include thickened liquids, a common intervention that aims to control the speed, direction, duration and clearance of a bolus and reduce the risk of aspiration. However, thickened fluids are often associated with patient dissatisfaction and poor compliance, which may lead to poor quality of life and reduced fluid intake and an

increased risk of malnutrition and dehydration. Thus, nurses must monitor this closely to prevent dehydration and seek to find products that suit the person's lifestyle and taste. Other strategies may include oral nutritional supplements, specialist dietary advice and/or enteral feeding (nasogastric tube or PEG). Educating carers involved in the care of people with dysphagia is essential in ensuring compliance.

Practice Assessment Document

Supports people with their diet and nutritional needs, taking cultural practices into account and uses appropriate aids to assist when needed
  Eating and drinking are activities of living that are key to health and well-being. When addressing this practice outcome, how might you undertake a robust and meaningful assessment of a person's diet and nutritional needs? In the care area where you are working, put together, with the help of your supervisor and other health and care staff, a fact sheet detailing the practices that nurses and others need to consider when ensuring people are offered culturally sensitive care that is appropriate and responsive to a person's individual needs.

Medicines Management

A patient receiving intravenous alteplase requires close neurological monitoring and observations, including observing for bleeding, orolingual angio-oedema (swelling starting in the tongue, which may rapidly progress to cause upper airway obstruction, which may be fatal) and signs of raised intracranial pressure.

A central part of recovery from stroke is to create a safe and therapeutic environment to ensure positive outcomes. The goal for the patient is to achieve as much independence as possible through learning to adapt to their disabilities. There should be early identification of problems and referral to relevant members of the multidisciplinary team, such as physiotherapists for exercise, posture and rehabilitation programmes; speech and language therapists for specialised swallowing (for those who fail a swallow screen) and speech assessments; and occupational therapists for evaluation and activities to remediate performance skill deficits, body structure and function impairment.

Patients with detected or suspected visual field defects should be referred for formal visual assessment. Patients with visual field defects experience difficulties with activities of living, such as eating, washing and dressing, and are at increased risk of falling and bumping into objects (see Chapter 33).

The Nursing Associate

A *Platform 6* Contribute to integrated care to meet the needs of people across organisations and settings. 6.1 understand the roles of the different providers of health and care (NMC, 2018b).

What the Experts Say

" 'Neurological rehabilitation following nervous system damage, e.g. TBI, stroke and multiple sclerosis, aims to facilitate neural recovery and prevent contractures. Splinting, the application of an external device to maintain a position of a limb, aims to prevent and correct contractures and improve function through an increased range of movement.'
Penny, occupational therapist

Post-stroke patients can suffer from a range of mood disturbances including depression, anxiety and emotional lability, which can have a significant and negative impact on functional recovery. Depression is a major issue after stroke, affecting approximately one-third of patients (Hackett & Anderson, 2014). Early identification and treatment of post-stroke depression may enhance functional recovery. The *National Clinical Guideline for Stroke* (Rudd *et al.*, 2017) advocates screening for mood disturbances following stroke. Nurses can make an active contribution to detecting mood symptoms with stroke survivors and refer to specialists for treatment and contribute to the monitoring and adjusting of medication.

Nurses can both promote and encourage participation in rehabilitation and exercise programmes to help prevent the wasting (atrophy) of leg muscles and restore function. Prevention is undeniably the most effective strategy to reduce the burden of stroke and at the forefront of stroke prevention is the role of nurses in initiating lifestyle modifications aimed at improvements in risk factors such as hypertension, hypercholesterolaemia, obesity and preventing a recurrence. This includes:

- Smoking cessation and low-to-moderate alcohol intake
- Consuming a healthy diet
- Moderate-to-vigorous exercise (NMC, 2018b).

Neurological Oncology

Central nervous system cancers comprise a group of nearly 100 different types of primary tumours, with different incidence rates, clinical behaviour and response to treatment and prognosis (Crocetti *et al.*, 2012). Some brain tumours can be cured by surgery, some are rapidly fatal despite treatment, and some do not require treatment.

Epidemiology

Overall, CNS tumours are relatively rare, accounting for about 2% of all cancers, and those arising from the neuroglia cells, known as gliomas, are the most common (6–8 per 100000 per year). However, brain tumours are the fourth most common tumour, the biggest cancer killer under the age of 40 years and the eighth most common under the age of 65. Survival rates for brain tumours have improved little over the last 40 years despite improvements in modern medicine, with 40% of adults diagnosed with a brain tumour surviving their cancer for 1 year or more (Cancer Research UK, 2021).

Glial tumours are subdivided and analysed following the WHO classification; gradings range from WHO low Grade I to high Grade IV (Louis *et al.*, 2016). Of all brain tumours, glioblastoma multiforme (Grade IV) is the most aggressive, characterised by rapid glial cell growth and spread throughout the CNS and resistant to radiotherapy and chemotherapy.

Pathophysiology

Brain tumours grow within and originating from the brain parenchyma, most of which are gliomas, but they can also arise from:

- Structures adjacent to the brain that can compress and distort it, for example meningiomas arising from the meninges, schwannomas from the cranial nerves and adenomas from the pituitary gland
- Metastatic tumours originating from outside the CNS; the most common sources are carcinomas of the breast, lung and kidney and malignant melanoma.

The concept of 'benign' and 'malignant' in the brain implies simple local expansion versus brain parenchymal invasion.

Risk Factors The cause of glioma is unknown, although previous exposure to ionising radiation is a known risk factor. Some patient groups have genetic abnormalities that convey a lifelong risk of glial or other tumours, e.g. neurofibromatosis, tuberous sclerosis.

Signs and Symptoms

Signs and symptoms are dependent on location, rate of growth and invasiveness. The brain can be divided into 'eloquent' and 'silent' areas.

- *Eloquent:* tumour with significant neurological signs and symptoms, including:
  - Speech areas in the temporal and frontal lobes
  - Primary motor cortex in the frontal lobe
  - Visual cortex in the occipital lobe.
- *Silent:* areas where the tumour may grow to a significant size without any obvious neurological signs and symptoms; includes frontal and non-dominant temporal lobes.

Presentations may be dramatic, with seizures or focal symptoms that reflect the site of the lesion in the brain. However, tumours in silent areas may produce only subtle focal symptoms (e.g. personality change, motivational impairment). Many tumours are not suspected until a patient complains of headache, usually worse in the morning, due to raised ICP caused by the space-occupying effect of the tumour mass and oedema; it may also be associated with vomiting. Other symptoms may include:

- Altered consciousness
- Changes in cognition and behaviour
- Epileptic seizures
- Limb weakness, hemiparesis, unsteadiness and abnormal gait
- Visual disturbances, e.g. diplopia (double vision) and loss of vision.

Diagnosis and Investigations

Along with a full medical and surgical history, a range of assessment measures appropriate to the location of the lesion and suspected type of tumour are carried out; these are summarised in Box 32.5.

> **Box 32.5 Summary of Investigations and Tests for Patients with Brain Tumours**
>
> · Karnofsky Performance Status scale: measures the patient's functional ability and general well-being.
> · MRI scan of the brain and spine, usually with intravenous injection of the contrast agent gadolinium.
> · Whole-body CT scan for persons with metastases or PET scan (to detect primary neoplasms).
> · Chest X-ray.
> · Blood tests: for example, germ cell tumours produce chemicals (tumour markers) that can be detected in blood.
> · Laboratory tests, such as staining of tissues and cells to microscopically determine type and proliferation of tumour cells, and erythrocyte sedimentation rate (ESR).
> · Genetic screening, for example in cases of neurofibromatosis and tuberous sclerosis.
> · Angiography: to visualise blood vessels near the lesion.
> · Intracarotid sodium amobarbital (WADA) presurgical test to determine cerebral language localisation; this is useful in deciding how much tissue can be safely removed.
> · Brainstem auditory evoked responses and visually evoked responses.

Nursing Care and Management

Treatment options are varied and depend on the tumour histology, grade and location, and patient's functional level, assessed using the Karnofsky Performance Status which measures the patient's functional ability and general well-being.

Surgery

· Tumour biopsy: the removal of a sample of tissue to examine under a microscope, enabling a diagnosis to be made.
· Partial resection or debulking (partial removal of the tumour when it cannot be completely removed) or total resection (complete removal of the tumour).

· Methods to maximise resection of malignant gliomas include intraoperative visualisation using 5-aminolevulinic acid (5-ALA), a dye that makes brain tumour cells glow red under ultraviolet (UV) light, which then helps the surgeon to check they are removing as much brain tumour as possible, or intraoperative MRI.
· Insertion of biodegradable wafer impregnated with carmustine (Gliadel®), a chemotherapeutic agent that slowly releases into residual tissue; the wafer is placed into the resection cavity following glioma removal.

Radiotherapy and Chemotherapy

After surgery (biopsy or resection), the use of external beam radiotherapy and/or chemotherapy is dependent on the grade and location of the tumour.

· *Radiotherapy*: includes stereotactic radiation therapy (Gamma Knife®) and robotic radiation therapy (CyberKnife®), often used to treat small tumours close to very important structures in the brain; and proton beam radiotherapy.
· *Chemotherapy*: for example, temozolomide (TMZ), often used in conjunction with radiotherapy.

Steroids

Cerebral oedema is a common feature of cerebral tumours and contributes greatly to the neurological deterioration of the patient and causes symptoms of raised ICP. Corticosteroids, such as dexamethasone, are used to treat oedema, although side-effects increase with dose and duration of treatment; thus doses are carefully considered.

A brain tumour diagnosis could signal the start of a long period of uncertainty and fear about the future for those involved. Additionally, patients may have neurological and cognitive, behavioural and emotional deficits that they and their families/carers have to cope with before and/or after surgery. Patients may also experience side-effects from chemotherapy and following radiotherapy (these are covered in more detail in Chapter 15). More specific side-effects related to the treatment therapies and how these might be managed are described in Table 32.5.

Table 32.5 Treatment therapies and how these might be managed.

TREATMENT	SPECIFIC SIDE-EFFECTS	NURSING CONSIDERATIONS
Cranial radiotherapy	Worsening of presenting neurological signs and symptoms due to cerebral oedema Accumulative fatigue as the treatment progresses Hair loss (alopecia) due to damage to the hair roots during therapy; tends to occur 2–3 weeks after treatment Hypersensitivity to taste and smell due to stimulation of the olfactory nerve endings during treatment	Reassurance and support when the symptoms occur Steroids may be prescribed to counter cerebral oedema Observe for headaches and manage with analgesia, such as paracetamol Inform the patient that they are entitled to a wig on NHS prescription Changes in taste and smell may reduce appetite, so ensure that the patient receives adequate nutrition
Corticosteroid therapy, e.g. dexamethasone	Increased susceptibility to infections Disturbances in behaviour, e.g. irritability, insomnia, agitation Metabolic and endocrine changes, e.g. hyperglycaemia, increased appetite, Cushing syndrome	Ensure that patient has written information regarding steroid side-effects and management of side-effects Advise the patient that steroids cannot be stopped abruptly due to suppression of adrenal gland production of cortisol Monitor blood glucose for hyperglycaemia

Apart from postsurgical or radiotherapy care, the key aspects of nursing management are the same as for the patient with a TBI and/or raised ICP (see earlier).

Specific Nursing Considerations

- Observe for signs of diabetes insipidus, the production of a large quantity of urine with low specific gravity caused by decreased secretion of antidiuretic hormone (ADH), because of surgical manipulation of the pituitary gland.
- Maintain an accurate fluid balance.
- Assess the patient for serum electrolyte levels, urine osmolality, urine specific gravity and urine sodium level.
- Observe cranial wound site for signs of infection and CSF leakage.
- Assess the level of pain (headache) related to stretching and cutting of the brain tissues following surgery and increase in ICP using a validated rating scale and administer analgesics as prescribed.

The diagnosis of an intracranial tumour brings anxiety and feelings of uncertainty about the future. Both the patient and family members are likely to be apprehensive and require education and emotional support. Clear, relevant and timely information is important and may include:

- An overall treatment plan, procedures and investigations along with management of deficits and/or disabilities
- Referral to a neuro-oncology specialist nurse for additional support information and guidance.

Infections of the CNS

The list of pathogens that infect the CNS is limitless and includes viruses, bacteria, parasites and fungi. Infections can be broadly categorised into three groups, depending on the part of the CNS tissue affected and the extent of the infection. Infection of the meninges is called meningitis and that of brain tissue is called encephalitis. A localised collection of pus in the brain is called a brain abscess.

Epidemiology

Bacterial meningitis is common worldwide, with an annual incidence rate of 5 per 100 000, and is a notifiable disease, whereas brain abscesses and encephalitis are rare conditions affecting all ages and both sexes. Despite its rarity, encephalitis is of public healthcare importance because of its high morbidity and mortality rates.

Pathophysiology

Infectious agents that cause meningitis enter the CSF via fractures of the skull or circulating blood and breaching of the BBB. The inflammatory response within the subarachnoid space may result in pus, affecting the flow of CSF and causing a subsequent rise in ICP. The infection may spread down the spinal cord and the sheaths of the cranial nerves.

Over 100 different infectious agents may cause encephalitis, although the aetiology of encephalitis remains unknown in most cases. The most commonly identified pathogen in the UK is the herpes simplex virus (HSV or the cold sore virus). Encephalitis is caused by brain cell dysfunction due to direct infective invasion and associated inflammatory changes.

Abscesses begin as a localised area of cerebritis that later evolves into a pus-filled area, which then becomes encapsulated with vascularised tissue and collagen fibre; this is visible on a CT scan with contrast as a white ring.

Risk Factors

- *Meningitis*: impaired immune system caused by other diseases or in patients receiving cytotoxic therapy; infection elsewhere within the body, e.g. penetrating head injury; neurosurgical procedures, e.g. lumbar puncture or epidural anaesthesia.
- *Encephalitis*: mosquito and tick bites enhance the likelihood of encephalitis virus spread.
- *Brain abscess*: solitary or multiple; may occur following brain surgery or penetrating injury, or by haematogenous spread of infection from nearby structures, e.g. middle ear or frontal sinuses.

Signs and Symptoms

A person with meningitis may present with a variety of symptoms.

- Fever
- Restlessness, irritability and agitation
- Meningeal irritation: cervical rigidity and head retraction due to widespread muscular rigidity, photophobia
- Raised ICP
- Seizures
- Petechial rash (small spots) (in meningococcal meningitis)
- Kernig's sign and Brudzinski's sign, thought to be caused by irritation of motor nerve roots passing through inflamed meninges.

Patients with encephalitis typically present with fever, headache and alteration of consciousness. However, the diversity of neurological symptoms can make it difficult to distinguish encephalitis from other infectious and non-infectious CNS conditions.

Brain abscess typically begins with fever, focal neurological signs and headaches and later raised ICP may occur due to enlargement of the lesion and surrounding localised swelling.

Diagnosis and Investigations

Computed tomography scan with contrast may show the extent of inflammation in the brain in encephalitis and help differentiate encephalitis from other conditions; CT may also show abscesses. Lumbar puncture, providing there are no signs of raised ICP, allows collection of CSF for culture and identification of causative organisms in cases of meningitis and some cases of encephalitis. Genetic material from HSV, varicella zoster virus (chickenpox) and enteroviruses can also be detected by a specific CSF test (polymerase chain reaction, PCR).

Nursing Care and Management

Central nervous system infections are associated with high morbidity and mortality and therefore early recognition and treatment are critical to preventing neurological deterioration and life-threatening complications. Patients may be extremely ill, requiring basic nursing care in addition to constant monitoring.

Nursing care associated with altered LOC, raised ICP and seizures is also appropriate for the person with a CNS infection.

Specific Nursing Management
- Isolation/barrier nursing considerations (if required for bacterial meningitis); see Chapter 16 for further information.
- Care of the intravenous site for the administration of intravenous antibiotics or antivirals.
- Provision of information and prophylaxis (treatment, screening) to close family/carers, e.g. to eliminate nasopharyngeal carriage of organisms.

Epilepsy

Epilepsy is a common chronic disorder characterised by an abnormal, unpredictable and often unprovoked, recurrent, excessive and self-terminating electrical discharge from brain neurones. This abnormal transient neuronal activity may involve all or part of the brain and disturbs skeletal motor function, sensation, the autonomic function of the viscera, behaviour and/or consciousness. Epilepsy is the name given to the diverse group of conditions all having in common the presence of at least one seizure and its neurobiological, cognitive, psychological and social consequences.

Epidemiology
Epilepsy is the most common serious neurological condition in the world, affecting up to 50 million people. In the UK, there are 600 000 people with epilepsy and one in every 220 children has a diagnosis of epilepsy (Epilepsy Action, 2021). Epilepsy carries a risk to life; in the UK, approximately 1000 people every year will die due to epilepsy, with most premature deaths associated with accidents and injuries.

Pathophysiology
A full understanding of epilepsy is not known. However, it is recognised that epilepsy occurs when brain neurones produce an abnormal rhythmic and repetitive hypersynchronous discharge, referred to as the *epileptogenic focus*. This electrical discharge can be recorded with EEG scalp electrodes. Neurotransmitters play an important part in the balance between excitation and inhibition in the CNS. During a seizure, the metabolic needs of the brain increase dramatically, resulting in an increased demand for glucose and oxygen by as much as 60%. If CBF cannot meet these increased needs, cellular exhaustion and cellular destruction may result. Seizures are generally self-limiting, although in some cases generalised seizures continue for 30 minutes or more; this is termed *status epilepticus* and is a major life-threatening medical emergency.

Epileptic seizures may also occur after an acute CNS insult from structural, systemic, toxic, metabolic or genetic causes. Approximately 60% of epilepsies have no identifiable cause.

Diagnosis and Investigations
- Comprehensive clinical history from patients/eyewitnesses to the attack.
- Diagnostic testing to detect any abnormal structures that may be treatable, e.g. skull X-ray, MRI or CT scan.
- Electroencephalogram (EEG) helps to localise the epileptogenic focus and confirm diagnosis.
- Blood tests to exclude any metabolic causes, e.g. hypoglycaemia.
- CSF examination for CNS infections.
- Other tests may be carried out to explore cardiac or psychogenic causes.

There are currently over 60 different types of epilepsy with no agreed universal classification system but they can be categorised into focal (or partial) seizures, generalised seizures, and unknown onset (Fisher *et al.*, 2017).

- *Focal or partial seizures*: result from abnormal neuronal activity that is localised, causing partial or focal seizures, usually involving one part or several different parts of the brain at the onset.
- *Generalised seizures*: affect all or most of the brain and consciousness is always impaired.

Signs and Symptoms
Clinical signs of seizures depend on the location of the epileptogenic focus and the extent and pattern of the epileptic discharge. Typical signs include:
- Temporary changes in mental status and LOC
- Abnormal behaviour
- Sensory disturbance.

Non-epileptic Seizures (NES) or Non-epileptic Attack Disorder These are events that resemble epileptic seizures and are relatively common. There are other names for this condition, such as pseudo-seizures and psychological seizures, but they are not used today. There are two major types of NES.

- *Psychogenic NES (PNES)*: episodes of altered movement, sensation or experience caused by a psychological process, not by abnormal electrical signals in the brain or by brain damage (Doss & LaFrance, 2017). The cause of PNES is unknown but it is often associated with previous trauma, for example childhood abuse or neglect, and is often triggered by stressful/challenging life events or changes in physical or mental health.
- *Physiological NES*: caused by physiological dysfunction, e.g. cardiac arrhythmias, hypotensive episodes or cerebrovascular disease, that may result in loss of consciousness with or without motor signs such as twitching.

Non-epileptic seizure can be difficult to differentiate from events due to epilepsy, and misdiagnosis leads to inappropriate treatment with antiepileptic drugs. The gold standard for the diagnosis of PNES is video-electroencephalography (video-EEG), whereby behavioural events are observed and recorded along with simultaneous ECG recording, often carried out in specialised epilepsy monitoring centres. The absence of epileptic activity on the EEG before, during or after an event suggests a diagnosis of PNES. A correct diagnosis is important to ensure appropriate interventions and improvement in the person's quality of life. Table 32.6 illustrates the difference between NES and epilepsy.

Table 32.6 Different behaviours and observations during psychogenic non-epileptic seizures and epileptic seizures.

FEATURE	NON-EPILEPTIC SEIZURES	EPILEPTIC SEIZURES
Response to verbal commands	Yes	No
Pupil reaction to light	Yes	No
Eyes	Shut and resist eyelid opening	Open, with gaze straightforward or deviated
Avoids danger	Yes	No
Synchronised purposeful movements	Yes (side-to-side head and body movement is common)	No
Seizures occurring in medical settings or in front of an audience	Yes	Uncommon
Postictal recovery	Rapid recovery and accompanied by shallow, quiet and irregular breathing	Stertorous breathing

Nursing Care and Management

Medicines Management

Most people with epilepsy are treated with antiepileptic drugs (AEDs) which are aimed at:
· Reducing or controlling seizure activity without impairing cognitive function by raising the seizure threshold in the motor cortex or by limiting the spread of rapidly firing epileptic foci in the brain.
· Preventing irreversible complications because of a seizure.
Where possible, the lowest possible dose of a single medication that will control the seizures is prescribed on an individual basis.

Some people may not achieve full control of their epilepsy despite receiving AEDs, and alternative treatments may be offered, including:

- Surgery to remove the epileptogenic focus via stereotactic radiotherapy (GammaKnife), neurostimulation therapy such as deep brain stimulation, or surgical resection
- Vagal nerve stimulation, designed to prevent seizures by transmitting regular small pulses of electrical energy to the brain via the vagus nerve.

Whether a person has established epilepsy or has been admitted after their first seizure, the nurse has an important management and education role. Observing and providing a written account during an attack should include the following.

Before the seizure (preictal)
Was there any warning (aura) that may have preceded the generalised seizure activity, e.g. sense of uneasiness or an abnormal gustatory, visual, auditory or visceral sensation? Seizures often occur without auras.

During the seizure (ictal)
- Was there a loss of postural control? The patient may fall to the floor with muscle rigidity, jaw clenched.
- Was there a sudden loss of consciousness?
- Was there any urinary incontinence or bowel incontinence?

After the seizure (postictal)
- Is there any confusion and/or disorientation?
- Any amnesia of the seizure and the events just before the seizure activity?

Seizure recognition, seizure management and awareness of the associated risks are important nursing care issues. In the hospital setting, the following should be considered for a patient known to have epilepsy: call bell near to hand, bedside oxygen and suction equipment, and lowering the bed to near the floor. Immediate care of a patient during a seizure includes the following.

- Do not restrain the patient or put anything into their mouth.
- Provide a safe environment to protect the patient from unnecessary harm.
- Secure airway and administer oxygen.
- Assess cardiorespiratory function.
- Stay with the patient to reassure and reorientate.
- Prevent the patient from injuring themselves, loosen clothing around the neck, place in the recovery position (after the clonic phase, suctioning if excessive salivation).
- Administer rescue AEDs, such as nasal/buccal midazolam or rectal diazepam, to abort the seizure and prevent status epilepticus.
- Record and report the seizure (start and stop time, activity during the seizure) on a seizure chart.

Case Study

Bianca, a 27-year-old accountant with no previous medical history of note, experiences a generalised seizure. Following admission to hospital and tests (MRI and EEG), she is diagnosed with epilepsy and commenced on AEDs and is due for discharge home soon. Bianca lives with her partner and enjoys socialising at the weekends.

As Bianca is newly diagnosed, she will need help and support in coming to terms with her diagnosis. Being aware of the stigma and psychosocial effects of having, or fear of having, recurrent seizures is important, allowing time and opportunities for her to discuss her fears and anxieties.

Providing opportunities to discuss general health and safety advice is important; for example, it is safer to shower rather than use a bath, as this reduces the risk of drowning if patients have a seizure; avoiding sports activities, such as rock climbing and hang gliding. Advise Bianca of triggers that may precipitate a seizure such as

(Continued)

603

excessive alcohol, poor general health, excessive stress and the importance of keeping an epilepsy diary as a means of recording information about her epilepsy. Bianca has been driving to work before her seizure. The nurse has a responsibility to raise awareness of the legal requirement for her to stop driving and inform the Driver and Vehicle Licensing Agency (DVLA).

Headaches

Headaches are among the most common neurological disorders. The Headache Classification Committee of the International Headache Society (2018) classifies headaches into 14 groups and lists 200 headaches, which can be broadly divided into three main groups:

- *Primary*, unrelated to an underlying condition and constituting approximately 98% of all headaches, for example migraine and tension and cluster headaches
- *Secondary*, due to underlying conditions such as trauma to the brain, raised ICP, vascular and structural pathologies, CNS infections and medication overuse
- *Neuropathies and facial pains* and other headaches, for example, trigeminal neuralgia.

Many headaches are disabling, reduce the patient's quality of life and are a substantial public health problem. Migraine is ranked second amongst the world's leading causes of disability (GBD, 2019).

Epidemiology

Headache affects people of all ages, races and socio-economic statuses and is more common in women. Migraine is a common occurrence, affecting one in seven people, and most 'migraineurs' will have their first attack before they are 35 years old. Peak incidence is in the late teens and early twenties. Tension-type headaches are common and affect up to 80% of people from time to time; in adults, incidence seems higher in women than men and they are mostly episodic.

Pathophysiology

Headache is experienced when there is traction, pressure, displacement, inflammation or dilation of nociceptors in areas sensitive to pain within the cranium, including facial and scalp structures, meninges and cerebral vessels. There are several causes of secondary headaches.

- Vascular: subarachnoid haemorrhage, strokes.
- Non-vascular:
  - Post-traumatic brain injury
  - Tumours and other space-occupying lesions causing raised ICP
  - Benign intracranial hypertension
  - Infections in the nasal or sinus passages and CNS infections (meningitis, encephalitis)
  - Headaches due to medications
  - Postlumbar puncture headache
  - Toxins and other substances

- Headaches due to metabolic disturbances
- Headaches related to psychiatric disorders, e.g. depressive disorders, anxiety.

Diagnosis and Investigations

Diagnosis is made following a good medical history. In some cases, neuroimaging may be necessary to exclude structural causes but for primary headache disorders (tension, migraine or cluster), this rarely reveals important intracranial pathology. A headache diary, recording frequency, duration and severity of headaches, may assist the doctor in the diagnosis.

Secondary headaches should be considered in those patients who present with new-onset headaches or changes in features of their usual headaches. Warning signs that require further investigation by a specialist and which are suggestive of a secondary headache are highlighted in the Red Flag box.

Red Flag

- Change in characteristics of headache, i.e. increased frequency, severity or associated symptoms
- New onset of headache, particularly in those aged <10 and >50 years
- New onset of headache in patients with pre-existing cancer, HIV infection or head trauma
- Progressive headache worsening over weeks or longer
- Persistent morning headache with nausea
- Headache associated with postural changes, physical exertion, coughing or Valsalva manoeuvre and fever
- Thunderclap headache (intense, sudden onset)

Signs and Symptoms

Signs and symptoms of headaches vary according to the cause, type and precipitating symptoms.

Nursing Care and Management

Chronic daily headache, consisting of chronic migraine and chronic tension-type headache, occurs on 15 or more days per month for 3 months or more (Murinova & Krashin, 2015) and is the most challenging to treat. Ultimately, the goal of treatment is to restore the patient's ability to function with minimal adverse effects. Headache treatment is either:

- Abortive, aimed at managing the acute headache, for example with triptans, or
- Prophylactic, aiming to reduce the frequency or severity of the attacks, for example anticonvulsants, beta-blockers and selective serotonin reuptake inhibitors (SSRIs).

Botulinum toxin A is an effective, safe, and generally well-tolerated prophylactic treatment of chronic migraine headaches, at a dose of 155 units divided among 31 injection sites across seven specific head and neck muscles. This dose is repeated after 12 weeks, providing two cycles of treatment and may reduce the number of migraine days (Herd *et al.*, 2018).

Symptom management includes:

- Simple analgesics such as aspirin, paracetamol and ibuprofen, which may be effective in relieving pain symptoms
- Antiemetics such as prochlorperazine, and fluid replacement for nausea, vomiting and subsequent dehydration.

Multiple Sclerosis

Multiple sclerosis (MS) is the most common non-traumatic disabling disease in young people in the UK. MS is an incurable and unpredictable chronic inflammatory disease associated with brain atrophy. The needs of people with MS shift over time and they can experience many disabling symptoms that result in emotional, psychological and physical burdens for themselves and their families.

Epidemiology

Multiple sclerosis affects an estimated 100 000 people in the UK and 2.5 million people globally. The worldwide prevalence of MS correlates positively with latitude (Simpson *et al.*, 2019). MS prevalence increases the greater distance from the equator, the highest prevalence being found in temperate zones of the world, for example Europe and North America. Onset is usually between 20 and 40 years of age, with a peak age of onset at 28–31 years. It is more common in women than men, with a male to female ratio of 1:1.7.

Pathophysiology

Although the exact cause remains unknown, there is evidence to suggest that it starts as dysregulation of the immune system triggered by an interaction between genetic and environmental factors (Waubant *et al.*, 2019). It is thought that the initial trigger involves damage to the BBB, resulting in lymphocytes (T and B cells) entering the CNS and triggering an immune response, these cells then releasing substances that attack the myelin sheath that surrounds the nerves This results in damage and loss of the nerve axon and the formation of localised inflammation called plaques and eventual nerve death.

Multiple sclerosis is characterised by periods of exacerbation or relapse (return to old symptoms or the appearance of new ones; patients often refer to these as 'attacks') and periods of remission (recovery from relapse), during which the damaged myelin sheath undergoes remyelination. In the early stages, the disease is commonly a relapsing and remitting condition but over time, during the remission period the myelin sheath is unable to repair itself completely and patients are left with residual deficits. Repeated healing and inflammation can lead to scarring (gliosis) and loss of axons, evidenced on MRI scans as 'black holes'. As the disease progresses, remissions become shorter and fewer, and patients become more disabled physically and a new clinical stage called secondary progressive MS is initiated.

There are four main types of MS.

1. Relapsing-remitting (most common type), accounting for approximately 85% of patients from onset
2. Primary progressive
3. Secondary progressive
4. Progressive–relapsing

Risk Factors

- Environmental risks include:
  - Born and living in high-latitude regions: reduced UVB radiation
  - Vitamin D deficiency or variations in DNA sequence of vitamin D gene: vitamin D has a central role in modulation of the immune response
  - Postviral infections, e.g. Epstein–Barr virus
  - Cigarette smoking.
- Genetic factors.
- Family history: maternal and first-degree relatives have a 10-fold increased chance of developing MS.
- Dysbiosis; reduction in gut microbiota.
- Female sex.

Signs and Symptoms

Signs and symptoms are determined by the location and number of demyelination plaques in the CNS and represent a balance between inflammation, progressive neurodegeneration and reparative processes in the brain.

A wide range of symptoms are associated with MS, with common symptoms and signs including:

- Visual dysfunction, such as diplopia and blurred vision due to optic neuritis (demyelination of the optic nerve)
- Brainstem symptoms including dysarthria and dysphagia
- Mobility-related symptoms:
  - Spasticity is common
  - Ataxia and tremor
  - Transient muscle weakness (commonly occurring in the lower limbs)
- Sensory disturbances
- Bladder, bowel and sexual dysfunction
- Fatigue: most disabling complex symptom
- Cognitive impairment
- Psychiatric and psychological dysfunction, such as depression, psychosis
- Pain: due to inflammation or neuropathic pain related to the CNS lesion or secondary to spasticity and spasms
- Sleep disorders.

Diagnosis and Investigations

Early diagnosis, based on clinical history, examination and laboratory findings, is important in facilitating the exclusion of alternative diagnoses and early implementation of treatment. MS is diagnosed after tests to exclude alternatives have been carried out and no feature is suggestive of another diagnosis; this may require repeated tests before a conclusive diagnosis is given. Investigations that provide information to aid diagnosis include:

- *MRI scans*: may reveal plaques within the CNS
- *CSF examination*: may reveal the presence of oligoclonal bands (i.e. immunoglobulins, suggesting inflammation of the CNS), which are present in over 95% of patients with MS

- *Evoked response testing (visual, auditory and somatosensory)*: may show delayed conduction (slowing of the nerve messages).

Nursing Care and Management

Management of patients with MS varies according to the acuteness of exacerbations (relapses), and the presenting signs and symptoms. MS management generally is divided into treating the symptoms of the disease and those that target the disease mechanism; however, both require an interdisciplinary individualistic approach.

Although there is no cure for MS, disease-modifying therapies are available that can reduce disability and improve quality of life. However, these therapies have only been found to be effective in preventing relapses in relapsing-remitting MS and for some people with secondary progressive MS.

The three main treatment categories are:

- Disease-modifying therapies using medication
- Disease-suppressing therapies
- Corticosteroids.

Jot This Down

What specific aspects of medication management might need to be considered with patients receiving treatment for their MS?

In this exercise, you might have considered some of the following.

- The availability of different formulations, including injections, infusions or tablets.
- Degree of patient flexibility in administering medications themselves, e.g. taking tablets or self-injections.
- Understanding the patient's home life; the availability and support of the family.
- Ability to cope with treatment that requires administration by a healthcare professional.
- Monitoring the degree of compliance with medication.
- Awareness of side-effects and ways to mitigate them; the importance of follow-up.
- Emphasising that it is important for women who are pregnant, or planning to become pregnant, to discuss any medications they are taking and any new medications, with their specialist.

Being diagnosed with MS may cause uncertainty about the future and worry about the possibility of becoming disabled. MS can potentially have a future impact on employment, income, relationships and activities of living. Patients must understand that early treatment can delay the development of disability, but that treatment will need to be continuous and long term. As integral members of the multidisciplinary team, nurses can play a major role in supporting and educating patients and their families in selecting treatment options. Nurses may be faced with adherence challenges with patients with MS and should seek strategies for optimising patient adherence, which may include:

- Patient education, including an understanding of the disease, need for treatment and potential benefits of treatment
- Management of the patient's expectations

- Providing information on therapeutic options, potential side-effects and how these can be managed
- Ensuring that the patient is appropriately trained, e.g. in injection technique
- Use of reminder systems, such as drug diaries, pillboxes or alarms, especially for patients experiencing cognitive impairment
- Helping the patient to seek assistance from family members and/or friends
- Providing information on support networks.

It is also important that nurses remain informed about the potential risks and benefits and special considerations (e.g. long-term safety data, dosing and frequency) of all MS therapies, to ensure that patient information is accurate. Careful regular monitoring is also important, as symptoms change throughout the disease.

Specific Symptom Management: Spasticity (High Muscle Tone)

Spasticity, common in MS patients and many other neurological conditions such as TBI and stroke, is a motor disorder characterised by increased stretch reflexes leading to exaggerated muscle resistance (increased muscle tone) with exaggerated tendon jerks. Spasticity can range from muscle stiffness to severe painful uncontrolled muscle spasms and restricted, excessive or inappropriate movement, and may be associated with pain. It can affect a single muscle or multiple muscles, for example a whole limb. Spasticity can affect an individual's ability to carry out activities of living and may result in complications, such as contractures because of prolonged spasticity and the development of pressure sores. Spasticity can lead to treatment and management difficulties and can be very distressing for the individual with spasticity and their family.

The degree to which spasticity affects mobility is dependent on the severity of symptoms. For example, severe spasticity in lower limbs may result in the involuntary crossing of the legs (often referred to as scissoring reflex) or the legs being forced into extension due to extensor spasms and this poses an increased risk of falling out of chairs or bed.

Early identification and initiating referral to either hospital or community-based neurorehabilitation teams are important in preventing and managing complications of spasticity. Management requires assessment and the formulation of a management plan, depending on the underlying pathology, that is aimed at maximising function, relieving pain and preventing complications and injury.

Physical interventions include:

- Splinting/casting regimes
- Minimising noxious stimuli that can activate flexor reflex afferents that may trigger spasms, such as skin irritation (e.g. tight clothing, ingrowing toenails), sudden movements, constipation, urinary infection and retention, inappropriate moving and handling
- Passive limb exercises to prevent contractures and loss of muscle bulk
- Early involvement of the physiotherapist to assess and provide positioning and manual handling management plans
- Referral to the occupational therapist for assistive devices
- Careful positioning to maintain neural assignment to prevent primitive reflexes being triggered, which may stimulate spasms (e.g. tonic neck reflexes when the neck or head is tilted); this may include a postural management plan

- Assessing for and treating any underlying pain
- Educating and empowering the patient to self-manage their condition. Reinforcement of safety information provided by the multidisciplinary team, e.g. physiotherapist.

Medicines Management

The most common medication for spasticity is generalised antispasticity agents, e.g., baclofen. Other medications may include gabapentin (an anticonvulsant drug) and Sativex® , a cannabis-based drug. Local treatment may include intrathecal baclofen and injection of botulinum toxin type A (Botox® or Dysport®) directly into the affected muscle.

Parkinson's Disease

Parkinson disease (PD) is a common, slowly progressive neuro-degenerative disorder of the CNS, usually affecting the older adult, which eventually leads to disability. PD is the second most common neurodegenerative disorder after Alzheimer disease.

Epidemiology

Approximately 1 in 500 people in the UK has PD. As this disease primarily affects older adults, its prevalence is expected to dramatically increase in the future. The incidence rates increase exponentially in people in their 70s and 80s. The mean age of onset is 55–60 years. PD is slightly more common in men than women and the prevalence increases with age and duration of symptoms (Parkinson's UK, 2017).

Risk Factors There is no cure and in most cases, the cause is not known. However, there are several factors linked to PD: genetics; prolonged use or misuse of neuroleptics (e.g. haloperidol and chlorpromazine) and antiemetics (e.g., prochlorperazine) is known to induce drug-induced Parkinsonism; prolonged exposure to pesticides or herbicides.

Pathophysiology

Parkinson disease involves the death of dopamine-releasing neurones in a group of structures called the substantia nigra and the striatum located in the diencephalic area of the brain called the basal ganglia, and the formation of Lewy bodies, small spherical protein deposits found in neurones.

Signs and Symptoms

Parkinson disease exhibits progressive development of motor and non-motor symptoms. Onset is insidious, often making it difficult for the family to notice when the signs start and progress. Non-motor symptoms often present well before motor symptoms occur (5–10 years) and are referred to as the premotor phase. Common symptoms are summarised in Table 32.7.

Patients may experience extreme fluctuations in the severity of their symptoms, which are often difficult to predict and control and are subsequently accompanied by a reduction in motor function. These fluctuations in symptoms are the cause of reduced psychological well-being and caregiver distress and

Table 32.7 Motor and non-motor signs and symptoms in PD.

MOTOR IMPAIRMENT	NON-MOTOR SYMPTOMS
Repetitive tremor (pill rolling)	Early prodromal signs, including loss of smell (anosmia), constipation, rapid eye movement
Akinesia: inability to initiate a willed movement	Sleep disturbances
Bradykinesia: slowness of movement or difficulty in starting to move	Dysphagia
Dyskinesia: abnormal involuntary movements of the limbs, trunk or face	Excessive salivation, dribbling and drooling
Rigidity	Communication problems: voice softening, slurring and slowness of speech
Postural instability	Constipation and bladder dysfunction
Gait disturbances: shuffling and festinant gait	Apathy
Dystonia: sustained and painful muscle contractions	Cognitive impairment
	Dementia
	Depression
	Restless leg syndrome
	Pain

burden. When the patient has severe worsening of parkinsonian signs and symptoms, with very severe motor deterioration, this is considered an 'off' situation. Other common motor fluctuations include:

- Early 'wearing-off' (emergence of motor and non-motor symptoms before the next scheduled levodopa dose)
- The 'on–off' phenomenon (severe fluctuations in motor function)
- Dyskinesias.

Diagnosis and investigations

Diagnosis of PD is based primarily on a thorough history and physical examination and is usually made based on the presence of any two of the following signs and symptoms: tremor at rest, bradykinesia, rigidity and postural instability.

Nursing Care and Management

Once a diagnosis of PD has been made, nursing interventions are based on a holistic assessment to include intensity, frequency and duration of symptoms and those symptoms that cause distress. This assessment will identify symptoms that need to be targeted and the necessary interventions to address those symptoms to improve disability and quality of life.

The aim of nursing interventions is primarily to support and encourage patients to maintain independence as far as possible. Regularly evaluating the effectiveness of these interventions on the targeted symptoms is an important aspect of the nurse's role in managing people with PD.

A range of medications are available to treat PD and should be prescribed on an individual basis, aiming to balance patient preference with control and management of their symptoms (NICE, 2017). PD medication is aimed at alleviating symptoms and, if possible, slowing the progression of the disease by increasing the levels of dopamine, or mimicking its effect to stimulate areas of the brain where dopamine works.

Red Flag

Abrupt withdrawal of medications can result in:
· Sudden development of symptoms
· Increased risk of falling
· Prolonged hospital stay that may be life-threatening.

As well as ensuring that prescribed medications are administered at the prescribed time, supporting patients to self-medicate (patients control their medication) is an important aspect of nursing care, ensuring a constant therapeutic level of symptom control for PD patients.

Other treatment options include:

- Dopaminergic stimulation therapies, such as deep brain stimulation non-destructive surgery, which is reversible
- Restorative therapies, although still in their experimental stage, include foetal nigral transplantation and stem cell therapies.

What To Do If . . .

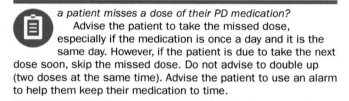

a patient misses a dose of their PD medication?
Advise the patient to take the missed dose, especially if the medication is once a day and it is the same day. However, if the patient is due to take the next dose soon, skip the missed dose. Do not advise to double up (two doses at the same time). Advise the patient to use an alarm to help them keep their medication to time.

Alzheimer Disease and Related Disorders

Dementia is widely recognised as a major, rapidly increasing epidemic and a global healthcare challenge. Dementia is a chronic progressive mental disorder and Alzheimer disease (AD), a degenerative cerebral disease with characteristic neuropathological and neurochemical features, is the most common form. Other common causes include Lewy body dementia (accompanied by PD symptoms), vascular dementia and frontal lobe dementia.

Epidemiology

Alzheimer disease is the leading cause of disability in old age. In the UK, approximately 850 000 people are living with dementia (Alzheimer's Research UK Dementia Statistics Hub, 2021), and the number of cases is expected to rise, with women being more susceptible to dementia than men, primarily because they live longer. It is estimated that 5% of cases have been diagnosed with young-onset dementia, usually between 30 and 65 years old (Alzheimer's Society, 2014).

Risk Factors Several risk factors have been identified that affect the likelihood of developing some form of dementia. These include advancing age, female, ethnicity and genetics and family history.

Modifiable factors include:

- Vascular disease
- Smoking and excessive alcohol use

- Diet
- History of stroke, particularly in the presence of vascular risk factors
- Serious TBI, especially repeated cerebral concussions.

Pathophysiology

The neuropathology of AD is the extracellular insoluble amyloid plaques and intracellular dense neurofibrillary tangles (NTF), mainly composed of Tau proteins. Currently, a definitive diagnosis requires pathological confirmation at autopsy. These plaques and NTF lead to synaptic dysfunction, synapse plaques, neuronal cell death and subsequent brain atrophy (DeTure & Dickson, 2019). Death typically occurs 3–15 years after the onset of AD.

Vascular dementia is associated with small blood vessel narrowing in the brain resulting in hypoperfusion and leading to brain damage.

Signs and Symptoms

Typically, the symptoms of AD progress from mild memory problems to severe cognitive impairment, affecting reasoning, judgement, planning and execution of familiar tasks. Several behavioural symptoms are characteristics of AD, including apathy (affecting up to 70%), agitation (occurring in 60%), and anxiety and depression (affecting 50%). Disinhibition occurs in up to one-third of all AD patients and delusions and hallucinations occur in up to 25% and 10%, respectively. Other features of dementias include disturbances to sleep patterns, wandering, language production and verbal expression and urinary urgency, frequency and incontinence.

The progression of dementia varies but as the disease progresses, the patient exhibits a range of signs and symptoms that are individual to the person and not manifest in everyone.

Diagnosis and Investigations

Clinical diagnosis is more difficult and as there are no specific tests for AD, the diagnosis is based on excluding other conditions with similar signs and symptoms. Detailed history taking and appropriate screening, to exclude other possible causes for the patient's signs and symptoms such as infections and side-effects of medications, are necessary. Families/carers should be involved in the history taking, as they may be extremely useful in providing information patients may have forgotten. Imaging is crucial in helping to diagnose any changes such as atrophy. Referral to clinical psychology for more detailed cognitive assessment and behavioural management strategies may be helpful, along with genetic screening.

Nursing Care and Management

Alzheimer disease is profoundly life-changing for both the individual and their family/carers. The behavioural and psychological symptoms are challenging and a source of considerable distress, anxiety and strain for families and carers. Nursing care is centred on an individual approach and some key points are summarised in Box 32.6.

Despite there being no cure for AD, if the disease is diagnosed early, medication has been developed that can help to improve, slow or stabilise the symptoms and promote a better quality of life.

When caring for patients with dementia who are vulnerable or incapable, nurses need to work in partnership with both the patient and their family/carer to:

Gain a comprehensive person-centred picture of the person with dementia

Identify patient and family/carer needs in a framework of person-centred care and respect for human rights.

Alzheimer disease patients have altered dietary preferences, taste patterns and cognitive impairment, which may make it difficult to obtain a healthy diet. Thus, early nutritional screening and providing nutritional support and advice to the patient and their carer are important to prevent adverse eating behaviours that may be detrimental to the patient.

Box 32.6 Key Points in the Nursing Management of Patients with Alzheimer Disease

- Regularly structured assessments, and evaluation to identify, plan and meet the needs of the individual.
  - Mini-Mental State Examination (MMSE).
  - Holistic problem-solving approach.
  - Behavioural analysis using the 'ABC' (A, Antecedents, triggers and causes; B, Behaviour; and C, Consequences of that behaviour) evaluation of behaviour to identify possible precipitating factors and devise effective management plans.
  - Consider the possibility of maintaining a familiar environment that is stimulating and supports individual lifestyles.
- Engage in specific training to enable:
  - Safe and effective management of problems as they occur
  - Effective management strategies to be deployed; may include music therapy, reminiscence therapy, reality orientation, validation therapy and purposeful activity
  - Multidisciplinary input and referral to relevant agencies that can offer assistance and support, e.g. Admiral Nurse Services (based on NMC, 2018a).

Peripheral Neuropathy

Peripheral neuropathy (PN) refers to damage to the peripheral sensory, motor and autonomic nerves, often affecting them distally. There are over 100 different conditions, each with its specific pattern of development and prognosis.

Epidemiology

Peripheral neuropathy (PN) is common; in the UK, it is estimated that almost 1 in 10 people aged 55 or over is affected by peripheral neuropathy. Diabetic peripheral neuropathy eventually affects nearly 50% of adults with diabetes (Hicks & Selvin, 2019).

Pathophysiology

Peripheral neuropathy may be either inherited, collectively referred to as Charcot–Marie disease, or acquired, with causes including:

- Pathological reaction, e.g. inflammatory, demyelinating neuropathy such as multiple sclerosis and Guillain–Barré syndrome
- Physical trauma, e.g. physical damage to nerves due to accidents, falls
- Nerve entrapment: compression of the median nerve (carpal tunnel syndrome) and ulnar nerve palsy. Spinal nerves, as they emerge from the spinal cord, can be trapped by bony spurs or intervertebral discs and give rise to sensory and motor disturbances commonly affecting the cervical and lumbar nerves
- Disease, metabolic and endocrine: diabetes mellitus, hypothyroidism; malnutrition and vitamin deficiency, e.g. B1 (thiamine)
- Kidney conditions, in which abnormal levels of toxins can severely damage nerve tissue
- Infectious processes, e.g. HIV, herpes simplex and syphilis
- Cancers that invade nerves
- Exposure to toxins, such as heavy metals (lead, mercury), anticancer agents, anticonvulsants and antiviral drugs
- Medications, e.g. digoxin, phenytoin, statins.

Diagnosis and Investigations

Diagnosis involves establishing the presence of the neuropathy via history (i.e. onset, duration and course) and neurological examination, and tests are used to confirm the anatomical and pathological pattern of the neuropathy. The objective of the investigations is to localise the PN to a part of the PNS. Tests may include nerve conduction studies, electromyography (EMG), CSF evaluation, radiological studies, imaging and blood tests including fasting blood glucose, comprehensive metabolic profile, erythrocyte sedimentation rate/C-reactive protein (ESR/CRP) and thyroid-stimulating hormone levels. Nerve biopsy may be considered if the diagnosis remains uncertain after other tests.

Signs and Symptoms

Because every peripheral nerve has a highly specialised function in a specific part of the body, the patient may present with a wide array of symptoms, depending on the type and distribution of nerves affected. Sensory nerve damage may cause numbness, tingling and pricking sensations (paraesthesia), sensitivity to touch or loss of position sense, inability to feel pain or changes in temperature. In the early stages of the condition, these symptoms affect the distal limbs, often described as a 'glove and stocking' distribution. Others may suffer more extreme symptoms, including burning, stabbing and shooting pains. Pain is the most common presentation of PN associated with diabetes mellitus.

Motor nerve damage causes muscle wasting, paralysis or organ or gland dysfunction. Symptoms of autonomic nerve damage are diverse, depending on the organ affected, but may include the inability to sweat normally, digest food easily, maintain safe levels of blood pressure or experience normal sexual function.

Nursing Care and Management

Inherited PN has no specific treatment or cure. Regardless of the cause, there are no effective medications available. However, peripheral nerves can regenerate, and thus many people have resolution of their symptoms over time; however, if the damage is too severe, patients may have persistent symptoms. Symptoms can often be controlled and eliminating the causes of specific forms of neuropathy can often prevent new damage. By encouraging a proactive and personalised approach to promoting self-initiated strategies such as massage, heat therapy, cold therapy, exercise, walking, rest, and transcutaneous electrical nerve stimulation (TENS), nurses can help to reduce symptoms and improve aspects of quality of life.

Peripheral neuropathy often causes neuropathic pain, which can manifest as burning, shooting and tingling due to damage or dysfunction of the peripheral nerves and abnormal processing of stimuli; for example, non-painful stimuli such as touch are painful and this is called allodynia.

Pharmacological options to treat neuropathic pain may include anticonvulsants, such as gabapentin, and antidepressants, such as amitriptyline.

Primary Care

Primary prevention measures include adopting a healthy lifestyle: avoiding toxins, correcting vitamin deficiencies, limiting alcohol intake and weight reduction.
Advise and teach the patient self-care skills:
· Regular meticulous foot care, inspecting feet and toes for blisters and sores that may appear on numb areas of the foot, because pressure sores or injury may go unnoticed
· Report any changes in cuts, calluses, ulcers, etc.
· Suitable footwear, in particular protective footwear to protect against injury, may also be necessary
· Use of a bed cradle to lift the bedclothes off hyperaesthetic skin
· Referral to the community physiotherapist for walking aids (NMC, 2018a).

Conclusion

This chapter begins with a brief overview of the organisation, structure and functions of the central and peripheral nervous systems. Critical to nursing a patient with a neurological condition is an accurate and comprehensive neurological assessment, the key principles of which have been outlined, including clinical, non-invasive and invasive assessment techniques and tools, such as the GCS. The principles of caring for a patient with raised ICP have been discussed, along with the main conditions that may present with raised ICP: traumatic brain injury, stroke, brain tumours and CNS infections. Common neurological conditions and disorders have been outlined, along with their associated nursing care and management principles. This care is not only complex but challenging and requires the acquisition of a wide range of skills and experience. The principles of care outlined in this chapter will support a nurse in caring for a patient with any neurological condition and not just those discussed in this chapter.

Key Points

· The neurological system is both complex and challenging and to ensure effective and competent nursing care for neurological patients, nurses need the necessary skills and experience.
· Nursing care of conditions related to the neurological system requires an understanding of the anatomy and physiology of the nervous system.
· Nursing care for this vast, diverse patient group requires a collaborative approach with other healthcare professionals, the patient and/or their relatives/informal carers.

References

Alzheimer's Research UK Dementia Statistics Hub (2021) *Statistics about dementia*. www.dementiastatistics.org/statistics-about-dementia/ (accessed December 2021).

Alzheimer's Society (2014) *Dementia UK*, 2nd edn. Alzheimer's Society, London.

Brain Trauma Foundation (2016) *Guidelines for the Management of Severe Traumatic Brain Injury*, 4th edn. https://braintrauma.org/uploads/03/12/Guidelines_for_Management_of_Severe_TBI_4th_Edition.pdf (accessed December 2021).

Braine, M.E. & Cook, N. (2016) The Glasgow Coma Scale and evidence-informed practice: a critical review of where we are and where we need to be. *Journal of Clinical Nursing*, 26(1/2), 280–293.

Cancer Research UK (2021) *Brain tumours: survival*. www.cancerresearchuk.org/about-cancer/brain-tumours/survival (accessed December 2021).

Crocetti, E., Trama, A., Stiller, C., *et al.* (2012) RARECARE working group. Epidemiology of glial and non-glial brain tumours in Europe. *European Journal of Cancer*, 48, 1532–1542.

DeTure, M.A. & Dickson, D.W. (2019) The neuropathological diagnosis of Alzheimer's disease. *Molecular Neurodegeneration*, 14(32).

Doss, R.C. & LaFrance, W.C. (2017) Psychogenic non-epileptic seizures. *Epileptic Disorders*, 18(4), 337–343.

Epilepsy Action (2021) *Epilepsy facts and terminology*. www.epilepsy.org.uk/press/facts (accessed December 2021).

Fisher, R., Cross, J., D'Souza, C., *et al.* (2017) Instruction manual for the ILAE 2017 operational classification of seizure types. *Epilepsia*, 58(4), 531–541.

GBD 2019 Diseases and Injuries Collaborators (2020) Global burden of 369 diseases and injuries in 204 countries and territories, 1990–2019: a systematic analysis for the global burden of disease study 2019. *Lancet*, 396, 1204–1222.

Hackett, M.L. & Anderson, C.S. (2014) Part I: frequency of depression after stroke: an updated systematic review and meta-analysis of observational studies. *International Journal of Stroke*, 9(8), 1017–1025.

Headache Classification Committee of the International Headache Society (2018) The International Classification of Headache Disorders, 3rd edn. *Cephalalgia*, 38(1), 1–211.

Herd, C.P., Tomlinson, C.L., Rick, C., *et al.* (2018) Botulinum toxins for the prevention of migraine in adults. *Cochrane Database of Systematic Reviews*, 6, CD011616.

Hicks, C.W. & Selvin, E. (2019) Epidemiology of peripheral neuropathy and lower extremity disease in diabetes. *Current Diabetes Reports*, 19(10), 86.

Lin, B., Zhang, Z., Mei, Y., *et al.* (2021) Cumulative risk of stroke recurrence over the last 10 years: a systematic review and meta-analysis. *Neurological Sciences*, 42, 61–71.

Louis, D.N., Ohgaki, H., Wiestler, O.D. & Cavenee, W.K. (2016) *International Agency for Research on Cancer, World Health Organization Histological Classification of Tumours of the Central Nervous System*, 4th edn. International Agency for Research on Cancer/World Health Organization, Lyon.

Murinova, N. & Krashin, D. (2015) Chronic daily headache. *Physical Medicine Rehabilitation Clinics of North America*, 26(2), 375–389.

National Institute for Health and Care Excellence (2017) *Parkinson disease in adults*. NG71. *NICE*, London.

NHS (2021) FAST. www.nhs.uk/actfast/Documents/Act-FAST-A5-leaflet-white-man.pdf (accessed December 2021).

Nursing & Midwifery Council (2018a) *Future nurse: Standards for proficiency for registered nurses*. NMC, London.

Nursing & Midwifery Council (2018b) *Standards for proficiency for nursing associates*. NMC, London.

Parkinson's UK (2017) The prevalence and incidence of Parkinson's in the UK. www.parkinsons.org.uk/sites/default/files/2018-01/Prevalence%20%20Incidence%20Report%20Latest_Public_2.pdf (accessed December 2021).

Pollock, A., Hazelton, C., Rowe, F.J., *et al.* (2019) Interventions for visual field defects in people with stroke. *Cochrane Database of Systematic Reviews*, 5(5), CD008388.

Rudd, A.G., Bowen, A., Young, G. & James, M.A. (2017) *National Clinical Guideline for Stroke*, 5th edn. www.strokeaudit.org/SupportFiles/Documents/Guidelines/2016-National-Clinical-Guideline-for-Stroke-5t-(1).aspx (accessed December 2021).

Simpson, S. Jr, Wang, W., Otahal, P., Blizzard, L., Van Der Mei, I. & Taylor, B. (2019) Latitude is significantly associated with the prevalence of multiple sclerosis: an updated meta-analysis. *Journal of Neurology, Neurosurgery and Psychiatry*, 90(11), 1193–1200.

Teasdale, G. & Jennett, J. (1974) Assessment of coma and impaired consciousness. A practical scale. *Lancet*, ii(7872), 81–84.

Waubant, E., Lucas, R., Mowry, E., *et al.* (2019) Environmental and genetic risk factors for MS: an integrated review. *Annals of Clinical and Translational Neurology*, 6(9), 1905–1922.

Wilkins, E., Wilson, L., Wickramasinghe, K., *et al.* (2017) European Cardiovascular Disease Statistics Brussels: European Heart Network. www.ehnheart.org/images/CVD-statistics-report-August-2017.pdf (accessed December 2021).

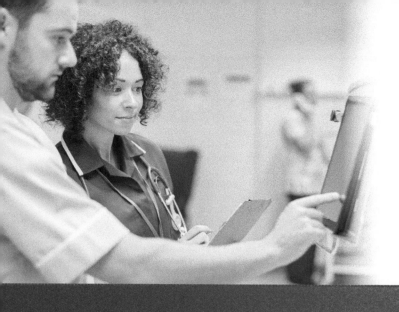

33

The Person with an Ear or Eye Disorder

Sara Meakin and Mahesh Seewoodhary

University of West London, UK

Learning Outcomes

On completion of this chapter you will be able to:

- Demonstrate and apply knowledge of body systems by outlining the anatomy and physiology and key functions of the ears and the eyes
- Understand and apply a person-centred approach to the nursing care of the person with an ear or eye disorder, demonstrating shared assessment, planning, decision making and goal setting when working with people, their families, communities and populations of all ages
- Demonstrate knowledge of epidemiology, demography, genomics and the wider determinants of health, illness and well-being of ear and eye problems and apply this to an understanding of global patterns of health and well-being outcomes
- Understand the importance of effective communication skills and apply a range of skills and strategies with people with ear and eye problems

Proficiencies

NMC Proficiencies and Standards:

- Communicate effectively using a range of skills and strategies with colleagues and people at all stages of life and with ear and eye problems
- Demonstrate the skills and abilities required to support people at all stages of life who are emotionally or physically vulnerable
- Provide and promote non-discriminatory, person-centred and sensitive care at all times, reflecting on people's values and beliefs, diverse backgrounds, cultural characteristics, language requirements, needs and preferences, taking account of any need for adjustments
- Understand and apply a person-centred approach to nursing care, demonstrating shared assessment, planning, decision making and goal setting when working with people, their families, communities and populations of all ages with ear and eye problems
- Demonstrate the knowledge, communication and relationship management skills required to provide people, families and carers with accurate information that meets their needs before, during and after a range of interventions

 Visit the companion website at www.wiley.com/go/peate/nursingpractice3e where you can test yourself using flashcards, multiple-choice questions and more.

Nursing Practice: Knowledge and Care, Third Edition. Edited by Ian Peate and Aby Mitchell.
© 2022 John Wiley & Sons Ltd. Published 2022 by John Wiley & Sons Ltd.
Companion website: www.wiley.com/go/peate/nursingpractice3e

Introduction

In this chapter, an overview of the anatomy and physiology of the ears and the eyes is presented, along with the functions of these sensory organs. Several common disorders related to hearing and vision will be outlined employing a patient-centred holistic approach.

The sensing organs send information to the brain to help us understand and perceive the world around us. The ears and the eyes are the means by which visual and auditory stimuli reach the brain. These special senses, often taken for granted, are key to human survival; the sudden loss of vision or an eye disorder with visual impairment can impact negatively on a person's health and well-being. The senses of smell, taste and touch are discussed in other chapters.

When diseases or trauma of these organs occur, there is potential to affect the person's ability to maintain a safe environment and this can limit the ability to carry out the activities of living. Mobility becomes restricted which, coupled with an impact on the ability to communicate, may lead to social isolation and loneliness and difficulties with safety, independence, communication and relationships with others. Hearing and vision provide us with the opportunity to hear people laugh, to see the people we love and to participate in the communication process.

When impairment or deficit occurs, the responsibility of the nurse is to support patients to carry out the activities of living that they are unable to carry out and, above all, to help them maintain a safe environment and be independent. It is important that nurses draw on best-practice communication strategies with patients who have impairment (Davis, 2019).

The nurse will be able to support in a more competent manner when they have an understanding of the anatomy and physiology of the ears and eyes. The RCN (2016) document on the nature, scope and value of ophthalmic nursing clearly states that the primary aim of eye care is to promote a high standard of ocular health that necessitates a holistic, patient-centered approach supported with evidence of knowledge and understanding of normal and altered anatomy, physiology, the manifestation of eye disease and the impact on a person's well-being. The key aim is to provide care that is safe and effective for patients with an eye or ear disorder.

Anatomy and Physiology of the Ear

Hearing is one of the major senses and, like vision, is essential for distant warning and communication. It can be used to alert and to communicate pleasure and fear. Hearing is an appreciation of vibration perceived as sound. For this to happen, the appropriate signal must reach the higher parts of the brain. In the ear, the vibration is converted into a nervous impulse, which is then processed by the central auditory pathways of the brain.

There are two key functions associated with the ears: hearing and the maintenance of equilibrium. The anatomy and physiology of the ears, as well as both functions, will be discussed prior to describing a few common ear conditions and the care required for people with ear problems.

For further information on anatomy and physiology of hearing, please see Peate & Evans (2020).

The ears (Figure 33.1) are paired organs, one on each side of the head, with the sense organ itself, which is called the cochlea, buried

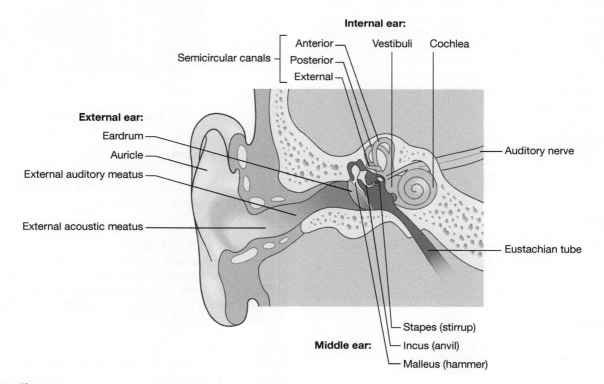

Figure 33.1 The ear.

deep within the temporal bones. There are three anatomical parts associated with the ear:

1. External ear
2. Middle ear
3. Inner ear.

The External Ear

The external ear can be divided into two structures:

- The auricle
- The external acoustic meatus.

The Auricle

Also known as the pinna, the auricle is an external, lateral paired structure (Figure 33.2). Its function is to capture and transmit sound to the external auditory meatus. In the centre of the auricle is a hollow depression called the concha of the auricle which continues as the external acoustic meatus. The role of the concha is to direct sound into the external acoustic meatus.

The External Acoustic Meatus

The external acoustic meatus (ear canal) is a sigmoid-shaped tube extending from the deep part of the concha to the tympanic membrane (Figure 33.3). It is covered with skin which contains hair and modified sweat glands producing cerumen (earwax).

The external acoustic meatus travels in an S-shaped curve with a varying diameter, being wider laterally and narrow medially, and terminates at the tympanic membrane. The tympanic membrane is translucent which allows structures located within the middle ear to be seen, such as the handle of malleus which attaches to the tympanic membrane at a point called the umbo.

The Middle Ear

The middle ear sits within the temporal bone, extending from the tympanic membrane to the lateral (side) wall of the internal ear. The key function of the middle ear is to transmit vibrations from the tympanic membrane (the eardrum) to the inner ear and it does this via the three bones of the ear. The tympanic cavity contains the majority of the bones of the middle ear.

The bones of the middle ear, also called the auditory ossicles, are:

- The malleus (hammer)
- The incus (anvil)
- The stapes (stirrup).

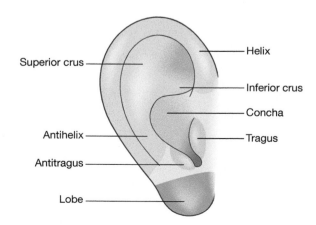

Figure 33.2 **The auricle.**

Labels:
- Superior crus
- Helix
- Inferior crus
- Concha
- Antihelix
- Tragus
- Antitragus
- Lobe

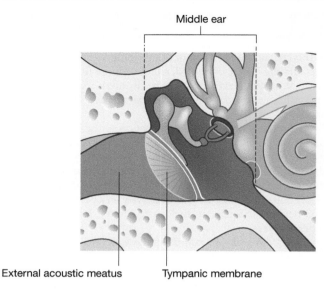

Middle ear

External acoustic meatus   Tympanic membrane

Figure 33.3 **The external acoustic meatus.**

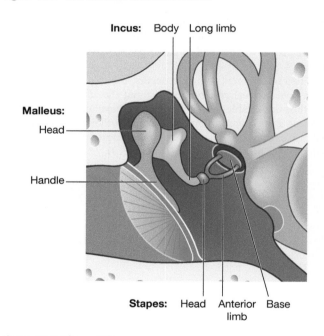

Incus: Body   Long limb

Malleus:
Head

Handle

Stapes: Head   Anterior   Base
limb

Figure 33.4 **The ossicles.**

The bones (Figure 33.4) are connected in a chain-like manner and link the tympanic membrane to the oval window of the internal ear.

The Muscles of the Middle Ear

The tensor tympani and stapedius are two muscles that act to protect the middle ear. These muscles contract in response to loud noise, inhibiting the vibrations of the malleus, incus and stapes and reducing the transmission of sound to the inner ear. This action is called the *acoustic reflex*.

Mastoid Air Cells

The mastoid air cells are a collection of air-filled spaces in the mastoid process of the temporal bone. They act as a buffer system of air, discharging air into the tympanic cavity when the pressure is too low.

The Eustachian Tube

The eustachian tube, a cartilaginous and bony tube, connects the middle ear to the nasopharynx. Its function is to equalise the pressure of the middle ear to that of the external auditory meatus.

The Inner Ear

Auditory transduction (conversion of mechanical vibrations entering the ear canal into electrical signals) occurs in the inner ear. The inner ear is composed of several different structures (Figure 33.5).

The vestibule is associated with vestibular function (balance). Receptors present in the vestibule provide sensations of gravity and linear acceleration.

Three semicircular canals are also associated with vestibular function. Receptors in the semicircular canals are stimulated when the head moves (rotates). Together with the vestibule, this is called the *vestibular complex*. The fluid-filled chambers within the vestibule are usually continuous with those of the semicircular canals.

The cochlea is a coiled tube (*cochlea* is derived from Greek, meaning 'snail') and is concerned with hearing and the detection of sound waves. The sense of hearing is provided by receptors within the cochlear duct where two perilymph-filled chambers can be found. The oval window separates the perilymph of the cochlear chambers from the air-filled middle ear.

The Organ of Corti

Located in the cochlea, the organ of Corti is often referred to as the receptor organ of hearing. Hair cells within the organ of Corti sense mechanical forces and communicate with cranial nerve VIII.

Table 33.1 provides a summary of the structures and functions of the ear.

Physiology of Hearing

Hearing is the faculty of perceiving and interpreting sound; the physiology of hearing is complex. It is essential to understand the anatomy and physiology of the ear prior to discussing the physiology of hearing.

Sound waves enter the external auditory canal, and this then causes the tympanic membrane to vibrate at the same frequency. The ossicles (the bones in the ears) communicate the motion of

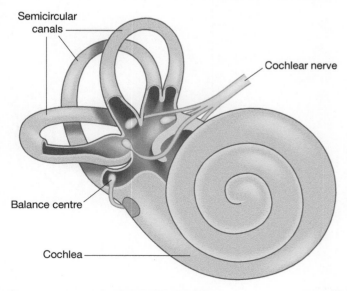

Figure 33.5 The structures of the inner ear.

the tympanic membrane to the oval window, amplifying the energy of the sound wave. As the stapes moves against the oval window, the perilymph (a fluid located in the vestibule) is set in motion; this then generates action potentials that are transmitted to cranial nerve VIII and then onward to the brain for interpretation (Figure 33.6) (Campbell & Shoup, 2019).

Equilibrium and Balance

The other function of the inner ear is to provide information concerning the position of the head; this helps to synchronise body movements, maintaining balance and equilibrium. Several types of receptors send information to the brain to maintain position and balance; the eyes and proprioceptors in muscles are important in informing the brain about equilibrium.

So far, this chapter has provided you with an overview of the anatomy and physiology of the various functions and structures of the ear, as well as a brief understanding of hearing and how equilibrium is maintained. There are a number of ways in which the nurse can undertake a holistic assessment of the needs of people with problems associated with the ear. The use of various diagnostic tests can help the nurse gather objective data that will be essential for the planning and implementation of high-quality, safe and effective care. Before performing these tests, the ear should be examined, a detailed history taken, and the patient should be assessed with otoscopy to check for obvious ear pathology.

When the tests have been carried out, the nurse must ensure the findings and any treatment are clearly documented in the person's notes. The patient should also be advised of the findings and any further treatment or tests that may be required.

Assessing the Person with an Ear Problem

History Taking

History taking may be part of an overall health assessment, or it may be carried out in response to a specific complaint the person may have, for example a buzzing noise in the ears. The nurse should set out to gather as much relevant subjective data as possible.

The nurse should ask when the problem started, what are the features of the problem and how it has progressed. They should assess the severity, factors that exacerbate the condition and factors that offer relief. Consideration should be given to hearing problems and occupational or social exposure to loud noises. Ask the patient if there has been any previous trauma such as diving or cotton bud use. Ask about redness, discharge, odor, fever and pain. A full history should be gathered, taking note of the past medical history and medications, to assess if they are ototoxic.

The skills required to inspect the ear are:

- Communication skills
- Inspection, external and internal
- Palpation.

Inspecting the External Ear

You must inspect and palpate the external structures. Observe the ears for position and symmetry. Both ears should be the same

Table 33.1 Summary of the structures and functions of the ear. *Source*: Adapted from Goddard & Lee (2019) and Campbell & Shoup (2019).

NAME	STRUCTURE	FUNCTION
Auricle (pinna)	Composed of folds of skin over cartilage	Collects sound, channelling it down the ear Helps to determine the direction of sound Protects internal aspects of the ear
External acoustic meatus (ear canal)	A tube (about 2.5 cm) leading from the pinna to the tympanic membrane	Directs sound waves towards the tympanic membrane Secretes cerumen (a waxy substance) and sebum to protect and lubricate the ear
Tympanic membrane	Located between the external ear and the middle ear	Vibrates with the same frequency as the sound wave that hits itProvides airtight protection between the external and middle ear
Ear ossicles	Three bones in the middle ear: malleus, incus and stapes	Transfer the vibrations from the tympanic membrane to the middle of the ear to the oval window
Oval window	A thin membrane situated between the middle and inner ear	Receives the vibration from the tympanic membrane via the ossicles
Round window	Sited just below the oval window	Acts like a piston, transferring the vibration from the oval window to the fluid in the inner ear
Cochlea	A long tube wound around itself and filled with liquid	The fluid in the cochlea transfers the vibrations to the hairs in the organ of Corti
Organ of Corti	Situated inside the cochlea Contains receptors and hair cells connected to nerves	Hairs are tuned to a certain wave frequency. When the waves pass over the hairs, an electrical signal is triggered
Auditory nerve VIII	A bundle of nerve fibres	Sends the electrical signals to the brain for interpretation
Eustachian tube	A long narrow tube opening into the middle ear, leading to the pharynx	Equalises the pressure between the outer and inner ear

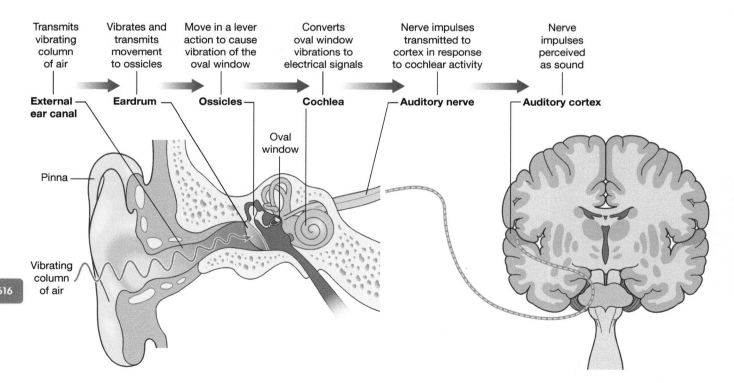

Figure 33.6 **The mechanism of hearing.** *Source*: Munir & Clarke 2013/John Wiley & Sons.

shape, and the same colour as the face. Look for obvious signs of abnormality; consider:

- The presence of any nodules or redness
- Size and shape of the pinna
- Extra cartilage tags/pre-auricular sinuses or pits
- Signs of trauma to the pinna
- Suspicious skin lesions on the pinna, including neoplasia
- Skin conditions of the pinna and external canal such as eczema
- Infection/inflammation of the external ear canal, with discharge
- Signs/scars of previous surgery.

Gently pull the helix back, determining if it is tender. Inspect and palpate the mastoid area behind the auricles, noting tenderness, redness and heat. Palpate the tragus for tenderness as this can be a sign of otitis externa.

Inspecting the Ear Canal and Eardrum

To inspect the ear canal and eardrum, an otoscope with its own light source is used to perform the examination. The otoscope (Figure 33.7) provides a good view of the tympanic membrane magnification.

Check that the batteries are fully operational to permit optimal light during the examination.

- The person should be asked to sit (or be supported) with the back straight and the head tilted slightly away from the examiner.
- Gently grasp the pinna, pulling posteriorly and superiorly (upwards and outward); this helps to straighten the ear canal for inspection of the tympanic membrane.
- Hold the otoscope with the thumb and finger, near to the eyepiece rather than at the end; this helps to reduce the patient's discomfort due to hand movements, which are exaggerated in the ear. Right hand on otoscope to patient's right ear and vice versa, handle pointing away from the patient (see Figure 33.8).
- Insert the speculum one-third of its length gently down and forward into the ear canal.
- Otoscopes are designed to use a disposable speculum. Choose the correct size of speculum to achieve the best view.

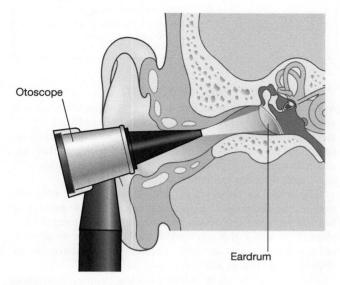

Figure 33.7 The otoscope.

Otoscope

Eardrum

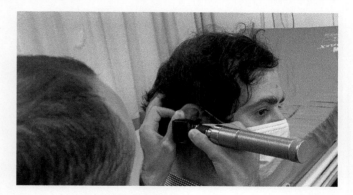

Figure 33.8 Holding the otoscope.

Note the condition of the canal skin and the presence of wax, foreign body or discharge, redness and malodour. If there is discharge, consider taking a swab using local guidelines and policy.

Nursing Fields Children

The infant's ear canal is directed downward, therefore pull the auricle gently downward and outward.

What the Experts Say

> Yemisi, a general practice nurse, says: 'For children, use stabilising and support techniques appropriate to age. As with adults, a full explanation of the procedure should be given to the child and if possible, allow the child to touch or handle the otoscope prior to the procedure'.

Jot This Down

Look at the picture in Figure 33.8 for the correct positioning for the otoscope. The benefits of the correct technique are examination comfort, stability and obtaining a good view of the canal and tympanic membrane. Can you list the adverse effects of incorrect positioning?

Inspecting and Viewing the Tympanic Membrane

The eardrum is roughly circular (about 1 cm in diameter). The tympanic membrane should be pearl grey, glistening and transparent; it may have a pink tinge. Observe for signs of bulging, retraction, bleeding, lesions, redness and perforations.

Primary Care Ear Irrigation

Ear irrigation may be recommended in primary care or community ear care services (NICE, 2019) for adults with earwax that is contributing to hearing loss or other symptoms or preventing ear examination or ear canal impressions being taken. It involves using a pressurised flow of water to remove the build-up of earwax.

(Continued)

An electronic ear irrigator is used by a trained healthcare professional; the intention is to avoid damaging the ear. The irrigator has an adjustable pressure control, so that syringing can commence with the minimum pressure. During the procedure, a controlled flow of water is instilled into the ear canal to clean out the earwax. The water used is at body temperature.
Ear irrigation should be a painless procedure. Manual ear irrigation should not be performed (NICE, 2019).

Red Flag Ear Irrigation

Ear irrigation is not recommended if the person has:
- Previously had problems with irrigation, such as pain in the ear or severe vertigo
- A perforated eardrum, or a perforated eardrum in the last 12 months
- A discharge of mucus from the ear
- A middle ear infection in the past 6 weeks
- A grommet
- Undergone ear surgery within the last 18 months
- A cleft palate
- A foreign body in the ear
- Otitis externa.

Hearing Acuity Tests

Detailed hearing tests are usually performed in audiology clinics. People who have normal hearing should hear equally well in both ears. See Box 33.1 for an overview of four tests used to assess hearing acuity in general practice.

Box 33.1 The Four Tests Used to Test Hearing Acuity		
Whisper test		Stand behind the patient at 40–60 cm distance facing towards one of the ears; ask the patient to occlude the opposite ear by pressing lightly on the tragus. Whisper something simple like 'tennis ball' and ask the patient to repeat what you have said. Repeat on the opposite ear. This is a gross whisper test and if the patient cannot hear it further testing or referral should be sought
Tuning fork tests A tuning fork is used to conduct these tests (Figure 33.9)	Weber's Test	This test checks for lateralisation. A 512 Hz vibrating fork is placed in the middle of the forehead and the patient is asked whether any sound is heard and, if so, whether it is equally heard in both ears. In a patient with normal hearing, the tone is heard centrally (equally in both ears). If the patient has unilateral hearing loss, the sound is louder in the weaker ear; this suggests a conductive hearing loss. If the sound is louder in the better ear, it is more likely to be a sensorineural hearing loss
	Rinnes's Test	Apply a 512 Hz tuning fork to the mastoid bone and ask the patient if they can feel the vibration. Once confirmed, ask the patient to tell you when the vibration stops. Once confirmed, without dulling the vibration or touching the prongs, place the tuning fork with the prongs positioned towards the external auditory meatus and ask the patient if they can hear anything. Air conduction should be greater than bone conduction and the patient should still be able to hear the vibration. If the patient cannot hear, this may suggest conductive hearing loss
	Pure tone audiometry	This can be performed in primary care or when the patient is referred to audiology. Hearing is measured over a range of pure tones in each ear. Frequencies vary from low pitches (250 Hz) to high pitches (8000 Hz). It measures the threshold for air and bone conduction and can determine whether it is due to conductive or sensorineural loss, or mixed Each ear is tested at octave intervals from 250 to 8000 Hz and plotted on a pure-tone audiogram with the test frequency along the horizontal axis and the thresholds of hearing on the vertical axis. This is in decibels of hearing level (dB HL), which ranges from minus 10 (at the top) to 120 (the loudest that most audiometers can generate)

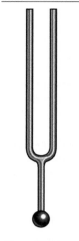

Figure 33.9
A tuning fork.

Physiological Measurement

Audiology services may include assessment of patient needs and selection of appropriate care pathways and offer hearing assessment and rehabilitation of hearing loss, including counselling, fitting and programming of hearing aids and advice on their use and management. They offer a range of different hearing aids and clinics for more specialist needs.

The results of physiological and other diagnostic tests will support the diagnosis of a particular injury, disease process or hearing problem. The aim is to reveal information required to identify or adjust the appropriate medications or to provide hearing devices and to help monitor patient outcomes in response to treatment and care provision.

The role of the nurse when assisting people undergoing diagnostic testing, regardless of the kind of test, is to offer the person an explanation of the proposed procedure and to advise if there is any special preparation needed.

Physiological measurement tests related to hearing are carried out in several care areas. Nurses may be required to undertake the test, or they may be involved in the delivery of some elements of the diagnostic test components (e.g. the decision to investigate or, in more complex testing or in reporting and interpreting, assisting the patient and technician). It is essential that the nurse is competent and confident if they are required to undertake these tests. Any physiological measurement that is undertaken must:

- Be patient centred
- Make use of the benefits of new technology
- Be streamlined and efficient
- Be delivered closer to home
- Provide excellent patient information
- Be accessible to primary as well as secondary care
- Be evidence based.

> ### Jot This Down
> Bhupi Singh is a 72-year-old man who wears an analogue hearing aid. He seems rather withdrawn and less responsive than usual. His wife is asking you if his hearing aid is working. How would you test if his hearing aid was working correctly?

Person-centred Care

Any treatment and care must consider people's needs and preferences. People with hearing problems should have the opportunity to make informed decisions about their care and treatment in partnership with the person providing that care.

> ### Nursing Fields Learning Disabilities
> If a person with a learning disability does not have the capacity to make decisions, the nurse should follow the advice given in Chapters 2 and 9, as well as the guidance offered by the four UK countries' Departments of Health and Social Care. Nurses must always act in the best interests of the patient. Any information offered to people should also be accessible to those with additional needs, such as physical, sensory or learning disabilities.

Communication should be supported by evidence-based written information that has been tailored to the individual's needs. Treatment and care and the information that people are given about it should be culturally appropriate and provision made for people who do not speak or read English.

If the person being cared for agrees, families and carers should have the opportunity to be involved in decisions about treatment and care. The nurse should also ensure that families and carers are given the information and support they need.

Red Flag Ototoxicity

Medicines that may cause hearing loss include the following.

- Certain antibiotics, especially aminoglycosides, may be ototoxic (e.g. gentamicin, streptomycin and neomycin). Hearing-related side-effects from these antibiotics are most common in people who have renal disease or who already have underlying ear or hearing problems.
- Other ototoxic medicines include loop diuretics used to treat hypertension and heart failure, such as furosemide or bumetanide, and medicines used to treat cancer, including cyclophosphamide and cisplatin.

Common Conditions of the Ear

Gaining an understanding of the key issues concerned with assessment of hearing can help you offer care that is safe and appropriate.

Presbycusis

Also known as age-related hearing loss or presbyacousia, this condition is progressive and is usually bilateral, occurring in older people as they age. The hallmark of presbycusis is the progressive symmetrical loss of high-frequency hearing (microwave beeping, phone ringing) over many years, with normal hearing in childhood (Tawfik *et al.*, 2020). Presbycusis is the most common cause of sensorineural hearing loss (see Table 33.2 for a discussion of the types of deafness). Age-related diseases can be viewed as accelerated aging stemming from genetics during life interacting with environmental and social/lifestyle factors (Franceschi *et al.*, 2018).

The condition can range from being bothersome to severely debilitating in its effects. It can lead to the older person becoming isolated and depressed and has the potential to significantly exacerbate age-related disability/cognitive impairment and dementia. The condition is correctable using rehabilitative measures and when treatment is successful, this can improve quality of life for the older person

It is essential that the nurse can communicate effectively with the patient. Box 33.2 provides some simple steps to reduce communication problems.

Hearing loss is a major public health issue. Figures from the World Health Organization (WHO) *World Report on Hearing* (2021) are concerning, with over 5% of the world's population needing rehabilitation to address their 'disabling' hearing loss (432 million adults and 34 million children); over 65% of adults above 60 years of age experience hearing loss.

Signs and Symptoms of Presbycusis

These are some of the symptoms people may experience (RNID, 2021):

- Other people sound like they are mumbling
- Asking people to repeat things for you often
- Having difficulty understanding what is being said in noisy places
- Finding it hard to keep up with group conversation
- Getting tired from having to concentrate so much
- Other people saying your TV or music is too loud
- Often have difficulty hearing on the telephone.

Table 33.2 Types of deafness. *Source*: Adapted from RNID (2021).

CONDUCTIVE HEARING LOSS	SENSORINEURAL HEARING LOSS
Occurs with problems in the transmission of sound waves from the external ear through the middle ear. The disease processes, which may be congenital or acquired, include conditions such as excess earwax, trauma, otitis externa or otitis media with effusion and otosclerosis	Refers to problems occurring in the cochlea (the most common site of disease), cochlear nerve or brainstem resulting in abnormal or absent neurosensory impulses. There are also several congenital and acquired conditions, the most common being *presbycusis*

Box 33.2 Some Simple Steps the Nurse Can Take to Enhance Communication with People Who are Deaf

- Ask the patient how they prefer to communicate: do not assume that if the patient is wearing a hearing aid they can automatically follow what you are saying. Ask if they prefer to lip-read and have pen and paper handy
- Sit in good lighting and, if possible, away from noise and distractors
- Make sure you have the listener's attention before you start speaking
- Do not turn your face away when speaking
- Speak clearly but not too slowly or using exaggerated mannerisms
- If they do not understand what you have said, do not just repeat it but try saying it in a different way
- Do not waffle; avoid jargon and abbreviations
- Check that the person is following what you are saying
- If the patient can use British Sign Language (BSL), consider using a suitably trained interpreter or 'Sign Translate' via a computer live webcam

Pathophysiology

There are many factors that contribute to hearing loss in the older person. Histological changes associated with ageing occur throughout the auditory system, from the hair cells of the cochlea to the auditory cortex in the temporal lobe of the brain. The nerves or hair cells in the inner ear, where the cochlea starts to deteriorate, die off or become damaged. The loss of the hair cells makes it harder to hear. Presbycusis can also result from changes in the middle ear as a person ages or from changes in the nerve pathways to the brain.

Practice Assessment Document

Confidently assesses needs and plans person-centred care. Uses skills of active listening, questioning, paraphrasing and reflection to support therapeutic interventions using a range of communication techniques as required

Demonstrate knowledge and understanding of communication skills with your practice assessor by role play. Ask them or a colleague to occlude their ears with headphones or ear plugs, carry out a simple interaction, apply what you have learnt and understood by going through the simple steps the nurse can take to enhance communication with people who are deaf. Ask the assessor for feedback.

Risk Factors

There are multiple risk factors that influence the onset and severity of presbycusis (Box 33.3).

Box 33.3 Risk Factors Associated with Presbycusis

- Noise exposure, e.g. exposure to industrial, urban, armament noise without ear protection
- Ototoxic medication, e.g. loop diuretics.
- Family history/genetic factors
- Hypertension
- High cholesterol
- Diabetes
- Smoking
- High BMI

Sources: Gopinath (2021); Tawfik *et al.* (2020).

Investigations and Diagnosis

The diagnosis of presbycusis should be suspected based on a history of slowly progressive, symmetrical hearing loss in the older person. A simple gross whisper test can be used to screen for hearing loss. Observing the person during conversation can often highlight hearing problems. Audiometry may be used to screen patients and/or to confirm the diagnosis.

Primary Care

The World Health Organization has developed the hearWHO app (HearX Group, 2019). It can be used by people to self-screen or by healthcare professionals as a primary screening tool (it does not replace diagnostic tests). If abnormalities with hearing are detected, the person can be referred for diagnostic testing.

QR code for hearWHO app

Download the app

Source: hearWHO app/World Health Organization/Public Domain.

A careful history of associated factors, such as family history, ototoxic medications, trauma and concurrent otological symptoms, can help explain potential aetiologies. Asymmetrical hearing loss should lead to evaluation for other conditions such as otitis media, tumours, trauma or asymmetrical noise exposure (as often occurs from firearms exposure or the long-term use of power tools on one side).

Nursing Care and Management

Presbycusis is not curable but the effects of the condition on the person's life can be alleviated. Simple recognition of the problem can be a significant positive step, as hearing loss in the older person can often be mistaken for cognitive impairment. The identification of hearing loss can be reassuring for many patients.

- *Amplification devices*: properly fitted and working hearing aids may contribute to the rehabilitation of a patient with presbycusis. Those with arthritis in their fingers and visual difficulties need extra help in learning to use hearing aids. Speech discrimination in noisy situations may remain supoptimal.
- *Lip reading*: may help patients with diminished speech discrimination and may help hearing aid users who have difficulty in noisy environments.
- *Assistive listening devices*: these range from a simple amplification of the telephone signal to a device on the television that sends a signal across the room to a headset worn by a patient with hearing loss. The patient can amplify the sound without disturbing other people with normal hearing who are in the same room.
- *Cochlear implants*: some people with presbycusis benefit from cochlear implants. Patients with cochlear changes and relatively intact spiral ganglia and central pathways appear to be most suited to this type of intervention.

Health Promotion

Some sensory presbycusis is inevitable but avoiding noise exposure and using ear protection in noisy environments will prevent some progressive damage. A balanced diet and general health and fitness may reduce the cardiovascular contribution to hearing loss.

Chronic Suppurative Otitis Media

Chronic inflammation of the middle ear and the mastoid cavity is known as chronic suppurative otitis media (CSOM). While the condition primarily affects children, it can also occur in adults. CSOM is a chronic inflammation and infection, often with polymicrobial infection of the middle ear and mastoid cavity, typified by ear discharge (otorrhoea) through a perforated tympanic membrane (Chong *et al.*, 2021). There is no universally accepted definition of CSOM and it may be defined as having a duration of discharge of more than 2 weeks or more than 6 weeks (WHO, 2004).

Pathophysiology

Diseases of the tympanic membrane may also be included within the definition of CSOM, such as tympanic perforation without a history of recent ear discharge, or the disease cholesteatoma (a growth of the squamous epithelium of the tympanic membrane).

Investigations and Diagnosis

Patients presenting with CSOM should be referred to ENT specialists. Microsuctioning or debridement is performed to allow examination of the tympanic membrane perforation. An audiogram will usually reveal conductive hearing loss. Mixed hearing loss may suggest more extensive disease and possible complications. Imaging studies such as CT may be useful for failed treatment and may show occult cholesteatoma, foreign body or malignancy.

Signs and Symptoms

CKS (2017) advises that CSOM should be suspected if:

- Ear discharge persists for more than 2 weeks, without ear pain or fever
- There is hearing loss in the affected ear
- There is a history of acute otitis media (AOM), ear trauma, or glue ear and grommet insertion
- There is a history of allergy, atopy and/or upper respiratory tract infection
- There is tinnitus and/or a sensation of pressure in the ear.

Nursing Care and Management

Conservative treatment of CSOM consists of three elements:

- An appropriate antibiotic, usually administered topically
- Microsuction to remove debris
- Control of granulation tissue.

Medication Topical antibiotics are often given in combination with a steroid; this is always carried out in a specialist setting. There is debate regarding the effectiveness of topical antibiotics (Brennan-Jones *et al.*, 2020; Chong *et al.*, 2021).

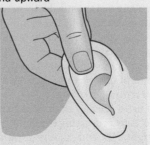

(Continued)

621

8. Place the correct number of drops in the ear. Gently press on the small skin flap over the ear to help the drops to run into the ear canal

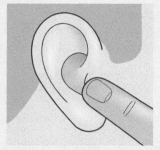

9. Keep the ear tilted up for a few minutes. Gently swab any leakage; avoid plugging the ear with cotton wool or gauze as this may soak up the medication
10. Replace and tighten the cap or dropper right away
11. Wash hands to remove any medication

What to Do If . . . Administering Ear Drops to a Child

If instilling ear drops in a child younger than 3 years of age, pull the ear backward and downward to open the ear canal.

Surgery Surgical intervention and type depend on the severity of the disease process and may involve myringoplasty (repair of the eardrum perforation alone) or tympanoplasty (repair of the eardrum and surgery involving the bones of the inner ear).

If cholesteatoma is present, radical mastoidectomy, modified radical mastoidectomy or the combined approach tympanoplasty (anterior tympanotomy plus extended mastoidectomy) may be used depending on the extent of cholesteatoma. The aim of surgery is to remove all disease and to give the person a dry and functioning ear.

Anatomy and Physiology of the Eye

In this section, an overview of the anatomy and physiology of the eyes will be presented. The function of the eye will be discussed prior to describing a few common eye conditions and the care required for people with eye problems.

For further information on the anatomy and physiology of the eyes, visit Peate & Evans (2020).

The eye is the organ of sight which reacts with light and allows light perception, colour vision and depth perception (Yanoff & Duker, 2014). It provides us with the sense of sight, letting us observe and learn about the surrounding world, more than with any of the other special senses. The eyes are used in most activities we carry out and sight is the sense that people usually value most. Eighty percent of our perception, learning, cognition and activities is mediated through vision.

The eye allows us to see and understand shapes, colour and dimensions of objects by processing the light they reflect or emit. The eye detects bright light and colours or dim light due to specialised photoreceptors known as rods and cones in the retina. Vitamin A is an essential component of these photoreceptors.

The eye is formed by week 5 of gestation, and by age 3 years the diameter of the eye is about 22.5–23 mm (Vaughan, 2017). By the late teens, the eye has attained its full size.

The eye is a complex structure that gathers information about the environment. Structures associated with the eye are outlined in Box 33.4. A cross-section of the eye is detailed in Figure 33.10.

The Protective Structures of the Eye

The Orbit
The bony orbits are pyramid-shaped cavities located at the front of the skull (Marsden, 2017), known as the 'sockets', which protect the eyes. Each has a wider opening anteriorly (towards the front) narrowing to a small opening posteriorly known as the optic foramen where the optic nerve exits to connect with the visual pathways and the brain (Figure 33.11). Orbital fat and connective tissue surround and support the eye. The orbital bones are thin but have a strong rim to protect the eye against the impact of blunt trauma. The orbit surrounds and supports the posterior segment of the eye but the anterior cornea extends beyond the orbital rim and is protected by the eyelids.

The Eyelids, Eyelashes, Eyebrows and Extrinsic Ocular Muscles
These are known as ocular adnexal structures; positioned external to the eyeball, they provide integrity and protection to the eye. Other protective structures include the conjunctiva and the lacrimal apparatus which contributes to tear formation which is essential for clear vision.

In order for an individual to have normal vison, the extrinsic muscles must work well in a co-ordinated manner, otherwise double vision (diplopia) will occur. There are six extrinsic eye muscles, which allow the eye to move into different positions (Marsden, 2017). There are four recti muscles:
1. Medial
2. Lateral
3. Superior
4. Inferior

and two obliques:
1. Superior
2. Inferior.

Box 33.4 Structures of the Eye

The important structures of the eye
- The bony orbit
- The eyelids
- The eyelashes and eyebrows
- The lacrimal apparatus
- The sclera

The anterior segment of the eye
- The cornea and the tear film
- The aqueous humour
- The iris
- The lens and ciliary muscle

The posterior segment of the eye
- The retina
- The vitreous humour

The visual system pathways to the brain
- The optic nerves and optic tracts
- The visual cortex

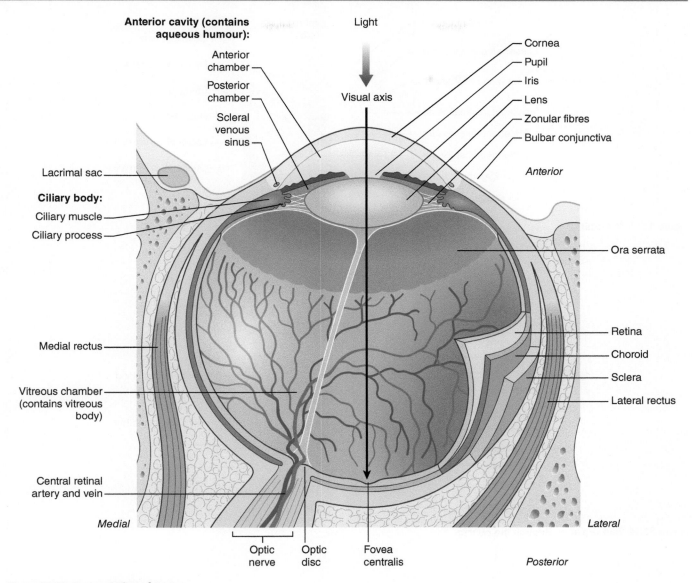

Figure 33.10 Cross-section of an eye.

The action of these muscles is controlled by the third, fourth and sixth cranial nerves to ensure that the image of the object falls on the macula and a single image is seen with both eyes (Vaughan, 2017). This is known as binocular single vision which is essential for depth and perception. If there is a weakness in one of the muscles, a squint will occur, resulting in double vision in an adult.

A muscle imbalance in a child under 7 years of age will result in a 'lazy eye'. A lazy eye with poor vision is known as an amblyopic eye in a child. It is important to note that in a young child, the brain should be stimulated by clear vision in order to learn to see. The child's brain switches off the blurred vision arising from a squint so it is essential to manage a squint as early as possible to prevent amblyopia (Yanoff & Duker, 2016). The vision in an amblyopic eye is blurred which may have consequences for the child later on in life with the choice of certain occupations, such as pilot or engineer.

The eyelids (palpebrae) are thin loose folds of skin covering the anterior eye, protecting the eye from foreign bodies and excessive light. They also spread tears by blinking. They contain the puncta, through which the tears flow (Figure 33.12).

The eyelids (Figure 33.13) are protective to the eye and protect the cornea against dryness. The cross-sectional view in Figure 33.13 shows important lid structures, that is, the various muscles which assist in lid closure and opening. The meibomian glands are inside the tarsal plate and produce sebaceous fluid to lubricate the eye. Rows of lashes are situated on the lid margin and are lubricated by the oily gland known as Zeis.

The eyebrows provide shade and keep perspiration and other debris away from the eyes. Warren (2013) suggests that the periorbital region is the most expressive part of the face.

The eyelashes are short hairs projecting from the top and bottom borders of the eyelids. An unexpected touch to the eyelashes initiates the involuntary blinking reflex. Blinking also assists in the movement of tears across the eye (Yanoff & Duker, 2014).

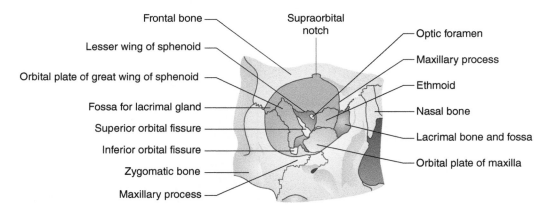

Figure 33.11 **The orbit.**

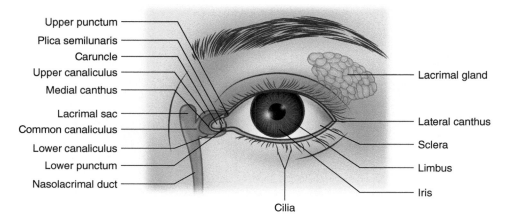

Figure 33.12 **Tear drainage through the puncta.**

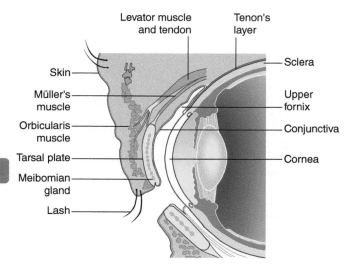

Figure 33.13 **The eyelid.**

The Lacrimal Apparatus

The lacrimal apparatus (Figure 33.14) produces and drains tears (lacrimal fluid) and is composed of:

- The lacrimal gland
- The puncta
- The lacrimal sac
- The nasolacrimal duct.

The surface of the eye is continuously bathed in tears that are primarily secreted by the lacrimal gland. The conjunctiva produces mucin and immunoglobulin IgA which keep the cornea wet and protect the eye against pathogens. These structures secrete, distribute and drain tears to cleanse and moisten the eye's surface for clarity of vision (Seewoodhary & Awelewa, 2014). Each time an individual blinks, tears are pumped into the lacrimal sac and cleared via the nasolacrimal duct.

The Sclera

The sclera is the fibrous outer protective coat of the eye. It is dense and white and is continuous with the cornea anteriorly and with the dural layer of the optic nerve posteriorly.

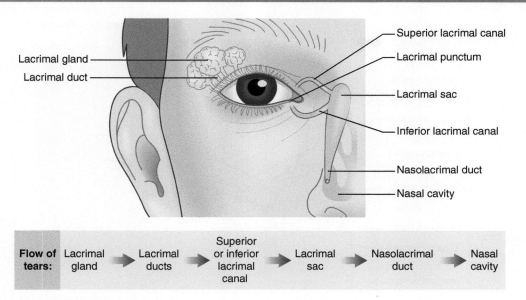

Figure 33.14 The lacrimal apparatus.

The Anterior Segment of the Eye

The Cornea

The cornea is the main refractive medium of the eye and is a transparent window which allows light to enter the retina; it does not contain any blood vessels. It is approximately 11 mm in diameter and 550 μm thick in the centre, thickening to around 750 μm at the periphery, curved anteriorly and has six layers. The outer epithelial layer heals well, the middle stromal layer is collagenous and its inner endothelial layer controls its water content rigidly to maintain clarity (Vaughan, 2017). The cornea and lens refract light rays to the retina macular region. The cornea also protects the inner ocular structures. It is very sensitive to touch and is innervated by the trigeminal nerve.

The Aqueous Humour

The area between the cornea and the front surface of the lens is called the anterior chamber. This contains a transparent fluid (the aqueous humour) that provides oxygen and nutrients to the lens and cornea. Its vitamin C content is 20 times higher than that of plasma (Marsden, 2017). It is important for the maintenance of normal intraocular pressure which ranges between 12 mmHg and 20 mmHg. Its rate of formation must be equal to the rate of drainage through the trabecular meshwork (Vaughan, 2017). It also refracts light rays.

The Iris

This is the coloured aspect of the eye and is known as the anterior uvea. It is shaped like a flattened doughnut. It controls the amount of light entering the retina, similar to the aperture on a camera. The round opening in its center is the pupil. There are two sets of muscles in the iris that dilate and constrict the pupil size. The iris and chambers of the eye are shown in Figure 33.15.

The colour, texture and patterns of each person's iris are as unique as a fingerprint. The colour pigments are deposited around 6 months after birth and are genetically inherited.

The Lens and Accommodation

The lens is a clear structure which lies posterior to the pupil and the iris. It changes its shape in order to increase or decrease the amount of refracting power applied to light rays coming into the eye, a process known as *accommodation*. Throughout life, the lens continues to grow (Marsden, 2017); its main function is to bend light rays for accuracy of sight. The lens refractive power is stronger in the very young and diminishes with age.

The lens is held in place by a suspensory ligament known as the zonule. It is composed of numerous fibrils that arise from the muscular ciliary body and insert into the lens equator. The ciliary muscle is innervated by the oculomotor nerve which enables the ciliary body to contract or relax to change the shape of the lens for far and near vision.

The ciliary body is the middle portion of the uveal tract and is divided into three parts as shown in Figure 33.16.

- The ciliary muscle
- The ciliary processes (pars plicata)
- The pars plana

The Choroid

The choroid forms the posterior part of the uveal tract, situated next to the ciliary body. It has a rich blood supply which nourishes the retina. It is heavily pigmented in order to absorb excess light rays that enter the eye. It acts as a coolant for the retina, which is metabolically a very active tissue.

The Posterior Segment of the Eye

The Retina

The retina is a complex photosensitive structure. It is a transparent thin tissue which captures photons of light and initiates processing of the image by the brain. The average thickness of the retina is 250 μm and it consists of 10 layers (Figure 33.17).

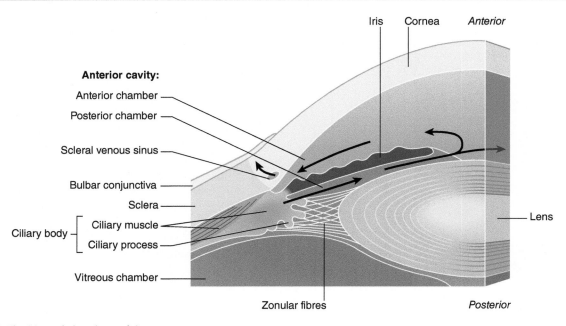

Figure 33.15 The iris and chambers of the eye.

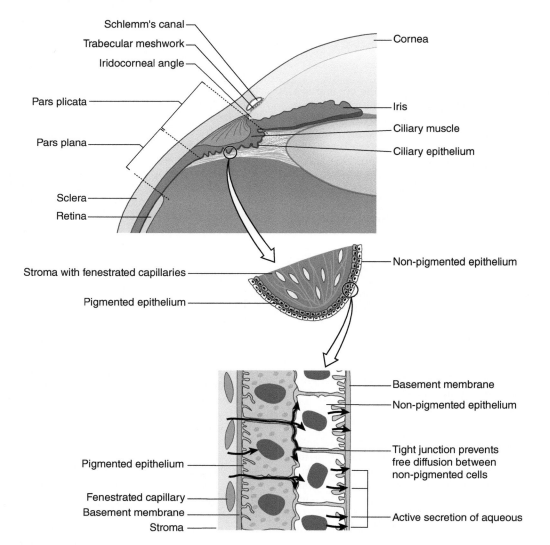

Figure 33.16 Anatomy of the ciliary body.

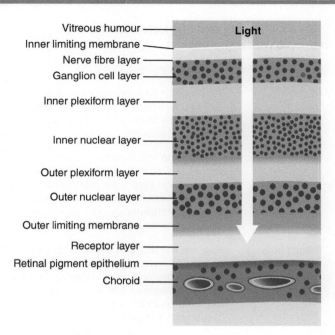

Figure 33.17 **Retinal layers.**

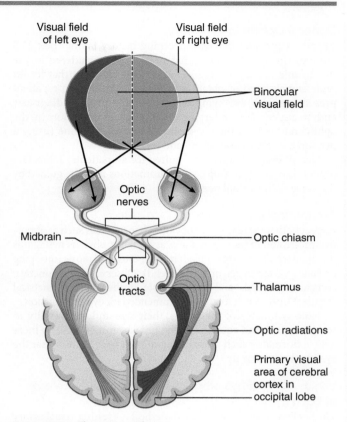

Figure 33.18 **The optic pathway.**

There are two types of photoreceptors in the retina: rods and cones (named for their shape). The outer segment of the photo-receptors contains the light-sensitive visual pigment molecules called opsins in stacked discs (rods) or invaginations (cones). Vitamin A is essential for visual pigments. There are approximately 7 million cones and 120 million rods in the retina. Cones provide the ability to discern colour and to see fine detail, and are more concentrated in the macula, the central retina. Rods are mainly responsible for peripheral vision and vision under low light conditions and are more prevalent in the midperipheral and peripheral retina. Rod cells do not discern colours.

The Visual System Pathways to the Brain

The Optic Nerve and Optic Tracts

The retinal nerve fibres leave each eye as the optic nerve (the 2nd cranial nerve) and meet at the optic chiasm, anterior to the pituitary gland in the brain (Figure 33.18).

At the optic chiasm, the crossing of the axons results in each optic tract carrying information from both eyes (see Figure 33.18).

There is an overlap of the visual fields, with each eye seeing a slightly different image. As a result of this overlap, along with the crossing of the axons, information from both eyes reaches both sides of the visual cortex. The information is then fused into one image (binocular single vision).

The Visual Cortex

The visual cortex in the occipital lobe of the brain is where the final processing of the neural signals from the retina takes place and vision occurs. The occipital lobe is in the most posterior portion of the brain (see Chapter 32). There are a total of six separate areas in the visual cortex, known as V1, V2, V3, V3a, V4 and V5.

The Nursing Associate

Nursing associates should be able to demonstrate and apply knowledge of body systems, human anatomy and physiology when delivering care (NMC, 2018b). If a patient asked you to give a simple description of the structures of the eye and how the eye perceives light, how would you describe it? Have a go saying this out loud to yourself or to a friend/family member to practise. How much did you recall?

Assessing Vision

Reaching an ophthalmic diagnosis is dependent on a good history and detailed examination.

Red Flag Competence

Only nurses who have demonstrated that they have the competence and confidence to take the history and undertake the examination should carry out visual activity tests.

There are a number of visual acuity tests available that assess the ability to see fine detail. Vision assessment is an organised procedure for gathering information about the health and function of the visual system. The assessments can be done in a number of venues by specialist practitioners, for example nurses, ophthalmologists and optometrists.

General Ophthalmic History

Chapter 4 provides details concerning history taking. Box 33.5 outlines the specific issues that need to be considered in the ophthalmic history. Gibbons *et al.* (2010) highlight that health professionals need to obtain a thorough history from a patient presenting with eye symptoms to enable prompt diagnosis and treatment. To undertake a thorough examination in the ophthalmic setting, the nurse should inspect, examine (using a pen torch or ophthalmoscope) and test the eye.

Not all examinations are required for all patients. Table 33.3 provides some suggestions, but examinations must be guided by the person's individual needs.

Anatomical Examination

Inspect both eyes, noting any obvious abnormalities such as abnormal protrusion of the eye, redness, asymmetry, obvious nystagmus (involuntary, to-and-fro oscillation of the eyes) and ptosis (drooping or falling of the upper or lower eyelid). Observe the conjunctiva, cornea, iris, pupils and eyelids; note if they are symmetrical (Figure 33.19). A pen torch is recommended for eye examination.

Note symmetry of the pupils, their size and their ability to react normally and equally to light and accommodation. Is there a lid abnormality such as drooping of the eyelid? Check that the eyelids close correctly.

Visual Acuity (Physiological Testing of Central Vision of Each Eye)

The Snellen chart is the standard method for testing visual acuity (Figure 33.20). The chart contains rows of letters in varying sizes; there are standardised numbers at the end of each row. If the person is unable to read or does not read English, the E-chart (a set of random tumbling Es) can be used, or the Gardiner Sheridan

Table 33.3 History and suggested examination in people with eye problems.

CONDITION	EXAMINATION/INVESTIGATION
All patients	Take a history, undertake a visual acuity and pen torch assessment. A slit lamp eye examination is important for all ophthalmic patients
Red/painful eye	Examine the lids, lacrimal system, conjunctiva, cornea, pupils, anterior chamber and intraocular pressure if possible (if not and no obvious cause, refer to ophthalmology/emergency eye clinic as per local guidelines)
Foreign body	Examine the lids, conjunctiva and cornea. If there is a presenting high-velocity injury, a full detailed anatomical examination of the eye is required. Use a cotton bud to evert the upper lid to examine and remove a subtarsal foreign body if present
Reduced vision	Examine the cornea, anterior chamber and beyond. Undertake functional testing of visual field, pupils, optic nerve and macula
Double vision/ orbital problems	Examine the fundus, optic nerve function, extraocular muscle function; undertake X-ray or CT scan
Headache/eye pain in absence of red eye	Examine the fundus, optic nerve, pupillary reaction, blood pressure; carry out a full neurological examination including a colour vision test

Box 33.5 Key Points and the Ophthalmic History

Think about the symptoms carefully.
- Determine how long the symptoms have been present.
- Are the symptoms continuous or intermittent?
- What triggered them?
- Does anything make them better or worse?
- Describe how the symptoms are changing.
- Are there any related symptoms?
- Is there a previous eye or related systemic disease?
- Ascertain if there is a:
  ○ Past ophthalmic history (e.g. cataract, iritis, dry eye, blepharitis); recurrence is quite common
  ○ Past medical history (e.g. diabetes, hypertension, thyrotoxicosis)
  ○ Drug history (any drugs being taken that may cause visual disturbance, i.e. eye drops, and many medications do affect sight, such as steroids, antidepressants). Do enquire about drug allergy or allergy to eye drop preservative
  ○ Family history (inherited visual problems, i.e. glaucoma, cataract)
  ○ Social history (smoking, alcohol use, recreational drug use, exposure to chemicals).
- Is the person registered blind or do they have a known visual impairment?
- Are there any adaptations in the home?
- Does the person need assistive devices, such as Braille?

Source: Adapted from Gleadle (2012); Olver *et al.* (2014); Watkinson (2009).

Redness

Ptosis

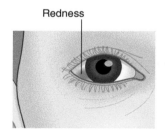
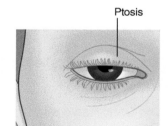

Pupils
- Symmetry
- Size, shape
- Reaction to light
- Reaction to accommodation
- PERRLA (pupils equal round and reacting to light and accommodation)

Figure 33.19 **Inspection of the eyes.**

chart is used for letter or picture matching. The Snellen chart provides a standardised test of visual acuity and can be handheld at 3 m or placed at 6 m from the person.

The nurse asks the person to cover one eye, avoiding pressing the eye. The problem eye should be tested first. The person is then asked to read each row of letters; they should move from the largest to the smallest letters that they can see. The same approach is used to measure visual acuity in the other eye. Each eye must

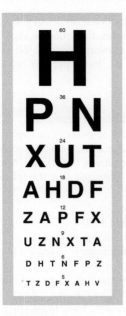

Figure 33.20 The Snellen chart.

be tested separately. Ask the person to wear their corrective glasses or note if they use contact lenses according to the distance of the Snellen chart used. This will test best corrective vision, and this is recorded in the patient's medical notes, ensuring local policy and procedure are adhered to.

The Cardiff testing chart is useful in young children as illustrated in Figure 33.21.

Nursing Fields Children: Testing Visual Acuity

· Very young children are observed to see if they can follow or pick up objects such as scattered 'hundreds and thousands' cake decorations.
· A chart called the Cardiff card can be used instead of the Snellen chart (Figure 33.21).
· The older child should be able to identify or match single pictures and letters on charts held in their hands with those of varying sizes presented to them at a distance.

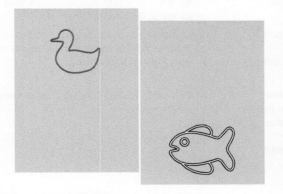

Figure 33.21 Cardiff cards.

Source: Adapted from James & Bron (2011).

Other tests include the Ishihara chart for colour vision. Visual fields are tested using a variety of methods; confrontation visual field testing is a common approach.

Pupillary Reactions

The pupils should be of equal size: 3–5 mm. Assess direct and consensual pupil response. Ask the person to look straight ahead and shine a light obliquely into one eye at a time and observe for constriction of the pupil in the illuminated eye. Carry out this test for both eyes. The normal direct and consensual pupillary response is constriction. Consensual response is achieved by shining the light into one pupil and observing the constriction of the pupil in the other eye.

In order to test for accommodation, the nurse holds an object at a distance of about 60 cm from the person; pupils should dilate. Ask the person to follow the object as you bring it to within a few centimetres of their nose. The pupils should constrict, and the eyes converge as they change focus to follow the object.

Examination with an Ophthalmoscope

Examination of the internal eye using the ophthalmoscope should only be undertaken by a skilled practitioner. This allows visualisation of the lens, vitreous humour and retina. Opacity (whiteness) of the pupil caused by a cataract or a haemorrhage into the vitreous humour can be seen with an ophthalmoscope.

On examination, the normal lens should be clear. There should be no visible haemorrhages, discharge or white patches when inspecting the retina. The optic disc should be round to oval with clear, well-defined borders. Inspecting the blood vessels of the retina can reveal glaucoma, caused by increased intraocular pressure. Hypertension can result in a narrowing of the arteries and veins and retinal bleeding. Diabetes, atherosclerosis and blood disorders can cause engorged veins to occur. The retina is usually a constant red-orange colour; it is lighter around the optic disc. The macula should be visible on the temporal aspect 3 mm distant from the optic disc. There should be no tenderness, excessive tearing or discharge over the lacrimal glands, puncta and nasolacrimal duct. Presence of a red reflex when the light is shone in the retina is a normal finding. Both eyes should be assessed and absence of a red reflex may signify a retinal disorder or an intraocular tumour.

Common Conditions of the Eye

Understanding the anatomy and physiology of the eye, along with an awareness of the various ways of assessing those with eye disorders, can assist you when you offer care to people that is safe, evidence based and person-centred.

Acute or chronic conditions can affect the eye and its protective structures. Often, eye disorders are minor and have minimal or no effect on vision, but there are some that can cause permanent vision impairment, cause discomfort and impact negatively on a person's body image. Either temporary or permanent visual impairment can ensue after eye surgery or as a result of minor trauma.

Inflammation of the Eyelids: Blepharitis

Blepharitis is a common inflammation of the lid margins that may be acute or chronic. The true prevalence is unknown and studies trying to estimate this have been unsatisfactory (American Academy of Ophthalmology, 2018). The predisposing factors are skin disorders, environmental pollution or diabetes.

Blepharitis can be classed as anterior or posterior (College of Optometrists, 2021). Anterior blepharitis involves the lid margin and lashes. Posterior blepharitis is caused by dysfunction of the meibomian glands in the inner eyelid margin. Some patients can present with a mixture of both types.

Pathophysiology

There are several pathological causes associated with blepharitis. Direct bacterial infection can result in a response against bacterial toxins which will destabilise the tear film, causing soreness and dryness, and can threaten the corneal integrity leading to corneal ulcer.

There may be structural alterations and secretory dysfunction of the meibomian glands which can lead to dry eye.

Investigations and Diagnosis

The American Academy of Ophthalmology (2018) reports that the diagnosis of blepharitis is usually based on patient history and slit-lamp findings. Additional testing such as taking swabs of the eyelid and conjunctiva, and dynamic meibomian gland imaging may be undertaken. A biopsy is required where crustiness is accompanied by a suspicious lesion on the lid margin to rule out malignancy. The AAO suggests a slit-lamp biomicroscope to check for *Demodex folliculorum* worms in the base of the lash follicles.

Signs and Symptoms

The person usually complains of sore eyes, itchiness, burning and a gritty sensation with crusting to the lids and lashes on waking; this is usually bilateral and chronic. The eye(s) may be red and sometimes people complain of epiphora (excess tears) or dry eye and photophobia.

Blurred vision may occur secondary to epiphora. If the person wears contact lenses, they may be unable to tolerate them, and this may cause corneal infection. Blepharitis can wax and wane (there may be long periods of exacerbations and remissions).

Nursing Care and Management

There is good evidence to make definitive recommendations for the management of blepharitis. A cure is not possible in most cases. The College of Optometrists (2021) and American Academy of Ophthalmology (2018) suggest that the following treatments are helpful:

- Warm compresses
- Eyelid hygiene (Table 33.4)
- Antibiotics (topical and/or systemic)
- Topical anti-inflammatory agents (e.g. corticosteroids, ciclosporin)
- Healthy diet (e.g. vegetables, fruits and oily fish rich in omega 3 and 6).

Initially treat patients who have blepharitis with a regimen of warm compresses and eyelid hygiene, carried out twice daily during the acute phase and then daily. A topical antibiotic such as chloramphenicol can be prescribed for 1 week to treat the infection, such as for those with staphylococcal blepharitis. For those with meibomian gland dysfunction, where chronic symptoms and signs are not adequately controlled with eyelid hygiene, oral tetracyclines can be prescribed. A brief course of topical corticosteroids may be helpful for eyelid or ocular surface inflammation. The minimal effective dose of corticosteroid should be used and long-term corticosteroid therapy avoided.

The person should be advised not to wear contact lens, especially during acute inflammatory episodes, as this may be a source of reinfection. Reassurance should be given that the condition is seldom sight-threatening, and it should not prevent their usual activities, e.g. swimming, unless there is an acute infection. The use of make-up and eyeliner should be avoided.

Table 33.4 Lid hygiene.

ACTIVITY	TECHNIQUE	REASONING
Warm compresses	Soak a flannel in warm water: apply to closed lid of each eye for 5–10 minutes. Keeping the eyelid closed is important	Softening the crusts and the meibomian glands, making subsequent cleansing easier and more comfortable
Lid massage	Close lids and gently rotate a clean finger along lid, ending in a downward stroke (upper lid) and upward stroke (lower lid). Move along the length of each lid. Repeat several times daily	Loosening meibomian gland content and expressing this through the meibomian openings on the lid margin
Lid cleansing	Dip a clean Q-tips bud in boiled but cooled water, and gently scrub the lid margin, starting from the nasal side to remove crusts from the lash base Hypoallergenic soaps such as baby shampoo diluted with sterile water or sodium bicarbonate are useful in seborrhoeic blepharitis with its frequency tailored according to severity. Commercial lid scrubs may also be used	Removing lid debris helps to heal margin inflammation

Health Promotion and Discharge

This condition rarely fully resolves (American Academy of Ophthalmology, 2018). However, symptomatic control can be gained with patient education and empowering the patient to adhere to lid hygiene.

There are several everyday steps that the person can take to prevent blepharitis.

- Keeping the hands and face clean.
- Avoiding rubbing the eyes with dirty fingers or a dirty towel, for example.
- Removing all eye make-up before bedtime.
- Avoiding the use of eye make-up to prevent further irritation.
- Not to share make-up.

What the Experts Say

'There is always the risk of reinfection with blepharitis, and I suggest that when the patient starts to use make-up again, they replace the products they have been using in or near the eyelids, as these may be contaminated.'
Kelly, practice nurse

Cataract Surgery

A cataract occurs when the lens becomes opaque and vision is affected. The majority of cataracts occur in older people, developing gradually. Cataracts are usually treated as a day-case in a day surgery unit; the cloudy lens is removed and is replaced with an intraocular lens. However, in low-income countries where treatment is not available, cataracts are a major cause of blindness.

The Royal College of Ophthalmologists' (2017) project The Way Forward predicts a growth in cataracts, anticipating an increase in cataract operations of around 50% by 2035; it reported that 35% of people over 65 years old have visually significant cataract.

Pathophysiology

Globally, cataract is the most common cause of treatable and preventable blindness. Fibres and proteins in the lens undergo chemical changes and degenerate as the person ages. Proteins agglutinate, causing clouding of the lens and reducing light transmission to the retina. As the cataract continues to develop, the whole lens gradually becomes opaque.

A cataract scatters the light as it passes through the lens, preventing a sharply defined image from reaching the retina. As a result, vision becomes blurred. The cause of cataract is varied, for example ageing, underlying eye disease, trauma, systemic disease, ultraviolet radiation, environmental, social, congenital and developmental (CKS, 2020).

Nursing Fields Children

In the UK, all babies are screened for congenital cataracts at birth (as part of the physical examination of newborn babies) and again when they are 6–8 weeks of age (CKS, 2020). Causes of paediatric cataracts include the following

- Congenital: hereditary/genetic, metabolic (e.g. galactosaemia, a metabolic disorder)
- A result of *in utero* infection (e.g. rubella, cytomegalovirus, herpes simplex)
- Developmental: genetic, metabolic (e.g. galactokinase deficiency)
- Acquired: metabolic (e.g, diabetes mellitus), traumatic, post radiotherapy
- The most common cause of congenital cataract is infection. These include rubella (most common), measles, chickenpox, cytomegalovirus, herpes simplex and herpes zoster.

Sources: Royal College of Ophthalmologists (2010); CKS (2020)

Investigation and Diagnosis

Sometimes cataracts are diagnosed during a routine examination. A medical history should be obtained, and the person will be asked to describe the symptoms they are experiencing.

- A visual acuity test is performed.
- A slit-lamp is used to magnify and examine the eye. This apparatus allows the practitioner to see the structures at the front of the eye under magnification. The slit permits viewing of these structures in small sections, making it easier to detect any abnormalities. Using the slit-lamp or an ophthalmoscope allows the practitioner to examine the lens for signs of a cataract.
- Retinal examination is performed using eye drops that cause dilation of the pupils.

Signs and Symptoms

The cataract causes painless loss of vision. The person may report glare and a change in refraction.

In some people, visual acuity is reduced, depending on the severity of the lens opacity. There may be no symptoms with early cataracts. As the cataract develops, decrease in clarity of vision, not fully correctable with glasses, is noticed. Haloes may be observed around lights. Night vision will be diminished and night driving becomes hazardous. In some types of cataracts, uniocular diplopia may be noted in the affected eye.

Nursing Care and Management

Surgical removal of the cataract remains the only effective treatment available to restore vision. Non-surgical management includes counselling patients about cataract-related visual symptoms, offering reassurance concerning the cause of the visual disability and prescribing new eyeglasses where appropriate. A healthy diet rich in antioxidants may retard the progression of cataracts.

Cataract management requires a multiprofessional approach that involves nurses, ophthalmologists, optometrists and technicians. Usually, only one eye at a time is operated on.

Chapter 14 provides detailed information concerning the role of the nurse with regard to preoperative care. The procedure can be performed on a day-case basis, using a locally injected anaesthetic or even with the use of anaesthetic eye drops.

The following should be considered prior to surgery.

- General health evaluation including blood pressure check.
- No blepharitis is present.
- Biometry and keratometry tests to ensure best vision with correct intraocular lens power.
- Note of current medication.
- Record of allergies.
- Assessment of hearing and understanding of English.
- Assessment of patient's ability to co-operate with the procedure and lie reasonably flat during surgery.
- Identification of social problems that may hinder recovery.
- Instruction on eyedrop instillation.
- Clear explanation of the procedure.
- Opportunity to ask questions.
- Informed consent.

It is the role of the nurse to act as the person's advocate (NMC, 2018a) and this may mean having to explain and educate the patient regarding preoperative, perioperative and postoperative care in detail. The nurse, acting on the person's behalf, will ask the surgical team to provide the person with more details in order for informed consent to be made.

The most widely used, safest and most effective technique for cataracts is phacoemulsification (NICE, 2017) (Figure 33.22). Prior to surgery, adequate pupillary dilation is needed.

An incision is made at the limbus approximately 2–3 mm in diameter. A round rupture on the anterior lens capsule approximately 5 mm in diameter is made using a microscope. The hard lens nucleus is liquefied using an ultrasonic probe inserted through the hole and the lens matter is then extracted, leaving the clear capsule intact. The replacement intraocular lens is placed folded into the empty capsular bag, where it unfolds. No sutures are required to close the surgical incision; this heals without sutures.

Complications from cataract surgery that could threaten a person's sight or require further surgery are low, occurring in about 2% of cases (CKS, 2020).

Although the risk is low, surgery does involve the risk of partial to total vision loss. Some complications can be treated and vision loss reversed; however, others cannot. Complications that may occur with cataract surgery include:

- Endophthalmitis (infection in the eye)
- Swelling and fluid in the macula
- Corneal oedema
- Hyphaema (bleeding in the anterior chamber)
- Rupture of the posterior lens capsule
- Retinal detachment
- Glaucoma
- Iritis.

Topically applied antibiotics and an anti-inflammatory agent will be prescribed postoperatively, and the patient will be reviewed in an eye clinic.

Chapter 14 discusses postoperative care in detail. When caring for a person who has undergone eye surgery, the following points should be considered.

- If possible, explain carefully to the person what the outcome of surgery was.
- When approaching the person, let them know and approach from the unaffected side. This enables eye contact, enhancing communication.
- Observe and assess the eye dressing for bleeding or drainage, documenting your findings.
- Explain to the patient the purpose of the protective eye patch (Cartella shield) and the need to keep it in place, and that it is to help prevent unintentional injury to the operative site.
- When safe to do so, elevate the head of the bed and encourage the person to lie on the unaffected side as this reduces the possibility of intraocular pressure in the affected eye. Undertake an assessment of needs, for example assess and provide analgesia as required for pain.
- If the person complains of sudden, sharp eye pain, lacrimation and visual disturbance, this should be reported immediately as it may indicate an ocular emergency.
- Ensure you place personal articles and the nurse call bell within easy reach.
- Administer all prescribed medications.
- Document and record all activity in line with local policy and procedure.

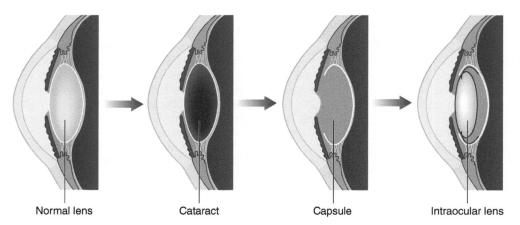

Normal lens   Cataract   Capsule   Intraocular lens

Figure 33.22 **Phacoemulsification.**

Care, Dignity and Compassion Assisting the Person Who is Blind or Visually Impaired: Eating and Drinking

- When serving a meal, offer to describe the location of food on the person's plate as corresponding to the numbers on a clockface. For example, tell the person that their fish is at 3 o'clock, their carrots are at 9 o'clock.
- This method can also be used to describe the location of other items on the table; for example, if the dinner plate is directly in front of the person, you can say that the mustard is above the plate at 1 o'clock and the person's glass is at 2 o'clock.
- Ask the person whether they would like you to refill their cup before doing so. If you refill it without telling them, it may cause a spill.
- If you are filling up a person's glass or cup, do not fill it to the brim in case it spills as they lift it.

Practice Assessment Document

Participates in providing and evaluating person-centred care. Supports people with their diet and nutritional needs, taking cultural practices into account and uses appropriate aids to assist when needed

Demonstrate this by discussing with your practice assessor how you would support a blind or visually impaired person who is additionally hearing impaired with eating a meal. Utilise the skills you have learnt in care, dignity and compassion to assist the person who is blind and visually impaired and additionally the simple steps the nurse can take to enhance communication with people who are deaf (see Box 33.2).

Health Promotion and Discharge

The person is discharged home, based on meeting certain criteria that may include the following.

- Vital signs are stable.
- Preoperative mental state is restored.
- Nausea and vomiting are controlled.
- Pain is absent or minimal.
- An escort is available.
- Postsurgical care has been reviewed with the patient and/or escort and written postoperative instructions have been provided.
- A follow-up appointment has been made.

Some people need reading glasses after cataract surgery, but some may choose to have different lens implants in their eyes so that one eye can be used for distance vision and the other for near vision.

The person should arrange for someone to take care of them for the first 24 hours postoperatively. Full vision may take days to return, though sensation usually returns to the eye within a few hours. Complete healing may take several weeks. The nurse should ensure the person (and/or carer) understands the correct method of instilling eye drops and when they are to be administered.

Medicines Management Instilling Eye Drops: Information for Patients

1. Read the instructions carefully before using eye drops.
2. Store eye drops at room temperature and away from heat, moisture and direct light (or as directed).
3. Do not use the drops if they change colour or turn cloudy .
4. Do not use the drops if they have debris (bits) floating in them.
5. Wait 5 minutes before instilling a different eye drop.
6. Wash hands before and after instilling eye drops.
7. Gently shake the bottle.
8. Do not touch the tip of the bottle to the eye.
9. Tilt the head back and pull down the lower eyelid with the index finger.
10. Gently squeeze the bottle and do not exceed more than one drop into the eye.
11. Keep medication away from children.
12. Replace the cap on the bottle.
13. Close the eye and press the index finger on the inside corner of the eye for 1 minute to prevent the drop entering the tear duct.
14. Gently wipe away any extra liquid with a tissue.
15. Do not rub the eyes.

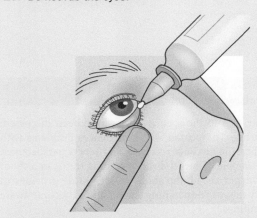

The person should be advised that they can bend, carry light shopping, wash their face and hair and carry on with their usual activities of living.

The person is offered advice on the following.

- Try not to touch or rub the eye.
- Keep soap and shampoo out of the eyes.
- Do not wear eye make-up for 1 week after surgery.
- Wear a Cartella shield for eye protection at bedtime for 4–6 weeks.
- Eat healthily.
- Do not swim for 4 weeks after surgery.
- Avoid lifting heavy objects.
- Avoid playing contact sports for about 4 weeks.
- Implement actions to avoid constipation and straining at stool.
- Wear sunglasses with side shields when outdoors.
- Keep a daily diary record of visual progress for the first 2–3 months.

The person will be able to read and watch television almost immediately if they have reading glasses; however, vision may be blurry as the healing eye gets used to its new lens. Driving can take place when the person can read a number plate 20.5 m away. There may be a need for new eye lens prescription to be able to do this.

What to Do If . . .

If the person experiences severe eye pain or loss of vision postoperatively, or if the eye starts to go red, they should contact the hospital immediately for advice. Other symptoms to report include blurred vison, lacrimation, the appearance of floaters or flashes of light, or haloes around bright objects.

Highlight the significance of attending follow-up appointments. Provide referral to the community nursing services for assistance with home care after discharge (if appropriate).

Jot This Down

Mrs Alicia Joaquin is 62 years old and has developed very poor vision in both eyes due to diabetic retinopathy for the past 6 months. She has been admitted to your ward for surgery to her hip; understandably she is anxious. How would you help Mrs Joaquin with:

- Eating and drinking?
- Mobilising?
- Washing and dressing?

Conclusion

In this chapter, two of the special senses have been discussed: sight and hearing. The person who experiences problems with their sight or hearing can be at risk from a variety of perspectives. Hearing, for example, allows to hear oncoming traffic or a shout that there is danger ahead; the ability to see clearly provides us with the ability to see the oncoming danger and to become aware of our surroundings.

In this chapter a brief overview of the anatomy and physiology and assessment of the ear and eye has been presented. A few common problems have been discussed giving insight into the care of people who may experience problems with their sight or hearing. This has highlighted the important role of the nurse in ensuring tat the person, aided or independently, can maintain a safe environment and that they are empowered and educated using a patient-centred approach.

There are several special investigations and tests associated with assessment of the person's sight and hearing. This chapter has offered an overview of some of them. It takes time to develop the knowledge, skills and behaviours that will enable you to undertake these assessments in a competent and confident manner.

When a threat to a person's ability to see or hear occurs, or there is potential for this to occur, the person needs the nurse to be able to offer them support and comfort. You will only be able to do this if you have developed an in-depth understanding of the person, their condition, the pathophysiology and the holistic care required.

Key Points

- A brief overview of the normal and altered anatomy and physiology of the ear and eye has been provided.
- In delivering care that is patient centred and safe and effective, the nurse needs to use an evidence-based systematic approach.
- The nurse should develop an understanding of the assessment of needs using a range of screening/diagnostic tools, make inferences from the data collected, plan care with the person, ensuring that person is central to all that is done, deliver care that is sensitive to the needs of the individual (and their family if appropriate) and undertake an evaluation of care delivered, making changes where required.
- Risk factors related to the senses of sight and hearing have been discussed. The nurse must understand these risk factors as preventive measures may be put in place to avoid harm or deterioration in the person's condition.
- It is essential to work in partnership with the person and other healthcare professionals. The nurse should aim to practise in a holistic manner, respect the individual's choices, act as an advocate, support health and well-being and uphold the rights and dignity of people.

References

Action on Hearing Loss (2014) *Hidden Disadvantage.* https://rnid.org.uk/about-us/research-and-policy/social-research-reports/ (accessed December 2021).

American Academy of Ophthalmology (2018) *Blepharitis: Preferred Practice Pattern 2018.* www.aao.org (accessed December 2021)

American Academy of Ophthalmology (2011) *Cataract in the Adult Eye.* www.aao.org/clinical-education (accessed December 2021).

Brennan-Jones, C.G., Head, K., Chong, L., Burton, MJ., Schilder, A.G.M. & Bhutta, M.F. (2020) Topical antibiotics for chronic suppurative otitis media. *Cochrane Database of Systematic Reviews,* 1, CD013051.

Campbell, K. & Shoup, A. (2019) Audiology. In: Y. Chan & C. Goddard (eds) *KJ Lee's Essential Otolaryngology, Head and Neck Surgery,* 12th edn. McGraw Hill, New York.

Chong, L-Y., Head, K., Webster, K.E., *et al.* (2021) Systemic antibiotics for chronic suppurative otitis media. *Cochrane Database of Systematic Reviews,* 1, CD013052.

CKS (2017) *Otitis media – chronic suppurative.* https://cks.nice.org.uk/topics/otitis-media-chronic-suppurative/have-i-got-the-right-topic/ (accessed December 2021).

CKS (2020) *Cataracts.* https://cks.nice.org.uk/topics/cataracts/management/adults/ (accessed December 2021).

College of Optometrists (2021) *Blepharitis (lid margin disease).* www.college-optometrists.org (accessed January 2022).

Davies, A. (2019) Hearing loss: essential knowledge and tips for nursing practice. *Nursing Times,* 115(11), 60–62.

Franceschi, C., Garagnani, P., Morsiani, C., *et al.* (2018) The continuum of aging and age-related diseases: common mechanisms but different rates. *Frontiers in Medicine,* 5, 61.

Gibbons, H., Amro, R. & Cox, C.L (2010) Ocular history-taking skills in primary care. *Practice Nursing,* 24(1), 41–43.

Gleadle, J. (2012) *History and Clinical Examination at a Glance,* 3rd edn. John Wiley & Sons, Oxford.

Goddard, J. & Lee, K. (2019) Anatomy of the ear. In: Y. Chan & C. Goddard (eds) *KJ Lee's Essential Otolaryngology, Head and Neck Surgery*, 12th edn. McGraw Hill, New York.

Gopinath, B., McMahon, C., Tang, D., Burlutsky, G. & Mitchell, P. (2021) Workplace noise exposure and the prevalence and 10-year incidence of age-related hearing loss. *PLoS One*, 16(7), e0255356.

HearX Group (2019) *hearWHO* (version 1.1.6). Mobile app (accessed December 2021).

James, B. & Bron, A. (2011) *Ophthalmology Lecture Notes*, 11th edn. John Wiley & Sons, Oxford.

Marsden, J. (2017) *Ophthalmic Care*, 2nd edn. M&K Publishers, Keswick.

National Institute for Health and Care Excellence (2017) *Cataracts in adults: management*. NICE, London.

National Institute for Health and Care Excellence (2019) *Hearing loss in adults*. QS185. NICE, London.

Nursing & Midwifery Council (2018a) *Future nurse: Standards of proficiency for registered nurses*. NMC, London.

Nursing & nmcMidwifery Council (2018b) *The Code: Professional standards of practice and behaviour for nurses, midwives and nursing associates*. NMC, London.

Olver, J., Jutley, G., Crawley, L. & Cassidy, L. (2014) *Ophthalmology at a Glance*, 2nd edn. Wiley Blackwell, Oxford.

Peate, I. & Evans, S. (eds) (2020) *Fundamentals of Anatomy and Physiology for Nursing and Healthcare Students*, 3rd edn. Wiley, Oxford.

Royal College of Nursing (2016) *The Nature, Scope and Value Of Ophthalmic Nursing*. RCN, London.

Royal College of Ophthalmologists (2010) *Cataract Surgery Guidelines*. www.rcophth.ac.uk/wp-content/uploads/2014/12/2010-SCI-069-Cataract-Surgery-Guidelines-2010-SEPTEMBER-2010.pdf (accessed January 2022).

Royal College of Ophthalmologists (2017) *The Way Forward. Options to help meet demand for the current and future care of patients with eye disease. Cataract*. www.rcophth.ac.uk/wp-content/uploads/2021/12/RCOphth-The-Way-Forward-Cataract-300117.pdf (accessed January 2022).

Royal National Institute for Deaf People (RNID) (2021) *Types and causes of hearing loss*. https://rnid.org.uk/information-and-support/hearing-loss/types-of-hearing-loss-and-deafness/ (accessed December 2021).

Seewoodhary, M. & Awelewa, C. (2014) Cited in Watkinson, S. (ed) (2014) *Older People with Visual Impairment. Clinical management and care*. M&K Publishing, Keswick.

Tawfik, K.O., Klepper, K., Saliba, J. & Friedman, R.A. (2020) Advances in understanding of presbycusis. *Journal of Neuroscience Research*, 98. 1685–1697.

Vaughan, D. (2017) *Vaughan and Asbury's General Ophthalmology*. McGraw Hill Medical, New York.

Warren, R.J. (2013) Forehead rejuvenation. In: P.C. Neligan & G.C. Gurtner (eds) *Plastic Surgery, Vol. 2. Aesthetic*, 3rd edn, pp. 93–107. Elsevier Saunders, Philadelphia, PA.

Watkinson, S. (ed.) (2009) *Issues in Ophthalmic Nursing: Current and future challenges*. M&K Publishing, Keswick

World Health Organization (2004) *Chronic Suppurative Otitis Media: Burden of Illness and Management Options*. World Health Organization, Geneva.

World Health Organization (2021) *World Report on Hearing*. www.who.int/teams/noncommunicable-diseases/sensory-functions-disability-and-rehabilitation/highlighting-priorities-for-ear-and-hearing-care (accessed January 2022).

Yanoff, M. & Duker, J.S. (2014) *Ophthalmology*, 4th edn. Elsevier, Philadelphia, PA.

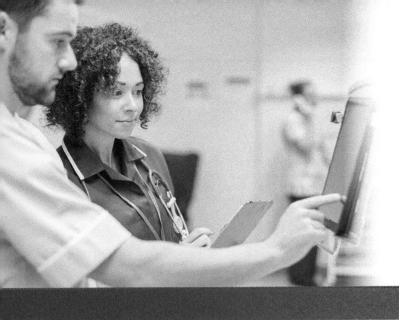

34

The Person with a Musculoskeletal Disorder

Nadine Manfred

School of Health Studies, Gibraltar

Learning Outcomes

On completion of this chapter, you will be able to:

- Provide an overview of the musculoskeletal system
- Discuss the structure of the musculoskeletal system
- Outline the function of the musculoskeletal system
- Explain the normal and abnormal changes that may occur in the musculoskeletal system
- Describe some disorders and impairments associated the musculoskeletal system
- Use the nursing process as a framework for care provision

Proficiencies

NMC Proficiencies and Standards:

- Work in partnership with patients to address their needs
- Assess physical and psychological needs
- Practise in a holistic manner
- Respect individual choice
- Support and promote the person's health and well-being
- Offer information and advice to people relating to the musculoskeletal system

 Visit the companion website at www.wiley.com/go/peate/nursingpractice3e where you can test yourself using flashcards, multiple-choice questions and more.

Nursing Practice: Knowledge and Care, Third Edition. Edited by Ian Peate and Aby Mitchell.
© 2022 John Wiley & Sons Ltd. Published 2022 by John Wiley & Sons Ltd.
Companion website: www.wiley.com/go/peate/nursingpractice3e

Introduction

The musculoskeletal system is composed of all the bones, cartilage, muscles, joints, tendons and ligaments in the body. It is the bones that provide the body with a framework; the bones give the body its shape and support and serve as protection for internal organs, for example, the lungs and heart. Muscles are fibres that help to make deliberate movement of a body part or involuntary movement within an internal organ possible. The muscles are the active part of the apparatus of locomotion. In some cases, the musculoskeletal system is seen as two body systems in one or two systems that work very closely with each other, with one being the muscular system and the other the skeletal system. Without the skeleton to pull against, contracting muscle fibres could not make us sit, stand, walk or run.

A detailed discussion of the anatomy and physiology of the musculoskeletal system is provided in Peate & Evans (2020). Having an undertaking of the anatomy and physiology of bones and muscles can help the nurse provide care that is informed, evidence based and patient centred.

Musculoskeletal Conditions

'Musculoskeletal conditions' is a broad term which encompasses over 200 disorders which can affect bones, muscles, tendons, connective tissue and ligaments. Musculoskeletal conditions range from those that arise suddenly and are short-lived, such as fractures, sprains, and strains, to those that are often progressive and lifelong. There are three main groups of musculoskeletal conditions:

- Osteoarthritis and back pain
- Osteoporosis and fragility fractures
- Inflammatory conditions.

These conditions are typically characterised by pain, stiffness, loss of movement and dexterity resulting in loss of function and the individual's ability to participate in activities of living.

Musculoskeletal conditions can also have an impact on mental health, as living with a painful condition, by its very nature, will be associated with negative emotions and psychological distress. It has been reported that depression is four times more common for those in persistent pain and two-thirds of individuals with osteoarthritis report symptoms of depression when pain is at its worst (Zheng *et al.*, 2021).

Jot This Down

How do you think the administration of medicines to control pain and inflammation can also help the person carry out their activities of living in a more effective way, promoting independence?

With an ageing population, increasing numbers of people are living with multiple long-term conditions. Among those living with multimorbidity, musculoskeletal conditions such as osteoarthritis and back pain are very common.

Musculoskeletal conditions have a great impact on society in terms of morbidity, long-term disability and economics. In 2017, an estimated 18.8 million people across the UK were affected by a musculoskeletal condition (Versus Arthritis, 2019). Estimates from the Health and Safety Executive (2020) suggest that in Great Britain for the period 2019–20, 480 000 workers were affected by work-related musculoskeletal disorders, accounting for 30% of all work-related ill health cases. This resulted in an estimated 8.9 million working days lost.

The rate of work-related musculoskeletal disorders in 2019–20 was similar for males and females. Skilled trades occupations, such as process, plant and machine operatives, and caring, leisure and other service occupations all had statistically significantly higher rates of work-related musculoskeletal disorders than the rate for all occupations Most of these work-related musculoskeletal disorders affect the upper limbs or neck (44%) or the back (37%), with the remaining 19% of cases affecting the lower limbs.

Primary Care

One in five GP consultations is for a musculoskeletal condition.

Many people with a musculoskeletal condition are referred to other health professionals forming part of the multidisciplinary team such as physiotherapists, occupational therapists, dietitians and podiatrists. Referral is also made to medical specialists such as clinical nurse specialist, orthopaedic surgeon or rheumatologist.

Assessing the Musculoskeletal System

Assessment is the first stage of the nursing process, and the nurse must be able to undertake a holistic assessment of the person's needs in a competent and confident manner. Nursing staff need knowledge and assessment skills to care for patients with musculoskeletal conditions effectively and make appropriate referrals to other members of the healthcare team, as needed.

The assessment consists of two components: taking a patient history and a physical examination. The patient history is the most crucial aspect of the examination as it helps to determine the severity, irritability and nature of the problem. Good questioning will help guide the physical examination and develop a hypothesis. The physical examination encompasses what the nurse sees or measures and helps in confirming the nature of the problem.

When performing an assessment, it is more realistic for nurses to adopt a classification scheme and to utilise the information gained from the patient history and physical examination to place the patient's problems within the classification (Versus Arthritis, 2021).

The five key questions which need to be answered are:

1. Does the problem arise from the joint, tendon or muscle?
2. Is the condition acute or chronic?
3. Is the condition inflammatory or non-inflammatory?
4. What is the pattern of affected areas/joints?
5. What is the impact of the condition on the patient's life?

Table 34.1 **History taking.**

PATIENT FACTOR	REMARKS
Age	How might this relate to the potential for pathology?
Onset of symptoms	Sudden or gradual? If there was an injury, what was the mechanism?
Duration of symptoms	How long have they had the problem?
Progression of symptoms	Have symptoms remained the same, got worse or better since onset?
Previous symptoms	Any previous similar problems or injuries? If so, did they receive any treatment and what was the outcome?
Location of symptoms	Where exactly is their pain?
Description of symptoms	Is the pain sharp, stabbing, aching, burning, shooting or throbbing? Is the pain deep or superficial?
Associated symptoms	Pins and needles, numbness
Intensity	Using a visual or numerical analogue scale for the patient to rate the intensity of their symptoms
Aggravating/easing factors	What makes their symptoms worse or better?
24 hour/diurnal pattern	How do the symptoms behave over a 24-hour period? Is it worse at a particular time of day? Is there night pain? Is there morning stiffness? How long does the stiffness last?
Special questions	Screening for red flags
Current general health	Any other current medical issues?
Past medical history	Patient's own past medical history and is there any family history of musculoskeletal disorders?
Drug history	What medication do they take? This will give you information on their past medical history. If they are taking any medication for the current symptoms, do they help?
Social history	Occupation, sports, hobbies. Any changes in occupation or level of activity

Patient History

Chapter 4 discusses patient history taking in detail. When taking a patient history from a person with a musculoskeletal condition, the points covered in Table 34.1 should also be considered.

Physical Examination

When performing a physical assessment of a patient with a musculoskeletal condition, the points covered in Table 34.2 should be considered. Table 34.3 outlines muscle grading which forms part of the physical examination.

Table 34.2 **Physical examination.**

PATIENT FACTOR	REMARKS
Posture	Observe body alignment in general; are there any asymmetries? Look more specifically at area of issue: · Bony deformity – alignment, asymmetry? · Colour changes – bruising, redness, any discolouration? · Wasting – muscle bulk, asymmetry? · Swelling – soft tissue joint, thickened joints? · Temperature – is the area warm to touch?
Gait	It is preferable to assess gait barefoot; if this is not possible, make note of the type of shoes being worn. Do they use insoles? Are they weight bearing equally? Is there a limp? Are they using an assistive device? Is there a lack of movement at the kip, knee, ankle or toes?
Range of movement	Assess actively and passively. The use of a goniometer will provide you with an objective measurement in degrees
Muscle strength	Grading of muscle strength (see Table 34.3)
Palpation	· Skin temperature · Muscle · Bony articulations · Tenderness or pain

Table 34.3 Grading of muscle strength.
Source: Adapted from Kendall *et al.* (2005).

SCORE	DESCRIPTION
0/5	No contraction is present. Occurs when a muscle is paralysed, e.g. after a stroke, spinal injury. Pain can also prevent a muscle from contracting
1/5	The muscle can perform a palpable contraction. Occurs when muscle contraction is noted but no visible movement occurs
2/5	This muscle-strength grade is given when muscles can contract; the muscle is able to complete a range of motion in a plane that is parallel to gravity, but cannot move the body part fully against gravity
3/5	This grade means that the person can fully contract the muscle and move the body part through its full range of motion against the force of gravity. When resistance is applied, however, the muscle is unable to maintain the contraction
4/5	Signifies that the muscle can withstand a moderate degree of resistance, but yields to maximum resistance
5/5	Indicates the muscle is functioning normally and can maintain its position even when maximum resistance is applied

Carrying out a competent and confident assessment of the musculoskeletal system takes much practice. The nurse should be deemed competent prior to undertaking assessment. Documentation of findings should be undertaken as soon as the assessment has been completed and should comply with local policy and procedure.

Practice Assessment Document

Whilst on clinical placement, the nursing student will need to demonstrate and apply knowledge of commonly encountered presentations to inform a holistic nursing assessment.

You may show your supervisor your knowledge and understanding by carrying out an assessment of a patient considering all six aspects of the holistic assessment: physiological, psychological, sociological, developmental, spiritual and cultural.

Arthritis

There are several different types of arthritis, with the main ones being:

- Osteoarthritis
- Gout and calcium crystal diseases
- Rheumatoid arthritis
- Spondylarthritis.

Arthritis affects people of all ages, including children and teenagers. Around 10 million people in the UK are thought to have arthritis (Versus Arthritis, 2019).

Osteoarthritis

Osteoarthritis (OA) is the most common form of arthritis and is one of the leading causes of pain and disability globally. Although it can affect any joint in the body, it most commonly affects those that bear most of our weight or that we use a lot in everyday life, such as hips, knees and hands (NICE, 2014). There is an estimated overall prevalence in the general adult population of 10.9% for hip OA and 18.2% for knee. The risk of developing OA increases with age, with a higher prevalence in women than in men.

Pathophysiology

The pathogenesis of OA is complex, with biomechanical factors, proinflammatory mediators and proteases playing an important role. The interaction of these processes results in changes in the composition and mechanical properties of the articular cartilage which is composed of water, collagen and proteoglycans (proteins). OA is viewed as an inflammatory disease with multiple phenotypes (Van Spil, 2019). The clinical disease results from an imbalance between damage and repair of the cartilaginous tissue. Symptoms are not normally due to damage to the cartilage alone but to the combination of changes in the subchondral bone, joint margins and articular tissues (Sandiford *et al.*, 2020)

The consequences associated with deterioration and changes to the articular cartilage result in formation of new bone (osteophytes) at the surfaces of the joints (known as spurs). The weight-bearing joints, which include the spine, hip, knee and ankle, are the joints that are commonly affected. Other joints affected include the small bone joints of the hands and feet. During the early stages, the cartilage is frequently thicker than normal but as the condition progresses to OA, the joint surface becomes thinner and the cartilage softens; this causes disruption in the integrity of the surface and clefts begin to develop. The outcome of this is the formation of ulcers extending deep into the bones, leading to increased degenerative changes and an abnormal repair response. Repair of the cartilage does occur, but the subsequent repair is substandard and, as such, is unable to tolerate mechanical stress. Cartilage is metabolically active and as stress on the joints continues, the cartilage becomes hypocellular (lacking the chondrocytes to help rebuild and maintain integrity) (Figure 34.1).

Risk Factors

Osteoarthritis has several risk factors, of which only a few are modifiable. The risk of developing OA throughout life increases with rising BMI (Wang & He, 2018). The risk of developing knee OA is affected by occupations that require squatting and kneeling, whereas the need to sit or stand for prolonged periods will increase the risk of hip OA. Hand OA is more frequent in people with occupations requiring increased manual dexterity (Clemence *et al.*, 2016). It is thought that at least 30% of the risk of OA is genetically determined (Warner & Valdes, 2016). Box 34.1 outlines the risk factors for OA.

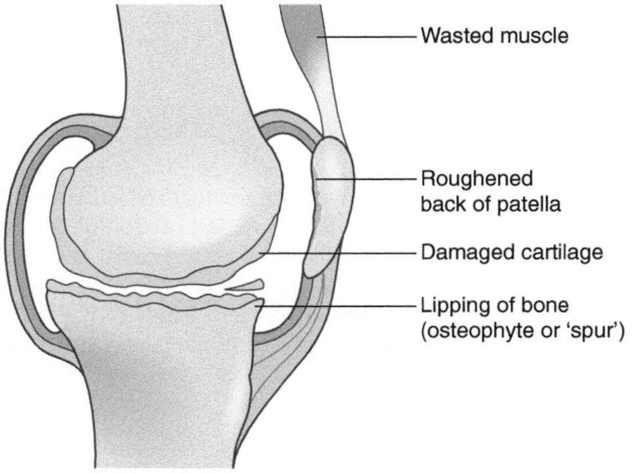

Figure 34.1 **Osteoarthritis.**

Labels:
- Wasted muscle
- Roughened back of patella
- Damaged cartilage
- Lipping of bone (osteophyte or 'spur')

Box 34.1 Risk Factors for OA

- **Age:** those aged 50 and over
- **Joint injury:** a bone fracture or cartilage or ligament tear
- **Overuse:** using the same joints over and over in a job or sport
- **Obesity:** excess weight adds stress and pressure on a joint, and fat cells promote inflammation
- **Musculoskeletal abnormalities:** malalignment of bone or joint structures
- **Weak muscles:** if muscles do not provide adequate joint support, there will be poor alignment
- **Genetics:** people with family members who have OA are more likely to develop it
- **Gender:** women are more likely to develop OA than men
- **Environmental factors:** modifiable environmental risk factors include things like someone's occupation, level of physical activity, diet, sex hormones and bone density

---

Signs and Symptvoms

Structural changes may occur in OA with no associated symptoms.

Pain is the main symptom, associated with functional impairment and disability. Usually, the pain associated with OA develops slowly. With mild-to-moderate OA, the pain typically worsens with use of the joint and improves with rest.

Pain in the joint is made worse by exercise and alleviated when resting. When there is advanced disease, night pain may occur. If there is knee pain due to OA, this is often bilateral and is experienced in and around the knee. Hip pain due to OA is felt in the groin and anterior or lateral thigh. Hip OA pain can also be referred to the knee and, in men, to the testicle on the side that is affected.

Joint stiffness can occur in the morning or after a period of rest. There will be a reduction in function and participation in activities is restricted (NICE, 2020).

The person is likely to experience a reduced range of joint movement. When moving, pain in the joint or at the extremes

of the joint can be felt. The joints can become oedematous and there may be synovitis (the joint often feels warm and there may be an effusion and evidence of synovial thickening).

Tenderness surrounding the joint (periarticular tenderness) may be present; on palpation, there may be crepitus.

As a result of osteophyte formation, bony swelling can occur. This may be present in the fingers, occurring as swelling at the distal interphalangeal joints (called Heberden's nodes); when swelling occurs at the proximal interphalangeal joints, this is known as Bouchard's nodes.

Joint instability is possible, where joints can be easily displaced or dislocated, leading to injury. Muscle weakness/wasting around the affected joint may be seen.

Investigations and Diagnosis

There is a poor link between the symptoms of OA and the changes that can be seen on an X-ray, MRI or ultrasound. Minimal joint changes can cause substantial pain whereas modest structural changes can cause minimal symptoms.

NICE (2014) states that OA can be clinically diagnosed without the need for investigations if the person:

- Is 45 years of age or older **and**
- Has activity-related joint pain **and**
- Has either no morning joint-related stiffness or morning stiffness that lasts no longer than 30 minutes.

This reduces the need for further investigations and consequently the harm from X-ray exposure as well as limiting unnecessary imaging procedures.

Nurses need to be aware of atypical features, such as a history of trauma, prolonged morning joint-related stiffness, rapid worsening of symptoms or the presence of a hot, swollen joint, as these may be indicative of an alternative or additional diagnosis.

Nursing Care and Management

Care provided must reflect the individual needs of the person and should be carried out after a detailed holistic health assessment has been undertaken and an individual treatment package formulated. NICE (2014) provides details about management strategies.

Osteoarthritis can have a significant impact on a person's ability to function, their quality of life, their ability to pursue an occupation, their mood, relationships and leisure activities. The nurse must determine how OA affects the individual's ability to carry out the activities of living. OA is a condition that causes pain; it is a progressive joint disorder which leads not only to physical symptoms but also anxiety and depression (El Monaem et al., 2017). Many people with the condition may have trouble sleeping and carrying out their everyday activities; quality of life may deteriorate, the person may lose their job and they may become socially isolated.

Education and Self-management

The person should be offered accurate verbal and written information to enhance their understanding of the condition and its management as well as to tackle common misconceptions regarding OA (NICE, 2020). The education should be an ongoing process and not just at the time of diagnosis. There should also be an agreed self-management plan specific to the individual.

By the time they register, nursing associates are required to promote preventive health behaviours and provide information to support people to make informed choices to improve their mental, physical and behavioural health and well-being (NMC, 2018, p.8), for example helping the patient understand OA and how they can best manage it.

You may show your supervisor your knowledge and understanding of the importance of self-management in OA by discussing the benefits of exercise in improving strength, physical function, pain and depression. You could liaise with the physiotherapist to devise a local muscle-strengthening programme for a patient with OA of the knee.

Exercise NICE (2014) suggests that exercise should be a core treatment for those with OA, regardless of the person's age, co-morbidity, pain severity or disability. Exercise should include local muscle strengthening along with general aerobic fitness.

Maintaining fitness can help to improve endurance and suppleness, which can help to build confidence, enhance independence and improve quality of life. Exercise can help to relieve pain; fitness also has a positive influence on postoperative recovery for those people who have had joint replacements (Versus Arthritis, 2021).

The nurse, as a member of the multidisciplinary team working with physiotherapists, can give advice about exercise. The key aim is to encourage the person to keep fit and active. Improvements in physical function and pain can lead to improvements in depression (Katz *et al.*, 2020).

Interventions to Help Weight Loss Obesity is a significant risk factor in OA. Weight loss advice should be offered if the person is overweight/obese. This will help to reduce the load on their joints and to improve pain. Weight reduction is one of three core interventions in guidance on OA, along with information and the promotion of exercise (NICE, 2014).

Other Non-pharmacological treatments Thermotherapy, which is the use of heat or cold, can be applied locally and used as an adjunct to core treatment. The nurse must ensure that no harm from the application of heat or cold comes to the person.

Occupational therapists can offer advice to people whose OA affects their activities of daily living. They may require assistive

Jot This Down

If the occupational therapist has assessed the needs of the person and has provided assistive devices. What can you do to ensure that these are included in the person's care plan, so that they can be used appropriately?

devices such as a helping hand, leg lifter, jar opener or tap turners. Physiotherapists can provide walking aids, supports or braces. A walking stick held in the hand of the unaffected side may reduce the load through the affected joint and help with pain relief

and function. A wrist splint may support the damaged joint to increase stability and thus improve function. Transcutaneous electrical nerve stimulation (TENS) may be used as an adjunct to core treatment for pain relief.

Pharmacological Interventions Pain can be responsible for the debilitating impact OA may have on a person (and their family); this should be managed using several techniques. Chapter 22 discusses the management of pain in detail. Pain assessment should be undertaken, and the nurse should assess any self-help strategies the person is using, and current drugs being used, including dose, frequency and route of administration, timing and any possible side-effects.

Paracetamol, NSAIDs and opioids may be used to help control the pain the person is experiencing (Stewart *et al.*, 2018).

Cyclo-oxygenase (COX)-2 inhibitors can be used if paracetamol and/or topical NSAIDs are not providing sufficient pain relief. They should be co-prescribed with a proton pump inhibitor (to prevent gastric irritation). They can be prescribed in addition to paracetamol. The lowest effective dose for the shortest period should be prescribed. In the older person, risks and benefits should be considered; if the patient is already taking low-dose aspirin, then other analgesics should be considered prior to adding an NSAID/COX-2 inhibitor.

Medicines Management

When taken at doses of less than 4000 mg per day, ibuprofen is a relatively safe drug; however, it may cause gastric irritation if it is taken in high doses over a long period.

The risk of adverse events related to the use of NSAIDs decreases significantly when topical gels are used as opposed to oral preparations. Topical NSAIDs, according to NICE (2014), are being suggested as first-line treatment for managing osteoarthritic pain.

Opioids can be very effective in the management of pain. However, they can cause side-effects, such as nausea, vomiting, dizziness and constipation, which affect several people who use these drugs.

What to Do If . . .

If a patient with knee OA who takes ibuprofen comes to see you complaining of vomiting, which is dark brown in colour, advise them immediately to stop taking the ibuprofen and arrange for them to be seen by a doctor.

Surgical Intervention Replacement of the hip or knee joint can be an effective management strategy. Joint surgery should be considered for those people with joint symptoms such as pain, stiffness and reduction in function if these have a substantial impact on their quality of life or if they have not responded to non-surgical treatment.

Surgery can be helpful in terms of pain reduction and restoration of function, but improvement is not guaranteed. Most people benefit from it but there are variations in health-related quality-of-life outcomes.

Health Promotion and Discharge

Health promotion and prevention of OA centre on weight control, increasing physical activity and avoiding injury. It is essential to learn as much about OA as possible. The use of expert patient programmes should be considered in improving education about OA. These programmes teach people about OA, its treatments, exercise and relaxation. People who understand more about their condition and those who participate in expert patient programmes are more likely to have positive outcomes.

Staying active and engaging in regular physical activity are key aspects in self-care and wellness. Strengthening exercises can help to maintain or increase muscle strength. Aerobic conditioning exercises improve cardiovascular fitness, help with weight control and improve overall function. Range-of-motion exercises can help reduce stiffness and maintain or increase joint movement and flexibility.

There is no specific diet that will make OA better. Eating a well-balanced diet and controlling weight can help by minimising stress on the weight-bearing joints.

Case Study

Alfred is a 77-year-old man with a recent diagnosis of OA of the right knee and is awaiting a consultation with an orthopaedic surgeon.

Alfred was a keen hockey player up until his early 40s. It was an injury to his right knee that forced him to retire from playing hockey.

Despite co-morbidities including hypertension, type 2 diabetes and heart disease, Alfred has been very active until the onset of the COVID-19 pandemic. During periods of lockdown, Alfred was engaged in minimal amounts of exercise at home and he has gained a significant amount of weight. As a result of the weight gain and reduced activity levels, he has developed significant right knee pain which is now affecting his quality of life.

The physiotherapist has provided Alfred with a walking stick, which he uses in his left hand to offload the right knee when walking. He also has specific knee-strengthening exercises and uses ice on his knee to help with pain relief.

The occupational therapist has raised the sofa and issued a toilet raise to make sitting to standing less effortful. He also has a helping hand to help with picking small objects from the floor and a perching stool which allows him to assist with preparing meals as he is unable to stand for long periods of time.

Gout

Gout is a type of arthritis that causes sudden, severe joint pain (often in the big toe). Attacks usually come on very quickly and often during the night. The attack will usually settle after 5–7 days.

Gout is a metabolic disease due to deposition of monosodium urate monohydrate crystals within joints causing acute inflammation and eventual tissue damage. It is four times more common in men than in women. It can affect men of any age, but the risk is greater as they get older. Women tend to develop gout after menopause when oestrogen levels drop and as a result, urate levels rise (Versus Arthritis, 2020).

The condition is classified into primary or secondary gout, depending on the cause of hyperuricaemia. Primary gout predominantly occurs in men aged 30–60 years presenting with acute attacks. Secondary gout is often due to chronic diuretic therapy.

Pathophysiology

Usually, a balance exists between the production and excretion of uric acid (uric acid is the breakdown product of purine metabolism). Uric acid levels in the blood are normally maintained between 3.4 and 7.0 mg/dL in men and 2.4 and 6.0 mg/dL in women. When levels rise above 7.0 mg/dL, monosodium urate crystals can form. How the crystals of monosodium urate are formed and deposited in joints is not fully understood.

The monosodium urate crystals can form in the synovial fluid or synovial membrane, cartilage or other joint connective tissues. It is also possible for the crystals to form in the heart and kidneys. These crystals stimulate the inflammatory system and neutrophils respond by ingesting the crystals. As a result of neutrophil activity (release of their phagolysosomes), tissue damage can occur, continuing the inflammatory process.

Gout affects the upper and lower limbs with acute attacks. Less often, it presents with painful tophaceous deposits (with or without discharge) in Heberden's and Bouchard's nodes.

Most people with hyperuricaemia never develop gout, and gouty patients may not have hyperuricaemia at presentation. Patients can overexcrete uric acid, secrete normal amounts of uric acid or underexcrete.

A study of UK general practice in 2012 found that the incidence of gout per 1000 person-years was 1.77, with the overall ratio of men to women being 4.3:1 (Kuo *et al.*, 2015).

What the Experts Say Stuart's Story

'After several nights of eating out with friends, I woke up with my foot on fire. My toe and the whole side of my foot were as red as a beetroot. I couldn't even get out of bed.'

Stuart states he has now learned how to keep his gout under control through medication, pain management strategies and diet modifications.

'When I get gout, it keeps me off my feet for about a week. During this time, I take over-the-counter pain relievers and I have a prescription for colchicine which I take at the first sign of an attack.'

Risk Factors

The following have been identified as risk factors.

- Obesity
- High blood pressure
- Type 2 diabetes
- High cholesterol
- Male
- Postmenopausal women
- Use of diuretics, beta-blockers and ACE inhibitors
- Chronic kidney disease
- Osteoarthritis

Signs and Symptoms

There is synovitis (inflammation of the lining of the joints) and swelling and extreme tenderness with overlying erythema. The person may not be able to move the joint; there may be pyrexia and tachycardia.

Uncharacteristic attacks can occur with tenosynovitis (inflammation of the sheath surround the tendon), bursitis (inflammation of the synovial fluid), cellulitis (infection of the deepest layers of the skin and underlying tissue) or mild discomfort without swelling lasting a day or two.

Chronic tophaceous gout is a condition where large crystal deposits produce irregular firm nodules occurring mainly around extensor surfaces of the fingers, hands, forearms, elbows, Achilles' tendons and ear. Usually, tophi are asymmetrical with a chalky appearance beneath the skin. Damage is most often found in the first metatarsophalangeal joints, midfoot, small finger joint and wrist, with restricted movement, crepitus and deformity.

Investigations and Diagnosis

A full physical examination and a patient history are required to ensure that an evidence-based approach to investigation is taken. A clinical diagnosis can be made with reasonable accuracy for typical presentations such as inflammation of the first metatarsophalangeal joint with hyperuricaemia; however, this is not definitive unless the presence of uric acid crystals can be demonstrated. Demonstration of monosodium urate crystals in synovial fluid or tophi will confirm the diagnosis of gout.

It must be remembered that gout may present atypically. All samples of synovial fluid aspirated from joints should be analysed for the presence of monosodium urate crystals.

The use of serum uric acid as a diagnostic test is limited (even though a raised serum uric acid level is a key risk factor for gout), as this can be normal during the acute phase of gout, while people with hyperuricaemia may never develop an attack.

Renal uric acid secretion (as detected by a 24-hour urine sample) can be helpful in diagnosis. Such patients are likely to be overexcreters of uric acid.

Radiographs may be useful in chronic gout. The first lesions usually occur in and around the first metatarsophalangeal joint. CT may be helpful in less accessible areas. In early gout or during an acute attack, radiography is less helpful.

Nursing Care and Management

The nurse's key objective in an acute attack is to relieve pain and inflammation as quickly as possible. Referral to a specialist nurse or doctor may be required.

Arthritis Research UK (2016) suggests that an ice pack may help with the relief of pain and the promotion of comfort. Elevation of the limb may help to ease pain and the nurse should ensure that the limb is protected from any potential trauma.

There is a range of pharmacological therapeutic options available, including the administration of non-steroidal anti-inflammatory drugs (NSAIDs). Commencing NSAIDs within 24 hours can produce rapid relief. Diclofenac, naproxen and indomethacin are generally preferred. The dose should be tailored to meet the needs of the patient and consideration should be given to the person's age, co-morbidity and interactions with other drugs. Colchicine works by reducing the number of white blood cells that travel into the inflamed areas, helping to break the cycle of inflammation (reducing swelling and pain).

Colchicine and/or NSAIDs are recommended as the first-line option for acute gout (NICE, 2018a). Lifestyle changes should be discussed with the patient and should include issues such as weight loss, exercise, diet, alcohol consumption and fluid intake.

Medicines Management

Corticosteroids can be given orally, intramuscularly, intravenously or intra-articularly. They are useful where NSAIDs or colchicine are contraindicated (British Society for Rheumatology, 2017). Compound analgesics (a combination of two different drugs in one tablet, usually paracetamol/aspirin and codeine hydrochloride) may also be considered.

Health Promotion

The nurse should identify factors that cause the person to have gout symptoms. Eliminating these triggers may reduce the chances of having gout again. Gout can be prevented from recurring by making changes to the diet and taking medicines if needed.

The patient should be advised to reduce the number of foods that contain purine. Some foods are very high in purines and may increase the amount of uric acid in the blood. These include:

- Liver and kidneys
- Oily fish, such as mackerel, sardines and anchovies
- Shellfish, including mussels, crab and shrimp
- Some vegetables, such as asparagus, cauliflower, lentils, mushrooms and spinach
- Oats and oatmeal.

Eating a well-balanced diet will help to manage symptoms.

If the person drinks alcohol, they should aim to drink less and should consider cutting out beer, stout, port and fortified wines as these can have the greatest effect on causing gout symptoms. Drinking enough water every day will help to dilute blood and urine and, in so doing, lower the uric acid levels in the body. Encourage the person to drink about 2–4 L of fluid each day, with at least half being water.

As well as making changes to the diet and reducing the amount of alcohol consumed, the person may need to take medicines to prevent gout. The nurse should explain how the medications work, i.e. helping to control the levels of uric acid in the blood with the aim of preventing the person getting gout again or, if the person does get gout again, it should be for a shorter period and be less severe. Some medications will need to be taken daily, for example allopurinol (or the alternative, febuxostat). These medicines prevent gout by stopping the formation of uric acid. When they are first taken, allopurinol and febuxostat may cause more symptoms of gout. NSAIDs, colchicine or steroid tablets may be prescribed along with allopurinol or febuxostat for up to 3 months.

Osteoporosis

Osteoporosis is a fragile bone disease that puts people at risk of fractures from everyday activities. A fragility fracture is one which results from a force that would not ordinarily result in a fracture, such as a fall from standing height or less (NICE, 2017). It can also occur as a result of simple daily activities such as hugging a grandchild or reaching for a cupboard.

The most up-to-date data suggest that in the UK, the estimated number of individuals aged 50+ with osteoporosis in 2019 was 3.75 million (International Osteoporosis Foundation, 2021) with over 527 000 fragility fractures occurring annually.

Reduced bone density is a major risk factor for fragility fracture. Other factors that may affect the risk of fragility fracture include the use of oral or systemic glucocorticoids, age, sex, previous fractures and family history of osteoporosis. The prevalence of osteoporosis increases with age from 2% at 50 years to more than 25% at 80 years in women. This is further aggravated by increased bone loss after the menopause in women. With an ageing population, the incidence of osteoporosis and fragility fractures will increase.

Fractured Neck of Femur

The femoral neck connects the femoral head with the femoral shaft. Femoral neck fractures are intracapsular and the most common site for a hip fracture.

According to the National Hip Fracture Database Annual Report 2020, 67 302 people presented to trauma units with hip fracture in the UK in 2019. Hip fracture is a serious and costly injury, which affects mainly the elderly, in particular women. It usually results from the combination of osteoporosis and a fall. People who fracture their neck of femur tend to have other co-morbidities which contributes to the high mortality rate associated with this injury. With an average age of over 75 years and a 1 in 10 chance of dying within 1 month, people with a fractured neck of femur represent some of the frailest patients the nurse may care for. Caring for people who experience a fracture relies on close multidisciplinary relationships. Persons presenting with hip fractures tend to be among the frailest and sickest with complex medical problems and co-morbidities.

Surgical intervention is usually needed to help mend the fracture. There are several types of operative procedure that can

be used, and the procedure of choice depends on where the fracture is and whether the bones have moved out of their normal position (Figures 34.2 and 34.3). If surgical intervention is inappropriate (e.g. if the fracture has seriously affected the person's health), options other than surgery may be made available, for example a palliative care approach.

Surgical intervention is usually carried out on the day of admission or as soon as possible thereafter. Delays in surgery have the potential to cause the person distress as well as being associated with an increase in morbidity and mortality.

The administration of analgesia is a key element in fracture care. Effective, holistic and patient-centred pain control, in the early stages of care, will enhance and promote comfort as well as confidence. Poorly controlled acute postoperative pain is associated with increased morbidity, delayed recovery time, prolonged duration of opioid use, functional impairments and higher healthcare costs (Gan, 2017).

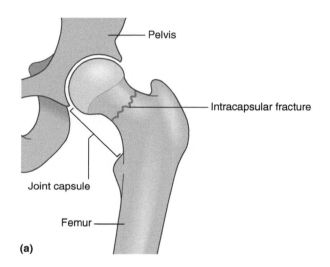

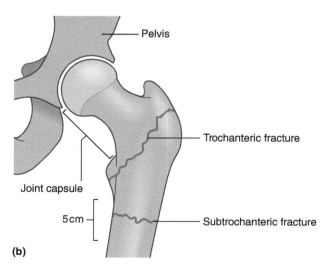

Figure 34.2 Types of fracture: (a) intracapsular; (b) extracapsular.

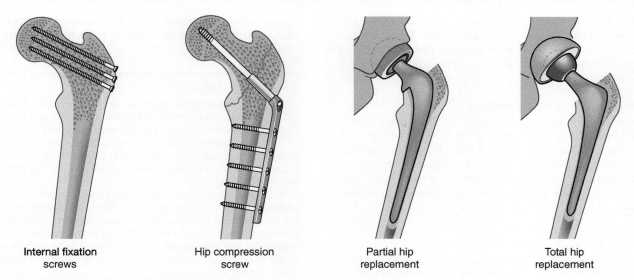

| Internal fixation screws | Hip compression screw | Partial hip replacement | Total hip replacement |

Figure 34.3 Types of fixation and implantation for hip fracture.

See Table 34.4 for some common complications associated with fractures.

Signs and Symptoms

The classic visible signs of a fractured neck of femur include shortening and external rotation of the affected leg, associated with contraction of the femoral musculature. The person may complain of pain that may radiate to the knee, or there may be knee pain present with no pain on movement of the hip. The person may be unable to lie on the injured side. In the older person who is confused or who has other forms of cognitive impairment such as dementia, there may be no history of injury.

What to Do If . . .

You have accompanied Mrs Bhatti to the bathroom and gone back to her locker to grab her toiletries.
On your return to the bathroom, you find Mrs Bhatti on the floor, conscious and in pain; you notice her right leg is externally rotated and noticeably shorter than the left leg. What do you do?

Investigations and Diagnosis

Radiography, for example anteroposterior (AP) pelvic and lateral hip X-rays, are required to confirm diagnosis and type

Table 34.4 Some complications associated with fractures. *Source:* Adapted from Whitening (2008).

INTERMEDIATE	EARLY	LATE
Immobility	Immobility	Immobility
Damage to soft tissue	Infection	Malunion of fracture
Nerve injury	Neurovascular complications	Delayed union of fracture
Haemorrhage	Fat and pulmonary embolism	Non-union of fracture
	Deep vein thrombosis (DVT)	Osteoarthritis
	Compartment syndrome (bleeding or swelling within an enclosed bundle of muscles)	Avascular necrosis (death of bone tissue due to lack of blood supply)
	Pressure ulcers	
	Chest infection	

of fracture. MRI should be performed if a hip fracture is suspected but the AP pelvic and lateral hip X-rays are not showing a fracture. NICE (2014) suggests that if MRI is not available within 24 hours, or if this is contraindicated, then CT should be carried out.

Nursing Care and Management

There should be early identification of the person's goals for multidisciplinary rehabilitation to recover mobility and independence. Discharge planning should commence within the first 48 hours after admission. Throughout the hospital stay, the nurse should assess the person's activities of living, ensuring that needs are met and, when needed, assistance provided.

Red Flag Fat Embolism

Fat embolism is a common occurrence for patients following trauma or surgery to the lower limbs. Fat from the bone marrow can escape into the bloodstream and form emboli (collections of fat droplets). Many patients will not even be aware that they have fat emboli as the symptoms may be minor. In a small number of people, however, these emboli block small blood vessels in the lungs, skin or brain and this triggers a cascade of events that leads to the illness known as fat embolism syndrome.

The most severe problem in fat embolism syndrome is acute respiratory distress syndrome – the lungs are unable to absorb oxygen properly and patients become severely hypoxic. It is this group of patients who will be admitted to the intensive care unit.

The nurse should be aware of the following.

· Fat embolism syndrome is usually evident 24–72 hours after an injury and involves the lungs, brain and skin.
· Symptoms can include:
   – An altered mental state: irritability, agitation, headache, confusion, seizures or coma
   – Lung problems, including rapid breathing, dyspnoea and a low oxygen level
   – A rash on the skin (petechiae): blockages in small blood vessels lead to small pinpoint haemorrhages, often in the upper torso. These haemorrhages also occur in the eye.

The nurse should report any of the symptoms immediately.

Preoperative Care The nurse will play an important role in preparing the person for surgical intervention by carrying out the following.

• Investigations include blood tests (full blood count and cross-match). Initial assessment of renal function, glucose, ECG and chest X-ray. Depending on history and general examination, other investigations may be required.
• Intravenous access and commencing intravenous infusion.
• Administration of analgesia (including opiates) sufficient to allow the movements necessary for investigations and for nursing care and rehabilitation.
• An early assessment is carried out of any cognitive impairment and any treatable co-morbidities such as anaemia, fluid volume depletion, electrolyte imbalance, uncontrolled diabetes,

uncontrolled heart failure, correctable cardiac arrhythmias or ischaemia, acute chest infection or exacerbation of chronic chest conditions.

The Nursing Associate

 By the time they register, nursing associates are expected to demonstrate the knowledge and skills required to support people with commonly encountered symptoms including anxiety, confusion, discomfort and pain (NMC, 2018, p.10), for example supporting a patient admitted with a fractured neck of femur, awaiting theatre.

You may show your supervisor your knowledge and understanding by discussing factors which will contribute to the patient being confused and anxious; the importance of good analgesia to control pain and help reduce patient discomfort and anxiety; the need to liaise with the patient and family to keep them informed about what is happening during this stressful time.

Jot This Down

When on your next orthopaedic placement, find out what protocols are being used in relation to good hip fracture care.

The nurse must ensure that the patient and family are kept informed about what is happening during this stressful and anxiety-provoking time. Nurses are ideally placed to give advice and offer information; they can offer comfort and provide explanations concerning ward routines, processes and procedures.

Postoperative Care The first concern with all postoperative patients is to assess and maintain an effective airway; the use of anaesthesia has the potential to impact on respiratory function of the older person.

Postoperative care will be directed according to the type of surgery that has been performed. Depending on the nature of the facture, the nurse must act as advocate and play a key part in the multidisciplinary team approach to the care of the person with femoral fracture. Riemen & Hutchison (2016) discuss the role of the multidisciplinary team in hip fracture before and after surgery.

Integrated care pathways (ICPs) are often used for the care of the person with a fractured neck of femur. These draw on a sound evidence base and are usually adapted to meet local needs.

Pain Relief Analgesia is an important aspect in the care and management of the person with a hip fracture. If pain is controlled in the early stages of care, this will encourage comfort and confidence; conversely, if pain is poorly controlled, then early mobilisation can be delayed, and dependency can result in complications associated with prolonged bedrest.

The nurse must involve the wider acute pain team based in many acute care settings. It must, however, be remembered that addressing the analgesic needs of the person is the responsibility of the nurse caring for the person; the nurse must determine the presence of pain and provide analgesia (see Chapter 22).

Diagnosing pain in people who may be cognitively impaired as a result of dementia, for example, may be difficult; therefore, addressing the needs of these people requires familiarity with the person and also information from carers (Achterberg *et al.*, 2020).

In the immediate postoperative period, many people will be given opiates; these are the mainstay of treatment, given orally or intramuscularly.

Jot This Down

Nurses have a unique role as they can assess the pain a person is experiencing in their daily interaction with patients in a way that doctors cannot. Think about why this may be case.

Regular paracetamol and other analgesia (e.g. codeine phosphate or tramadol) should be provided to all patients. The objective is to pre-empt pain and to promote comfort when resting and during active rehabilitation. The nurse should offer analgesia in anticipation of active rehabilitation.

Red Flag

Intravenous opiates may be used for pain control in the older person, but they should be given only in small incremental doses due to the unpredictable response in this client group.

Wound Care Surgical site infections can range from a relatively trivial wound discharge with no other complications to a life-threatening condition. Clinically, surgical site infections can result in scarring, persistent pain and itching, restriction of movement, particularly when over joints, and a significant impact on emotional well-being. Surgical site infections can double the length of time a patient stays in hospital and thereby increase the costs of healthcare.

Chapter 18 discusses wound infection and management.

Pressure Ulcer Formation The nurse has the responsibility to address pressure ulcer prevention at the earliest opportunity, identifying those at risk and implementing strategies to reduce risk of pressure sore formation. The following factors contribute to pressure sore formation.

- Time spent lying on the floor at home after falling.
- Delays in the accident and emergency department.
- Hard surfaces on accident and emergency department trolleys.
- Hard mattresses on the ward.
- Poor nutrition.
- Anaemia.
- Delays from admission to surgery.
- Prolonged surgery.
- Failure to mobilise the person immediately after surgery.

Good anticipatory care can reduce the risk of pressure sore formation. Chapter 18 discusses pressure sore prevention.

Early mobilisation in the postoperative period will reduce the risk of pressure ulcer formation. A formal pressure area risk assessment is recommended for all patients, with pressure area skin inspection on admission and at least twice a day while patients are immobile. The finding of early or superficial skin damage should trigger an immediate response and the implementation of appropriate care. Risk factors such as pressure, shearing forces, friction, incontinence, pain and malnutrition should be addressed and if problems do arise, the nurse should refer the person to a tissue viability nurse.

Thromboprophylaxis The use of cyclic leg compression devices and foot pumps can help to reduce the incidence of thrombosis. Graduated stockings (compression stockings) are effective; however, these are painful to put on when there is a hip fracture and bring with them a risk of foot ulcers in those who have fragile skin or vascular insufficiency. Chemical prophylaxis reduces the incidence of deep vein thrombosis and pulmonary embolism considerably, but also carries the risk of introducing bleeding complications as well as increasing the rates of wound healing complications.

Early surgical intervention and immediate postoperative mobilisation, as well as avoiding prolonged operations and overtransfusion, will help to reduce the incidence of clinical thrombosis.

Jot This Down

Early mobilisation is effective in lowering the risk of clinical thrombosis. Describe the signs and symptoms of thromboembolism.

Nutritional Needs One of the most powerful risk factors for hip fracture is poor nutrition. Practical challenges associated with feeding pose a major threat to recovery. People with hip fracture are at risk of failing to receive the recommended daily energy, protein and other nutritional requirements. The nurse must liaise and communicate with all members of the clinical and operational services teams – nutrition is an interdisciplinary concern.

All staff caring for people recovering from a hip fracture should understand the importance of adequate dietary intake and ensure that specific attention is given to helping people to eat at mealtimes. An integral aspect of routine nursing care should be assessment of nutritional intake, using a tool such as the Malnutrition Universal Screening Tool, and, where appropriate, referral should be made to the dietitian for specialist advice to ensure appropriate nutritional intake. See also Chapter 17 for further discussion on nutrition.

Early Rehabilitation Postoperatively, it is usual practice to sit the person out of bed and begin to help them stand on the day after surgery. This progress will vary significantly, depending on the individual and the type of fracture. Those people with an extracapsular fracture tend to take longer to mobilise than those with intracapsular fractures. The care pathway can assist with early rehabilitation.

Jot This Down

Efforts to institute supervised full weight-bearing mobilisation should usually commence on the first day following surgery. Why is this important in the older person?

Weight-bearing There should be very few occasions on which weight-bearing is restricted. Most people will bear weight as pain allows and become fully weight-bearing as the fracture heals. The nurse working with the physiotherapist can help the person to bear weight.

Hip Movements Hip movements will depend on the surgical intervention. Customary practice was to restrict hip flexion after an arthroplasty to prevent prosthetic dislocation. This meant that the patient required a raised bed and chairs and was restricted from getting in and out of a car or bath. These measures are still used for a total hip replacement, but they should no longer be required for a hemiarthroplasty introduced via an anterolateral approach. As surgical technique has become more refined and with a more careful repair of the hip joint capsule, the risk of dislocation is reduced, making any restrictions on hip movements unnecessary.

Practice Assessment Document

Whilst on clinical placement, the nursing student should assess the need for support in caring for people with reduced mobility and demonstrate understanding of the level of intervention needed to maintain safety and promote independence.

You may show your supervisor your knowledge by accessing the medical notes to ascertain the recommended postoperative weight-bearing status, speaking to the patient, family or carers to ascertain the preadmission level of mobility and liaising with the physiotherapist to support the patient with their mobility.

Discharge and Community Rehabilitation

Early supported discharge and community rehabilitation schemes are being implemented that will allow the more able person with a fracture to be discharged directly to their home from the orthopaedic ward. It is essential, however, that a multidisciplinary assessment of needs is undertaken with the involvement of older person consultant nurses, geriatric physicians, community nurses and community physiotherapists and occupational therapists. The multidisciplinary team will carry out a detailed assessment, ensuring optimal patient selection. Such ongoing rehabilitation will allow patients to progress from using a frame to a stick, and to walking unaided if appropriate. Advice and practice about walking outside and, if appropriate, a return to driving may also be given.

Primary Care

Nurses form an integral part of the multidisciplinary primary care teams, which are well placed to deal with chronic disease management.

With an ageing population, there is an increased proportion of the population living for longer with multimorbidity. This places increased demands on the healthcare system as well as socioeconomic costs.

Nurses are ideally placed to educate, advise and help manage those presenting to primary care with chronic conditions.

Health Promotion

In early adulthood, healthy lifestyle choices can help to build a higher peak bone mass and reduce the risk of osteoporosis in later years; this may lower the risk of falls and improve overall health if adopted at any age.

Exercise strengthens bones and improves balance. Weight-bearing exercises, for example walking, result in increased bone density. Exercise also increases overall strength, reducing the risk of falling. The nurse can suggest exercising for 30 minutes a day on most days of the week.

Drinking too much alcohol can impair balance and make the person more prone to falling. Avoiding excessive use of alcohol and not smoking preserve bone density.

The nurse can suggest an assessment of the person's home to identify any fall hazards.

Primary Care

Before discharging patients, nurses should offer information on the following strategies to reduce the risk of falls.

- Mop up spillages straight away.
- Remove clutter, trailing wires and frayed carpet.
- Use non-slip mats and rugs.
- Use high-wattage light bulbs in lamps and torches to help see clearly.
- Organise the home so that climbing, stretching and bending are kept to a minimum and to avoid bumping into things.
- Encourage the person to ask for help with things that they are unable to do safely on their own.
- Avoid walking on slippery floors in socks or tights.
- Do not wear loose-fitting, trailing clothes that could result in a trip.
- Wear well-fitting shoes that are in good condition, supporting the ankle.
- Make referral to a chiropodist about any foot problems, taking care of the feet by trimming toenails regularly.
- Refer to an optician to check the eyes every other year or more often if the person has diabetes or an eye disease.
- Monitor the effects of medication.

Red Flag

Be aware that the side-effects of some medicines can result in the person feeling weak and dizzy and this could increase their risk of falling.

Rheumatoid Arthritis

Rheumatoid arthritis (RA) is an autoimmune disease characterised by inflammation and swelling of the synovium of the joint which in the long term results in destruction of the articular structures. It affects around 430 000 adults aged 16 and over in the UK (Arthritis Research UK, 2019). The inflammatory activity can cause irreversible damage very quickly so early diagnosis and intensive treatment are essential.

Rheumatoid arthritis affects adults of any age. However, prevalence increases with age, with peak onset being between 40 and 60 years and women are 2–3 times more at risk than men (National Rheumatoid Arthritis Society, 2019).

The exact cause of RA is unknown, although the initiation of the disease seems to be linked to a combination of genetic susceptibility and environmental triggers. There is some evidence to suggest that eating too much red meat and not consuming enough vitamin C may increase the risk of developing RA.

Pathophysiology

Inflammation of the synovium is key to the pathogenesis of RA. Blood-derived cells such as T cells, B cells, macrophages and plasma cells infiltrate the sublining of the synovium. The local invasion of the synovial tissue goes on to cause the erosions that are seen in RA (BMJ Best Practice, 2021).

Signs and Symptoms

The main symptoms of rheumatoid arthritis are:

- Joint pain
- Joint swelling, warmth and redness
- Stiffness that lasts more than 30 minutes, especially first thing in the morning or after sitting still for a long time.

In the early stages, the person may not experience redness and swelling but rather tenderness and pain. Adults with active RA also experience systemic inflammation, which can result in other symptoms that include:

- Fatigue
- Poor appetite
- Weight loss
- Low-grade fever
- Sweating
- Eyes: dryness, pain, inflammation, redness, sensitivity to light and trouble seeing properly
- Mouth: dryness and gum inflammation, irritation or infection
- Skin: rheumatoid nodules – small lumps under the skin over bony areas
- Lungs: inflammation and scarring that can lead to shortness of breath and lung disease
- Blood vessels: inflammation of blood vessels that can lead to damage in the nerves, skin and other organs
- Blood: a lower than normal number of red blood cells
- Heart: inflammation can damage the heart muscle and the surrounding areas.

Painful joints can make it hard to exercise, leading to weight gain. Being overweight may make people with RA more likely to develop high cholesterol, diabetes, heart disease and high blood pressure.

Rheumatoid arthritis can affect any joint in the body, although it is often felt in the small joints in the hands and feet first. Both sides of the body are usually affected at the same time, in the same way, but this does not always happen.

Investigations and Diagnosis

Once a clinical diagnosis has been made, several laboratory tests will help with determining prognosis. NICE (2018b) recommends the following.

- Blood test for rheumatoid factor (RF): this should be tested at presentation but does not need to be repeated if positive. The higher the value, the worse the prognosis.
- Blood test for anti-CCP antibodies in adults with suspected RA if they are negative for rheumatoid factor.

- X-ray of the hands and feet to help with diagnosis and determine disease severity. However, a plain radiograph does not show early signs of the disease. An MRI or ultrasound is more sensitive at detecting early changes such as synovitis (Takase-Minegishi et al., 2018).

Nursing Care and Management

The nurse may be involved in the care of a patient with RA at various points of the disease. This could be as a first contact in a GP practice, in clinic when a diagnosis has been given or on a ward when the patient presents with systemic problems secondary to RA.

Education is an integral part of the standard care for a patient with RA. The education should be tailored specifically to the needs of the patient but available throughout the course of the disease. Education should focus on knowledge and management of the disease, non-pharmacological treatments, pain control and self-help methods, prevention of structural damage and deformity, activity regulation, exercise and behaviour change to enable maintenance of an acceptable lifestyle.

The nurse may need to refer on to the wider multidisciplinary team to assist with the above. Physiotherapists can help with the exercise aspect of care. During an acute phase, rest is very important. Once this has settled, exercise is essential to maintain a good range of movement with strong muscles to protect the joints. An occupational therapist will be able to provide advice on joint protection or the provision of aids for the home to allow the person to maintain function.

What the Experts Say

'Wearing a wrist or thumb splint can help you to rest and support joints that are painful or unstable. There are different types of splints available to support your joints while you are working and to keep your joints in a stable position while you are resting. Your occupational therapist or hand therapist may make a custom-made splint for you or prescribe a ready-made one.'
Mair, occupational therapist

Case Study

Grace is a 44-year-old married mother of three very active boys aged 8, 10 and 13 years. She works part time as a hairdresser and enjoys running around taking her sons to after-school sports clubs.

Six months ago, Grace noticed stiffness in both her hands in the morning. Initially the stiffness lasted 10–15 minutes, recently it lasts more than 1 hour, and it now affects her hands, wrists and ankles. Grace also noticed difficulty standing in work for long periods due to ankle and foot pain. She began taking ibuprofen 800 mg three times daily and found it helped her get through the day.

Two months ago, Grace started noticing pain in her shoulders when drying her client's hair. She also began feeling extremely tired and short-tempered. Grace found that the ibuprofen was no longer effective for her pain and stiffness.

One morning, Grace woke up and found she could not lift her arms without extreme pain. She knew it was time to get help. Grace saw her GP who examined her, ran some blood tests and requested X-rays of her hands and feet. The blood results revealed a positive rheumatoid factor and CCP antibodies. Plain X-rays showed marginal erosions in the metacarpophalangeal joints of the hands.

The GP has completed an urgent referral for Grace to see a rheumatologist.

Conclusion

This chapter has provided some insight concerning musculoskeletal conditions. It has not been possible in this chapter to provide all the information that you may need to care competently and confidently for people with a wide range of conditions that impact on the person's health and well-being. However, it has given you an overview of the common musculoskeletal conditions people may present with.

The nurse should aim to provide people who have musculoskeletal conditions with care that responds to their individual needs, to prevent further injury or deterioration, to reduce the risk of complications and to promote healing. The nurse working in partnership with the patient and other members of the health and social care team can minimise dependence and enhance optimal rehabilitation.

The nurse may be required to care for people with musculoskeletal conditions in a variety of settings, including primary, secondary and tertiary care, and as such, they will need to have some understanding of the common conditions that have been discussed in this chapter.

Key Points

- This chapter has presented an overview of the disorders and impairments associated with the musculoskeletal system. It has also highlighted the impact of musculoskeletal conditions on a person's physical and psychological well-being, as well as on society.
- The first stage of the nursing process when caring for a person with a musculoskeletal condition is a comprehensive holistic assessment. This allows for appropriate referrals to other members of the multidisciplinary team, as needed.
- Nursing care must reflect the individual needs of the person. The nurse needs to establish the impact of the condition on the person's perception of their quality of life, how this relates to their ability to function in society and ultimately engage in activities of daily living.
- Nurses may be required to care for persons with musculoskeletal disorders in a variety of settings. This places them in an ideal position to play a vital role in the health promotion of those with musculoskeletal conditions.
- Nursing care for patients with musculoskeletal conditions requires a collaborative approach with other healthcare professionals, relatives and carers to establish management in line with the individual's holistic needs and goals.

References

Achterberg, W., Lautenbacher, S., Husebo, B., Erdal, A. & Herr, K. (2020) *Pain in dementia*. www.painreportsonline.com (accessed December 2021).

Arthritis Research UK (2016) *What treatments are there for gout?* www.arthritisresearchuk.org/arthritis-information/conditions/gout/treatments.aspx (accessed December 2021).

Arthritis Research UK (2019) *The Musculoskeletal Calculator*. www.versusarthritis.org/media/13130/wandsworth-back-pain.pdf (accessed January 2022).

BMJ Best Practice (2021) *Pathophysiology of Rheumatoid Arthritis*. https://bestpractice.bmj.com/topics/en-gb/105 (accessed December 2021).

British Society for Rheumatology (2017) *Guideline for the Management of Gout*. www.rheumatology.org.uk/goutguideline (accessed December 2021).

Clemence, P., Nguyen, C., Lefevre-Colau, M., Rannou, F. & Poiraudeau, S. (2016) Risk factors and burden of osteoarthritis. *Annals of Physical and Rehabilitation Medicine*, 59(3), 134–138.

Department of Health and Social Care (2021) *The NHS Constitution for England*. www.gov.uk/government/publications/the-nhs-constitution-for-england/the-nhs-constitution-for-england (accessed January 2022).

El Monaem, S.M.A., Hashaad, N.I. & Ibrahim, N.H. (2017) Correlations between ultrasonographic findings, clinical scores and depression in patients with knee osteoarthritis. *European Journal of Rheumatology*, 4(3), 205–209.

Gan, T.J. (2017) Poorly controlled postoperative pain: prevalence, consequences and prevention. *Journal of Pain Research*, 10, 2287–2298.

Health and Safety Executive (2020) *Work related musculoskeletal disorder statistics (WRMSDs) in Great Britain 2020*. www.hse.gov.uk/statistics/causdis/msd.pdf (accessed December 2021).

International Osteoporosis Foundation (2021) *Epidemiology, Burden and Treatment of Osteoporosis for 29 European Countries*. www.osteoporosis.foundation/facts-statistics/key-statistic-for-europe (accessed December 2021).

Katz, P., Andonian, B.J. & Huffman, K.M. (2020) Benefits and promotion of physical activity in rheumatoid arthritis. *Current Opinion in Rheumatology*, 32(3), 307–314.

Kendall, F.P., Provance, P. & McCreary, E.K. (2005) *Muscles: Testing and Function with Posture and Pain*, 5th edn. Lippincott, Williams and Wilkins, Baltimore, MD.

Kuo, C., Grainge, M., Mallen, C., *et al* (2015) Rising burden of gout in the UK but continuing suboptimal treatment: a nationwide population study. *Annals of Rheumatic Diseases*, 74(4), 661–667.

National Institute for Health and Care Excellence (2011) *Hip Fracture: Management*. CG124. www.nice.org.uk/guidance/cg124 (accessed December 2021).

National Institute for Health and Care Excellence (2014) *Osteoarthritis: Care and Management*. CG177. www.nice.org.uk/guidance/cg177 (accessed December 2021).

National Institute for Health and Care Excellence (2017) *Osteoporosis: Assessing the Risk of Fragility Fracture*. CG146. www.nice.org.uk/guidance/cg146 (accessed December 2021).

National Institute for Health and Care Excellence (2018a) *Gout: Scenario: Acute Gout*. https://cks.nice.org.uk/topics/gout/management/acute-gout/ (accessed December 2021).

National Institute for Health and Care Excellence (2018b) *Rheumatoid Arthritis in Adults: Management*. NG100. www.nice.org.uk/guidance/ng100 (accessed December 2021).

National Institute for Health and Care Excellence (2020) *Osteoarthritis: Care and Management*. www.nice.org.uk/guidance/cg177/chapter/1-Recommendations#education-and-self-management-2 (accessed December 2021).

National Rheumatoid Arthritis Society (2019) https://nras.org.uk/resource/what-is-ra/ (accessed January 2022).

Nursing & Midwifery Council (2018) *Standards of Proficiency for Nursing Associates*. www.nmc.org.uk/globalassets/sitedocuments/standards-of-proficiency/nursing-associates/nursing-associates-proficiency-standards.pdf (accessed December 2021).

Peate, I. & Evans, S. (eds) (2020) *Fundamentals of Anatomy and Physiology for Nursing and Healthcare Students*, 3rd edn. Wiley, Oxford.

Riemen, A.H.K. & Hutchison, J.D. (2016) The multidisciplinary management of hip fractures in older patients. *Orthopaedics and Trauma*, 30(2), 117–122.

Sandiford, N., Kendoff, D. & Muirhead-Allwood, S. (2020) Osteoarthritis of the hip: aetiology, pathophysiology and current aspects of management. *Annals of Joint*, 5(8).

Stewart, M., Cibere, J., Sayre, E.C. & Kopec, J.A. (2018) Efficacy of commonly prescribed analgesics in the management of osteoarthritis: a systematic review and meta-analysis. *Rheumatology International*, 38, 1985–1997.

Takase-Minegishi, K., Horita, N., Kobayashi, K., *et al.* (2018) Diagnostic test accuracy of ultrasound for synovitis in rheumatoid arthritis: systematic review and meta-analysis. *Rheumatology*, 57(1), 49–58.

Van Spil, W.E., Kubassova, O., Boesen, M., Bay-Jensen, A.C. & Mobasheri, A. (2019) Osteoarthritis phenotypes and novel therapeutic targets. *Biochemical Pharmacology*, 165, 41–48.

Versus Arthritis (2019) *The state of musculoskeletal health 2019*. www.versusarthritis.org/about-arthritis/data-and-statistics/state-of-musculoskeletal-health-2019/ (accessed December 2021).

Versus Arthritis (2020) *Gout*. www.versusarthritis.org/media/23086/gout-information-booklet.pdf (accessed December 2021).

Versus Arthritis (2021) *Keep moving*. www.versusarthritis.org/media/1310/keep-moving-information-booklet-with-poster.pdf (accessed December 2021).

Wang, T. & He, C. (2018) Pro-inflammatory cytokines. The link between obesity and osteoarthritis. *Cytokine Growth Factor Reviews*, 44, 38–50.

Warner, S.C. & Valdes, A.M. (2016) The genetics of osteoarthritis: a review. *Journal of Functional Morphology and Kinesiology*, 1, 140–153.

Whitening, N. (2008) Fractures: pathophysiology, treatment and nursing care. *Nursing Standard*, 23(2), 49–57.

Zheng, S., Tu, L., Cicutini, F., *et al.* (2021) Depression in patients with knee osteoarthritis: risk factors and association with joint symptoms. *BMC Musculoskeletal Disorders*, 22, 40.

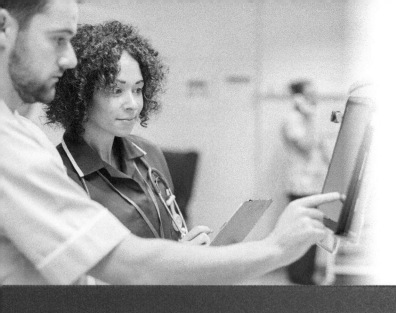

35

The Person with a Skin Disorder

Melanie Stephens

University of Salford, UK

Learning Outcomes

On completion of this chapter you will be able to:

- Review the holistic assessment of the patient with a skin disorder
- Recognise the effect of the psyche on the skin
- Explain the importance of using correct terminology in the assessment and management of skin disorders
- Review the investigations that can be undertaken to aid diagnosis and management of skin disorders
- Recognise and review common skin conditions, their clinical management and the involvement of members of the multidisciplinary team

Proficiencies

NMC Proficiencies and Standards:

- Use evidence-based, best practice approaches for meeting the needs for care and support with hygiene and the maintenance of skin integrity, accurately assessing the person's capacity for independence and self-care and initiating appropriate interventions
  - observe, assess and optimise skin and hygiene status and determine the need for support and intervention
  - use contemporary approaches to the assessment of skin integrity and use appropriate products to prevent or manage skin breakdown
  - identify and manage skin irritations and rashes.

 Visit the companion website at www.wiley.com/go/peate/nursingpractice3e where you can test yourself using flashcards, multiple-choice questions and more.

Nursing Practice: Knowledge and Care, Third Edition. Edited by Ian Peate and Aby Mitchell.
© 2022 John Wiley & Sons Ltd. Published 2022 by John Wiley & Sons Ltd.
Companion website: www.wiley.com/go/peate/nursingpractice3e

Introduction

A skin disorder can be defined as a disease affecting the skin and involves one in five babies and 54% of the population (All Party Parliamentary Group on Skin, 2013). Often, a skin disorder has a visible dramatic impact on the lives of both the patients and their families (Changing Faces, 2021). Most skin conditions are self-managed, with only 14% utilising healthcare resources, such as a practice nurse, GP, pharmacist or dermatologist. Often there is no cure; the condition is long term and follows periods of remission and exacerbation. Many nurses will only see patients at their worst, and therefore it is essential that those who provide care focus not only the physical aspects of care but provide psychological input too.

Anatomy and Physiology

Revisit Chapter 18 to remind yourself of the structure and functions of the skin, hair and nails.

> ### Nursing Fields
> The potential for skin disorders spans all fields of practice and requires healthcare practitioners to provide extra health education on the care of skin, hair and nails. Think about how you might do this for the following cases:
> - A new parent whose 10-month-old baby has developed facial eczema whilst teething
> - A teenager who presents with acne
> - An adult with learning disabilities who presents with rosacea
> - An adult with dark skin who presents with vitiligo from depigmentation
> - An older adult with dry and friable skin.
>
> Which members of the multidisciplinary team including those from voluntary organisations could provide further advice and support to both the patient?

Assessment

Assessment of the skin uses both subjective and objective data, including a full physical assessment of a patient and an assessment interview. According to Lawton (2001), this should take into consideration four main sections: a detailed history of the patient's skin condition, a general assessment of the patient, an assessment of the patient's knowledge and a physical assessment.

Patient Assessment Interview

On first meeting a patient, the nurse would carry out a comprehensive holistic health assessment (collection of subjective data). Data collected includes when the person first noticed the skin disorder, how long it has been present, how often it occurs or recurs, the characteristics of the disorder, what route the disorder has taken, whether it is affected by seasonal changes, the severity of the disorder, any precipitating or predisposing factors (e.g. family history of the condition), what relieves the disorder if at all (pharmacological and non-pharmacological), and any related symptoms.

> ### Jot This Down
> Why would a nurse ask a patient with a skin disorder about their occupation and hobbies?

Questioning of the patient about their skin disorder would focus on skin, hair, nails and patient knowledge. Table 35.1 highlights issues a nurse would consider as part of the patient assessment.

It is important to ask the patient questions about their knowledge of the disorder, as this may mean that further health promotion and education is required at the end of the assessment.

The next stage is to conduct a full medical history, so that a holistic picture of the patient and their skin disorder can be obtained. Questions would centre on previous problems, any allergies, prior lesions or moles. Questions that explore the patient's past medical and surgical history help explore symptoms linked to other disorders. Questions could focus on neurological, cardiovascular, respiratory, gastrointestinal, genitourinary, musculoskeletal, reproductive, haematological, immunological and endocrine issues. Interviewing would also focus on current and past medication and treatments and activities of daily living, for example communication, work and play, sleep and how the condition affects the patient's current lifestyle.

Risk of skin cancer and malignant melanoma would also be explored, including factors such as the presence and number of moles on the skin, and prior exposure to radiation, X-rays, coal, tar or petroleum-based products. Record the age, sex and gender of the patient, and any previous personal or family history of skin cancer or malignant melanoma; their routine in relation to exposure to sunlight; their predisposition to sunburn or an inability to tan; the presence of any previous skin trauma; the presence of freckles; and the colour of hair and eyes.

Examination of the Skin

Examination of the skin includes a general assessment and a physical skin assessment, and can be part of a total assessment or a focused assessment for those patients with a known or suspected problem, perhaps a referral from a GP to a dermatology service.

> ### Care, Dignity and Compassion
> The place in which the examination takes place should be considered prior to commencement. As the patient may be removing all their clothes in front of strangers, it is necessary to ensure both that an explanation is provided as to why this is necessary and that the venue should be an area full of bright natural light, private and warm. Consideration should be given to
> *(Continued)*

Table 35.1 Questions to consider when questioning a patient about their skin disorder.

ANATOMICAL PART OF THE INTEGUMENTARY SYSTEM	QUESTIONS A NURSE WOULD CONSIDER
Skin	*What recent changes in skin have occurred?* Has there been development of any rashes? Are they in the same place or different ones? Is there any itching? Is this worse at any particular time during the day? Have there been any changes in colour of the skin or the skin disorder? Is there increased dryness or oiliness? *Has the patient noticed any lesions, warts, or moles?* Have these changed in colour or size? *What might have triggered the skin disorder?* Has there been any change in the use of cosmetics, soaps, skin care agents? Have they recently acquired a new pet, travelled to a different country, changed their diet or experienced high levels of stress?
Hair	*What recent changes in hair have occurred?* Is there excessive hair loss, thinning or baldness? Has the distribution of hair changed across the body? Has there been a recent change in hair products? Has the patient recently commenced a diet?
Nails	*What recent changes in the nails have occurred?* Is there any splitting, breakage or discoloration? Are there visible signs of infection? Have there been recent changes to the diet, dieting or exposure to chemicals?

any religious or cultural beliefs in relation to undressing in front of others. Curtains should be closed, dignity should be maintained and, as all clothing should be removed, a gown should be worn by the patient so as not to expose areas of the body that do not need revealing. Depending on where the skin disorder is, the patient may be assessed standing, sitting or lying down, so equipment to accommodate all these positions is required and explained to the patient with clear instructions.

Personal protective equipment should be worn when assessing open lesions, infections or infestations or when wounds or mucous membranes are oozing discharge. Some lesions may need measuring or photographing, others visualising more accurately. Therefore, it is imperative to have torches, rulers, grids and tape measures available and consent forms for photography to hand.

General Assessment

The skin conveys a wealth of information about the patient and often reflects their health status. Often, the general appearance during initial interview indicates the patient's self-caring abilities, state of mind and existence of support.

Jot This Down

What signs and symptoms from a patient's general appearance can tell us about their health status?

Physical Assessment

This assessment provides the opportunity to touch the patient and their skin and should occur in a clinical area with bright natural light. This can be embarrassing and uncomfortable, but the ability to touch the skin can tell a lot about the patient and their skin disorder. Vital clinical information gathered includes the colour of the skin both in relation to race and the skin disorder; skin texture and temperature; moisture; turgor and presence of oedema. Record other findings, such as scars, missing fingers, toes and limbs, and the presence of any open wounds. The skin tells a narrative about the patient; assess the distribution, character and shape of any lesions, their site and location (Table 35.2).

Table 35.2 Questions to ask about the character, distribution and shape of lesions.

	QUESTIONS
Character	Is there redness, scaling, crusting, exudate? Are there excoriations, blisters, erosions, pustules, papules? Are the lesions all the same (monomorphic), e.g. drug rash, or variable (polymorphic), e.g. chickenpox?
Shape	Are the lesions small, large, ring-shaped, linear? Do they have a border? Are they flat, fluid-filled, indurated?
Distribution	Is the disorder on the hands, feet, extremities of ears and nose, in light-exposed areas or mainly confined to the trunk? Is it localised or widespread? If widespread, is it symmetrical and is this central or peripheral? Is the disorder linear, regional (in a groin) or following a dermatomal pattern, such as shingles?

In patients with darkly pigmented skin, some disorders present differently, and it is important for a nurse to be aware of these differences (Lang, 2000).

Colour Lesions that appear red or brown on light skin often present as black or purple on dark skin. Always assess an area of skin that is not affected by the skin disorder and compare that with the skin disorder, highlighting any abnormalities. Mild inflammatory reactions may not be visible so use touch to detect heat on an area of skin (indicator of a reaction). However, prolonged inflammation can lead to hyperpigmentation and hypopigmentation.

Pigmentation An obvious difference is the change in pigmentation in Asian and Afro-Caribbean patients compared with Caucasians. This is categorised as a normal variant, i.e. pigmentary demarcation, and midline primary conditions, i.e. vitiligo, and secondary conditions, i.e. postinflammatory hypopigmentation, and hyperpigmentation (darkening of the pigment of the skin) in atopic eczema.

Reaction Patterns Darker skins show reaction patterns such as follicular (affecting hair follicles), papular (elevations of the skin) and annular (ring-like skin conditions), and keloid scarring.

Terminology Used for Describing Lesions

Use terminology correctly when describing lesions on a body plan of care. Common terminology can include descriptions of primary lesions, i.e. those that occur at onset of a skin disorder, and secondary lesions, i.e. those that occur over time as a consequence of the disease progressing, manipulation (scratching, rubbing, picking) and treatment. These terms can be found in Tables 35.3 and 35.4.

Professional and Legal Issues

It is crucial that the nurse describes the lesions correctly as this may affect the general management and treatment of a patient by the nurse and other members of the multidisciplinary team. The NMC (2018) states that nurses must keep clear and accurate records relevant to their practice.

During the physical assessment, skin lesions should be palpated between the finger and thumb (unless widespread) as this helps assess if the lesion is soft, firm, hard, raised or irregular and its texture. Then the lesion should be given a colour, i.e. pink,

Table 35.3 Terminology of primary lesions.

NAME		PRESENTATION	EXAMPLE
Macule		A flat circumscribed area of colour change: can be brown, red, white or tan	Vitiligo
Papule		An elevated 'spot'; palpable, firm, circumscribed, less than 5 mm in diameter	Scabies or bite from an insect
Nodule		Elevated, firm, circumscribed, palpable, larger than 5 mm in diameter	Erythema nodosum
Plaque		Elevated, flat-topped, firm, rough, superficial papule, greater than 2 cm in diameter. Papules can coalesce to form plaques	Psoriasis
Wheal		Elevated, irregular area of cutaneous oedema: red, pale pink or white	Urticaria

(Continued)

Table 35.3 (Continued)

NAME	PRESENTATION	EXAMPLE
Vesicle	Elevated, circumscribed, superficial, fluid-filled blister, less than 5 mm in diameter	Herpes simplex
Bulla	Vesicle greater than 5 mm in diameter	Bullous pemphigoid
Pustule	Elevated, superficial, similar to vesicle but filled with pus	Impetigo

Table 35.4 Terminology of secondary lesions.
Source: **Adapted from Lawton (2002).**

NAME	PRESENTATION	EXAMPLE
Scale	Thickened, flaky exfoliation, irregular, thick or thin, dry or oily, variable size, silver, white or tan in colour	Psoriasis
Crust	Dried serum, blood or purulent exudate; slightly elevated; size variable	Impetigo discoid
Excoriation	Loss of epidermis caused by scratching	Atopic eczema
Lichenification	Rough thickened epidermis, accentuated skin markings due to scratching	Lichen simplex

solitary (a single lesion), satellite (a single lesion in close proximity to a larger group), grouped (a cluster of lesions), generalised (total body area) and localised (a limited area of involvement that is clearly defined).

Skin disorders can be extremely distressing so assess the degree of discomfort the patient may be experiencing from itching, pain and soreness. Identification of the underlying cause of the pruritus is the most important factor, with appropriate management and treatment of the condition.

The Nursing Associate

 According to the NMC (2018) standards of proficiency, nursing associates will work with registered nurses to provide care and support with hygiene and the maintenance of skin integrity of patients. This will include the use of topical treatments for skin disorders, explaining how topical medicines act (across patient groups/life span), mechanism of action, therapeutic action, how doses are determined, and how they are prescribed, stored and administered safely.

Assessment of the Nails, Hair and Mucous Membranes

A skin assessment should end with a review of the nails, hair and mucous membranes. This would include any blistering, scarring and erosions of the mucous membranes and colour, shape, capillary refill and pigment changes of the nails. Finally, note any hair loss, erythema and scale of the scalp.

Jot This Down

What are the most common causes of pruritus in both skin disorders and systemic diseases?

red, purple and mauve (due to blood); brown, black and blue (due to pigment); white (due to lack of blood or pigment); or yellow and orange (due to bilirubin levels).

Describe correctly the type of lesion and its spatial relationship with other lesions on the body. Lesions can be termed as

Skin and The Psyche

Emotional trauma can occur from the development of many a skin disorder leading to stress, low self-esteem, social isolation, depression and even suicide (Zaidi & Lanigan, 2010).

As social beings, humans need interaction with each other both verbally and physically to survive; when something affects this, psychological consequences can occur. Scars can be both physical and psychological, as witnessed in acne vulgaris in teenagers (Thomas, 2005). However, it is also known that psychological illnesses such as depression, anxiety and stress can trigger or exacerbate a skin disorder. Because of this link between emotions and the skin, a new clinical field or subspecialty of dermatology has developed – psychodermatology – and within this there has been identified a four-group classification of disorders connecting the skin and the mind. These groups are:

- Psychophysiological: emotional stress causing inflammatory skin reactions
- Primary psychiatric: self-induced injury of the skin (iatrogenic)
- Secondary psychiatric: emotional consequences such as anxiety, anger and depression developing as a result of an existing skin disease
- Cutaneous sensory disorders: patients with no apparent dermatological skin or medical condition presenting with disagreeable skin sensations, such as itching, soreness and pain, and negative sensory symptoms, such as numbness and hypoaesthesia.

Assessment is key. Does the patient have a skin disorder? Is the skin disorder having a psychological impact on the patient?

Is the emotional stress suffered a constant trigger of the skin disorder itself? Is the skin disorder self-induced? Once assessed, either the nurse can measure the impact the skin disorder is having on the quality of a patient's life or referrals can be made to other members of the multidisciplinary team for psychological interventions such as relaxation, meditation, hypnosis and self-hypnosis, psychotropic medications, biofeedback and focused psychiatric care and psychotherapy.

Assessment and monitoring of the impact of a skin disorder during a patient episode of care (before, during and after treatment) can be achieved through quality of life tools. Reliable and validated tools include the Dermatology Life Quality Index, the Cardiff Tool and the SF-36 (available for adults and children).

Patient-reported experience and outcome measures are also collated to allow staff to measure not only a patient's health status but also how patients feel about the care they received (Department of Health, 2008).

Investigations

Further investigations in conjunction with other members of the multidisciplinary team may be necessary. Investigations aid the nurse in supporting the diagnosis of a skin disease, condition or injury and management or modification of treatment used to optimise repair of the hair, nails, skin and conditions for healing. Table 35.5 highlights some of the most common tests used.

Table 35.5 **Dermatological investigations.**

TYPE OF TEST	REASON FOR TEST
Oxygen saturation	A test used to measure the oxygenation of a person's haemoglobin; a lack of oxygen can lead to cell death and tissue breakdown
Toe blood pressure monitoring	A test used to measure the systolic pressure of blood in the toe; aids detection of poor vascular flow
Sinogram/fistulogram	An X-ray examination of a wound used to detect tracking, undermining and tunnelling of a wound
Urinalysis	A test used to detect and/or screen for metabolic and kidney disorders
Blood sugar	Used to determine the plasma glucose level. Mainly used as a diagnostic or screening tool for diabetes
Body mass index (BMI)	A tool to assess the weight and height of a person, which aids assessment of factors such as nutritional status and risk of pressure ulcer development and is linked to numerous illnesses and child development
Blood tests	Various blood tests assess the function of the liver, kidneys and lungs and also aid screening for issues such as anaemia, infections, immune problems and platelet levels
Magnetic resonance imaging (MRI)	A non-invasive medical imaging technique used to visualise the internal structures of the body
Computed tomography (CT)	A medical imaging procedure that uses computer-processed X-rays to produce tomographic images or 'slices' of specific areas of the body
Sonography	An ultrasound-based diagnostic imaging technique used for visualising subcutaneous body structures, including tendons, muscles, joints, vessels and internal organs; also used in obstetrics to visualise the unborn foetus

(Continued)

Table 35.5 (*Continued*)

TYPE OF TEST	REASON FOR TEST
Phlebography	A test that provides X-ray images of the venous system when radio-opaque dye is injected into the veins of the lower limbs
Photoplethysmography	A non-invasive test used to measure blood volume changes in microvascular bed of tissues using infrared light source and transducer light probe. Often used to assess venous reflux
Duplex ultrasonography	A form of medical ultrasonography that incorporates two elements: grey-scale ultrasound to visualise the structure or architecture of the body part and colour Doppler ultrasound to visualise the flow or movement of a structure, e.g. to image blood within an artery
X-rays	A medical imaging test to detect problems such as osteomyelitis
Allergy testing	Can help confirm or rule out allergies and consequently reduce adverse reactions and limit unnecessary avoidance and medications. Tests can involve the taking of blood or skinprick tests
Wood's lamp, immunofluorescent studies, potassium hydroxide and Tzanck test	A variety of tests used to identify infections, i.e. to look for chickenpox, fungal and bacterial infections
Culture	A test used to identify infections from collections of tissue samples, serum, pus, exudates and drainage. In sepsis, serum will be obtained
Skin biopsy	Allows the clinician to differentiate a benign skin lesion from a cancer or to determine an infection that cannot be obtained through routine swabbing. Techniques of biopsy can be punch, incision, excision and shaving
Genetic testing	A test used to examine the structure of a person's DNA, gene products and chromosomes

Skin Infections: Viral, Bacterial and Fungal

Epidemiology

Sebum, the immune system and skin flora protect the skin from infections; however, if a breach of the skin occurs, the immune system is impaired or a potent mediator falls onto the skin, then these normal functions are weakened and the skin may be at risk of disorders such as viral, bacterial and fungal infections. Minor skin infestations and infections are often self-managed by patients but skin conditions are major causes for consultation in primary care (Schofield *et al.*, 2011). Skin infections such as cellulitis affected nearly 317 000 people in England in 2017–2018 (NHS Digital, 2019), many of whom required admission to hospital for intravenous antibiotics and further investigation.

Viral Skin Infections

A virus is a micro-organism smaller than a bacterium and consists of an RNA or DNA core surrounded by a protein coat. It cannot grow or reproduce unless it is inside a living cell. The skin lesions that occur as a consequence have attacked the keratinocyte, reproduced and caused either cell death or growth.

Common viral skin infections have recently increased and it is thought that this is due to numerous causes: antibiotics, contraceptive medication, corticosteroids, any medication that causes immunosuppression and the COVID-19 coronavirus.

Common viral infections of the skin include the following.

Warts

The human papillomavirus (HPV) (over 60 types) is the cause of warts or verrucae. Often found on non-genital and genital areas of the skin and mucous membranes. Present as flat, tapered at both ends and round in shape, with a rough grey surface. Table 35.6 highlights the most common warts, their location and appearance.

Table 35.6 **Common warts.**

TYPE OF WART	LOCATION	APPEARANCE
Verruca vulgaris (common wart)	Anywhere on the skin and mucous membranes, most common on fingers	Dome-shaped with ragged borders
Plantar warts	Pressure points on the feet	Inward-growing wart due to pressure of shoes and walking; often painful
Verucca plana (flat wart)	Forehead or back of hand	Small flat lesion
Condylomata acuminata (HPV or venereal warts)	Glans of the penis, anal region, vulva and cervix	Cauliflower-like, pink and purple in colour

Herpes simplex

Herpes simplex virus (HSV) is a common virus that affects much of the population (cold sore). Initial infection is often the most severe and may be accompanied by fever and sore throat; in the under-5s, the virus may cause inflammation of the gums. Once a primary infection has occurred, the virus lives in the nerve ganglia and is usually reactivated by sunlight, menstruation, stress, injury or low immunity. Herpes simplex is caused by two viruses:

- *HSV-1*: attributed to simplex lesions of the face, lips and mouth, transmitted through kissing, oral sex and physical contact
- *HSV-2*: commonly attributed to genital infections.

Signs and Symptoms Include a tingling or burning sensation followed by reddening of the skin or membranes and formation of a painful vesicle. The vesicle advances through pustules, ulcers and crusting, and healing occurs between 10 and 14 days after initial symptoms. If the eyes are affected, conjunctivitis can occur. Secondary infection can occur, mainly in patients with skin breakdown such as active eczema; in extreme cases, the ulcers can spread rapidly and affect the lungs, brain and heart (eczema herpeticum) (Linh, 2011).

Nursing Care For mild and uncomplicated HSV infection, no treatment or management is necessary. An antiviral cream such as aciclovir may help ease some of the symptoms but should be applied at the tingling stage to shorten the eruption. Patients who experience recurrent eruptions may be offered long-term antiviral therapy.

Severe infection may require hospitalisation and oral antiviral therapy. With eye infections, antiviral eye drops can be prescribed.

Health Promotion Prevention is key and the nurse's role is to provide education and advice in relation to the wearing of sunscreen, avoiding stressors that trigger HSV, eating a healthy diet and taking exercise, all activities that create a healthy immune system. Other advice is not to kiss or have oral sex with someone who has signs and symptoms of HSV.

Herpes Zoster

Known as shingles, the chickenpox (varicella zoster) virus remains dormant in the dorsal root ganglion of a nerve. Reactivation of herpes zoster triggers a reaction, a rash in the dermatome section of the skin, coinciding with illnesses that cause immunosuppression, such as HIV or infections, malignancy such as leukaemia, lymphoma and Hodgkin disease, or during or after a course of radiotherapy or chemotherapy. Can occur at any age but common in the over-50s, affecting one in five people.

Signs and Symptoms A period of hypersensitivity precedes an outbreak of shingles, with complaints of feeling under the weather, headache, fever, burning and pain; this is called the pre-eruptive phase. In the eruptive phase, blisters develop in a unilateral area, and take 3–4 weeks to clear.

Complications include secondary infection and postherpetic neuralgia lasting 3–6 months; this is named the chronic phase.

Rare but serious complications include impairment or loss of vision if the ophthalmic division of the trigeminal nerve is affected, facial paralysis and, in the immunocompromised individual, visceral lesions and encephalitis, which potentially result in death.

Nursing Care Cool tap water compresses and calamine lotion can ease blistering and petroleum jelly aids healing. Early antiviral therapy within 72 hours of the rash developing can reduce the duration of the rash and any potential postherpetic neuralgia. Loose-fitting cotton clothing reduces the risk of irritation. Regular pain relief such as paracetamol or paracetamol and codeine derivatives are useful. If a patient is experiencing postherpetic neuralgia, then topical capsaicin cream and antidepressants may be prescribed. In severe cases, steroids may be prescribed. Referrals to other members of the medical team may be needed if shingles affects the eye and brain.

Medicines Management

Research over the years has shown that using ibuprofen in children who have chickenpox may lead to a masking of symptoms and an increased risk of serious skin infection – a condition called necrotising fasciitis.

Health Promotion Studies have shown that providing the over-60s with varicella zoster vaccine boosts immunity (Tseng *et al.*, 2011) and prevents herpes zoster disease (Gagliardi *et al.*, 2012). The person with shingles is infectious to others when the rash appears, but only if the person coming into contact has not had chickenpox. Women who are pregnant should avoid anyone with shingles until the vesicles have dried up. Patients should not share towels, play contact sports, or go swimming while they have a shingles rash.

COVID-19 Skin Manifestations

Since the emergence of COVID-19, there have been case reports worldwide documenting five cutaneous (skin) signs and symptoms: these include acral areas of erythema named 'Covid toes' (pseudo-chilblains), urticarial lesions (hives and wheals rash), maculopapular eruptions, a skin rash that contains flat discoloured areas and raised bumps in adults, vesicular eruptions (chickenpox-like rash) and livedo (mottling of the skin). Since the first list in May 2020, other skin manifestations include acroischaemia and necrosis, petechiae and purpuris eruptions, intertriginous and flexural (skinfold) exanthems (viral rashes), pityriasis rosea-like eruptions, erythema multiforme-like eruptions, unspecified erythematous facial eruptions and androgenic alopecia.

Bacterial Skin Infections

The most common bacterial skin infections are caused by Gram-positive *Staphylococcus aureus* and beta-haemolytic streptococci. Infections may be primary, caused by a single pathogen from the skin, or secondary, occurring in diseased or traumatised skin. Treated quickly, the infections can be easily cleared. Severe complications such as septicaemia can occur if treatment is delayed or inadequate. Table 35.7 highlights the

Table 35.7 Common types of bacterial skin infections.

BACTERIAL INFECTION OF THE SKIN	MOST COMMON CAUSATIVE BACTERIA	SIGNS, SYMPTOMS AND COMPLICATIONS	SITE
Folliculitis: bacterial infection of the hair follicle	*Staphylococcus aureus* and *Pseudomonas aeruginosa*	Inflammation, pustules and lesions seen at the hair follicle. Discomfort ranging from slight burning to intense itching. Complication of abscess formation	Scalp, face of bearded men (sycosis barbae), eye (stye) and extremities on the legs of women who shave
Furuncles (boils): inflammation of the hair follicle	*Staphylococcus aureus*	Deep, firm, red, painful nodule 1–5 cm in diameter. After few days the nodule changes to a large painful cystic nodule draining infected, purulent pus	Any part of the body that has hair, particularly neck, face, flexures and buttocks
Carbuncles: group of infected hair follicles	*Staphylococcus aureus*	Firm mass located in the subcutaneous tissue and lower dermis. Mass becomes painful and swollen and has multiple openings to the skin surface. Patient may experience chills, fever and malaise	Neck, back and lateral thighs
Cellulitis: localised infection of the dermis and subcutaneous tissue	*Streptococcus pyogenes*	Red, swollen and painful area. Vesicles may form over the cellulitic area, accompanied by chills, fever, malaise, headache and swollen lymph glands	Anywhere on the body. Common areas are lower legs in adults and eye and perianal area in children
Erysipelas: infection of the skin	*Streptococcus pyogenes*	Chills, fever and malaise (4–20 hours) precede a skin lesion appearing. Lesion(s) appear as firm red spots enlarging to form a circumscribed, bright red, raised, hot lesion. Petechiae, necrosis and blistering can occur if not treated early	Face, ears and lower legs

common types of bacterial skin infections, the causative bacteria and their signs and symptoms. Contributing factors for the development of bacterial skin infections include no apparent cause, poor hygiene, poor nutrition, prolonged skin moisture or excessive moisture from perspiration, trauma to the skin (including trauma from shaving), systemic diseases such as diabetes mellitus and haematological malignancies, and heavy fabrics on the upper legs.

Nursing Care
All bacterial infections need to be monitored carefully, taking vital observations, noting the spread of inflammation, and marking and measuring this clearly on a body map. In emergency situations, the ABCDE (Airway, Breathing, Circulation, Disability, Exposure) approach to patient management should be applied.

Folliculitis No treatment is advised in mild cases, although emollients may improve the condition of the skin. Topical antibiotics

may be prescribed once culture and sensitivity of the causative organism has been identified.

Furuncles and carbuncles Warm compresses may ease the pain and draw a boil or carbuncle to a head. If it bursts, cleansing with normal saline and the application of ointments and dressings may be necessary. Large boils and carbuncles may be lanced by a trained nurse who has extended their skill in this area. Antibiotics are often not necessary unless the inflammation extends around the boil or carbuncle, or lymphadenopathy, fever or multiple boils are present. A urinalysis for glucose levels should be performed in patients who return with frequent boils.

Cellulitis Mild or moderate cellulitis is treated with antibiotics for 7 days. More serious cases may need hospitalisation. Orbital cellulitis is a medical emergency that can lead to loss of sight and cerebral complications.

Erysipelas This is a medical emergency and the patient would receive antibiotics for the first 7 days; often patients are hospitalised.

> ### Case Study
>
> Aubrey aged 78 was admitted with a red, tender, oedematous left leg after banging it on the corner of the coffee table. Aubrey reported feeling feverish and had also developed an ulcerated area to the pretibial area. The GP had prescribed oral antibiotics 48 hours previously, but a rash had spread to the whole lower leg. A diagnosis of Class II cellulitis (CREST, 2005) was made. The outline of inflammation was marked using a skin pen (to observe spread or receding of infection) and IV antibiotics, analgesia, leg elevation and a wound swab were prescribed. Initial dressing of the leg was with a hydrofibre and secondary dressing to the ulcer, with toe-to-knee stockinette, wool and crepe. After 48 hours an ABPI was performed (0.9) and compression bandaging was applied.

Health Promotion

Health education should be related to contributing factors of the bacterial infection such as personal hygiene, nutritional intake, weight management and choice of clothing.

Fungal Skin Infections

Dermatophytoses, candidiasis and mycoses are fungi that cause superficial skin infections. Many people have a fungal infection without even knowing it and it is often only when they access healthcare resources that the infection is identified and treated (Nazarko, 2011).

Common fungal infections are caused by two main groups: dermatophytoses (tinea or ringworm) and candidiasis (yeasts). Patients most at risk are those who take antibiotics, either orally or intravenously, as antibiotics not only treat the invading infection but kill the bacteria and disturb the normal flora on the body. Increased risk exists with those patients who already have an underlying medical condition, such as diabetes mellitus, leukaemia or HIV, and the elderly. Fungi love a moist environment so areas of the skin between the toes and under folds of skin are at risk. Patients who have poor nutritional status, are obese, take oral contraception, are pregnant, iron deficient or immune suppressed are equally at risk.

Candidiasis

Candida albicans is the yeast-like infection generally found on mucous membranes, the skin, vagina and gastrointestinal tract. *Candida* intertrigo (sweat rash) occurs due to perspiration being trapped in skinfolds or tight clothes and the sweat being unable to evaporate.

Signs and Symptoms *Candida albicans* start as a pustule that extends under the stratum corneum. The pustule habitually burns, causes itching and has a red and swollen base. As infection develops, a white curd-like substance appears. This is the shedding of the surface cells and accumulation of inflammatory cells, such as white blood cells. Satellite lesions can be seen outside the boundaries of the original site.

Candida intertrigo occurs in folds of skin under the breasts, in the groin or in the apron/peduncular (overhang of skin from the abdomen).

Dermatophytoses (Tinea and Ringworm)

Superficial fungal infections are known as dermatophytoses and are identified by the body part that they are invading (Table 35.8). The organism can be transmitted by direct contact with an animal, another person or an inanimate object. Contact can occur from the sharing of towels, pillowcases and combs. Dermatophytoses like moist environments.

Nursing Care

Local fungal infections are treated with topical antibiotics as a cream, powder or solution. Antibiotic use varies from 1 to 4 weeks and can continue for an extra week once the infection has cleared. If the infected area is very sore, red and painful, topical steroids can be used in conjunction with the antibiotic treatment, treating and soothing the skin.

> ### Case Study
>
> Charlie was 53 and was invited for breast screening. On arrival, it was noted that Charlie has a BMI of 28 and had intertrigo under the breasts. Charlie found the mammogram painful and felt a stinging sensation under the breasts during the investigation. On examination, there were two small tears, one in each fold of the skin under the breasts. The mammographer completed a clinical incident report and referred Charlie to the radiology nurse for advice. The skinfolds and wounds were cleaned with normal saline and non-adherent dressings were applied. Charlie was advised to see the GP for some antifungal and steroid cream. Once healed, Charlie was also advised to wash the area morning and night and pat dry, wear a well-fitting supportive bra and use a barrier cream.

Health Promotion

Fungal infections are often embarrassing and uncomfortable. Preventive methods include weight loss, attention to personal hygiene (washing and drying folds and creases well), and the wearing of natural fibres such as cotton and linen to enable perspiration and evaporation, keeping the skin dry and cool.

Infestations

Skin irritations and disorders can be a result of infestations affecting anyone, regardless of social class or standing. However, they are often associated with crowded or unsanitary conditions. The most common infestations seen in the UK are lice, scabies, fleas and bedbugs.

Lice

There are three types of lice infestation, named according to the part of the body affected: pediculosis corporis (body lice), pediculosis pubis (pubic lice) and pediculosis capitis (head lice). A typical louse is 2–4 mm in length and oval in shape.

Table 35.8 Signs and symptoms of dermatophytoses.

NAME OF DERMATOPHYTOSIS	AREA AFFECTED	SIGNS AND SYMPTOMS
Tinea pedis (athlete's foot; Figure 35.1)	Sole of foot, space between the toes and toenails	Lesions that can appear as scaliness to fissures with drainage, accompanied by pruritus and foul-smelling odour. Occurs more frequently in summer due to feet perspiring
Tinea capitis (infection of the scalp)	Scalp	Grey, round, bald spots with erythema and crusting. Temporary hair loss. More common in children than adults
Tinea corporis (infection of the body)	Anywhere on the body	Large circular patches with raised red borders; can include vesicles, papules or pustules. Very itchy
Tinea versicolor (infection of the upper chest, back and arms)	Upper chest, back and arms	Yellow, pink or brown lesions that are like sheets of scaling skin. The patches of skin contain no pigment and do not tan in sunlight
Tinea cruris (infection of the groin, thighs and buttocks)	Groin, thighs and buttocks (jock itch)	Signs and symptoms as tinea pedis. Occurs in the physically active, obese and those who wear tight clothing

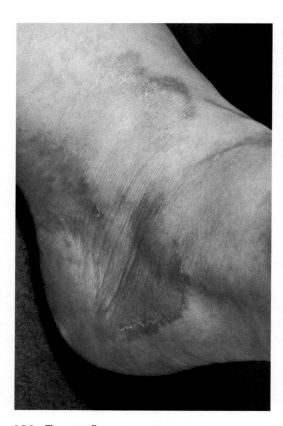

Figure 35.1 Tinea pedis. *Source:* Buxton & Morris-Jones (2013). Reproduced with permission of John Wiley & Sons Ltd.

It possesses a stylet that enables it to pierce the skin to feed on the host; an anticoagulant contained within the louse's saliva prevents clotting. While living on the host, the female louse lays eggs on the hair shafts. These eggs are pearl-grey or brown in colour. Once hatched, the louse quickly reaches the reproductive stage of adulthood, lays eggs and then dies. The normal life cycle of a louse is 30–50 days. The spread of lice requires hair-to-hair contact. Signs and symptoms include the following.

- *Head lice*: an itchy scalp; on closer observation the scalp may contain sores and the eggs and the louse may be seen, especially behind the ears and on the nape of the neck.
- *Body lice*: itching, scratch marks, eczema, discoloured skin and urticaria.
- *Pubic lice*: itchy, small red spots in the pubic area and the hair mats.

Secondary infections can occur in all cases.

Scabies

The *Sarcoptes scabiei* mite burrows into the skin to lay eggs each day for a month; 3–5 days later, the eggs hatch, travel to the surface of the skin and then burrow back down for food and security. Back in the safety of the skin, the mites lay larvae and the cycle repeats itself. Scabies tends to leave lesions 2 mm in length that are small and reddish brown in colour and often found in webspaces of the fingers, wrists and elbow, axillae, nipple, penis, belt line and gluteal crease. Common signs and symptoms include pruritus that is worse at night and urticaria (an allergic response to the mite droppings). Immunocompromised elderly patients are at risk of developing Norwegian scabies, where thousands of mites are present on the body. If this is diagnosed, the Health Protection Agency must be notified. The spread of scabies requires skin-to-skin contact.

Fleas

There are many different types of flea (Siphonaptera); however, those that most commonly affect humans are *Ctenocephalides* (cat and dog flea) and *Pulex irritans* (human flea). A flea, like lice, feeds on the blood of humans by piercing the skin and sucking the blood. The female lays eggs on bedding, soft furnishings or carpets. After 2 weeks, the eggs hatch into larvae that feed on organic matter around them. They then pupate into a cocoon and the flea hatches. The flea can leap some distance to source its host. The life cycle of a flea is 3–4 weeks. Signs and symptoms include a clustering of irritating, inflamed papules, which if consistently scratched can become infected. On assessment of the skin, especially the skin olds of the waist and flexures (knees and elbows), a darkened red spot with a surrounding reddened area is seen.

Bed Bugs

Cimicidae (bed bug family) spend most of their life in dark places near hosts, for example the settee, chair or bed. They do this so that at night, they can feed on the host, either animal or human. Bed bugs are 6–9.5 mm in size. Their bodies are flattened, oval in shape and rust coloured and they possess small wings. Once mature, a female bed bug will lay 2–3 eggs per night. The eggs take 10–20 days to hatch and this cycle is then replicated. To mature, a bed bug must pass through five moults, which occur commonly after a feed. The bite of a bed bug leaves a firm white swelling. Signs that bed bugs are present are small spots of blood on the sheets in the morning and an almond-like smell in the room if there is a large infestation.

Nursing Care

The nursing care of infestations is as follows.

Head Lice

Wet combing can be done every 4 days for 4 weeks, with each wet comb taking 30 minutes per occasion (not a stand-alone treatment). Parasiticidal preparations may be applied to the hair, following the manufacturer's guidance, and repeated after 7 days. Dimethicone, a silicone oil, can be rubbed into the hair or scalp and left for 8 hours. It coats, suffocates and kills the lice but has no effect on the nits, so treatment has to be repeated after 7 days, when they have hatched (Burgess et al., 2005).

Body Lice

Washing clothes and bedding in a hot wash and tumble-drying kills body lice and their eggs. Close family members and partners need treating with a parasiticidal preparation, which is repeated after 7 days. Oral antihistamines should be prescribed to help reduce itching and damage to the skin.

Pubic Lice

Once diagnosed with pubic lice, the affected area should be shaved, or groomed with a fine comb. A pediculicide is used following manufacturer's instructions and repeated 7 days later.

Scabies

How scabies is managed depends on whether it is a single case or outbreak. Usual treatment is to apply to the whole body, paying particular attention to areas to which the scabies tend to migrate but avoiding the eyes, using either a 5% permethrin cream or a lotion containing 0.5% malathion, which kills the mites. The preparation is left on the skin as per manufacturer's instructions and then showered off. Treatment is repeated 7 days later to kill any eggs that survived and hatched into mites. Clothes, bedding and towels are washed in a hot wash and tumble-dried. Antihistamines may be prescribed to reduce the itching and damage to the skin.

Fleas

Antiseptic soaps and creams are used to prevent a secondary infection. Calamine lotion or 1% hydrocortisone may be used to ease the itching. Other treatments are aimed at killing the fleas, including spraying an insecticide (following manufacturer's guidance) and then vacuuming the carpets, beds, chairs, settee and soft furnishings and disposing of the vacuumed material when finished. This is to kill the eggs and pupae. Animals may need to be treated and veterinary advice should be sought.

Bed Bugs

Advice from the pest control unit can help decide which company to use to treat the house. Cleanliness is paramount, so laundering of all bed linen, meticulous cleaning of cupboards, drawers and bed frames with hot water and vacuuming of carpets and soft furnishings are advised.

Health Promotion

Household cleanliness is a key factor in the prevention of many infestations; however, some infestations occur from touching or sitting close to another person who owns pets. Advice should be provided to patients and their significant others about personal hygiene, household maintenance and care of animals.

Acne

One of the most common skin disorders in the UK, acne can cause significant psychological distress. However, it is both treatable and preventable if managed early. A skin condition most commonly found on the face, back and chest, acne is the partial or total obstruction of pilosebaceous ducts due to the hypercornification of cells (atypical accumulation of keratinocytes) lining the ducts.

Acne can be both non-inflammatory and inflammatory. Non-inflammatory acne is thought to arise from the movement of melanin into the duct from adjacent epidermal cells, leading to the development of lesions called comedones, which can be open, such as blackheads, or closed, such as pimples and whiteheads. Inflammatory acne, on the other hand, consists of comedones, erythematous pustules and cysts. These are thought to develop from the obstructed ducts being colonised by bacteria, in particular *Propionibacterium*, which produces substances along with the fatty acid constituents of sebum that irritate the skin. Cytokines (inflammatory mediators) are released that attract white cells, such as polymorphs and lymphocytes, to the area and pus formation occurs as a consequence. Rupture of the comedones can occur.

There are many forms of acne: the most common are acne vulgaris and acne conglobata. Table 35.9 highlights the common forms and their signs and symptoms.

Nursing Care

Nursing care requires a full assessment of the severity of the acne. Many dermatology specialists use the Leeds Acne Scale (Cunliffe, 1994), medical photography and a quality-of-life indicator. General principles of care include washing twice daily with a mild cleanser or antiseptic wash. Spots should not be picked or scratched. If the pustules are tense, the 'traffic light' guide should be used: red pustules means stop; yellow means get ready and squeeze gently; green means go to the doctor. Oral antibiotics may be ineffective if patients do not take the full course. Early topical treatment can prevent scarring. Advise the patient to avoid irritant oils and non-comedogenic cosmetics and that all

Table 35.9 Common signs and symptoms of acne.

TYPE OF ACNE	SIGNS AND SYMPTOMS
Acne vulgaris	Common in teenagers and young to middle-aged adults Cause unknown but possible androgenic influence on sebaceous glands Can be: • *Mild*: a few scattered comedones and occasional papules • *Moderate*: presence of comedones, macules, papules and pustules • *Severe*: comedones, papules and pustules, painful nodules and cysts that scar and cause pigment changes
Acne conglobata	Occurs in middle years Cause unknown Serious skin lesions occur, with discharge ranging from serous to purulent. Has a foul odour

acne treatments are slow to respond and improvements may not be seen until 2–3 months later.

Referrals to other members of the multidisciplinary team may be advisable for further support – counselling and therapies, both skin and psychological.

Health Promotion

Health promotion would be to consider a healthy nutritious diet, take exercise and avoid triggers such as stress. There is an increasing link between aggravation of acne and a diet with a high glycaemic load and dairy products (Smith *et al.*, 2007).

Rosacea

Rosacea is a persistent reddening or flushing of the skin, accompanied by visible superficial facial capillaries (telangiectasia). It is often mistaken for a side-effect of the excess consumption of alcohol. It is an under-reported skin disorder, mainly affecting middle-aged and older adults. It is a chronic skin condition that affects women more than men, usually aged between 36 and 50 years, with fair skin. Its cause is unknown but suggestions include damage to dermal connective tissue caused by the sun, which may result in damage to the endothelium of blood vessels or abnormal vascular reactivity, and an association with those who suffer with migraine (Berth-Jones, 2010). Rosacea has many subtypes and characteristics. Symptoms and areas affected are as follows.

- *Erythematotelangiectatic*: signs of redness and visible superficial blood vessels, with stinging and soreness around the central zone of the face.
- *Papulopustular*: signs of redness, flushing, papules, pustules and transient oedema. The face stings, has a burning sensation and is sore and sensitive to facial products and topical creams. This can appear on the face, chest, ears and scalp (bald men).
- *Phymatous*: the patient has a visibly distorted nose, redness and pustules on the face. The symptoms are the same as erythematotelangiectatic, but only the nose is affected.

- *Ocular*: only the eye is affected and this is often sore, red and can have conjunctivitis and blepharitis. The patient complains of a gritty feeling in the eyes, with blurred vision. Often, eye problems can occur before a flare-up of the skin.

Nursing Care

Rosacea can be very distressing and have a dramatic effect on a patient's mental well-being. With a full assessment and completion of a dermatology quality-of-life index, care should then focus around factors that trigger and exacerbate the skin disorder. This can include keeping the face cool, avoiding overheating from warm rooms, baths and showers, and protection of the face all year with a good sun block no less than factor 30. The nurse should also discuss the limiting of alcohol and spicy food. Skin care would focus around gentle washing with emollient face washes, avoiding soap products and the application of light, non-greasy moisturisers between treatments. Any oil-based products, both skin care and cosmetic, should be avoided. Treatment usually takes 3 months before any visible changes are noted, but is effective in the long term; topical treatments such as metronidazole and azelaic acid are prescribed and used as per dermatologist guidance. Oral antibiotics may also be prescribed.

Referrals may be made to other members of the multidisciplinary team, in particular cosmetic camouflage, dermatologists who offer laser therapy, plastic surgery for severe rhinophyma, and ophthalmology if keratitis (eye pain, sensitivity to light and blurred vision) is suspected.

Health Promotion

Health promotion for patients with rosacea focuses on general skin care and guidance. However, the nurse must explore the side-effects of the topical agents, treatments and options to ensure informed consent. Changing Faces is a charity that can offer support to patients affected by rosacea and their families.

Psoriasis

Affecting 2–3% of the population, psoriasis is a common non-infectious inflammatory skin disorder, which offers the patient and nurse many challenges due to its unpredictable periods of exacerbation and remission (Ryan, 2008).

The phase of epidermal cell proliferation is hastened in psoriasis, reducing from 28 days to only 4 days. This acceleration does not allow the cell to mature; the nucleus remains and keratinisation does not occur. A build-up of keratin transpires and the classic scales seen in a patient with psoriasis result. As the epidermis becomes thickened, blood flow to the subcutaneous layer increases and gives the psoriasis the reddened appearance that accompanies the scaly plaque. The cause of psoriasis is unknown but causative factors can include genetic predisposition and environmental triggers such as trauma, infection, stress, smoking, hormones, medication and sunlight.

The psychological impact of psoriasis cannot be overstated: not only are the plaques and scales visible to others but when they fall off on bedding, clothes and furniture, they are a constant reminder of the chronic condition. Psoriasis can occur anywhere on the body, either as a single lesion or multiple – the

Table 35.10 **Different presentations of psoriasis.**

PRESENTATION OF PSORIASIS	SITE OF PRESENTATION	CLINICAL APPEARANCE
Plaque psoriasis	Elbows, knees and scalp	Red, well-defined plaques with silver scales
Guttate psoriasis	Upper trunk and extremities, usually preceded by a throat infection	Small erythematous plaques in the shape of a raindrop
Scalp psoriasis	Scalp	Dry scaly skin to thick plaques
Flexural psoriasis	Axillae, submammary area and groin	Well-demarcated smooth plaques
Erythroderma	Entire skin	Reddening all over the body. A medical emergency as the patient will feel generally unwell
Localised pustular psoriasis	Palms and soles	Inflamed skin with yellow pustules that dry to form brown patches
Generalised pustular psoriasis	Entire skin	Inflamed skin with clusters of pustules that join together. A medical emergency. The patient may appear toxic with severe pain. Often precipitated by a course of high-dose steroids (topical or systemic)

areas most commonly affected are elbows, knees and scalp. The nail and gluteal cleft can also be affected. The different presentations of psoriasis are outlined in Table 35.10.

Nursing Care

Treatment is classified according to the severity of the skin disorder: topical for mild-to-moderate disease, phototherapy for moderate-to-severe disease and systemic for severe disease. Patients often receive a combination of treatments.

Topical treatments include emollients, vitamin D analogues, tar, dithranol and topical steroids which are messy and offensive smelling.

Phototherapy involves irradiation with UVB, whereas photo-chemotherapy necessitates the use of a photoactive drug (psoralen) in combination with UVA irradiation (Van Onselen, 2001). During treatment, patients will attend hospital 2–3 times per week for 6 weeks and documentation of the patient's lifetime of exposures is required, as there is a risk of cutaneous malignancy with this treatment.

Patients who require systemic treatment include those who, for example, have had repeated hospital admissions, pustular psoriasis and extensive disease.

Health Promotion

Health promotion centres on reducing trigger factors for the exacerbation of psoriasis and encouraging the patient to apply the topical therapies and attend for phototherapy. Keeping the skin soft and moist can offer comfort as well as avoiding itching and the use of irritating cosmetics and soaps.

Eczema

Eczema is reported to affect one in nine of the population. Often described as an itchy, inflammatory skin disorder, eczema can have unfavourable effects on the sufferer and their significant others. There are many different types of eczema, each caused by different factors. *Atopic eczema* has no known cause, although research suggests the patient has a predisposition to develop an allergic response to various substances (Stanway, 2011). Many patients with atopic eczema have asthma and/or hay fever: 15–20% of children and 2–10% of adults are affected. Flare-ups can often be triggered by allergies, the seasons, infection and even teething in small children (British Association of Dermatologists, 2009). Other types of eczema include irritant eczema, allergic contact eczema, food allergy, xerosis (dry skin), lichen simplex from repeated scratching, gravitational eczema, discoid eczema and seborrhoeic eczema.

Signs and symptoms of atopic eczema differ with age; early in the acute phase of eczema, the rash can be inflamed, weeping and blistering, in the subacute phase dry, scaly and burning, and in the chronic phase the skin becomes dry, thickened, fissured and excoriated. Atopic eczema can start as early as 4 months of age and can commence as a dry, scaly rash on the face and possibly on the rest of the body. The British Association of Dermatologists (2009) has developed guidance on diagnosing atopic eczema and suggests that the patient can present with three of the following in conjunction with a dry itchy rash:

- Previous history of rashes to the back of the knees and elbows
- Family history or medical history of asthma and/or hay fever
- Tendency to dry skin
- Onset under 2 years of age.

Nursing Care

A full history is required when assessing a patient with eczema. This will help identify the type of eczema, the triggers and causative factors in order to focus treatment and management. The nurse should also be aware of the possibility of complications resulting from a secondary infection with bacteria, a virus or fungi, as this can often become a medical emergency. Once the type and cause have been ascertained, the treatment will focus on removing the trigger factors, keeping nails short and avoiding scratching.

The most important aspect of management is regular use of emollients to moisturise the skin. This can be supplemented with topical steroids to reduce inflammation, antibiotics to treat infection and antihistamines to reduce pruritus. More serious cases may need referral for immunomodulatory treatments, phototherapy and immunosuppressive drugs. Patients may need other therapies in relation to body image and psychological issues.

Health Promotion

Health promotion focuses around removing the causative factors, moisturising of the skin, a well-balanced diet and self-help and support.

> ### What the Experts Say
>
> 'Having eczema on the hands really affected my 9-year-old's life. Previously Lei was a really happy child, apparently always putting their hand up at school and joining in activities. One day, I was rung by the school who were asking what had happened to my child. They had noticed a dramatic change in their behaviour. Lei was now quiet, did not get involved in activities and was always tucking their hands in their jumper or cardigan. They asked if anything was going on at home and wanted me to come in to speak with them about Lei. We agreed on a group meeting and Lei just blurted it out; Lei was ashamed of their hands and wished they would heal up. I could not believe that I had missed something so simple.
>
> Jian, parent of Lei aged 9

> ### Jot This Down
> What advice can you give to patients with a skin disorder in relation to nutrition? Which nutrients are essential to optimise the skin's condition and why?

Skin Tumours

Some lesions found on the skin are malignant in aetiology due to long-term exposure to the environment and sun. The three main types of malignant lesion are actinic keratosis, non-melanoma skin cancer and melanoma.

Actinic Keratosis

Premalignant epidermal lesions that occur due to long-term exposure to the sun are known as actinic keratosis. The lesions are small, shiny but scaly, erythematous rough macules found on the face, upper trunk, forearms and dorsa of the hands in patches. They are considered as premalignant lesions and signs that suggest transformation include enlargement or ulceration.

Non-melanoma Skin Cancer

Basal cell and squamous cell cancer are malignant tumours of the skin. Found in adults over the age of 30, in men more than women, and in those with fair hair and blue eyes. Rates of new cases are rising, and it is suggested that almost 152 000 new cases of these types of skin cancer occur each year (Cancer Research UK, 2019). Other risk factors include red hair, freckles, green eyes, family history of skin cancer, unprotected or repeated exposure to the sun, radiation treatment, occupational exposure (coal, tar, pitch, asphalt), sunburn as a child and lowered immunity due to medication.

Basal Cell Cancer

Basal cell cancer is the most common, the most likely to recur, but the least aggressive; 75 of every 100 cases of skin cancer are basal cell in origin (Cancer Research UK, 2019). Basal cells are found in the basal layer of the epidermis and the cancer that originates from them is thought to develop because the cells have an impaired ability to mature into keratinocytes. This causes a solid neoplasm to grow, destroying around it skin, nerves, blood vessels, lymphatic tissue, cartilage and bone. This type rarely metastasises, it can destroy body parts such as the nose or eyelid. There are different types of basal cell cancer: nodular, superficial, pigmented, morpheaform and keratotic.

Nodular cancers are the most common and initially look like a smooth pimple that is itchy. This papule progressively grows, doubling its size every 6–12 months. The epidermis thins but remains intact as the cancer grows, often with the skin having a pearly white appearance that is shiny with visible telangiectasia. As the cancer grows, ulceration may occur either in the centre or at the periphery. This may bleed when knocked; it has well-defined borders.

Superficial cancers appear as flat erythematous papules or plaques. These too can ulcerate and can appear covered with crusts or erosions. They are often found on the trunk and extremities.

Pigmented basal cell cancer occurs on the face, neck and head and concentrates the melanin pigment from the skin into the centre of the lesion; thus the appearance of this form of skin cancer is dark brown, blue or black with a shiny well-defined border.

Morpheaform basal cell cancer is very rare; it resembles a flesh-coloured scar along a tissue plane and is usually found on the head and neck.

Keratotic basal cell cancer is a square-like lesion located on the groove at the front of and behind the ear.

Squamous Cell Cancers

Squamous cell carcinoma develops from proliferating keratinising cells of the squamous epithelium. It permeates the epidermis, over-runs the dermis and grows into irregular-shaped lesions. Pre-existing skin disorders such as scars and actinic keratosis can develop into squamous cell carcinoma. Metastases are common via the lymphatic system and the development of secondaries is dependent on the size and site of the initial tumour.

Skin exposed to sunlight and weather such as on the legs, arms and face is most commonly where squamous cell cancers occur. This malignant cancer of the squamous epithelium (either skin or mucous membranes) is more aggressive than its basal cell counterpart and has the potential to metastasise. It can also occur on skin that has been burned or had periods of chronic inflammation. The cancer initially starts as a small red nodule, which may or may not have crusts on it; as the cancer develops, it can bleed and become painful and indurated.

Malignant Melanoma

Melanocytes (cells that produce the pigment melanin in the basal layer of the skin) are where melanomas occur, one-third of them originating in pre-existing moles. The characteristics of a melanoma are a slow-developing, symmetrical, flat lesion, more than 6mm in diameter. Initially, they are classified as malignant melanoma *in situ*. These are considered benign but have the potential to infiltrate the dermis and metastasise by spreading through the blood and lymph network. The melanoma's characteristics change to a raised nodular appearance with satellite lesions around the margins.

People with fair skin are 10 times more at risk of melanoma than those with dark skin and those who have had prolonged exposure to the sun. Other risk factors include people with lots of freckles and precursor moles, regular use of sunbeds, family history, previous history of skin cancer, lowered immunity, being a woman over 50, higher body mass index in men and working with chemicals.

Melanomas account for 10% of all skin cancers and 79% of skin cancer deaths (Cancer Research UK, 2019). Several factors determine the prognosis for patients with a melanoma; these include tumour thickness, presence of ulceration, site, age, gender and metastasis.

Malignant melanomas are classified using Clark's five levels of staging, from level 1, where the melanoma grows parallel to the skin surface, to grade 5, where there is invasion of the epidermis, dermis and subcutaneous tissue increasing the risk of metastasis (vertical growth phase). Table 35.11 highlights the types of melanoma and their clinical presentations.

Table 35.11 Types and clinical presentations of malignant melanomas.

TYPE OF MELANOMA	CLINICAL PRESENTATION
Superficial spreading melanoma	2cm in diameter, flat, scaly and crusty lesions, found on the trunk and back of men and legs of women. Begins as mixture of tan, brown and black in colour in the radial phase and red, white and blue in the vertical phase
Nodular melanoma	Raised, dome-shaped, blue, black or red nodules found on the head, neck and trunk. Looks like a blood blister, which can ulcerate and bleed. Only has a vertical growth phase, which makes this an aggressive form of melanoma, and metastasises usually before diagnosis
Acral lentiginous melanoma	Usually commences as a flat tan, brown or black lesion to an elevated nodule approximately 3cm in diameter. Found on the soles of the feet, palms of the hands, mucous membranes and nailbeds. Affects men and women equally, usually in their 50s and 60s

Nursing Care

Treatment for skin cancers depends on whether the skin cancer is diagnosed at an early, medium or advanced stage. After medical examination and assessment, treatment options are as follows.

Early Stage (Clark's Level 1) Wide local excision of the lesion under local or general anaesthesia, depending on how large the lesion is, with or without sentinel lymph node biopsy. A small amount of dye or radioactive substance is injected into where the cancer was removed. The dye drains away into the lymph glands and the surgeon can see when the dye reaches the lymph glands or measure the radioactivity of the glands with a scanner. Those nodes that are visible or measurable are called sentinel nodes and are excised and sent for testing to see if they contain melanoma cells. If the results are positive, other lymph nodes are removed at a later date.

What To Do If . . .

the patient refuses treatment for the melanoma.
Patients are within their rights to refuse treatment, but it is important that they are aware of what they are refusing. There are different stages of melanoma, some more dangerous than others and requiring different treatment. It is important to ensure that patients fully understand the treatments available and prognosis with and without treatment. Then they can make a rational informed decision.

Medium Stage (Clark's Levels 2 and 3) Same surgery as level 1 (wide local excision and sentinel node biopsy with potential lymph node removal), with adjuvant treatment such as chemotherapy, radiotherapy and biological therapy (the use of interferon only in rare instances because of the side-effects).

Advanced Stage (Clark's Levels 4 and 5) The treatment and management of these stages of cancer will depend on the spread of metastasis, symptoms currently experienced by the patient and prior treatments. Surgery and adjuvant therapies may be offered, although palliation may be the only plan with symptom control. Other members of the multidisciplinary team would be involved, including specialist nurses (skin cancer, Macmillan, district), GP and oncologist. Plans for end-of-life care may need to put in place with support for the family and significant others.

Health Promotion

Health promotion will focus on attending follow-up, checking the skin on a regular basis for other moles, lesions, growths and swellings, and checking lymph nodes. Discussions will include care of the skin in the sun, eating a well-balanced diet, taking exercise, returning to work or social activities, giving up any habits that impact on the patient's health and well-being, and offering support and referral to others for emotional well-being. For advanced stages of melanoma, health promotion will focus around quality of life and symptom management issues.

Vascular Disorders (Including Naevi)

Benign vascular skin disorders are much more common than malignant ones, so it is imperative that a nurse can recognise and differentiate between the various types of lesions to offer support and guidance to patients. Many require identification and the reassurance that no clinical treatment is required.

Angiomas

Angiomas, otherwise known as haemangiomas (abnormal proliferation of capillaries), and naevi (moles, i.e. flat or raised macules and papules with well-rounded and defined borders) commonly appear on child and adult skin in various forms.

- *Venous lakes*: found on the back of the hands, ears and lips of older adults, present as small, flat, blue blood vessels.
- *Spider angiomas (small red papules with radiating lines)*: occur on the face, neck and upper chest. They are superficial dilated arteries and are usually associated with puberty, pregnant women, those on the contraceptive pill and patients with hepatic disease.
- *Telangiectases*: appear like broken veins on the nose and cheeks. They are commonly found in older adults and are the result of photoaged skin.
- *Cherry angiomas*: occur at any age and appear as small, red to purple, rounded papules. They are most common in the over-40s and increase in number as a person ages.
- *Naevus flammeus (port-wine stain)*: a vascular lesion that develops congenitally. The light red to dark purple lesion appears on the face and upper body as macular patches, is often present at birth and grows proportionately with the child.
- *Mongolian blue spot*: a variant of blue naevus and resembles a large bruise over the lumbosacral area of babies, especially from Asian and Afro-Caribbean families. Most fade but they can be mistaken for accidental injuries.
- *Blue naevus*: begins from melanocytes in the basal layer of the epidermis. It appears as a smooth, round, raised, blue-black lesion in late childhood on the hands, face or feet and is only 1 cm in diameter. These remain for the life of the patient.
- *Spitz naevus*: a fast-growing lesion that appears on the face of children or pregnant women. The lesion is single, red or orange in colour and, because of its rapid growth, is almost always excised.
- *Becker's naevus*: affects the skin of men in puberty on the chest and shoulders. It is visible as a faint pigment with hypertrichosis (abnormal amount of hair growth) and often occurs after being burnt by the sun.
- *Strawberry naevus*: a raised haemangioma that grows rapidly in the first year of life. There are two types: capillary superficial, which fades and disappears by the age of 5–7 years, and cavernous, which can impair function of organs such as the eye, nose, mouth and genitals, and can often itch or bleed.

Nursing Care

Nursing care is often just supporting and educating patients to understand that many of the lesions are benign and do not require any treatment. If the lesions are unsightly, causing emotional and psychological distress and affecting the patient's quality of life, then referral to a dermatologist, cosmetic camouflage team or psychologist may be of benefit. Occasionally some benign vascular lesions do require further management, and this can involve surgical excision, cryosurgery, laser therapy, cold point cautery and shave biopsy.

Health Promotion

The focus of health promotion for patients with vascular lesions is to offer advice on skin protection in the sun and support from other services in relation to cosmesis and body image.

Disorders of the Hair and Nails

Nails

When assessing a patient clinically, *always* take note of the nails, as an underlying condition or problem may be highlighted. Common conditions that affect the nailbed are listed in Table 35.12.

Table 35.12 **Common conditions and the effect on the nailbed.**

CONDITION	EFFECT ON NAIL BED
Anxiety, depression or compulsive disorders	Nail biting, paronychia, periungual warts
Median nail dystrophy usually caused by an underlying psychological condition	Longitudinal depression along the nailbed with an enlarged lunula
Psoriasis	Pitting of the nail plate, onycholysis (separation of the free edge of the nail plate which whitens) and dystrophy (thickened, opaque and discoloured nail)
Alopecia areata, eczema, Reiter syndrome and pemphigus	Pitting of the nail plate
Eczema, lichen planus, periungual warts, fungal infections of the nail, iron deficiency anaemia, thyrotoxicosis and sarcoidosis	Onycholysis
Psoriasis acrodermatitis continua of Hallopeau	Dystrophy
Eczema	Nail shedding
Trauma, rheumatoid arthritis and bacterial endocarditis	Splinter haemorrhages
Systemic lupus erythematosus, dermatomyositis, sarcoidosis and HIV	Periungual erythema
Terry's half-and-half nail (proximal part whitens)	Renal failure, liver cirrhosis, congestive cardiac failure, type 2 diabetes

Hair

During a normal life cycle, hair is constantly falling out and new hairs growing. However, when changes to the hair occur that have the potential to dramatically affect hair growth, the consequences may cause significant psychological problems. There are many hair problems that can occur, from disproportionate oiliness to a dry flaky scalp. Some are due to infections, others to allergic responses, but all have some level of inflammation; hair loss can occur consequently. Table 35.13 highlights common diseases and disorders of the scalp.

Table 35.13 Common disorders of the scalp.

NAME OF HAIR DISORDER/DISEASE	SIGNS AND SYMPTOMS
Seborrhoea: excessive production of sebum	Excessive oiliness of hair and scalp
Seborrhoeic dermatitis: dermatitis of the scalp	Seen as cradle cap in babies. Flaking of whitish to brown scales from the scalp, greasy crusts on the scalp that turn yellow brown when they fall off, inflamed boggy patches under the crusts, extension of inflammation to ears, eyebrows, eyelids, cheeks and nostrils, and pruritus
Tinea capitis: a fungal infection of the scalp (Figure 35.2)	*Non-inflammatory:* hairs appear grey because of the dusting of fungi, the scalp has reddish patches and scaling, hairs break just above the follicle *Inflammatory:* hair follicles are inflamed with moist patches and broken hairs; discharge and pus may be visible, itching is intense *Black dot:* black dots of infected hairs are seen in the scalp, these are broken hairs just above the follicle; accompanied by inflammation
Bacterial and viral infections of the scalp	*Bacterial infections:* abscesses can occur, the scalp is inflamed and painful; folliculitis can be present *Viral infections:* can be caused by herpes simplex or zoster and inflamed oozing lesions can appear
Head lice	Red swollen patches in areas. Louse may be visible as may brown or silvery white nits attached to the hair shaft, particularly around the nape of the neck and ears
Psoriasis	Red, scaly, silvery white lesions and plaques to the scalp
Lichen planus: inflammatory disorder of the mucous membranes and skin	Violet papules, 2–10 mm in size, that are intensely itchy, thicken over time and become dark red and form hypertrophic lichen planus
Lupus erythematosus: autoimmune condition of the skin and organs	Patchy skin inflammation, scaling of the skin, plugging of the follicles and telangiectasia
Alopecia areata: an autoimmune disorder of the scalp	Small localised patches of hair loss to scalp and beard to complete hair loss, including eyebrows
Androgenic alopecia: male and female pattern hair loss	Begins with thinning of the hair with a receding hairline at the frontotemporal area
Trauma traction alopecia: alopecia developing at the site of a hairstyle that constantly pulls on the hair	Bald areas between plaits and ponytails
Trichotillomania: self-inflicted hair loss	Patches of hair loss which are geometrical, small or single patches without scarring. Usually psychological cause to the hair pulling
Telogen effluvium: hair loss following childbirth, chemotherapy or drugs	Can vary from thinning to complete loss of all body hair
Acne	The scalp may be affected by acne that is: *Mild:* a few scattered comedones and occasional papules *Moderate:* presence of comedones, macules, papules and pustules *Severe:* comedones, papules and pustules, painful nodules and cysts that scar and cause pigment changes
Allergic or irritant dermatitis of the scalp	Itchy inflammation of the scalp caused by a reaction to an external agent

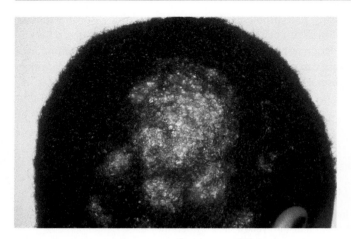

Figure 35.2 **Tinea capitis.** *Source:* Buxton & Morris-Jones (2013). Reproduced with permission of John Wiley & Sons Ltd.

Nursing Care

Nursing care of hair and nails will always concentrate around treating and managing the causative factor. This may require taking nail clippings for further investigation, treatments varying from topical applications to phototherapy and systemic treatments, referral to other members of the multidisciplinary team for advice and psychological support and, in some instances, the obtaining of wigs and hairpieces. General care of hair and nails in most skin disorders is to ensure that hair is kept clean and styles are altered accordingly, and nails are kept short.

Health Promotion

The nurse would focus on promoting a well-balanced diet, avoiding trigger factors, and ensuring that the patient complies with treatment options.

Connective Tissue Disorders

Connective tissue disorders comprise a wide range of autoimmune diseases and are often associated with specific autoantibodies (blood proteins) that aid their diagnosis. They occur when the body's own immune system mistakenly attacks the body tissues, causing an inflammatory reaction. Connective tissue is found in all body organs and its role is to support the organs, as it is made from elastin and collagen. If attacked by the immune system, the tissue becomes inflamed and can consequently result in cell death.

The most common connective tissue disorder that affects the skin is *discoid lupus erythematosus* (DLE). DLE is considered a chronic long-term condition and affects 12–48 per 100 000 people. It is most common in women aged between 20 and 40 years of age and is thought to be triggered by underlying genetic factors, smoking, exposure to UV light and certain medications such as non-steroidal anti-inflammatory drugs. Of patients with DLE, 5% may develop systemic lupus erythematosus (SLE).

At the outset, the patient presents with symptomless erythematous plaques or papules that can merge and spread to sun-exposed areas of the skin. The lesions then become thickened and scaly, often with hypopigmentation, follicular plugging and hyperpigmentation

of the lesion's edges; the lesions can then become itchy and painful. Once the lesions resolve, they leave scars.

Nursing Care

Care of the patient with DLE concentrates on controlling the rash and preventing spread and recurrence by reducing exposure to the triggering factors. Topical steroids are prescribed, usually beginning with quite potent levels and reducing these on a sliding scale over weeks of treatment to moderate and then mild steroids. Antimalarial drugs such as hydroxychloroquine (200 mg daily) should also be offered as first-line treatment, increasing to twice daily when tolerated, reminding the patient that any visible change will not be noticed for 4–6 weeks. It is important for the nurse and patient to look out for potential side-effects of the medication, such as retinal toxicity and visual disturbances, and inform the doctor of these immediately.

Red Flag

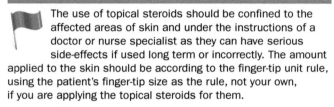

The use of topical steroids should be confined to the affected areas of skin and under the instructions of a doctor or nurse specialist as they can have serious side-effects if used long term or incorrectly. The amount applied to the skin should be according to the finger-tip unit rule, using the patient's finger-tip size as the rule, not your own, if you are applying the topical steroids for them.

Affected Body Area	Quantity of Cream/Ointment
Both sides of one hand	1 finger-tip unit
One foot	2 finger-tip units
One arm	3 finger-tip units
One leg	6 finger-tip units
Chest and abdomen	7 finger-tip units
Back and buttocks	7 finger-tip units

Health Promotion

Health promotion is aimed at reducing the trigger factors, such as cessation of smoking, avoiding exposure to UV by wearing protective clothing, using factor 30 sunscreen, and avoiding going outdoors when it is sunny between 11 a.m. and 3 p.m. As with most dermatological conditions, consider referral to other members of the multidisciplinary team such as psychologists and the cosmetic camouflage team.

Practice Assessment Document

If a PAD requires the assessment of performance, for example 'Assesses skin hygiene status and demonstrates knowledge of appropriate products to prevent and manage skin breakdown', this can be achieved through holistic assessment of the patient, including a detailed history of the skin condition, a general assessment of the patient, an assessment of the patient's knowledge and a physical assessment. Using this information and reading this chapter and Chapter 18, you will be able to discuss with your practice supervisor/assessor your assessment and decisions. This may include products to prevent skin breakdown or treatment with topical agents or referral to other members of the MDT for advice.

Conclusion

Dermatology conditions are a major part of the primary care workload, and the incidence of skin conditions is rising. Skin conditions affect all age groups and although problems such as eczema and acne can be considered minor in biomedical terms, they actually present the patient with considerable psychological challenges (Rumsey *et al.*, 2002). The role of the nurse in caring for patients with skin disorders involves use of the nursing process, in particular a thorough assessment, planning and implementation of smart, realistic and patient-centred care and regular evaluation.

Key Points

- This chapter has provided the reader with an overview of the structures of the skin, hair and nails.
- An understanding of the processes involved in the way wounds heal has been offered.
- The nurse is required to undertake a holistic assessment of the patient with a skin disorder in order to provide care that is safe and effective, as well as meeting the individual needs of the person and recognising the effect of the psyche on the skin.
- The importance of using correct terminology in the assessment and management of skin disorders has been emphasised.
- A number of investigations can be undertaken to aid diagnosis and management of skin disorders and the nurse should assist the person before, during and after investigation, explaining the rationale for the investigations and the care required after the investigation has been completed.
- This chapter has provided a review of common skin conditions, the care required, clinical management and the involvement of members of the multidisciplinary team.
- High-quality care requires the nurse to promote health and well-being, self-care and independence, by teaching and empowering people and carers to make choices in coping with the effects of treatment.

References

All Party Parliamentary Group on Skin (2013) *Priority Workstreams for 2014–15*. www.appgs.co.uk/wp-content/uploads/2013/12/APPGS-2014_15-Strategy.pdf (accessed January 2022).

Berth-Jones, J. (2010) Rosacea, perioral dermatitis and similar dermatoses. In: T. Burns, S. Breathnach, N. Cox & C. Griffiths (eds) *Rook's Textbook of Dermatology*, 8th edn, pp. 1–6. Wiley Blackwell, Oxford.

British Association of Dermatologists (2009) *Guidelines for the Management of Atopic Eczema*. British Association of Dermatologists, London.

Burgess, I.F., Brown, C.M. & Lee, P.N. (2005) Treatment of head louse infestation with 4% dimethicone lotion: randomised controlled equivalence trial. *British Medical Journal*, 330(7505), 1423.

Buxton, P.K. & Morris-Jones, R. (2013) *ABC of Dermatology*, 5th edn. John Wiley & Sons Ltd, Chichester.

Cancer Research UK (2019) *Skin cancer – How common is it?* www.cancerresearchuk.org/about-cancer/skin-cancer/about-skin-cancer (accessed January 2022).

Changing Faces (2016) *Look at Me: Integrated Care for People with Skin Conditions. Second Campaign Report and Recommendations*. www.changingfaces.org.uk/ (accessed January 2022).

Cunliffe, W. (1994) *New Approaches to Acne Treatment*. Martin Dunitz, London.

Department of Health (2008) *Guidance on the Routine Collection of Patient Reported Outcome Measures (PROMs)*. Department of Health, London.

Gagliardi, A.M., Gomes Silva, B.N., Torloni, M.R. & Soares, B.G. (2012) Vaccines for preventing herpes zoster in older adults. *Cochrane Database of Systematic Reviews*, 10, CD008858.

Lang, P.G. (2000) Dermatoses in African-Americans. *Dermatology Nursing*, 12(2), 87–98.

Lawton, S. (2001) Assessing the patient with a skin condition. *Journal of Tissue Viability*, 11(3), 113–115.

Lawton, S. (2002) *Assessing the patient with a skin condition*. www.worldwidewounds.com/2002/may/Lawton/Skin-Assessment-Dermatology-Patient.html (accessed January 2022).

Linh, C.Y. (2011) *Eczema herpeticum*. https://dalieu.vn/wp-content/uploads/2018/11/Eczema-Herpeticum-1.pdf (accessed January 2022).

Nazarko, L. (2011) Fungal skin infections and HCAs: identify, treat and act. *British Journal of Healthcare Assistants*, 4(11), 551–553.

NHS Digital (2019). *Hospital admitted patient care activity 2018–19*. https://digital.nhs.uk/data-and-information/publications/statistical/hospital-admitted-patient-care-activity/2018-19 (accessed January 2022).

Rumsey, N., Clarke, A. & Musa, M. (2002) Altered body image: the psychosocial needs of patients. *British Journal of Community Nursing*, 7(11), 563–566.

Ryan, S. (2008) Psoriasis: characteristics, psychosocial effects and treatment options. *British Journal of Nursing*, 17(5), 284–290.

Schofield, J.K., Fleming, D., Grindlay, D. & Williams, H. (2011) Skin conditions are the commonest new reason people present to general practitioners in England and Wales. *British Journal of Dermatology*, 165(5), 1044–1050.

Smith, R.N., Mann, N.J., Braue, A., Makelainen, H. & Varigos, G.A. (2007) A low-glycemic-load diet improves symptoms in acne vulgaris patients. *American Journal of Clinical Nutrition*, 86(1), 107–115.

Stanway, A. (2011) *Causes of atopic dermatitis*. https://dermnetnz.org/topics/causes-of-atopic-dermatitis/ (accessed January 2022).

Thomas, D.R. (2005) Psychosocial effects of acne. *Journal of Cutaneous Medicine and Surgery*, 8(Suppl. 4), 3–5.

Tseng, H.F., Smith, N., Harpaz, R., Bialek, S.R., Sy, L.S. & Jacobsen, S.J. (2011) Herpes zoster vaccine in older adults and the risk of subsequent herpes zoster. *Journal of the American Medical Association*, 305(2), 160–166.

Van Onselen, J. (2001) Psoriasis. In: E. Hughes & J. Van Onselen (eds) *Dermatology Nursing: A Practical Guide*. Churchill Livingstone, Edinburgh.

Zaidi, Z. & Lanigan, S.W. (2010) *Dermatology in Clinical Practice*. Springer Verlag, London.

Appendix A List of Units

cm	centimetre
mm	millimetre
L	litre
mL	millilitre
kg	kilogram
g	gram
mg	milligram
µg	microgram
ng	nanogram
pg	picogram
mol	mole
mmol	millimole
µmol	micromole
mEq	milliequivalent
mosm	milliosmole
mmHg	millimetres of mercury
kcal	kilocalorie

Nursing Practice: Knowledge and Care, Third Edition. Edited by Ian Peate and Aby Mitchell.
© 2022 John Wiley & Sons Ltd. Published 2022 by John Wiley & Sons Ltd.
Companion website: www.wiley.com/go/peate/nursingpractice3e

Index

Page numbers in *italic* refer to figures. Page numbers in **bold** refer to tables.

Nursing Practice: Knowledge and Care, Third Edition. Edited by Ian Peate and Aby Mitchell.
© 2022 John Wiley & Sons Ltd. Published 2022 by John Wiley & Sons Ltd.
Companion website: www.wiley.com/go/peate/nursingpractice3e